The ESC Textbook of
Acute and Intensive Cardiac Care

The multiple choice questions accessible through the online version of *The ESC Textbook of Acute and Intensive Cardiac Care* have been approved by the ESC Working Group on Acute Cardiac Care. The knowledge assessment as part of the accreditation process in Acute Cardiac Care will be based on the results of the online formative testing using the MCQs in the book together with the summative MCQ testing session organized by the Working Group.

The ESC Textbook of
Acute and Intensive Cardiac Care

Edited by

Marco Tubaro

Nicolas Danchin

Gerasimos Filippatos

Patrick Goldstein

Pascal Vranckx

and

Doron Zahger

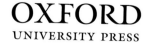

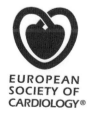

EUROPEAN
SOCIETY OF
CARDIOLOGY®

OXFORD

UNIVERSITY PRESS

Great Clarendon Street, Oxford OX2 6DP

Oxford University Press is a department of the University of Oxford.
It furthers the University's objective of excellence in research, scholarship,
and education by publishing worldwide in

Oxford New York

Auckland Cape Town Dar es Salaam Hong Kong Karachi
Kuala Lumpur Madrid Melbourne Mexico City Nairobi
New Delhi Shanghai Taipei Toronto

With offices in

Argentina Austria Brazil Chile Czech Republic France Greece
Guatemala Hungary Italy Japan Poland Portugal Singapore
South Korea Switzerland Thailand Turkey Ukraine Vietnam

Oxford is a registered trade mark of Oxford University Press
in the UK and in certain other countries

Published in the United States
by Oxford University Press Inc., New York

British Library Cataloguing-in-Publication-Data

Data available

Library of Congress Cataloging-in-Publication-Data

Data available

Typeset by Glyph International, Bangalore, India
Printed in Spain
on acid-free paper by
Grafos S. A

ISBN 978–0–19–958431–4

10 9 8 7 6 5 4 3 2 1

Oxford University Press makes no representation, express or implied, that the drug dosages in
this book are correct. Readers must therefore always check the product information and clinical
procedures with the most up-to-date published product information and data sheets provided by
the manufacturers and the most recent codes of conduct and safety regulations. The authors and
the publishers do not accept responsibilityor legal liability for any errors in the text or for the
misuse or misapplication of material in this work. Except where otherwise stated, drug dosages
and recommendations are for the non-pregnant adult who is not breastfeeding.

Foreword

The current Intensive Cardiac Care Units (ICCU) and Coronary Care Units (CCU) developed from the original concept presented by Desmond Julian in 1961. Initially the CCU was a spe-cial unit in the hospital to monitor the heart rhythm of patients with evolving myocardial in-farction, at risk for sudden death from ventricular fibrillation, heart block, or asystole. It was a special unit with dedicated nurses and physicians trained to treat such arrhythmias. Over the years the CCU evolved, particularly in the cardiac centres with facilities for cardiac thoracic surgery, interventional cardiology, and clinical electrophysiology to a complete intensive care unit for patients with heart disease. In addition to the heart rhythm, current monitoring sys-tems provide information on invasive- or non-invasive circulatory pressures, cardiac output, oxygen saturation, fluid balance, and ventilatory parameters. Furthermore, a great variety of treatment options are provided when appropriate, including circulatory and ventilatory sup-port, such as extra corporal membrane oxygenation (ECMO) and haemodialysis.

This *Textbook of Intensive and Acute Cardiac Care* by The European Society of Cardiology provides extensive, complete, and detailed information about the recommended structure and facilities of the ICCU and CCU and its relation to pre-hospital and hospital emergency care. The textbook gives an overview of monitoring systems and the diagnostic methods used in cardiac patients including non-invasive imaging by echocardiography, computer tomography and magnetic resonance imaging, as well as the therapeutic procedures.

Most patients admitted to an ICCU or CCU suffer from acute coronary syndromes, acute heart failure, or severe cardiac arrhythmias. The diagnosis, classification, risk-stratification, and therapy of these conditions, as well as important concomitant disorders such as diabetes and bleeding complications, are described in detail.

The Intensive Cardiac Care Unit and Coronary Care Unit are pivotal units in any department of cardiology, often operating in close collaboration with the cardiac surgery intensive care unit. Since the introduction of these units in the 1960's, the outcome for patients with acute cardiac conditions has remarkably improved and continues to improve. Dedicated and skilled physicians, nurses, and other staff are essential to the success of the ICCU and CCU. This ESC textbook provides students, nurses, and physicians with a wealth of information to de-velop and maintain their knowledge.

I recommend this book to all who are interested in acute and intensive cardiac care and only regret that I could not read it earlier, at the time that I was personally responsible for the ICCU in my hospital.

Maarten L. Simoons, MD PhD
Professor of Cardiology,
Thoraxcenter, Erasmus University Medical Center
Rotterdam, The Netherlands
President European Society of Cardiology 2000—2002

Contents

Symbols and abbreviations

➲	cross reference	AHF	acute heart failure
📷	additional online material	AHFS	acute heart failure syndrome
℘	website	AI	adrenal insufficiency
AA	amino acids	AIH	amiodarone-induced hypothyroidism
AAR	AST/ALT ratio	AIVR	accelerated idioventricular rhythm
ABC	airway, breathing, and circulation	AKI	acute kidney injury
ABG	arterial blood gases	AKIN	Acute Kidney Injury Network
ABIM	American Board of Internal Medicine	ALI	acute lung injury
ABP	aortic balloon pump	ALT	alanine aminotransferase
ACC	American College of Cardiology	AMC	acute myocarditis
ACC	acute cardiac care	AMI	acute myocardial infarction
ACCP	American College of Chest Physicians	ANC	absolute neutrophil count
ACE	angiotensin converting enzyme	ANP	atrial natriuretic peptide
ACEF	age, creatinine value, and ejection fraction	AP	antero-posterior
ACGME	Accreditation Council for Graduate Medical Education	APAH	associated pulmonary arterial hypertension
		APC	activated protein C
ACHD	adult congenital heart disease	APTT	activated partial thromboplastin time
ACLS	advanced cardiac life support	AR	aortic regurgitation
ACPE	acute cardiogenic pulmonary oedema	ARB	angiotensin receptor blocker
ACS	acute coronary syndrome	ARDS	acute respiratory distress syndrome
ACT	activated clotting time	ARF	acute renal failure
ACTH	adrenocorticotropic hormone	ARVD	arrhythmiogenic right ventricular dysplasia
ADA	adenosine deaminase	AS	aortic stenosis
ADH	antidiuretic hormone	ASA	acetylsalicylic acid (aspirin)
ADHF	acute decompensated heart failure	ASD	atrial septal defect
ADP	accelerated diagnostic protocols	AST	aspartate aminotransferase
ADQI	Acute Dialysis Quality Initiative	ATLS	advanced trauma life support
ADV	adenovirus	AUC	area under the curve
AED	automatic external defibrillation	AV	atrioventricular
AF	atrial fibrillation	AVNRT	atrioventricular nodal re-entrant tachycardia
AFE	amniotic fluid embolism	AVR	aortic valve replacement
AFP	α-fetoprotein	AVRT	atrioventricular reciprocating tachycardia
AG	anion gap	AVSD	atrioventricular septal defect
AGE	advanced glycation end	BAER	brainstem auditory evoked responses
AHA	American Heart Association	BAL	bronchoalveloar lavage

BBB	bundle branch block
BIS	bispectral index
BLS	basic life support
BMI	body mass index
BMS	bare metal stents
BNP	B-type natriuretic peptide
BSA	body surface area
BTS	British Thoracic Society
BUN	blood urea nitrogen
C&S	culture and sensitivities
CABG	coronary artery bypass grafting
CAD	coronary artery disease
CAM	cell adhesion molecule
CAP	community-acquired pneumonia
CAV	cardiac allograft vasculopathy
CBF	cerebral blood flow
CBV	cerebral blood volume
CBV	Coxsackie B virus
CC	core curriculum
CCA	conventional coronary angiography
CCB	calcium channel blockers
CCTA	coronary CT angiography
CCU	cardiac care unit, coronary care unit, or critical care unit
CEA	combination of epithelial membrane antigen or carcinoembryonic antigen
CFM	cerebral function monitor
CHD	congenital heart disease or coronary heart disease
CHF	chronic heart failure or congestive heart failure
CHP	continuous haemoperfusion
CI	cardiac index or confidence interval
CIH	cardiogenic ischaemic hepatitis
CIN	contrast medium induced nephropathy
CK	creatine kinase
CKD	chronic kidney disease
CME	continuing medical education
CMR	cardiac magnetic resonance
CMV	continuous mandatory ventilation or cytomegalovirus
CO	cardiac output
COSTR	Consensus on Science and Treatment Recommendations
COX	cyclooxygenase
CP	chest pain
CPAP	continuous positive airway pressure
CPB	cardiopulmonary bypass
CPI	cardiac power index
CPM	continuous passive motion

CPO	cardiac power output
CPP	cerebral perfusion pressure
CPR	cardiopulmonary resuscitation
CPU	chest pain unit
CRF	case record form
CRP	C-reactive protein
CRRT	continuous renal replacement therapy
CRS	cardiorenal syndromes
CRT	cardiac resynchronization therapy
CS	cardiogenic shock
CSA	compressed spectral array
CSF	cerebrospinal fluid
CSM	carotid sinus massage
CT	computed tomography
CTA	CT angiography
CTEPH	chronic thromboembolic pulmonary hypertension
CTL	cytotoxic T lymphocytes
CTO	chronic total coronary artery occlusion
CUS	cardiac ultrasound
CV	coefficient of variation or curriculum vitae
CVC	central venous catheter
CVD	cardiovascular disease
CVHF	continuous volume constant hemofiltration
CVP	central venous pressure
CVR	cerebral vascular resistance
CVST	cerebral venous and sinus thrombosis
CVVH	continuous venovenous haemofiltration
CVVHD	continuous venovenous haemodialysis
CVVHDF	continuous venovenous haemofiltration
CXR	chest radiograph
DCM	dilated cardiomyopathy
DCMi	inflammatory cardiomyopathy
DES	drug-eluting stents
DIA	digital image analysis
DIC	disseminated intravascular coagulation
DM	diabetes mellitus
DNR/DNAR	do not resuscitate
DSA	density spectral array
DSE	dobutamine stress echocardiography
DTI	direct thrombin inhibitors
DVT	deep vein thrombosis
DWI	diffusion-weighted images
EACTS	European Association of Cardio-Thoracic Surgery
EAPCI	European Association for Percutaneous Cardiovascular Interventions
EAPCI	European Association of Percutaneous Cardiovascular Interventions

EBCT	electron beam CT		FV	flow velocity
EBM	evidence-based medicine		FVII	factor VII
EBSC	European Board for the Specialty of Cardiology		FWD	free water deficit
EBV	Epstein–Barr virus		FWR	free wall rupture
ECF	extracellular fluid		GABA	γ-aminobutyric acid
ECG	electrocardiogram, electrocardiography		GAPDH	glyceraldehyde-3-phosphate dehydrogenase
ECM	extracellular matrix		GBS	Guillain–Barré syndrome
ECMO	extracorporeal membrane oxygenation		GCS	Glasgow Coma Scale
ED	emergency department		GFR	glomerular filtration rate
EDTA	ethylene diamine tetra-acetic acid.		GGT	γ-glutamyl transpeptidase
EEG	electroencephalogram		GH	growth hormone
EF	ejection fraction		GIK	glucose–insulin–potassium
EGDT	early goal-directed therapy		GISEN	Gruppo Italiano di Studi Epidemiologici in Nefrologia
EMB	endomyocardial biopsies		GLA	γ-linolenic acid
EMS	electrical muscle stimulation *or* emergency medical services		GPI	glycoprotein IIb/IIIa inhibitor
EMT	emergency medical technician		GRACE	Global Registry of Acute Coronary Events
EN	enteral nutrition		H&E	haematoxylin & eosin staining
EOL	end-of-life		HAART	highly active antiretroviral therapy
EP	evoked potential		Hb	haemoglobin
EPA	eicosapentaenoic acid		HBV	hepatitis B virus
EPAP	expiratory pressure		HCT	haematocrit
ERC	European Resuscitation Council		HCV	hepatitis C virus
ERO	effective regurgitant orifice		HDL	high-density lipoprotein
EROA	effective regurgitant orifice area		HE	histological examination
ERS	European Respiratory Society		HES	hydroxyethyl starch
ES	electrical storm		HF	heart failure
ESA	European Society of Anaesthesiology		HFNEF	heart failure with normal ejection fraction
ESC	European Society of Cardiology		HFO	high-frequency oscillation
ESICM	European Society of Intensive Care Medicine		HFOV	high-frequency oscillatory ventilation
ESPEN	European Society for Clinical Nutrition and Metabolism		HFpEF	heart failure with preserved LVEF
			HHS	hyperosmolar hyperglycaemic state
ESR	erythrocyte sedimentation rate		HHV	human herpesvirus
ESRD	endstage renal disease		HIPA	heparin-induced platelet activation
ESRF	endstage renal failure		HIT	heparin-induced thrombocytopenia
ESVI	end-systolic volume index		HIV	human immunodeficiency virus
ETI	endotracheal intubation		HPV	hypoxic pulmonary vasoconstriction
ETT	exercise treadmill testing		HR	hazard ratios
EV	enterovirus		HRS	Heart Rhythm Society
FABP	fatty acid binding protein		HRV	heart rate variability
FAST	focused assessment with sonography for trauma		HSV	herpes simplex virus
			HU	Hounsfield unit
FBC	full blood count		IA	immunoadsorption
FBI	fast, broad, irregular		IABP	intra-aortic balloon pumping
FFA	free fatty acids		IACC	intensive and acute cardiac care
FLAIR	fluid-attenuated inversion recovery		iv	intravenous
FOB	fibreoptic bronchoscopy		IBW	ideal body weight
FRC	functional residual capacity		ICAM	intercellular cell adhesion molecule
			ICCU	intensive cardiac care unit

ICD	implantable cardioverter/defibrillator		LAD	left anterior descending artery
ICF	intracellular fluid		LAFB	left anterior fascicular block
ICH	intracerebral haemorrhage		LAVI	left atrial volume index
ICIS	integrated cardiology information system		LBBB	left bundle branch block
ICP	intracranial pressure		LDH	lactate dehydrogenase
ICU	intensive care unit		LDL	low-density lipoprotein
IE	infectious endocarditis		LED	light-emitting diode
IFN	interferon		LFA-1	lymphocyte function antigen-1
Ig	immunoglobulin		LGE	late gadolinium enhancement
IHD	intermittent haemodialysis		LIMA	left internal mammary artery
IIT	intensive insulin therapy		LIS	lung injury score
ILCOR	International Liaison Committee on Resuscitation		LMWH	low-molecular-weight heparin
			LNAA	large neutral amino acids
ILVT	idiopathic left ventricular tachycardia		LOS	length of stay
IM	intramuscular		LOV	length of ventilation
IMA	internal mammary artery or ischaemia-modified albumin		LOX	lipoxygenase
			LPFB	left posterior fascicular block
IMD	immunomodulating diet		LPS	lipopolysaccharide
IMH	intramural haematoma		LQTS	long QT syndrome
IMR	ischaemic mitral regurgitation		LV	left ventricle, left ventricular
IMV	intermittent mandatory ventilation		LVAD	left ventricular assist device
INO	inhaled nitric oxide		LVEDD	left ventricular end-diastolic diameter
INR	international normalized ratio		LVEDP	left ventricular end-diastolic pressure
INTERMACS	Interagency Registry for Mechanically Assisted Circulatory Support		LVEDVI	left ventricular end-diastolic volume index
			LVEF	left ventricular ejection function
IP	intrapericardial		LVESD	left ventricular end-systolic diameter
IPAH	idiopathic pulmonary arterial hypertension		LVF	left ventricular failure
IPAP	inspiratory pressure		LVH	left ventricular hypertrophy
IPPB	intermittent positive pressure breathing		LVMI	left ventricular mass index
IPPV	intermittent positive pressure ventilation		LVOT	left ventricular outflow tract
IPV	intrapulmonary percussive ventilation		LVSWI	left ventricular stroke work index
IRA	infarct-related artery		MACE	major adverse cardiovascular events
IRAD	International Registry of Acute Aortic Dissection		MAP	mean arterial pressure
			MARS	molecular adsorbents recirculation system
IRI	ischaemia and reperfusion injury		MBG	myocardial blush grade
IS	incentive spirometry		MC	myxoedema coma
ISHLT	International Society for Heart and Lung Transplantation		MCS	mechanical circulatory support
			MDCT	multidetector CT
ISTH	International Society for Thrombosis and Haemostasis		MEGX	monoethylglycinexylidide
			MEP	multimodality evoked potential
ITA	internal thoracic artery		MHI	manual hyperinflation
ITP	idiopathic thrombocytopenic purpura		MI	myocardial infarction
IVC	inferior vena cava		MICU	mobile intensive care unit
IVIG	intravenous immunoglobulin		MIP	maximum intensity projections
IVUS	intravascular ultrasound		MMF	mycophenolate mofetil
JVP	jugular venous pressure		MMI	methimazole
KDOQI	Kidney Outcome Quality Initiative		MMP	matrix metalloproteinases
KIM	kidney injury molecule		MODS	multiple organ dysfunction syndrome
LA	left atrium		MPI	myocardial perfusion imaging

MPO	myeloperoxidase
MPR	multiplanar reconstruction
MPS	myocardial perfusion scintigraphy
MRA	magnetic resonance angiography
MRSA	meticillin-resistant *Staphylococcus aureus*
MS	mitral stenosis
MSF	multisource feedback
MTHFR	methylenetetrahydrofolate reductase
MV	mitral valve
MVO	microvascular obstruction
MVR	mitral valve replacement
MVS	mitral valve surgery
NAC	*N*-acteylcysteine
NACB	National Academy of Clinical Biochemistry
NAFLD	nonalcoholic fatty liver disease
NAG	*N*-acetyl-β-(D)-glucosaminidase
NASH	nonalcoholic steatohepatitis
NCDR	National Cardiovascular Data Registry
NEFA	nonessential fatty acids
NGAL	neutrophil gelatinase-associated lipocalin
NHAAP	National Heart Attack Alert Program
NHBOD	non-heart-beating organ donation
NICM	nonischaemic cardiomyopathy
NIH	National Institutes of Health
NIPSV	noninvasive pressure support ventilation
NIST	National Institute of Standards and Technology
NIV	noninvasive ventilation
NMDA	N-methyl-D-aspartate
NNT	number needed to treat
NP	natriuretic peptide
nPCR	nested polymerase chain reaction
NPV	negative predictive value
NPV	negative pressure ventilation
NRMI	National Registry of Myocardial Infarction
NRS	numeric rating scale
NS	not significant
NSAID	nonsteroidal anti-inflammatory drug
NSTE	non-ST-segment elevation
NSTEMI	non-ST-segment elevation myocardial infarction
NSVT	nonsustained ventricular tachycardia
NTG	nitroglycerine
NTP	nitroprusside
NYHA	New York Heart Association
OFR	oxygen free radicals
OoHCA	out-of-hospital cardiac arrest
OPCAB	off-pump coronary artery bypass
OPS	orthogonal polarization spectroscopy
OR	odds ratio
OSCE	objective structured clinical examination
PA	postero-anterior
PA	pulmonary artery
PAC	pulmonary artery catheter
PAD	peripheral arterial disease
PAF	platelet activating factor
PAH	pulmonary arterial hypertension
PAOP	pulmonary artery occlusion pressure
PAP	pulmonary artery pressure
PAV	percutaneous balloon aortic valvuloplasty
PAV	proportional assist ventilation
PCA	patient-controlled analgesia
PCC	prothrombin complex concentrates
PCI	percutaneous coronary intervention
PCPS	percutaneous cardiopulmonary support
PCR	polymerase chain reaction *or* protein/creatinine ratio
PCT	procalcitonin
PCV	pressure control ventilation
PCWP	pulmonary capillary wedge pressure
PD	peritoneal dialysis
PDA	posterior descending coronary artery
PDD	pleural drainage device
PDE	phosphodiesterase
PDGF	platelet derived growth factor
PE	pulmonary embolism *or* pericardial effusion
PECS	prehospital emergency care systems
PEEP	positive end-expiratory pressure
PEP	positive expiratory pressure
PESI	Pulmonary Embolism Severity Index
PET	positron emission tomography
PFO	PFO, patent foramen ovale
PDGF	platelet derived growth factor
PH	pulmonary hypertension
PI	protease inhibitors
PIFGI	percutaneous intrapericardial fibrin glue injection
PL	plasmapheresis
PLGF	placental growth factor
PMC	percutaneous mitral commissurotomy
PMCS	portable mechanical circulatory support
PMI	perioperative myocardial infarction
PMK	pacemaker
PMN	polymorphonuclear leucocyte
PMR	papillary muscle rupture
POC	point of care
PPAR	peroxisome proliferator-activated receptors

PPC	peripartum cardiomyopathy		SC	subcutaneous
PPV	positive predictive value *or* positive pressure ventilation		SCCM	Society of Critical Care Medicine
			SCD	sudden cardiac death
PRVC	pressure-regulated volume control		SCPC	Society of Chest Pain Centers
PS	P-selectin *or* phosphatidylserine		SCUF	slow continuous ultrafiltration
PT	prothrombin time		SD	standard deviation
PTA	angioplasty		SDF	side stream dark field
PTCA	percutaneous transluminal balloon coronary angioplasty		SFAR	Société Française d'Anesthésie et de Réanimation
PTT	prothrombin time		SIADH	syndrome of inappropriate antidiuretic hormone hypersecretion
PTU	propylthiouracil			
PUFA	polyunsaturated fatty acid		SIMV	synchronized intermittent mandatory ventilation
PVE	prosthetic valve endocarditis			
PVR	pulmonary vascular resistance		SIRS	systemic inflammatory response syndrome
PWI	perfusion-weighted images		SLED	sustained low-efficiency dialysis
PWP	pulmonary wedge pressure		SLEDD	slow low-efficiency daily dialysis
qPCR	quantitative PCR		SMC	smooth muscle cells
RA	right atrium		SNF	systemic nephrogenic fibrosis
RAAS	renin–angiotensin–aldosterone system		SNO	*S*-nitrosothiol
RASS	Richmond Agitation-Sedation Scale		SOD	superoxide dismutase
RBBB	right bundle branch block		SPAD	single pass albumin dialysis
RBC	red blood cell		SPECT	single photon emission computed tomography
RBF	renal blood flow			
RCA	right coronary artery		SSC	Scientific and Standardization Committee
RCM	restrictive cardiomyopathy		SSEP	somatosensory evoked potentials
RCT	randomized clinical trial		SSFP	steady-state free precession
RCV	reference change value		STEMI	ST-elevation myocardial infarction
REE	resting energy expenditure		STICH	spontaneous intracerebral haemorrhage
REM	rapid eye movement			
RF	respiratory failure		STS	Society of Thoracic Surgery
RHC	right heart catheterization		SV	stroke volume
RIFLE	Risk Injury Failure Loss Endstage classification		SVC	superior vena cava
			SVR	surgical ventricular remodelling *or* systemic vascular resistance
ROC	receiver operating characteristic			
ROS	reactive oxygen species		SVT	supraventricular tachycardia
ROSC	restoration of spontaneous circulation		TASH	transcoronary alcohol ablation of septal hypertrophy
RPP	renal perfusion pressure			
RR	relative risk		TAVI	transcatheter aortic valve implantation
RRT	renal replacement therapy		TCD	transcranial Doppler
RV	right ventricle, right ventricular		TCPC	total cavo-pulmonary connection
RVA	right ventricular apex		TD	tissue Doppler
RVAD	right ventricular assist device		TdP	torsades des pointes
RVOT	right ventricular outflow tract		TEE	transesophageal echocardiography
RVOTO	right ventricular outflow tract obstruction		TE	Thromboelas tometry
SAECG	signal averaged ECG		TEVAR	thoracic endovascular aortic repair
SAH	subarachnoid haemorrhage		TF	tissue factor
SAMU	service d'aide médicale urgente		TGA	transposition of the great arteries
SBP	spontaneous bacterial peritonitis *or* systolic blood pressure		TGC	tight glycaemic control
			TIA	transient ischaemic attacks
			TnT	troponin T

TOE	transoesophageal echocardiography		VCI	inferior vena cava
TOF	time-of-flight		VCV	volume controlled ventilation
TOR	termination of resuscitation		VEP	visual evoked potentials
TPG	transpulmonary pressure gradient		VF	ventricular fibrillation
TPP	transpulmonary pressure		VHD	valvular heart disease
TS	thyroid storm		VKA	vitamin K antagonist
TSH	thyroid stimulating hormone		VPD	valvular prosthesis dysfunction
TT	thrombolytic therapy		VRS	verbal rating scale
TTE	transthoracic echocardiography		VSD	ventricular septal defect
TTP	thrombotic thrombocytopenia purpura		VSR	ventricular septal rupture
TV	tidal volume *or* tricuspid valve		VT	ventricular tachycardia
UA	unstable angina		VTE	venous thromboembolism
UAG	urinary anion gap		VTI	time velocity integral
UEMS	Union Européenne des Médecins Spécialisés		VWF	von Willebrand factor
UFH	unfractionated heparin		VZV	variccella zoster virus
UO	urine output		WBC	white blood cell
UPA	urokinase-type plasminogen activator		WCC	white cell count
URL	upper reference limit		WGACC	Working Group on Acute Cardiac Care
VAD	ventricular assist device		WHF	World Heart Federation
VADT	Veterans Affairs Diabetes Trial		WHO	World Health Organization
VALI	ventilator-associated lung injury		WPW	Wolff–Parkinson–White syndrome
VAP	ventilator-associated pneumonia		XMRV	xenotropic murine leukaemia virus related virus
VAS	visual analogue scale			
VASP	vasodilator-stimulated phosphoprotein		ZEEP	zero end-expiratory pressure
VCAM	vascular cell adhesion molecule			

Contributors

Dr Gihan Abuella
Specialist Registrar
Anaesthesia & Intensive Care
St George's Hospital
Blackshaw Road
London UK

Professor Frédéric Adnet
Urgences - SAMU 93
Hôpital Avicenne
125 rue de Stalingrad
93009 Bobigny Cedex
FRANCE

Dr Benedetta Agnoli
Department of Obstetrics and Gynaecology
Policlinico, Mangiagalli e Regina Elena
IRCCS
Milan
ITALY

Dr Ömür Akhavuz
Heartcenter
Leipzig University
Struempelstrasse 39
04289 Leipzig
GERMANY

Dr Joakim Alfredsson
Department of Cardiology
University Hospital
SE 58185 Linkoping
SWEDEN

Professor Joseph Alpert
University of Arizona College of Mediciine
Tuscon A2
USA

Dr Diego Ardissino
Divisione di Cardiologia
Azienda Ospedaliero Universitaria di Parma
Via Gramsci 14
43126 Parma
ITALY

Dr Nisha Arenja
Universitatspital Basel
Petersgraben 4
4031 Basel
SWITZERLAND

Dr Hans-Richard Arntz
Charite: Campus Benjamin Franklin
Department of Cardiopulmology
Hindenburgdamm 30
12200 Berlin
GERMANY

Dr Arthur Atchabahian
Department of Anesthesiology
NYU Medical Center
301 East 17th St, C2-222
New York, NY 10003
USA

Professor Lina Badimon
Director, Cardiovascular Research Center (CSIC-ICCC)
Institut Català de Ciències Cardiovasculars
Hospital de la Santa Creu i Sant Pau,
Av. Sant Antoni M. Claret 167
08025 Barcelona
SPAIN

Dr Sean Bagshaw
Intensive Care Unit
University of Alberta Medical Center
Edmonton
Alberta
CANADA

Dr Jan Bahr
Universitätsmedizin Göttingen
Zentrum Anaesthesiologie, Rettungs- und Intensivmedizin
Robert-Koch-Str. 40
37075 Göttingen
GERMANY

Dr Andrea Ballotta
Postop Intensive Care - Heart Surgery Department
IRCCS Policlinico San Donato
Via Morandi, 30
20097 San Donato Milanese
ITALY

Professor George Baltopoulos
Chairman
Department of Critical Care
University of Athens
GREECE

Professor Jean Pierre Bassand
Head, Cardiology Department
University Hospital Jean Minjoz
Boulevard Fleming
25000 Besancon
FRANCE

Dr Jeroen J Bax
Department of Cardiology C5P
Leiden University Medical Centre
Albinusdreef 2
2333 ZA Leiden
THE NETHERLANDS

Professor Rinaldo Bellomo
Department of Intensive Care
Austin Hospital
Studley Road
Heidelberg VIC 3084
AUSTRALIA

Dr Vanessa Belpomme
Médecine Générale
Hôpital Beaujon
100 bd du Général Leclerc
92110 Clichy
FRANCE

Dr Ruxandra Beyer
Institutul Inimii 'Prof. Dr. Nicolae Stancioiu'
Calea Motilor, Nr. 19-21
400001 Cluj-Napoca
ROMANIA

Dr Dionyssia Birmpa
Research Fellow
Heart Failure Unit
Attikon University Hospital
Athenes
GREECE

Prof Dr Eric Boersma
Department of Cardiology   Erasmus MC
Gravendijkwal 230 3015 CE Rotterdam
THE NETHERLANDS

Dr Bernd Böttiger
Chairman, Department of Anaesthesiology and Postoperative
Intensive Care Medicine
University of Cologne
Kerpener Straße 62
50937 Köln
GERMANY

Professor Leo Bossaert
Faculty of Medicine
University of Antwerp
Heuvelstraat 31
BE2530 Boechout
BELGIUM

Professor Jens Bremerich
Department of Radiology
University Hospital Basel
Petersgraben 4
CH 4031 Basel
SWITZERLAND

Dr Dirk Brutsaert
A.Z. Miiddelheim Hospital, Univ. of Antwerp
Department of Cardiology
Lindendreef 1
BE-2020 Antwerpen
BELGIUM

Prof Dr Michael Buerke
Department Of Medicine Iii
Martin-Luther-University
Ernst-Grube-Str.40
06097 Halle/Saale
GERMANY

Dr Eleonora Carlesso
Dipartimento di Anestesiologia, Terapia Intensiva e Scienze
Dermatologiche
Università degli Studi
Via F. Sforza 35
Milan
ITALY

Dr Valeria Caso
Consultant Neurologist
Stroke Unit and Division of Cardiovascular Medicine
University of Perugia
Santa Maria della Misericordia Hospital
Sant'Andrea delle Fratte
06126 Perugia
ITALY

Dr Serenella Castelvecchio
Division of Cardiac Surgery
Division of Cardiothoracic and Vascular Anaesthesia
IRCCS Policlinico San Donato
Via Morandi 30
20097 San Donato Milanese
Milan
ITALY

Dr Guillaume Cayla
Department of Cardiology
University Hospital Caremeau
30000 Nîmes
FRANCE

Dr Aures Chaib
Hopital Georges Pompidou
Cardiology Department
20 rue Leblanc
75015 Paris
FRANCE

Dr Pierre-Géraud Claret
Division anesth.,crit.care, pain & emergency
SAMU 30
University Hospital Caremeau
30000 Nîmes
FRANCE

Dr Peter Clemmensen
Department of Cardiology
The Heart Center
Rigshospitalet - Copenhagen University Hospital
9, Blegdamsvej
DK-2100 Copenhagen
DENMARK

Dr Charlotte Cordonnier
Associate Professor of Neurology
Department of Neurology
Univ Lille Nord de France, CHU Lille
Lille
FRANCE

Dr Sonja Curac
Service d'Anesthésie-Réanimation-SMUR
Hôpital Beaujon
100 Bld du Général Leclerc
92100 Clichy
FRANCE

Dr Nicolas Danchin
Service de Cardiologie
Hopital Europeen Georges Pompidou (HEGP)
20 rue Leblanc
75015 Paris
FRANCE

Dr Yves Debaveye
Department of Intensive Care Medicine
University Hospital Gasthuisberg
B-3000 Leuven
BELGIUM

Dr Cathy de Deyne
Department of Anesthesiology
Campus St Jan
Schiepsebos 6
3600 Genk
BELGIUM

Dr Laurent de Kerchove
Cardiothoracic and vascular surgery
Cliniques Universitares Saint-Luc,
Av. Hippocrate 10,
1200 Brussels
BELGIUM

Professor Jean Emmanuel de la Coussaye
Division anesth.,crit.care, pain & emergency
SAMU 30
University Hospital Caremeau
30000 Nîmes
FRANCE

Dr Demetrios Demetriades
Department of Surgery
Division of Trauma & Surgical Intensive Care
Keck School
University of Southern California
Los Angeles
USA

Dr Gregory Ducrocq
Cardiology Department
Hopital Bichat
46 rue Henri Huchard
75018 Paris
FRANCE

Dr Eric Durand
Service de Cardiologie HEGP
20 rue Leblanc
75908 Paris cedex 15
FRANCE

Dr Alain Durocher
Réanimation Médicale
Hôpital Calmette
CHRU de Lille
59037 Lille cedex
FRANCE

Dr Henning Ebelt
Department of Medicine III
University Clinics of the Martin-Luther-University
Halle-Wittenberg
Ernst-Grube-Str. 40
D-06097 Halle(Saale)
GERMANY

Dr Joachim Ehrlich
Assistant Professor of Medicine
Department of Cardiology, Div. of Clinical Electrophysiology
Intensive Coronary Care Unit
Goethe-University Hospital
Theodor Stern Kai 7
60590 Frankfurt
GERMANY

Dr Gébrine El Khoury
Cardiothoracic and vascular surgery
Cliniques Universitaires Saint Luc
10 av. Hippocrate
1200 Brussels
BELGIUM

Dr Wesley Ely
Health Services Research Center
6109 Medical Center East
Vanderbilt University School of Medicine
Nashville TN 37232-8300
USA

Dr Raphaël Favory
Réanimation Médicale
Hôpital Calmette
CHRU de Lille
59037 Lille cedex
FRANCE

Dr Gerasimos Filippatos
Department of Cardiology
University of Athenes Hospital
Athenes
GREECE

Prof Dr Frank Flachskampf
Med Klinik 2
University of Erlangen
Ulmenweg 18
91054 Erlangen
GERMANY

Dr Nazzareno Galiè
Institute of Cardiology
University of Bologna
Via Massarenti, 9
40138 Bologna
ITALY

Professor Luciano Gattinoni
Dipartimento di Anestesiologia, Terapia Intensiva e Scienze
Dermatologiche
Università degli Studi
Via F. Sforza 35
Milan 20122
ITALY

Dr Etienne Gayat
Anesthesie Department
Hôpital Lariboisière
2, rue Ambroise Paré
FR-75475 Paris cedex 10
FRANCE

Dr Mihai Gheorghiade
Northwestern Univ Feinberg School of Medicine
676 North St. Clair Street
Suite 600
Chicago IL 60611
USA

Prof Dr Med Evangelos Giannitsis
Medizinische Klinik III
Im Neuenheimer Feld 410,
69120 Heidelberg
GERMANY

Dr Marijke Gielen
Department of Intensive Care Medicine
University of Leuven
Herestraat 49
B-3000 Leuven
BELGIUM

Prof Dr Matthias Girndt
Department of Medicine III
University Clinics of the Martin-Luther-University Halle-Wittenberg
Ernst-Grube-Str. 40
D-06097 Halle(Saale)
GERMANY

Dr Anselm Gitt
Klinikum Ludwigshafen
Bremserstraβe 79
67063 Ludwigshafen
GERMANY

Dr Patrick Goldstein
Emergency Department
Lille University Hospital
59037 Lille Cedex
FRANCE

Dr Bulent Gorenek
Eskisehir Osmangazi Universitesi
Tip Fakultesi Hastanesi
Kardiyoloji Poliklinigi
2. Kat
TURKEY

Professor Rik Gosselink
Faculty of Kinesiology and Rehabilitation Sciences
Catholic University of Leuven
Tervuursevest 101 - bus 01500
B-3001 Heverlee
BELGIUM

Dr Erik Grove
Department of Cardiology
Aarhus University Hospital
Skejby
8200 Aarhus N
DENMARK

Dr Olga Gurjeva
Emergency Cardiology Department
National Scientific Center -Institute of Cardiology
5 Narodnogo Opolchemia Str
01151 Kiev
UKRAINE

Dr David Hasdai
Department of Cardiology
Rabin Medical Center
Beilinson Campus
39 Jabotinsky St.
49100 Petah-Tikva
ISRAEL

Professor Yonathan Hasin
Head, Cardiovascular Institute
Poria Medical Center
MP Lower Galilee 15208
ISRAEL

Dr Magda Heras
Head, Secció de Cardiologia Clínica
ICT
Hospital Clínic
Villarroel, 170
08036 Barcelona
SPAIN

Dr Sanne Hoeks
Thoraxcenter/ Klep Group/ Ba559
Erasmus MC
Dr Molewaterplein 40
3015 GD Rotterdam
THE NETHERLANDS

Dr Stefan Hohnloser
Professor of Medicine
Head, Division of Clinical Electrophysiology, Department of
Cardiology, Division of Clinical Electrophysiology, Intensive
Coronary Care Unit
Goethe-University Hospital
Theodor Stern Kai 7
60590 Frankfurt
GERMANY

Prof Dr Kurt Huber
Director, 3rd Department of Medicine
Cardiology and Emergency Medicine Wilhelminenhospital
Montlearstr. 37
1160 Vienna
AUSTRIA

Dr Anne-Mette Hvas
Head, Department of Clinical Biochemistry
Aarhus University Hospital
Skejby
8200 Aarhus N
DENMARK

Dr Zaza Iakobishvili
Department of Cardiology
Beilinson Campus
Clalit Health Services
ISRAEL

Professor Bernard Iung
Cardiology Department
Bichat Hospital
46, rue Henri Huchard
75877 Paris Cedex 18
FRANCE

Professor Allan Jaffe
Mayo Clinic
200 First Street SW
Rochester, MN 55905
USA

Dr Ilya Kagan
Institute for Nutrition Research
Rabin Medical Center
Beilinson Hospital
Petah Tikva 49100
ISRAEL

Dr Konstantinos Karatolios
Klinik für Innere Medizin-Kardiologie
Universitätsklinikum Giessen und Marburg GmbH
Standort Marburg Baldingerstr
35043 Marburg
GERMANY

Dr Hugo Katus
Department of Internal Medicine and Cardiology
University of Heidelberg
Im Neuenheimer Feld 410
D-69120 Heidelberg
GERMANY

Dr Brian F. Keogh
Consultant Anaesthetist
Royal Brompton & Harefield NHS Foundation Trust
Sydney Street
London SW3 6NP
UK

Dr Leslie Kobayashi
Department of Surgery
Division of Trauma & Surgical Intensive Care
Keck School
University of Southern California
Los Angeles
USA

Dr Viktor Kočka
Cardiocenter of 3.Medical School of Charles Universit
Šrobárova 50
Prague 10
CZECH REPUBLIC

Prof Dr Stavros Konstantinides
Department of Cardiology
Democritus University of Thrace
University General Hospital
68100 Alexandroupolis
GREECE

Dr Emmanuel Koutalas
Cardiology Department
Heraklion University Hospital
Heraklion
Crete
GREECE

Dr Steen Kristensen
Department of Cardiology
Aarhus University Hospital
Skejby
8200 Aarhus N
DENMARK

Dr Lucia J Kroft
Department of Radiology
Leiden University Medical Center
Albinusdreef 2
2333 ZA Leiden
THE NETHERLANDS

Dr Christian Laplace
Département d'anesthésie-réanimation chirurgicale
CHU de Bicêtre, assistance publique-hôpitaux de Paris
78, rue du Général-Leclerc,
94275 Le Kremlin-Bicêtre, Cedex
FRANCE

Dr Frédéric Lapostolle
Urgences - SAMU 93
Hopital Avicenne
125 rue de Stalingrad
93009 Bobigny, Cedex
FRANCE

Dr Carlo Lavalle
Department of Cardiology
San Filippo Neria Hospital
via Michele di Lando, 60
00162 Rome
ITALY

Dr Enri Leci
Institute of Cardiology
University of Bologna
Via Massarenti, 9
40138 Bologna
ITALY

Professor Didier Leys
Professor of Neurology
Service de neurologie et pathologie neuro-vasculaire
Univ Lille Nord de France, CHU Lille
Lille
FRANCE

Dr Daniela Lina
Divisione di Cardiologia
Azienda Ospedaliero Universitaria di Parma
Via Gramsci 14
43126 Parma
ITALY

Professor Bertil Lindahl
Uppsala Clinical Research Center
Department of Medical Sciences
Uppsala Science Park
751 83 Uppsala
SWEDEN

Dr Pablo Loma-Osorio
Coronary Care Unit
Hospital Josep Trueta
Av. Francia sn
17007 Girona
SPAIN

Professor Bernhard Maisch
Director, Department of Internal Medicine & Cardiology
Philipps Universitaet Marburg
Baldingerstrasse
D-35043 Marburg
GERMANY

Dr Alan Maisel
Veterans Affairs Medical Center
Cardiology 111-A
3350 La Jolla Village Drive
San Diego CA 92161
USA

Dr Alessandra Manes
Institute of Cardiology
University of Bologna
Via Massarenti, 9
40138 Bologna
ITALY

Dr P M Mannucci
A. Bianchi Bonomi Hemophilia and Thrombosis Center
Department of Medicine and Medical Specialties
Via Pace, 9
20122 Milan
ITALY

Dr Josep Masip
Associated Professor of Cardiology, University of Barcelona;
Critical Care Department Director,
Hospital Sant Joan Despí, Consorci Sanitari Integral,
University of Barcelona,
Jacint Verdaguer 90,
08970 Sant Joan Despí, Barcelona
SPAIN

Dr John McPherson
Health Services Research Center
6109 Medical Center East
Vanderbilt University School of Medicine
Nashville TN 37232-8300
USA

Professor Alexandre Mebazaa
Anesthesie Department
Hôpital Lariboisière
2, rue Ambroise Paré
FR-75475 Paris cedex 10
FRANCE

Dr Nicolas Meneveau
Department of Cardiology
Pôle Coeur-Poumons
University Hospital Jean-Minjoz
3 Boulevard Fleming
FR-25000 Besançon
FRANCE

Dr Dieter Mesotten
Department of Intensive Care Medicine
Herestraat 49
B-3000 Leuven
BELGIUM

Dr Marco Metra
Department of Expermental and Applied Medicine
University Section of Cardiovascular Diseases
C/O Spedali Civili
P.zza Spedali Civili 1
25123 Brescia
ITALY

Dr Fred Mohr
Heart Center Leipzig
University of Leipzig
Clinic of Cardiac Surgery
Struempellstrasse 39
DE-04289 Leipzig
GERMANY

Professor Christian Mueller
Departement Innere Medizin
Universitätsspital Basel
Petersgraben 4
CH-4031 Basel
SWITZERLAND

Dr Wilfried Mullens
Heart Failure And Cardiac Transplantation
Cleveland Clinic
9500 Euclid Avenue
Cleveland OH 44195
USA

Dr Pavlos Myrianthefs
ICU
KAT Hospital
Nikis 2
14561 Athens
GREECE

Dr Menachem Nahir
Cardiovascular Institute
Poria Medical Center
MP Lower Galilee 15208
ISRAEL

Dr Francesca Notarangelo
Divisione di Cardiologia
Azienda Ospedaliero Universitaria di Parma
Via Gramsci 14
43126 Parma
ITALY

Dr Michel Noutsias
Department of Cardiology
University Hospital of Marburg - UKGM GmbH
Baldinger Strasse 1
D-35033 Marburg
GERMANY

Dr Julian Arias Ortiz
Erasme Hospital
Free University of Brussels
Route de Lennik 808
B-1070 Brussels
BELGIUM

Dr Teresa Padro
Cardiovascular Research Center (CSIC-ICCC)
Institut Català de Ciències Cardiovasculars
Hospital de la Santa Creu i Sant Pau
Av. Sant Antoni M. Claret 167
08025 Barcelona
SPAIN

Dr Massimiliano Palazzini
Institute of Cardiology
University of Bologna
Via Massarenti, 9
40138 Bologna
ITALY

Dr Sabine Pankuweit
Department of Internal Medicine/Cardiology
Philipps-University Marburg
Baldinger Str.
35043 Marburg
GERMANY

Dr John T Parissis
Heart Failure Unit,
Attikon University Hospital,
Navarinou 13,
15122 Maroussi
Athens
GREECE

Professor Alexander Parkhomenko
Emergency Cardiology Department
National Scientific Center -Institute of Cardiology
5 Narodnogo Opolchemia Str
01151 Kiev
UKRAINE

Dr Tomislav Petrovic
Urgences - SAMU 93
Hopital Avicenne
125 rue de Stalingrad
93009 Bobigny Cedex
FRANCE

Dr Manuel Pirotte
Cardiothoracic and vascular surgery
Cliniques Universitares Saint-Luc,
Av. Hippocrate 10,
1200 Brussels
BELGIUM

Dr Antonis Pitsis
Thessaloniki Heart Institute
St. Luke's Hospital
Thessaloniki
GREECE

Dr Kenneth Planas
Critical Care Department,
Hospital Moisès Broggi Sant Joan Despí,
Consorci Sanitari Integral
Barcelona 08025
SPAIN

Dr Mario Plebani
Department of Laboratory Medicine
University Hospital
Padova
ITALY

Dr Don Poldermans
Erasmus MC
Department of Surgery, Room H 805,
's Gravendijkwal 230
3015 CE Rotterdam
THE NETHERLANDS

Professor Piotr Ponikowski
Center for Heart Diseases, Department of Cardiology,
Military Hospital Wroclaw;
Department of Cardiac Diseases, Wroclaw Medical University
ul. Weigla 5
50981 Wroclaw
POLAND

Dr Patrizia Presbitero
Istituto Clinico Humanitas
Via Manzoni n 56
Rozzano (Milan)
ITALY

Dr Susanna Price
Consultant Cardiologist & Intensivist
Royal Brompton & Harefield NHS Trust
ENGLAND

Dr John Prowle
Department of Intensive Care
Austin Hospital
Heidelberg
Melbourne ViC
AUSTRALIA

Professor Tom Quinn
Professor of Clinical Practice
23DK04, Duke of Kent Building
Division of Health and Social Care
Faculty of Health and Medical Sciences
University of Surrey
Guildford
UK

Dr Pam Rajendram
UCSD Medical Center
Division of Cardiology
200 West Arbor Drive
San Diego, CA 92103-8411
USA

Dr Marco Ranucci
Director of Clinical Research
Department of Anesthesia and Intensive Care
IRCCS Policlinico S.Donato
Via Morandi 30
20097 San Donato Milanese (Milan)
ITALY

Dr Ardawan Rastan
Herzzentrum der Universität Leipzig
Struempellstr. 39
04289 Leipzig
GERMANY

Dr Andrew Rhodes
Consultant
Intensive Care Medicine
St George's Hospital
Cranmer Terrace
London
ENGLAND

Dr Agnes Ricard-Hibon
Department of Anaesthesiology
University Hospital
100 Bld du Général Leclerc
92110 Clichy
FRANCE

Dr Renato Ricci
San Filippo Neri Hospital
Department of Cardiology
Via G. Martinotti, 20
00135 Rome
ITALY

Professor Arsen Ristic
Department of Cardiology
University of Belgrade
Koste Todorovica 8
11000 Belgrade
SERBIA

Dr Jean Roeseler
Cliniques Universitaires St Luc
Soins intensifs & Urgences
Av Hippocrate 10
1200 Bruxelles
BELGIUM

Dr Martin Russ
Cardiology Department
University of Halle
Ernst-Grube-Strasse 40
06120 Halle
GERMANY

Professor Massimo Santini
Director, Cardiovascular Department
S. Filippo Neri Hospital
Via G. Martinotti, 20
00135 Rome
ITALY

Dr François Schiele
Department of Cardiology
Pole Coeur-Poumons
University Hospital Jean-Minjoz
Boulevard Fleming
25000 Besançon
FRANCE

Dr Andreas Schneider
Department of Anaesthesiology and Postoperative Intensive Care
Medicine
University of Cologne
Kerpener Straße 62
50937 Köln
GERMANY

Dr Joanne D Schuijf
Department Cardiology C5-P
Leiden University Medical Center
Albinusdreef 2
2333 ZA Leiden
THE NETHERLANDS

Professor Jurg Schwitter
Director Cardiac MR Center of the CHUV
University Hospital Lausanne - CHUV
rue de Bugnon
CH-1011 Lausanne
SWITZERLAND

Dr Sofia Sederholm-Lawesson
Department of Cardiology
University Hospital
SE 58185 Linkoping
SWEDEN

Dr Maria Sejersten Ripa
Department of Cardiology Rigshospitalet
Copenhagen University Hospital
Nørregade 10
1165 Copenhagen
DENMARK

Dr Kevin Shah
Department of Cardiology 111A
Veterans Affairs San Diego Healthcare System
3350 La Jolla Village Dr
San Diego CA 92161
USA

Professor Alexander Shpektor
Chief, Cardiology Department
Moscow State University of Medicine and Dentistry
11 Yauskaya Str
Moscow 109240
RUSSIA

Dr Emmanuel Simantirakis
Cardiology Department
Heraklion University Hospital
Heraklion
Crete
GREECE

Professor Pierre Singer
Institute for Nutrition Research
Rabin Medical Center
Beilinson Hospital
Petah Tikva 49100
ISRAEL

Dr Peter Sinnaeve
Department of Cardiology
University of Leuven
Herestraat 49
B-3000 Leuven
BELGIUM

Dr Alessandro Sionis
Consultant, Intensive Cardiac Care Unit
Cardiology Department
Thorax Institute
Hospital Clínic
08036 Barcelona
SPAIN

Dr Thenral Socrates
Interne Medizin
Universitatsspital
Petersgraben 4
CH 4031 Basel
SWITZERLAND

Dr Martin Strueber
Department of Cardiothoracic, Transplant, and Vascular Surgery
Hannover Medical School
Carl-Neuberg-Str. 1
30625 Hannover
GERMANY

Professor Eva Swahn
Department of Cardiology
University Hospital
SE 58185 Linkoping
SWEDEN

Dr Lorna Swan
Cardiology Department
Royal Brompton Hospital
Sydney Street
London
ENGLAND

Dr Karim Tazarourte
Pôle Urgence
SAMU 77-SMUR -SAU-Réanimation Polyvalente
Hôpital Marc Jacquet
77000 Melun
FRANCE

Dr Peter Teschendorf
Department of Anaesthesiology and Postoperative Intensive Care
Medicine
University of Cologne
Kerpener Straße 62
50937 Köln
GERMANY

Dr Franck Thuny
Département de Cardiologie
Unité Valvulopathies et Insuffisance Cardiaque
Hôpital de la Timone
Marseille
FRANCE

Professor Kristian Thygesen
Department of Medicine and Cardiology
Aarhus University Hospital
Tage-Hansens Gade 2
DK-8000 Aarhus C
DENMARK

Professor Adam Torbicki
Department of Chest Medicine
Institute of Tuberculosis and Lung Disease
ul. Plocka 26
01-138 Warszawa
POLAND

Dr Petr Tousek
3rd Medical Faculty
Ruska 87
100 00 Prague
CZECH REPUBLIC

Dr Marco Tubaro
Intensive Cardiac Care Unit
Cardiovascular Department
San Filippo Neri Hospital
Rome
ITALY

Professor Alec Vahanian
Service de Cardiologie
Hôpital Bichat
46 rue Henri Huchard
75018 Paris
FRANCE

Dr Greet Van den Berghe
Head, Department of Intensive Care Medicine
University of Leuven
Herestraat 49
B-3000 Leuven
BELGIUM

Dr Jeroen Vandenbrande
Department of Intensive Care Medicine
University Hospital Gasthuisberg
B-3000 Leuven
BELGIUM

Dr Frans Van de Werf
Department of Cardiovascular Diseases
University of Leuven
Herestraat 49
B-3000 Leuven
BELGIUM

Dr Joëlla E van Velzen
Leiden University Medical Centre
Cardiology
Albinusdreef 2
2300 RC Leiden
THE NETHERLANDS

Dr Yoo-Mee Vanwijngaerden
Department of Intensive Care Medicine
Herestraat 49
B-3000 Leuven
BELGIUM

Professor Panos Vardas
Head, Cardiology Department
Heraklion University Hospital
Heraklion
Crete
GREECE

Professor Elena Vasilieva
Department of Cardiology
Moscow State University of Medicine & Dentistry
Yauzskaya Street,11
109240 Moscow
RUSSIA

Dr Antoine Vieillard-Baron
University Hospital Ambroise Paré
Intensive Care Unit
9 avenue Charles de Gaulle
92104 Boulogne
FRANCE

Dr Johan Vijgen
Cardiology Department
Virga Jesse Hospital
Stadsomvaart 11
3500 Hasselt
BELGIUM

Dr Gemma Vilahur
Cardiovascular Research Center (CSIC-ICCC)
Institut Català de Ciències Cardiovasculars
Hospital de la Santa Creu i Sant Pau
Av. Sant Antoni M. Claret 167
08025 Barcelona
SPAIN

Professor Jean-Louis Vincent
Head Department of Intensive Care
Erasme Hospital
Free University of Brussels
Route de Lennik 808
B-1070 Brussels
BELGIUM

Dr Aikaterini Visouli
St. Luke's Hospital
Thessaloniki Heart Institute
Panorama, Thessaloniki
55131 Thessaloniki
GREECE

Dr Pascal Vranckx
Hartcentrum Hasselt
Campus Virga Jesseziekenhuis
Stadsomvaart 11
BE-3500 Hasselt
BELGIUM

Dr Chad Wagner
Health Services Research Center
6109 Medical Center East
Vanderbilt University School of Medicine
Nashville TN 37232-8300
USA

Professor Karl Werdan
Director, Department of Medicine III
University Clinics of the Martin-Luther-University Halle-
Wittenberg
Ernst-Grube-Str. 40
D-06097 Halle(Saale)
GERMANY

Professor Harvey D White
Auckland City Hospital
Auckland
NEW ZEALAND

Professor Petr Widimski
Head of the Cardio Center
University Hospital Vinohrady
3rd Medical School, Charles University,
Srobarova 50
100 34 Prague 10
CZECH REPUBLIC

Dr Doron Zahger
Associate Professor of Cardiology
Faculty of Health Sciences
Ben Gurion University of the Negev
Beer Sheva
ISRAEL

Dr Martina Zaninotto
Department of Laboratory Medicine
University Hospital
Padova
ITALY

Dr Dennis Zavalloni
Istituto Clinico Humanitas
Via Manzoni n 56
Rozzano (Milan)
ITALY

CHAPTER 1

Intensive and acute cardiac care: an introduction

Nicolas Danchin, Gerasimos Filippatos, and Marco Tubaro

Cardiovascular diseases (CVDs) are the leading cause of death in the Western world and for most of them rapid (within minutes) diagnosis and intervention are necessary to improve patient prognosis. Cardiologists must be trained and cardiovascular institutions equipped accordingly, to deal with the emergencies in cardiology. That is why intensive and acute cardiac care (IACC) is the core of cardiology. IACC is carried out in many different settings—from the patient's home to the ambulance, hospital emergency department (ED), intensive cardiac care unit (ICCU), and cardiology ward—and patient care also includes hospital discharge and implementation of secondary prevention strategies. Complex cases (with renal failure, diabetes, respiratory insufficiency, or sepsis) are nowadays treated by different specialists, without proper cardiological training: the knowledge, skills, and training of IACC cardiologists are essential to the provision of high quality care.

The history of IACC in modern cardiology began with the early experiences of open-chest defibrillation, demonstrating the feasibility resuscitating a patient from cardiac arrest; subsequently, Zoll introduced the external defibrillator, which was used in combination with mouth-to-mouth ventilation and chest compression to perform cardiopulmonary resuscitation (CPR) in patients with ventricular fibrillation. Desmond Julian was the first to suggest the concept of the coronary care unit (CCU) to the British Cardiothoracic Society in 1961; in 1962 he set up the first CCU in Sidney for the monitoring of patients with acute myocardial infarction (AMI), and in 1964 he established the first CCU in Europe (in Edinburgh). A few years later, Killip and Kimball demonstrated a reduction in mortality from 28 to 7% in AMI patients without shock treated with 'aggressive' pharmacological therapy in a CCU.

To begin with, CCUs were particularly devoted to the identification and treatment of ventricular arrhythmias. In the 1970s, the role and importance of CCUs began to be recognized, together with the development of seminal experiences of fibrinolytic therapy in humans. In 1980, the seminal paper of De Wood *et al.* demonstrated that the vast majority of AMIs were caused by a thrombotic obstruction of a coronary artery. Consequently, thrombolytic therapy was considered to be the best possible approach, and after the GISSI and ISIS-2 studies thrombolytic therapy became the accepted standard treatment of AMI. These megatrials led the way to an extremely active development of clinical trials in acute heart diseases, particularly in the field of antithrombotic therapy, and there is no doubt that CCUs have been the port of entry of many new medications now widely used in cardiology.

The first comparison between primary percutaneous coronary intervention (PCI) and thrombolysis (in this case, intracoronary thrombolysis) date from the same year (1986) as the seminal GISSI paper: in the following years, several studies were carried out, showing the advantage of mechanical over pharmacological coronary reperfusion.

Driven by the wider use of interventional cardiology, in more recent years CCUs have been integrated into systems of care: the beginning of the treatment of ST-elevation myocardial infarction (STEMI) moved from the CCUs to ED and then to the pre-hospital stage (with pre-hospital thrombolysis) and networks between peripheral hospitals and STEMI-receiving centres were implemented, linked to the emergency medical service (EMS) operated by physicians and/or paramedics and nurses. Parallel to these changes in the early management of patients with STEMI, changes could be observed in the definition of myocardial infarction, based on the more and more widespread use of troponin measurement; the use of these new highly sensitive biological tools has led to a reclassification of many patients from unstable angina to non STEMI.

In the meantime, the transition from CCUs to ICCUs was in progress. The proportion of elderly patients with acute coronary syndromes (ACS) increased: patients with complex and multiorgan diseases, who need recourse to high-tech treatment and interventional/surgical procedures represent a large proportion of the ICCU population. Moreover, ageing of the population and better management of patients

with heart disease increased the number of patients admitted to the ICCU with acute decompensated heart failure (ADHF). As in the case of ACS, the use of new biomarkers, such as natriuretic peptides, has helped reascertain the diagnosis of acute heart failure; in addition, these new markers are potent discriminators of outcomes and are now used as prognostic tools in many different clinical settings. ADHF patients are admitted to the ICCU if they are poor responders to first line therapies, with low cardiac output, oliguria, myocardial ischaemia, or cardiogenic shock: they require complex and intensive care, high-tech equipment, skilled ICCU staff, and a prolonged stay. Patients with ADHF deserve more knowledgeable, skilful, and better-trained ICCU physicians and multispecialty treatment, with the use of complex equipments such as intra-aortic balloon pumping (IABP), renal replacement therapy (RRT), implantable cardioverter-defibrillators (ICD), cardiac resynchronization therapy (CRT), and ventricular assist devices (VAD). Other diseases are also becoming more commonly seen in the ICCU, such as acute pulmonary embolism, severe dysrhythmias, electric storms and ICD malfunctions, sepsis, and multiorgan failure. An example of the case mix in modern ICCUs is shown in ➔ Fig. 1.1.

The combination of elderly patients, severe multiorgan diseases, and technically demanding diagnostic and therapeutic strategies provides the treating staff with a special challenge, requiring dedicated training. To accomplish this task, the Working Group on Acute Cardiac Care (WGACC) of the European Society of Cardiology (ESC) established

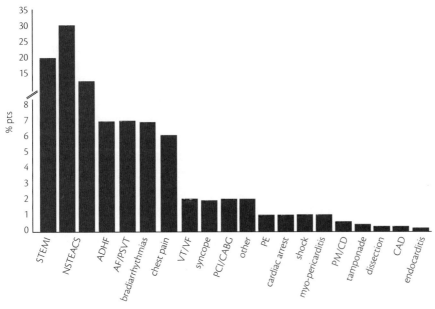

Figure 1.1 BLITZ 3. Italian registry of ICCUs, conducted for 15 days (7–21 April 2008) in 332 out of 409 (81%) Italian ICCUs.

Diagnosis at ICCU discharge

a training programme and an accreditation process in IACC. The aim was to properly train cardiologists to offer state-of-the-art treatment for severe cardiac diseases throughout the many countries belonging to the ESC, reducing inequalities of care and improving overall outcome. IACC is a new and important subspecialism in cardiology, and the role of intensive care cardiologist is depicted in a new core curriculum (CC) in IACC, based on a comprehensive combination of knowledge, skills, and attitudes: this CC outlines the education and training for cardiologists working in ICCUs, with log books, a written examination, and final accreditation (and re-certification) (see ➲ Chapter 11 for details).

Application of evidence-based medicine to complex high-risk cardiac patients in the ICCU needs a formal, intensive training in the field; moreover, both the provision of a very high quality of care and the need for reporting and audit make necessary to establish a process of accreditation of ICCU cardiologists by the scientific societies.

This book has been written with the purpose of serving IACC accreditation: all the various aspects of this pivotal subspecialty of cardiology are treated in a comprehensive way.

The first two sections are devoted to the first points where acute cardiac diseases are treated: the pre-hospital setting and the ED. Particularly in ACS the treatment must be initiated as soon as possible, and the main field of operation is the heart attack site: cooperation with other professional figures is pivotal in this setting.

The ICCU is the main cardiological institution performing IACC, and its structure, equipment, staff, and operations are addressed, as well as monitoring and procedures. Patients are monitored more closely in the ICCU than in other departments, not only for cardiovascular function is concerned, but also for brain, pulmonary, and renal function: close monitoring allows the implementation of intensive treatments for acute diseases, with the important help of imaging techniques, particularly echocardiography.

The need for a shift from CCUs to ICCUs is also linked to the application of several complex therapeutic techniques, such as ventilation (both noninvasive and mechanical), cardiac support (IABP and VAD), and RRT, among others.

Laboratory medicine is widely used in IACC, both for prompt diagnosis of acute conditions and for prognostic stratification, which frequently drives patient allocation and treatment strategies.

ACS, ADHF, and serious arrhythmias deserve a whole section each, being the three most important groups of diseases managed in ICCUs: they are dealt with in great detail, including pharmacological and nonpharmacological treatments. As well as the three main groups of acute diseases, many other cardiovascular acute conditions are treated in ICCUs, and a whole section of the book is devoted to myocardial, valvular, and aortic emergencies, among many others.

The largest section of the book is dedicated to the many acute noncardiovascular conditions that contribute to the patients' case mix in ICCU and widen the concept of IACC: the acute and intensive management of this vast variety of acute illnesses requires a deep and at the same time wide clinical training, not only in acute cardiac care, but in acute medical care in broad terms.

Each chapter has been written by a real expert in the field, and is fully in agreement with the ESC guidelines and the CC in IACC; multiple choice questions (MCQs) on many of the chapters are available for continuing medical education (CME).

A particular asset of this textbook is the online edition, which includes many more figure and tables, a long reference list for each chapter and original material like photos and videos, to better show diagnostic and therapeutic techniques and procedures in IACC.

We believe that this textbook will be very useful in establishing a common basis of knowledge and a uniform and improved quality of care in all European countries, for the benefit and better care of our patients.

SECTION I

Prehospital phase

CHAPTER 2

Sudden cardiac death: epidemiology and prevention

Hans-Richard Arntz

Contents

Summary

Sudden cardiac death (SCD) is considered to be the most frequent mode of death in adults in industrialized countries, but its incidence varies widely depending on definition and the source and quality of underlying data. It is estimated that about 80% of cases are due to coronary heart disease (CHD). The remaining 20% are attributable to a wide variety of inborn, genetically determined, or acquired diseases including a small group with hitherto undefined background.

Prevention primarily encompasses treatment of cardiovascular risk factors to avoid manifestation of CHD. Furthermore, preventive strategies are targeted to define groups of patients with an increased risk for SCD. A major target group are patients with impaired left ventricular function, especially due to myocardial infarction. These patients and some less clearly defined patient groups with nonischaemic cardiomyopathy and heart failure may profit from insertion of an ICD. With regard to pharmacological prevention, treatment of the underlying condition is the mainstay since no antiarrhythmic medication—with the exception of β-blockers in some situations—has shown to be efficacious.

The problem of definition

Although several definitions of the term 'sudden cardiac death' have been used, in more recent investigations it is usually defined as a natural death due to cardiac causes, heralded by abrupt loss of consciousness within 1 h after onset of acute symptoms [1]. Regrettably, the existence of different definitions of SCD make comparisons of many studies difficult if not impossible. Even the generally accepted definition, as above, is hampered by several problems. One is the mostly unproven definitive cardiac cause of death and another is the unclear duration of symptoms, particularly in unwitnessed arrests. Indeed, a prolonged time delay from first signs of change in clinical status to definitive loss of consciousness and cardiac arrest, for example as used in the Maastricht study [2], may increase the number of SCD cases but at the cost of lowering the proportion of deaths due to definitive cardiac causes. In a recently published study signs of change or cardiac symptoms preceding cardiac arrest were present for less than 1 h in only 116 of 323 patients and were present for up to 10 h in the majority of unexpected cardiac deaths according to of eye-witness observations [3]. Bypassing the problem of unwitnessed arrest by requiring an observation of the victims alive within 24 h of their death is therefore not very reliable. Finally, the notoriously low autopsy rates remain a major obstacle to the exact definition of the burden of the problem.

Incidence of sudden cardiac death

The incidence of SCD is varying widely depending on the data source, e.g. data from rescue services [4, 5] or from death certificates, the definition of SCD, and the population investigated [6] (➲ Table 2.1). The geographic area of the investigation may play a role. In addition, secular changes in the frequency and presentation of SCD have been observed.

The estimations for the 300 million population of the United States vary between 180 000 and 450 000 SCD cases/year. The highest numbers are derived from death certificates, which may lead to a significant overestimate. In prospective studies [7, 8] the SCD rate is noticeably less than 100/100 000 population/year. In an ongoing study in Oregon, which tried to use a multimodality approach (EMS data, coroner's and hospital reports) the incidence was 53/100 000 population per year [9]; similar findings were reported in Europe [10, 11]. In contrast, in the Maastricht study which included witnessed and unwitnessed sudden arrests of assumed cardiac origin, the incidence was 100/100 000 in the population aged 20–75 years [2]. In former West Berlin, with a population of 2.1 million, we observed 89 EMS-initiated resuscitation attempts per 100 000 population per year in witnessed and unwitnessed

arrests of assumed cardiac origin in the years 1987–1989 [12]. For the total European population of 730 million, this incidence would result in a burden of about 500 000–650 000 SCD cases per year in the whole of Europe.

Causes of sudden cardiac death

The incidence of SCD increases with age and is more frequent in males than in females. The same is true of CHD, which is the most common cause of SCD; it is estimated that about 80% of cases of SCD are attributed to this condition [13]. Since CHD becomes manifest in women about 10–15 years later than in men, the proportion of women with SCD increases in the old and very old population [42]. SCD may be triggered by acute ischaemia clinically presenting as an acute coronary syndrome due to a plaque rupture or erosion and partial or complete obstruction of a coronary artery. Alternatively, SCD may be caused by re-entry loops due to post-infarction scars often initiated by additional ischaemia [14]. The probability of the latter mechanism increases with impaired (left) ventricular function. Although CHD is the cause of SCD even in the majority of cases in younger adult victims of SCD, several other conditions expose predominantly younger people and some specific groups to risk. These conditions may be related to drugs; trauma; inflammatory, infiltrative, dilated and structural cardiomyopathies; a wide variety of genetically determined abnormalities; and, finally, a smaller group of as yet undefined background.

Several drugs with different indications may increase the risk of sudden arrhythmic death. Diuretics, for example, may lead to critical loss of potassium; tricyclic antidepressants may prolong the QT interval, especially in women and individuals with a genetic disposition; the same may be observed even with cardiac medications, e.g. sotalol. Other cardiac medications may lead to high degree atrioventricular block; amphetamines may induce ventricular

Table 2.1 Incidence of sudden cardiac death: dependency on the source of the data underlying the calculation

Study and reference	Incidence (per million population per year)	Source of data
USA (2001) [9]	1250–1500	Death certificates
USA (1967–1988) [23]	410–890	EMS
Maastricht, Netherlands (1997) [2]	900–1000	Death certificates, private physician
Oregon Sudden Unexpected Death Study (2006) [9]	530	EMS, hospital reports, coroners' reports
Ireland (2002) [11]	510	Out-of-hospital SCD, EMS coroners' reports
Canada (2004) [9]	560	Out-of-hospital SCD, EMS coroners' reports
Berlin, Germany(1987–1989) [12]	890	Resuscitation attempts in EMS

EMS, emergency medical services.

tachycardia (VT) or ventricular fibrillation (VF); cocaine abuse may provoke coronary spasm and subsequent fatal arrhythmia. Finally, many antiarrhythmic drugs also have proarrhythmic properties [15–17].

In rare cases SCD may be triggered by blunt thorax trauma (so-called commotio cordis), sometimes even without findings at autopsy [18, 19]. Inflammatory diseases causing sudden death are also seen especially in younger patients [20]. Several viruses have been identified as causing myocarditis, which often follows a recent viral syndrome. Enteroviruses are most common, but also adenoviruses. Cytomegalovirus, herpes simplex, Epstein–Barr and even HIV infections have been reported to cause myocarditis-associated SCD [21]. Specific subtypes of myocarditis, such as hypersensitivity and toxic myocarditis or giant cell inflammation of the heart, are other rarely observed causes

for SCD, as is cardiac involvement of sarcoidosis [22]. In isolated cases SCD may also be provoked by one of the rare storage diseases. Finally, in some patients coronary abnormalities are causative for SCD [23].

Arrhythmiogenic right ventricular dysplasia (ARVD) is a genetic cardiomyopathy characterized by right ventricular thinning and fat infiltration and may be the cause of SCD in younger victims. Interestingly, and in contrast to the findings in North America, ARVD accounts for most SCD cases in competitive athletes in northern Italy [24]. In the United States hypertrophic cardiomyopathy is the main cause of SCD in competitive athletes [18, 19]. This disease is mostly based on a variety of inherited abnormalities of sarcomeric protein synthesis.

So-called channelopathies (Brugada syndrome, long QT (⊃Fig. 2.1), or short QT syndrome and catecholaminergic

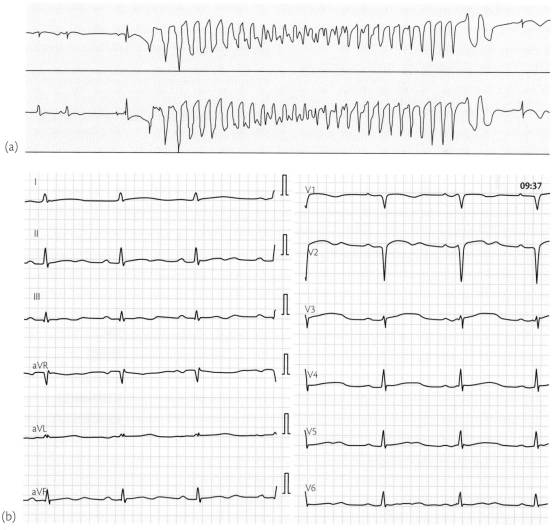

Figure 2.1 (a) Monitor recording of a spontaneously terminated episode of torsades de pointes in the same patient. (b) Long QT syndrome: ECG registered after cardiopulmonary resuscitation in an 18-year-old woman who collapsed shortly after awakening. Ventricular fibrillation was the first registered arrhythmia.

polymorphic VT) primarily represent genetic determined electrical disorders may be responsible for SCD especially in children and adolescents [20, 22, 25–29]. It is suggested that on the background of one of these diseases, similarly to patients suffering from CHD, additional triggers initiate the final catastrophic event. These triggers may be environmental conditions, physical or emotional stress, or endogenous factors such as circadian variation of blood pressure, hormonal levels, or endogenous fibrinolytic activity [30–35]. All the listed conditions and an additional small group of unexplained aetiology add up to about 20% of all SCD not related to CHD.

Underlying arrhythmia

VF or pulseless VT is thought to be the most frequent arrhythmia precipitating SCD in up to 80% of patients [36]. The proportion of patients with VF as documented initial arrhythmia varies widely in the literature, however [7, 36–41]. In recent years it has been repeatedly observed that the distribution of arrhythmia found in victims of SCD is changing, with a decreasing proportion of patients in VF and an increase in pulseless electrical activity and/or asystole (◐ Figs 2.2, 2.3). It is suggested that improved prevention of CHD [42, 43] and more widespread use of specific prevention measures in patients at high risk for SCD at least partially explains this observation, although it is not yet fully understood. The key problem of epidemiology and prevention of SCD is related to the fact that its incidence is high in a very small, well-defined, high-risk group of the total population, whereas the vast majority of cases will occur in a population with very low or almost no

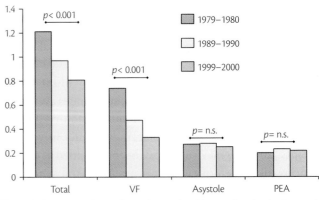

Figure 2.3 Age- and sex-adjusted rate of sudden cardiac death observed in the rescue service (Seattle, Washington, USA, 1979–2000). PEA, pulseless electrical activity; VF, ventricular fibrillation; n.s., not significant. Data from Cobb LA, Fahrenbruch CE, *et al.* Changing incidence of out-of-hospital ventricular fibrillation, 1980–2000. *JAMA* 2002;**288**(23):3008–3013.

definable risk. This fact, first pointed out by Myerburg [44], represents the key challenge in SCD prevention (◐ Fig. 2.4).

Prevention of sudden cardiac death

Preventive strategies are divided into primary prevention for patients at risk who have had no event to date, and secondary prevention for survivors of a cardiac arrest or life-threatening VT [45–47]. Both primary and secondary prevention basically encompass consequent treatment of cardiovascular risk factors, i.e. stopping smoking, appropriate exercise, keeping to a prudent diet and adequate treatment of hypertension, hyperlipidaemia, and diabetes according to the guidelines. In patients with signs of heart

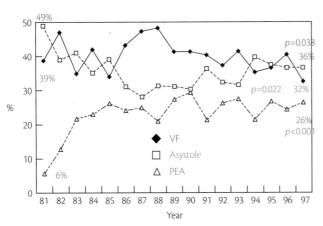

Figure 2.2 Prehospital sudden cardiac death in the rescue services (Gothenburg, Sweden, 1981–1997) according to the initial arrhythmia. PEA, pulseless electrical activity; VF, ventricular fibrillation.
Reproduced from Herlitz J, Andersson E, *et al.* Experiences from treatment of out-of-hospital cardiac arrest during 17 years in Goteborg. *Eur Heart J* 2000;**21**(15):1251–1258, by permission of Oxford University Press.

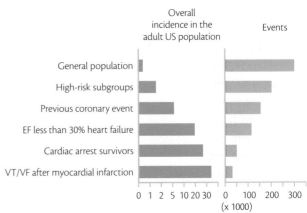

Figure 2.4 Sudden cardiac death among population subgroups: estimates of incidence (%/year left column) and total number of victims/year (right column). The increasing incidence is accompanied by a decrease in total numbers. EF, ejection fraction; VT/VF, ventricular tachycardia/ventricular fibrillation.
Reproduced with permission from Myerburg RJ, Kessler KM, *et al.* Sudden cardiac death. Structure, function, and time-dependence of risk. *Circulation* 1992;**85** (1 Suppl):I2–10.

failure, optimal treatment of this condition is equally important [47].

Achieving an increased awareness of the problem in the general public, and even more in patients at higher risk and their relatives, is also an important part of primary prevention. Learning the skills of basic life support, including the use of automated external defibrillators, should be part of education for schoolchildren and needs to be more widely implemented; recognition and prompt reaction on warning signs and symptoms of a heart attack by individuals at risk and their relatives is also important [3].

In a more specific sense, primary prevention targets a group of patients with a high risk of SCD by definition[44, 48]. Patients with a LVEF of less than 40%, of ischaemic or nonischaemic origin, represent a typical high-risk group. Electrophysiological testing may be helpful in further defining the risk in those patients and may guide catheter ablation of arrhythmic structures [46, 49, 50]. For ischaemic cardiomyopathy, every attempt should be made at revascularization to prevent ischaemia—the most important trigger for fatal arrhythmias.

Antiarrhythmic drugs for prevention of sudden cardiac death

Lidocaine has been tested for prophylaxis of SCD due to VF in acute myocardial infarction (MI) in several studies of different design. Even though the incidence of VF was reduced in some studies, a meta-analysis revealed a trend to higher mortality with lidocaine prophylaxis due to an increase of deaths due to asystole [51]. Primary prevention with β-blockers—mostly dating from the era before reperfusion—resulted in a significant reduction of SCD [32, 52, 53]. In the ISIS I study [53], intravenous initiation of β-blocker prophylaxis was advantageous, but later studies in patients receiving reperfusion treatment revealed no better results with this strategy[54]. In contrast, patients with heart failure at presentation may develop cardiogenic shock if treated with (high-dose) intravenous β-blockers [55]. Oral treatment after stabilization of the patient is therefore actually recommended.

In the CAST trials three class I antiarrhythmics (encainide, flecainide, and moricizine) were tested for prevention of SCD in post-MI patients [15, 16]. The studies resulted in an increased mortality (SCD and nonsudden death) with active treatment. With D-L-sotalol, a class III antiarrhythmic with some β-blocker properties, a significant reduction in re-infarctions was achieved but SCD rate was unchanged [56]. Amiodarone, another class III antiarrhythmic, was also tested in several studies for prevention of SCD. A reduction in

total mortality not was achieved either in the large EMIAT study [57] or the CAMIAT study [58], although a significant decrease in arrhythmic death was observed. Since amiodarone apparently has no proarrhythmic effect it has been successfully used in combination with β-blockers to suppress VF/VT episodes in patients treated with an ICD [59]. In summary, none of the available antiarrhythmic drugs—with the exception of β-blockers—has proved to be effective in the prevention of SCD [60].

Implantable cardioverter–defibrillators

ICD therapy is recommended as a class I, level of evidence A indication for patients with a functional NYHA class II or III with a LVEF of 30–40% in ischaemic and 30–50% in nonischaemic cardiomyopathy [45, 61–63]. Selecting patients for primary prevention is difficult, however, since no clinical test or electrophysiological study leads to definitive results [14, 26, 46, 48, 64, 65]. With respect to outcomes of randomized clinical studies, one of the problems is that in some ICD trials [66] side effects of antiarrhythmic treatment in the control arm, e.g. amiodarone, may have led to worse outcome for the controls compared to the ICD group. The timing of ICD insertion is even more problematic. The MADIT I and MADIT II trials [67, 68] resulted in favour of primary prevention by ICD treatment. The device was implanted 6 months or later after the index infarction in more than three-quarters of the patients. In the VALIANT study [49], a secondary prevention study testing an angiotensin converting enzyme (ACE) inhibitor against an angiotensin receptor blocker, a high number of patients died from SCD shortly after the index event. Early insertion of the device within 6–40 days after a MI was therefore tested in patients with impaired ventricular function in the DINAMIT and IRIS studies [69–71]. In both trials SCD incidence was indeed reduced in the early phase of observation, but this was later counterbalanced by more deaths of nonarrhythmic causation [72]. A wearable defibrillator [73] may be considered as a bridging device until a definitive decision on ICD treatment is possible.

Another specific problem is primary prevention in patients suffering from nonischaemic cardiomyopathies with low EF. Until now studies including this group of patients resulted in encouraging results in NYHA class II patients but only in trends favouring ICD treatment in more severe heart failure [6, 74, 75]. Better outcomes were seen if an ICD is combined with cardiac resynchronization treatment [76].

A further problem is the efficacy of an ICD in elderly patients [77, 78]. Probably because of concomitant diseases, e.g. renal failure or COPD, the efficacy of ICD treatment is of limited efficacy in elderly patients. Concomitant diseases and life expectancy should therefore be a consideration in ICD therapy planning.

In patients with genetically determined arrhythmic syndromes, such as long QT or Brugada syndrome, an ICD may be indicated (together with β-blockers in LQT and catecholaminergic VT) in high-risk groups as well as in selected patients with inflammatory, infiltrative, or hypertrophic cardiomyopathy [26, 45]. Potentially lethal arrhythmias in these patients are often triggered by emotional or physical stress. Competitive sports or other stressful activities should therefore be avoided [25–28].

Since channelopathies demonstrate ECG abnormalities—spontaneous or provoked—awareness of typical alterations in routine ECG readings is decisive in identifying individuals at risk, and in primary preventive measures. The observation of these abnormalities also offers the potential for family screening, including the clarification of the genetic mutation in more than two-thirds of cases. Channelopathies do not show any structural or histological abnormality of the heart at autopsy, so it is of the utmost importance to keep these rare conditions in mind in order to identify other affected family members.

Secondary prevention refers to patients who have survived a SCD or a life-threatening sustained VT. If cardiac arrest occurs in patients beyond 48 h of the onset of an acute MI, the risk of a recurrent event may also be high [79]. Early implantation of an ICD in these patients, however, resulted in a trend of reduction of SCD but not a reduction in total cardiovascular mortality [70, 71]. All patients with an ischaemic cause of arrest should have optimal treatment for this condition. In patients suffering from structural heart disease as well as from heart failure, targeted treatment of the specific condition is necessary to reduce the risk of future events. Principally, regardless of the underlying heart disease, implantation of an ICD is indicated for all survivors of an cardiac arrest for secondary prevention [45].

Conclusion

SCD is the most frequent mode of death in industrialized countries even if numbers differ widely depending on definition and sources of data. CHD and its complications is the commonest cause of SCD, specifically in the presence of impaired left ventricular function. Inflammatory diseases, trauma, and genetically determined disorders represent a minor group of causes of SCD but are particularly meaningful since they affect preferentially younger patients.

Primary strategies for prevention of SCD should focus on general measures to prevent CHD and optimal treatment of the sequelae of this disorder. However, primary prevention also targets a group of patients with manifest heart disease defined by a reduced LVEF of less than 40 %. Since antiarrhythmics are of limited value for this high-risk group and since VF is the most frequent arrhythmia precipitating SCD, implantation of a cardioverter–defibrillator is indicated. These devices are life-saving for patients with an EF of 30–40% with ischaemic heart disease, and an EF of 30–50% with nonischaemic heart disease. These well-defined target groups, however, include only a small percentage of potential victims in the general population. To successfully reduce the burden of SCD, we need to increase awareness of the problem among the general public, especially high-risk patients and their relatives. Widespread training in basic life support, including the use of automated external defibrillators (AEDs), is of outstanding importance.

Personal perspective

The problem of SCD is far from being solved. Specifically, primary prevention awaits targeted strategies in the whole population. These strategies must include not only medical treatment but also increased awareness of the problem in the general population and better education. Most cases of SCD occur in patients with a known but not very high risk for SCD, at home, in the presence of relatives. This scenario offers an excellent chance for bystanders to help—a chance that is all too seldom used. For the high-risk population we urgently need better criteria for ICD with or without cardiac resynchronization therapy.

Further reading

Bunch TJ, Hohnloser SH, *et al*. Mechanisms of sudden cardiac death in myocardial infarction survivors: insights from the randomized trials of implantable cardioverter-defibrillators. *Circulation* 2007;**115**(18):2451–2457.

Chugh SS, Reinier K, *et al*. Epidemiology of sudden cardiac death: clinical and research implications. *Prog Cardiovasc Dis* 2008;**51**(3):213–228.

de Vreede-Swagemakers JJ, Gorgels AP, *et al*. Out-of-hospital cardiac arrest in the 1990s: a population-based study in the Maastricht area on incidence, characteristics and survival. *J Am Coll Cardiol* 1997;**30**(6):1500–1505.

Echt DS, Liebson PR, *et al*. Mortality and morbidity in patients receiving encainide, flecainide, or placebo. The Cardiac Arrhythmia Suppression Trial. *N Engl J Med* 1991; **324**(12):781–788.

Goldberger JJ, Passman R. Implantable cardioverter-defibrillator therapy after acute myocardial infarction: the results are not shocking. *J Am Coll Cardiol* 2009;**54**(22):2001–2005.

Huikuri HV, Castellanos A, *et al*. Sudden death due to cardiac arrhythmias. *N Engl J Med* 2001;**345**(20):1473–1482.

Kadish A, Dyer A, *et al*. Prophylactic defibrillator implantation in patients with nonischemic dilated cardiomyopathy. *N Engl J Med* 2004;**350**(21):2151–2158.

Moss AJ, Zareba W, Hall WJ, *et al*. Multicenter Automatic Defibrillator Implantation Trial II Investigators. Prophylactic implantation of a defibrillator in patients with myocardial infarction and reduced ejection fraction. *N Engl J Med* 2002;**346**:877–883.

Myerburg RJ. Implantable cardioverter-defibrillators after myocardial infarction. *N Engl J Med* 2008;**359**(21):2245–2253.

Steinbeck G, Andresen D, *et al*. Defibrillator implantation early after myocardial infarction. *N Engl J Med* 2009;**361**(15):1427–1436.

⊃ For additional multimedia materials please visit the online version of the book (✍ http://www.esciacc.oxfordmedicine.com).

CHAPTER 3

Cardiopulmonary resuscitation and the post-cardiac arrest syndrome

Andreas Schneider, Peter Teschendorf, and Bernd W. Böttiger

Contents

Summary

Cardiac arrest is a state of whole-body ischaemia. It leads to brain injury and myocardial dysfunction, as well as systemic coagulation and inflammation. Management of cardiac arrest consist of two steps: first, restoration of spontaneous circulation by means of cardiopulmonary resuscitation; second, post-cardiac arrest care. Cardiopulmonary resuscitation comprises chest compressions and mechanical ventilation, electrical defibrillation, and drug therapy. Detailed algorithms have been developed and published in international guidelines. After successful resuscitation, maintenance of physiological homeostasis, i.e. normotension, normoglycaemia, and normocapnia, represents the basic goal. In addition, therapeutic hypothermia has been shown to improve both survival and neurological outcome.

Introduction

Resuscitation from cardiac arrest remains challenging. Restoration of spontaneous circulation (ROSC) can be achieved in up to 50% of the patients, yet only 2–15% survive to hospital discharge [1–3]. These data point out that management of cardiac arrest consists of two different steps of equal importance: cardiopulmonary resuscitation (CPR) *per se* and post-cardiac arrest care. Only optimal therapy in both phases will lead to favourable outcome.

Basic principles of modern CPR were developed 50 years ago [4–6]. Since then, our knowledge has continuously increased, and is still increasing. Guidelines on CPR are released by the European Resuscitation Council (ERC) every 5 years, most recently on October 18, 2010 [7] (see ⊃ Online resources www.erc.edu). Those 'new' guidelines basically followed the tone of the previous version from 2005, yet a number of details were subject of reconsideration:

- The importance of continuous and effective chest compressions was further emphasised, chest compression depth was increased to now 5–6 cm.

- The compression/ventilation ratio was left unchanged at 30:2.

- Early electrical defibrillation is now recommended without necessarily a pre-specified period of chest compression.

- Drug administration via a tracheal tube is no longer recommended.

- Routine use of atropine is no longer recommended.

- After ROSC, inspired oxygen should be titrated.

- Tight glucose control in the post-cardiac arrest period was abandoned, and blood glucose levels >180 mg/dL should be treated.

- Therapeutic hypothermia is now recommended not only for adults and childrens after cardiac arrest, but also for newborn infants suffering from peripartal asphyxia

Pathophysiology of cardiac arrest and the post-cardiac arrest syndrome

Causes of cardiac arrest

Many different pathologies can lead to cardiac arrest (➲ Table 3.1). Acute myocardial infarction is responsible for 40–60% of the cases of out-of-hospital cardiac arrest [8–11]. Pulmonary embolism represents a second important cause of out-of-hospital cardiac arrest.

For in-hospital cardiac arrest, aetiologies are slightly different. In general, patients in hospital have more severe comorbidities, so other internal pathologies gain in importance. Cardiac arrest frequently develops more subacutely, with respiratory insufficiency or haemodynamic instability being present before the final event [3, 12].

Table 3.1 Causes of cardiac arrest

Cardiac	Noncardiac
Myocardial infarction	Pulmonary embolism
Cardiomyopathy	Bleeding
Valvular diseases	Lung diseases
Congenital heart defects	Stroke
Primary electrophysiological abnormalities	Metabolic or electrolyte disorders
	Trauma
	Intoxication

Adopted from Pell JP, Sirel JM, Marsden AK, et al. Presentation, management, and outcome of out of hospital cardiopulmonary arrest: comparison by underlying aetiology. Heart 2003; 89 :839–842 and Zipes DP, Wellens HJJ. Sudden cardiac death. Circulation 1998; 98 :2334–2351..

Whole-body ischaemia

Cessation of the cardiac pump function leads to an immediate and rapid decline of the arterial blood pressure and, subsequently, the antegrade blood flow [13–15]. Complete suspension of blood flow occurs within minutes, when arterial and central venous pressure have equilibrated. Tissue supply of oxygen and other substrates such as glucose is, therefore, interrupted, and metabolic products such as lactate and hydrogen ions remain uncleared. Further on, elimination of carbon dioxide is interrupted due to the cessation of respiration.

Neuronal death after cardiac arrest

The brain is particularly susceptible to ischaemia. Only 5–6 s after the onset of circulatory arrest, the patient loses consciousness [16]. Without a supply of blood, cerebral tissue oxygen tension declines continuously, reaching zero after about 2 min [17, 18]. Simultaneously, neuronal energy in terms of ATP is depleted and metabolites such as adenosine, lactate, and hydrogen ions accumulate [19–21]. Dysfunction of the cell membrane ion pumps leads to a severe breakdown in cellular homeostasis [22, 23]. One particular consequence is a massive accumulation of calcium in the cell cytosol when calcium efflux pumps fail, voltage-gated calcium channels open, and ligand-gated channels are activated by released excitatory amino acids such as glutamate and aspartate [23–26]. This calcium overload is considered a key factor in cellular toxicity [27, 28].

If the ischaemia persists long enough, neuronal necrosis ultimately ensues throughout the brain [29]. However, neuronal energy is recovered rapidly upon reperfusion due to CPR and ROSC [18, 20]. Reperfusion therefore stops neuronal degeneration to a certain degree; but it does not necessarily completely restore function. During reperfusion, free radicals form when the oxygen supply is restored, which might even aggravate cellular damage [30–32]. The main characteristic of the reperfusion period is that refuelling ATP gives the cell the opportunity to actively react to the damage. This is associated with the expression of immediate early genes, a complex machinery involving both cell survival and cell death cascades [33–37]. The morphological correlate of 'subnecrotic' cellular damage is delayed neuronal death, which shows typical signs of apoptosis and occurs mainly in so-called selectively vulnerable brain areas such as the CA-1 sector of the hippocampus, the nucleus reticularis thalami, or distinct layers of the cortex [33–36]. Clinical correlates of these lesions include impaired memory, attention, or executive functioning, which can be found in up to 50% of surviving patients [38–40].

Myocardial dysfunction after cardiac arrest

The heart is also severely affected by the circulatory arrest. After ROSC, a marked reduction of myocardial function can be observed [41–45]. Both systolic contractility and diastolic relaxation are affected, leading to pronounced haemodynamic instability. The underlying pathophysiology of this myocardial stunning is often complex. Just like the brain, the myocardium is particularly susceptible to the state of global ischaemia [46]. Furthermore, if there is a specific cardiac cause of the circulatory arrest, e.g. myocardial infarction, this of course contributes to the cardiac damage [41, 43, 44]. Finally, it has been suggested that further damage to the heart could even be caused by therapeutic interventions during CPR, e.g. electrical defibrillation [47–49] and administration of adrenaline [50]. However, if post-arrest myocardial stunning can be treated effectively with inotropic agents, it is usually self-limiting within 72 h [42, 43].

Inflammation and coagulation after cardiac arrest

Cardiac arrest leads to expression of cytokines such as interleukins or tumour necrosis factor both systemically and locally, e.g. in the brain [51–53]. Local cytokine expression leads to leucocyte accumulation and infiltration, mediated by specific endothelial adhesion molecules [33, 53–57]. It has been suggested that leucocytes contribute to organ damage after cardiac arrest, e.g. by jamming of microcirculation or through the release of destructive enzymes like elastase. In addition to cytokine release and leucocyte migration, activation of complement [54] and an increase in endothelial permeability [55, 57] are observed after cardiac arrest. A majority of patients after cardiac arrest fulfil the criteria of a systemic inflammatory response syndrome (SIRS) [58].

Both plasmatic coagulation and platelets are activated during cardiac arrest and reperfusion [59–61]. There is also a slight increase in endogenous fibrinolysis, but this seems inadequate to counterbalance hypercoagulability [60, 62]. Coagulation disorders might play an important role in emergence of the so-called no-reflow phenomenon, i.e. circumscribed regional reperfusion failures despite sufficient systemic circulation [63–65].

Mechanical cardiopulmonary resuscitation

Chest compressions

External chest compressions restore antegrade blood flow by increasing the intrathoracic pressure and by directly compressing the heart [66–68]. Data from patients undergoing CPR show that mean arterial blood pressure during CPR (with the use of vasopressors) can be expected at about 30–50 mmHg [18, 66, 69, 70]. CPR is therefore able to produce a small yet critical amount of coronary and cerebral blood flow [15, 18, 69, 70].

The available data on ideal chest compression are scarce and ambiguous. Some studies found haemodynamic variables to improve with increasing compression rate [70, 71], whereas others found a decrease [72]. The ERC guidelines recommend giving 100–120 compressions per minute. It has been shown that too weak compressions impair defibrillation success and survival [73, 74]. The new guidelines ask for compressions which are 5–6 cm deep. After each compression, the chest should be allowed to recoil completely.

The ERC again, after 2005, does emphasize the importance of continuous and effective chest compressions, which are regarded more important than any other measure during resuscitation efforts. Interruptions, e.g. for electrical countershocks, airway management, or drug administration, possibly impair resuscitation success [73, 75–77] and must be kept to a minimum. Since providing effective chest compression is exhausting within short time [78], the person delivering chest compressions should be changed every 2 minutes.

Ventilation

Bag-mask ventilation suffers from several drawbacks. First, there is the risk of distending the stomach which might lead to regurgitation and aspiration [79, 80]. Second, chest compressions must be interrupted during bag-mask ventilation.

Both limitations can be overcome by tracheal intubation or placement of a supraglottic airway device such as a laryngeal mask airway or laryngeal tube. The tracheal tube represents the gold standard, but its placement requires a certain amount of skill and experience. It has been repeatedly shown that there is a considerable risk of tube misplacements when emergency intubation is attempted by less experienced staff [81– 83]. In addition, the time needed to perform intubation may be critical [84]. Supraglottic airway devices should always be considered as an easy to use and safe alternative [79, 80, 85]. Their use is highly encouraged by the ERC guidelines.

Too aggressive ventilation during CPR seems to impair the outcome [86–88]. Excessive tidal volumes should be avoided, the ERC guidelines recommend to give enough volume to produce a normal chest rise (or 500–600 ml). During CPR, the patient should be ventilated with 100% oxygen, if it is available. After ROSC, inspired oxygen should be titrated (see below).

Compression/ventilation ratio

Chest compressions have to be interrupted for bag-mask ventilation. However, all interruptions of chest compressions probably reduce resuscitation success [73, 75–77]. On the other hand, arterial oxygen stores deplete within minutes during CPR without ventilation [89]. The compression/ventilation ratio has, therefore, been discussed repeatedly. In 2005, it was increased to 30:2, which was largely based on animal experimental data [90, 91] and mathematical considerations [92].

In the meantime, several studies have suggested that CPR with chest compression only might not be inferior to classic CPR [93-97]. However, these studies suffer from several methodological drawbacks. Other groups have investigated modified CPR protocols with a 50:2 ratio [98] or three cycles of 200 uninterrupted initial chest compressions prior to tracheal intubation [99, 100]. Still, the 30:2 ratio has been confirmed in the 2010 ERC guidelines (◑Fig. 3.1). Compression-only CPR might be performed, if no airway equipment is available and the lay rescuer is reluctant to provide mouth-to-mouth ventilation.

After endotracheal intubation or insertion of advanced supraglottic airway devices, compressions can be delivered continuously. A ventilation rate of 10/min is then regarded adequate by the guidelines.

Electrical defibrillation

In cases of ventricular fibrillation (VF) or ventricular tachycardia (VT), electrical countershocks mean a causal therapy. The electrical discharge is able to fully terminate all electrical activity within the heart for a short period [101–103], which then gives the sinus node the chance to resume control. However, electrical countershocks are not appropriate in asystole and pulseless electrical activity.

The success of defibrillation is largely dependent on time. With every minute that passes until defibrillation is attempted, the chance of survival decreases by 10–15% [104, 105]. The importance of delivering defibrillation rapidly is emphasized by two randomized clinical trials on the use of automated external defibrillators (AEDs) [106, 107]. When basic CPR as performed by laypersons before the arrival of medical emergency service is complemented by public AEDs, survival after out-of-hospital events can be improved. Not surprisingly, improvement diminishes as the benefit in time to the arrival of the emergency medical service decreases [107].

There are currently two different types of defibrillators available, delivering shocks with monophasic or biphasic waveforms. Biphasic defibrillators seem to attain higher defibrillation success or require less energy for successful defibrillation [108–112]. However, none of these studies found a difference in survival after monophasic or biphasic defibrillation.

The ERC guidelines do not specifically recommend either waveform. Appropriate energy levels are stated as 360 J for monophasic shocks and >150 J for biphasic shocks (◑Fig. 3.1). It is recommended to attempt defibrillation as soon as possible. However, until the defibrillator is available and charged, basic CPR measures must be performed. Only one shock should be applied at once and CPR should afterwards be resumed immediately without checking the rhythm.

Recent research aims at determining the ideal waveform of biphasic countershocks to improve defibrillation success [113, 114]. For AEDs, rhythm analysis during ongoing chest compressions will be established by different filtering techniques to reduce no-flow times [115 –117].

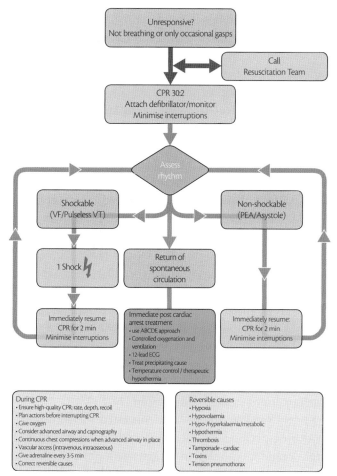

Figure 3.1 Advanced cardiac life support algorithm.
Reproduced From the European Resuscitation Council guidelines for resuscitation 2010. Resuscitation 2010; in press.

Drugs during cardiopulmonary resuscitation

Adrenaline

Adrenaline is used during CPR because of its α-adrenergic properties. It leads to peripheral vasoconstriction, resulting in increased blood pressure and improved myocardial and cerebral perfusion [118–120]. Data from animal experiments suggest that the use of adrenaline (or other vasopressors) is very important for successful resuscitation [121–123]. However, there remains much controversy about adrenaline. It has been suggested that as a result of its β-adrenergic properties, myocardial oxygen consumption increases and is not necessarily balanced by increased blood flow [124, 125]. In epidemiological studies, higher doses of adrenaline correlate with increased mortality [126]. However, a possible explanation for this observation could be that higher doses of adrenaline simply reflect a longer duration of cardiac arrest and CPR, which is of course associated with worse outcome.

Adrenaline has been compared with other vasopressors such as noradrenaline [127] and vasopressin [128–132] in randomized clinical trials. However, no difference was found in terms of survival.

The need for adrenaline has further been addressed by a recent randomized clinical trial which compared standard CPR to CPR without intravenous drugs [133]. While the rates of ROSC (40% vs 25%, p <0.001) and hospital admission (43% vs 29%, p < 0.001) were significantly higher in the group receiving standard CPR including adrenaline, this did not translate into higher survival to hospital discharge (10.5% vs 9.2%, p = 0.61).

The ERC guidelines specify adrenaline as the standard vasopressor during CPR. 1 mg should be administered every 3–5 min.

Amiodarone

Amiodarone is the only antiarrhythmic drug for which a (short-term) benefit has been demonstrated in cardiac arrest. It has been investigated in out-of-hospital cardiac arrest with refractory ventricular fibrillation by two randomized clinical trials [134, 135]. The first study compared 300 mg amiodarone to placebo, the second amiodarone 5 mg/kg to lidocaine 1.5 mg/kg. In both studies, patients receiving amiodarone were more likely to survive to hospital admission than the patients of the control group. However, neither of the two studies could detect differences in survival to hospital discharge.

Recently, two retrospective analyses have questioned the value of amiodarone compared to lidocaine in in-hospital cardiac arrest [136, 137]. However, since both studies were highly susceptible to confounding (e.g., amiodarone was administered later in the arrest than lidocaine), amiodarone presently remains the first line antiarrhythmic drug.

The ERC guidelines recommend 300 mg amiodarone in refractory ventricular fibrillation.

Magnesium

Although intravenous magnesium does not help to control ventricular fibrillation [138–141], it remains the first line treatment in patients with torsades de pointes [142, 143]: 8 mmol (2 g magnesium sulphate) are recommended by the ERC guidelines.

Bicarbonate

Buffering agents were once considered standard drugs in CPR. However, their value has repeatedly been questioned. In a large randomized clinical trial, patients with out-of-hospital cardiac arrest received either a combined buffer agent (bicarbonate/Tris/phosphate/acetate) or saline during CPR [144]. There were no differences in resuscitability between the two groups. In a more recent randomized clinical trial, patients with out-of-hospital cardiac arrest received bicarbonate (1 mmol/kg) or saline [150]. Overall, there was no difference in survival. However, in the subgroup of patients with prolonged cardiac arrest (>15 min), survival increased twofold in the bicarbonate group.

According to the ERC guidelines, bicarbonate should be used reluctantly during CPR, only in cases of severe metabolic acidosis, hyperkalaemia, or tricyclic antidepressant overdose. Excessive buffering might lead to alkalosis [146].

Thrombolytics

Cardiac arrest is caused by acute myocardial infarction or pulmonary embolism in 50–70% of patients [8–11]. Thrombolysis represents an effective and causal therapy of both myocardial infarction and pulmonary embolism (without cardiac arrest). Combining CPR with thrombolysis therefore seems a promising approach. Furthermore, there is evidence that disordered coagulation [60, 62] is involved in the emergence of microcirculatory disorders after cardiac arrest [147, 148].

Several smaller studies have suggested that thrombolysis during prolonged CPR might be beneficial [149–151], while a randomized trial in patients with pulseless electrical activity did not show a benefit [152]. The largest body of data has recently been provided by the Thrombolysis in

Cardiac Arrest (TROICA) trial [153]. 1050 patients with witnessed out-of-hospital cardiac arrest of presumed cardiac origin were randomized to receive a bolus of 30–50 mg tenecteplase (adjusted to body weight) or placebo during early CPR. There was no difference in overall outcome. However, patients with confirmed pulmonary embolism only survived when they had received tenecteplase.

The ERC guidelines recommend that thrombolysis should be considered during CPR, when pulmonary embolism is suspected.

Algorithms for cardiopulmonary resuscitation

Basic cardiac life support

After confirmation of cardiac arrest, CPR must be initiated immediately. Chest compressions and ventilations should be delivered at a ratio of 30:2. It is recommended to start with chest compressions rather than initial rescue breaths. While oxygen content of peripheral tissues is rapidly consumed during cardiac arrest, arterial oxygen tension remains high [154, 155]. Therefore, initial ventilation would only delay chest compressions without having any advantages. If possible, the person delivering chest compressions should be changed every 2 minutes to prevent decreasing CPR quality due to fatigue [78].

While initiating CPR, help must be requested in terms of both manpower and technical equipment. In particular, a defibrillator must be provided as soon as possible. During ongoing CPR, the defibrillations pads have to be applied for immediate rhythm analysis. Further management of cardiac arrest differs between shockable and non-shockable rhythms. Rhythm analysis is repeated every 2 minutes.

In addition, an advanced airway device and an intravenous or intraosseous access have to be established. However, neither measure should interfere with basic CPR. Even short interruptions in chest compressions can be associated with bad outcome [73, 75-77].

Advanced cardiac life support – shockable rhythms

In shockable rhythms (VF, VT), electrical defibrillation represents the causal therapy [101-103]. The countershock should be applied as soon as possible after diagnosis has been established. However, the time needed for charging the defibrillator should be used for further chest compressions.

When VF develops in monitored patients, e.g. on intensive care units, a single precordial thump might be successful to terminate cardiac arrest [156-158] and can be given before mechanical CPR. However, it is not recommended in any other situations.

After the defibrillation attempt, CPR should be resumed immediately. It is not recommended to use more than one countershock at once, i.e. stacked sequences. Neither should there be an immediate rhythm check. On the one hand, a pulse can rarely be palpated immediately after defibrillation [159], on the other hand, on-going CPR is unlikely to cause any harm even if an organized rhythm is present [160].

Rhythm analysis is done every 2 minutes. When there is a potentially perfusing rhythm, the pulse should be palpated, followed by measuring blood pressure. When VF or VT is still present, the next countershock should be applied, again followed by immediate continuation of CPR. When asystole or PEA is present, CPR should be resumed immediately according for the algorithm for non-shockable rhythms.

After the third defibrillation attempt, 1 mg adrenaline and 300 mg amiodarone should be administered. Adrenaline is then repeated every 3–5 minutes, i.e. every second 2-minutes cycle.

Advanced cardiac life support—non-shockable rhythms

When rhythm check reveals asystole or PEA, CPR must be resumed immediately. Defibrillation is not a therapeutic option here. Different from shockable rhythms, 1 mg adrenaline should be given immediately.

After 2 min, the next rhythm analysis is done. Adrenaline is repeated every two CPR cycles. No other drugs (including atropine) are recommended for routine use.

Critical care after restoration of spontaneous circulation

Normotension

After cardiac arrest, many patients are haemodynamically unstable due to myocardial dysfunction, arrhythmias, and peripheral vasodilation [41, 43, 44]. Furthermore, most patients after cardiac arrest completely or partially lack autoregulation of cerebral blood flow [161]. In healthy individuals, cerebral blood flow remains constant during decreased arterial blood pressure. In patients after cardiac arrest, however, cerebral perfusion can drop critically.

Blood pressure management in the post-resuscitation period has not yet been tested in clinical studies. Epidemiological studies suggest that hypotensive periods are associated with poor outcome [126]; animal experimental data suggest that elevation of blood pressure might produce better outcome [162]. However, with regard to the lack of clinical data, the ERC guidelines recommend aiming the blood pressure at the patient's normal levels. Hypotension should be avoided.

Haemodynamic optimization starts with adequate volume substitution. Even though patients after cardiac arrest show myocardial dysfunction, intravenous fluids are tolerated well. In one study, an average of 8000 mL within the first 72 h was necessary for stabilization of the patients [43]. The reason for this is probably the systemic inflammatory response after cardiac arrest leading to vasodilation and fluid extravasation. When volume load fails to stabilize haemodynamics, vasopressors and inotropics should be used.

It seems reasonable to adopt the concept of early goal-directed therapy, as known from sepsis [163]. However, this has not yet been tested in patients after cardiac arrest.

Normoglycaemia

Hyperglycaemia after cardiac arrest is associated with both increased mortality and impaired neurological recovery in survivors [126, 164]. It has been suggested that tight glucose control (80–110 mg/dL vs 180–200 mg/dL) might improve outcome in the critical care setting [165]. However, recent studies focusing on patients after cardiac arrest suggest that only slightly elevated blood glucose (<150 mg/dL) might not be associated with poorer outcome [166, 167]. It is possible that during tight glucose control with insulin, periods of hypoglycaemia that could impair outcome might not be recognized.

Normocapnia

The need for sufficient ventilation in the post-resuscitation period is obvious, but hyperventilation must be avoided, too. Hypocapnia due to hyperventilation causes cerebral vasoconstriction [168]. The consecutive reduction of cerebral blood flow can possibly induce further cerebral ischaemia. Ventilation parameters should therefore be adjusted to maintain normocapnia.

Normoxaemia

During CPR, patients should be ventilated with 100% oxygen, if available. However, hyperoxia leads to increased oxidative stress and might therefore be detrimental [169-171]. In one recent descriptive study, hyperoxaemia in the post-resuscitation period was associated with increased in-hospital mortality compared with either normoxaemia or hypoxaemia [172]. The ERC guidelines recommend to lower inspired oxygen after ROSC as soon as blood gas analysis or pulse oxymetry is available. It should be titrated to maintain the arterial blood oxygen saturation between 94–98%.

Therapeutic hypothermia

Two randomized clinical trials have shown benefits of mild therapeutic hypothermia after cardiac arrest [173, 174]. In both studies, comatose adult patients after out-of-hospital cardiac arrest with ventricular fibrillation as the initial rhythm were cooled to 32–34°C for 12 h or 24 h, respectively. Compared to normothermia, mild therapeutic hypothermia led to both improved survival and improved neurological recovery. These results have been confirmed by subsequent meta-analyses [175, 176]. The number needed to treat (NNT) to allow one additional patient to leave the hospital with no or only minimal neurological damage was calculated at 6. Hypothermia is therefore clearly recommended by the 2005 guidelines for comatose adult patients after out-of-hospital cardiac arrest due to VF. Furthermore, it seems reasonable not to withhold therapeutic hypothermia from patients suffering from in-hospital cardiac arrest or non-shockable rhythms. This view is also encouraged by the ERC guidelines, even though conclusive data are still missing.

Hypothermia can be induced by different methods, e.g. surface cooling, ice-cold infusions, or endovascular cooling catheters. Although there are great differences in efficacy and invasiveness among them, it is currently not clear whether one particular technique should be preferred to the others. No studies are available that have compared different cooling devices in terms of survival.

Possible adverse effects of hypothermia include electrolyte and volume changes [177–179], impaired immune defence [180–182], and impaired coagulation [183–185]. However, these complications can usually be managed by intensive care strategies. The two large randomized clinical trials did not find a significant increase in severe complications as compared to normothermia [173, 174]. The safety of hypothermia treatment has also been confirmed by newer observational studies [186].

A contentious topic is when to start cooling. Experimental data shows that hypothermia is more effective when induced with minimal delay after cardiac arrest [187, 188]. In cases of out-of-hospital cardiac arrest, cooling should therefore be initiated in the field. In one randomized clinical trial, patients were assigned to either receiving 4°C normal saline or not in the prehospital setting [189]. After arrival at the hospital, patients were treated according to the local preferences, i.e. patients were cooled or not regardless of the randomization. Survival rates tended to be higher in patients who had received prehospital cooling treatment. The investigators have therefore initiated a second randomized clinical trial with a larger number of patients [190]. It has even been considered to start cooling during ongoing CPR [181, 192]. Experimental data suggests that mild hypothermia might improve defibrillation success [193].

Coronary revascularization

Acute myocardial infarction is responsible for 40–60% of the cases of out-of-hospital cardiac arrest [8–11]. In these patients, coronary revascularization by means of catheter intervention or thrombolysis has to be considered. It has been shown that ST-segment elevation after ROSC is a good predictor of myocardial infarction, whereas serum troponin lacks specificity [8].

Coronary interventions can be coupled with therapeutic hypothermia. When hypothermia is induced by noninvasive means such as cold infusions and surface cooling, it does not lead to a delay in door-to-balloon-time [194]. Catheterization is even possible during ongoing CPR with the help of automated CPR devices [195].

Prognostication

Predicting outcome after cardiac arrest is complex. Although pre-cardiac arrest factors (age, gender, health status) and intra-arrest factors (duration of cardiac arrest, initial rhythm) must be considered, prognostication is largely based on post-cardiac arrest evaluation of the patient. Absent brainstem reflexes 24 h after the arrest [196], myoclonus status [197], absent median nerve somatosensory evoked potentials [198], or elevated serum levels of neuron-specific enolase (NSE) and astroglial protein S-100 [199] have been associated with poor outcome. However, there is an ongoing discussion on the reliability of these parameters. In particular, none has been evaluated in patients treated with therapeutic hypothermia.

Conclusion

In October 2010, new CPR guidelines have been published by the ERC. Particular emphasis has again been laid on continuous and effective chest compressions during CPR. Pushing hard and fast with minimized interruptions is the key to save our patients' lives.

Personal perspective

Despite 50 years of development, there are still remarkable knowledge gaps in CPR science. Many steps of CPR have never been tested in larger clinical trials. Scientific evaluation of our current practice will continue in the next decade and might lead to slight adaptation of the treatment recommendations.

Recently, we have seen the introduction of therapeutic hypothermia after cardiac arrest. Scientific evidence for this therapy is considerable, but its use in daily clinical routine is at least in part still poor. This example shows that the survival of our patients depends not only on scientific progress, but also on all our efforts on education and implementation.

Further reading

European Resuscitation Council. European Resuscitation Council guidelines for resuscitation 2010. *Resuscitation* 2010; in press.

Online resource

✍ European Resuscitation Council guidelines for resuscitation 2010. http://www.erc.edu

➲ For additional multimedia materials please visit the online version of the book (✍ http://www.esciacc.oxfordmedicine.com).

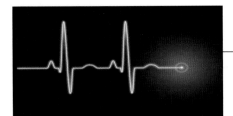

CHAPTER 4

Comparison of prehospital emergency care systems in Europe and the United States

Frédéric Adnet, Tomislav Petrovic, and Frédéric Lapostolle

Contents

Summary

Health care systems are well defined in most countries worldwide. Whereas intrahospital emergency departments benefit from standardized organization, prehospital care systems still vary from one country to another, and even within the same country.

Usually, telephone calls for out-of-hospital emergency problems are routed to dedicated call centres by means of nationwide unique numbers. But there are many different approaches to the triggering of responders, from systematic dispatch by a switchboard operator to regulated dispatch of medical crews by emergency medical dispatchers.

In the past, differences were observed essentially between two diametrically opposed visions of prehospital: the Anglo-Saxon system of taking the patient to the nearest hospital as fast as possible vs the Germano-French system of stabilizing the patient on site before transfer to a suitable medical ward. It is now becoming more and more obvious that both approaches can be necessary and even complementary, depending on many factors such as the type of pathology, human, financial or technological resources, training and even socio-cultural factors. In fact, through the world prehospital care systems can vary from none at all (no call centre, no ambulance system, no hospital emergency system) to the highest level of integration of both systems with medicalized dispatching of calls, regulation of responders, on-site stabilization and treatment if necessary, and optimization of the final destination for critical patients.

Finally, to achieve the highest possible level, the training has to be adapted to each category of prehospital emergency practitioner, from EMTs (emergency medical technicians) to physicians, regardless of what type of system is or will be implemented. The policy has to be as close as possible to the needs and available means to reach an optimal usage of the resources.

Specific knowledge of prehospital emergency medicine may not be necessary if its teaching is integrated into a more general curriculum of a true emergency medicine specialism, as already recognized in United States and some other countries.

Introduction

A fundamental aspect for evaluating health systems and especially emergency systems is the organization of the first link in the chain of health care: prehospital emergency care systems (PECS). The type and training of practitioners, the means used (ambulances, helicopters, planes) and their equipment, the coordination and the reliability of the communication network are critical elements in assessing the effectiveness of the prehospital emergency chain. PECS are the subject of heated debate between two systems of care responding to two different philosophies, a situation which is not encountered within intrahospital emergency departments. Thus, it is conventional to contrast the Anglo-Saxon system, based on quick uplift and transfer of the victim to a hospital ('scoop and run') and the Germano-French-inspired system, which takes the hospital beyond its walls to make available to the patient, at the scene, health care on the same level as would be offered in the hospital itself ('stay and stabilize') [1]. The Anglo-Saxon system is based on auxiliary health workers, 'paramedics', while the Germano-French system is based on teams staffed by physicians.

Outside the United States, the North American 'paramedics' model is more or less implemented in four countries: Canada, New Zealand, Australia, and the United Kingdom [2]. The usage of the Germano-French model through Europe is very variable, however, so it is not a question simply of two different systems. The situation is often complex: PECS varies betweeen countries and even within the same country [2] The range of prehospital care may vary from near absence (Bosnia-Herzegovina) to a nationwide, uniform, and fully medicalized system (France). Between these two extremes exists a variety of systems that can mix medicalized, paramedicalized, or even nonmedicalized PECS. A similar lack of homogeneity holds for dispatch systems, which may be nonexistent in some areas (rural Russia), nonmedicalized (USA), run by nurses (Denmark), or fully medicalized, staffed by physicians (France). The complexity extends even further: some Anglo-Saxon systems may employ medicalized teams (staffed by physicians) for secondary transfers from a hospital structure to another (Life-Flight in the USA). Helicopters can be used in PECS

(Switzerland, USA) but are usually staffed by specific crews, even if dedicated to the same type of mission. Finally, some countries have a partially medicalized PECS, making its description difficult.

The differences between prehospital care systems within Europe have their origins in the history of prehospital emergency care itself. Emergency care systems first appeared in Europe during the 11th century when orders of chivalry such as the Knights of Malta and St John created rescue systems for victims. In France, the establishment of autonomous prehospital care dates back to the Napoleonic wars (late 18th century). The Red Cross (1859) and the Geneva Convention (1864) instituted actions leading to the organization of rescue systems outside the hospital. Thus, each European country independently developed prehospital care systems in which the voluntary sector has more or less influence, sometimes leading to regional and organizational variations within the same country (e.g. Switzerland).

The main types of organization on which prehospital emergency systems depend are shown in ➲Table 4.1. These include government or institutional agencies (Ministry of Health, EMS (emergency medical services), firefighters, etc.), but also membership organizations (Red Cross, St John's Ambulance, Alpine Rescue, etc.) [3].

Currently, two major areas of development and research in trying to harmonize European systems are the introduction of a single telephone number for emergency calls ('112') and the distribution of equipment for automatic external defibrillation (AED) to all staff involved in the chain of survival [4].

The purpose of this chapter is not to evaluate the two different types of organizations, but to describe the PECS used in Europe and, by extension, in North America.

Triggering the rescue

A unique call number for medical emergencies and exclusively dedicated to this function is not universally used. In Europe, there are at least 10 different telephone numbers for medical help [5].

In the United States, the unique number for emergency calls is '911', with a centralized reception regardless of the type of request. Thus, calls requiring police response, firefighters, or those relating to a medical emergency are all answered in '911' call centres. These centres then direct the call according to the nature of the request.

In Europe, a call number for medical emergencies exists in most countries. This number may be national (France) or regional (Spain). These numbers are shown in ➲Table 4.2.

Table 4.1 Main organizations responsible for prehospital emergency care systems in selected countries

Country	Organizations (in order of importance)		
	1	2	3
Austria	Red Cross	Arbeiter Samariter Bund[a]	Ordre de Malte[a]
Belgium	Red Cross	Hospital	Fire services
Denmark	FALCK[b]	Fire services	Roskilde
Eastern Europe	Ministry of Health	Red Cross	
Finland	Fire services	EMS/Hospital	Red Cross
France	SAMU	Fire services	Red Cross
Germany	Red Cross	Fire services	Arbeiter Samariter Bund[a]
England	National Health Service	Red Cross	St John's Ambulance[a]
Greece	National Insurance Foundation	Red Cross	First Aid Center
Iceland	Life Saving Association	Scouts[a]	Coast Guards
Italy	Red Cross	Regional Green Cross[a]	Alpine Rescue[a]
Norway	National Health Organization	Regional organizations	Red Cross
Portugal	NIEM	Fire services	Red Cross
Sweden	Medical care system	Fire services	Police
Switzerland	ACLC	REGA	SLSA
Turkey	Ministry of Health	Red Cross	

[a] Associations responsible for prehospital emergency care systems.

[b] A private rescue company that has the monopoly on ambulances in Denmark, except in Copenhagen.

ACLC, Ambulance Corps of Large City; EMS, emergency medical services; NHS, National Health Service; NIEM, National Institute of Emergency Medicine; REGA, Swiss Air Rescue Guard; SAMU, Service d'Aide Médicale Urgente; SLSA, Swiss Life Saving Association.

On 29 July 1991 the Council of the European Community proposed the creation of a European unique telephone number, '112'. The founding document envisages the introduction of this call number in addition to national dedicated call numbers, if they exist [6]. Such a number, like '911' in the United States, aims to deal with all urgent requests for police, firefighters, and medical problems. However, only 10 European countries currently use this number as a single number. The other countries have specific call numbers for specific emergencies or health problems (➲ Table 4.2). The first analysis of the reasons for calling this number clearly shows that calls relating to a true health emergency are not very frequent, between 10 and 15%. A recent survey, conducted by the French SAMU 68 (Service d'Aide Médicale Urgente), noted that only 13% of the calls received through '112' were related to health problems [7].

Regulation of calls and dispatching

Around the world, call centres for medical problems are not, in general, staffed by physicians (➲ Table 4.2). In France, all the medical calls coming in to the dedicated call centre (nationwide call number, '15') are first answered by specially trained operators and then transferred to emergency medical regulators (physicians). After having evaluated the level of emergency, envisaged a diagnosis, and possibly given advice (regulation), they choose the most suitable way of responding to the situation (decision-making and dispatching of means of intervention). This kind of organization is exceptional [8, 9].

In the Anglo-Saxon system, specialized nonmedical staff decide what kind of response has to be given. The mode of questioning and the type of dispatching/triggering are based on predetermined decision-making algorithms. In general, two types of decisions are taken: (1) sending an ambulance for a simple medical reason, where the ambulance crew maybe made up of paramedics or ambulance drivers (emergency medical technicians, EMTs), and (2) in cases of life threatening distress or a major accident, sending an ambulance staffed by paramedics and a fire vehicle at the same time. This type of decision, whatever the type of need and in the absence of any triage of the calls, probably creates an excessive use of resources and an overcrowding of emergency departments. Recognizing the dysfunction relating to the absence of triage, some North American call centres have tried to make their dispatching more focused by transferring some calls to a hospital nurse (paramedicalized regulation). A study showed that 31% of calls received by the nurses did not need an ambulance to be sent and

Table 4.2 Telephone numbers for medical emergencies, and existence or otherwise of medicalized regulation

Country	National number for medical emergencies	Number	Medicalized regulation
Austria	Yes	122/112	
Belgium	Yes	100/112	No
Bulgaria	Yes	150	
Cyprus	No	199/112	
Czech Republic	Yes	155/112	Yes[a]
Denmark	No	112	Yes[b]
Estonia	Yes	03/112	Partly
Finland	No	112	
France	Yes	15/112	Yes
Germany	No	112	
Greece	Yes	166/112	
Hungary	Yes	105/112	
Ireland	Yes	999/112	
Italy	Yes	118/112	Partly
Latvia	Yes	03/112	
Lithuania	No	112	
Luxembourg	No	112	No
Malta	No	112	
Netherlands	Yes	0611/112	
Norway	Yes	003/112	
Poland	Yes	115/112	No
Portugal	No	112	Yes
Romania	No	112	
Russia	Yes	3/112	Yes[a]
Slovakia	Yes	155	
Slovenia	No	112	
Spain	No	Regional/112	Yes
Sweden	No	112	
Switzerland	Yes	144/112	No
Turkey	Yes	77	No
UK	Yes	999/112	No
USA	Yes	911	No

[a] Specifically trained nurses.
[b] Nurses/paramedics.

telephone advice was given in 41% of cases. This system, still experimental, could change '911' call centres to a more 'medicalized' call regulation [10]. Similarly, the comparable '999' dispatch system in the United Kingdom was recently been the subject of similar discussions when a considerable increase in the number of transfers by ambulances to emergency departments was observed [11].

In some countries (Denmark, urban Russia, Czech Republic), health-related calls are regulated by nurses who decide what type of response is required. These staff are also authorized to give advice to the caller before the ambulance arrives [12].

Other European countries (e.g. Belgium) do not use medicalized triage or decision-making algorithms. Either a nonmedicalized or a medicalized ambulance is dispatched, depending on the evaluation of the severity of the call. In Austria, a regulating structure for calls exists but only for air medical transfers. The search for available beds at hospitals for prehospital emergency care is virtually nonexistent [5].

The structure of the regulation system can also vary from one region to another. In Switzerland, the regulation for urgent medical calls may be assigned to different staff categories ranging from a secretary to specifically dedicated and trained staff [13].

Prehospital care

Most PECS are highly dependent on the density differences existing between rural and urban areas (Russia), on the importance of the involvement of the voluntary sector (Switzerland, Germany) or on geopolitical circumstances (Spain). In some countries, the prehospital system is considered as an extension of a referral hospital and entirely dependent on it (Belgium, Finland, Italy, Austria, Switzerland) whereas other countries provide totally independent PECS (France, Spain, Portugal, United Kingdom) [14]. The characteristics of PECS in major European countries and the United States are summarized in ➲ Table 4.3.

The organization of PECS in Europe can be classified into four levels, as follows.

No prehospital emergency care

In these countries, patients generally go to hospital by their own means or are transferred by private transports. Until recently Bosnia-Herzegovina had no organized system of prehospital emergency care. However, in urban areas, some patients may be transported to a hospital by ambulances with unskilled crews that have no function other than transport [15].

One-level rescue system with basic skills for Basic Life Support resuscitation

The rescue is provided by EMT or paramedics who are authorized to practice basic first aid actions (mask ventilation, thoracic compressions). Some teams may be

Table 4.3 Characteristics of prehospital emergency care systems in European countries and the United States

| Country | 1st level | 2nd level | Responsible nonmedical staff during intervention | | | Medicalized interhospital transfers |
			Paramedics	Nurse	EMTs/firefighters	
Austria	EMTs/firefighters	Medicalized[a]	No	No	Yes	Yes
Belgium	Firefighters	Medicalized	No	Yes	Yes	Yes
Czech Republic	FACT/firefighters	Medicalized	No	No	Yes	Yes
Denmark	EMTs	Nurses	No	Yes	No	Yes
Estonia	EMTs/firefighters	Medicalized[a]	No	No	Yes	
Finland	EMTs/firefighters	Medicalized[a]	Yes	Ho	Yes	
France	Firefighters	Medicalized	No	Partly	Yes	Yes
Germany	EMTs	Medicalized[a]	Partly	Yes	Yes	Yes
Greece		Medicalized[a]	Yes	Yes		
Hungary	Firefighters	Medicalized	No	No	Yes	Yes
Iceland	EMTs	Medicalized[a]	No	No	Yes	
Ireland		Paramedics	Yes	Yes		
Italy	EMTs/firefighters	Medicalized[a]	Partly	Partly	Yes	Yes
Slovakia	EMTs/firefighters	Medicalized	No	No	No	Yes
Luxembourg	Firefighters	Medicalized	No	No		
Netherlands	EMTs	Nurses	No	Yes		
Norway	EMTs	Medicalized[a]	Ho	Ho	Yes	
Poland	EMTs	Medicalized				
Portugal	EMTs/firefighters	Medicalized[a]	Ho	Yes	Yes	Yes
Russia	EMTs	Medicalized	Yes	No	No	Yes
Spain	EMTs	Medicalized[a]	No	Yes	Yes	Yes
Sweden	EMTs/firefighters	Paramedics	Yes	Yes	Yes	
Switzerland	EMTs	Medicalized	No	No	Yes	Yes
Turkey	EMTs/firefighters	Medicalized[a]	No	Yes	Yes	No
UK	Paramedics	Paramedics	Yes	No	No	Yes
USA	Paramedics	Paramedics	Yes	No	Yes	Yes

[a] Partly.

authorized to use an AED (EMT-D, D = defibrillation). Most Spanish territories meet these criteria. The education of these specialized ambulance staff differs from one country to another: the duration of the training varies from 20 to 520 h [14].

Two-level rescue system with Advanced Cardiac Life Support resuscitation by paramedics or nurses

Some European countries (e.g. the United Kingdom, Finland, the Netherlands, Sweden) are using this kind of system, similar to that in the United States [16]. In general, the first level is undertaken by ambulances and/or fire vehicles whose crews are staffed by paramedics authorized to practice ACLS-type resuscitation. In Europe, paramedics

have a 2-year training [17]. When the call suggests a life-threatening emergency, a second response (fire service) can be dispatched simultaneously (USA). For calls without emergency characteristics, an ambulance with an EMT crew or a fire vehicle can be sent.

In the United Kingdom the prehospital system was largely inspired by the United States. Of the 15 180 ambulances recorded in 1997, 42% were staffed by paramedics. Their training is similar to that provided in the United States. After having graduated as EMTs, they receive further training to enable them to practice advanced resuscitation (intubation, venous access, emergency drug injections) [16]. However, these personnel do not seem to gain much experience of vital distress management: of the 1350 calls received every day by London Ambulance Service only two or three relate to trauma patients. Thus, the frequency of trauma patient management by a paramedic team in London is estimated at one or two call-outs per year [18].

Finland has second-level paramedics, although some ambulances staffed by firefighters (first level) may have ACLS clearance. A supervising physician (one per city) can be sent out if necessary, but in fact this rarely happens [17].

Two-level rescue system with a medicalized second level

This is the most common system in Europe (France, Germany, Belgium, Czech Republic, Norway, Estonia, Russia, Switzerland, Hungary, Island, Finland, partially Italy, Portugal, Turkey, and Greece). Some regional differences exist, depending on call centres or human or technical means [13, 19–23]. The most complete system seems to be that used in France, where the PECS is uniform from the reception of the emergency call to the admission of the patient to hospital, after medicalized regulation and care [21].

In Italy, most ambulances are not staffed by physicians or paramedics. Crews are made up of first-aid rescuers, able to provide at least basic life support. However, since 1992, ambulances including nurses have come into use in some regions. These nurses may, subject to written protocols, practise advanced resuscitation (intubation, injection of drugs). In regions where prehospital care systems are more sophisticated, an emergency physician or anaesthesiologist may reach the ambulance in a light vehicle. Finally, helicopters can be staffed by medicalized teams consisting of a physician, a nurse and two pilots [24].

Switzerland has a partially medicalized system. There are three structures for prehospital emergencies: air (helicopter) rescue, land rescue, and marine rescue. The medicalized helicopter service consists of 13 helicopters and is designed to cover the whole national territory within 15 min [13]. Voluntary mountain rescue associations (e.g. the Swiss Alpine Club) complete the system. For a minor emergency, a team of two paramedics can be sent to the scene. Paramedics were only recently equipped with AED: the Red Cross and firefighters are less involved in this scheme. In case of a serious emergency, a medicalized team with a physician and two paramedics can be sent to the scene [13].

Belgium uses medicalized care for severe prehospital emergencies. The composition of the ambulance crew is similar to a mobile intensive care unit (MICU), including an emergency physician (sometimes an anaesthetist), a nurse, and ambulance drivers. It is a two-level system, giving the ability to send a nonmedicalized ambulance or a fire vehicle at the same departure time, supplemented if necessary by a medical team.

Some countries have a system where nonmedicalized and medicalized prehospital care coexist. In Russia, there is a system seemingly identical to the French model, with regulation (usually nurse-led) deciding for the level of the response to be sent. This may be a nonmedicalized ambulance or an ambulance with a physician and a nurse. This system exists mainly in urban areas where medical density is quite high (75 doctors per 10 000 inhabitants) but is almost nonexistent in rural areas where medical density is less (10 doctors per 10 000 inhabitants) [20].

Helicopters staffed by medicalized crews are used in Austria, Germany, Switzerland, Iceland, Norway, and partly in France and Italy [3].

Although there is still a debate, mostly based on the duration of management, between supporters of the different PECS, it is difficult to favour one system over another. A prospective cohort registry of adult trauma patients transported by EMS agencies in North America recently showed that the time elapsed from the on-scene arrival of an ambulance to its final destination was not correlated to mortality [25]. Thus, even if time is still crucial, particularly for trauma patients, the argument that on-scene treatment should be minimized to decrease mortality [26] is no longer valid. To be pragmatic and impartial, we should consider that for life threatening situations, prehospital personal (including physicians) should have to be skilled at the highest possible level to perform all necessary procedures for stabilizing and treating patients as fast as possible, before and even during transfer. For situations that are not life threatening, the type of crew involved should be chosen according to the initial evaluation (medicalized regulation?), in order to match the level of emergency as closely as possible to the level of performance. That means that some compromise between Anglo-Saxon and Germano-French systems must probably be found in the future to adapt the response more closer to the requirments, and fulfil the guidelines for prehospital care.

Training

The effectiveness of prehospital care system depends heavily on the training of emergency practitioners. Many countries have legislation and a certification system in emergency medicine in order to standardize the level of competence of health care staff, including for prehospital emergency care. The United States and the United Kingdom have developed an educational system with national certification for prehospital emergency care. Conversely, in Germany, the teaching of emergency medicine for physicians does not include any specific program for prehospital emergency care [27]. In France, the teaching of emergency medicine is holistic and nonmodular, and a large part of the programme is dedicated to prehospital emergencies.

As in the United States, training modules such as advanced trauma life support (ATLS) and advanced cardiac life support (ACLS) have sometimes been promoted. They are taught in parallel with the academic training but are not always intended for physicians [28]. Other modules more specifically oriented towards particular prehospital situations have also emerged: prehospital trauma life support, pediatric advanced life support, advance disaster life support, trauma nurse core curriculum, wound care courses, integrated management of childhood illnesses, and prehospital cardiac life support. Finally, the increasing integration of bedside clinical ultrasound in emergency medicine has necessitated the creation of numerous local, national, or international training schemes [29]. In practice, emergency medicine is taught in the medical curriculum in a vast majority of European countries and in the United States, where internships for students in emergency medical wards are specifically suggested [30].

The length of the training for different staff (EMTs, paramedics, nurses, physicians) involved in PECS varies widely. The minimum training level of EMTs ranges between 20 and 520 hours, specifically organized for paramedics in the United Kingdom and Germany [14]. The training of a paramedic is in fact a specialization of EMT training, lasting approximately 2 years [17]. Emergency physicians are specialists in their own right only in some countries (USA, Italy, Turkey, Croatia, UK, France) [16, 24, 31]. In France, Switzerland, Austria, Finland, Spain, Slovenia, and the Czech Republic, there is additional training and certification [30]. In addition, eastern European countries, Germany, France, and Spain provide specific training in prehospital emergency care for emergency physicians [14].

Conclusion

There are obvious and important organizational disparities in PECS between Europe and North America, and even within European countries. This variety can be interpreted as a result of socio-cultural, economic, geographical, political, and even religious factors in each country. But despite this diversity, convergent evolution is perceptible. Some basic principles are spreading throughout all these countries, especially for cardiac arrest management. Thus, first level rescuers, whatever the means used for intervention, must have the benefit of AED. This technology is now even spreading to lay bystanders or other nonmedical personnel.

Some medicalization of the regulation of emergency calls seems to be necessary, but is not common in Europe. It helps to decrease the flow of patients to emergency departments, as confirmed by experiments carried out in North American '911' call centres to evaluate regulation by nurses. Although medicalization of prehospital care now appears to be well accepted (except in the United Kingdom), it remains incomplete and there are still many who oppose it. But more and more physicians are involved in prehospital care, even in English-speaking countries.

Rather than trying to promote the advantages of one system rather than another, we should probably search for a way to use both approaches, depending on the specific situation, to optimize medical care systems in out-of-hospital scenarios, particularly in acute cardiac pathologies.

Personal perspective

In Europe and the United States, PECS correspond to two different philosophies. Some countries favour intrahospital medical care with extensive training of nonmedical practitioners for out-of-hospital care (Anglo-Saxon system). Others have adopted the Germano-French system, which advocates medicalization at the scene. It is risky to compare these systems in terms of efficiency, since they depend on very different medico-economic logic, and patients themselves are not really comparable. We believe that the prospects of prehospital medicine lie in being developed as an essential component, a subspecialism, of emergency medicine. If we consider emergency medicine as the 'science of the acute', the corollary is the need to offer, as quickly as possible, the most appropriate care to patients in distress. This involves pursuing specific technical and academic research on the potential benefits of specific care for acute patients before their arrival at hospital. The benefits may be felt only if some upstream sorting and grading exists, implying the medicalized regulation of distress calls. Debates about emergency medicine should consider the answers given by various models of emergency call centres ('911', '112', '15', etc.). The nature of the dispatcher would then probably be seen as an essential component of medical decision-making.

Further reading

Arnold JL, Dickinson G, Tsai MC, Han D. A survey of emergency medicine in 36 countries. *Can J Emerg Med* 2001;**3**:1–13.

Bossaert LL. The complexity of comparing different EMS systems—a survey of EMS systems in Europe. *Ann Emerg Med* 1993;**22**:99–102.

Bossaert L, Handley A, Marsden A, *et al*. European Resuscitation Council guidelines for the use of automated external defibrillators by EMS providers and first responders: A statement from the Early Defibrillation Task Force, with contributions from the Working Groups on Basic and Advanced Life Support, and approved by the Executive Committee. *Resuscitation* 1998;**37**(2): 91–94.

Carli PA, Orliaguet GA. Prehospital trauma care. *Curr Opin Anesthesiol* 1995;**8**:157–162.

Dick WF. Does prehospital care by physicians result in a better outcome than resuscitation by other EMS personnel? *Resuscitation* 1993;**26**(2):109–110.

Herlitz J, Bahr J, Fischer M, *et al*. Resuscitation in Europe: a tale of five European regions. *Resuscitation* 1999;**41**(2):121–131.

Lechleuthner A, Emerman C, Dauber A, *et al*. Evolution of rescue systems: a comparison between Cologne and Cleveland. *Prehosp Disaster Med* 1994;**9**:193–7.

Nemitz B. Advantages and limitations of medical dispatching: the French view. *Eur J Emerg Med* 1995;**3**:153–159.

Sikka N, Margolis G. Understanding diversity among prehospital care delivery systems around the world. *Emerg Med Clin North Am* 2005;**23**:99–114.

Smith JP, Bodai BI, Hill AS, Frey CF. Prehospital stabilization of critically injured patients: a failed concept. *J Trauma* 1985;**25**(1):65–70.

➲ For additional multimedia materials please visit the online version of the book (🔗 http://www.esciacc.oxfordmedicine.com).

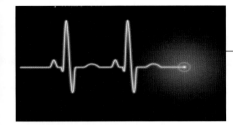

CHAPTER 5

Telemedicine

Peter Clemmensen and Maria Sejersten Ripa

Contents

Summary

Telemedicine has become an important tool for optimizing treatment in the individual patient within the field of cardiology. It allows exchange of information for the purpose of consulting, and the initiating of medical procedures, examinations, and therapy. Teletransmission of ECGs from the prehospital setting to the receiving hospital is the most widespread technology within prehospital cardiac care. Providing a diagnostic ECG from patients with acute coronary syndromes (ACS) to health care professionals with decision making power has proved pivotal for an early diagnosis, ideal triage, and initiation of reperfusion therapy of the large group of patients presenting with ST-segment elevation acute myocardial infarction (STEMI) each year. Using ECG teletransmission, the treatment delay is significantly reduced allowing fibrinolysis to be administered in less than 30 min and primary percutaneous coronary intervention (pPCI) to be provided in less than 120 min, as mandated by STEMI guidelines, improving the case fatality rate and morbidity of STEMI.

Introduction

Definition of telemedicine

Telemedicine can be defined as:

> the practise of diagnostic procedures, decision support, and patient care in any form at a distance, and supported by some means of multimedia communications.

Telemedicine thus has the ability to provide interactive health care using modern technology and telecommunications. It has been in rapid development as technology has evolved, and involves the exchange of medical information though the phone, Internet, or other networks for the purpose of consulting and initiating therapy or even guiding medical procedures or examinations. Accordingly, the concept of telemedicine can be used for a simple contact between two health care professionals by phone, or for more complex technology such as video-conferencing or satellite communications in remote areas.

Despite the broader definition given above, the present chapter focuses on the ECG in the setting of acute coronary care. However, at the end we describe some of the ongoing evaluations of telemedicine in the prehospital phase as well as possible future developments.

The prehospital ECG in telemedicine

History of ECG in telemedicine

ECG tracings were first transmitted over a phone line in the early 1960s [1]. In those days, where coronary care units in hospitals had recently been introduced, the ECG diagnosis focused on arrhythmia detection and treatment. Certainly, with the need for very early action with defibrillation of ventricular tachycardia (VT) and ventricular fibrillation (VF), the time delay involved in consultations rendered telecommunication for this purpose obsolete. Consequently, most ambulances were equipped with ECG monitors using a single lead or a few leads for arrhythmia detection [2, 3]. After the introduction of fibrinolysis in the 1980s and 1990s, there was renewed interest in the 12-lead ECG since many studies showed the importance of early fibrinolysis, and several studies of prehospital fibrinolysis were published [4, 5]. During the following decade many countries adopted a strategy of prehospital fibrinolysis, especially in remote and mountainous areas [6, 7]. The focus on a reliable prehospital diagnosis of STEMI in recent years has been the possibility of rerouting patients to hospitals with the capacity to perform percutaneous coronary intervention (pPCI) [8–10]. Because of the issue of safety in transporting STEMI patients over long distances, often bypassing local hospitals, and the cost involved in activation of a cardiac catheterization suite with its doctor(s) and nurses, a correct prehospital diagnosis is mandatory.

Wireless transmission of ECG

The technology of cellular telephonic transmission of prehospital 12-lead ECGs from the ambulance to hospital receiving stations has been available for more than 20 years [10, 11]. Currently, wireless transmission systems for recording prehospital ECGs are commercially available from four companies: Phillips Healthcare (Andover, MA, USA), Physio-Control Inc. (Redmond, WA, USA), Ortivus (Danderyd, Sweden), and Zoll Medical (Chelmsford, MA, USA).

The number of ambulances carrying equipment to record and transmit 12-lead ECGs is increasing, with more than one-third of all ambulances in Europe and the United States possessing this ability [12]. This technology allows high quality remote diagnosis and facilitates early triage of patients with STEMI to reperfusion therapy (prehospital fibrinolysis, hospital fibrinolysis, or pPCI), and initiation of adjunctive therapies even in the prehospital setting. In addition, the receiving hospital receives early notification of incoming patients, and can either prepare for immediate hospital fibrinolysis or activate the catheterization laboratory.

A 12-lead ECG can be transmitted from the ambulance to a receiving station located within the hospital, where it can be stored, displayed, and printed. Simultaneously, the ECG can be forwarded to the on-call cardiologist's mobile phone and a fax in the emergency department [8]. A model for the use of prehospital electrocardiographic recording and triage of ACS patients is shown in ➲ Fig. 5.1.

Success and quality of ECG transmission

The general availability of the global system for mobile communication (GSM) network has enabled successful ECG transmission from most locations. However, failure is still common in areas with poor GSM coverage, including locations where (e.g.) mountains or buildings interfere with the signal. Technical errors or lack of patient cooperation have also been reported to cause unsuccessful ECG transmission [13]. However, increased acquaintance with the system, technical developments, widespread and dependable GSM networks, and further optimization of standard operating procedures may increase the transmission success rate. The quality of the transmitted ECG depends on several variables including where the ECG is recorded (on scene, in the ambulance, during transport), the patient's condition (calm, agitated), the accuracy with which both precordial and limb electrodes are placed, the equipment, and the expertise of the person recording the ECG. In general, a very high quality of prehospital recorded ECG has been reported, with 98–99.7% of the recorded ECGs being acceptable for diagnostic purposes [13, 14]. Although these studies report a high success rate it is important to have internal quality control and performance measures for routine use of this technology. A high transmission failure rate is likely to result in lower acceptance and thus reduced use of the technology.

Reduction of prehospital and hospital delays by telemedicine

Delay in initiation of reperfusion therapy is a great problem in the treatment of STEMI patients, because mortality rates increase with time to therapy [5, 15, 16]. To facilitate this challenge the European Society of Cardiology, the American Heart Association, and the American College of Cardiology

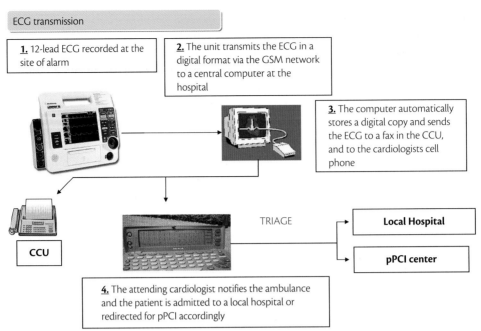

Figure 5.1 A four-step model for the implementation of prehospital recording of a 12-lead ECG. In the present figure the Copenhagen model is displayed, but in other health care systems similar routines are used for decision support regarding prehospital fibrinolysis. The cellphone displayed is a Nokia Communicator but other technologies can be used including PDAs, etc. The 12-lead recorder is an integrated part of the defibrillator in the LifePak 12 (Physio-Control Inc., Redmond, WA, USA).

Table 5.1 Important studies demonstrating the reduction in treatment delay among ST-segment elevation myocardium infarction (STEMI) patients diagnosed in the prehospital phase using prehospital ECG recording with interpretation on site or supported by teletransmission of the ECG to a cardiologist

	N	Year of publication (study year)	Transport time to hospital (min)	Reduction in time to needle	Reduction in time to balloon
EMIP [32]	5469	1993 (1988–1992)	35	55[a]	
REPAIR [7]	749	1995 (1988–1994)	11	50[b]	
Lamfers et al. [22]	744	2003 (1995–1999)	–	57[b]	
MITI [23]	360	1993 (1988–1991)	<23	33[a]	
GREAT [33]	311	1992 (1988–1991)	47	130[a]	
Pedersen et al. [21]	1437	2009 (2005–2008)	–		20[c]
Sejersten et al. [8]	565	2008 (2003–2005)	12		63[c,d]
Adams et al. [27]	277	2006 (2001–2005)	–		51[c,e]
Terkelsen et al. [9]	161	2005 (2002–2004)	37		81[c]
Wall et al. [10]	77	2000 (1995–1996)	–		29[c]

[a] By going from prehospital diagnosis combined with hospital thrombolysis to prehospital diagnosis and thrombolysis.
[b] By going from hospital diagnosis and thrombolysis to prehospital diagnosis and thrombolysis.
[c] By going from hospital diagnosis to prehospital diagnosis and direct transfer to a tertiary hospital for primary percutaneous coronary intervention.
[d] Time to a. femoralis puncture.
[e] Time for thrombolysis in myocardial infarction 3 flow.

have listed goals for transportation and initiating reperfusion treatment in STEMI patients [17, 18]. Generally thrombolysis should be started within 30 min and pPCI within 90 min from first medical contact. These should be considered the longest acceptable delays, and every effort should be made to keep the total ischaemic time less than 120 min, ideally 60 min, from symptom onset to initiation of reperfusion therapy. However, while time delays reported by clinical studies may meet guideline recommendations, real world data from registries often give a completely different picture with time delays by far exceeding recommendations [19–21].

Several studies have demonstrated a reduction in time to reperfusion therapy with rapid ECG availability [8–10, 22–27]. Accordingly, time to both thrombolysis and pPCI is significantly reduced in patients with the STEMI diagnosis established in the ambulance rather than on arrival at hospital. ➲Table 5.1 gives an overview of some of the important studies which have demonstrated the time savings made possible using prehospital diagnosis in patients with STEMI. However, transmission of an ECG to a fixed receiving station within the hospital requires that the physician on call must be near the receiving station in

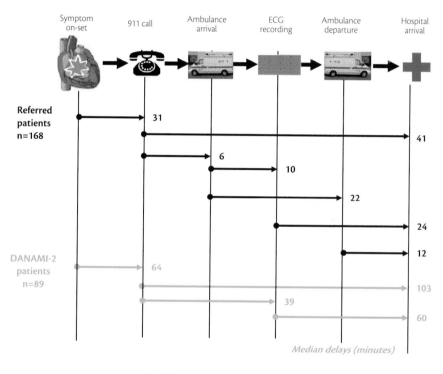

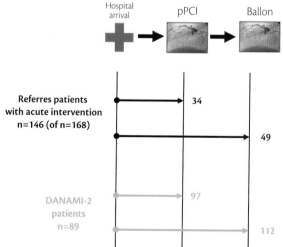

Figure 5.2 Time savings obtained in one study comparing historic controls in urban Copenhagen to the era where teletransmission of the ECG occurred. The controls had participated in the DANAMI-2 trial where patients with STEMI were not diagnosed in the field, but rather transported to the emergency department for ECG recording and diagnosis, then followed by activation of the cardiac catheterization laboratory with the resultant time delays. Note that the time line is not chronological, and if the time from ECG recordings are compared it is important to realize that in the 'referred patients' the ECG is taken in the field compared to the emergency department in the DANAMI-2 trial, which actually leads to an underestimation of the time saved.
Reproduced from Sejersten M, Sillesen M, Hansen PR, *et al.* Effect on treatment delay of prehospital teletransmission of 12-lead electrocardiogram to a cardiologist for immediate triage and direct referral of patients with ST-segment elevation acute myocardial infarction to primary percutaneous coronary intervention. *Am J Cardiol* 2008;**101**:941–946, with permission from Elsevier.

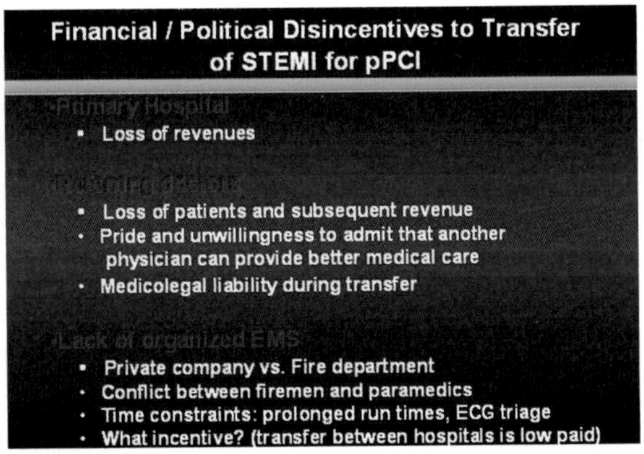

Figure 5.3 Potential financial and political disincentives to transferring patients and bypassing spoke hospitals in order to reach larger hubs for more specialized care.

Table 5.2 Future developments in telemedicine surrounding the prehospital phase of acute coronary care

ECG and algorithms for early diagnosis and triage	Improved predictive instruments
Implantable devices	Transmission of biological data to receiving stations/monitoring facility
GPS tracking	Online tracking of EMS vehicles or patients
Point of care biomarkers	Early cardiac markers for diagnosis and triage
Echocardiography	Diagnostic refinement

EMS, emergency medical service; GPS, Global Positioning System.

order to quickly view and interpret the ECG to ensure an early triage decision. Transmission to a receiving station in the emergency department may also require cardiology consultations on arrival, which can create further delays [28]. A solution would be to transmit the ECG directly to the cardiologist's phone or handheld computer [8, 29, 30]. With transmission to a handheld device the cardiologist would be available for a consultation, including ECG analysis, even if located remote to the receiving station within or outside the hospital (➲ Fig. 5.1).

The great advantage of this technology is the direct contact with an ECG specialist with real decision-making competence and ability to activate the catheterization laboratory. With the cardiologist's expertise it may also be possible to reduce the number of times the catheterization laboratory team is activated unnecessarily because of an incorrect diagnosis. ➲ Figure 5.2 shows the time savings obtained in one study comparing historic controls in urban Copenhagen to the era where there was teletransmission of the ECG. The controls participated in the DANAMI 2 trial where patients with STEMI were not diagnosed in the field, but rather were transported to the emergency department for ECG recording and diagnosis, followed by activation of the cardiac catheterization laboratory [31].

Telemedicine in other diagnostic fields for cardiovascular patients

The greatest benefit with telemedicine is obtained in areas where there may be a long distance between patients and qualified health care professionals, as mentioned above. Although the prehospital phase is the focus of this chapter, other application of telemedicine deserves some mention, since it is often used in the evolution of patients with cardiovascular disease. 'Real time' is the most common mode in telemedicine and requires the presence of all parties involved at the same time for interaction and communication. An example is live video, where all involved can communicate together and determine type of therapy, for example. 'Store-and-forward' telemedicine, on the other hand, does not require simultaneous presence of the involved parties; instead, medical data like echocardiographic CT images can be forwarded for evaluation by a specialist, or second opinion, at the earliest convenience. 'Home health telemedicine' is a third modality which can be used for remote monitoring of patients outside the hospital and thereby assists optimal patient care, including shared care as seen in the pacemaker/ICD field and heart failure management.

Conclusion

Telemedicine in the form of routine 12-lead standard ECG recording in the prehospital phase and transmission of this pivotal diagnostic test to hospitals from patient suffering ACS has had a major impact in reducing the treatment delays, especially in STEMI. Whether the treatment of choice is prehospital fibrinolysis or emergency transfer to a tertiary hospital for pPCI, telemedicine has been a major contributor to improved organization and collaboration between the emergency medical service with its emergency physicians and the cardiology community. Overall, these advanced has resulted in time savings ranging from 20 min to more than 1 h from symptom onset to reperfusion therapy, thus contributing to the historically low mortality of STEMI.

Personal perspective

Many obstacles have been encountered during the implementation of telemedicine including prehospital ECG recording and transmission to hospitals. Some of the financial and political disincentives of transferring patients with STEMI for pPCI are shown in ➲ Fig. 5.3. Best practice in cardiology demands governance from the political and hospital administrative leadership. One of the implications of rerouting patients directly to pPCI hubs is lower acute admissions in spoke hospitals leading to both financial and educational challenges. In some regions this development can even lead to closure of smaller hospitals.

In regions with large distances to hospitals and in the more densely populated area where small hospitals are being closed, there needs to be a continued development of prehospital care, often supported by helicopters. Other diagnostic modalities are either being developed or currently tested in the prehospital setting. Point-of-care testing including biomarkers or echocardiography is likely to evolve with telemedicine in the future. Some possible fields of improvement and developments in the field of prehospital care and telemedicine is listed in ➲ Table 5.2.

Further reading

Garvey JL, MacLeod BA, Sopko G, Hand MM. Pre-hospital 12-lead electrocardiography programs: a call for implementation by emergency medical services systems providing advanced life support—National Heart Attack Alert Program (NHAAP) Coordinating Committee; National Heart, Lung, and Blood Institute NHLBI); National Institutes of Health. *J Am Coll Cardiol* 2006;**47**:485–491.

Sejersten M, Sillesen M, Hansen PR, *et al*. Effect on treatment delay of prehospital teletransmission of 12-lead electrocardiogram to a cardiologist for immediate triage and direct referral of patients with ST-segment elevation acute myocardial infarction to primary percutaneous coronary intervention. *Am J Cardiol* 2008;**101**:941–946.

Ting HH, Krumholz HM, Bradley EH, *et al*. Implementation and integration of prehospital ECGs into systems of care for acute coronary syndrome: a scientific statement from the American Heart Association Interdisciplinary Council on Quality of Care and Outcomes Research, Emergency Cardiovascular Care Committee, Council on Cardiovascular Nursing, and Council on Clinical Cardiology. *Circulation* 2008;**118**:1066–1079.

Online resources

🙨 International Society for Telemedicine and eHealth. http://www.isft.net/cms/index.php?starting_point

🙨 American Telemedicine Association. http://www.americantelemed.org/i4a/pages/index.cfm?pageid=1

➲ For additional multimedia materials please visit the online version of the book (🙨 http://www.esciacc.oxfordmedicine.com).

SECTION II

Emergency department

CHAPTER 6

Chest pain and chest pain units

Eric Durand, Aures Chaib, and Nicolas Danchin

Contents

Summary

In the last decade, patients visiting the emergency department with suspected acute coronary syndrome (ACS) were classically admitted in cardiology resulting in expensive and time-consuming evaluations. Despite this, 2–5% of patients with ACS were discharged home, resulting in increased mortality. To address the inability to exclude an ACS diagnosis, chest pain units (CPUs) were developed particularly in the United States. These units provide an environment where serial ECGs, cardiac marker testing, and provocative test can be performed to rule out ACS. Eligible candidates are the majority of patients with nondiagnostic ECG and normal troponin measurements. The results have been impressive. CPUs have markedly decreased adverse events, while simultaneously increasing the safe discharge rate by 36%. Despite evidence to suggest that care in CPU is more effective for such patients, the percentage of emergency or cardiology departments in Europe setting up CPUs remains very low.

Introduction

In the United States, it was recently estimated that 8% of all emergency department (ED) visits may be for chest pain (CP). Acute coronary syndrome–ST elevation (ACS-STE), rapidly diagnosed by ECG, clearly identifies the higher risk population. However, a diagnostic ECG is found in not more than 4% of all CP presentations [1]. In the United States, before the creation of chest pain units (CPU), patients presenting to hospital with suspected ACS were classically admitted to the coronary care unit (CCU) for expensive and time-consuming evaluations. Despite this, 2–5% of patients with ACS were discharged home, resulting in increased mortality [1, 2]. With the addition of rapid troponin assays, identification of high risk patients became more objective. However, it suffers from a critical sensitivity deficit as an early isolated troponin measurement can discriminate only the highest risk patients [3]. A positive troponin identifies the patient with an ACS, but an undetectable troponin does not exclude an event.

CPUs were developed to address the inability to exclude an ACS diagnosis. Eligible candidates are the majority of patients with nondiagnostic ECG and normal troponin measurements. CPUs have markedly decreased adverse events, while simultaneously increasing the safe discharge rate.

Why do we need chest pain units?

In the United States in 2005, 13.9 million people were admitted to the emergency department (ED) for CP. Only 20% were discharged with diagnoses of ACS, suggesting that the other 80% were not related to coronary artery disease (CAD) [4]. From the physicians' perspective, failure to diagnose or treat acute myocardial infarction (MI) represents the largest percentage of malpractice claims paid on behalf of emergency physicians for any one condition [5]. This largely because some patients experiencing an ACS do not present in a typical manner, particularly when they are older, female, diabetic, and have a history of heart failure. Less than half of MI patients will present with diagnostic cardiac markers on arrival, and roughly half will not have a diagnostic ECG. As a result of this, studies have reported that 2–8% of patients with an acute MI are inadvertently discharged home from the ED [1, 2]. Short-term mortality rate for MI patients mistakenly discharged from the ED is about 25%, which is almost twice what would be expected if they were admitted [6].

Although the clinical and medico-legal risks of CP patients might drive one to simply admit all patients to the hospital as inpatients, there is evidence that this is not the optimal solution. Studies have demonstrated that the approach of admitting CP patients is associated with a length of stay of roughly 2–3 days, with lower rates of completed testing than care in a CP observation unit. The American College of Emergency Physicians has therefore recommended an expansion of what has been called 'observation medicine' to improve the use of limited hospital resources in order to avoid unnecessary admissions and inappropriate discharges. Similarly to the trauma centre concept, CP centres include protocols related to the timely diagnosis and reperfusion of STEMI patients, CP diagnostic protocols to avoid inadvertent discharge of ACS patients, public outreach efforts to bring patients suffering with ACS to the hospital sooner, appropriate staffing and resources, and an effective interface with both emergency medical services and hospital administration. In 1998, the Society of Chest Pain Centers (SCPC; see ➲ Online resource) was established, involving a collaboration of physicians, nurses, and health care experts from cardiology, emergency medicine, nuclear medicine, and clinical pathology. The society has developed standardized criteria for accreditation of CP centres.

The CPU is generally where patients at low to intermediate risk of having an ACS are managed. Different models can be used for this approach. The unit may be located in the ED or adjacent to the it, or may be located remotely in an inpatient unit. It may be managed by emergency physicians alone, cardiologists or internists alone, or a combination of these specialties. ED is frequently the preferred location in the United States and the United Kingdom since the ED is where most CP patients enter the hospital. The unit may be a pure CPU or a unit where CP is one of the several conditions managed in a general 'observation unit' or a 'clinical decision unit'. CPUs generally use a standardized approach that includes initial ED risk stratification or patient selection, admission to the CPU with CPU protocol orders that include serial testing (cardiac markers and ECGs) to identify MI, followed by some type of provocative testing (stress test with or without imaging) to identify unstable angina [7–12].

There are several good reasons, listed in ➲ Box 6.1, why a hospital should consider having a CPU. Earlier studies of CPU protocols evaluated the outcomes of these patients and reported extremely low rates of mortality or morbidity [7, 9, 11, 13]. A multiple site registry study of CPUs has been compared with previous studies on CP evaluation with standard care [14]. A total of 23 407 patients were included, representing 5.3% of ED visits. In the CPUs, 153 of 2229 patients (6.9%) had an acute MI. Most of the patients admitted in the CPUs (76%) were discharged home without hospital admission. Compared to previous studies of CP patients, a higher proportion of patients underwent

---

Box 6.1 Potential advantages in having a chest pain unit

- Reduction in mortality and morbidity risk for ACS patients
- Reduction in unnecessary inpatient admissions, costs, and length of stay for CP patients
- Improved patient satisfaction and quality of life with a CPU
- Improved physician satisfaction
- Improved hospital resource utilization
- Economic benefits

a 'rule-out MI evaluation' (67 vs 57%), a lower proportion of MIs was missed (0.4 vs 4.5%), and final hospital admission rate was lower (47% vs 57%) [14]. Formal evaluation in the CPU resulted in a noticeable cost reduction ($124/patient) as compared to standard care [14]. Additionally, studies have shown that patients enrolled in a CPU diagnostic protocol are more likely to receive stress testing prior to discharge than if they were admitted to a general inpatient bed. This increases the likelihood that patients with unstable angina will be detected [15]. The impact of a CPU on inpatient admissions has also been demonstrated in other studies documenting the beneficial impact of a CPU on cost, admission avoidance, and length of stay. Interestingly, these studies demonstrated that mandatory stress testing was a frequent (84% of patients), safe, cost-effective, and valuable diagnostic and prognostic test in CPU patients [15]. In one study patients were allocated randomly to either an inpatient admission or a CPU admission [16]. MI or unstable angina occurred in 6% of patients within 30 days. No diagnoses were missed. The hospital stay was shorter and charges were lower in the CPU than with routine care. Among patients in whom ischaemia was ruled out, those assigned to CPU had a shorter hospital stay, and less initial hospital charges than did patients in routine care [16]. Before the study began, historical control data were collected. Historical control subjects had an even longer hospital stay and higher charges [16]. In 1998, a prospective randomized trial evaluated the safety, efficacy, and cost of admission to a CPU in the ED (n = 212) as compared to standard care in a cardiology department [17]. There was no significant difference in the rate of cardiac events between the two groups. All the patients assigned to the CPU and directly discharged home were free of adverse event at 6 months [17]. More resources were used for patients assigned to hospital admission than for those assigned to the CPU admission. A CPU located in the ED can therefore be a safe, effective, and cost-saving alternative to inpatient admission in cardiology [17]. In a 2004 cluster-randomized controlled trial [18], 442 days were randomized to either CPU care days or routine care days. The objective was to compare the effectiveness and cost-effectiveness of CPU compared with routine care for patients with acute and undifferentiated CP. This British study included 972 patients. The use of a CPU reduced the proportion of CP patients admitted from 54% to 37%, and the proportion discharged with ACS from 14% to 6%. Care in CPU was associated with improved health quality during follow-up, and financial savings [18]. Interestingly, despite evidence from the United States and the United Kingdom to suggest

that care in a CPU is more effective, the percentage of emergency or cardiology departments setting up CPUs is very low elsewhere in Europe. The poor development of CPUs in Europe greatly contrasts with their expansion in the United States, where more than 1500 CPUs are currently available [19]. In Spain, where EDs are chronically overcrowded, the Spanish Society of Cardiology recommended in 2002 that CPUs should be set up in all EDs to provided fast and efficient care for patients with CP. However, by 2008, only four centres had followed this advice. The CPU Task Force of the German Society of Cardiology recently introduced prerequisites for a CPU certification programme to evaluate CPUs across the country in October 2008. The aim is to ensure a network of fully resourced centres which meet or exceed quality-of-care measures in order to improve the standard of care of patients with acute CP.

Initial presentation and risk stratification in the emergency department

Patients with suspected ACS may present to the ED via emergency medical services or self-transport. In Europe, and particularly in France, prehospital care of these patients is often performed by a mobile intensive care unit (MICU).

Typical presentation of acute coronary syndromes

The initial evaluation of a patient with a suspected ACS commonly includes assessing the presence of the major risk factors for CAD. Although these have been shown to be rather poor predictors of ACS, their presence, along with the history and physical examination, ECG, and cardiac markers, forms the basis for risk stratification. Unstable angina is defined as angina that (1) is of new onset, (2) occurs at rest for prolonged periods (>20 min), or (3) is crescendo angina The recognition of unstable angina is extremely important because of the high risk for MI associated with this condition. Prinzmetal's angina is caused by coronary artery vasospasm. It commonly exhibits a circadian pattern, with most episodes occurring in the early hours of the morning. The pain may be associated with palpitations or syncope secondary to arrhythmia. It is usually relieved by nitroglycerine (NTG). The ECG reveals classically transient ST-segment elevation relieved by NTG. During MI CP is usually persistent (>20 min), more severe, and sometimes associated with symptoms of dyspnoea, diaphoresis, or nausea. It is typically not or incompletely relieved by rest or NTG.

Atypical presentation and differential diagnosis

Many patients present with atypical symptoms such as dyspnoea, nausea, diaphoresis, syncope, or pain in the arms, epigastrium, shoulder, or neck. Pain perception and descriptions vary widely among patients and are influenced by numerous factors, including include older age, diabetes mellitus, female gender, and nonwhite ethnicity. Interestingly, in a multicentre study of patients with documented ACS, 13% had pleuritic CP and 7% had pain reproducible with palpation [20]. Moreover, it is estimated that approximately 50% of patients with ACS will not have CP as a chief complaint. Unfortunately, patients with atypical presentations are more difficult to diagnose and have poorer outcomes. These patients are also less likely to receive adjunct therapies shown to reduce mortality [21].

The emergency physician should use a thorough history and physical examination, not only to help determine the risk of possible ACS but also to recognize and distinguish anginal CP from other serious and life-threatening conditions (e.g. aortic dissection, pulmonary embolism, pericarditis with pericardial tamponade, oesophageal perforation, and spontaneous pneumothorax).

ECG

The ECG is the single most important diagnostic test in the evaluation of patients with CP, to identify as soon as possible patients with acute myocardial infarction (AMI) who will benefit from early reperfusion therapy. It is currently recommended that EDs establish a triage protocol for ECG recording within the first 10 min upon the presentation of a patient with chest discomfort or symptoms consistent with ACS [22]. Furthermore, ECGs must be immediately presented to a treating physician for interpretation.

The ECG will provide a specific diagnosis in only about 5% of ED patients with CP [23]. However, there are many findings on an initial ECG that carry prognostic significance and allow for risk stratification. In a large retrospective study, specific findings on the initial ECG were shown to predict an increased risk of 30-day death or reinfarction. These findings included isolated T wave inversions, ST-segment elevation, ST-segment depression of more than 0.05 mV, and combined ST-segment elevation or depression. ST-segment elevation correlated with higher rates of early morbidity and mortality, while ST depression was associated with later events [24] (⊙ Fig. 6.1).

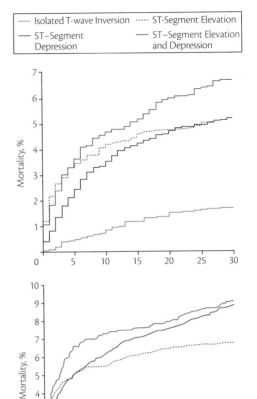

Figure 6.1 Kaplan–Meier curves evaluating the probability of death according to ECG abnormalities at presentation.
From Savonitto S, Ardissino D, Granger CB, *et al.* Prognostic value of the admission electrocardiogram in acute coronary syndromes. *JAMA* 1999;**281**:707–13. Copyright 1999 American Medical Association. All rights reserved.

The consequences of missed critical ECG findings in patients presenting with symptoms suggestive of ACS can be significant. In a retrospective study of patients with documented MI, high risk ECG findings were not documented in 12% of patients. T wave inversions are nonspecific and occur in many conditions, but in the setting of CP may be an indication of cardiac ischaemia. T wave inversion may also represent reperfusion of a completed infarct. Wellens' warning is a biphasic T wave with terminal T wave inversion in the anterior leads V2–V4 [25]. This finding is a highly specific in predicting proximal to mid- left anterior descending (LAD) lesions. Pathologic Q waves often indicate ischaemia or dead myocardium. Pre-existing Q waves from a previous MI should not be ignored in patients presenting with CP, as they demonstrate strong evidence of CAD. New left branch bundle block (LBBB) should be also considered a potential sign of acute MI in the setting of acute CP. New rhythm disturbances in the setting of

CP are disturbing and warrant investigation. While serial ECGs are critical to look for dynamic ST-segment changes, they may miss acute changes due to intermittent ischaemia. Continuous ST-segment monitoring may also be used to detect asymptomatic transient ischaemia.

Initial risk stratification: history, physical, ECG, and scoring systems

Initial triage of patients into appropriate risk categories, after obtaining a patient's initial history, physical examination, and ECG, is the most difficult part of CP evaluation. Usually patients are stratified according to their probability (i.e. low, intermediate, and high) of presenting an ACS (➲ Table 6.1).

Many scoring systems have been proposed for risk stratification of patients with suspected ACS, e.g. the Goldman criteria, ACI-TIPI instrument, TIMI (➲ Box 6.2, ➲ Table 6.2), PURSUIT, and GRACE scores [26–31]. There is robust evidence that these risk scores are predictive of acute and long term adverse outcomes. However, they are of limited interest for ruling out ACS in the ED. In 1997, The Medical College of Virginia detailed an elegant five-level approach to ACS risk stratification utilizing the initial ECG, CP characterization, and history [32]:

- Level 1 is defined as ECG criteria of ACS–STE requiring immediate reperfusion and CCU admission.

Box 6.2 TIMI risk score

- Age 65 years or older
- Three or more traditional risk factors for CAD
- Prior coronary stenosis of 50% or more
- ST-segment deviation on presenting ECG
- Two or more angina events prior to presentation
- Aspirin use within 7 days prior to presentation
- Elevated cardiac markers

CAD, coronary artery disease.

- Level 2 patients have a high probability for ACS–NSTE manifested by abnormal ECG or known CAD with typical symptoms. These patients are considered for admission to the CCU for further evaluation and treatment.
- Level 3 patients have a high probability of unstable angina, but low probability of MI. They are defined by >30 min of typical symptoms, a nondiagnostic ECG, and no prior history of CAD.
- Level 3 patients undergo a 'fast-track' protocol to confirm myocardial necrosis.
- Level 4 patients have a low to moderate probability of unstable angina manifested by <30 min of typical symptoms or prolonged atypical symptoms, a nondiagnostic ECG, and no history of CAD. In practice, level 3 and 4 indicate patients with CP without evidence of ischaemia. These patients are often evaluated in CPUs in the United States.
- Level 5 implies noncardiac CP defined by a clear diagnosis not related to ACS.

This strategy was reported to be a safe and effective method for rapid triage in 1187 consecutive patients [32].

Table 6.1 Stratification of risk of presenting an acute coronary syndrome for patients presenting to the emergency department with acute chest pain. Patients with low to moderate probability of presenting an acute coronary syndrome are usually candidates for evaluation in the chest pain unit

Variables	Low probability	Intermediate probability	High probability
History of CAD including MI	No	No	Yes
Other localization of atherosclerosis	No	Yes	Yes
Risk factors Including diabetes	<2 No	≥2 Yes	– –
Typical CP	No	No	Yes
Hypotension or CHF	No	No	Yes
ECG	Normal	± Normal	Abnormal
ST-segment elevation	No	No	Yes
ST-segment depression	No	No	Yes
Negative T wave	No	Yes	No
Elevated cardiac troponin	No	No	Yes

CAD, coronary artery disease; CHF, congestive heart failure; MI, myocardial infarction.

Table 6.2 Relative risk of composite outcome for each TIMI risk score component

TIMI variables	RR	95% CI
Age >65	1.3	0.92–1.88
Prior CAD	3.1	2.26–4.24
>3 cardiac risk factors	2.1	1.54–2.92
ST-segment deviation	5.3	3.81–7.23
Aspirin use	2.3	1.64–3.10
≥2 anginal events in 24 h	1.7	1.22–2.30
Elevated cardiac markers	6.3	4.64–8.45

Role of the chest pain unit in the management of chest pain

Eligible candidates for CPU evaluation are the majority of patients with nondiagnostic ECG and initial normal troponin measurement. Frequently, the first troponin measurement is performed in the ED. These patients are then admitted to CPU for further evaluation. The first step is an observational phase including serial ECGs and troponin measurements to identify transient ischaemia and to rule out myocardial necrosis using cardiac markers. Abnormal findings in this period involve admission to CCU. Patients presenting without evidence of ischaemia and normal troponin measurements remain in the CPU. The second step consists in performing provocative testing or CT to rule out unstable angina and CAD.

First step: to rule out myocardial necrosis: cardiac markers

Cardiac biomarkers are critical for risk stratification assessment of patients presenting with nontraumatic CP to rule out myocardial necrosis. Cardiac troponin T (cTnT) and troponin I (cTnI) are the preferred marker for diagnosis of MI, for risk stratification of suspected ACS patients, and for guidance of therapy and intervention. Troponin I and T are structural proteins, so some hours are frequently required for their release and detection in circulation. Thus a critically important point when utilizing cardiac troponin is timing of blood sample collection. In general, blood should be obtained at hospital presentation in the ED, followed by serial sampling based on the clinical circumstances in the CPU. For most patients this includes sampling upon presentation and several hours later (➲ Fig. 6.2). A cardiac troponin value on at least one occasion during the first 24 h after the acute event above the maximal concentration exceeding the 99th percentile of values for reference control group is indicative of myocardial necrosis consistent with MI [33]. Although cTnT and cTnI are found only in myocardium, troponin elevation is not specific of ACS (other aetiologies are listed in ➲ Box 6.3).

Relying solely on troponin testing for disposition strategy is not adequate to evaluate patients presenting for CP because it cannot safely rule out unstable angina. In a prospective longitudinal study in 266 patients at low risk for ACS, with a normal creatine kinase-isoenzyme subunit MB (CK-MB) index, admitted to a CPU, troponin T levels were measured at baseline and at 4, 8, and 16 h after admission [3]. Troponin testing identified only 2 (9.5%) of 21 patients

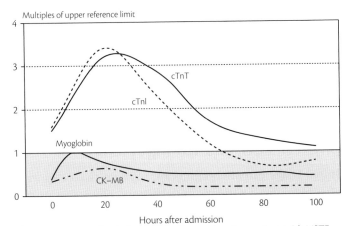

Figure 6.2 Example of release of cardiac markers in a patient with NSTE–ACS (shaded area indicates normal range). CK-MB, MB subunit of creatine kinase; cTnT, cardiac troponin T; cTnI, cardiac troponin I.

who developed an adverse event. The sensitivity and specificity were 9.5% and 99.2%, respectively, at the index visit, and 0% and 98.4% at 6 months. The positive and negative predictive values were 50% and 93%, respectively, at the index visit; and 0% and 92% at 6 months [3].

Box 6.3 Noncoronary aetiology of cardiac troponin elevation

- Severe congestive heart failure: acute and chronic
- Aortic dissection, aortic valve disease, or hypertrophic cardiomyopathy
- Cardiac contusion, ablation, pacing, cardioversion, or endomyocardial biopsy
- Inflammation diseases, e.g. myocarditis or myocardial extensions of endocarditis/pericarditis
- Hypertensive crisis
- Tachy- or bradyarrhythmias
- Pulmonary embolism, severe pulmonary hypertension
- Hypothyroidism
- Takotsubo syndrome (apical ballooning syndrome)
- Acute neurological disease, including stroke or subarachnoid haemorrhage
- Infiltrative disease, e.g. amyloidosis, haemochromatosis, sarcoidosis, scleroderma
- Drug toxicity, e.g. adriamycin, 5-fluorouracil, herceptin, snake venoms
- Burns, if affecting >30% of body surface area
- Rhabdomyolysis
- Critically ill patients, especially with respiratory failure or sepsis

Although conventional necrosis markers have a high diagnostic value, their sensitivity is weak within the first hours after the onset of CP. To overcome this limitation, a new generation of sensitive assays for cardiac troponins with a 10% coefficient of variation for levels below the 99th percentile has been introduced recently. Very recently, in a multicentre study, sensitive troponin I was compared to traditional myocardial necrosis markers (troponin T, myoglobin, CK and CK-MB) in 1818 consecutive patients with CP and suspected ACS, on admission and 3 and 6 h after admission [34]. The diagnostic accuracy was higher with the sensitive troponin I assay (area under the receiver operating characteristic curve [AUC], 0.96), as compared with the troponin T assay (AUC 0.85) and traditional myocardial necrosis markers (➲ Fig. 6.3). Sensitivity and specificity were higher than 90%. In patients presenting within 3 h after onset of CP, a single sensitive troponin I assay had a negative predictive value of 84% and a positive predictive value of 87%. A troponin I level of more than 0.04 ng/mL was independently associated with an increased risk of an adverse outcome at 30 days [34]. Similar results have been obtained with other sensitive troponin assays [35] Therefore, sensitive troponin assays might further enhance the accuracy of the diagnosis of MI and improve diagnostic sensitivity and specificity, even in patients presenting early after the onset of CP.

Of the numerous inflammatory markers that have been investigated over the past decade, C-reactive protein measured by highly sensitive assays (hsCRP) is the most widely studied and linked to higher rates of adverse events, even among patients with troponin-negative NSTE-ACS [36–38]. However, hsCRP has no role in the diagnosis of ACS.

Neurohumoral activation of the heart can be monitored by measurements of systemic levels of natriuretic peptides secreted from the heart (B-type natriuretic peptide [BNP] or its N-terminal prohormone fragment) which are highly sensitive and fairly specific markers for the detection of LV dysfunction. In NSTE-ACS, patients with elevated BNP or NT-proBNP levels have a three- to fivefold increased mortality rate when compared with those with lower levels [39]. However, these markers of long-term prognosis have limited value for diagnosis and initial risk stratification, and hence for selecting the initial therapeutic strategy in NSTE-ACS.

A considerable number of patients can still not be identified as being at high risk by today's routine biomarkers. Accordingly, a great number of novel biomarkers have been investigated in recent years to explore their usefulness as diagnostic tools and for risk stratification in addition to established markers. These include markers of oxidative stress (myeloperoxidase), markers of thrombosis and inflammation (e.g. soluble CD40 ligand) or markers involved further upstream in the inflammation cascade,

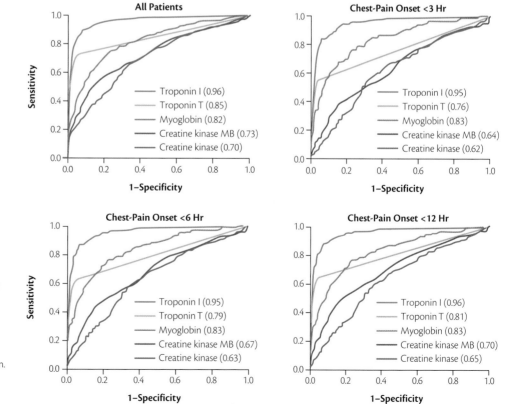

Figure 6.3 Receiver operating characteristic (ROC) curves and the corresponding areas under the curve (AUC) for baseline measurements of troponin I with the sensitive assay (troponin I), troponin T, myoglobin, creatine kinase MB, and creatine kinase, according of the time of the onset of chest pain. The sensitivity and specificity of these measures are also shown.
From Keller T, Zeller T, Peetz D, *et al.* Sensitive troponin I assay in early diagnosis of acute myocardial infarction. *N Engl J Med* 2009;**361**:868–877.

i.e. markers specific of vascular inflammation [40–42]. All have shown their incremental value over troponins in retrospective analyses, but have not been tested prospectively and are not yet available for routine use.

Second step: to rule out unstable angina and coronary artery disease: provocative testing and multislice CT

Patients presenting with CP with normal or inconclusive ECG and initial normal cardiac markers may still have ACS. After a period (3–9 h) of clinical observation, serial 12-lead ECGs, continuous telemetry monitoring, and serial measurement of cardiac injury markers are usually performed to rule out myocardial necrosis. In most institutions, accelerated diagnostic protocols (ADPs) have incorporated additional 'provocative' diagnostic testing to rule out unstable angina after myocardial necrosis has been excluded [1]. Diagnostic tests typically include exercise treadmill testing (ETT), stress myocardial perfusion imaging (MPI) or stress echocardiography. The decision to use echocardiography or radionuclide myocardial imaging in a CPU depends largely on local expertise with either of these two imaging modalities. Patients with a positive provocative test are generally admitted for further evaluation, most often coronary angiography, and those with a negative result are discharged to outpatient follow-up.

The selection of a specific diagnostic test, and whether or not imaging is incorporated, is most commonly dependent upon the patient's ability to exercise and the ability to interpret the stress ECG. ETT is the most frequently used strategy in current ADPs. ETT is recommended as a first line test unless the clinical circumstances described below preclude its use. The largest study evaluating the feasibility of this strategy included 1000 patients [43]. In this study, ETT was negative in 64%, positive in 13%, and nondiagnostic in 23%. There were no complications of testing and 80% of patients were safely discharged home from the ED. Compared to a negative exercise test, the relative risk of a cardiac event or the diagnosis of CAD was 38-fold for a nondiagnostic test and 114-fold for a positive test. What emerges from these studies is a recognition of the common occurrence and excellent predictive value of negative ETT in identifying patients at low risk [16, 17, 30]. Furthermore, although the positive predictive value is modest, positive tests are infrequent and result in the need for further evaluation in only small numbers of patients. Therefore, the utility of a strategy incorporating ETT into an ADP was confirmed by its ability to safely and efficiently reduce

unnecessary admissions in low risk patients while avoiding inappropriate discharge of patients with ACS not identified by routine measurement of cardiac injury markers and ECGs.

In patients who cannot exercise because of physical limitations, peripheral arterial disease, or pulmonary disease, pharmacological stress testing with either MPI or echocardiography is usually indicated. Pharmacological stress MPI can be performed with either a vasodilator (dipyridamole or adenosine) or dobutamine, with vasodilators considered to be the preferred agents. Sensitivities and specificities for diagnosing CAD are similar to that of exercise stress MPI [44]. The other common indication for using imaging in conjunction with stress testing is baseline ECG abnormalities that preclude accurate interpretation of the stress ECG: LBBB, left ventricular hypertrophy with significant ST-segment changes, ventricular paced rhythm, or preexcitation [45, 46]. In the patient with baseline ECG abnormalities who can exercise, stress echocardiography is an equally appropriate test, so that the ultimate test selected is often dependent upon institutional or operator expertise. Unlike all other imaging techniques, it is noninvasive and poses no risk from radiation exposure. Several studies have examined the incremental value of stress MPI compared with ETT in patients with a normal rest ECG [47, 48]. In a study of 1659 low risk patients without known CAD, it was found that MPI results did not add additional information over pretest data in the subgroup of 1451 patients who had a normal rest ECG [47]. Similarly, another report analysed outcomes of 3058 consecutive patients with a normal rest ECG who underwent exercise dual isotope MPI [48]. There were 70 adverse events (2.3%) during a mean follow-up of 1.6 ± 0.5 years. After adjusting for pretest indicators of risk, stress MPI yielded incremental value to predict adverse events, but not in low risk patients. Patients with a low pretest probability of CAD had an adverse event rate of only 0.4%, suggesting that stress MPI would be unlikely to be cost-effective.

Coronary CT angiography (CCTA) has great promise for expediting the triage of acute CP patients. Indeed, CCTA allows direct visualization of the coronary anatomy, has the ability to simultaneously image the rest of the thorax to exclude aortic dissection and pulmonary embolism, and the ability to provide alternate causes of CP, such as pneumonia, pericardial fluid, and oesophageal inflammation. Examples of CCTA are shown in ➔ Figs 6.4 and 6.5. At least six recent studies have evaluated the safety and diagnostic accuracy of 64-slice CCTA for triage of ED patients with acute CP [49–54]. In aggregate, 376 patients with low to

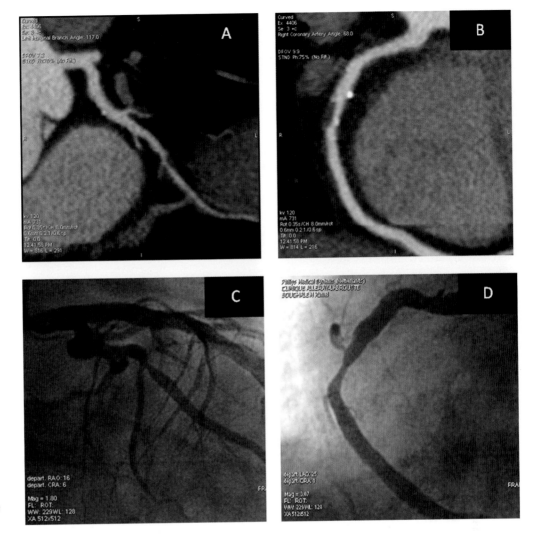

Figure 6.4 Visualization of noncalcified significant stenosis of left marginal (A) and moderate calcified significant stenosis of the right coronary artery (B) by 64-slice coronary CT angiography (CTTA) in patients admitted with suspected acute coronary syndrome with normal ECG and troponin measurements. Invasive coronary angiography of the same arteries (C, D).

intermediate pretest probability of ACS were prospectively followed over a 30-day to 15-month follow-up period after diagnosis by CCTA. All six studies excluded patients with abnormal cardiac biomarkers or ischaemic ECG changes, and two of the six studies excluded patients with pre-existing CAD [49–54]. Overall, an adjudicated diagnosis of ACS occurred in 72 (19.1%) of the 376 study patients. The absence of significant coronary artery stenosis by CCTA accurately excluded the presence of ACS in 373 of the 376 patients, resulting in a combined study mean negative predictive value of 99%. Interestingly, these results were recently confirmed in a large observational cohort study in 368 patients with normal initial troponin and nonischaemic ECG. Sensitivity and negative predictive value for ACS were 100% [55]. This suggests that CCTA can identify a subset of ED CP patients who can be safely discharged home on the basis of CT findings. In one of these studies, 197 low risk acute CP patients were evaluated by either early CCTA or by a standard diagnostic protocol

(MPI) [54]. The two groups were compared for safety, diagnostic accuracy, and efficiency. Among patients randomized to CCTA, 75% had decisive triage by CCTA alone (67% were immediately discharged and 8% were referred for immediate catheterization, which revealed significant disease in 7 of 8 referred cases). Importantly, CCTA alone was not considered adequate for diagnosis in 24 of 99 cases, owing either to lesions of unclear haemodynamic significance in 13 patients or to nondiagnostic quality scans in 11 patients. Among the patients discharged immediately, none had a major cardiac event or subsequent diagnosis of CAD over a 6-month follow-up period. The overall diagnostic accuracy of CCTA was 94% and the negative predictive value was 100%. Diagnostic efficiency, defined as time from randomization to definitive diagnosis, showed that the CCTA approach was more rapid (3.4 vs 15.0 h) and reduced costs by 15% [54].

Given the robust clinical performance of CCTA for exclusion of ACS in ED patients, as well as the widespread use

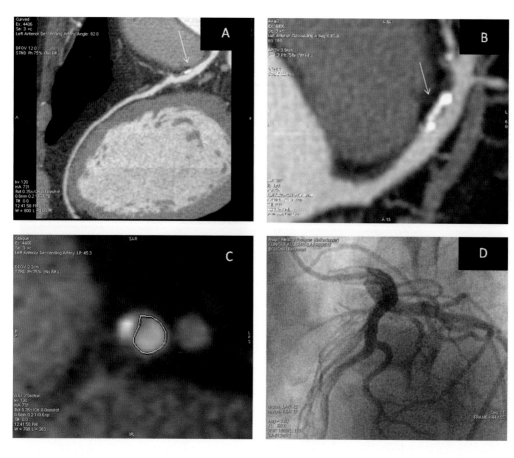

Figure 6.5 Visualization of calcified nonsignificant stenosis of proximal left anterior descending (LAD) artery (A–C) by 64-slice coronary CT angiography. Transversal view of the same lesion indicating nonsignificant stenosis. Invasive coronary angiography of the same artery (D).

and proven clinical accuracy of CT angiography for diagnosis of acute aortic dissection and pulmonary embolism, a 'triple rule-out' scan protocol to simultaneously exclude all three potentially fatal causes of acute CP with a single scan is an attractive option [56, 57]. A conventional cardiac CTA 'field of view' already includes the anatomy between the carina and the diaphragm. A triple rule-out protocol has to achieve high and consistent contrast intensity in all three vascular beds. Combined simultaneous evaluation for the pulmonary and coronary arteries and thoracic aorta requires a carefully tailored imaging and injection protocol. Although feasibility studies of this and similar protocols are promising, large-scale clinical trials assessing the clinical accuracy of such triple rule-out protocols are not yet available. In spite of these technical advances, important radiation safety concerns remain that should limit indiscriminate application of a triple rule-out scan protocol. Compared to the usual radiation dose of a standard CCTA (generally ranging from 8 to 22 mSv), the effective radiation dose of a triple rule-out scan is often 50% more, simply because of the increased field of view. By comparison, rest-stress radionuclide scans typically involve exposures in the range of 8–16 mSv, while diagnostic invasive angiography doses range from 5 to 13 mSv. Further, among patients who undergo CCTA as a primary triage test in the ED, a subset may require additional diagnostic and interventional invasive angiographic procedures, thus increasing the radiation dose.

In patients who undergo a dedicated CCTA, images of noncardiac thoracic structures (in addition to aortic and pulmonary arterial pathology) are contained in the field of view and therefore available to the expert reader. Previous studies have demonstrated that up to one in six patients without coronary abnormalities detected on CT was diagnosed with noncardiac findings that could explain their presenting symptoms [58].

Conclusion

Each year, millions of people visit the ED for acute CP. At one end of the spectrum are a minority of patients presenting with ST-segment elevation and thus definite ACS who require immediate reperfusion therapy and admission to CCU. At the other end of the spectrum are patients with atypical and noncardiac chest discomfort and normal ECG who can be safely discharged home. Between these two extremes are numerous patients with atypical presentation and nondiagnostic ECG who might have an ACS. CPUs have been designed for the triage of such patients. They use

ADPs including serial ECGs, troponin measurements, and provocative testing to rule out ACS and CAD in order to reduce unnecessary admissions and to avoid inappropriate discharge.

Personal perspective

Despite evidence to suggest that care in a CPU is more effective for such patients, the percentage of emergency or cardiology departments setting up CPUs remains very low in Europe, although Spain and the German Society of Cardiology promote such units. To our mind, the discrepancies in the organization of care between the United States and Europe require further investigation. In particular, observational registries in patients visiting the ED for acute CP would be helpful in order to evaluate the percentage of admission, inappropriate discharge, and cost of care for such patients in Europe.

Further reading

Bassand JP, Hamm CW, Ardissino D, *et al*. Guidelines for the diagnosis and treatment of non-ST segment elevation acute coronary syndromes. *Eur Heart J* 2007;**28**:1598–1660.

Canto JG, Shlipak MG, Rogers WJ, *et al*. Prevalence, clinical characteristics, and mortality among patients with myocardial infarction presenting without chest pain. *JAMA* 2000;**283**:3223–3229.

Farkouh ME, Smars PA, Reeder GS, *et al*. A critical trial of a chest pain observation unit for patients with unstable angina. Chest Pain Evaluation in the Emergency Room (CHEER) investigators. *N Engl J Med* 1998;**339**:1882–1888.

Gibbons RJ, Balady GJ, Bricker JT, *et al*. ACC/AHA 2002 guideline update for exercise testing: summary article: A report of the American College of Cardiology/American Heart Association Task Force on practice guidelines (committee to update the 1997 exercise testing guidelines). *J Am Coll Cardiol* 2002;**40**:1366–1374.

Keller T, Zeller T, Peetz D, *et al*. Sensitive troponin I assay in early diagnosis of acute myocardial infarction. *N Engl J Med* 2009;**361**:868–877.

Lee TH, Goldman L. Evaluation of the patient with acute chest pain. *N Engl J Med* 2000;**342**:1187–1195.

Peacock WF, Emerman CL, McErlean ES, *et al*. Prediction of short and long term outcomes by troponin-T in low risk patients evaluated for acute coronary syndromes. *Ann Emerg Med* 2000;**35**:213–220.

Pope JH, Aufderheide TP, Ruthazer R, *et al*. Missed diagnoses of acute cardiac ischemia in the emergency department. *N Engl J Med* 2000;**342**:1163–1170.

Renaud B, Maison P, Ngako A, *et al*. Impact of point-of-care testing in the emergency department evaluation and treatment of patients with suspected acute coronary syndromes. *Acad Emerg Med* 2008;**15**:216–224.

Thygesen K, Alpert JS, White HD. Joint ESC/ACCF/AHA/WHF Task Force for the Redefinition of Myocardial Infarction. Universal definition of myocardial infarction. *Circulation* 2007;**116**:2634–2653.

Van de Werf F, Bax J, Betriu A, *et al*. Management of acute myocardial infarction in patients presenting with persistent ST-segment elevation: the Task Force on the Management of ST-Segment Elevation Acute Myocardial Infarction of the European Society of Cardiology. *Eur Heart J* 2008;**29**:2909–2945.

Online resource

Society of Chest Pain Centers (SCPC). http://www.spcp.org

➲ For additional multimedia materials please visit the online version of the book (⌕ http://www.esciacc.oxfordmedicine.com).

CHAPTER 7

Acute dyspnoea

Nisha Arenja, Thenral Socrates,
and Christian Mueller

Contents

Summary

Acute dyspnoea is a very common symptom in the acute cardiac care setting. The rapid and accurate identification of the cause of dyspnoea is difficult, albeit critical to the initiation of specific and effective treatment. In the emergency department, the prevalence of acute heart failure in patients with acute dyspnoea is about 50%. A detailed patient history, physical examination, blood tests including natriuretic peptides and C-reactive protein, ECG, and chest radiograph help the clinician to make a diagnosis in the vast majority of patients. Once pulmonary embolism (PE) is suspected, the diagnostic work-up combines clinical assessment by a prediction rule, D-dimer measurement, and CT angiography in patients with an elevated D-dimer level or a high clinical probability of PE. Transthoracic echocardiography should be performed immediately in all patients with acute dyspnoea and shock, and in those patients in whom the diagnosis remains uncertain even after initial work-up.

Definition and epidemiology

Dyspnoea is the perception of an inability to breathe comfortably. Acute dyspnoea is a very common symptom in acute cardiac care. The chief complaint of dyspnoea or shortness of breath makes up 3–5% or more than 10 million visits to the emergency department (ED) in Europe and the United States. Among the more than 30 possible diagnoses that may be responsible for the acute dyspnoea, heart failure is very common and therefore particularly important [1, 2]. Unfortunately, the reliability of a clinical diagnosis of heart failure and other common causes of dyspnoea is poor [3–6]. Moreover diagnostic uncertainty delays the initiation of adequate treatment; and increases hospitalization rates, cost and most importantly morbidity.

Pathophysiology

Dyspnoea is a complex syndrome and the pathophysiological mechanisms are still poorly understood. Mismatch between efferent signals (motor output) from the brain to the respiratory muscles and the afferent feedback from mechanoreceptors and chemoreceptors of the lung and chest wall (sensory input) seems to play a major role [7–9]. Many disorders resulting in dyspnoea are associated with increased work of breathing or a sense of increased breathing (as in hyperinflation).

In 1963 Campbell and Howell [8] postulated the association between dyspnoea and structures of the central nervous system in the theory of 'length–tension inappropriateness'. According to their theory, dyspnoea arises from a disturbance in the relation between the force or tension generated by the respiratory muscles and the resulting changes in muscle length and lung volume. The theory is designed to include information about the mismatch between respiratory motor command and afferent feedback. Experimental data are also consistent with the concept of afferent mismatch [10–12].

The current understanding of dyspnoea still assumes a mismatch between central respiratory motor activity and incoming afferent information from respiratory mechanoreceptors, which are localized in the airways, lungs, and chest wall structures or chemoreceptors. Changes in arterial blood gas and acid–base metabolism are observed by peripheral chemoreceptors in the aorta and in the carotid sinus, or alternatively by the brainstem. When stimulated by bronchospasm, mechanoreceptors in the lungs lead to a sensation of chest tightness; other receptors are activated by interstitial oedema or pulmonary artery hypertension [10–12]. The respiratory centre in the medulla oblongata is abnormally activated by stimuli derived by alterations in respiratory muscles, ventilator impedance, breathing patterns, and blood gases. All of these factors play a role in the onset of dyspnoea [9].

Prevalence of the most common disorders underlying acute dyspnoea

Acute heart failure is the most common disorder responsible for acute dyspnoea, with prevalence in the ED of about 50% [2–6, 13–16]. Other common causes of acute dyspnoea include exacerbation of chronic obstructive pulmonary disease (COPD) or asthma (20%), pneumonia or bronchitis (15%), pulmonary embolism (PE) (5–10%), anxiety disorders (5%), and other causes such as malignancy,

interstitial lung disease, upper airway obstruction, or anaemia in 5–10%. In about 10% of patients two disorders will be present at the same time (e.g. acute heart failure and pneumonia).

We estimate the prevalence of acute heart failure in other health care settings as follows: primary care 30%, intensive care units 50%, and coronary care units 85% [2–9, 13–24].

Triage and initial management

It is important to stress that immediate assessment of vital signs including oxygen saturation and application of supplemental oxygen is mandatory. Airway, breathing, and circulation (ABC sequence) are the primary focus when beginning management of the patient with acute dyspnoea. Once these parameters are stabilized, further clinical investigation and treatment can proceed. In cases of severe respiratory failure, immediate unspecific treatment including noninvasive ventilation or intubation must precede further diagnostic measures. The severity of respiratory failure and the response to the initial measures of bed rest, upright positioning, and supplemental oxygen needs to be carefully monitored particularly within the first minutes to decide whether the patient needs noninvasive ventilation, intubation, and transfer to an intensive care unit (➲ Fig. 7.1).

The first contact with the patient may be at the patient's home. It is important to check all medications or devices such as inhalers, as they may be the only clue regarding the previous medical history in an acute dyspnoeic patient unable to speak. In many European countries ambulances are staffed with emergency physicians trained in intubation. In these circumstances, a number of patients with severe respiratory failure therefore arrive intubated and under analgosedation at the hospital. Giving the hospital team

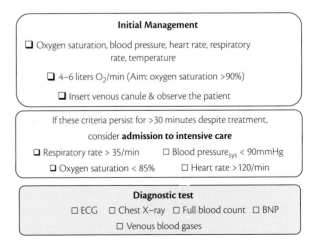

Figure 7.1 Initial management of dyspnoea.

early information about the patient's cardiorespiratory condition will allow timely preparation of a ventilator in the intensive care unit ('forewarned is forearmed'). Also, if it has not been possible to definitely secure the airway in a critically ill patient before arrival at hospital, it is mandatory to get expert support to the ED before the ambulance arrives.

From symptom to diagnosis

Detailed patient history and physical examination remain the basis for the diagnosis of patients with acute dyspnoea. As specific treatment for heart failure may be detrimental to pulmonary disorders and vice versa, rapid and accurate diagnosis is key for effective patient management.

A history of dyspnoea in the past, caused by any of the above-mentioned diseases commonly resulting in acute dyspnoea, increases the likelihood that the current episode is a relapse. For example, in patients with a history of heart failure the likelihood ratio for acute heart failure is about 5.

Current evidence regarding the diagnostic performance of symptoms, signs, and other individual diagnostic tests is largely based on studies performed in the ED setting. As patient characteristics, severity of dyspnoea, incidence of heart failure, and physician experience differ considerably between the ED and (e.g.) private practice or the intensive care unit, these findings should only cautiously be applied to other settings.

Heart failure

Acute dyspnoea may be the presenting symptom of acute myocardial infarction, particularly in women and elderly people.

Symptoms and signs

It is currently unclear whether the exact wording used by the patient to describe dyspnoea may help to differentiate the cause. Most symptoms are rather unspecific. ➲ Figure 7.2 shows symptoms and ➲ Fig. 7.3 signs that help to differentiate cardiac from pulmonary causes of acute dyspnoea [20, 25].

Most classical clinical signs associated with acute heart failure (HF) are not very sensitive (➲ Table 7.1) [20, 25].

ECG

An ECG should be performed in every patient with acute dyspnoea [6]. Electrocardiographic changes are common in patients with acute HF (➲ Table 7.2). However, an abnormal ECG has little predictive value for the presence of HF. If the ECG is completely normal, acute HF, especially with left ventricular systolic dysfunction, is unlikely.

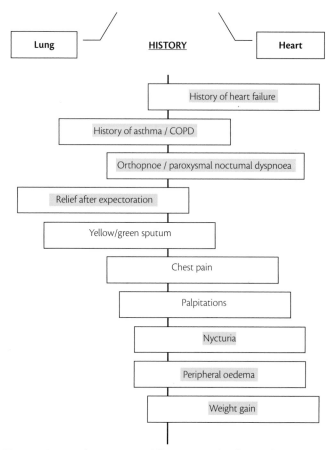

Figure 7.2 Use of symptoms to differentiate cardiac from pulmonary causes of acute dyspnoea. The less central the position of the box, the more helpful is the symptom. The presence of paroxysmal nocturnal dyspnoea, orthopnoea, nycturia, peripheral oedema, and weight gain increases the likelihood of acute heart failure.

In patients with acute HF the ECG may immediately help in identifying common causes of the acute decompensation such as tachycardiac atrial fibrillation, ventricular tachycardia (VT) or ST-elevation myocardial infarction (STEMI). The immediate identification of these conditions holds high priority in the diagnostic process of any patient, as therapeutic measures should not be delayed.

Chest radiograph

Chest radiography is an established, easily available, non-invasive, and inexpensive method, which should be part of the initial work-up in all patients with dyspnoea. Whenever possible, chest radiographs should be obtained in the erect position in two planes. The chest radiograph quantifies cardiac size and shape and directly visualizes pulmonary congestion. Findings of cardiomegaly, cephalization, interstitial signs including peribronchial cuffing, septal lines and hilar blurring, pleural effusions, or alveolar oedema suggest the presence of acute HF (➲ Fig. 7.4) [26–29].

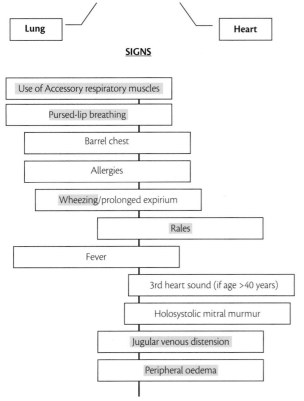

Figure 7.3 Use of signs to differentiate cardiac from pulmonary causes of acute dyspnoea. The less central the position of the box, the more helpful is the sign.

Table 7.1 Sensitivity of findings on physical examination

Sign	Sensitivity (%)
Third heart sound	10
Jugular venous distension	40
Lower extremity oedema	50
Rales	60

It is important to note that up to 20% of patients with acute HF may have no radiographic signs of congestion. On the other hand, bronchitis and pneumonia may mimic many of the radiographic findings of congestion. Therefore, all radiographic findings need to be integrated to obtain an overall impression. The overall impression then has moderate to high accuracy in the diagnosis of acute dyspnoea.

Natriuretic peptides

Natriuretic peptides (BNP and NT-proBNP as well as mid-regional proANP and proANP) are considered quantitative markers of haemodynamic cardiac stress and HF. BNP is a 32-amino acid polypeptide that is co-secreted with the inactive N-terminal proBNP (NT-proBNP) from the left and right cardiac ventricles in response to ventricular volume expansion and pressure overload [21].

Recent data suggest that left ventricular end-diastolic wall stress and wall stiffness may be the predominate triggers of BNP and NT-proBNP synthesis and release. B-type natriuretic peptides are released into the blood in relation

Table 7.2 Common ECG abnormalities in heart failure

Abnormality	Cause	Clinical implication
Sinus tachycardia	Decompensated HF, anaemia, fever, hyperthyroidism	Clinical assessment, laboratory investigation
Sinus bradycardia	β-Blockade, digoxin Antiarrhythmics, hypothyroidism, sick sinus syndrome	Evaluate drug therapy, laboratory investigation
Atrial tachycardia/flutter/fibrillation	Hyperthyroidism, infection, mitral valve diseases, decompensated HF, infarction	Slow AV conduction, medical conversion, electroversion, catheter ablation, anticoagulation
Ventricular arrhythmias	Ischaemia, infarction, cardiomyopathy, myocarditis, hypokalaemia, hypomagnesaemia, digitalis overdose	Laboratory investigation, exercise test, perfusion studies, coronary angiography, electrophysiology testing, ICD
Ischaemia/infarction	Coronary artery disease	Echo, troponins, coronary angiography, revascularization
Q waves	Infarction, hypertrophic cardiomyopathy, LBBB, pre-excitation	Echo, coronary angiography
LV hypertrophy	Hypertension, aortic valve disease, hypertrophic cardiomyopathy	Echo/Doppler
AV block	Infarction, drug toxicity, myocarditis, sarcoidosis, Lyme disease	Evaluate drug therapy, pacemaker, systemic disease
Microvoltage	Obesity, emphysema, pericardial effusion, amyloidosis	Echo, chest radiograph
QRS length >120 ms of LBBB morphology	Electrical and mechanical dyssynchrony	Echo, CRT-P, CRT-D

AV, atrioventricular; CRT-D, cardiac resynchronization therapy with pacemaker/defibrillator; CRT-P, cardiac resynchronization therapy with pacemaker; HF, heart failure; ICD, implantable cardioverter–defibrillator; LBBB, left bundle branch block; LV, left ventricular.

Reproduced with permission from Dickstein K, Cohen-Solal A, Filippatos G, et al. ESC Guidelines for the diagnosis and treatment of acute and chronic heart failure 2008: the Task Force for the Diagnosis and Treatment of Acute and Chronic Heart Failure 2008 of the European Society of Cardiology. *Eur Heart J* 2008; **29** (19):2388–2442.

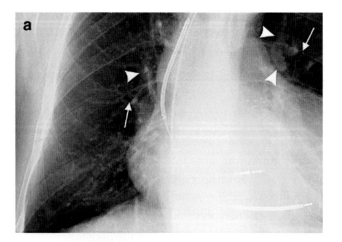

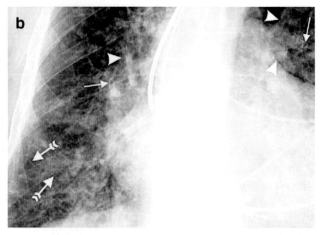

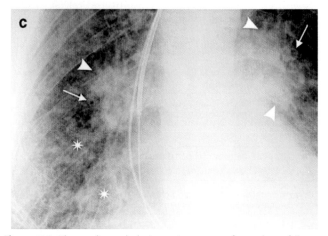

Figure 7.4 Chest radiograph during various stages of acute heart failure showing different radiographic findings and degrees of congestion: (a) Close-up view of a PA radiograph reveals clearly visible bronchial walls (arrows) without blurring of the margins (no peribronchial cuffing). Hilar vessels (arrowheads) are sharply outlined (no hilar changes). Redistribution of flow is present. (b) Close-up view of a PA radiograph from the same patient with increasing signs of congestion. Prominent thickening of bronchial walls (plain arrows) with partially indistinct outlines are present (peribronchial cuffing), as well as hilar enlargement together with blurred vascular margins. Septal lines (tailed arrows) appear between indistinct vessels in the basal region. (c) Close-up view of an AP radiograph obtained in the supine position. There is now a complete loss of the bronchial interface (arrows, peribronchial cuffing). The density and size of the hila have further increased (arrowheads), and the margins of hilar vessels are indeterminable. Alveolar oedema is present (asterisks).

to disease severity and correspond to the New York Heart Association (NYHA) functional classification system. A natriuretic peptide (NP) level can be used to quantify the severity of HF, reflecting the combined haemodynamic consequences of systolic and diastolic left ventricular dysfunction, as well as valvular heart disease and right ventricular dysfunction [21].

The clinical importance of a specific disease marker is related to the overall importance of the disease or biological signal it quantifies, the availability of alternative methods to reliably diagnose the disease and quantify disease severity, and of course the performance of the marker. NPs, as quantitative markers of cardiac stress and HF, owe their enormous clinical importance to the fact that HF is a major public health problem, the uncertainty in the clinical diagnosis and management of HF, and their excellent diagnostic and prognostic utility.

Two important principles underlie the clinical use of NPs. First, a NP level is not a stand-alone test. It is always of greatest value when it complements the physician's clinical skills along with other available diagnostic tools. Second, NP levels should be interpreted and used as continuous variables in order to make full use of the biological information provided by the measurement.

NPs have consistently been shown to have high accuracy in the diagnosis of HF in patients presenting with acute dyspnoea to the ED. NP levels are very high in patients with dyspnoea due to HF and low in patients with other causes of dyspnoea[14–17, 21, 22].

Numerous observational studies, including patients presenting with dyspnoea, have validated NPs against a gold standard diagnosis of HF and have shown convincingly that NPs have a very high diagnostic accuracy [14, 16–24]. The higher the NP level, the higher the probability that dyspnoea is caused by HF. Overall, BNP, NT-proBNP and mid-regional proANP seem to have similar accuracy in the diagnosis of HF [21, 22].

The clinical impact of using the diagnostic and prognostic information provided by BNP or NT-proBNP has also been demonstrated in several randomized controlled studies [15, 23, 30–32]. In the BASEL study the BNP group showed a significant reduction in time to adequate therapy, admission rate, and time to discharge. Hence, if we diagnose the cause of dyspnoea earlier and with higher accuracy, we initiate appropriate treatment earlier, patients improve more rapidly and are able to be discharged sooner from the hospital. These findings were confirmed by two additional randomized controlled studies [23, 32]. The initial reduction in total treatment costs associated with the use of NPs in the ED still exists after 360 days [30, 31].

Easily applicable algorithms for the interpretation of BNP and NT-proBNP applying specific cut-off levels have been developed (➲ Table 7.3).

As NPs are quantitative markers of HF, the use of cut-off levels is only the second-best approach. Yet, NPs can be helpful in the busy ED. In a patient presenting with dyspnoea, BNP levels below 100 pg/mL strongly argue against HF [14–17, 21, 22]. On the other hand, a BNP above 400 pg/mL has a high positive predictive value for HF being not only present but also the major cause of dyspnoea. When using NT-proBNP, 300 pg/mL should be used as the 'rule-out' cut-off level [24]. The 'rule-in' cut-off level is 450 pg/mL in patients below 50 years of age, 900 pg/mL in patients 50–75 years of age, and 1800 pg/mL in patients above the age of 75 years [24]. In patients with NP levels above the upper cut-off level and therefore with substantial cardiac haemodynamic stress, we can be quite certain that HF is the predominate cause of dyspnoea and it is imperative to promptly initiate appropriate treatment such as nitrates, diuretics, and ACE inhibitors. It is important to remember that NPs are also secreted from the right ventricle. Therefore, severe PE with resulting right ventricular stretch will also result in NP secretion and should always be included into the differential diagnosis of elevated NP levels.

BNP levels need to be adjusted in obese patients and those with severe kidney disease, but do not have to be adjusted for gender or age [21]. When using NT-proBNP the use of an age-adjusted upper cut-off level largely obviates the need for further adjustments for renal function [24]. For patients presenting with NP levels in the grey zone, other diagnostic tools including CT scans and bedside echocardiography have particular additional value.

Echocardiography

Transthoracic echocardiography with Doppler imaging should be done immediately in all patients with acute dyspnoea and shock and in those patients in whom the diagnosis remains uncertain after the initial work-up. In patients diagnosed with acute HF, echocardiography is critical to determine the structural cardiac disease underlying acute HF. In most cases of acute HF, echocardiography can safely be delayed until dyspnoea has improved sufficiently to allow the patient to remain in the supine position for some time (usually day 2–4).

Routine assessment includes determination of atrial and ventricular size, ventricular thickness, regional and global left and right ventricular function including tissue Doppler analyses, valvular structure and function, possible pericardial pathology, and mechanical complications of myocardial infarction. About 50% of patients with acute HF will be found to have HF with preserved ejection fraction, so detailed evaluation of left ventricular diastolic function including tissue Doppler is critical. In addition, increased left atrial volume is a relevant and valuable indicator of left ventricular diastolic dysfunction in patients with preserved left ventricular ejection fraction.

Obstructive pulmonary disease

Exacerbations of COPD can present with acute shortness of breath. Most often, a viral or bacterial respiratory infection exacerbates the patient's underlying illness. PE may be responsible for up to 25% of apparent 'COPD exacerbations' and should be suspected when the patient has no signs of acute infection or fails to improve with standard COPD treatment measures. Oxygen must not be withheld from patients with COPD. The target oxygen saturation in such patients is 90–92%.

Pneumonia and other pulmonary infections

Lung infections such as severe bronchitis or pneumonia can cause shortness of breath and hypoxia. Productive cough, fever, and pleuritic chest pain are common but indiscriminate signs. The onset of dyspnoea in these patients is generally not acute unless underlying chronic pulmonary disease is present. A chest radiograph is generally necessary for diagnosis. It is important to remember that small infiltrations may not be seen by standard chest radiography but only become visible on CT scanning.

Pulmonary embolism

The diagnosis of PE should be considered in any patient with acute dyspnoea. Risk factors include a history of deep venous thrombosis or PE, prolonged immobilization, recent trauma or surgery (particularly orthopaedic),

Table 7.3 Decision limits for natriuretic peptides

	No CHF	'Grey zone'[a]	Yes CHF
BNP (pg/ml)	<100	100–400	>400
NT-proBNP (pg/ml)			
Age <50 years	<300	300–450	>450
Age 50–75 years	<300	300–900	>900
Age >75 years	<300	300–1800	>1800

CHF, congestive heart failure
[a] More information required.

pregnancy, malignancy, stroke or paresis, and a personal or family history of hypercoagulability. Presentation varies widely, but dyspnoea at rest and tachypnoea are the most common signs. A sizeable minority of patients have no known risk factor at the time of diagnosis. Other embolic phenomena include fat embolism, especially after a long bone fracture, and amniotic fluid embolism. Once PE is suspected, the diagnostic work-up combines clinical assessment by a prediction rule, D-dimer measurement, and CT angiography in patients with an elevated D-dimer level or a high clinical probability of pulmonary embolism.

Uncommon but important causes of dyspnoea

Upper airway disease

Any disease that results in a narrowing of the upper airways may result in acute dyspnoea, often accompanied with an inspiratory stridor. These include tracheal foreign objects such as food, dentures, and medication tablets; angioedema; anaphylaxis; and infections.

Poisoning

As with other presenting symptom, poisoning should also always be included in the differential diagnosis of patients with acute dyspnoea. Several toxins, including carbon monoxide, can cause derangements in respiratory function, leading to acute dyspnoea.

Carbon monoxide is a potentially lethal toxin that impairs oxygen metabolism leading to tachypnoea and acute dyspnoea. Extrapulmonary symptoms include altered mental status, headache, malaise, and chest discomfort.

Organophosphate poisoning causes an increase in airway sections and bronchospasm.

Salicylate overdose leads to stimulation of the medullary respiratory centre, causing hyperventilation and respiratory alkalosis initially, followed by metabolic acidosis. Additional symptoms include tinnitus, vertigo, vomiting, diarrhoea, and in more severe cases mental status changes.

Diabetic ketoacidosis

This can cause tachypnoea and acute dyspnoea from the involuntary respiratory correction of metabolic acidosis. Additional symptoms include polyuria, polydipsia, and progressive weakness.

Anaemia

This may result in dyspnoea due to the lack of oxygen-carrying capacity. Usually, other symptoms including fatigue predominate.

Neuromuscular disease

Neuromuscular diseases such as Guillain–Barré syndrome or myasthenia gravis may lead to weakness of the respiratory muscles and acute respiratory failure.

Risk stratification

Risk stratification of patients with acute dyspnoea presenting to the ED is challenging, as the range and urgency of the cause for breathlessness is vast. Logically a clinician should proceed in a stepwise manner, first assessing the vital signs of a patient, monitoring, and then looking at certain lab values. The first step in approaching this scenario is determining the mental status of the patient. A patient who is conscious and can communicate clearly is likely to be at less risk of a serious event than a patient who is unconscious or delirious. Easily observable and measurable vital parameters such as heart rate, respiratory rate, and temperature are also very important in distinguishing whether the dyspnoeic patient is at high risk. Monitoring of oxygen saturation and blood pressure can also help the clinician to determine the status of the patient. Recent evidence shows that these easy to measure parameters are important factors in risk stratification of these patients. Currently biomarkers such as BNP, NT-proBNP, MR-proANP, MR-proADM, and ST2 have been shown to also help in the risk stratification of patients with acute dyspnoea presenting to the ED.

End of life

Acute dyspnoea may occur at the end of life in patients with various cancers, chronic lung disease, and HF. Although the details of palliative care go far beyond the scope of this chapter, it is important to stress that patient management in an end of life situation should of course be very different from the management of other patients. Ideally, patients and their relatives should be prepared for this scenario in advance, to ensure that the health care professionals involved in the acute dyspnoea episode are immediately aware of the end of life situation. We think that patient history and physical examination should search for easily treatable causes like upper airway obstruction due to secretions that could potentially be resolved, e.g. by tracheal suctioning. As the end of life is often a period rather than a time point, these measures should whenever possible be tailored according to the patient's wish. Close physical contact with family members and continuous intravenous infusion of morphine might be considered helpful in terminal patients (see also ➲ Chapter 13).

Personal perspective

The introduction of rapid testing for NPs has significantly improved the clinical management of patients presenting with acute dyspnoea. We expect that the use of these tools will in the near future become widespread, with routine use outside of the ED; including private practice and the ambulance service. The effectiveness of noninvasive positive pressure ventilation is very high regardless of the specific cause: it should be applied with a low threshold. The patient's acceptance of this technique can be increased by applying it early rather than later.

Further reading

Dickstein K, Cohen-Solal A, Filippatos G, *et al*. ESC Guidelines for the diagnosis and treatment of acute and chronic heart failure 2008: the Task Force for the Diagnosis and Treatment of Acute and Chronic Heart Failure 2008 of the European Society of Cardiology. Developed in collaboration with the Heart Failure Association of the ESC (HFA) and endorsed by the European Society of Intensive Care Medicine (ESICM). *Eur Heart J* 2008;**29**(19):2388–2442.

Dyspnea. Mechanisms, assessment, and management: a consensus statement. American Thoracic Society. *Am J Respir Crit Care Med* 1999;**159**(1):321–340.

Maisel A, Mueller C, Adams K, Jr, *et al*. State of the art: using natriuretic peptide levels in clinical practice. *Eur J Heart Fail* 2008;**10**(9):824–839.

Maisel AS, Krishnaswamy P, Nowak RM, *et al*. Rapid measurement of B-type natriuretic peptide in the emergency diagnosis of heart failure. *N Engl J Med* 2002;**347**(3):161–167.

McCullough PA, Nowak RM, McCord J, *et al*. B-type natriuretic peptide and clinical judgment in emergency diagnosis of heart failure: analysis from Breathing Not Properly (BNP) Multinational Study. *Circulation* 2002;**106**(4):416–422.

Moe GW, Howlett J, Januzzi JL, Zowall H. N-terminal pro-B-type natriuretic peptide testing improves the management of patients with suspected acute heart failure: primary results of the Canadian prospective randomized multicenter IMPROVE-CHF study. *Circulation* 2007;**115**:3103–3110.

Mueller C, Scholer A, Laule-Kilian K, *et al*. Use of B-type natriuretic peptide in the evaluation and management of acute dyspnea. *N Engl J Med* 2004;**350**:647–654.

Studler U, Kretzschmar M, Christ M, *et al*. Accuracy of chest radiographs in the emergency diagnosis of heart failure. *Eur Radiol* 2008;**18**(8):1644–1652.

Wang CS, FitzGerald JM, Schulzer M, *et al*. Does this dyspneic patient in the emergency department have congestive heart failure? *Jama* 2005;**294**(15):1944–1956.

Wright SP, Doughty RN, Pearl A, *et al*. Plasma amino-terminal pro-brain natriuretic peptide and accuracy of heart-failure diagnosis in primary care: a randomized, controlled trial. *J Am Coll Cardiol* 2003;**42**:1793–1800.

➲ For additional multimedia materials please visit the online version of the book (🔗 http://www.esciacc.oxfordmedicine.com).

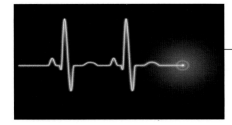

CHAPTER 8

Arrhythmias in the emergency department

G. Cayla, P. G. Claret, and J. E. de La Coussaye

Contents

Summary

Cardiac arrhythmias are a daily problem in the emergency department (ED) but not all arrhythmias need rapid intervention. Management of these arrhythmias is quite simple, based on clinical evaluation and ECG information. Cardiac arrhythmias can occur in patients with or without underlying heart disease. Acute ischaemia, one of the main causes of arrhythmia must be systematically suspected, especially in the prehospital setting, in order to dispatch the patient directly to a catheterization lab in the case of acute myocardial infarction (MI). Indeed, the earliest and successful reperfusion therapy remains the best antiarrhythmic therapeutic method in these patients.

Schematically, all haemodynamically unstable patients with symptomatic tachycardia should be treated by immediate cardioversion and patients with no pulse must be treated as cardiac arrest according to guidelines. Treatment should not be systematically considered in the ED or in the mobile intensive care unit (MICU) for haemodynamically stable patients.

Bradycardia associated with symptoms of poor perfusion should be considered for treatment in the MICU or the ED. Atropine is the first line treatment of nodal block and transcutaneous pacing of third-degree block.

Introduction

Cardiac arrhythmias are a common cause of sudden death. Arrhythmias in the emergency department (ED) remain a daily problem and require a rapid diagnosis and sometimes rapid intervention. The treatment appears to be quite simple if the patient is haemodynamically unstable: immediate cardioversion should be considered in the case of tachycardia and a transcutaneous or transvenous pacing in the case of bradycardia. If the patient is haemodynamically stable, no urgent treatment is usually required and the diagnosis of arrhythmia can be performed using physical examination, 12-lead surface ECG, and response to manoeuvres or drugs.

Tachycardia

Tachycardia occurs in individuals with or without cardiac disorder. General findings are listed in ⊃ Box 8.1. Tachycardia can be classified in several ways, based either on the regularity or on the width of QRS complexes (⊃ Table 8.1 ⊃ Fig. 8.1). Supraventricular tachycardia remains the most frequent tachycardia, and is usually not life threatening. In contrast, ventricular tachycardias need to be quickly recognized and treated. The tachycardia algorithm for evaluation and treatment of tachycardia with pulses is summarized in ⊃ Fig. 8.2.

Table 8.1 Classification of tachycardia

Narrow QRS tachycardia (QRS <0.12 s)	Wide QRS tachycardia (QRS >0.12 s)
Sinus tachycardia	Ventricular tachycardia
AF	Supraventricular tachycardia with aberrancy or bundle branch block or metabolic disturbances
Atrial flutter	Pre-excited tachycardia
AV nodal re-entry tachycardia AVNRT (typical and atypical)	
AV re-entry tachycardia AVRT (accessory pathway mediated)	
Atrial tachycardia	
Focal atrial tachycardia	
Junctional tachycardia	

AF, atrial fibrillation; AV, atrioventricular; AVNRT atrioventricular nodal reciprocating tachycardia; AVRT, atrioventricular reciprocating tachycardia.

Ventricular arrhythmias

A classification of ventricular arrhythmias has been proposed [1], according to clinical presentation and ECG (⊃ Table 8.2). Most patients who suffer from ventricular tachycardias have underlying heart disease (⊃ Box 8.2). Acute coronary ischaemia remains one of the leading cause of ventricular arrhythmias and should be systematically suspected in patients with ventricular arrhythmia, specifically in the prehospital setting. Indeed, the earliest and successful reperfusion therapy remains the best antiarrhythmic therapeutic method in patients with acute MI. These patients should be directly dispatch from the MICU to the catheterization laboratory of PCI-capable hospitals.

Management of ventricular tachycardia

The evaluation of the haemodynamic status of the patient remains the first step in the management of ventricular tachycardia.

Ventricular tachycardia with circulatory arrest must be immediately treated by defibrillation as cardiac arrest according to the international guidelines for cardiopulmonary resuscitation and emergency cardiovascular care [2].

Hemodynamically unstable ventricular tachycardia (i.e. tachycardia associated with hypotension and poor tissue perfusion) must be also treated by a cardioversion. If the patient is conscious, sedation must be given (class I, level C) [1].

Hemodynamically stable ventricular tachycardia is frequently associated with sensations of palpitation and chest discomfort. It should be rapidly treated even if ventricular tachycardia is well tolerated. Correction of aggravating conditions such as hypokalaemia, hypoxemia, or ischaemia should be considered as a priority. Three different options are available if the termination of tachycardia appears urgently required:

1 The intravenous administration of antiarrythmic drug. In the acute phase, intravenous amiodarone is the first line treatment (other antiarrythmic drugs such as lidocaine were used in the past and might be efficient especially in the case of acute ischaemic disease) and should be administered as 150 mg over 10 min followed by a repeated dose as needed [3] or by a continuous infusion. Hypotension [4] secondary to the detergent in intravenous amiodarone is a specific complication and can be avoided by using a slower rate of infusion.

2 Transvenous catheter termination (overdrive pacing) can be done only in a hospital setting (expert cardiologist's consultation).

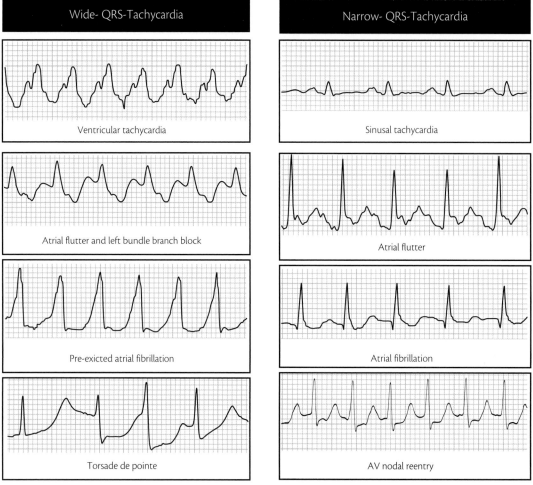

Figure 8.1 Examples of electrocardiograms: Wide-QRS-Tachycardia and Narrow-QRS-Tachycardia.

3 Direct current (DC) cardioversion with appropriate sedation is recommended at any point in the treatment cascade in patients with ventricular tachycardia with haemodynamic compromise (class I, level C) [1].

Torsade de pointes

Torsades de pointes correspond usually to nonsustained, morphologically distinctive polymorphic ventricular tachycardia associated with a marked QT interval prolongation. They can occur in different settings: congenital long QT syndrome (LQTS), or, especially, acquired long QT syndrome. Acquired LQTS is due to severe bradycardia (heart block), some drugs, or electrolyte abnormalities associated particularly with hypokalaemia and hypocalcaemia.

If the patient is unstable, specially when torsades de pointes become sustained, high-energy unsynchronized shock must be delivered immediately. If a monophasic defibrillator is used, a dose of 360 J is used; with a biphasic device, a 150–200 J shock should be considered. Recurrences must be immediately prevented: intravenous magnesium sulphate

(IV bolus with 1.5–3 g over 5–60 min, then infusion) must be firstly systematically considered (class IIa, level B) [1]. Then, the correction of electrolytes abnormalities and withdrawal of any offending drugs (i.e. medication known to prolong QT interval) should be considered (class I, level A) [1]. Acute pacing is recommended (class I, level A) for treatment of severe bradycardia in the ED. In absence of pacing devices, isoproterenol should also be considered as temporary treatment for patients with recurrent pause-dependent torsades de pointes (class IIa, level B) [1]. For patients with congenital LQTS 3, intravenous lidocaine may be considered (class IIb, level C) [1].

Other wide complex tachycardias

Supraventricular tachycardia in patients with a wide ECG complex can be confused with ventricular tachycardia. Several algorithms based on 12-lead ECG pattern have been proposed to differentiate these arrhythmias [5–8]. Among them, Brugada *et al.* [8] have proposed a simple approach to the differential diagnosis of a regular tachycardia with

Table 8.2 Classification of ventricular tachycardia by clinical presentation and ECG

(a) Classification by clinical presentation

Haemodynamically stable	Asymptomatic	The absence of symptoms that could result from an arrhythmia
	Minimal symptoms, e.g. palpitations	Patient reports palpitations felt in either the chest, throat, or neck described as follows: – Heartbeat sensations that feel like pounding or racing – An unpleasant awareness of heartbeat – Feeling skipped beats or a pause
Haemodynamically unstable	Presyncope	Patient reports presyncope described as follows: – Dizziness – Lightheadedness – Feeling faint – 'Greying out'
	Syncope	Sudden loss of consciousness with loss of postural tone, not related to anaesthesia, with spontaneous recovery as reported by the patient or observer. Patient may experience syncope when supine
	Sudden cardiac death	Death from an unexpected circulatory arrest, usually due to a cardiac arrhythmia occurring within an hour of the onset of symptoms
	Sudden cardiac arrest	Death from an unexpected circulatory arrest, usually due to a cardiac arrhythmia occurring within an hour of the onset of symptoms, in whom medical intervention (e.g. defibrillation) reverses the event

(b) Classification by ECG

Nonsustained		Three or more beats in duration, terminating spontaneously in <30 s
		VT is a cardiac arrhythmia of three or more consecutive complexes in duration emanating from the ventricles at a rate of greater than 100 beats/min (cycle length <600 ms)
	Monomorphic	Nonsustained VT with a single QRS morphology
	Polymorphic	Nonsustained VT with a changing QRS morphology at cycle length between 600 and 180 ms
Sustained VT		VT >30 s in duration and/or requiring termination due to haemodynamic compromise in less than 30 s
	Monomorphic	Sustained VT with a stable single QRS morphology
	Polymorphic	Sustained VT with a changing or multiform QRS morphology at cycle length between 600 and 180 ms
Bundle branch re-entrant tachycardia		VT due to re-entry involving the His–Purkinje system, usually with LBBB morphology; this usually occurs in the setting of cardiomyopathy
Bidirectional VT		VT with a beat-to-beat alternans in the QRS frontal plane axis, often associated with digitalis toxicity
Torsade de pointes		Characterized by VT associated with a long QT or QTc, and characterized on ECG by twisting of the peaks of the QRS complexes around the isoelectric line during the arrhythmia – 'Typical,' initiated following 'short–long–short' coupling intervals – Short coupled variant initiated by normal–short coupling
Ventricular flutter		A regular (cycle length variability 30 ms or less) ventricular arrhythmia approximately 300 beats/min (cycle length 200 ms) with a monomorphic appearance; no isoelectric interval between successive QRS complexes
Ventricular fibrillation		Rapid, usually more than 300 bpm/200 ms (cycle length 180 ms or less), grossly irregular ventricular rhythm with marked variability in QRS cycle length, morphology, and amplitude

VT, ventricular tachycardia.

Reproduced with permission from Zipes DP, Camm AJ, Borggrefe M, et al. ACC/AHA/ESC 2006 Guidelines for management of patients with ventricular arrhythmias and the prevention of sudden cardiac death. Europace 2006;8:746-837.

a wide QRS complex, summarized in ➲ Fig. 8.3. If the diagnosis of supraventricular tachycardia (SVT) cannot be proven or cannot be made easily, the patient should be treated as having ventricular tachycardia (VT).

For suspected supraventricular tachycardia with aberrancy, adenosine or ATP is recommended. Verapamil or diltiazem may be deleterious because they can precipitate

haemodynamic collapse for a patient with ventricular arrhythmias [9–11].

In pre-excited tachycardias associated or mediated by an accessory pathway, an antiarrhythmic drug (amiodarone 150 mg IV over 10 min) should be considered.

Tachycardias with narrow QRS complex

When the ventricular activation (QRS) is narrow (<120 ms), tachycardia is usually of supraventricular origin. Supraventricular tachycardia is a frequent cause of ED consultations [12, 13]. In order of occurrence: sinus tachycardia, atrial fibrillation, atrial flutter, atrioventricular (AV) nodal re-entry, accessory pathway-mediated tachycardia, other macro-re-entrant atrial tachycardia, focal and multifocal atrial tachycardias.

Sinus tachycardia

Sinus tachycardia is defined as an increased sinus rate (>100 beats/min). Sinus tachycardia accelerates and terminates gradually. It is very common in the ED setting and is usually the results of an appropriate physiological stimulus,

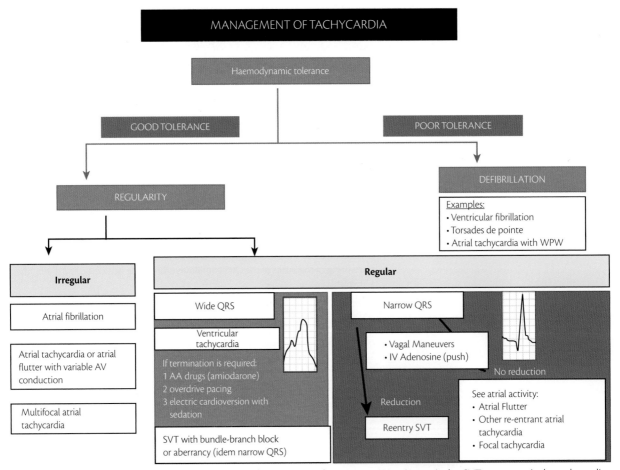

Figure 8.2 Initial evaluation and management of tachycardia in the emergency department. AV, atrioventricular; SVT, supraventricular tachycardia; WPW, Wolff–Parkinson–White syndrome.

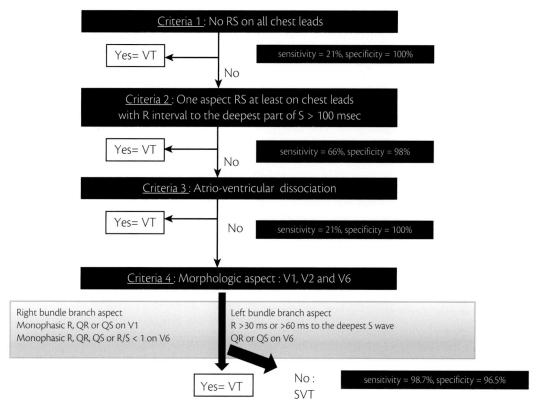

Figure 8.3 Differential diagnosis of a tachycardia with a wide QRS complex. SVT, supraventricular tachycardia; VT, ventricular tachycardia.

e.g. fever, anaemia, shock, or hyperthyroidism. Sinus tachycardia requires comprehensive evaluation, and specific treatment of the underlying cause. No specific drug treatment is required.

Atrial fibrillation and atrial flutter (macro-re-entrant atrial tachycardia)

Atrial fibrillation (AF) and atrial flutter are the most frequent arrhythmias observed in the ED and represent a specific challenge to emergency physicians. AF is easily recognized because of its irregular ventricular rhythm, while the common atrial flutter has a regular ventricular rhythm with atrial waves at about 300 beats/min and usually 2/1 AV conduction. Atrial flutter, which is classified as a macro-re-entrant tachycardia, includes isthmus-dependent atrial flutter (typical or atypical) and non-isthmus-dependent atrial flutter.

Both types of arrhythmia (i.e. atrial flutter and AF) may present as accidental findings in a patient who is admitted for other complaints. These arrhythmias are common in the general population, with the incidence increasing with advanced age [14]. It has been estimated that 4.5 million people in the European Union suffer from paroxysmal or persistent AF.

Patients with AF lasting more than 48 h are at increased risk for cardioembolic events and must first undergo anticoagulation before controlling rhythm. Pharmacological or electrical cardioversion should not be attempted in patients with AF with a duration of 48 h or longer, or when the duration is unknown, except in the case of haemodynamic compromise. In patients with AF lasting more than 48 h, heparin should be administered concurrently (unless contraindicated) by an initial intravenous bolus injection followed by a continuous infusion (class I, level C). For patients with AF of less than 48 h duration, cardioversion should be done without delay before anticoagulation is initiated (class I, level C).

When the patient is haemodynamically stable, a cardiologist should be consulted. However, when the AF is poorly tolerated (e.g. chest pain, dyspnoea), control of the ventricular rate using pharmacological agents should be considered (note that this is not the same as pharmacological cardioversion). In patients without hypotension, heart failure, or pre-excitation, the intravenous administration of β-blockers (esmolol, metopropol, or propranolol) or nondihydropyridine calcium channel antagonists (verapamil, diltiazem) is recommended (class I, level B). Intravenous magnesium [15] has also been shown to be effective for rate control in the prehospital setting. In patients with signs of heart failure without accessory pathway, intravenous administration of digoxin or amiodarone (150 mg over a 10-min period) is recommended (class I, level B).

Supraventricular tachycardia (re-entry supraventricular tachycardia)

Re-entry SVT includes atrioventricular nodal reciprocating tachycardia (AVNRT), typical and atypical, and atrioventricular reciprocating tachycardia (AVRT). The characteristics of re-entry SVT are episodes of regular and paroxysmal palpitations with sudden onset and termination. The rate of re-entry SVT exceeds 120 beats/min with or without discernible retrograde P waves.

In re-entry SVT or suspected re-entry SVT, efforts should be made to terminate tachycardia or modify AV conduction. Vagal manoeuvres [16] (Valsalva manoeuvre, carotid sinus massage, facial immersion in cold water), and adenosine or ATP are the preferred initial therapeutic options. Vagal manoeuvres alone will terminate about 20–25% of re-entrant SVT [17].

The use of intravenous adenosine or ATP has several advantages: it has rapid onset and short half-life and therefore it is the preferred agent in the absence of contraindications. Several studies have demonstrated that adenosine is effective and safe, especially in the prehospital setting, to terminate re-entry SVT [18–22]. Adenosine is also safe and effective in pregnancy [23]. Adenosine should be avoided in patients with severe bronchial asthma. Side effects are common but transient: flushing, dyspnoea, chest pain, and possible initiation of AF. The initial dose is 6 mg intravenously for adenosine (and 20 mg for ATP solution) as a rapid push into a running intravenous line (at least 18 gauge). If this is not effective, an increased dose of 12 mg bolus is required and a second 12-mg bolus may be administered 1–2 min after the first one.

Calcium channel blockers and β-blockers are longer acting agents. Calcium channel blockers may decrease myocardial contractility and reduce cardiac output in patients with severe ventricular dysfunction and therefore should not be given to patients with impaired ventricular function or heart failure. For diltiazem, the initial dose is 0.25 mg/kg intravenously over 2 min and for verapamil 2.5–5 mg intravenously over 2 min. Esmolol, which is a short acting β-blocker (9 min half-life), may also be used (0.5 mg/kg per min IV).

An ECG must be recorded during the vagal manoeuvres or drug administration and a defibrillator should be available. If the tachycardia is terminated, it was probably a re-entry SVT. If the tachycardia is not terminated, P waves (morphology, number, and coupling compared to QRS) will help to obtain the diagnosis.

Focal atria\l tachycardia

Focal atrial tachycardia is characterized by a regular atrial activation of 100–250 beats/min. The P waves are frequently obscured by the QRS complexes.

Focal tachycardias have different sites of origin: right or left atrium, and some unusual sites, e.g. coronary sinus, noncoronary aortic cusp, and superior vena cava.

When there are three or more different P-wave morphologies associated with an irregular atrial tachycardia, the diagnosis of multifocal atrial tachycardia is made.

Bradycardia

General findings

Bradycardia is defined as a heart rate of less than 60 beats/min. It is a common finding in the ED setting. The management of bradycardia depends on the severity of symptoms, the correlation of symptoms with the bradycardia, and the presence of possible reversible causes. Symptoms of poor perfusion are syncope, acute altered mental status, chest pain, hypotension, and other signs of shock.

First, a correlation must be established between symptoms of poor perfusion and bradycardia. Asymptomatic patients do not require any immediate treatment. Bradycardia can be a sinus bradycardia associated with an increased vagal tone or due to sinoatrial node or atrioventricular conduction dysfunction (➲ Fig 8.4).

Bradycardia can be caused by different factors (➲ Box 8.3). Specific treatment of contributing causes, such as hyperkalaemia or hypothermia, must be systematically considered.

Management

The initial approach to bradycardia should be to improve oxygenation, monitor ECG, establish venous access, and maintain a patent airway. Management of bradycardia with evidence of myocardial ischaemia in the prehospital setting is summarized in ➲ Fig. 8.5.

Acute bradycardia due to ST-elevation myocardial infarction

Sinus bradycardia is the most common bradycardia occurring during the early hours after MI [24] (especially in inferior or posterior infarction) resulting from an increase in vagal tone. Symptomatic bradycardia should be treated by an intravenous bolus of atropine sulphate.

The incidence of complete heart block during ST-elevation myocardial infarction (STEMI) is decreasing but data from randomized trial suggest that AV block still occurs in 7% of cases [25]. The AV and intraventricular block during STEMI is generally related to the extensive myocardial damage and associated with higher in-hospital mortality.

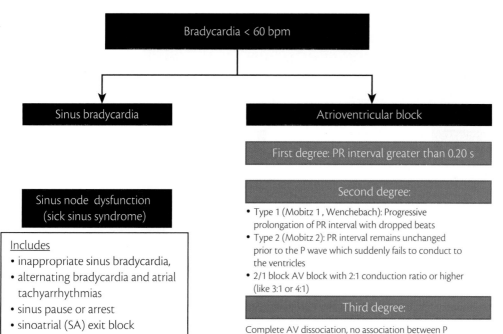

Figure 8.4 Different types of bradycardia. AV, atrioventricular; SA, sinoatrial.

Bradycardia < 60 bpm

Sinus bradycardia

Atrioventricular block

First degree: PR interval greater than 0.20 s

Second degree:
- Type 1 (Mobitz 1 , Wenchebach): Progressive prolongation of PR interval with dropped beats
- Type 2 (Mobitz 2): PR interval remains unchanged prior to the P wave which suddenly fails to conduct to the ventricles
- 2/1 block AV block with 2:1 conduction ratio or higher (like 3:1 or 4:1)

Third degree:
Complete AV dissociation, no association between P waves and QRS complexes

Sinus node dysfunction (sick sinus syndrome)

Includes
- inappropriate sinus bradycardia,
- alternating bradycardia and atrial tachyarrhythmias
- sinus pause or arrest
- sinoatrial (SA) exit block

Box 8.3 Main causes of bradycardia

- Ischaemia, myocardial infarction
- Idiopathic degeneration
- Drugs (β-blockers, calcium channel blockers, digoxin, antiarrhythmic agents)
- Hyperkalaemia, hypokalaemia
- Carotid sinus hypersensibility
- Neurocardiac syncope
- Situational disturbances (coughing, micturition, defecation, vomiting)
- Post cardiac surgery (valve replacement, etc.)
- Myotonic dystrophy (Steinert's disease, etc.)
- Hypothyroidism
- Hypothermia
- Infiltrative diseases (sarcoidosis, amyloidosis, haemochromatosis)
- Endocarditis
- Chagas' disease
- Autonomic nervous system disorders
- Systematic lupus erythematosus, scleroderma, rheumatoid arthritis, etc.

A new bundle branch block usually indicates an anterior infarction and is associated with significant myocardial necrosis and an increase risk of developing infranodal AV block, congestive heart failure, cardiogenic shock, ventricular arrhythmia, and sudden death. AV block related to anterior or anteroseptal wall infraction is located below the AV node (infranodal) caused by myocardial necrosis and associated with a wide (>0.12 s) and unstable QRS escape rhythm (often <30/min). In this case, administration of atropine sulphate is ineffective: transcutaneous pacing must be done as sooner as possible. Unlike the AV block related to inferior wall infarction, the intranodal block is mainly caused by excess of parasympathetic activity and associated with a narrow (<0.12 s) and stable QRS escape. In this case, atropine sulphate is usually effective.

In a patient with no evidence of ischaemia, treatment should be considered when bradycardia is associated with signs of poor perfusion.

Atropine sulphate

This remains the first line drug for acute symptomatic bradycardia. Atropine effectively removes the hyperparasympathetic tone and is useful for treating symptomatic bradycardia and AV block at the nodal level [26]. In patients with suspected infranodal third-degree AV block or type II second block, atropine sulphate should be avoided because of its inefficiency. and pacing (or isoproterenol or dopamine or adrenaline infusion) should be considered. Atropine sulphate (initial dose of 0.5 mg, repeated as needed to a total amount of 1.5 mg) is only effective for the treatment of unstable bradycardia due to hypervagal tone [27].

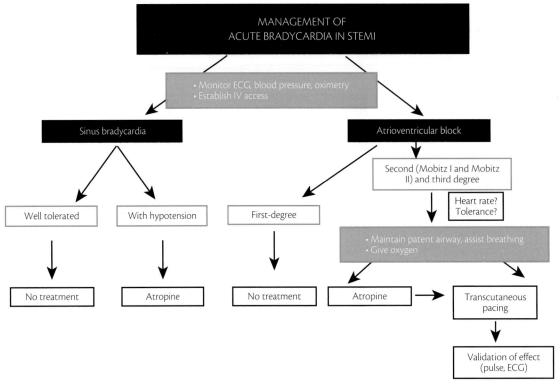

Figure 8.5 Management of bradycardia in STEMI (prehospital setting).

Pacing

For patients with a high degree AV block and with poor perfusion despite atropine sulphate, transcutaneous pacing should be considered and can be easily done even in the prehospital setting. This treatment may be painful and uncomfortable for the patient and therefore analgesia and light sedation should generally be used. Capture is confirmed electrically by the presence of a complex after each spike and mechanically by the presence of a palpable pulse. If this treatment is ineffective, transvenous pacing should be considered.

Other drugs

Other drugs can be used when the bradycardia is unresponsive to atropine. Isoprenaline or dopamine infusion or adrenaline can be considered until pacing is available.

Bradycardia with suspected hyperkalaemia

Specific management of hyperkalaemia with the administration of calcium gluconate, sodium bicarbonate, furosemide, and β_2-agonists should be considered.

Bradycardia associated with hypothermia

This requires rewarming the body core temperature and specific management in the prehospital and hospital settings.

Conclusion

The management of arrhythmia in the ED must be pragmatic and based on ECG and clinical evaluation. There are very few studies and no specific recommendations for patients admitted to the ED. Ischaemic disease remains one of the leading causes of arrhythmias in clinical practice, especially for ventricular arrhythmias. Early and successful reperfusion therapy remains the best antiarrhythmic therapeutic method in patients with acute myocardial infarction. The cardiological prognosis of patients admitted to the ED with arrhythmias depends mainly on the level of ventricular dysfunction.

Personal perspective

The prevalence of arrhythmias, like that of other cardiac diseases, is increasing as a result of growing life expectancy; this is particularly true for atrial arrhythmias. The management of atrial arrhythmias is now well standardized.

For ventricular arrhythmias, the improved availability of automated external defibrillators has improved the prognosis of sudden cardiac death. The implantation of internal automatic defibrillators has contributed to the reduction of cardiac deaths due to ventricular fibrillation or tachycardias.

Further reading

Zipes DP, Camm AJ, Borggrefe M, *et al.* ACC/AHA/ESC 2006 Guidelines for Management of Patients With Ventricular Arrhythmias and the Prevention of Sudden Cardiac Death: a report of the American College of Cardiology/American Heart Association Task Force and the European Society of Cardiology Committee for Practice Guidelines (writing committee to develop Guidelines for Management of Patients With Ventricular Arrhythmias and the Prevention of Sudden Cardiac Death): developed in collaboration with the European Heart Rhythm Association and the Heart Rhythm Society. *Circulation* 2006;**114**(10):e385–484.

Online resource

℠ European Resuscitation Council Guidelines for Resuscitation 2005. https://www.erc.edu/index.php/guidelines_download_2005/en/

⮕ For additional multimedia materials please visit the online version of the book (℠ http://www.esciacc.oxfordmedicine.com).

SECTION III

The intensive cardiac care unit

Recommendations for the structure, organization, and operation of intensive cardiac care units

Menachem Nahir and Yonathan Hasin

Contents

Summary

The modern intensive cardiac care unit (ICCU) receives older and more complicated patients, with multiple pathologies, combinations of diseases, side effects of new drugs, or complications of innovative procedures. The ICCU serves as the core and the basis of the whole cardiology layout in the hospital, receiving patients from the emergency department, internal wards, cardiac catheterization rooms, operations and procedures rooms, as well as other departments in the hospital. Patients are usually in an unstable condition, and always need immediate full attention and highly professional medical and nursing care. Sophisticated monitors and machinery must be handled by qualified expert medical staff or technicians, procedures must be performed rapidly, and prompt decisions must be made, with very narrow safety margins for mistakes.

The ongoing changes intrinsic to cardiology, partly due to modern technology and the increasing diversity of patients, required a combined effort from the Working Group on Acute Cardiac Care of the European Society of Cardiology (ESC) to write a paper on the structure and operation of the ideal ICCU. This chapter is based on the published paper. It deals with the requirements for adequate training and accreditation both for physicians and for nurses, as well as the structure of intensive and intermediate CCUs, considering in detail the number of beds, the standard equipment, including monitoring (invasive and noninvasive), additional equipment, medical devices, and computers. Also discussed is the functional recommendation considering which patient should be admitted to the CCUs, length of stay and relocation.

Introduction

The first description of an intensive cardiac care unit (ICCU) was presented to the British Thoracic Society in 1961 [1] and was based on monitoring patients with acute myocardial infarction (AMI) for the early diagnosis and treatment of ventricular fibrillation (VF). No significant benefit was obtained from these units until some decisive policy changes were made, including treatment protocols and structural organization [2]. The main objectives of ICCUs became the monitoring and support of failing vital functions in acute and/or critically ill cardiac patients, in order to implement adequate diagnostic measures followed by medical and invasive therapies. In more recent years a difference in the case mix of the patients and development of new treatment modalities has influenced the needs of the modern ICCU. Since the implantation of the policy of immediate percutaneous mechanical revascularization for high-risk acute coronary syndrome (ACS) patients, the catheterization laboratory and the ICCU have become more and more intimately associated. The European Society of Cardiology (ESC) Working Group on Acute Cardiac Care set up a task force to provide an updated guide indicating the minimal optimal requirements for the modern functioning ICCU. This was published in the *European Heart Journal* [3], and has been adopted by cardiology societies throughout Europe. As stated in the original paper, the authors recommend that local modifications should be implemented according to local special needs relating to specific patient case mix, available resources, and different laws and regulations.

Background

Two changes have occurred over the past two decades that demand distinctive alterations in the function of the ICCUs in the next decade. Changes will take place both in the patient population admitted to the ICCU and in the medical care supplied.

◆ Emergency reperfusion treatment policies (noninvasive or invasive) have now been adopted as an accepted standard of care in patients with AMI [4]. These policies dictate the necessity for special attention and immediate treatment of the patients early on; after the success of the initial treatment, the patients show immediate drastic improvement in many cases. Follow-up and management are simpler and easier than in the past, recovery is faster, the average length of stay is shorter, and therefore the turnover is larger.

◆ The medical profession has reached a level of specialization in which cardiologists and intensive care physicians must establish a long-term treatment policy for their patients rather than just taking care of the patient's immediate and urgent problems.

Patient population

ACS will probably remain the most frequently primary admission diagnosis in ICCU in the near future. Today these patients are treated effectively and quickly in different ways, so the length of stay both in the unit and in the hospital is expected to decrease. On the other hand, the ageing population, with increasing comorbidities, will probably change the ICCU population. Dramatic improvement in therapeutic measures will lead to a better outcome and prolonged survival for patients with coronary artery disease, with either normal or depressed left ventricular function. The case mix of patients in the ICCU will therefore change dramatically in the coming decades.

As the population ages, the ICCU will have to treat elderly patients who tend to suffer from multisystem diseases and the number of patients treated by multiple percutaneous or surgical revascularization procedures will increase. Moreover, the ICCU is becoming the treatment centre for patients suffering from severe cardiac arrhythmias and decompensated heart failure or different combinations of diseases of the heart and of other organs. As a result, it is likely that the ICCU will be utilized for more complex patients who require a relatively longer stay in the unit and will provide the staff with a special challenge. For these reasons, the ICCU requirements will increase, not decrease.

A special group of patients are those suffering from complications following invasive treatments in the catheterization laboratory. The still growing number of severe cases with multivessel disease, complex lesions, reduced left ventricular function, and a multitude of comorbidities treated in the catheterization laboratory may increase the number of complications during and after coronary intervention procedures. These patients represent a special group of patients admitted to the ICCU, and require specific cardiological nursing and medical expertise.

Treatment policies

Reperfusion in acute ST-elevation myocardial infarction (STEMI) patients is undoubtedly an emergency.

Direct mechanical revascularization is becoming increasingly popular [5], although its availability is still restricted by lack of trained staff and budget constraints. In the near future, the cooperation between catheterization laboratory and the ICCU will increase.

In the coming decade, cardiologists will continue to observe the pharmaceutical industry's constant efforts to improve reperfusion at the patient's bedside, with new, more efficient thrombolytics, anticoagulants, and antiplatelet agents, and more effective interventional therapy, which, in combination with newly developed drugs aimed at salvaging the microvasculature and the myocardium from ischaemia/reperfusion injury, will hopefully improve outcome in these patients. This scenario has clear implications for the necessity of constantly updating the ICCUs about novel methods for diagnosis and treatment, as well as preparing them to participate in multicentre research in order to determine the efficacy of the new therapeutic developments.

Specialization within the medicine profession is becoming more intense, with the need for cardiac patients to be treated preferentially by properly trained cardiologists. In hospitals where patients are transferred from the ICCU to the internal medicine ward, the physician in the ICCU is obliged to determine a long-term treatment policy, in addition to providing acute treatment. Thus, the different units will develop methods for prognostic stratification (index-risk stratification), which will most probably include a combination of clinical data (traditional risk factors, heart rate, blood pressure); ECG (ST-segment depression or elevation, T-wave inversion); cardiac biomarkers (especially myocardial troponin); evaluation of the left ventricular function; residual ischaemia; and electrical instability.

Staff

The changes in patient population and treatment policies necessitate appropriate staff training. An increase in the number of complex and/or elderly patients who may need respiratory support, intra-aortic balloon counter-pulsation, complex haemodynamic monitoring, or renal replacement therapy, and participation in multicentre research projects, require suitable training of the physicians as well as the nursing staff. It is reasonable that for specific specialization, there will be a requirement for adequate training and accreditation both for physicians (see ➲ Chapter 11) and for nurses, especially for the research nurses who will be an integral part of the ICCU's nursing staff.

Equipment

The standard monitoring equipment, including invasive and noninvasive ECG, haemodynamic, and respiratory assessment, will continue to be the basis of the ICCU [6]. Monitoring for the evaluation of autonomous function and electrical instability (heart rate variability, baroreceptor sensitivity, signal average electrocardiogram, and built-in continuous ECG Holter monitoring) is likely to be added to standard equipment. Noninvasive assessment of cardiac function such as cardiac output, systemic vascular resistance, and pulmonary congestion is becoming available and may be routinely used in the modern ICCU.

Computers are a part of the everyday monitoring of the patients; they are used for collecting and analysing patient's data. A uniform electronic database management system for different ICCUs is an important prerequisite for participation in large national and international registries, including at least basic demographic and clinical data, modes of intervention, and in-hospital outcome. It will make communication among the different ICCUs simpler, and could serve as a database with an enormous source of information both for research and for quality control purposes.

Functional recommendations

Intensive cardiac care unit patients

The decision to admit a patient should be made by the emergency department (ED) physician in agreement with the ICCU physician on duty; in case of disagreement, the decision will be made at the senior physician level. It is advisable for the following patients to be routinely admitted to the ICCU [7, 8]:

◆ Any patient with suspected acute STEMI, up to 24 h from the onset of symptoms, especially if suitable for thrombolytic or primary angioplasty treatment.

◆ Patients with AMI, presenting more than 24 h after onset of symptoms with complications, or unstable high-risk patients (heart failure that requires intravenous therapy or haemodynamic monitoring or support of an intra-aortic balloon, serious cardiac dysrrhythmias and conduction disturbances).

◆ Patients in cardiogenic shock.

◆ Patients with high-risk unstable coronary syndromes (e.g. ongoing or repeated anginal pain, heart failure, significant diffuse ST depression, dynamic ST shift, elevated troponins).

- Patients with life-threatening cardiac arrhythmias, from any cause.
- Unstable patients after a complicated percutaneous coronary intervention (PCI), who need special attention (at the discretion of the PCI operator).
- Patients with acute decompensated heart failure in need of continuous or frequent intravenous therapy and special haemodynamic monitoring.
- Patients with acute pulmonary oedema unresolved by initial therapy independent of the underlying conditions.
- Patients in need of haemodynamic monitoring for evaluation of therapy.
- Patients after a heart transplant with acute problem, e.g. infection, haemodynamic deterioration, electrolyte imbalance, suspected acute rejection.
- Patients with massive pulmonary embolism.

This list is not exhaustive and should be adapted according to each individual case.

Recommended length of stay

- The length of stay in the ICCU should be primarily planned for 2–4 days, dictated by the individual clinical presentation.
- Patients with STEMI without complications should continue the treatment in the ICCU for 48 h.
- Patients with unstable coronary syndromes with dynamic ST shift and elevated cardiac troponins should stay in the ICCU until 24 h after the last episode of ischaemia (non-invasive or planned invasive treatment, as recommended by the ESC guidelines).
- High-risk ACS patients after acute PCI (with GPIIb/IIIa antagonists) should stay in the ICCU until stabilization.

Relocation policy

- Once stabilized, patients are transferred from the ICCU to a cardiac intermediate care unit (with simple electrocardiographic monitoring and run by cardiology-oriented staff) or to the general ward, according to the local policy. After a short stay, a specialized out-of-hospital recreation facility is recommended prior to going back home. An alternative possibility is an outpatient rehabilitation clinic.
- It is advisable to discuss the following with the patient in the presence of a close family member: chronic medications, return to activities, risk factors and lifestyle modifications, and recommendations for future tests (invasive and noninvasive) including an appointment for the outpatient follow-up clinic; this should be done shortly before discharge from the ICCU.

Intermediate cardiac care unit patients

The decision to admit a patient to the intermediate ward is at the discretion of the referring or ED physician, and according to the local policy at the particular institution [9]. It is recommended that patients in the following categories should be considered:

- Intermediate risk unstable coronary syndrome patients.
- Patients in the first stages of recovery from myocardial infarction.
- Patients with decompensated cardiac insufficiency not responsive to regular oral therapy, especially those with comorbidities.
- Patients with heart disease in need of medical therapy adjustment, special cardiac investigations (e.g. electrophysiological study, cardiac catheterization), or some patients after special cardiac procedures (e.g. implantation of permanent pacemaker or internal cardiac defibrillators).

Intensive cardiac care unit and intermediate cardiac care unit

Number of beds

Intensive cardiac care unit

The number of beds in the ICCU must suit the size of the relevant population and the relative specific workload of the hospital. The hospital's specific workload can be evaluated in a number of ways: the simplest measure is the number of visits to the hospital's internal ED. The recommendation is that there should be 4–5 ICCU beds for each 100 000 inhabitants, or 10 ICCU beds for every 100 000 visits per year to the hospital ED. The number of beds will be determined according to the higher of these two figures.

Intermediate cardiac care unit

The desired ratio of beds between the ICCU and the intermediate CCU is 1:3.

Construction [10–12]

- The ICCU/intermediate cardiac care unit/cardiac ward should be constructed as an independent ward in the hospital [13].

- The desired standard is a separate room for each patient in the ICCU and up to two to three patients per room in the intermediate unit.

- There should be at least one single bedroom to allow the possibility of isolating patients with contagious infection.

- The architecture of the unit should be designed to make it possible to observe the patients from the nurses' monitoring station and to have easy and fast access.

- The station should be in a central position and well equipped, and the surrounding area should be spacious in order to afford optimal working conditions.

- The separate intensive care procedure room (➲ Fig. 9.1) should be spacious enough that it can contain all the clinicians (cardiologists, anaesthesiologists, nurses, technicians) and the large quantity of bulky equipment (X-ray machine, heavy monitoring, intra-aortic balloon pump device) necessary to initiate treatment for a complicated acute case. The minimal area should be 25 m^2. The room must have washable walls for 2 m in height. Construction should fit requirements for the use of X-ray fluoroscopy.

- The electrical equipment should have emergency back-up and a continuous power supply.

- Windows in the intensive care ward are desirable, but not a prerequisite.

- The lighting should be good, but not dazzling; lightning should be indirect.

- A dialysis facility (source of water and sewage outlet) should be established in several rooms as necessary.

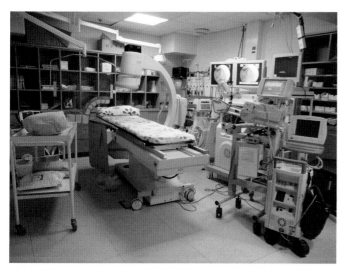

Figure 9.1 Procedure room within ICCU: the room includes mobile X-ray fluoroscopy, ECG and haemodynamic monitors, and essential equipment for coronary angioplasty. Also visible are the intra-aortic balloon pump device and mechanical ventilation machine.
Courtesy of Mr Alex Shochat, architect, Tel-Aviv, Israel.

- In larger units, consideration should be given to dividing the nurses' station into two or three according to the number of beds. It is advisable that one nurse's station should serve not more than six to eight beds.

- The ICCU should be situated as close as possible to the ED, catheterization laboratory, general intensive care unit, and operating theatres (if available in the institution) (➲ Fig. 9.2).

- It is also desirable for the intensive care ambulance to have direct access to the unit, so that in appropriate cases a patient may be directly admitted, bypassing the ED (➲ Fig. 9.3).

Other areas to be included

- Staff rooms (meeting the demands of the medical staff, nursing staff, patient relatives' interview, physician on-call dormitory, head nurse, and director of the unit)

- Meeting room.

- Family waiting room.

- Office (secretary).

- Storage rooms for equipment, laundry (taking into account electronic equipment that requires constant battery recharge).

- Computer communications—interdepartmental.

Intensive cardiac care unit equipment

Patient monitoring unit

The basic patient monitoring unit must include at least two ECG channels, invasive pressure channel, noninvasive blood pressure monitor, and SaO_2 meter. It is desirable that 50% of the beds include the following additional basic parameters: five ECG channels, two additional haemodynamic channels, end-tidal CO_2, noninvasive cardiac output, and indwelling thermometer.

Nurse station

This is to be used for central monitoring and analysis. At least one ECG lead from each patient as well as relevant haemodynamic and respiratory data should be continuously present on a central screen. Slave monitors should be installed to enable monitoring of patients from different sites within the unit, as well as working stations for retrospective analysis of index events, e.g. changes in heart rate, blood pressure, rhythm disturbances, ST events (ST-segment changes algorithm), O_2 saturation, and so on.

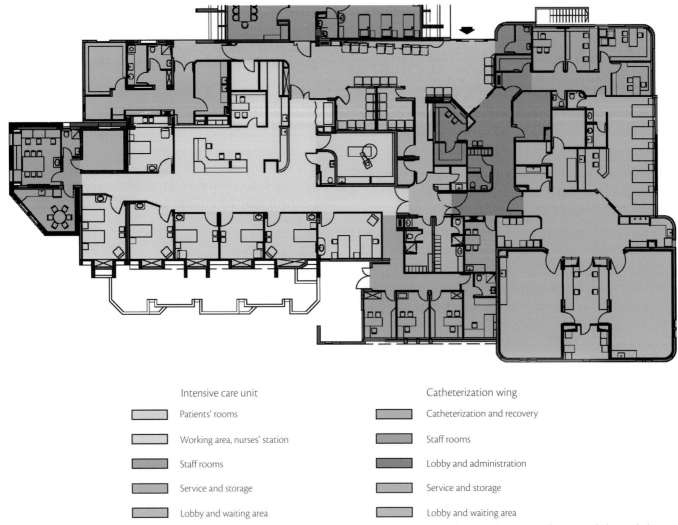

Intensive care unit

☐ Patients' rooms

☐ Working area, nurses' station

☐ Staff rooms

☐ Service and storage

☐ Lobby and waiting area

Catheterization wing

☐ Catheterization and recovery

☐ Staff rooms

☐ Lobby and administration

☐ Service and storage

☐ Lobby and waiting area

Figure 9.2 Intensive care unit and catheterization wing. The special procedure room is in proximity to the nurses' station, and any extra help needed during the procedure may be given immediately by the ICCU staff.
Courtesy of Mr Alex Shochat, architect, Tel-Aviv, Israel.

Patient beds

Beds in the ICCU have to allow vertical movement, with the possibility of up and down head and leg positioning. Every bed must be equipped with oxygen, vacuum, and compressed-air intakes. It is desirable for one of the beds to be suitable for the proper isolations of patients with active contagious infectious diseases (e.g. methicillin-resistant *Staphylococcus aureus*, cephalosporin-resistant enterobacter, HIV, tuberculosis, etc.) and filtered accordingly.

It is important to make sure that the patient can be radiographed on the bed.

Additional equipment [14]

◆ Volumetric pump/automatic syringe: 4–6 per bed.

◆ Mechanical respirators, including continuous positive airway pressure (CPAP) delivery system to use with face mask: 1 machine every 2 beds.

◆ Intra-aortic balloon pump: 1 console every 3 beds, up to the first 6 patients.

◆ Haemodyalisis/haemofiltration machine should be available (probably more cost effective if supplied by the nephrology department).

◆ Pacemaker defibrillator (preferable biphasic): 1 every 3 beds.

◆ External pacemaker: 1–2 every 6–8 beds.

◆ Temporary pacemakers: 3–4 VVI and one DDD every 6–8 beds.

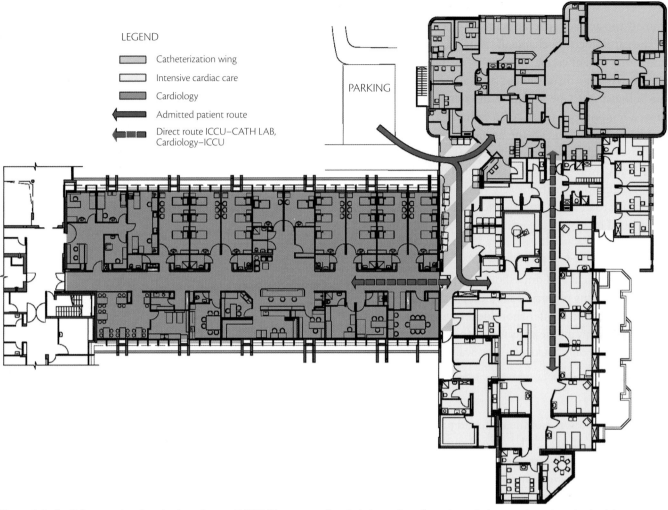

Figure 9.3 Cardiology ward, catheterization wing, and ICCU. Direct routes for admitting patients from the ambulance to the catheterization laboratory or ICCU (full arrow) and from the cardiology ward or catheterization laboratory to the ICCU (dotted arrows).

◆ Mobile echocardiography machine: 1 (consider a portable one, according to future technology development), including a TEE probe.

◆ Blood clot meter (ACT): 1.

◆ Biochemical markers kits, for myocardial infarction, optional (may be omitted if biochemistry tests are available from the central laboratory in <30 min).

◆ Glucose level measurement kit: 1.

◆ Blood gases and electrolyte analyser: optional (may be omitted if results of blood gas and electrolyte tests come back from the central laboratory within 10 min).

◆ X-ray system for fluoroscopy: digital cardiac mobile C-arm enabling coronary angiography is recommended.

◆ Ideally, a fully equipped catheterization and PCI laboratory should be in close association with the ICCU and ready to perform invasive procedures on a 24-h basis.

◆ Mechanical compression devices used for groin and radial homeostasis: optional.

Staff

◆ Physicians (daytime shift): cardiologists/residents in cardiology/cardiology fellows.

◆ Department head: a certified cardiologist, preferably with special accreditation in acute cardiac care.

◆ First 6 beds: one physician every 3 beds.

◆ If more than 6 beds: one physician every 4 beds.

The ICCU should be staffed by at least one physician for every three to four patients, including the unit director.

The director should be a board-certified cardiologist, specially trained and accredited as an acute cardiac care specialist.

The cardiologist in charge of the ICCU should be skilled in treating urgent cardiac situations, including rhythm and haemodynamic disturbances and acute ischaemia. The cardiologist must be skilled at inserting an endotracheal tube, a temporary pacemaker, a catheter in the pulmonary artery, and a balloon in the aorta for counter-pulsation. The cardiologist should be able to perform a transthoracic echo study on a basic level (i.e. evaluate the left ventricle systolic function, identify severe valvular heart disease, and find pericardial fluid) and should have further training in the general intensive care unit [15].

On-duty and on-call physicians

A skilled physician on duty should be present in the ICCU at all times. This physician should be able to handle acute cardiac emergencies after short local training and approval for night duties by the director of the unit. An attending cardiologist on call should always be available for consultation and assistance.

Nurses

Nurses are the essence of the unit, and proper nursing staff is the strength of the ICCU. A head nurse for the ICCU is appointed with authority and responsibility for the appropriateness of nursing care; he/she must have extensive experience in intensive care nursing and proper medical managerial skills, must be able to conduct routine nursing activity of the unit, must be involved in the ongoing training of the unit staff, and must take an active part in research activities. The ICCU will employ only registered nurses, at least 75% of whom should have completed formal intensive care training (which includes formal cardiology training) [16].

A unified recommendation for the size of the nursing staff is a complicated issue hampered by the divergence of nursing working habits and skills, case mix of patients, and different Therapeutic Interventions Scoring System levels [17]. The following recommendation is based on the estimated workload of an average ICCU, and the calculated whole time equivalents [18]. The allocation of nursing staff should take into account the number of shifts per day, the number of beds in the units, the desired occupancy rate, extra staff for holidays, and the ability to transfer nurses from one facility to the other (intensive to intermediate to cardiology and vice versa).

The nursing staff should consist of at least 2.8 nurses per bed, to cover three shifts per day, so that the minimal number of nurses in a given time will be at least one nurse per two beds during day time and one per three beds during the night shift [19, 20].

Cardiac intensive care nurses should have further training at least once in 5 years in the general intensive care unit. It is also advisable that further training courses be reciprocal, so that the nurses working in the general intensive care unit could work in the ICCU as well.

Intermediate cardiac care unit staff

- Department head: a certified cardiologist.
- First 12 beds: one physician per every 6 beds.
- If more than 12 beds: one physician per every 8 beds.
- Nurses: 1.8 nurses per bed.

Additional staff

- Secretary and nurse assistant full time.
- Dietitian, computer expert (hardware and software), ventilation technician, social worker, physiotherapist, porters, and cleaners (part time).

Database

It is recommended that the ICCU should use electronic charting routinely. This could facilitate patient admission, discharge, and follow-up as well as research and quality control. As several different hardware and software options are available, and many ICCUs in Europe have already implemented their own electronic charting, a common European electronic chart would be an impractical dream. Yet, some key items common to all electronic charts could be chosen, transmitted over the Internet, and used as a common European database for patients admitted to the different ICCUs.

The ESC launched the Cardiology Audit and Registration Data Sets (CARDS) initiative, under the auspices of the European Union [21]. One of the three main issues in CARDS is ACS, and the related Expert Committee on ACS published a report on the data standards for an ICCUs database on ACS. This data set can constitute the common basis for all the different databases in European ICCUs, allowing interoperability and data sharing.

Quality assurance should be an integral part of the organization and standards of an ICCU: processes currently considered effective for patients' outcome, such as adequately timed reperfusion and evidence-based care at discharge, should be monitored and quality control reviewed at least on an annual basis, together with the treating team and administrators.

Conclusion

The current recommendations have been written as guidelines for the functioning of a modern ICCU. The exponential speed of changes in technology, procedures, and treatment policies will undoubtedly provide a continual need to update these guidelines. For instance, what will be the effect on the ICCU of chest pain units (which are emerging throughout Europe—see ➲ Chapter 6)?

In the near future, reference centres for primary or facilitated PCI for STEMI, as well as for early intervention in patients with non-STEMI, will play a key role in the treatment of patients with ACS. The concept of computer networking for coordination among tertiary centres, community hospitals, EDs, and patient transport, might also result in a need for updating.

The lack of evidence-based recommendations on the structure and function of ICCUs demand properly designed studies looking at unresolved issues such as numbers of ICCU beds required for a given population size, specific equipment, required personnel, and such like.

Personal perspective

ICCUs continue to be essential and central to the proper care given to hospitalized cardiac patients. Recent years have seen a change in patient case mix, culminating in an evolution from intensive coronary care units to ICCUs. This transition has required upgrading of the units with respective caregiver expertise, equipment, structure and organization. In is our belief that the present chapter outlines the minimum requirements for the proper functioning of an ICCU that delivers suitable up-to-date care to its target patient population.

Further reading

Bone RC, McElwee NE, Eubanks DH, Gluck EH. Analysis of indications for intensive care unit admission. Clinical efficacy assessment project: American College of Physicians. *Chest* 1993;**104**:1806–1811.

Fuster V. 50th anniversary historical article. Myocardial infarction and coronary care units. *J Am Coll Cardiol* 1999;**34**:1851–1853.

Julian DG. The history of coronary care units. *Br Heart J* 1987;**57**:497–502.

Mangan B. Structuring cardiology services for the 21st century. *Am J Crit Care* 1996;**5**:406–411.

Quinio P, Baczynski S, Dy L, *et al.* Evaluation of a medical equipment checklist before intensive care room opening. *Ann Fr Anesth Reanim* 2003;**22**:284–290.

Wedel S, Warren J, Harvey M, *et al.* Guidelines for intensive care unit design. *Crit Care Med* 1995;**23**:582–588.

Online resource

℘ Accreditation of acute cardiac care physicians: ESC website. http://www.escardio.org/communities/Working-Groups/acute-cardiac-care/accreditation/Pages/aims.aspx

➲ For additional multimedia materials please visit the online version of the book (℘ http://www.esciacc.oxfordmedicine.com).

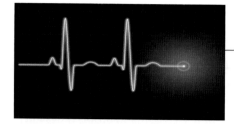

CHAPTER 10

The intensive cardiac care unit team

Tom Quinn and Eva Swahn

Contents

Summary

Effective, safe health care is a multidisciplinary undertaking. From its inception almost half a century ago, the concept of intensive coronary (now cardiac) care has drawn on the expertise of a range of professionals, particularly physicians working closely with nurses. As the evidence base for some aspects of care in the intensive cardiac care unit (ICCU) has developed, the traditional role of the ICCU has been devolved in many instances to other parts of the healthcare system such as emergency department (ED) or prehospital care, and the concept of critical care 'outreach' has been further developed to take expertise to the patient on the general ward. With more aggressive treatment policies for older people becoming the norm, the range of multipathology problems to be addressed by the clinical team requires input from a range of other specialties. Moreover, increasing complexity of diagnostic and interventional techniques requires close collaboration with laboratory and imaging personnel. Thus the ICCU team arguably extends beyond staff working solely within the physical structure of the ICCU to encompass a range of other professional and support staff both within and outside the hospital setting.

Introduction

The advent of the intensive coronary (now cardiac) care unit ([I]CCU) in the 1960s followed Julian's observations that close observation and early resuscitation in patients judged at high risk of complications from acute myocardial infarction (AMI), nursed in a defined clinical area, was associated with improved outcome [1]. Despite some controversy concerning the true benefits and cost-effectiveness of the (I)CCU, such facilities are almost universally available in hospitals across the developed world, although their precise structure and staffing depends on a range of factors including the patient case mix and whether secondary or tertiary care facilities are available (⊃Box 10.1).

The core team

The 'core' ICCU team consists of physicians and nurses providing immediate, bedside observation and care on a 24-h basis. Supporting professional, administrative, and auxiliary staff are discussed later in this chapter.

The director

The ICCU team is preferably directed by a cardiologist, specially trained and appropriately certified as an acute cardiac care specialist. The range of skills required will depend on the type of patients the ICCU caters for (e.g. secondary or tertiary care population). The ICCU team should be skilled in treating the range of urgent cardiac problems, including rhythm and haemodynamic disturbances, and acute ischaemia, and competent to undertake procedures ranging from endotracheal intubation, temporary transvenous pacing, pulmonary artery catheterization and insertion of an aortic balloon pump. Basic ECG skills are also required, and within the team further knowledge of general intensive care will be necessary depending on the type of unit [2].

Physicians

The European Society of Cardiology (ESC) recommends a physician to patient staffing ratio of 1:3–4, and that a skilled 'duty physician' be easily available at the ICCU at all times, to manage acute cardiac emergencies, supported by an 'on call' attending (consultant) cardiologist, available for consultation and assistance [2].

That patients with acute cardiological conditions should expect to have better outcomes when admitted under the care of a cardiologist than under a physician from another specialty seems a statement of the obvious, but establishing the true relationship between staffing levels, available clinical expertise, and outcomes for patients is a complex undertaking, not readily amenable to exploration through randomized trials, for practical and ethical reasons. In a large observational study of 88 782 patients with AMI admitted to hospitals in England and Wales, patients cared for by cardiologists were more likely to receive guideline-directed treatments and had lower 90-day mortality; however, cardiologist-treated patients had less comorbidity, and differences in use of interventional procedures were dependent largely on the type of facilities available at the hospital [3]. A systematic review of physician staffing concluded that outcomes were better in 'high intensity' staffed ICUs (pooled estimate of relative risk for hospital mortality of 0.71 (95% CI 0.62–0.82), pooled estimate of relative risk for ICU mortality of 0.61 (95% CI 0.50–0.75) [4]), reinforcing the need to ensure adequate numbers of physicians on the unit.

Nurses

Nurses are as important as physicians [2], and adequate numbers of appropriately trained nurses are essential to high quality care. That nurses are the strength of the ICCU has long been recognized:

> We felt that unless the nurse could develop these abilities [recognition of arrhythmias, understanding of treatment for complications and be able to perform life saving techniques by her/himself] the entire system of coronary care would be much less valuable [5].

A hallmark of the ICCU over the past half-century has been the development of specialist knowledge and skills, including empowerment of nurses to undertake decision-making and procedures that might previously have been regarded as responsibilities of the physician, such as arrhythmia monitoring and institution of treatments such as defibrillation, intravenous drug administration, and titration of intravenous medications to achieve pre-determined haemodynamic and other parameters, timely reduction of sedation and weaning from ventilation. This recognition of the 'extended role' of nurses can be traced back to the earliest days of the ICCU, although the degree of autonomy of the nurse differs between countries depending on national regulations:

> In our opinion, optimal treatment ... cannot be attained unless certain prerogatives hitherto reserved for the physician are delegated to the nurse [6].

It is important that all members of the ICCU team recognize and respect the experience and knowledge of colleagues from all disciplines. In some instances, for example, the ICCU nurse may often have encountered and managed many times, over several years, situations that the junior physician may be encountering for the first time. For example, errors in ICU transfer reports written by physicians are frequent and may be potentially harmful. ICU nurses may help to effectively and accurately intercept those inaccuracies, and therefore reduce the export of errors from the ICU to the ward [7].

The precise scope of nursing practice depends on a range of factors, not least national regulations and cultures, and individual training and experience. A survey of ICUs revealed variations in nurse staffing patterns among European countries and in their systems of training and education. Nurse autonomy also varied widely between countries [8], although the data are old and there is a need for more research to describe contemporary practices. In the United Kingdom, for example, legal advances have empowered appropriately trained nurses to undertake a range of responsibilities including administration of thrombolytic treatment, without the need to first consult with a physician [9]. Exploiting the full potential of the critical care nurse can benefit patients by using patient-centred care, proactive management and vigilance, coping with unpredictable events, and providing emotional support for patients and families [10]. Prompt and skilled intervention in the event of sudden patient deterioration is a further key nursing responsibility.

Head nurse

Strong, effective leadership of the ICCU team is an essential requirement. The head nurse must be clinically credible and possess managerial and leadership skills. Because ICCU patients are often enrolled in clinical trials and other studies, the head nurse must be familiar with the research process and associated regulations such as International Conference on Harmonisation (ICH)/Good Clinical Practice (GCP). The head nurse should have ongoing, 24-h responsibility for the nursing team, including working with these staff to address continuing professional development needs in a dynamic environment.

Shift leaders

Nurse leadership is required throughout the 24-h period, even in the absence of the head nurse, to ensure that appropriate levels of supervision and advice are available to nurses providing bedside care. The nurse taking 'shift leader' responsibilities requires substantial knowledge and experience of critical care in addition to organizational and leadership skills [11]. Because fulfilling these responsibilities

will frequently distract the nurse from focusing on an individual patient, it is recommended that direct patient care responsibilities should not be allocated to the shift leader.

Nursing assistants

The ESC have previously recommended that the ICCU employ only registered nurses (RNs) [2]. However, in some countries health care assistants are regarded as making an important contribution to patient care, supporting the work of RNs. Where such staff are employed, it is essential that they are not introduced merely to reduce staffing costs, and must work under the supervision of RNs, who retain responsibility for assessment, planning, and evaluation of patient care. Appropriate training, assessment, and supervision are required for assistant staff [12].

Nurse staffing levels

There is considerable evidence of an association between nurse staffing levels and patient outcomes. In the Cooperative Cardiovascular Project of 118 940 Medicare patients hospitalized with AMI, after adjustment for patient demographic and clinical characteristics, treatment, and hospital volume, technology index, and teaching and urban status, patients treated in environments with higher RN staffing were less likely to die in hospital [13].

Increased RN staffing was associated with lower hospital-related mortality in intensive care units (ICUs) (odds ratio [OR] 0.91; 95% confidence interval [CI], 0.86–0.96), with institutional and patient characteristics considered likely influences on this relationship [14]. This relationship, and the need for 'round the clock' physician staffing, was also demonstrated in a study of 27 372 ICU patients discharged from 42 tertiary and 194 secondary hospitals. In tertiary hospitals, a greater likelihood of dying was found among patients admitted to a mixed ICU (OR 1.61, 95% CI 1.14–2.26) and where there was no board-certified physician present for 4 or more hours per day (OR 1.56, 95% CI 1.20–2.01). In secondary care hospitals, every additional patient per RN was associated with a 9% increase in the odds of dying (OR 1.09, 95% CI 1.04–1.14). Nurse experience had no significant relationship to mortality [15].

Determining nurse staffing levels for the ICCU is a complex undertaking. The ESC recommend a nurse:patient ratio of at least 2.8 nurses per bed, covering three shifts per day so that at a minimum there is at least one nurse for every two patients during the day and one per three patients at night [2]. Other authorities, however, suggest that the complexity of patients' needs and the physical environment of the ICCU are important additional factors to consider, as well as the available 'skill mix' of nursing and other staff expertise, needs of patients' relatives and friends, the requirement to support patients being transferred to other wards for investigations off the ICCU (or even to another hospital), risk management, and patient safety [12]. Staffing levels also need to take into account the rapid alteration in patient dependency levels characteristic of the ICCU, including emergency admission of new patients.

The importance of teamwork

Effective teamwork is crucial for providing optimal patient care in the ICCU. In particular, team leadership has been acknowledged as vital for guiding the way in which team members interact and coordinate with others [16].

Teamwork plays an important role in causation and prevention of adverse events. Staff perceptions of teamwork and attitudes towards safety are related to quality and safety of patient care [17].

Quality improvement is an important activity for all members of the interdisciplinary critical care team. Success depends not only on committed interdisciplinary work that is incremental and continuous but also on strong leadership. Further research is needed to refine the methods and identify the most cost-effective means of improving the quality of health care received by critically ill patients and their families [18].

There has been considerable interest in the lessons that can be learnt from the aviation and motor sport industries to improve safety through better teamwork in health settings, including critical care. From aviation, Crew Resource Management (CRM) theory addresses six key areas: managing fatigue, creating and managing teams, recognizing adverse situations (red flags), cross-checking and communication, decision-making, and performance feedback [19].

Critical care outreach

Care of critically ill patients extends beyond the physical boundaries of the ICCU. In several countries critical care outreach services have been reported to have a positive impact on the delivery and organization of patient care, bringing the expertise of critical care staff to acute ward and other settings. However, a balance needs to be struck between the aims of service delivery and education—a tension that is partly resolved by sharing skills in the clinical and organizational context of direct patient care. First, on the organization of patient care: it was suggested that care was more timely, there were fewer referrals to the ICU, and

ICUs felt more able to discharge patients to hospital wards. There were also perceived to be improved links between ward nurses and medical teams. Second, on the confidence and skills of ward staff: increased contact on the wards resulted in more opportunities to share critical care skills. However, there remained concerns about the sustainability of improved skills and some respondents felt that junior doctors were becoming de-skilled [20].

The wider team

The ICCU team includes a wide range of other personnel working in support of the cardiologists and nurses. For example, the ICCU could not function without adequate administrative staffing, and the role of cleaning staff is essential in maintaining the ICCU environment and helping to reduce the incidence of hospital-acquired infections.

Other clinicians are important—for example, physicians from other specialties such as nephrologists and neurologists, anaesthetists, and general intensivists all play a role, as do those from crucial diagnostic and imaging disciplines including radiology and echocardiology, and the laboratory-based experts.

Non-medical professionals such as respiratory and physical therapists are important on a day-to-day basis, and in supporting patients as they recover from their critical state. Pharmacists support medicines management and safety, their expertise being a valuable resource. Similarly, social work staff have a key role in supporting patients and their families, as do language and cultural interpreters, and bereavement officers will be required when patients die. Hospital chaplains from many faiths bring spiritual support to those patients and families who seek it at times of distress and anxiety, so common to the critical care environment.

The role of ED and ambulance staff should not be underestimated within the context of the ICCU team. Their role in ensuring patients are managed speedily and receive guideline-directed care is essential, and liaison between these staff and the ICCU team is vital, e.g. in supporting decision-making before the patient even reaches hospital, and feedback afterwards [21] and where interhospital transfer is required (to or from the ICCU).

Conclusion

The effective ICCU team of today is dependent on all staff categories working around the patient. The team must also be able to work efficiently with all other actors dealing with the acute cardiac patient in need of intensive care. These partners involve not only hospital departments and service stations but also prehospital health care personnel and organizations.

An ICCU team working in a way outlined in this chapter can not only contribute to the individual patient's good health but also be cost effective for the society as a whole.

Personal perspective

The development of coronary care units (CCUs) during the 1960s was a landmark in the care of myocardial infarction patients. The intense monitoring of the ECG rhythm and prompt handling of the events reduced the in-hospital mortality to almost half. With new treatment possibilities, β-blockers during the 1970s, fibrinolysis and platelet inhibitors during the 1980s, and early revascularization in the 1990s, the mortality has continuously decreased, as has the incidence of myocardial infarction.

During the decades the patients admitted to CCUs have also changed. In some instances the CCU has become a chest pain unit, and mostly a good one as the skill of the staff has made it possible to sort and treat the patients early and adequately, thus sparing time, suffering, and money. On the other hand, the monitoring of chest pain patients with lower risk can safely be done in less intensive wards, with backup from CCU.

The initial aim of the CCU has undergone a shift from coronary patients only to intensive care of all cardiac patients who need it. Thus it has also become evident that the organization of the unit, its staffing, and the education of the staff has changed. The ICCU of today is focused on patients in need of intensive treatment given by highly skilled staff trained not only in high technology but also in early diagnosis, treatment without delay, and safety. They also need to have empathy, a high stress threshold and a good sense of teamwork.

Further reading

Birkhead JS, Weston C, Lowe D. Impact of specialty of admitting physician and type of hospital on care and outcome for myocardial infarction in England and Wales during 2004–5: observational study. *BMJ* 2006;**332**(7553):1306–1311.

Hasin Y, Danchin N, Filippatos GS, *et al*. Recommendations for the structure, organization, and operation of intensive cardiac care units. *Eur Heart J* 2005;**26**(16):1676–1682.

Kane RL, Shamliyan TA, Mueller C, *et al*. The association of registered nurse staffing levels and patient outcomes: systematic review and meta-analysis. *Med Care* 2007;**45**(12):1195–1204.

Manser T. Teamwork and patient safety in dynamic domains of healthcare: a review of literature. *Acta Anaesthesiol Scand* 2009;**53**(2):143–151.

⊃ For additional multimedia materials please visit the online version of the book (✎ http://www.esciacc.oxfordmedicine.com).

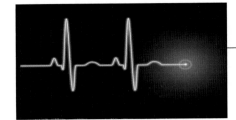

CHAPTER 11

Clinical competence and accreditation in intensive and acute cardiac care

Alessandro Sionis, Pablo Loma-Osorio, and Magda Heras

Contents

Summary

Advances in the treatment of cardiovascular diseases have changed their natural course and resulted in improved outcomes with prolongation of life. There is therefore a growing demand for intensive cardiac care from a sicker and older population with comorbidities, and a great need for trained cardiologists in this specialized area. This chapter describes the concept of clinical competence and its assessment, and highlights the competences that society demands from physicians. It also details the core curriculum and accreditation process established by the Working Group on Acute Cardiac Care of the European Society of Cardiology to train and accredit physicians in intensive and acute cardiac care (IACC). This specialized area of knowledge and skills has been largely neglected by cardiologists; however, the growing demand makes it necessary to establish this process. The success of this project requires the recognition and implementation throughout Europe, ideally with the endorsement of national societies.

Introduction

Cardiovascular medicine is a constantly evolving field in which new discoveries at molecular, cellular, and physiological levels have led to the development of novel therapeutic approaches and improved diagnostic methods. These advances have allowed physicians to change the course of the disease and prolong the lives of their patients. Intensive and acute cardiac care (IACC) has always been at the forefront of this process, striving to incorporate new medical and technological advances into the management of heart disease.

Four stages in the history of acute coronary care have been described [1]:

1 Clinical observation phase. Herrick's classic description of acute myocardial infarction (MI) was published in 1912. At the time the infarcted heart was considered a wounded organ for which the main treatment was bed rest. Clinical observation, electrocardiographic documentation, and empirical application of treatments resulted in an in-hospital mortality that approached 30%.

2 Coronary care unit phase. The first description of a coronary care unit (CCU) dates from 1961 [2]. Soon after, the first CCU was established in the United States, followed shortly by a landmark study [3] confirming the importance of the CCU as a beneficial tool in the management of patients with acute MI. Patients with MI were hospitalized in areas with continuous ECG monitoring, availability of external defibrillation, and resuscitation trained staff. This strategy was highly successful and halved in-hospital mortality.

3 Technological phase. In the early 1970s several landmark advances in diagnostics, such as the pulmonary artery catheterization and coronary angiography, provided new valuable insights in the pathophysiology of MI and its complications that lead first to the widespread use of β-blockers and then to the concept of early reperfusion and myocardial salvage, first with thrombolysis and later with primary Percutaneous Coronary Intervention (PCI).

4 Evidence-based phase. This phase is characterized by the concept that it is no longer acceptable to base the use of diagnostic tests and therapeutic measures on anecdotal experience or on the results of retrospective cohort studies. Randomized trials form the basis for treatment recommendations that are now codified in guidelines such as the ones sponsored by the European Society of Cardiology (ESC), among others.

As a result of this evolution, together with prolonged life expectancy, the landscape of today's CCU has radically changed from that of its beginnings. CCUs have evolved into units specialized in the care of highly complex patients including those with complicated and uncomplicated MI, decompensated heart failure and cardiogenic shock, severe valvular heart disease, high-grade conduction disturbances, incessant ventricular arrhythmias, complications of percutaneous procedures, and device-related infections [4, 5]. Furthermore, these conditions are seen in the context of numerous additional comorbidities. Thus, the distinctions between CCUs and traditional intensive care units (ICUs) have become increasingly blurred. Nowadays CCU

cardiologists, apart from providing highly specialized, state-of-the-art cardiological treatment, must be proficient in the management of a wide range of complications seen in other intensive care settings (➲ Boxes 11.1 and 11.2).

Additionally, cardiology remains at the forefront of clinical and translational research and CCUs represent a privileged and active area for quality research because of the high level of instrumentation, the favourable patient:clinician ratio, and the high incidence of cardiovascular events. Moreover, these units frequently act as coordinators of cardiac emergency networks, particularly in MI reperfusion strategies. CCUs of tertiary hospitals play a central role in keeping continuous and close relationships with peripheral hospitals and emergency systems, in order to ensure that highly specialized treatment is given in a timely way to patients in their area.

In summary, CCUs are no longer merely observation units for MI complications, but rather have become specialized intensive cardiac care units (ICCUs), training and research centres, and emergency hubs for patients with cardiovascular disease. Adaptation to such changes means that the CCU enter into a new stage that could be known as the 'ICCU phase' (➲ Fig. 11.1).

Professionals working in these areas are exposed to a highly technical and rapidly changing environment, and there is a direct relationship between clinical competence

---

Box 11.1 Techniques currently used in CCU

Cardiological techniques

◆ Invasive and noninvasive monitoring

◆ Transthoracic and transoesophageal echocardiography

◆ Temporary pacing

◆ Electrical cardioversion

◆ Pericardiocentesis

◆ Intra-aortic balloon counterpulsation

◆ Ventricular assist devices

General techniques

◆ Intubation and mechanical invasive ventilation

◆ Noninvasive ventilation

◆ Percutaneous tracheostomy

◆ Central venous line placement

◆ Renal replacement therapy

◆ Resuscitation (includes hypothermia)

Box 11.2 Complications commonly seen in ICCU

Cardiological complications

- Acute heart failure and cardiogenic shock
- Mechanical complications of MI
- Conduction disturbances
- Ventricular arrhythmias

Complications of percutaneous procedures

- Device-related complications

General ICU complications

- Acute lung injury
- Prolonged ventilation and weaning
- Delirium
- Acute renal failure
- Venous thrombosis
- Gastrointestinal haemorrhage
- Infections and septic shock

and outcomes in these settings. Training and accreditation in different critical care settings, including MI [6, 7], translate into a benefit in terms both of mortality and of the more efficient use of expensive medical resources.

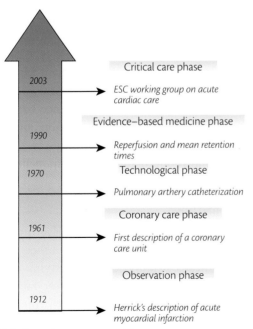

Figure 11.1 Stages in coronary care history.
Data from Braunwald E, Antman EM. Evidence-based coronary care. *Ann Intern Med* 1997;**126**(7):551–553.

Clinical competence

Background

There is a widespread consensus that evidence-based medicine (EBM) should constitute the core medical body of knowledge. The application of EBM to medical practice, however, presents some unique problems that can be viewed in terms of four basic competencies:

1 Recognition of a patient problem and construction of a structured clinical question.

2 Ability to efficiently and effectively search the medical literature to retrieve the best available evidence to answer the clinical question.

3 Critical appraisal of the evidence.

4 Integration of the evidence with all aspects of individual patient decision-making to determine the best clinical care for that particular patient.

It must be noted that EBM education programmes focus almost exclusively on the third item, thus neglecting key steps for the application of EBM in clinical practice [8]. Cardiologists, like other health care professionals, are increasingly exposed to an overwhelming amount of medical literature that forms the base of an enormous pyramid of knowledge, unreachable by the individual clinician, however industrious, critical, and self-directed.

Assessment

In 1990 the psychologist George Miller proposed a framework for assessing clinical competence [9]. At the lowest level of the pyramid is knowledge (knows), followed by competence (knows how), performance (shows how), and action (does) (➲ Fig. 11.2). Unfortunately, the assessment of medical competence in a specific field, as still performed today, is almost systematically based on the numerical evaluation of a body of knowledge, an inheritance from the 19-century philosophy [10]. Instead, the assessment of clinical competence should ideally embrace all levels, albeit focusing on the top 'action' level.

The assessment and maintenance of physician competence has been given worldwide attention, partly in response to concerns about physician performance as well as demands for accountability to patients and funding agencies. These concerns have shifted the concept of competence from a narrow definition of the ability to perform technical medical acts into much broader aspects of competence. For example, the Accreditation Council for Graduate Medical Education (ACGME), the body responsible for the accreditation for

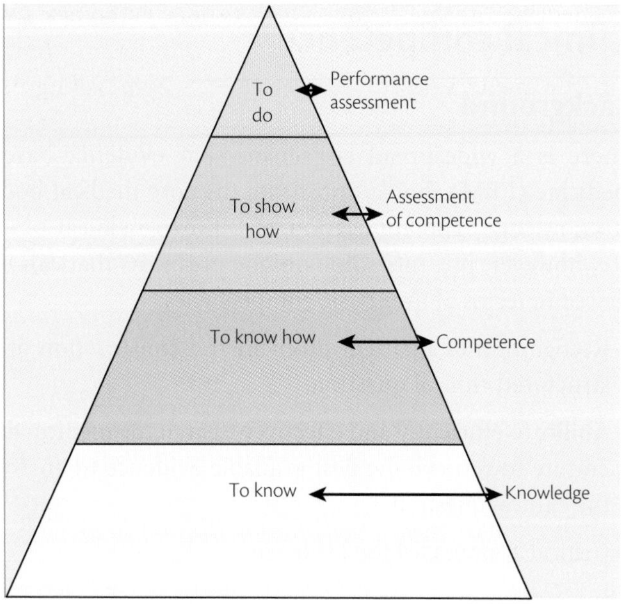

Figure 11.2 Miller's pyramid.
Adapted with permission from Miller GE. The assessment of clinical skills/competence/performance. *Acad Med* 1990;**65**:S63–7. Copyright Wolters Kluwer Health 1990.

postgraduate medical training programs for medical doctors in the United States, has declared that physicians need to attain competence in six domains: patient care, medical knowledge, practice-based learning and improvement, interpersonal and communication skills, professionalism, and systems-based practice [11, 12]. Physicians are encouraged to continue improving their medical skills and knowledge and asked to reflect on the care they provide; collaborate with other members of the health care team; recognize their roles within overall systems of care; and deliver their services with integrity, honesty, and compassion, exhibiting appropriate personal and interpersonal professional behaviours. New ways of thinking about competence have resulted in a quest to find new approaches to assess practising physicians and guide their development.

Tools for assessment

Multisource feedback evaluation

The concept of multisource feedback (MSF) evaluation (also known as 360° evaluation) was initially developed to support employee decision-making and quality improvement in industry [13]. The goal of MSF is to look at a person's work from a variety of perspectives, including those at the same level in the organizational chart, those above, and those at lower levels. The view from all perspectives helps to frame a more complete picture of performance. As medical services are provided increasingly within organizational systems that demand accountability to funding

agencies and patients, it is not surprising that the tools used to assess managers may also be seen as ways to provide physicians with feedback in areas such as communication skills and interpersonal relationships. At the same time, licensing and professional organizations struggle to ensure that the practice of medicine includes collegiality, communication skills, and professionalism, as well as medical expertise. MSF has been identified as a mechanism to provide this feedback in medical settings to the physician, his colleagues (peers), coworkers and patients. Besides, MSF is a survey-based method with flexibility. Questionnaire items and domains can be changed quickly to encompass new perspectives and needs. For example, the American Board of Internal Medicine (ABIM) has instruments for patient and peer assessment as part of its maintenance of certification programme [14]. Its patient instrument focuses on professionalism and interpersonal and communication skills, whereas the peer instrument covers professionalism, medical knowledge, and patient care. So, although it is unlikely that a single tool will be found to guide physician improvement or to satisfy all funding agencies that physicians are achieving satisfactory levels of performance, MSF shows promise as a means of assessing physician competence across a broad range of competencies [15–18].

Objective structured clinical examination

Objective structured clinical examination (OSCE) is a form of performance-based testing used to measure candidates' clinical competence [19, 20]. During an OSCE, candidates are observed and evaluated as they go through a series of stations in which they interview, examine, and treat standardized patients who present with some type of medical problem. Because OSCEs have been shown to be feasible and have good reliability and validity, their use has become widespread as a standard for performance-based assessment, particularly in undergraduate examinations.

Several of the medical Royal Colleges in the United Kingdom have introduced an OSCE component into their postgraduate membership examinations.

Traditional methods

Medical knowledge and practice-based learning competencies are probably better assessed by other tools such as traditional means. Multiple choice questions, essays, and oral examinations could be used to test factual recall and applied knowledge [21–23]. Similarly, medical audit and third-party data sharing techniques offer more specific information about quality of care provided in clinical situations [24].

Accreditation in IACC

European Board for the Specialty of Cardiology accreditation

The European Board for the Specialty of Cardiology (EBSC) was created in 1992 as a joint initiative from the ESC and the Union Européenne des Médecins Spécialistes (UEMS) Cardiology Section. The EBSC is the coordinating body for subspecialty accreditation of the ESC. A seminal paper on subspecialty accreditation was published in 2007; the process of accreditation described in this chapter follows its recommendations closely [25].

Core curriculum

The purpose of the core curriculum is to present a formal education plan for a training programme in IACC where the knowledge, skills, and attitudes that trainees must acquire are described. The core curriculum includes the core syllabus plus the structure on learning materials, teaching, and assessment methods for cardiologists who want to be accredited as a specialist in IACC. The core syllabus is the framework of the core of knowledge that cardiologists who want to become specialists must know.

The need for well-trained specialists in IACC has been highlighted earlier. Although the number of patients with acute cardiovascular disorders or severe cardiac comorbidities requiring special treatment is increasing, there is to date no pan-European standardized and accepted training programme for physicians in charge of the ICCU. In this chapter, the program to accredit ICCU physicians proposed by the Working Group on Acute Cardiac Care (WGACC) for training and credentialling is explained.

The physician in charge of the ICCU should be able to recognize and treat a wide variety of acute and chronic cardiac conditions leading to cardiac decompensation. Moreover, such a physician should be able to investigate and manage resulting organ system failure, in addition to determining more long-term management following stabilization. ICCU physicians should be well acquainted with the diagnostic and therapeutic techniques available to the modern cardiologist including ECG, echocardiography, nuclear cardiology, haemodynamic measurements and their interpretation, cardiac and coronary angiography, cardiac pharmacotherapy, and interventional cardiology. They should be familiar and confident in the operation of the available equipment including monitoring (invasive and noninvasive), cardiac pacemakers, defibrillators, artificial respirators (invasive and noninvasive), renal replacement therapy, and mechanical cardiac support. A comprehensive knowledge of interventions to treat cardiac pathology and also associated conditions such as liver and renal dysfunction is mandatory, in addition to knowledge regarding the management of infection, nutrition, sedation, and analgesia. To meet these requirements demands training in cardiology (all applicants must be fully certified cardiologists) with additional training in intensive care medicine.

The aims of the learning process detailed in this chapter are:

◆ To provide guidance on the training requirements for cardiologist in charge or working in the ICCU.

◆ To delineate the core competencies and curriculum for such physicians.

◆ To define the techniques in which the ICCU cardiologist should be proficient.

◆ To describe the minimum numbers of procedures that trainees must have done before applying for accreditation.

The main expected outcome is to have appropriately trained cardiologists in the subspecialty of acute cardiac care to support state-of-the-art treatment for patients with severe cardiac dysfunction and comorbidities. It is expected that the proposed programme contained in this document will be accepted by all national cardiology societies in Europe in the near future. This will result in a more uniform treatment of critically ill cardiac patients all over Europe, reducing inequalities among countries and improving outcomes.

Learning objectives

Cardiologists wishing to be trained appropriately to manage an ICCU and applying for accreditation in acute cardiac care must achieve during their learning process the objectives outlined in ➲ Table 11.1, for each of the listed syndromes.

All the skills outlined in this core curriculum are supplementary to those expected from general cardiologists not working regularly in an ICCU.

Definition of levels of competence

The levels of competence required are defined as follows:

◆ Level I: Experience of selecting the appropriate diagnostic modality and interpreting the results or choosing and appropriate treatment. Does not include the performance of a technique.

◆ Level II: Practical experience, but not as an independent operator (the technique is performed under the guidance of a superior).

Table 11.1 Learning objectives

	Number of patients	Competence level
General, core intensive medicine	All patients admitted to ICCU	III
Acute coronary syndrome	300	III
Acute heart failure and cardiogenic shock	100	III
Myocarditis	10	III
Cardiac tamponade	20	III
Acute valvular disease	20	III
Trauma and acute diseases of the aorta	10	III
Respiratory insufficiency Respiratory support Endotracheal intubations	100 30	III III
Arrhythmias Ventricular tachychardia Supraventricular tachycardia Atrioventricular block	20 50 20	III III III
Pulmonary embolism	10	III
Primary pulmonary hypertension	10	III
Sepsis and inflammatory syndromes	50	III

◆ Level III: Able to independently perform a technique unaided.

Objectives

To understand the pathophysiology, clinical presentation, investigation, differential diagnosis, treatment options, complications and secondary prevention measures for: general, core intensive care medicine, acute coronary syndromes (ACS), acute heart failure (AHF) and cardiogenic shock, myocarditis, cardiac tamponade, acute valvular disease (endocarditis, degenerative valve, artificial valves, chest trauma and complicated acute myocardial infarction), trauma and acute diseases of the aorta, respiratory insufficiency, arrhythmias, pulmonary embolism and primary pulmonary hypertension, sepsis and inflammatory syndromes. In all of them, a complete theoretical knowledge of the principles underlying general care of the ICCU patient are expected. ⊃ Table 11.1 lists the application of this theoretical knowledge in the management of a minimum of patients required during the learning process.

Special skills

It is expected that during the learning process, the trainee will undertake the following techniques to the level of competence requested, as listed in ⊃ Table 11.2.

Teaching and learning methods

The trainee will assume appropriate responsibility in obtaining the theoretical knowledge outlined in the syllabus (see ⊃ Online resources).

To do this, it is advisable to use the core curriculum book of cardiology from the ESC (CD, tutorials on the ESC web page), recent ESC guidelines, and other teaching materials from the different and relevant Working Groups and Associations of the ESC, especially the present textbook from the WGACC. Reference to training materials from the European Society of Intensive Care Medicine (ESICM; see ⊃ Online resources) and/or national intensive care societies may also be useful. The trainee will therefore be required to engage in continuous, independent self-directed learning and self-assessment. Other learning opportunities are also advised (ward rounds, case presentations, lectures, journal clubs, meetings of scientific societies, working groups, and associations).

Assessment methods

The accreditation committee (⊃ Fig. 11.3) is responsible for ensuring that the theoretical examination is based on the curriculum and that the questions asked are relevant. Thus, to assess the proficiency in acute cardiac care, several methods will be used to ensure that both the theoretical and practical skills have been mastered by the applicant. The trainees must prove that they have undergone the appropriate training (listed above) in an accredited unit under the guidance of accredited staff. They will be required to provide a logbook in which all procedures and patients have been listed, and signed by the trainee's tutor. They will also need to provide a list of other educational activities in which they have actively participated. This documentation must be provided before applying for the examination. Only trainees with an adequate CV are allowed to sit the written examination, which is in English and consists of a 100-question multiple choice questionnaire (MCQ).

In the near future, it is intended to create a web-based platform that will provide a continuous evaluation of the learning and techniques done by the applicant as well as a continuous assessment of the trainee's performance, making the examination unnecessary.

Organization of the accreditation process

The accreditation structure comprises:

◆ The working group nucleus, which oversees the process to ensure that it complies with the defined objectives of accreditation.

Table 11.2 Skills and level of competence required

Technique	Minimum number of cases in logbook	Level of competence (Accreditation)	Level of competence (Revalidation)
Primary angioplasty	50	I	II
Right heart catheterization	20	III	III
Invasive and noninvasive haemodynamic monitoring	100	III	III
Intra-aortic balloon pump	10	III	III
Advanced renal support	30	III	II
Noninvasive ventilation	50	III	III
Endotracheal intubation	30	III	III
Mechanical ventilation	50	III	III
Pericardiocentesis	10	III	III
Temporary pacemaker implantation	50	III	III
Current ACLS certificate	N/A	N/A	N/A
Care of the post resuscitation patient[a]	20	III	III
Extracorporeal cardiopulmonary support	10	I	I
Transthoracic and transoesophageal echocardiography	125 (TTE) 50 (TOE)	Level III (TTE) Level III (TOE)	II

ACLS, advanced cardiac life support
[a] Including the process of arranging organ donation.

- An accreditation committee: its mission is to establish the core curriculum and the syllabus and to organize the whole process of accreditation.
- Knowledge and skills committees, which assist in the preparation of the examination and audit merits presented by accreditation candidates.

The training programme

This training is reserved to board-certified or country-recognized cardiologists. A comprehensive cardiological background is necessary not only to master the technical aspects of the invasive techniques, but also to recognize the indications and the contraindications of different treatments for patients in need of intensive acute cardiac care. In addition, the trainee will need to obtain experience in the field of intensive care medicine.

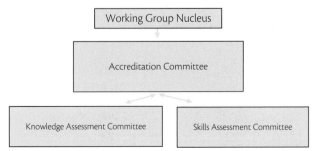

Figure 11.3 Structure of the accreditation committees on IACC.

In order to achieve these objectives:

- The trainee will be a fully trained cardiologist who will have been working for a minimum of a 1-year period in a centre authorized to give this training, and participate fully and regularly in formal and informal training provided by the centre.
- The trainee will have been an on-call junior cardiologist responsible for the ICCU for the equivalent of at least 1 night per week for at least 3 years.
- The trainee will undertake a 1-year period of at least 6 months as an ICCU attending physician, 3 months in a general intensive care unit, 1 month in intensive pulmonology/respiratory unit, 1 month in nephrology and 1 month in anaesthesia. The trainee should keep a logbook to register the patients he/she has taken care of, and invasive and noninvasive diagnostic and therapeutic procedures used in each patient. The logbook will be verified by the supervisor.

Entry requirements for cardiologists

Applicants for accreditation must have followed the above training programme. They also need to submit the following:

- A cardiology specialist qualification issued by a national health authority (or equivalent) or the European Union or, in the future, by the UEMS. Similarly, accreditation will be contemplated for those professionals who hold a cardiology specialist qualification issued by a non-European country, provided that it is homologated by an equivalent in Europe.

- Theoretical and practical training in the diagnosis and treatment of all types of cardiac pathologies, as described in this chapter.

- Theoretical and practical training in ACC. At least 1 year full-time training, in a centre which is recognized and accredited; this is in addition to training time in ICCU during cardiology specialization.

- Continuous online information on the training procedures and continuous assessment by the tutor. Until this online system is implemented, a theoretical 100-MCQ examination in IACC is set on a yearly basis.

Accreditation procedure

All practical details and documents required can be found on the ESC website (see Online resources).

Professionals

Applications must include:

- MD degree (or equivalent).

- Licence to practice medicine.

- Standard form completed with records and a recent photograph.

- Receipt showing payment of accreditation fees.

- CV.

- Certified photocopy of the cardiology specialist qualification issued by the national health authority or the European Union (or equivalent).

- Original letter signed and stamped by the director of the ICCU accredited for training, as well as the head of the cardiology department/service of the corresponding centre, certifying that the applicant has completed a full-time stay of at least 1 year in the unit detailing the activities undertaken, and the degree of competence attained.

- The logbook.

After evaluation, the accreditation committee will send candidates a letter indicating the result of their application and setting a date and place for the examination. The accreditation committee retains the right to investigate any application.

Requirements for training centres and training supervisors

Training centres will be located in hospitals certified by the local/national authorities to train general cardiologists. The ICCU must be part of the cardiology department and directed by a cardiologist who has been accredited by the WGACC. The hospital may also have other ICUs where trainees may complete their training. Training centres must be able to offer minimum capacity for training which will be evaluated by the accreditation committee in accordance with the following recommendations:

- Patient care capacity: a staff level that includes at least two cardiologists who hold ACC accreditation and a minimum of four beds.

- Research capacity: maintain a minimum level of scientific activity and interest in ACC.

Recertification

Professionals and centres must recertify their accreditation at least every 5 years. The specific requirements are still being defined. However, it is intended that recertification could be done using the web-based platform that ideally would capture their clinical and research work and continuing medical education (CME) hours.

Conclusion

The growing demand for intensive and acute cardiac care has created a need for cardiologists specifically trained in this area. This challenge can only be met by a joint effort of the European Society of Cardiology and national societies. Obtaining clinical competence in this area of knowledge requires the implementation of specific training. As outlined in this chapter, the assessment of skills must rely on a solid accreditation programme that includes continuous recertification on a regular basis.

Personal perspective

Clinical competence and skills evaluation are the cornerstones of excellence in practice. The accreditation program outlined in this chapter must be fully developed using web-based technologies that will allow continuous registration of the knowledge acquired, and documentation of skills as well as evaluation from the tutor on the trainees' attitudes. Evaluation from peers, other hospital-related staff, and patients is also fundamental. Attention to recertification is mandatory because of the continuous developments in knowledge and skills in ACC. CME and training done by certified professionals must be easily captured to provide recertification on a regular basis; this process should be done using technologies that will help professionals with the whole procedure.

It is important that this process, initiated by the ESC WGACC, should be endorsed by European national cardiology societies recognizing the need for intensive cardiac physicians. All countries should strive to have cardiologists who can deliver state-of-the-art treatment and this can only be done if their physicians are clinically competent in this specialized area.

Further reading

Higgins RS, Bridges J, Burke JM, *et al*. Implementing the ACGME general competencies in a cardiothoracic surgery residency program using 360-degree feedback. *Ann Thorac Surg* 2004;**77**:12–17.

Katz JN, Turer AT, Becker RC. Cardiology and the critical care crisis: a perspective. *J Am Coll Cardiol* 2007;**49**(12):1279–1282.

López-Sendón JL, Mills P, Weber H, *et al*. Recommendations on sub-specialty accreditation in cardiology. *Eur Heart J* 2007;**28**:2163–2171.

Lynch DC, Surdyk PM, Eiser AR. Assessing professionalism: A review of the literature. *Med Teach* 2004;**26**:366–373.

Miller G, Miller GE. The assessment of clinical skills/competence/performance. *Acad Med* 1990;**65**:S63–67.

Online resources

🖰 European Society of Cardiology Working Group on Acute Cardiac Care. http://www.escardio.org/communities/Working-Groups/acute-cardiac-care/accreditation/Pages/aims.aspx

🖰 European Society of Intensive Care Medicine. http://www.esicm.org/

➲ For additional multimedia materials please visit the online version of the book (🖰 http://www.esciacc.oxfordmedicine.com).

CHAPTER 12

Databases, registries, and quality of care

Eric Boersma, Anselm K. Gitt,
and Bertil Lindahl

Contents

Summary

During the last few decades, the understanding of coronary heart disease has considerably improved, and major progress has been achieved in (acute) patient management and outcome. One of the challenges for contemporary medicine is to rationally implement the available therapies in clinical practice, in the appropriate patients at the appropriate time. Before certain therapy is initiated, a physician must consider the probability that the patient will improve or deteriorate without such therapy, the chances of improvement if the therapy is initiated, the risks of adverse events, and, last but not least, the therapy-related costs. Consequently, predictive thinking plays an important role in cardiovascular medicine, and the improvement of our ability to make accurate predictions is one of the driving forces behind clinical research. In this respect, databases of systematic clinical observations are useful for the prediction of patient prognosis. Clinical experiments are necessary to obtain valid information on treatment effects. Surveys and registries are useful to monitor the quality of the applied care in routine clinical practice, as well as for benchmarking and quality improvement.

Introduction

The dominating philosophy in modern medicine dictates that patient management should be based on the best available evidence of its effectiveness, safety, and efficacy. The proof of the efficacy of clinical management is preferably derived from systematic patient-oriented research. Based on data that are obtained in cohorts of patients, relations are studied between the incidence and prognosis of diseases and their determinants. The concept of determinant–outcome relationships forms the central idea in this so-called evidence-based medicine (EBM) philosophy. The discovery of determinant–outcome relationships is not a goal in itself. It is the first step in a process to influence these relationships, with the ultimate goal of improving patient outcome. This is why clinical researchers keep searching for modifiable, preferably causal, determinants.

The obvious question that now arises is how to obtain insight in determinant–outcome relationships. What kind of data will provide a solid basis for EBM? An often defended statement is that each patient is a unique person who should be assessed individually. However, if that were really true, then medical schools should be closed down, as there is no general medical knowledge to transfer. Indeed, in some respect a patient should be considered a unique case, and medical treatment should be tailored to his or her individual needs. But in many other respects, a 'unique' patient can be viewed as a member of a group of congeners, who have a similar health problem, face a similar prognosis, and may benefit from a similar approach. Therefore, determinant–outcome relationships can be revealed by systematic analyses of patient-oriented databases, which form the cornerstone of EBM.

Clinical observations and clinical experiments

In view of the large number of physiological processes within the human body, it is not practically feasible to explain outcome of diseases and results of patient management on a fully deterministic basis. Still, that will not invalidate the EBM approach, as long as determinant–outcome relationships are interpreted probabilistically. An example may be useful here. The Global Registry of Acute Coronary Events (GRACE) is an observational study of acute coronary syndrome (ACS) patients, who are being enrolled in 247 hospitals in 30 countries worldwide [1]. By 2005 a total of 24 165 patients had been included, and 1342 had died during hospitalization. For each individual patient of this cohort one might state that the probability of in-hospital death was 1342/24 165 = 5.6%. Furthermore, 1072 deaths had occurred in the 12 971 patients above the age of 65 years. Hence, the probability of in-hospital death in this cohort was 8.3%, apparently higher than average. The probability of in-hospital death in patients below 65 years was 2.4%, apparently lower than average. Thus, age is revealed as a determinant of the outcome 'in-hospital death'.

Databases of routine clinical practice observations, such as GRACE, are particularly useful to help gain insight in determinants of patient prognosis. The GRACE investigators have developed a model to estimate patients' probability of

in-hospital death in relation to their characteristics (➲ Fig. 12.1). Following the EBM strategy, such estimates might then be used for clinical decision-making. Many risk evaluation models have been developed for ACS patients, and the question of their reliability and accuracy is relevant. In general, prognostic models accurately separate patients at low risk of clinical events from those at high risk. However, the estimation of the actual level of risk is often suboptimal, mainly due to poor representativeness of the model development data sets for routine clinical practices. Sophisticated statistical techniques must be applied to adjust the model parameters, so that the output matches with local practice. Information from the local past provides the best mirror of today's patient, so there is no doubt that such local databases should be created, maintained, and made accessible to treating physicians.

Observational data are less useful to obtain reliable, unbiased estimates of treatment effect. Another example from GRACE will be illustrative in this respect. In GRACE, 2407 patients underwent coronary angiography (CAG) within 24 h after hospital admission. In-hospital mortality in these patients was 3.5%, almost 2 times higher than the mortality figure of 1.8% that was observed in the 6446 patients who underwent CAG after 24 h (2005 report) [3]. Thus, at first glance, it seems justifiable to conclude that the strategy of early CAG (followed by early coronary revascularization if judged necessary) does not result in improved outcome compared with delayed CAG. On further consideration, however, we realize that the decision to opt for early CAG was made by the treating physician, who considered the individual characteristics and clinical course of particular patients, and judged them to be candidates for early intervention. In general, patients who are being selected

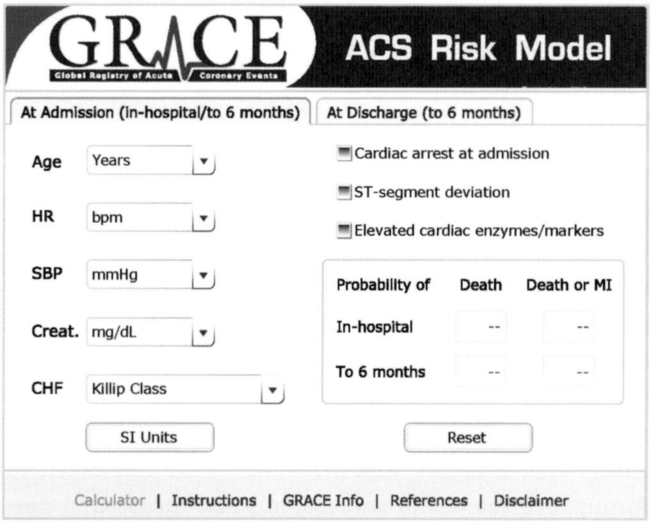

Figure 12.1 GRACE data entry screen.

for early management are in more urgent clinical need than those for whom treatment can be postponed. Thus, it is unfair to relate their outcomes directly to the applied treatment strategy. It is true that propensity analyses might be conducted, to adjust for factors that are associated with the decision to apply certain treatment. Also multivariate statistical analyses might be applied, to adjust for potential confounders. Still, these statistical techniques will only provide a suboptimal solution of the problem of selection and confounding, since unmeasured variables that might have influenced estimates of treatment effect remain, by definition, out of sight.

More reliable estimates of clinical treatment effects can be obtained by clinical experiments, particularly randomized clinical trials (RCTs). In patients who participate in an RCT, treatment decisions are not based on doctor or patient preferences, but depend only on drawing lots. In this way, separate patient cohorts are constructed with identical baseline characteristics, and their clinical course can directly be related to the allocated treatment. A total of six RCTs have been conducted to study the effectiveness of early CAG [4]. Altogether in these trials, patients who were allocated to early CAG had better clinical outcomes than their counterparts who were selected for conservative treatment: the incidence of in-hospital death or myocardial infarction (MI) was reduced by a factor of 0.84 (from 11.1% to 9.4%) [4].

In summary, systematic clinical observations are useful for the prediction of patient prognosis. Observational research may also result in estimates of treatment effects, but these should preferably be confirmed by clinical experiments.

Monitoring of quality of care, benchmarking, and quality improvement

To ensure that a diagnostic procedure, treatment, or intervention is really beneficial to patients in everyday clinical practice, a whole chain of functions is required (⊃Fig. 12.2). In recent years much focus has been on the earlier links in the chain: systematic research including RCTs, systematic reviews, and guidelines. Less attention has been given to the later links in the chain: implementation and follow-up of outcome and side effects in clinical practice. In order to ensure that evidence-based treatments are implemented throughout the health care system, that the desired outcomes are achieved, and that no unexpected side effects

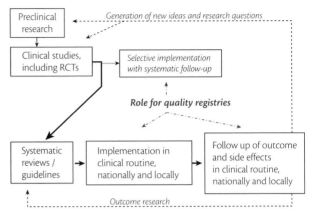

Figure 12.2 Functions needed for establishing an Evidence Based Health Care system and for systematic evaluation of the system. RCTs, randomized controlled trials.

appear, systematic registration of diagnostic and interventional procedures and patient outcome is critical. A description of the population in question is also necessary, to enable us interpret the results appropriately. In addition, studying and evaluating the health care in the 'real life' situation might generate important knowledge ('outcome research', see above), but also generate new research questions and ideas that can be a starting point for a new translational cycle.

Two different methods of obtaining such information are discussed next: surveys and continuous registries.

Surveys

A survey is here defined as a registration performed for a limited time, at a limited number of sites. The number of registered variables might vary. Provided that the patients included in the survey are a random sample of the centre-specific population, and provided the sample size is large enough, the results of the survey can be regarded as representative for that centre. Provided that the participating centres in a region/country are chosen randomly and there are enough of them, the results might be considered representative for that region/country. Surveys provide a 'snapshot' of a population at a particular point in time, and can be used to assess the prevalence of risk factors, acute or chronic conditions, applied treatments, and short-term outcomes.

Surveys have several advantages. Most important, a survey is an efficient way of collecting information from a large number of respondents, since they can easily be traced, and the collection and administration data is straightforward and inexpensive. Surveys are flexible in the sense that a wide range of information can be collected in a standardized way. Thus, surveys might be suitable for benchmarking of adherence to guidelines between countries, if enough patients in each country are included in order to get robust estimates.

Surveys also have several disadvantages. Since the participation in surveys of health care often is voluntary and the centres are not chosen randomly, it often remains uncertain to what extend the results can be generalized. Furthermore, surveys are less suitable for monitoring of adherence to guidelines on the hospital level, simply because it is seldom possible to include a sufficient number of cases at one hospital to get a statistically robust and representative sample. Finally, surveys usually do not include follow-up of outcomes and side effects outside the index hospitalization phase, nor are they suitable for supporting local quality improvement initiatives.

Many surveys that have been conducted in the recent past have provided valuable descriptions of the characteristics of different populations, as well as information on the use of diagnostic procedures and treatments. For example, the Euro Heart Surveys have given unique information on the use of diagnostic procedures and treatments in cardiology throughout Europe, and temporal trends in practice [5].

Continuous quality registries

In contrast to a survey, the aim of a continuous registry is to measure the 'total' population of interest. As for a survey, a continuous register might include a small or a large number of variables. In case of a national quality registry, the aim is to cover all units that manage patients with a certain disease or perform a certain intervention. The Swedish registry for coronary angiography and PCI is an example of a registry that covers 100% of all units and nearly 100% of all patients undergoing coronary angiography and/or PCI. The strength of a continuous registry with complete coverage is that there is no uncertainty in the results, because it covers the entire population. For example, in two hospitals the registry might show that in a given year 5 out of a total 50 patients with acute myocardial infarction (AMI) died within 30 days at one of the hospitals, and 15 out of 300 patients died in the other hospital. Thus the mortality in that particular year for these two hospitals was 10% and 5%, respectively. No less, no more. Obviously, however, factors unrelated to the quality of care might be very important for explaining the results, e.g. a few extra elderly patients with cardiogenic shock at presentation that particular year at the first hospital might explain the higher mortality.

From another perspective, a continuous registry can in some instances be regarded as a 'sample'. For example, the results of AMI treatment in Sweden might be regarded as a sample of the results of AMI treatment in Europe, and the out-come results after PCI in the year 2009 might be regarded as a sample of the outcome after PCI in the whole decade. Thus, the results derived from a continuous registry in one hospital or one region might give information that is valuable for other regions or hospitals. Still, it must be kept in mind that the sample is seldom random, and interpretation must be cautious.

Continuous data collection can be cumbersome and resource intensive. There is therefore currently much emphasis is on efforts to automate the data collection process by integrating the registries with electronic patient records.

Monitoring of quality of care and benchmarking

The health care system includes actions or processes undertaken by professionals that might influence patient outcome, including diagnostic procedures and pharmacological and nonpharmacological treatments. That is why process measurements, such as the adherence to guideline recommendations, are commonly used for monitoring of quality of care. When constructing a process indicator it is important to consider the target population for the process. For example, when assessing the adherence to ACE inhibitor treatment after AMI, the indicator should not show the proportion that receives an ACE inhibitor among all AMI patients, but only among those patients for whom the guidelines recommend its use.

Monitoring of the quality of care can be done on different levels, ranging from a whole nation to a local hospital unit. ⮞ Figure 12.3a gives an example of an outcome quality indicator. It shows that 30-day mortality after AMI has decreased steadily over the last decade, both in Sweden as a whole and at the local hospital level. ⮞ Figure 12.3b illustrates a process quality indicator: the application of reperfusion in ST-elevation AMI. It nicely demonstrates that the use of primary PCI has increased and the use of thrombolysis has decreased.

The possibility of benchmarking is an important feature of most quality registries and surveys (⮞ Table 12.1), since it stimulates clinicians and centres to improve their performance. Ideally the quality that is delivered by local health care systems—and thus benchmarking—should be assessed by its effect on relevant outcomes, such as mortality, morbidity, and quality of life. However, since patient outcome also depends on factors that cannot be modified by the system, including age and socio-economic factors, the interpretation of outcome measures is a major challenge. Generally, it is easier to compare process measures than outcome measures. For centre-to-centre outcome comparisons, appropriate adjustments of case mix are mandatory [5]. There are several methods for adjusting case mix; for an example of an useful and illustrative method see [6].

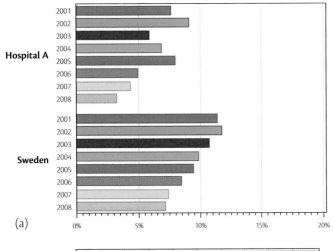

(a)

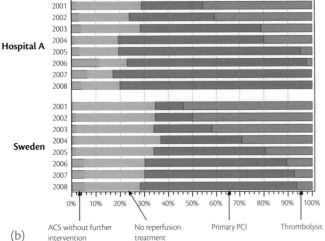

(b)

Figure 12.3 Monitoring of the quality of care: (a) 30-day mortality after AMI (outcome indicator) from 2001 to 2008 at an individual hospital and nationwide, respectively. (b) Use of different reperfusion treatments in acute ST-Elevation Myocardial Infarction (process indicator) from 2001 to 2008 at an individual hospital and nationwide, respectively. ACS, acute coronary syndrome; PCI, percutaneous coronary intervention.

Table 12.1 Reoperations due to bleeding after primary heart surgery during the year 2008

Centre	Patients	Reoperations	
	N	N	%
A	1215	99	8.1
B	342	16	4.7
C	690	32	4.6
D	1056	51	4.8
E	1111	51	4.6
F	824	40	4.9
G	653	55	8.4
H	496	32	6.5
Sweden (total)	6387	376	5.9

Source: Swedish Registry for Heart Surgery.

Management of care

Quality registries might be used for assisting in the management of health care, on both a local and a national level. In a cardiology department regular compilations of relevant quality indicators derived from the registry may help to identify areas that need special attention. ➔ Figure 12.4 shows a compilation of 11 quality indicators that are provided in every participating hospital on a monthly basis. It is immediately obvious that this particular cardiology department needs to focus on a faster delivery of primary PCI, since only 40% of the target patients receive primary PCI within the goal of 60 min, whereas satisfactory results are observed for several other indicators. On a regional or national level health authorities might use compilations of relevant quality indicators derived from registries to identify areas that prompt special efforts.

Supporting quality improvement

In order to be able to deliver the best possible quality of the health care within the available resources, a profound knowledge of medical and organizational issues is required. In all quality improvement work it is essential to measure the performance before and after a change is implemented, and to feed back the results immediately. Therefore, continuous registries might be valuable tools in local quality improvement efforts. However, the registry must provide reports that give immediate feedback of the local performance in a form that supports the quality improvement work. Control charts are most useful for this purpose [6], showing the performance in the target population over time. Examples of a control chart

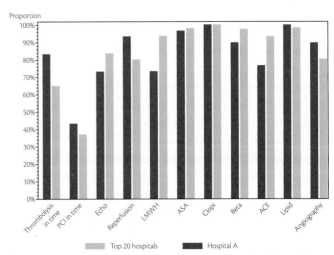

Figure 12.4 Quality at a glance: comparison of the results of 11 quality indicators in a local hospital with the results of the best 20 hospitals in the country. LMWH, low molecular weight heparin; ASA, aspirin; Clopi, clopidogrel; ACE, ACE inhibitor; Lipid, lipid lowering therapy.

available in the Swedish registry for AMI (RIKS-HIA) are shown in ➲ Fig. 12.5. Apparently, the change implemented resulted in improved adherence to treatment. There are several other examples of successful quality improvement initiatives that used a quality registry for the measurements [5].

Pitfalls

The quality of measurements in surveys and continuous registries depend on the informants' motivation, honesty, memory, and ability to respond. Failure to include a patient in the survey or registry might bias the results, especially if patients with certain characteristics are systematically excluded. It goes without saying that selection bias is deleterious when the data are used for benchmarking. Likewise, missing data weakens the validity and reliability of the results. In some instances the informants might in fact, be motivated to give answers that present themselves or their hospital in a favourable light. Efforts should be made to optimize the quality of the data in the registry. This might be achieved by having compulsory variables and logical controls of the data built in to the computer system, but regular manual review of a random sample of registrations by independent monitors is also a possibility.

Tips and tricks for running registries and building databases

As we have seen, systematic documentation of clinical practice by surveys or registries can provide important insights into the transferability of RCT results to groups of patients who have been excluded from trials, and can play a key role in quality assurance. Systematic documentation also allows verification of guideline implementation, whereas regular benchmarking can help to improve guideline adherence. Obviously, the quality of the surveys or registries, and thus the usefulness of the observed results, depends on the methods that are used to collect the appropriate data. In this section, we summarize the main steps in successfully designing and conducting a survey or registry (summarized in ➲ Table 12.2).

Identification of relevant topics, and of objectives

The first step in the design of a survey or registry is the identification of the topic of interest. In contrast to epidemiological studies such as the Framingham Study, which are population based, surveys and registries in cardiology focus on specific diseases. As in RCTs, a scientific committee should define the objectives of the survey or registry. These objectives might be more general, such as the documentation of applied treatment of ACS in clinical practice, or

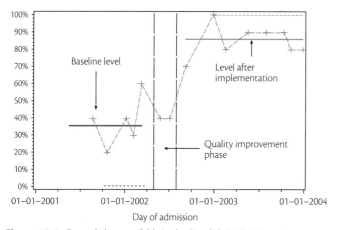

Figure 12.5 Control chart available in the Swedish RIKS-HIA registry showing the percentage of patients with Acute Myocardial Infarction at a particular hospital receiving clopidogrel at discharge before, during and after an intervention aiming at increasing the adherence to the national guidelines.

Table 12.2 Checklist for creating and running registries

To do	Example
Identification of topic	ACS
Definition of objectives	Documentation of current treatment/adherence to practice guidelines
Definition of inclusion/exclusion criteria	Consecutive patients with ACS Ideally no exclusion criteria to reflect current practice
Design of CRF	Ideally Internet-based data capture Use existing data standards/definitions Reflect that data captured can address the objectives
Design of study protocol	As short as possible including: Brief introduction Objectives Inclusion/exclusion criteria CRF Publication policy
Privacy and confidentiality	Anonymized data Ethical votes based on local needs
Selection of participating centres	Representative sample if possible Random choice
Data validation	Front-end quality checks Quality control programs as prelude to the finalized analysis data set
Audits	Predefined sample of randomly selected centres Audit consecutive enrolment and correctness of data entry

ACS, acute coronary syndrome; CRF, case record form.

more specific, such as the report of bleeding complications in relation to different treatment patterns of ACS patients. The expert committee ideally consists of clinical investigators who provide content expertise and leadership, and of methodologically and statistically aware investigators, who provide guidance on all aspects of statistical analysis even in this planning phase.

Funding

The expert committee should take care of the funding of the survey or registry. Possible resources might be public funds or industry sponsors. Beside the central costs for running the survey or registry, the expert committee has to decide if reimbursement of the centres is needed, dependent on the workload associated with the enrolment of patients. Independent of the resources of funding, the expert committee will be responsible for the scientific analysis of the data, avoiding any influence from sponsors.

Definition of inclusion and exclusion criteria

As the results that any survey or registry will obtain depend on how the data is collected, concise inclusion criteria have to be defined by the expert committee. Dependent on the disease to be documented, the complexity of the inclusion criteria will vary. As an example, it will be easy to define the inclusion criteria for an AMI registry (admission to hospital with MI), but more difficult to define inclusion criteria for an atrial fibrillation registry (new onset?, persistent?, permanent?, paroxysmal?). Ideally, surveys and registries should avoid excluding any patients, as enrolment of consecutive patients is one of their main strengths.

Design of the case record form

It is highly recommended that data are collected via a remote, web-based data management system. The electronic case record form (CRF) should reflect all necessary parameters to address the objectives of the survey or registry, but at the same time be as short and concise as possible to increase its acceptance by the investigators. In international surveys or registries, the software used should support multilingual CRFs. In some countries privacy laws prohibit certain questions or restrict the amount of identifying data that can be collected, so the electronic CRF may have to be adjusted to country-specific requirements. If available, international standards for data collection should be used, like the European 'Cardiology Audit and Registration Data Standards' (CARDS) [7], to ensure consistency and

comparability of data collected across the countries. Data on patients and procedures that are available in hospital information systems should ideally be copied automatically into the survey or registry database to avoid double data entry, and to avoid mismatch between the database and the source. To ensure the integrity and analytic utility of the study data, standardized data management procedures are necessary. Data quality assurance will include handling rules for missing or incomplete data, plausibility controls, and range checks, along with data transformations. In surveys or registries documenting newly approved medications, the CRF should fulfil the necessary requirements recommended by the regulatory authorities to adequately document possible complications of any new compound in clinical practice.

Follow-up

Data on clinical outcome of patients in daily practice is of the utmost importance. Therefore, surveys and registries should ideally collect follow-up information. The timing of the follow-up will be dependent on the disease monitored. Follow-up data might be collected by the enrolling centre and provided to the central database or collected centrally by a single institution responsible for the entire study population. Telephone contacts directly with the patient are a common and effective way to collect valid follow-up information. In case a patient cannot be reached, the investigator should try to obtain follow-up information from the patient's family or primary care physician.

Selection of participating centres

Which centres to invite for participation in a survey or registry depends on the patient population to be enrolled. For some questions outpatient clinics might be the best settings; in other cases hospitals would be the better choice. If representativeness is warranted, a randomized selection of hospitals or clinics should be strongly encouraged; community-wide data collection would even be better.

Data validation and quality

A site management team should be responsible for training the sites on all aspects of the study and being a resource for data collection questions and query resolution. This team will also closely monitor patient enrolment and data submission at each site and make calls, as necessary, to stimulate enrolment and data submission. We propose to develop two strategies for data quality checks: validations that occur at the time of data entry (i.e. front-end) and a second, more sophisticated quality control program that runs as a prelude to the creation of the analysis data set.

Front-end data checks are advantageous because mistakes are caught and corrected at the time of entry; a system that is efficient for data collectors as it minimizes any 'annoyance' factor to the user. Certain data elements can be required, while other variables may allow for missing values. Additionally, parameters will be defined to allow entry of only those records that meet inclusion criteria.

Data management and quality control

Before the analytic data is created, more extensive quality control processes are needed. These checks include parent–child edits, consistency edits, and data transformations that will facilitate analyses.

To ensure consecutive enrolment and correctness of data entry, randomly selected centres should be audited.

Confidentiality and privacy considerations

All surveys and registries should be conducted in accordance with the European Union Note for Guidance on Good Clinical Practice CPMP/ECH/135/95 and the Declaration of Helsinki. Ethical approval should be obtained according to the rules of national or local review boards if necessary. Usually, the patient data collected should not contain name, date of birth, or address information. The data that participating centres use to identify the patients is a case ID (pre-generated by the software), year of birth, and date of admission. The analysis data sets must be stored on secure servers, and access to the database should be limited to authorized personnel of the study. The data will be fully anonymized after database closure and final analysis. At this point, European privacy laws no longer apply to the data set and the data is considered destroyed.

Data analysis

The database should be analysed by experienced statisticians in close cooperation with the steering committee addressing the predefined objectives of the survey or registry. A report including descriptive statistics of all documented parameters will be generated for the overall patient population. Patients violating any inclusion/exclusion criteria will be deleted from the analysis data set.

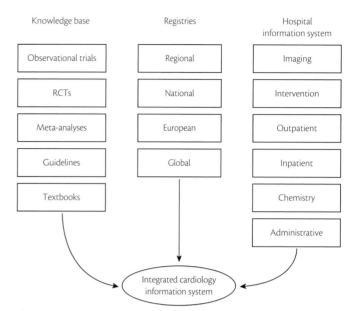

Figure 12.6 Integrated cardiology information system.

In order to avoid data-driven analysis (and the corresponding chance findings), all statistical analyses should preferably be specified in the protocol. Some of the methodological and statistical issues inherent to survey and registry analyses include selection bias, small sample sizes, and missing data.

Conclusion

Patient-oriented databases form the cornerstone of evidence-based medicine. Systematic clinical observations based on these data sets are useful for the development of risk-prediction tools. Observational research might also result in estimates of treatment effects, although these should preferably be confirmed by clinical experiments. Systematic registration of patient characteristics, applied diagnostic and interventional procedures, and patient outcome are essential not only for the development, but also for the implementation of evidence-based treatments. In the recent past, several instruments have been developed to attain both goals, including a wealth of local databases, national and international short-lived surveys, and continuous (quality) registries. We advocate the integration of these data depositories in order to provide practising physicians with a tool to deliver the best available treatment to each individual patient.

Personal perspective

Physicians base their patient management on knowledge obtained during their training. However, medicine in general, and clinical cardiology in particular, is rapidly evolving, and clinicians are challenged to keep their knowledge up to date with new research results. That is why cardiology professional associations, such as the European Society of Cardiology, intensively invest in the development and education of practical treatment guidelines, which summarize the evidence of the usefulness of treatment that has emerged from clinical research. Still, even with the guidelines at hand it might be quite a task to systematically apply EBM. For example, guidelines for ischaemic heart disease contain almost 500 recommendations [8], and it is unrealistic to assume that physicians will be able to adhere to all of these without further assistance.

The fundamental question that needs to be answered is, 'How can we translate results that are observed in well-designed clinical trials into everyday clinical practice, in the best interests of each individual patient?' We envisage that an 'intelligent' integrated cardiology information system (ICIS) may provide a solution. ➲ Figure 12.6 illustrates different sources of information that may be used by the practising clinician in an integrated manner. Clinical trials and meta-analyses provide information on expected treatment effects, registries provide data on patient prognosis, the local hospital information system provides details on the local situation, including the availability of resources. An ICIS may help the clinician to overcome problems with unawareness, accessibility, and interpretation of data sources. The system may force the clinician to notice (patient characteristics, treatment, and outcome), remember (results of past patients), learn (from what is remembered), interpret (models), and act (to improve patient management and outcome).

Further reading

Embi PJ, Kaufman SE, Payne PR. Biomedical informatics and outcome research: enabling knowledge-driven health care. *Circulation* 2009;**120**:2393–2399.

Fazel R, Krumholz HM, Bates ER, *et al*. National Registry of Myocardial Infarction (NRMI) Investigators. Choice of reperfusion strategy at hospitals with primary percutaneous coronary intervention: a National Registry of Myocardial Infarction analysis. *Circulation* 2009;**120**:2455–2461.

Gitt AK, Bueno H, Danchin N, *et al*. The role of cardiac registries in evidence-based medicine. *Eur Heart J* 2010;**31**:525–529.

Granger C, Gersh BJ. Clinical trials and registries in cardiovascular disease: competitive or complementary? *Eur Heart J* 2010;**31**:520–521.

Hersh WR. Medical informatics: improving health care through information. *JAMA* 2002;**288**:1955–1958.

Jenkins KJ, Beekman III RH, Bergersen LJ, *et al*. Databases for assessing the outcomes of the treatment of patients with congenital and paediatric cardiac disease—the perspective of cardiology. *Cardiol Young* 2008;**18**:116–123.

Kotseva K, Wood D, De Backer G, *et al*. EUROASPIRE Study Group. Cardiovascular prevention guidelines in daily practice: a comparison of EUROASPIRE I, II, and III surveys in eight European countries. *Lancet* 2009;**373**:929–940.

Motovska Z, Kala P. Benefits and risks of clopidogrel use in patients with coronary artery disease: evidence from randomized studies and registries. *Clin Ther* 2008;**30**:2191–2202.

Peterson ED, Roe MT, Rumsfeld JS, *et al*. A call to ACTION (acute coronary treatment and intervention outcomes network): a national effort to promote timely clinical feedback and support continuous quality improvement for acute myocardial infarction. *Circ Cardiovasc Qual Outcomes* 2009;**2**:491–499.

Scott IA. Why we need a national registry in interventional cardiology. *Med J* 2008;**189**:223–227.

Simoons ML, van der Putten N, Wood D, *et al*. The Cardiology Information System: the need for data standards for integration of systems for patient care, registries and guidelines for clinical practice. *Eur Heart J* 2002;**23**:1148–1152.

Stenestrand U, Lindbäck J, Wallentin L. RIKS-HIA Registry. Long-term outcome of primary percutaneous coronary intervention vs prehospital and in-hospital thrombolysis for patients with ST-elevation myocardial infarction. *JAMA* 2006;**296**:1749–1756.

Yusuf S, Flather M, Pogue J, *et al*. Variations between countries in invasive cardiac procedures and outcomes in patients with suspected unstable angina or myocardial infarction without initial ST elevation. OASIS (Organisation to Assess Strategies for Ischaemic Syndromes) Registry Investigators. *Lancet* 1998;**352**:507–514.

➲ For additional multimedia materials please visit the online version of the book (✏ http://www.esciacc.oxfordmedicine.com).

CHAPTER 13

Ethical issues in cardiac arrest and acute cardiac care: a European perspective

Leo Bossaert and Jan Bahr

Summary

Cardiac arrest constitutes a situation that focuses major ethical challenges in both the in-hospital and out-of-hospital settings. Although this situation is characterized by the necessity of immediate action and by the lack of reliable tools to predict outcome, the key ethical principles (autonomy, beneficence, nonmaleficence, justice) have to be considered, mainly in the context of withholding or withdrawing cardiopulmonary resuscitation (CPR). Advance directives may translate the ethical principles into practice; however, their application is often restricted by the need for timely interventions, especially in an out-of-hospital setting, and their legal power varies considerably throughout Europe. Important related ethical issues are euthanasia and organ donation.

Leading international resuscitation organizations such as the European Resuscitation Council (ERC) and the American Heart Association (AHA) have provided guidelines and recommendations on when to start or not to start CPR, and when to stop it. These guidelines are updated regularly and are easily accessible, but their implementation and application vary substantially, with local practice, culture, religion, society, and legislation being the main influencing factors.

The health care provider should understand the ethical principles and the context of individual, cultural, legal, social, and economic factors before being involved in a real situation where resuscitation decisions must be made. Therefore, this chapter deals with the key ethical principles and the factors that influence their implementation; the decision to start, withhold, or stop CPR; and the perspective of organ donation.

Ethics is dealing with how humans should act or behave. It is also about what is morally right or wrong, good or bad, which depends on time, place, culture, and other factors that are related to the patient and the caregiver and to external circumstances. This chapter will consider ethical aspects of emergency cardiac care when dealing with the acute situation of adult cardiac arrest and in situations where resuscitation efforts appear inappropriate or unsuccessful.

Sudden death, cardiac arrest, and the process of dying

Sudden cardiac death or cardiac arrest is the cessation of cardiac mechanical activity as confirmed by the absence of signs of circulation [1]. The nature, the mechanism, and the context of the potentially reversible sudden death syndrome should not be confused with the expected cessation of circulation and respiration at the end of a chronic condition.

Sudden death is a catastrophic unexpected event that may happen outside or inside the hospital. Outside the hospital, cardiac arrest is frequently initiated by ventricular fibrillation and has the potential to be successfully resuscitated, but the conditions are usually unfavourable: the arrest may or may not be witnessed by a partner or family member with some knowledge of cardiopulmonary resuscitation (CPR); the efficiency of the telephone call to the emergency number is variable; sometimes there is an automatic external defibrillator (AED) around; and after a more or less short time professional help will arrive with the EMS (emergency medical services) ambulance. Inside the hospital there is frequently comorbidity, but the external conditions are more favourable: expert health care professionals and resuscitation equipment are readily available within a short time, and the intensive care unit (ICU) is a short distance away.

Although the two settings are very different, the decision to start CPR or not, and to continue it or not, need to be made by the first health care provider. This is an individual responsibility to ensure the best chance of survival for those patients who may benefit but also to avoid prolonged suffering and waste of resources in cases where CPR is not indicated. These decisions are made in the perspective of scientific evidence, legislation, religion, culture, medical context, preferences and skills and beliefs of the rescuer, and preferences of the patient and the societal environment.

Nonmedical health care providers usually apply precise rules (standing orders), but medically qualified rescuers are expected to use their expert knowledge and judgement. It is their responsibility to use their judgement, not as an excuse for inconsequential behaviour or ad hoc decisions inspired by convenience or other nonmedical arguments, but with knowledge of current scientific evidence and according to the principles of ethical practice. These decisions should be guided by general ethical principles and modulated according to influencing factors.

Many national and international organizations have issued recommendations, but implementation of these recommendations among individual health care professionals, EMS systems, emergency departments (EDs), and hospitals is variable. Differences in national legislation and medical practice and social changes are obstacles to the production of uniform rules or flowcharts for starting or not starting CPR, continuing or not continuing it. This should not, however, serve as an excuse for not adhering to a consequentially implemented policy.

In Europe each year, between 4 and 10 per 10 000 inhabitants per year suffer out-of-hospital cardiac arrest (OoHCA): this represents between 350 000 and 700 000 people. Overall survival is low, with an average of less than 10%. The majority of these events occur at home, mostly in the presence of a witness. Cardiac arrest victims who are found in ventricular fibrillation have higher chances for survival: restoration of spontaneous circulation (ROSC) may be achieved in up to 50% of cases and eventual survival to hospital discharge may be up to 20% and even 30%, depending on the process of prehospital and in-hospital care [2, 3]. But the chance of survival decreases rapidly as time to defibrillation becomes longer.

Less accurate data are available about cardiac arrest *inside the hospital*. The incidence of cardiac arrest is estimated 0.175 per bed per year, or 1–5 per 1000 admissions per year. Although the underlying disease is different from OoHCA (comorbidity, endstage respiratory, neurologic, and metabolic disease), long-term survival from in-hospital cardiac arrest is similar to that for out-of-hospital cardiac arrest (average 20%).

More than 20% of hospital deaths follow admission to an ICU [4–7]. Frequently, patients unlikely to benefit from intensive care are admitted, leading to needless prolongation of the dying process, suffering for the patient and family, and unnecessary waste of resources.

In the in-hospital context more information is available about the medical condition, the prognosis, and the personal preferences, allowing a balanced decision to start or continue CPR.

Ethical principles are universal

Decisions on CPR and end of life are based on universally accepted ethical principles, but the implementation of these principles is influenced by the context and by individual, cultural, legal, social, and economic factors.

Health care providers should understand these ethical principles before being involved in a real situation where resuscitation decisions must be made. The key ethical principles of autonomy, justice, beneficence, and nonmaleficence [9] are the basis of the declarations of human rights [10, 11] (➲ Box 13.1) and reflect the principles of our individual behaviour in medical practice as expressed in the Hippocratic Oath [8].

Universal ethical principles

♦ Autonomy implies that a patient has the right to take informed decisions on future treatment. This implies also that the patient is adequately informed, competent, and free of pressure.

♦ Justice implies that the access to essential health care, including resuscitation, must be distributed equally within the society according to the available resources.

♦ Beneficence implies that health care must provide benefit to the individual or to society, taking into account the balance between benefit and risk.

♦ Nonmaleficence implies that no harm must be done. Resuscitation should not be applied if it is futile or if it is against the patient's wishes.

Definitions relating to end-of-life decisions

♦ Withholding a treatment is defined as a decision not to start a life-sustaining intervention, such as CPR.

♦ Withdrawing a treatment is defined as stopping a life-sustaining intervention that is currently provided.

Box 13.1 The Human Rights Conventions of the World Medical Association and of the Council of Europe

♦ The interests and welfare of the human being prevail over the sole interest of society or science.

♦ Parties shall take appropriate measures to provide equitable access to health care of appropriate quality.

♦ Any intervention in the health field, including research, must be carried out in accordance with relevant professional obligations and standards.

♦ Any intervention in the health field may only be carried out after the person (or representative) concerned has given free and informed consent to it.

♦ When because of an emergency situation the appropriate consent cannot be obtained, any medically necessary intervention may be carried out immediately for the benefit of the health of the individual concerned.

♦ The previously expressed wishes relating to a medical intervention by a patient who is not, at the time of the intervention, in a state to express his/her wishes shall be taken into account.

♦ Shortening of the dying process is defined as an act with the specific intention to actively shorten the dying process.

♦ Futility is defined as an intervention that cannot establish any increase in length or quality of life. If the purpose of a treatment cannot be achieved, the treatment is futile.

Definitions relating to advance directives and do-not-(attempt)-resuscitation orders

Advance directives, sometimes known as living wills, and do-not-(attempt)-resuscitation (DN(A)R) declarations, are a direct translation of these key principles and conventions into practice. But although all European countries and religions support the principle that resuscitation should not be attempted in case of endstage disease or injury, only a minority of countries have adopted a formal DN(A)R policy, and advance directives are more an exception than a rule.

Although the principles of advance directives and DNR orders are identical for the out-of-hospital and the in-hospital situation, the application in clinical practice will be fundamentally different according to this context:

♦ In out-of-hospital cardiac arrest the timely administration of CPR, defibrillation, and advanced resuscitation interventions is critical. Decisions need to be made in seconds, and delay of intervention is sanctioned by decreased outcome. CPR should be initiated unless there are evident contraindications of futility or refusal.

♦ Inside the hospital, there has been time to reflect and to ascertain the patient's well-informed preferences about end-of life decisions. In the critical care unit the medical history and the preferences of the individual patient are even better known and there has been time to place the treatment strategies in the appropriate legal, religious, individual, and medical perspective [12, 13].

There is considerable international variation in the medical attitude to written advance directives. In some countries they are considered legally binding; in other countries they are ignored if the doctor does not agree with the contents. However, in recent years there has been a growing tendency towards compliance with patient autonomy and a reduction in patronizing attitudes by the medical profession.

Predicting outcome

The objective of the key ethical principle of 'justice' implies giving the best care to the patients who are likely to benefit, and to avoid useless and costly interventions that prolong suffering in hopeless situations ('futility').

Many investigators have tried to develop a reliable algorithm for identifying those cardiac arrest patients who have a high potential and those who have only a dismal chance, or none, of survival. This might allow the health care provider to decide on starting or not starting, continuing or not continuing CPR. However, most methods seem to have good sensitivity but low specificity.

The OPALS study [14], for example, looked into the predictive value of termination of resuscitation (TOR) guidelines for identifying 'futility' in out-of-hospital cardiac arrest, defining 'futile' as an intervention with less than 1% chance of benefit. The following elements had a high predictive potential:

- Event not witnessed by EMS personnel.
- No AED or manual defibrillation applied in the out-of-hospital setting.
- No ROSC in the out-of-hospital setting.
- Arrest not witnessed by a bystander.
- No bystander-administered CPR.

The sensitivity of these guidelines for predicting futility was high (99%), but specificity was low (ranging between 10 and 53%); these findings where confirmed in other studies [15–20]. These data were generated in North America and extrapolation to other regions and EMS systems should be made with care, because of major differences in systems, organization, qualification, and legislation.

As a result, there are no validated reliable tools that allow us to predict early the outcome from cardiac arrest with an acceptable accuracy in an individual case.

Guidelines and recommendations

In the 2005 guidelines for CPR and emergency cardiovascular care, both the European Resuscitation Council (ERC) and the American Heart Association (AHA) provide recommendations for the care provider about starting, not starting, and stopping CPR. The guidelines are currently being updated and the 2010 CPR guidelines can be downloaded from the websites of the ERC (https://www.erc.edu/index.php/mainpage/en/) and AHA.

European Resuscitation Council guidelines

In its CPR guidelines [21], the ERC emphasizes that a well-informed, competent patient has the right to refuse treatment, but this does not imply that a patient has the right to demand any treatment in all circumstances.

ERC recommendations for withholding CPR and DN(A)R orders

- A physician is expected to provide treatment that is likely to benefit the patient and not to provide treatment that would be futile. Futility exists if resuscitation will be of no benefit in terms of prolonging life of acceptable quality. However, no validated tools for predicting non-survival after attempted resuscitation are available.

- Therefore, judgements will have to be made, and there will be grey areas where subjective opinions are required in patients with end stage disease, asphyxia or major trauma. The age of the patient is a weak predictor of outcome, but age is frequently associated with comorbidity.

ERC recommendation for stopping a CPR attempt

The ERC recommends to consider stopping a CPR attempt

- if it is evident that CPR is futile (not likely to be beneficial)
- if there is an advance directive
- if asystole persists after at least 20 min of full advanced life support.

This implies that in OoHCA CPR should be initiated while collecting information.

The decision to abandon the resuscitation attempt is made by the team leader, after consultation with the other team members. Many cases of out-of-hospital cardiac arrest are dealt with by emergency medical technicians or paramedics, who face dilemmas of when to determine if resuscitation is futile and when it should be abandoned. Clearly resuscitation is futile in cases of cardiac arrest with a mortal condition such as decapitation, incineration, rigor mortis, dependent lividity, and fetal maceration. In such cases the nonphysician is making a diagnosis of death but is not certifying death (which can only be done by a physician in most countries).

When considering abandoning the resuscitation attempt, the possibility of prolonging CPR and other resuscitative measures to allow organ donation to take place should be taken into account. The issue of initiating life-prolonging treatment with the sole purpose of harvesting organs is debated by ethicists and no consensus exists.

Also, it should be noted that the introduction of therapeutic hypothermia after cardiac arrest may have changed the predictive algorithms, and caution should be taken until new predictive values have been established for these patients.

In 2010 the ERC updated the CPR guidelines, after a systematic review by the International Liaison Committee on Resuscitation (ILCOR) of the scientific developments that have taken place since 2005. This science review is published as the ILCOR Consensus on Science and Treatment Recommendations (COSTR) document and provides ILCOR members with the common science on which to base their updated 2010 CPR guidelines. These documents are available on the ERC website (http://www.erc.edu).

American Heart Association guidelines

In the AHA guidelines for CPR and emergency cardiovascular care[22], guidance is provided to health care providers for making the decision to provide or withhold emergency cardiovascular care. This guidance is based on the goals of emergency cardiovascular care: to preserve life, restore health, relieve suffering, limit disability, and reverse clinical death.

The AHA emphasizes that truly informed decisions require that patients receive and understand accurate information about their condition and prognosis, the nature of the interventions, and the risks and benefits. When patients' preferences are uncertain, emergency conditions should be treated until those preferences can be clarified.

The Patient Self-determination Act of 1991 implies that health care institutions should inquire whether the patient has advance directives and that they facilitate the completion of these directives.

American College of Critical Care Medicine recommendations

The American College of Critical Care Medicine and the Society of Critical Care Medicine have published recommendations for end-of-life care in the ICU [23]. It is emphasized that ICU clinicians should be competent in all aspects of end-of-life care, including the practical and ethical aspects of withdrawing different modalities of life-sustaining treatment, and the use of sedatives, analgesics, and nonpharmacological approaches to easing the suffering of the dying person.

The key ethical principles for this care include the distinction between withholding and withdrawing treatment, between actions of actively terminating life and allowing to die, and between consequences that are intended versus those that are merely foreseen (the doctrine of double effect).

Implementation of universal principles in different European countries

Many investigators have studied the implementation of these principles, guidelines and recommendations in clinical practice. The plethora of reports underlines the wide divergence in the interpretation and application [12, 24–29].

Most European countries have signed the Oviedo Convention and the Declaration of Helsinki for the protection of human rights and dignity [10, 11]. However, so far, many countries have not introduced specific legislation to implement these recommendations. Some have rather progressive legislation, such as the Netherlands and Belgium, whereas others have more conservative legislation. As a result, it is still difficult in many countries to provide physicians with legal guidance on decisions about end-of-life caring, regarding limiting or withholding support in critically ill patients.

Baskett and Lim [24] reviewed the attitudes of experienced emergency health care providers about ethical issues in resuscitation in 20 European countries. They observed a widespread divergence of views on ethical aspects of resuscitation that are not always in line with the conventionally perceived national characteristics. Only a minority of countries had a formal DNAR policy, although virtually all reported not attempting resuscitation in patients with an endstage disease or injury. Advance directives were in use in only a minority of countries, and there is a considerable amount of individual variation. The majority felt that it is probably not possible in these critical situations to ensure really informed consent, and that doctors, nurses, patients, and relatives may have different perceptions of the situation. Active euthanasia was legal in three countries, but many responders reported on a liberal use of analgesia and sedation in patients with endstage disease or injury. In deciding to stop resuscitation attempts, almost all respondents abandoned resuscitation after 20 min of asystole in the absence of reversible causes; but the majority were also reluctant to leave the application of this rule to the responsibility of ambulance personnel who are not medically qualified.

Surveys in European ICUs by the European Society for Intensive Care Medicine (ESICM) documented that decisions to withdraw or withhold treatment vary substantially, depending on local practice, cultural and religious backgrounds, legal frameworks, organization of ICUs, national and societal guidelines, and even family or peer pressure [27, 30, 31]. The ETHICUS study [12] investigated patients admitted to ICUs in European countries. Of the admitted patients, 13.5% died and 10% had limitations of treatment. Substantial differences between countries were found in the limitation of therapy and in the manner of dying. Age, diagnosis, region, religion, and length of stay were most significantly associated with limitation of therapy versus continuation of life-sustaining treatment.

Specific information on end-of-life practice and law in European countries is also available in a series of articles in the journal of the ESICM and in national recommendations [32–37].

In recent studies a high involvement of intensive care nurses in the end-of-life (EOL) decision-making process in Europe has been reported. The opinions about practical modalities for EOL were consistent for many aspects such as oxygen treatment and presence of family, but were divergent for sedation and nutritional support. This is an encouraging evolution after the rather sobering findings in an earlier study, where the process of EOL decision-making was perceived as satisfactory by 73% of physicians but by only 33% of nurses [38, 39].

Others have investigated the wide variability in the acceptance of euthanasia by the general public. Religious beliefs, socio-demographic factors, and moral values (i.e. the belief in the right to self-determination) could largely explain the differences between countries, but national traditions and history were also major contributors. These variables might amount to the global 'culture' of a given population [25].

In most surveys, religion appears as a constant factor with a significant impact on the attitudes of patients and care providers. In 2005, the *Lancet* published a series of articles devoted to the position of religions on EOL care [40]. These positions were recently updated [41]: today, many religions have spread worldwide and with increasing mobility and globalization, health care providers should understand the religious beliefs of their patients well when dealing with EOL decisions. Religious authorities have expressed their opinions about decisions to withhold or to withdraw vital treatment, the principle of futility, the notion of brain death, the dual effect of analgesia and sedation, DNAR orders, advance directives, and euthanasia (⊃ Table 13.1). The purpose of medicine is to ensure 'a good life and a good death'. Religious doctrines and beliefs should therefore be considered as an important element in our medico-scientific approach to EOL care.

Save the patient, save the organs

Death and brain death

Diagnosis of death is essential if organ removal for transplantation is considered. This concept is also known as the 'dead donor' rule [42]. According to cardiorespiratory criteria, death is clinically defined as the irreversible loss of all cardiorespiratory activity. In the absence of external conditions (hypothermia, drugs) or in conditions indicating reversibility, cessation of oxygen delivery to the brain will lead within minutes to brain death. According to the Harvard neurologic criteria, brain death is defined as the irreversible and complete loss of all activity of the brain [43]. Diagnosis of brain death implies the following steps:

- Establish the aetiology of the underlying disease.
- Exclude potentially reversible conditions, such as hypothermia, metabolic disturbances or drugs that can lead to potentially reversible coma.
- Clinical diagnosis of coma, brainstem areflexia and apnoea.
- Confirmation procedure (repetition, multiple physicians, technical procedures such as EEG, evoked potentials, angiography, Doppler sonography, scintigraphy).

Table 13.1 Religious attitudes to end-of-life decisions

	Withhold	Withdraw	Organ donation	Dual effect	Euthanasia
Catholic	Y	Y	N	Y	N
Protestant	Y	Y	Y	Y	Y
Orthodox	N	N	Y	N	N
Muslim	Y	Y	Y	Y	N
Jew	Y	N	Y	Y	N
Buddhist	Y	Y	N	Y	N
Hindu	Y	Y	Variable	Y	N

Y, yes, accepted; N, no, not accepted.

Adapted from End-of-Life series, *Lancet* 2005;**366**: August–October, and Bülow H, *et al.* The world's major religions' points of view on end-of-life decisions in the intensive care unit. *Intensive Care Med* 2008;**34**:423–430.

This step-by-step approach and the principles for diagnosis of brain death are widely accepted in Europe. However, the application of these diagnostic steps in clinical and hospital practice is variable in individual European countries: there are variations in the repetition of the diagnostic tests, the methods for testing apnoea, the need of a confirmatory technical test, and the qualifications of the physician responsible for brain death diagnosis [44–46]. The responsible health care professional should have good knowledge of the diagnostic procedures in the country where he/she is professionally active.

Heart-beating organ donation

Accurate diagnosis of brain death has provided the possibility of harvesting of organs for transplantation in heart-beating conditions. In intensive care patients suffering disastrous brain damage (hypoxic or traumatic) with irreversible loss of brain function and with no hope for any meaningful recovery, the transport of oxygen to organs may be continued by artificial ventilation, intravenous feeding, and other intensive care treatment. After diagnosis of brain death according to the accurately defined procedures, this allows many patients with organ failure to benefit from the possibilities that are offered by transplant surgery.

The principles of organ donation and transplantation are also widely accepted throughout Europe. However, there is variability in the related legislation as to how an individuals can express their preferences about organ donation: in some countries (such as the United Kingdom, Ireland, Denmark, Netherlands, Germany) the individual may actively consent with organ donation ('opting in'); in other countries (such as Austria, Portugal, Belgium, Spain, Italy, France, Greece, Switzerland, the Scandinavian and most central European countries) the individual is assumed to agree with organ donation unless active disagreement ('opting out').

Non-heart-beating organ donation

Non-heart-beating organ donation (NHBOD) may be considered, in the absence of brain death, after the decision is made to stop the resuscitation efforts because of futility. If an injury is not compatible with life or if there is no response to CPR as defined by the current CPR guidelines for, organ harvesting may be considered after irreversible cardiorespiratory arrest has led to the death of the individual.

In these situations, after stopping CPR and after an observation period of several minutes (variable from country to country), the initiation of intravascular preservation methods with a view to organ harvesting and transplantation may be considered.

There is wide variation within Europe about the acceptance of NHBOD, about the selection of potential candidates, and about the procedures and protocols. Therefore, no general recommendation can be made.

Many reports have documented the good clinical results of this approach, mainly in kidney transplantation [47].

Conclusions

Although the general ethical principles are universal, their implementation and translation into practice throughout Europe is far from being uniform. A variety of factors are influential, including social, legal, religious, cultural and economic facts and conditions, most of which are rather stable and resistant to the short-term exercise of influence. Besides this, medical characteristics, especially in the context of cardiac arrest, make it difficult to always act clearly according to ethical rules. However, the core ethical principles are valid across borders and should be followed in any situation, and cardiac arrest and acute cardiac care, despite their very special conditions, are not ethics-free areas.

To act in an ethically competent way in a stressful and time-critical emergency situation such as cardiac arrest requires that the caregiver has reflected and thought about ethics in advance. If ethical considerations arise in such a situation for the first time they will be of no use. Thus, this subject should be included in any (continuing) education for personnel who will be confronted with such situations. Case conferences, debriefings, discussions with colleagues, etc. may further strengthen ethical competence.

Stating that implementation of ethical principles depends on many external factors and accepting those variables without criticism would fail to recognize that ethics is not stable, but a process subject to change. This implies that anyone involved should take any opportunity to actively participate in the debate, be it in the work environment, in scientific discussions, or at a political level. Ethics is not an end in itself but also serves the general purpose of applying the best possible care to our patients, their families, and their environment.

Personal perspective

This overview of ethical issues in cardiac arrest and acute cardiac care has revealed issues that may determine the discussion in the near future. Advance directives are of value for expressing wishes and preferences about EOL decisions; however, reliable mechanisms and tools are needed to facilitate their application especially in the out-of-hospital setting. Furthermore, international and intercultural approaches could identify strategies to promote their general acceptance and implementation.

Recent studies have shown that the involvement of nurses in EOL decisions has increased. This positive development might be further pursued and strengthened by ethical team discussions and by continuing interdisciplinary education, to improve integration of nurses into the decision-making process and thus to minimize team conflicts. Assuming that nurses' contact with patients and relatives is deeper and more frequent, they could play an important role in addressing ethical subjects, in the hospital as well as in society.

On a European level the debate on euthanasia is far from being harmonized, as a result of strongly differing historical, socio-cultural, and legal national backgrounds. It is hardly possible to predict whether there will be ever a rapprochement when we look at countries having enacted laws on euthanasia on the one hand, and on the other at countries where euthanasia meets with widespread societal disapproval, mainly based on religious convictions. Nevertheless, or perhaps just because of the divergence, the ethical dispute on this subject will continue.

The lack of validated reliable tools allowing us to predict the individual outcome from cardiac arrest is a major disadvantage in the field. Besides further studies on this issue that might reveal new insights and improve the specificity of TOR criteria, an open ethical debate could be helpful to identify within a given society what level of specificity could be acceptable for such TOR decisions.

Further reading

American Heart Association. 2005 Guidelines for cardio-pulmonary resuscitation and emergency cardiovascular care. *Circulation* 2005;**112**:1–211.

Azoulay E, Metnitz B, Sprung C, *et al*. End-of-life practices in 282 intensive care units: data from the SAPS 3 database. *Intens Care Med* 2009;**35**:623–630.

Baskett P, Lim A. The varying ethical attitudes towards resuscitation in Europe. *Resuscitation* 2004;**62**:267–73.

Beauchamp T, Childress J. *Principles of biomedical ethics*, 5th edition. Oxford University Press, Oxford. 2001.

Bülow H, Sprung C, Reinhart K, *et al*. The world's major religions points of view on end-of-life decisions in the intensive care unit. *Intens Care Med* 2008;**34**:423–430.

Carlet J, Thijs L, Antonelli M, *et al*. Challenges of end-of-life care in the ICU. *Intens Care Med* 2004;**30**:770–784.

European Resuscitation Council. ERC Guidelines for resuscitation 2005. *Resuscitation* 2005;**67**:S1–189.

Siegel M. End-of-life decision making in the ICU. *Clin Chest Med* 2009;**30**:181–194.

Sprung C, Cohen S, Sjokvist P, *et al*. End-of-life practices in European Intensive Care Units. The Ethicus study. *JAMA* 2003;**290**:790–797.

Truog P, Campbell M, Curtis J, *et al*. Recommendations for end-of-life care in the intensive care unit: a consensus statement by the American College of Critical Care Medicine. *Crit Care Med* 2008;**36**:953–963.

Wijdicks E, Rabinstein A, Manno E, *et al*. Pronouncing brain death: contemporary practice and safety of the apnea test. *Neurology* 2008;**71**:1240–1244.

Online resources

- American Heart Association. http://www.heart.org
- European Resuscitation Council. http://www.erc.edu
- European Society for Intensive Care Medicine. http://www.esicm.org

➲ For additional multimedia materials please visit the online version of the book (http://www.esciacc.oxfordmedicine.com).

SECTION IV

Monitoring and investigations in the intensive cardiac care unit

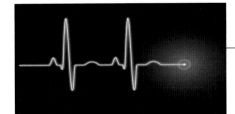

CHAPTER 14

Pathophysiology and clinical assessment of the cardiovascular system (including pulmonary artery catheter)

Etienne Gayat and Alexandre Mebazaa

Contents

Summary

Haemodynamic instability may be related to various mechanisms including hypovolaemia and heart and/or vascular dysfunction. Although acute heart failure (AHF) patients are often admitted for dyspnea, many mechanisms can be involved including left ventricular (LV) diastolic and/or systolic dysfunction and/or right ventricular (RV) dysfunction. Many epidemiological studies show that clinical signs at admission, morbidity, and mortality differ between the main scenarios of AHF: LV diastolic dysfunction, systolic dysfunction, RV dysfunction, and cardiogenic shock. Although echocardiography often helps to assess the mechanism of heart dysfunction, it can not be considered as a monitoring tool. In some cases, pulmonary artery catheter (PAC) can help to assess and monitor cardiovascular status and to evaluate response to treatments.

Introduction

Severe alteration in the cardiovascular system may lead to impairment in systemic blood pressure, stroke volume, and organ (lung, liver, kidney) function. As shown in ➲ Fig. 14.1, in the case of haemodynamic instability, one should assess which of the four most frequent causes (bradycardia, hypovolaemia, myocardial and vascular dysfunction) is involved. If both heart rate and volaemia seem adequate, haemodynamic instability is related to myocardial and/or vascular dysfunction. Note that a prolonged myocardial dysfunction may lead to an associated vascular dysfunction.

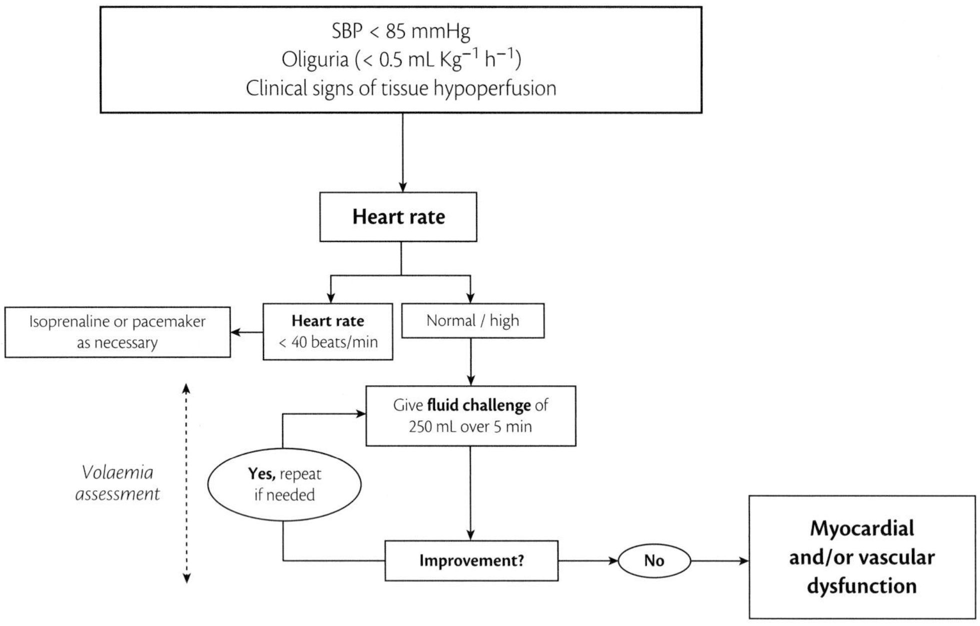

Figure 14.1 Algorithm for early management of haemodynamic instability. SBP, systolic blood pressure.

The present chapter describes the physiopathology and assessment of the four most frequent mechanisms and clinical scenarios of acute heart failure (AHF). They are:

- AHF with pulmonary oedema (left diastolic dysfunction).
- AHF with low stroke volume, often related to decompensated chronic heart failure (left systolic dysfunction).
- AHF with low blood pressure and low stroke volume often associated with organ dysfunction (cardiogenic shock).
- AHF with predominant RV failure (right ventricular failure).

Left ventricular diastolic dysfunction

Left ventricular (LV) diastolic dysfunction refers to abnormalities of diastolic distensibility, filling, or relaxation, regardless of whether LV ejection fraction is normal or abnormal and whether or not the patient is symptomatic [1].

Physiopathology

LV diastolic dysfunction can be defined as the inability of the LV chamber to fill up at low atrial pressures. This dysfunction can result either from an impairment in LV compliance (passive mechanism), or from an alteration in LV relaxation (active process). Of these two components, relaxation is usually the first to be altered in case of LV diastolic dysfunction and relaxation abnormalities can

occur abruptly especially in the context of anaesthesiology or critical care.

Myocyte energy imbalance

Zile and Brutsaert [2] defined relaxation as 'the time period during which the myocardium loses its ability to generate force and shorten and returns to an unstressed length and force'. From a mechanical point of view, the transition between systole and diastole has been described as the time of aortic valve closure. However, the transition between contraction and relaxation corresponds to the dissociation of actin–myosin cross-bridges that begins during the early phase of LV ejection, before aortic valve closure [3].

Alterations leading to diastolic dysfunction may involve phenomena that not only occur during the 'classic' diastole, but also earlier in the cardiac cycle, at the time when intracellular calcium falls.

Since relaxation is an energy-consuming process, it is adversely affected by myocardial ischaemia. Ischaemia precludes optimal calcium exchanges between cytosole and sarcoplasmic reticulum, and is rapidly associated with impairment in LV relaxation [4]. Sepsis is also likely to alter myocytes energetic balance and thus to alter LV relaxation [5].

Contraction–relaxation coupling

Relaxation begins early during systole [3, 6], indicating that relaxation and contraction are intimately coupled. As a consequence, LV relaxation is greatly affected by the lack of homogeneity in LV contraction. Both LV segmental coordination and atrioventricular (AV) synchronization are essential to guarantee efficient relaxation [7, 8]. The loss of atrial contraction associated with atrial fibrillation not only alters LV filling but also results in a slowing of myocardial relaxation.

Several other factors known to alter contractile function, including changes in afterload and the use of inotrope, markedly affect relaxation. On the other hand, the effect of preload variations on relaxation is still matter of debate.

In a failing heart, an increase in afterload induces a delay in the onset of relaxation and an increase in the time constant of isovolumic relaxation [8–10].

The afterload reserve

The afterload reserve is the capacity of the normal left ventricle to respond to afterload elevation without changes in LV end-systolic volume and LV pressure decline [11–13]. Ventricles with altered contractile function consistently show a decreased afterload reserve [14–18]. In such ventricles, even a small afterload elevation will markedly deteriorate LV relaxation parameters and increase LV systolic and diastolic volumes.

An alternative concept: end-systolic volume dependency

Chemla *et al.* recently proposed an alternative approach based on the suggestion that, at constant heart rate, relaxation might depend more on LV end-systolic volume than on afterload, namely LV systolic pressure [19]. Indeed, recoiling forces are generated when the LV contracts below its equilibrium volume (usually slightly higher than LV end-systolic volume) and therefore recoiling forces act during early diastole. Thus, since a healthy heart is able to respond to increased afterload without any change in its LV end-systolic volume, relaxation remains unaffected. On the contrary, in failing dilated ventricles, LV end-systolic volume might exceed the equilibrium volume, which deprives the LV of recoiling forces and decreases the rate of isovolumic relaxation.

How to assess left ventricular diastolic function in clinical practice

⮕ Table 14.1 shows the major differences between heart failure with reduced and preserved ejection fraction, regarding to the symptoms, physical examination, ECG abnormalities and radiographic findings. Diagnostic criteria are also proposed in ⮕ Table 14.2.

Cardiac catheterization

Diastolic heart failure is characterized by an elevated LV end-diastolic pressure (16–26 mmHg) in 92% of patients

Table 14.1 Differences between systolic and diastolic heart failure

	Systolic heart failure	Diastolic heart failure
Dyspnea	Chronic	Mainly transient
Heart rate	Increased	Increased
Mitral regurgitation	Present	Rare
S3/S4 gallop	S3>S4	S4 mainly
Rales	Present	Present
Peripheral oedema	Present	Rare
Cardiomegaly	Constant	Not constant
ECG abnormal	Constant	Not constant
LVEF	Reduced	>50%
LV dilatation	Nearly constant	Absent
BNP	Markedly increased	May be only mildly increased

BNP, B-type natriuretic peptide; LVEF, left ventricular ejection function.

[20, 21], while control patients had an average of 10 mmHg. Systolic and diastolic functions are best described using the LV pressure/volume relationship, represented graphically as P/V loops.

Using this mechanical approach, diastole begins at the closure of the aortic valve, and lasts until the closure of the mitral valve. Diastole can be divided into two phases. The first corresponds to the LV pressure decline at constant volume, called isovolumic relaxation, which lasts from the closure of the aortic valve until the opening of the mitral valve. The second, called auxotonic relaxation, corresponds to LV chamber filling and lasts until the closure of the mitral valve. LV filling mainly depends on the pressure gradient between left atrium (LA) and LV, which is mainly influenced by passive chamber properties (compliance), active relaxation, and, at end-diastole, by atrial contraction. Thus, impairment in LV compliance (which decreases the LA–LV pressure gradient) or the loss of atrial contraction directly impairs diastolic filling. Structural modifications (e.g. myocardial hypertrophy, fibrosis) mainly affect the passive, late phase of diastole and are more likely to develop chronically, whereas functional factors (e.g. ischaemia, sepsis) adversely affect active relaxation during early diastole. Consequently, for a given LV end-diastolic volume, LV end-diastolic pressure is increased and may result in pulmonary congestion.

Systolic dysfunction also affects the P/V loop: the end-systolic P/V slope is shifted downwards and to the right, indicating a reduction in contractility, while end-systolic and end-diastolic LV volumes are increased, which may also lead to upstream congestion. Patients with heart failure can have combined systolic and diastolic dysfunction. In such case, modest increases in end-diastolic volume may result in large increases in LV end-diastolic pressure.

Table 14.2 Criteria of diagnosis of diastolic heart failure (DHF)

Levels of evidence	Criteria	Objective evidence
Definite DHF	Definitive evidence of CHF AND	Includes clinical symptoms and signs, supporting laboratory tests (such as chest radiograph), and a typical clinical response to treatment with diuretics, with or without documentation of elevated LV filling pressure (at rest, on exercise, or in response to a volume load) or a low cardiac index
	Objective evidence of normal LV systolic function in proximity to the CHF event AND	LVEF ≥ 0.50 within 72 h of CHF event
	Objective evidence of LV diastolic dysfunction	Abnormal LV relaxation/filling/distensibility indices on cardiac catheterization
Probable DHF	Definitive evidence of CHF AND	Includes clinical symptoms and signs, supporting laboratory tests (such as chest radiograph), and a typical clinical response to treatment with diuretics, with or without documentation of elevated LV filling pressure (at rest, on exercise, or in response to a volume load) or a low cardiac index
	Objective evidence of normal LV systolic function in proximity to the CHF event BUT	LVEF ≥ 0.50 within 72 h of CHF event
	Objective evidence of LV diastolic dysfunction is lacking	No conclusive information on LV diastolic function
Possible DHF	Definitive evidence of CHF AND	Includes clinical symptoms and signs, supporting laboratory tests (such as chest radiograph), and a typical clinical response to treatment with diuretics, with or without documentation of elevated LV filling pressure (at rest, on exercise, or in response to a volume load) or a low cardiac index
	Objective evidence of normal LV systolic function, but not at the time of the CHF event AND	LVEF ≥ 0.50
	Objective evidence of LV diastolic dysfunction is lacking	No conclusive information on LV diastolic function

Adapted with permission from Vasan RS, Levy D. Defining diastolic heart failure: a call for standardized diagnostic criteria. *Circulation*. 2000 May 2;**101**(17):2118-21..

Kawaguchi *et al.* [22] recently demonstrated that in patients admitted for heart failure with a preserved LV ejection fraction, the diastolic portion of the P/V loop, although apparently normal at rest, became altered on exertion. Indeed, manoeuvres such as sustained isometric handgrips markedly impaired LV diastolic properties, increased LV end-diastolic pressure, and could reveal a diastolic heart failure.

In diastolic heart failure patients, LV pressure decline analysis reveals a significant increase in the time constant of isovolumic relaxation, τ [20, 21].

Zile *et al.* recently conducted a multicentre prospective study using cardiac catheterization and echocardiography to assess LV diastolic properties in 47 patients suffering from diastolic heart failure and 10 normal controls [23]. The authors demonstrated that insight into the respective roles of active relaxation and compliance could be gained using a detailed analysis of the LV diastolic pressure curve. The following measurements are of particular interest:

- τ, the time constant of the isovolumic relaxation

- P_{min}, the LV minimal pressure after the opening of the mitral valve

- P_{Pre-A}, the LV pressure just before atrial contraction

- LV end-diastolic pressure, just after the atrial contraction.

These authors showed that, in diastolic heart failure patients in contrast to normal subjects, isovolumic relaxation was incomplete at the time of P_{min}. Thus, τ was prolonged and P_{min} increased, resulting in a positive correlation between τ and P_{min}. Incomplete relaxation accounted for 7±1 mmHg of the measured increase in P_{min}. Among these patients, LV compliance was also significantly altered as supported by an increase in LV end-diastolic pressure despite a reduced LV end-diastolic volume.

Other investigations

Echocardiography findings are detailed elsewhere. Briefly, the mitral blood flow and tissue Doppler imaging are still a great help in suspected high left atrial pressure. Moreover, in cases of LV diastolic failure, B-type natriuretic peptide

(BNP) is now recognized as a specific marker of heart failure in patients presenting with acute dyspnoea [24]. It is important to keep in mind that BNP may be normal in some cases of acute hypertensive ('flash') pulmonary oedema in patients with preserved LV systolic function [25].

Left ventricular systolic dysfunction

Physiopathology

LV systolic dysfunction refers to impaired ventricular contractility. In chronic heart failure, the loss of cardiac inotropy results in a decrease in stroke volume and a compensatory rise in preload (often measured as ventricular end-diastolic pressure or pulmonary capillary wedge pressure). The rise in preload is considered compensatory because it activates the Frank–Starling mechanism to help maintain stroke volume despite the loss of inotropy. If the preload did not rise, the decline in stroke volume would be even greater for a given loss of inotropy. Depending on the precipitating cause of the heart failure, there will be LV hypertrophy, dilatation, or a combination of the two.

Loss of intrinsic inotropy is associated with an increase in end-systolic volume. There is also an increase in end-diastolic volume (compensatory increase in preload), but this increase is not as great as the increase in end-systolic volume. Therefore, the net effect is a decrease in stroke volume. Because stroke volume decreases and end-diastolic volume increases, there is a substantial reduction in ejection fraction (EF).

The reason for preload rising as inotropy declines is related to the increased end-systolic volume. Indeed, in the failing heart, at the beginning of diastole, there is already a 'high' end-systolic volume. The venous return is added to this, leading to an increase in end-diastolic volume and pressure. Thus, an important and deleterious consequence of systolic dysfunction is the rise in end-diastolic pressure. If the left ventricle is involved, then left atrial and pulmonary venous pressures will also rise. This can lead to pulmonary congestion and oedema.

It is important to realize that AHF may or may not be followed by ventricular remodelling. Indeed, in the case of AHF resulting from a large anterior myocardial infarct occurring in a previously healthy heart, a large portion of the anterior wall becomes functionally inactive within seconds and the rest of the ventricular myocardium is suddenly exposed to an increase in its haemodynamic load; it has to perform the work of the whole ventricle, including the ischaemic/infarcted area, under very unfavourable

biological conditions called 'biomechanical stress'. In this case, AHF simply results from an acute dysfunction of the cardiac pump as a whole, with an associated hyperfunction of the remote area that tries to compensate for the loss of function of the ischaemic/infarcted myocardial area. Another example of this situation of AHF with no previous cardiac remodelling is acute mitral regurgitation due to chordae rupture.

In the case of AHF occurring as a decompensation of a chronically failing heart, cardiac myocytes have been remodelled by years of biomechanical stress resulting from the originating disease. In such a situation, the heart is obviously placed in an unfavourable situation when, being previously weakened by a long process of detrimental remodelling, it is unable to compensate for the often mild insult at the origin of the acute decompensation, e.g. an episode of atrial fibrillation.

Clinical assessment

The commonest cause of chronic heart failure today is coronary heart disease. A previous history of myocardial infarction (MI) makes the diagnosis of heart failure more likely. Some patients, such as people with diabetes, may have had a silent MI. Other causes of heart failure include long-standing hypertension and alcohol excess. A smaller proportion of patients have valvular heart disease. In these patients symptoms and signs develop gradually, over days or weeks, and pulmonary and systemic congestion (jugular venous distension, pulmonary rales, and peripheral oedema) are usually present. They usually have a reduced EF. Despite high LV filling pressures they may present several degrees of pulmonary congestion (clinical and/or radiographic) but some may have minimal pulmonary congestion.

In western Europe the four most frequent causes of acute decompensation of chronic heart failure are ischaemia, arrhythmia, infection, and noncompliance with medication.

Investigations

An ECG can provide very useful information. LV systolic dysfunction was found to be unlikely in a primary care population if there was no major abnormality on the ECG (sensitivity 94%, negative predictive value (NPV) 98%) [26]. Thus, in patients with breathlessness and a normal ECG alternative causes might be considered first, although patients must be investigated further (e.g. with echocardiography) if heart failure is still thought to be the likely diagnosis.

A chest radiograph may provide useful information. Cardiomegaly may be present (cardiothoracic ratio (CTR) >0.50). It may also show pulmonary congestion or another explanation for breathlessness such as a lung tumour.

All patients in whom the diagnosis of heart failure cannot be excluded require an assessment of LV function. Patients in whom the diagnosis of heart failure is secure may also be considered for an assessment of LV function as an indicator of prognosis. Echocardiography is the most frequently used investigation, but may not be possible in approximately 10% of patients for technical reasons, and alternative investigation may be necessary. Atrial fibrillation also makes the assessment of LV function less reliable. Some patients may have had an alternative method of estimate of LV function in secondary care, e.g. gated heart scan, LV angiography during coronary angiography.

Cardiogenic shock

Physiopathology

Cardiogenic shock occurs when the heart is unable to deliver enough blood to maintain adequate tissue perfusion. It is one of the most challenging emergencies for the intensivist. The leading cause of cardiogenic shock is acute MI, and cardiogenic shock remains the most common cause of death in hospitalized patients with acute MI [27].

Cardiogenic shock usually results from an extensive acute infarction, although a smaller infarction in a patient with previously compromised LV function may also precipitate shock. Cardiogenic shock can also be caused by mechanical complications of infarction such as acute mitral regurgitation, rupture of the interventricular septum, or rupture of the free wall, or by large right ventricular (RV) infarctions.

A negative vicious cycle leads to myocardial hypoperfusion. Indeed, myocardial perfusion, which depends on the pressure gradient between the coronary arteries and the left ventricle and on the duration of diastole, is compromised by hypotension and tachycardia, exacerbating ischaemia. The increased ventricular diastolic pressures caused by pump failure further reduce coronary perfusion pressure, and the additional wall stress elevates myocardial oxygen requirements, further worsening ischaemia. Decreased CO also compromised systemic perfusion, which can lead to lactic acidosis and further compromise of systolic performance.

Another cause of a negative vicious cycle is the stimulation of sympathetic tone, which further impairs myocardial

contractility. Recent data show that systemic vascular resistance may even decrease, suggesting a systemic inflammatory response syndrome [28].

Clinical assessment

Patients with shock are usually cyanotic, and can have cool skin and mottled extremities. Cerebral hypoperfusion may cloud the sensorium. Pulses are rapid and faint, and may be irregular in the presence of arrhythmias. Jugular venous distension and pulmonary rales are usually present, although their absence does not exclude the diagnosis. The precordial heave resulting from LV dyskinesis may be palpable. The heart sounds may be distant, and third or fourth heart sounds are usually present. A systolic murmur of mitral regurgitation or ventricular septal defect may be heard, but these complications may occur without an audible murmur.

Documentation of myocardial dysfunction and exclusion of alternative causes of hypotension allows for the diagnosis of cardiogenic shock.

Investigations

An ECG should be performed immediately. Other initial diagnostic tests should include a chest radiograph and measurement of arterial blood gases, electrolytes, complete blood count, and cardiac enzymes.

Echocardiography is an excellent tool for confirming the diagnosis of cardiogenic shock and for sorting through the differential diagnosis, and should be performed as early as possible. Echocardiography is simple, safe, and permits systemic interrogation of cardiac chamber size, LV and RV function, valvular structure and motion, atrial size, and the anatomy of the pericardial space.

Invasive haemodynamic monitoring can confirm the diagnosis and can exclude volume depletion, RV infarction, and mechanical complications [29]. Right heart catheterization may reveal an oxygen step-up diagnostic of ventricular septal rupture or a large V wave that suggests severe mitral regurgitation. Right heart catheterization is most useful, however, to optimize therapy in unstable patients, because clinical estimates of filling pressure can be unreliable [30] and because changes in myocardial performance can change CO and filling pressures precipitously [31].

Right ventricular failure

Pathophysiologic changes in right heart failure vary according to the underlying cause. Often, patients experience RV failure secondary to various mechanisms including decreased RV contractility, increased RV pressure, and increased RV volume.

Physiopathology

Right ventricular contractile impairment

This condition occurs most often in cases of RV ischaemia and infarction. Usually, RV infarction is due to proximal occlusion of the right coronary artery (RCA). In this condition, the RV is unable to contract against normal pulmonary artery pressure (PAP) (see ➲ Fig. 14.2). Accordingly, RV ischaemia rapidly leads to RV dilatation with a concomitant rise in RV diastolic pressure. Such elevation causes a shift of the interventricular septum toward an already underfilled left ventricle. Accordingly, RV dilatation in the setting of limited pericardial compliance leads to increased intrapericardial pressures and an additional constraint on the RV but also on LV filling [32]. These changes in RV mechanic lead to depressed right-sided output, decreased LV preload, and subsequently a reduced overall cardiac output [33].

Effect of an increase in right ventricular afterload

As described above, increased PAP alters both coronary perfusion and ventricular function of the RV. In a patient with pulmonary hypertension, the RV dilates to maintain the stroke volume, though the EF is reduced and the peristaltic contraction is lost, causing an accelerated worsening in RV failure.

The increased afterload also prolongs the isovolaemic contraction phase and ejection time and, therefore, the increased myocardial oxygen consumption. In addition, RCA perfusion only occurs in diastole.

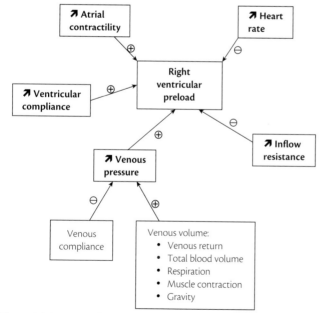

Figure 14.2 Factors determining right ventricular preload.

Accordingly, in a patient with further increase in PAP and decreased in RCA perfusion, it is important to rapidly reduce RV afterload to improve the oxygen supply/demand balance in the RV and maintain RV function.

Effect of an increase in right ventricular volume

Volume overload is common during RV failure, and volume loading may further dilate the RV, increase tricuspid regurgitation, and, consequently, worsen hepatic and renal congestion and RV failure. Accordingly volume management is a difficult but important task in the treatment of RV failure. Physiologically, volume loading may be useful in increasing preload, but in the large majority of patients with RV failure this compensatory mechanism is potentially limited beyond a mean PAP of 30 mmHg [34], and therefore caution is warranted when considering volume loading in any patient with suspected RV failure (➲ Fig. 14.2).

Ventricular interdependence

There is a high degree of ventricular interdependence due to the role of the interventricular septum in the contraction of both ventricles, which is pronounced because of the existence of pericardium [35]. This close association between the cardiac cavities can be seen in echocardiography images of the four chambers [36]. Indeed, increases in the end-diastolic volume of the left ventricle are transmitted to the right ventricle by movement of the interventricular septum toward the right cavity, increasing the end-diastolic pressure of the right ventricle [37]. Similarly, when RV end-diastolic volume is increased, the interventricular septum shifts toward the left cavity during diastole due to restrictions imposed by the pericardium on the RV as the cavity volume increases. This leftward shift impairs the function of the left ventricle due to the reduction in LV volume, decreasing both LV filling and compliance, manifested as increased LV muscle stiffness. Ventricular interdependence can also cause RV failure during LV assist device support. As the LV assist device unloads the left ventricle, the interventricular septum is shifted left. This alters the RV compliance, decreasing force and the rate of contraction together with a decreased afterload and increased preload. In a healthy heart, cardiac output may be maintained, but with pre-existing pathology, the decrease in contractility may result in RV failure [38]. It is therefore crucial to support RV function during the first few days following insertion of a LV assist device.

The vicious cycle of autoaggravation

Compared to the left ventricle, RV failure progresses quickly from compensated to endstage heart failure because of a vicious cycle of autoaggravation. This is unique to the right ventricle and is rarely seen in isolated LV failure. As seen in ⊃ Fig. 14.3, a sudden increase, although modest, in RV afterload (inhaled nitric oxide withdrawal, for instance) on an ischaemic right ventricle immediately dilates the ventricle, induces a tricuspid regurgitation, and decreases cardiac output.

Clinical assessment

The diagnosis of acute RV failure in patients in the intensive care unit (ICU) is complicated by the lack of specific clinical and biological signs. Some biological signs that may be indicative of cardiac dysfunction appear very early during acute RV failure. The organs most affected by RV failure-induced congestion are the liver and kidneys. Decreased perfusion of the kidneys is manifested as a reduction in both urine output and creatinine clearance. Decreased hepatic perfusion results in increased plasma lactate due to an impaired lactate clearance, a reduction in the synthesis of coagulation factors (observed as a decrease in prothrombin time), and hepatic cytolysis.

The sensitivity of conventional chest radiography techniques in identifying changes in RV form is limited by the unusual shape of the RV and the unpredictable manner in which it dilates. Inferential diagnosis may be possible by identification of other radiographic changes, such as the state of the pulmonary circulation and the position of the heart in the chest. Changes in the left ventricle may be apparent on chest radiograph, resulting from the decreased LV preload that is a consequence of RV failure.

Echocardiography is an alternative, more accessible technique for the diagnosis of RV failure and for the intermittent repetitive follow-up of the dynamics of therapeutic responses. Its advantage is that a qualitative conclusion can be reached instantaneously. When RV failure is secondary to an increase in afterload, the isovolaemic contraction phase and ejection time are prolonged, and increases in PAP and flow are accelerated. Echocardiography also provides information about the mechanisms of RV failure, such as pericardial effusion with or without tamponade, tricuspid insufficiency, pulmonary emboli, or RV ischaemia and the resulting acute cor pulmonale [39]. Additionally, echocardiography enables the simultaneous evaluation of LV function, a possible component of the RV failure. Because of the geometry and location of the RV, the accuracy and necessity of determining exact RV dimensions remains questionable and an experienced intensive care physician familiar with performing and evaluating echocardiography is essential. Although echocardiography can be repeated infinitely, the continuous flow of information provided by right heart catheterization is difficult to reproduce and when technical or human limitations render echocardiography impossible, right heart catheterization becomes the diagnostic tool of choice (see below).

Use of a pulmonary artery catheter in acute heart failure

The pulmonary artery catheter (PAC) is a monitoring device which is still widely used in critically ill patients. However, the attitude towards such an invasive monitoring system has evolved over the last decade. The motivation to find noninvasive or less invasive surrogate techniques has been partially successful: echocardiography, Doppler, and pulse contour techniques have been proposed as alternatives. The publication by Connors *et al.* [40] caused contention among intensivists and generated clinical trials to test the potential benefit of PAC use. This paper used a propensity score as a technique to compare the patients with and without PAC. In a mixed population of medical and surgical ICU patients, the authors found an increased mortality, length of stay, and costs associated with the use of PAC. In addition, many have claimed that there are no good data to support the use of PAC since no study has shown an outcome benefit in patients having a therapeutic strategy based on PAC data.

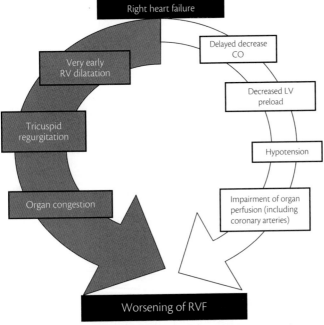

Figure 14.3 The vicious cycle of autoaggravation of right ventricular failure (RVF).

The approach for intensivists can be separated into three major issues:

♦ Has insertion a PAC a significant risk of complications?

♦ Can the data provided by the PAC improve the outcome of severely ill patients?

♦ Do we have data to better define the type of patients or diseases for which PAC may improve care quality and outcome?

Recommendations/indications for cardiac failure

Two major publications must be cited: the consensus conference from the Society of Critical Care Medicine (SCCM) [41] and the guidelines from the American Society of Anesthesiologists. The recent publication of guidelines for diagnosis and treatment of cardiac failure provides an opportunity to better position the use of PAC [42].

MI complicated by cardiogenic shock or progressive hypotension is a class I indication for PAC use in the American College of Cardiology/American Heart Association guidelines. This recommendation is also included in the PAC consensus conference of the SCCM in 1997 [41]. Such a recommendation is based on expert opinion and there is no conclusive proof that the PAC improves outcomes in this patient population [41]. The SCCM consensus conference also indicated that PAC was appropriate for patients with congestive heart failure refractory to empirical therapy.

The European Society of Cardiology (ESC) guidelines [42] published in 2005 insisted that invasive monitoring of the patient with AHF should be initiated as soon as possible after arrival at the emergency department, concurrently with ongoing diagnostic measures addressed at determining the primary aetiology. These guidelines, based on expert opinion, also explained that although the insertion of PAC for the diagnostic of AHF is usually unnecessary, it

could be used to distinguish between a cardiogenic and a noncardiogenic mechanism in complex patients with concurrent cardiac and pulmonary disease. The use of PAC is a class IIb recommendation (level of evidence C) in haemodynamically unstable patients who are not responding in a predictable fashion to traditional treatment, and in patients with a combination of congestion and hypoperfusion. In these cases, a PAC is inserted in order to ensure optimal fluid loading of the ventricles and to guide vasoactive therapies and inotropic agents.

It is recommended that, in cardiogenic shock and prolonged severe low output syndrome, the SvO_2 from the pulmonary artery must be measured and maintained above 65% [41].

Experts have stated that direct measurement of haemodynamic parameters can be helpful in patients for whom the physical examination is limited or discordant with symptoms. It may be particularly useful for determining the contribution of heart failure to a complex clinical picture, such as sepsis, acute renal failure, or acute coronary syndrome in the setting of chronic heart failure. Another common setting where PAC insertion may be helpful is the evaluation of dyspnoea and elevated right heart pressures in patients with concomitant pulmonary and cardiac disease.

In right heart failure, catheterization of the pulmonary artery is more invasive than echocardiography but useful to evaluate RV function and confirm the presence of RV failure in patients in the ICU [43].

These recommendations are summarized in ➲ Table 14.3.

Measurements derived from a pulmonary artery catheter

The PAC provides the physician with haemodynamic parameters (cardiac output, right atrial, pulmonary, and pulmonary artery occlusion pressures, and possibly RV volumes) and also with tissue perfusion variables (oxygen venous saturation, oxygen extraction, and the venous

Table 14.3 Recommendations for PAC use in acute cardiac care

Indications	Recommendations	Level of evidence	Society	Ref
Diagnosis of acute myocardial dysfunction	Usually unnecessary Can be useful to distinguish between a cardiogenic and noncardiogenic mechanism in complex patients with concurrent cardiac and pulmonary disease, especially when echo/Doppler measurements are difficult to obtain	B	ESC/ESICM	[48]
Monitoring and guiding therapy	PAC placement may be reasonable to guide therapy in patients with refractory endstage HF and persistently severe symptoms	C	ACC/AHA	[24]
	PAC may be useful in haemodynamically unstable patients who are not responding as expected to traditional treatments	B	ESC/ESICM	[48]

ACC, American College of Cardiology; AHA, American Heart Association; ESC, European Society of Cardiology; ESICM, European Society of Intensive Care Medicine; HF, Heart failure; PAC, pulmonary artery catheter.

Table 14.4 PAC-derived measurements

	Method/technique	Clinical usefulness
Cardiac output	Thermodilution: intermittent or continuous	Remains the gold-standard tool for measuring CO in the clinical settings
PAP (systolic and diastolic)	Invasive pressure measurements	In case of pulmonary hypertension, distinction between pre- and post-capillary pulmonary hypertension
Pulmonary artery occlusion pressure (PAOP)	The PAOP is the pressure obtained after inflating the distal balloon of the PAC and is assumed to reflect the pressure in a large pulmonary vein and thus left atrial pressure and the LV end-diastolic pressure [49]	For determining the cause of pulmonary oedema (cardiogenic vs noncardiogenic) [50] For assessing the pulmonary vasomotor tone [51] For assessing the mechanism of weaning-induced pulmonary oedema [52] For guiding fluid rescucitation/fluid restriction [53]
RV volumes	Only PAC with fast-response thermistor. Leads to evaluate RV EF [54]	Still unclear, even in the context of RV failure
Mixed venous oxygen saturation	By sampling the pulmonary arterial blood through the distal tip of PAC or by *in vivo* continuous monitoring (using fibreoptic spectrophotometry)	See Fig. 14.4.
Venoarterial carbon dioxide tension difference	Difference between PCO_2 in the mixed venous blood and the PCO_2 in the arterial blood	Normal value 2–5 mmHg. Due to the linear relationship between CO_2 content and tension, Pco_2 would be linearly related to CO_2 production and inversely related to cardiac output

PAC, pulmonary artery catheter; PAP, pulmonary artery pressure; RVEF, right ventricular ejection fraction; CO, cardiac output.

carbon dioxide pressure). These PAC-derived parameters are briefly summarized in ⊃ Table 14.4.

The particular case of right ventricular failure

Catheterization of the pulmonary artery is more invasive but useful to evaluate RV function and confirm the presence of RV failure in patients in the ICU. The Swan–Ganz catheter measures both mixed venous oxygen saturation and intravascular pressures or pressure changes in the RV as well as PAP and pulmonary capillary wedge pressure. Despite difficulties in the interpretation of mean intravascular pressure values, the tracings showing changes in pressure and flow enable the assessment of the impact of treatment on RV function. This cautious interpretation accounts for the almost constant reflux due to the tricuspid insufficiency, which can be observed by central venous and right atrial pressure changes. Such regurgitation could be used as a hallmark for RV failure and as a marker for treatment efficacy.

A more advanced pulmonary catheter, equipped with a fast-response thermistor, is another valuable diagnostic tool enabling clinical assessment of RV volume and haemodynamic parameters by thermodilution. It may also measure cardiac output more precisely even in the presence of tricuspid insufficiency, a particular problem during mechanical ventilation. Indeed, the more widespread introduction of thermodilution techniques to assess pump function has contributed to the recognition of the inherent pathology of RV failure. Values for cardiac performance obtained from

this technique compare favourably with those using radionuclides or two-dimensional echocardiography [44, 45].

If a central venous pressure or PAC is in place, haemodynamic parameters that can aid in the diagnosis of RV failure include an increase in right atrial pressure and a decrease in arterial blood pressure, cardiac output, and mixed venous oxygen saturation (⊃ Fig. 14.4), despite a usually preserved PAP and pulmonary capillary wedge pressure. For difficult cases, a technique often cited in the literature for the diagnosis of RV failure involves the administration of 250 mL of crystalloids or colloids over 10 min [46]. If the patient is suffering from RV failure, all the above haemodynamic parameters worsen, including a dramatic increase in right

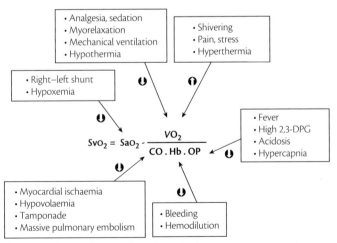

Figure 14.4 Main factors influencing mixed venous oxygen saturation. 2,3-DPG, 2,3-diphosphoglycerate; CO, cardiac output; Hb, haemoglobin rate; OP, oxygen-binding capacity of haemoglobin. SvO_2, mixed venous oxygen saturation; SaO_2, arterial oxygen saturation; VO_2, oxygen consumption.

atrial pressure with no change in cardiac output. This test should not be used in patients who are in acute RV failure, as there is a risk of severe aggravation of tricuspid insufficiency and organ congestion after volume loading.

Conclusion

In the case of haemodynamic instability, the right mechanism needs to be assessed rapidly. Indeed, the assessment will lead to the appropriate treatment. Impairment in blood pressure and heart rate may be due to various mechanisms including hypovolaemia and heart and/or vascular dysfunction. AHF may also be related to many mechanisms: LV diastolic and/or systolic dysfunction and/or RV dysfunction. Echocardiography is a great help in making the diagnosis. A PAC can help, in few cases, to monitor cardiovascular status while the patient is treated.

Personal perspective

Severe alteration in the cardiovascular system may lead to impairment in systemic blood pressure, stroke volume, and organ (lung, liver, kidney) function. If both heart rate and volaemia seem adequate, haemodynamic instability is related to myocardial and/or vascular dysfunction. It should be noted that a prolonged myocardial dysfunction may lead to an associated vascular dysfunction.

Further reading

Chemla D, Coirault C, Hebert JL, Lecarpentier Y. Mechanics of relaxation of the human heart. *News Physiol Sci* 2000;**15**:78–83.

Gillebert TC, Leite-Moreira AF, De Hert SG. Load dependent diastolic dysfunction in heart failure. *Heart Fail Rev* 2000;**5**(4):345–355.

Logeart D, Saudubray C, Beyne P, *et al*. Comparative value of Doppler echocardiography and B-type natriuretic peptide assay in the etiologic diagnosis of acute dyspnea. *J Am Coll Cardiol* 2002;**40**(10):1794–1800.

Mebazaa A, Karpati P, Renaud E, Algotsson L. Acute right ventricular failure—from pathophysiology to new treatments. *Intensive Care Med* 2004;**30**(2):185–196.

Reynolds HR, Hochman JS. Cardiogenic shock: current concepts and improving outcomes. *Circulation* 2008;**117**(5):686–697.

van Heerebeek L, Borbely A, Niessen HW, *et al*. Myocardial structure and function differ in systolic and diastolic heart failure. *Circulation* 2006;**113**(16):1966–1973.

Zannad F, Mebazaa A, Juilliere Y, *et al*. Clinical profile, contemporary management and one-year mortality in patients with severe acute heart failure syndromes: The EFICA study. *Eur J Heart Fail* 2006;**8**(7):697–705.

Zile MR, Brutsaert DL. New concepts in diastolic dysfunction and diastolic heart failure: Part I: diagnosis, prognosis, and measurements of diastolic function. *Circulation* 2002;**105**(11):1387–1393.

⊃ For additional multimedia materials please visit the online version of the book (🕮 http://www.esciacc.oxfordmedicine.com).

CHAPTER 15

The respiratory system

Antoine Vieillard-Baron

Contents

Summary

The respiratory system is key to the management of patients with respiratory and also haemodynamic compromise and should be monitored. The ventilator is more than just a machine that delivers gas: it is a true respiratory system monitoring device, allowing measurement of airway pressures and intrinsic positive end-expiratory pressure (PEEP) and plotting of pressure/volume (P/V) curves. For effective and reliable monitoring it is necessary to keep in mind physiology, such as the alveolar gas equation, heart–lung interactions, the equation of the movement, etc. Monitoring the respiratory system enables adaptation not only of respiratory management but also of haemodynamic management.

Introduction

A textbook on intensive and acute cardiac care should describe the mechanisms responsible for haemodynamic compromise, such as acute heart failure with its many aetiologies [1]. However, respiratory system status appears key to the management of such failure: first, because many causes of heart failure lead to pulmonary congestion and so respiratory failure; secondly, because changes in respiratory system properties may impact on haemodynamics; and finally, because mechanical ventilation, when required, may have beneficial but also deleterious effects on cardiac function [2].

Cardiologists and intensive care physicians have to be fully conversant with heart–lung interactions, with how their knowledge helps to understand changes in haemodynamics related to change in ventilatory settings or respiratory mechanics, and with how monitoring of the respiratory system can be done at the bedside.

Definitions—physiological reminders

Blood gas exchange

Blood gas exchanges occur passively through the alveola–capillary membrane, according to the gradient in gas concentration between the capillary blood and the alveolae. This gradient is mediated in part by the equilibrium between O_2 and CO_2 in the alveolae, depending on the alveolar gas equation (📷 15.1):

$$P_{AO_2} = P_{IO_2} - 1.2P_{ACO_2}$$

where P_{AO_2} is the alveolar pressure of O_2, P_{ACO_2} the alveolar pressure of CO_2 and P_{IO_2} the inspired pressure of O_2, calculated as $F_{IO_2} \times (760 - 47)$, where F_{IO_2} is the oxygen inspired fraction, 760 mmHg the atmospheric pressure and 47 mmHg the part of the inspired gas which is transformed into water.

Moreover, P_{ACO_2} is directly proportional to CO_2 production and inversely proportional to alveolar ventilation. Differences between P_{AO_2} and arterial pressure in O_2 (P_{aO_2}) are in part explained by the ventilation/perfusion ratio (V/Q). In a 'perfect' lung, i.e. a lung with $V/Q = 1$, P_{aO_2} is close to P_{AO_2}.

Then, in ambient air, oxygenation directly depends on alveolar ventilation. A decrease in alveolar ventilation will increase P_{ACO_2} and so decrease P_{AO_2}. Under oxygen, by contrast it is the F_{IO_2} that mainly determines the level of oxygenation. This explains why lung function must be evaluated using the P_{aO_2}/F_{IO_2} ratio. A patient with a 'perfect' lung has a ratio close to 500 mmHg, whereas acute lung injury is defined as a ratio below 300 mmHg.

Alveolar ventilation and dead space

Dead space (V_D) is defined as the volume of gas not usable for blood gas exchanges. The total dead space is also called the physiological dead space and is the sum of the alveolar dead space (part of the lungs with $V/Q > 1$) and the anatomical dead space (trachea, bronchae, etc.). Alveolar ventilation (L/min) is thus the difference between minute ventilation (tidal volume times respiratory rate) and the physiological dead space, and finally determines P_{aCO_2}. In healthy subjects in the supine position, the anatomical dead space has been reported as between 100–120 mL and the physiological dead space around 150 mL [3]. But dead space can also be expressed as a fraction of tidal volume (V_D/V_T).

Main causes of acute hypoxaemia

Hypoxaemia may occur if there is a mismatch between ventilation and perfusion, with $V/Q < 1$. This is described as a shunt effect, also called venous admixture. It occurs in many situations, including pulmonary oedema, whatever its cause, pneumonia, and pulmonary embolism. Interestingly, in these situations, changes in cardiac output, as induced by the treatment, may change blood gases. For instance, P_{aO_2} in the normal range at admission was reported in patients with massive pulmonary embolism, whereas the increase in cardiac output induced by dobutamine was secondarily responsible for its fall [4]. Conversely, low cardiac output induces an increase in peripheral oxygen extraction and so low oxygen venous saturation, leading to a sharp fall in P_{aO_2} which may be partially corrected after improvement in oxygen transport. This is why it is not rare for intensivists to note an increase in oxygen saturation after blood volume expansion in hypovolaemia.

The second cause of acute hypoxaemia, as explained above, is alveolar hypoventilation. This induces an increase in P_{aCO_2} and so a decrease in P_{aO_2}. Alveolar hypoventilation may be due, first, to an excessive alveolar dead space, as occurs in many situations such as acute exacerbation of chronic obstructive pulmonary disease (COPD), or, second, to a decrease in minute ventilation, as in comatose patients and in some cases of drug poisoning. Even if not classic, alveolar hypoventilation has also been reported in severe cardiogenic pulmonary oedema, especially in older patients. Increasing F_{IO_2} easily corrects P_{aO_2}, but does not change and may even mask and worsen alveolar hypoventilation, with deleterious consequences. The only way to improve the patient's condition is to correct hypoventilation.

Airway pressures and respiratory mechanics

There are, in fact, three 'airway pressures': pleural pressure (P_{PL}), alveolar pressure (P_{ALV}) and transpulmonary pressure (TPP) (see summary in 📷 15.2). In a spontaneously breathing patient, P_{PL} is negative throughout the respiratory cycle, whereas it is positive during tidal ventilation in a mechanically ventilated patient and also sometimes during expiration, depending on the PEEP. Changes in P_{PL} (ΔP_{PL}) are related to changes in tidal volume (TV), according to the compliance of the chest wall (C_{CW}):

$$C_{CW} = TV/\Delta P_{PL}$$

P_{ALV} is zero at end-expiration and at end-inspiration in a spontaneously breathing patient (📷 15.2). In a mechanically ventilated patient, airway pressure depends first on the end-expiratory pressure (PEEP), second on the resistive part of the pressure ($Q \times R$) and finally on the static part of the pressure (TV/CRS). It is expressed by the equation of the movement:

$$P\text{AIRWAY} = \text{PEEP} + QR + \text{TV}/C\text{RS}$$

where Q is the inspiratory flow, R the resistance to flow, and CRS the compliance of the respiratory system (lung + chest wall). When the flow is nil, during a pause, PAIRWAY represents the PALV at end-inspiration it represents the plateau pressure (PPLATEAU) and depends on the TV and on the compliance of the respiratory system. In normal subjects, PALV at end-expiration is zero. It can become positive either if a 'therapeutic' PEEP is applied or if dynamic hyperinflation is occurring, leading to an intrinsic PEEP.

Finally, TPP is the distending pressure of the lung, calculated as PALV – PPL. Changes in TPP (ΔTPP) are related to changes in TV according to the compliance of the lung (CL):

$$C\text{L} = \text{TV}/\Delta\text{TPP}$$

Any decrease in lung compliance will induce an increase in TPP for a given lung volume.

Heart–lung interactions

Briefly, any changes in respiratory mechanics, or passing from spontaneous ventilation to mechanical ventilation, will act on cardiac function by modifying the different airway pressures (📷15.2) [2].

An increase in PPL, due to a decrease in chest wall compliance, as in obese patients, or due to positive pressure ventilation, will decrease systemic venous return (➲ Fig. 15.1) [5]. This can explain the deleterious effect of PEEP in hypovolaemic patients or the beneficial effects of the same PEEP in a patient with cardiogenic pulmonary oedema.

What is true for therapeutic PEEP has also been described for intrinsic PEEP. Some studies have suggested that a positive PPL will help a failed left ventricle to act, by decreasing its afterload [6].

An increase in TPP due to severe alteration in lung compliance will induce systolic overload of the right ventricle [7]. This has been described especially in patients ventilated for severe acute respiratory distress syndrome (ARDS) [8].

What can and should be monitored at the bedside

In general, monitoring of the respiratory system is limited in spontaneously breathing patients, whereas in mechanically ventilated patients many tools are available to evaluate the properties of the respiratory system. In the first situation, the main aim of monitoring will be to identify patients and situations requiring invasive or noninvasive mechanical ventilation. In the second situation, the aims of monitoring will be to optimize respiratory settings (TV, respiratory rate, PEEP, etc.), to avoid excessive airway pressures, to limit the deleterious effect of positive pressure ventilation on cardiac function, and finally to optimize respiratory management.

The first requirement in monitoring the respiratory system is correct interpretation of the clinical signs of respiratory failure. These include polypnoea, cyanosis, tachycardia and intercostal, suprasternal or supraclavicular recession. Oxygen saturation can be noninvasively monitored by plethysmography (Spo$_2$), but some differences have been reported between Spo$_2$ and Sao$_2$ and the signal is not always optimal when shock is associated. Physicians should look especially for signs suggesting hypercapnia because they may require specific management, such as application of noninvasive mechanical ventilation. These signs include

ZEEP

PEEP 5

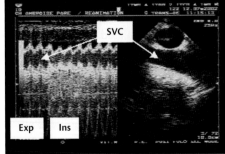
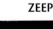
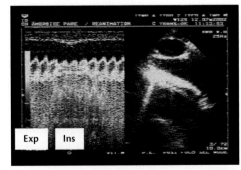

Figure 15.1 Transoesophageal echocardiography in a mechanically ventilated patient, at ZEEP (zero end-expiratory pressure) and 5 cmH$_2$O PEEP. Two-dimensional view of the superior vena cava (SVC), associated with the time–motion study, demonstrates collapse of the vessel during tidal ventilation in PEEP conditions, reflecting a decrease in systemic venous return. Exp, expiration; Ins, inspiration.

sweating, flapping tremor, and decreased consciousness. Blood gas analysis will confirm the clinical evaluation. In exacerbation of COPD, uncompensated respiratory acidosis will indicate the need for noninvasive mechanical ventilation [9]. Monitoring of blood gases, in accordance with the chest radiograph, may also help to clarify the effect of PEEP in a patient mechanically ventilated for acute lung injury, as illustrated in ➲ Fig. 15.2.

Monitoring of PPLATEAU is crucial in a sedated mechanically ventilated patient (➲ Fig. 15.5). It is used as a surrogate for TPP, but overestimates it. TPP is not available in clinical practice because PPL is difficult to record since it requires placement of a balloon in the oesophagus [10]. PPLATEAU has been reported to be strongly related to the risk of barotrauma and pneumothorax [11]. Strict limitation of PPLATEAU has been shown to save lives, especially in ARDS [12] and acute asthma [13]. A PPLATEAU below 30 cmH$_2$O, and much better below 27 cmH$_2$O, limits lung overdistension and pulmonary hypertension and their effects on the right ventricle [14]. However, respirators are not equipped with an alarm regarding PPLATEAU, but just peak pressure, i.e. the pressure reached before the end-inspiratory pause (👥 15.3). As recalled above in the equation of movement, a peak pressure alarm may reflect (1) an abrupt increase in intrinsic PEEP (does the patient have an expiratory flow limitation?), (2) an increase in flow resistance (is the endotracheal tube partially occluded?), and (3) a deterioration of lung mechanics (does the patient have pneumothorax, or abrupt-onset pulmonary oedema?). Intrinsic PEEP may be easily detected by performing an end-expiratory pause, as shown in 👥 15.3.

Recording of expiratory CO$_2$ is possible, especially in intubated patients, by sensors positioned between the proximal end of the endotracheal tube and the Y piece of the ventilator. Mean expiratory (PECO$_2$) and end-tidal (PETCO$_2$) CO$_2$ can thus be monitored, allowing calculation of the physiological dead space (VDphysiol/VT = 1 – PECO$_2$/PaCO$_2$) and the alveolar dead space (VDalv/VT = 1 – PETCO$_2$/PaCO$_2$). A decrease in VD/VT reflects improvement in respiratory mechanics and subsequently in the patient's status. This is true in acute exacerbation of COPD or in acute asthma, where decrease in VD/VT reflects decrease in expiratory flow limitation, but also in ARDS, where decrease in VD/VT mostly reflects decrease in lung overdistension. It has been suggested that in these patients even a slight decrease in PaCO$_2$ reflects functional lung recruitment induced by some procedures, such as prone positioning [15], and that this decrease is often associated with a better prognosis [16].

The pressure/volume (P/V) loop of the respiratory system has long been proposed as a means of evaluating respiratory

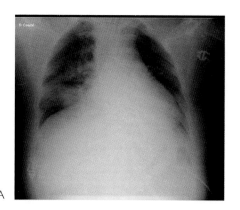

FiO$_2$ 0.7	12/01/09 14:57	12/01/09 15:21
	PEEP 5	**ZEEP**
		70.0
pH	7.46	7.50
PaCO$_2$	41	38
PaO$_2$	64	101

A

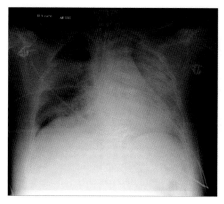

FiO$_2$ 0.7	13/01/09 15:24	13/01/09 16:20
	PEEP 5	**ZEEP$_{TEL}$**
pH	7.44	7.41
PaCO$_2$	41	45
PaO$_2$	108	57

B

Figure 15.2 Chest radiograph and blood gas analysis at ZEEP and PEEP (5 cmH$_2$O) in a patient on day 1 (panel A) and day 2 (panel B). On day 1, the chest radiograph showed unilateral injury of the lung. PEEP removal induced an increase in PaO$_2$ and a decrease in PaCO$_2$, reflecting overdistension of the lung related to PEEP. On day 2, lung injury was bilateral. PEEP removal induced a decrease in PaO$_2$ and an increase in PaCO$_2$, reflecting derecruitment of the lung.

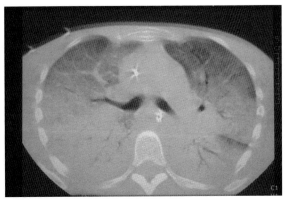

Figure 15.3 Lung CT scan in a ventilated patient with severe ARDS related to extensive pneumonia.

mechanics [17]. Whereas the curve is linear during inspiration in patients without lung injury (📷15.4), it includes a lower and a upper inflection point in ARDS (📷15.4). P/V loop pattern has been proposed for assessing the 'recruitability' of the system [18, 19] (📷15.4). However, this loop is difficult to use at the bedside.

Finally, a few words should be said about CT scanning of the lung. Although this is as yet unavailable at the bedside, many studies have demonstrated its utility in assessing the 'recruitability' of the lung in ARDS [20] and in evaluating the effect of PEEP in terms of lung overdistension and recruitment [21]. An example of a lung CT scan of a patient ventilated for severe ARDS is shown in ➲ Fig. 15.3. Whether lung ultrasonography can noninvasively give similar information remains to be confirmed [22].

Conclusion

The respiratory system is key to the management of patients with respiratory and also haemodynamic compromise. According to its properties, it may act differently on cardiac function. Because the most severely compromised patients in the intensive care unit are mechanically ventilated, it is mandatory for intensivists to understand fully that any change in ventilatory settings will also affect haemodynamics. It is clinically possible to monitor the respiratory system. The ventilator is more than just a machine that delivers gas; it is a true respiratory system monitoring device able to evaluate PPEAK, PPLATEAU, intrinsic PEEP, and expiratory flow limitation.

Personal perspective

Because most patients in the intensive care unit are mechanically ventilated, respiratory management, and so respiratory monitoring, is critical. Respirators are too often considered as simple machines that deliver gas, whereas they can be used as a true monitoring device. A serious effort has to be made to train intensivists better to understand how to monitor the respiratory system, and why. Recent studies in severely compromised patients, with ARDS or acute asthma, show that a rigorous approach to ventilation can save lives. Such studies should be used to increase intensivists' awareness of the importance of limiting plateau pressure, avoiding intrinsic PEEP, and adapting respiratory settings to respiratory mechanics. In the future, new methods will be available at the bedside for all intensivists: perhaps CT scanning and less 'aggressive' lung ultrasound.

Further reading

Brochard L, Mancebo J, Wysocki M, *et al.* Noninvasive ventilation for acute exacerbations of chronic obstructive pulmonary disease. *N Engl J Med* 1995; **333**:817–822.

Scharf SM, Caldini P, Ingram RH. Cardiovascular effect of increasing airway pressure in the dog. *Am J Physiol* 1977;**232**:H35–43.

Task Force on Acute Heart Failure of the European Society of Cardiology. Guidelines on the diagnosis and treatment of acute heart failure. *Eur Heart J* 2005;**26**:1115–1140.

Ventilation with lower tidal volumes as compared with traditional tidal volumes for acute lung injury and the acute respiratory distress syndrome. The Acute Respiratory Distress Syndrome Network. *N Engl J Med* 2000;**342**:1301–1308.

Vieillard-Baron A, Prin S, Chergui K, *et al.* Early patterns of static pressure-volume loops in ARDS and their relations with PEEP-induced recruitment. *Intensive Care Med* 2003;**29**:1929–1935.

Whittenberger JL, McGregor M, Berglund E, Borst HG. Influence of state of inflation of the lung on pulmonary vascular resistance. *J Appl Physiol* 1960;**15**:878–882.

Additional online material

📷 15.1 Schematic representation of blood gas exchange mechanisms

📷 15.2 Airway pressures in spontaneous ventilation and in mechanical ventilation during inspiration and expiration

📷 15.3 Recording of airway pressure

📷 15.4 Quasi-static P/V loop of the respiratory system in three mechanically ventilated patients

➲ For additional multimedia materials please visit the online version of the book (🔗 http://www.esciacc.oxfordmedicine. com).

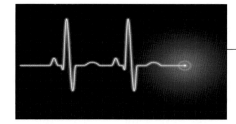

CHAPTER 16

Monitoring of the neurological condition of the acute cardiac care patient

Cathy S. De Deyne

Contents

Summary

Many techniques are currently available for cerebral physiological monitoring in the intensive care unit (ICU) environment. The ultimate goal of cerebral monitoring applied during the acute care of any patient with, or at risk of, a neurological insult is the early detection of regional or global hypoxic/ischaemic cerebral insults. Ideally, cerebral monitoring should enable the detection of any deterioration before irreversible brain damage occurs. Only those monitoring techniques that have been correlated with outcome, e.g. monitoring of intracranial pressure (ICP) and evoked potentials (EP), have found widespread acceptance in clinical practice. Most of the information that affects the bedside care of patients with acute neurological disturbances is now derived from clinical examination, and from the knowledge of pathophysiological changes in cerebral perfusion, cerebral oxygenation, and cerebral function. Online monitoring of these changes can be realized by many invasive (or even noninvasive) techniques estimating cerebral perfusion, cerebral oxygenation, and cerebral function, without neglecting clinical examination and basic physiological variables such as invasive arterial blood pressure monitoring or arterial blood gas analysis.

Neurological monitoring in the acute care setting offers an essential window into the 'brain' of the patient. Any patient in acute care needs special attention to brain function and moreover, if possible, preservation or restoration of normal brain function. Current cerebral monitoring techniques (invasive as well as noninvasive) can offer essential information on the patient's current neurological status, but knowledge of cerebral physiology and pathophysiology remains a keystone in the optimal interpretation and management of the patient's neurological condition. The main reasons for monitoring at-risk neuro-critical care patients are (1) to detect early neurological worsening before irreversible damage occurs; (2) to individualize patient care decisions; (3) to guide patient management; (4) to monitor therapeutic responses of some interventions and to avoid any consequent deleterious adverse effects; and finally (5) to improve neurological outcome in survivors of any acute neurological injury. In this chapter, most of today's bedside cerebral monitoring techniques are discussed, but the important role of neuroimaging should not be overlooked. However, despite its sometimes essential information, all neuroimaging techniques (CT, MRI) require transfer of the patient out of the ICU environment and can only offer intermittent information. Therefore, an additional role of cerebral monitoring in the acute care patient is to guide decisions on the need for additional neuroimaging examinations.

Clinical neurological monitoring

Neurological examination

Clinical neurological monitoring, by means of the neurological examination, assesses the depth of arousability, the content of consciousness, if awake, as well as more specific (focal) deficits. The general neurological examination always remains useful for additional aetiological questions and management. However, in the intensive care unit (ICU) environment, this clinical examination is often a challenging task as: (1) the patient may have received sedating or paralysing drugs; (2) drug pharmacokinetics may be altered by major organ dysfunction (liver, kidney); (3) the patient may be intubated, making communication difficult; and (4) more than one disease process may be going on: if multiple organ failure has occurred, this can contribute to the impairment of consciousness (particularly in the presence of septic encephalopathy).

In general, the neurological examination assesses the level of consciousness, the functioning of the cranial nerves, and the patient's motor function. Arousability is assessed by stimulating the patient, by speaking in their ear. It is far better to make an assessment of patient's activity and responsiveness than to use nonspecific terms such as semi-coma. Even within the context of coma (unrousable, unconscious) there may be different types of response (no response, posturing, purposeful movements, or abnormal posturing). Coma may obscure the evaluation of all but cranial nerves II, III and IV. Direct and consensual pupillary light reflexes are easily assessed with the patient's eyes passively held open looking for constriction of the ipsilateral and contralateral pupil.

With damage to cranial nerve III, the ipsilateral pupil is typically dilated and unreactive, the eye is turned outwards, and there is complete or nearly complete ipsilateral ptosis.

The presence of a normal pupillary light reflex indicates that its afferent and efferent limbs are intact. An early manifestation of brain herniation is the loss of pupillary reactivity, usually on the side of the mass effect.

Spontaneous movements in the ICU patient include posturing, purposeful movements, withdrawal movements, seizures, or myoclonus. A 'purposeful' motor response is one that avoids the noxious stimulus or attempts to push it away. Decerebrate or decorticate posturing indicates severe bilateral dysfunction deep in both hemispheres or in the brainstem.

Coma scales

Scoring systems were developed for the objective quantification of the severity of acute illness and for the prediction of outcome. The Glasgow Coma Scale (GCS) ⊃ Box 16.1) was introduced in 1974 aiming at standardizing assessment of level of consciousness in head-injured patients. It has been used mainly in evaluating prognosis, comparing different groups of patients, and monitoring neurological status. Today, the GCS is the most universal scale used in

---

Box 16.1 Glasgow Coma Scale

Best eye opening

E1 none

E2 to pain

E3 to voice

E4 spontaneously with blinking

Best motor response in unaffected limb

M1 no response to pain

M2 arm extension to pain (decerebrate posturing)

M3 arm flexion to pain (decorticate posturing)

M4 arm withdraws from pain

M5 hand localizes pain

M6 obeys commands

Best verbal response

V1 none

V2 sounds, no recognizable words

V3 inappropriate words

V4 confused speech

V5 normal, orientated

Lancet 1974;**ii**:81.

emergency departments (EDs) and ICUs and is by far the most common scale cited in the neuro-intensive care literature. It gives a maximum of 15 points: 6 points maximum for best motor response, 5 for best verbal response and 4 for eye opening. Problems with the use of the GCS arise when patients are intubated and cannot respond verbally, or if the eyes are swollen, preventing verbal response from the patient and ocular assessment, respectively. A theoretical disadvantage is the fact that the total GCS score is obtained by adding the values for three motor activities, namely eye opening, best motor response, and best verbal response. These are assumed to be independent variables, but they are not. Moreover, the GCS is often insufficiently sensitive for the detection of changes in the level of consciousness in ICU patients. The key concept in all literature data, however, is that even though GCS is not a perfect tool and other coma scales have been proposed, it seems destined to be incorporated in clinical decisions regarding coma for many years to come. Most recently, the GCS was reported as a simple and reliable method for clinical outcome assessment in patients treated with therapeutic hypothermia after cardiac arrest.

Specific neurological monitoring in the ICU

The reference standard for cerebral monitoring in the ICU environment is still the physical examination, most commonly a simple screening procedure such as the GCS. By the time any decrement in score has been noted, however, further brain injury that may or may not be reversible may have already occurred. In addition, management of any kind of acute neurological failure may necessitate sedation (and possible paralysis), thus negating the reliability of bedside examination as a screening tool. Ideally, cerebral physiological monitoring should provide the means of a continuous bedside assessment in the ICU, widely applicable to monitoring the course of various of disease processes, capable of detecting abnormalities before irreversible brain damage has occurred, and helpful in assessing therapeutic interventions known to influence outcome. Critical care monitoring (and management) of patients with acute severe brain injury (of any origin) has undergone tremendous advances. Today's armamentarium consists of invasive and noninvasive monitoring devices available to help detect secondary brain injury and guide therapy. In general, cerebral monitoring techniques applied in the ICU environment can be categorized into those measuring cerebral perfusion, cerebral metabolism (or cerebral oxygenation), and cerebral function.

Monitoring of cerebral perfusion

In terms of the neuro-ICU management of severely head-injured patients, the adequacy of cerebral perfusion is usually inferred, rather than measured directly, because of the relative complexity of cerebral blood flow (CBF) measurements. In an awake, normothermic man, CBF remains remarkably constant at 50 mL^{-1} 100 g^{-1} min^{-1}. If CBF decreases below a critical level (c.18 mL^{-1} 100 g^{-1} min^{-1}), cellular function is compromised, manifesting as a potentially reversible change in the EEG. Below 10 mL^{-1} 100 g^{-1} min^{-1} cellular integrity is affected irreversibly if the ischaemia even persists beyond a certain level.

CBF is determined by the formula:

$$CBF = CPP/CVR$$

where the cerebral perfusion pressure (CPP) is the mathematical difference between mean arterial pressure (MAP) and intracranial pressure (ICP), and CVR is the cerebral vascular resistance.

Normally, cerebral autoregulation adjusts CVR automatically and continuously such that global CBF remains constant over a wide range of MAP from 50 to 150 mmHg. In the presence of various diseases, such as head injury, subarachnoid haemorrhage, intracranial bleeding or post-reanimation status, however, autoregulation may be regionally impaired, resulting in a pressure-passive CBF and dictating the need for meticulous control of MAP. In these conditions, every decrease (as well as every increase) in MAP will induce the reciprocal decrease (or increase) in CBF, thereby reaching critical thresholds (for cerebral ischaemia in case of severe arterial hypotension, or for severe cerebral hyperaemia with the ensuing risk of breaking through the blood–brain barrier in case of severe arterial hypertension). This rigorous control of MAP is best accomplished using an intra-arterial catheter for invasive beat-to-beat control of blood pressure—noninvasive methods of blood pressure monitoring measure blood pressure only intermittently. A CPP threshold of 60–65 mmHg is the goal of blood pressure management. In case of normal ICP (10–15 mmHg), this implies a MAP threshold of 70–80 mmHg, but in case of increased ICP, MAP values of at least 90 mmHg should be aimed at. Calibration of the arterial pressure transducer to zero should ideally be done at the level of the external auditory meatus to account for differences in perfusion pressure between the level of the head and the thorax owing to alterations in head position.

In the absence of critical vascular stenosis, CVR is determined by cerebral autoregulation, the level of neural activity, blood viscosity, and arterial carbon dioxide and oxygen tensions. Acutely, incremental changes in $Paco_2$ cause corresponding directional changes in CBF, of the order of 4% change in CBF per 1 mmHg change in $Paco_2$. If intracranial compliance is reduced, as in the presence of any intracerebral bleeding, such an increase in CBF may be accompanied by a rise in cerebral blood volume (CBV) and ICP. Conversely, alterations in P_aO_2 cause directionally opposite changes in CBF. CBF increases abruptly as P_aO_2 falls below 40 mmHg, whereas a rise in P_aO_2 from the normoxic to the hyperoxic range results in a 15% decrease in CBF. This is offset by a corresponding increase in arterial oxygen content. Thus, monitoring of arterial blood gas tensions enhances the interpretation of changes in other parameters (e.g. ICP). This is accomplished either intermittently by sampling of arterial blood or continuously by measurement of transcutaneous peripheral oxygenation (pulse oximetry) or end-tidal CO_2 analysis (capnography).

In the past, techniques for accurate, quantitative measurement of regional CBF were tried out at the bedside in the ICU (e.g. based on clearance of the freely diffusible, poorly soluble, inert radioisotope xenon-133 from the brain tissue). However, technical complexity made it difficult to include this monitoring technique into the standard monitoring care of neuro-ICU patients. Moreover, few data are available to correlate CBF with clinical outcome in patients who have critical neurological illness. Clinical interpretation of CBF data is further hindered by the complex interaction between CBF, CBV, and ICP, intracranial compliance, and functional neural integrity.

A continuous, noninvasive, qualitative assessment of cerebral perfusion is available in the form of transcranial Doppler (TCD). This device utilizes 2-MHz pulsed Doppler ultrasound directed through the thin regions of the skull (e.g. the temporal area) to measure flow velocity (FV) rather than flow volume in the major intracranial arteries (mostly in the middle cerebral artery). Although the absolute measurements of FV correlate poorly with xenon-133 CBF measurements, FV measurements give an accurate indication of changes in CBF in individual patients. FV (in cm/s) varies directly with the absolute level of CBF and inversely with the square of the vessel diameter. In patients with SAH and cerebrovascular spasm, it was shown that FV elevations precede clinical signs of cerebral ischaemia. If TCD monitoring is performed on a frequent basis, the severity and time course of arterial narrowing can be monitored noninvasively, thus facilitating optimal timing e.g. for cerebral aneurysm surgery (best results if no cerebral vasospasm is already present) or for evaluation of medical treatment, while obviating the need

for repeat angiography. In closed head injury with raised ICP, TCD may aid distinction of patients with low CBF from those with high CBF and vasoparalysis (i.e. loss of autoregulation). A patient with high ICP and low CBF may suffer further ischaemia because of excessive hyperventilation (as a reduction in $Paco_2$ induces intense cerebral vasoconstriction). Nevertheless, hyperventilation was a therapy widely and empirically used in the past to reduce CBF (and ICP), but the application of bedside monitoring of cerebral perfusion completely changed this to the maintenance of strict normoventilation (with normal $Paco_2$ values).

Monitoring of intracranial pressure

Elevation of ICP is of major concern for two reasons; first, it is indicative of some ongoing change in the volume of intracranial contents (brain tissue, cerebrospinal fluid (CSF), and/or CBV) and second, it has adverse implications for cerebral perfusion. Any significant increase in ICP can reduce cerebral perfusion below the critical threshold of cerebral ischaemia. Direct measurement of ICP is indicated in circumstances in which intracranial hypertension is likely, either because of radiological findings or because of knowledge about the natural history of the disease. Direct measurement of ICP is not only applied in severe head injury (GCS <8 on hospital admission), but also in cases of severe stroke or severe encephalitis. Nevertheless, in patients with malignant middle cerebral artery infarction, it was reported that pupillary abnormalities and severe brain stem compression may be present despite normal ICP values. Therefore, in case of severe stroke, ICP monitoring cannot substitute for close clinical and radiological follow-up in the management of these patients.

In the setting of direct ICP monitoring, the concept of intracranial compliance must be clearly understood. A progressive increase in ICP suggests exhaustion of the compensatory ability of the semiclosed skull to absorb further volume increases. ICP increases cannot, therefore, be defined as an 'early warning sign' of reduced intracranial compliance. This increase in ICP is, however, superior to the classical clinical syndrome of pupillary dilation, bradycardia, hypertension, and decerebration, all of which may be absent despite significant ICP elevations.

Normal ICP is less than 10 mmHg in the supine position, and sustained baseline pressure greater than 15 mmHg is considered pathologic. The intraventricular catheter remains the reference standard to which other ICP monitoring devices are compared. Advantages include simplicity, low cost, and relative ease of insertion, although this may prove technically difficult if the lateral ventricles are compressed by interstitial oedema or by a space-occupying lesion. Through this intraventricular catheter, CSF can be drained, which can offer a therapy in the case of significant intracranial hypertension.

Monitoring of cerebral metabolism

Cerebral oxygen consumption ($CMRo_2$) is calculated from the product of mean global CBF and the cerebral arteriovenous oxygen content difference (a-vDo_2, normal 6 mL^{-1} 100 g^{-1} min^{-1}). Cerebral venous effluent is sampled from a catheter inserted percutaneously into the internal jugular vein and advanced in a retrograde fashion into the jugular bulb. Using this method, the value generated for a-vDo_2 is not global, because jugular venous oxygen tension is measured from a unilateral sample, but there is considerable mixing of the venous effluent from both hemispheres. Two-thirds of the blood supplied to one hemisphere through an internal carotid artery is drained through the ipsilateral jugular vein, whereas one-third drains contralaterally. Extracerebral contamination of blood in the jugular bulb accounts for around 3%.

Jugular bulb oximetry, by insertion of a fibreoptic catheter retrogradely into the internal jugular vein, until its tip reaches the jugular bulb, offers a continuous estimation of the adequacy of cerebral perfusion. Normal jugular bulb saturation values (S_jo_2) are between 50% and 80%. In particular, too low S_jo_2 values (<50%) indicate the presence of inadequate cerebral perfusion. Despite the relative simple technique and the clinical value of the information obtained, jugular bulb oximetry is currently only used now in the setting of multimodality monitoring for severe head injury.

Near-infrared spectroscopy is a noninvasive method of monitoring cerebral tissue oxygen saturation. It uses two or four wavelengths of LED or laser light to distinguish oxygenated haemoglobin from de-oxygenated haemoglobin, thereby providing the respective oxygen saturation of the cerebral tissue. This cerebral tissue oxygen saturation reflects arterial as well as venous (as capillary) components, and therefore straight comparison to S_jo_2 values remains difficult. It remains to be seen whether this noninvasive monitoring technique could become of any value e.g. to detect inadequate cerebral perfusion in the acute care patient.

The most recently introduced invasive monitoring techniques concern brain tissue oxygenation and brain metabolism. Invasive measurement of brain tissue Po_2 ($P_{bt}o_2$) enables continuous monitoring of brain oxygen tension by insertion of a specially designed oximetry probe into the brain tissue. This is an invasive, ultra-local monitoring technique, exclusively almost used in the multimodality monitoring of severe head injury. Cerebral microdialysis monitors the local cerebral metabolism by measuring interstitial glucose, lactate, pyruvate, glycerol, and glutamate. It is an invasive monitoring technique that relies on the insertion of a microdialysis catheter into the tissue of the cerebral cortex. As for brain oxygen tension monitoring, cerebral microdialysis is mostly used as part of multimodality neuromonitoring in severe head injury (or sometimes in cases of subarachnoid haemorrhage). Indeed, most of these techniques cannot be fruitfully used in isolation, but when combined with other monitoring methods they can provide unique insights into the biochemical and physiological derangements in the injured brain. The place and value of these invasive cerebral monitoring techniques in routine neurological monitoring in the critical care patient remains to be seen.

Electroencephalography

The standard electroencephalogram (EEG) is the summation of electrical activity generated in the pyramidal cells of the cerebral cortex. The EEG signal recorded at the scalp represents the activity of cortical cells to a depth of 1–2 cm only, because the high electrical impedance in the intervening bone and soft tissue attenuates the energy emanating from deeper brain structures. Typically, 16 leads are used, permitting considerable regional discrimination. These standardized leads are placed according to guidelines known as the international 10–20 system. Amplitude is measured from peak to peak and expressed in µV, normally ranging from 10 to 200 µV, with peak voltages of approximately 100 µV during seizure activity. The frequency spectrum of the EEG is categorized as follows: delta, <4 Hz; theta, 4–8 Hz; alpha, 8–13 Hz; beta, >13 Hz. In awake, relaxed adults, with eyes closed, the alpha rhythm predominates. Beta rhythm supervenes when the subject is stimulated (e.g. when the eyes are opened). Theta and delta waves are seen during normal sleep or sedation. Normally, some theta activity is detectable in awake patients, but persistent delta activity is considered abnormal. Visual, online interpretation of the raw EEG is confounded by many sources of electrical artefacts, including body movements, the ECG, and nearby electrical apparatus.

In the ICU setting, a premorbid tracing is seldom available for comparison, but cortical dysfunction is generally associated with slowing of EEG frequency and diminution of amplitude in the recorded signal, similar to that produced by cerebral ischaemia. Comparisons between the two hemispheres are usually helpful in clinical interpretation, particularly in patients with focal cerebral lesions.

Cerebral dysfunctions, accompanied by disturbed consciousness will result in some nonspecific slowing of EEG frequency and diminution of amplitude, but these changes in EEG cannot differentiate as to the exact aetiology of the respective cerebral dysfunction (e.g. metabolic, anoxic, toxic, infectious, or degenerative origin). Although no particular EEG pattern is related to a specific aetiology or prognosis, EEG monitoring can be used in comatose patients to assess the depth of coma and the reactivity to stimulation. Observation of rapid eye movement (REM) sleep and spontaneous variability in patterns of EEG activity over extended periods of time are associated with improved outcome in comatose patients, as compared to those with an invariant pattern. When EEG recordings are made over time, an improved EEG (higher EEG frequency and increased amplitude) can be one of the first signs pointing to a better neurological outcome.

Additionally, in paralysed patients, EEG monitoring may enable detection of seizures, prompting institution of anticonvulsant therapy and reversal of a potentially deleterious hypermetabolic state. It is noteworthy that recognition of seizure patterns is still hampered by computer processing of the EEG, emphasizing the need for immediate access to the raw data. In case of barbiturate therapy for intracranial hypertension, the drug infusion rate of barbiturates can be titrated against the EEG signal to produce a burst suppression pattern rather than a isoelectric signal, allowing maximum potential benefit without additional risk of drug overdosage.

In recent years years, EEG interpretation has been simplified by computer processing of the raw signal, which reduces the amount of data to be examined and facilitates interpretation by relatively inexperienced personnel. Several forms of EEG processing have been used in critical care practice including the cerebral function monitor (CFM), compressed spectral array (CSA), and density spectral array (DSA). The most recent computerized processed analysis of the raw EEG consists of a bispectral analysis of the EEG, offering a bispectral index (BIS) with a numerical value between 0 and 100. The recent literature has revealed the unique value of BIS in assessing depth of hypnosis during surgical anaesthesia and especially in preventing intraoperative awareness during anaesthesia. Likewise, BIS has been used in the ICU setting to assess depth of sedation, revealing satisfactory correlation with all clinical scoring systems (used to assess depth of ICU sedation, e.g. Ramsay sedation score, agitation sedation scale). Nevertheless, the exact value of BIS monitoring in patients with acute neurological disturbances is not yet established.

Future evolution of EEG monitoring in the ICU setting will surely focus on the application of continuous EEG monitoring (cEEG). cEEG monitoring offers advantages over intermittent EEG monitoring. Its main advantage is the possibility to detect nonclinical seizures, which are frequently reported in critical care patients. The future introduction of computerized algorithms for continuous EEG monitoring may render this monitoring even more feasible, at it should allow readily interpretation of any epileptic activity present in the raw EEG tracing.

Monitoring of evoked potentials

The major value of evoked potential (EP) monitoring is that signals are resistant to alterations by pharmacological agents such as barbiturates, so changes can be attributed correctly to genuine functional derangement. In addition, under conditions of cerebral hypoxia, the evoked responses are a more sensitive marker of irreversible hypoxic cellular damage than the EEG. Importantly, EP responses can be ascribed to specific anatomical structures not readily amenable to clinical assessment. The measurement and recording of EP requires computer-assisted analysis, because the amplitude of the EP signal is so low (0.12 µV) that it cannot readily be differentiated from the background EEG activity. Computer analysis is facilitated by the fact that EP signals occur at a predictable interval after a standardized stimulus, so many responses can be averaged. The information derived from interpretation of an EP response includes the poststimulus latency (in ms) and the peak amplitude (in µV) of the various waveforms in the tracing. Abnormalities are classified as absence of certain waveforms, prolonged latency, or reduced amplitude. Several neural pathways lend themselves to EP monitoring, but the three commonly used in clinical practice are somatosensory evoked potentials (SSEP), brainstem auditory evoked responses (BAER), and visual evoked potentials (VEP).

The stimulus for SSEP is supplied by electrical stimulation of nerves in any of the four limbs. Because SSEP monitor supratentorial elements that are affected early by shift of intracranial structures, they can be used diagnostically to detect expansion of space-occupying lesions. Prognostic information based on SSEP is extremely accurate in that absence of certain waveform components bilaterally in comatose patients is uniformly predictive of a persistent vegetative state or death.

Future developments will focus on using a variety of electrophysiological monitoring tools to follow patients clinically and formulate a prognosis. This concept has been termed multimodality evoked potential (MEP) monitoring, and consists of a combination of VEP, SSEP, and BAER. In patients with severe head injury, MEP measurements are highly predictive of outcome and improve the prognostic reliability of information derived from clinical examination.

⮕ For additional multimedia materials please visit the online version of the book (✇ http://www.esciacc.oxfordmedicine.com).

CHAPTER 17

Monitoring of kidney, liver, and other vital organs

K. Werdan, M. Girndt, and H. Ebelt

Contents

Summary

The prognosis of critically ill cardiac patients in the critical care unit (CCU) and intensive care unit (ICU) depends not only on the underlying cardiac disease but also on the development of secondary organ complications and failures. Therefore, close monitoring of vital organs is mandatory in all critically ill cardiac patients to detect the development of noncardiac organ failure as early as possible.

Introduction

Severe cardiac disease not only affects the heart, but also impairs other vital organs of the cardiac patient, like the kidneys, the liver, the gastrointestinal tract, and coagulation. Furthermore, acute heart failure and cardiogenic shock impair systemic microcirculation and may trigger the development of multiorgan dysfunction syndrome (MODS) and sepsis. These organ functions and systemic states have therefore to be carefully monitored in cardiac patients on the critical care unit (CCU) and intensive care unit (ICU).

Kidney

Monitoring of renal function

Though in critically ill patients the kidney is often just one of a number of failing organ systems, the presence of acute kidney injury (AKI) confers a disproportionate disadvantage in terms of survival and leads to an increased risk of developing 'nonrenal' complications such as bleeding and sepsis [1].

A number of clinical measures and biomarkers are in use for the monitoring of renal dysfunction (◉ Box 17.1). The routine measures of AKI have some severe limitations, however. In complete AKI, serum creatinine increases daily by 0.9–2.9 mg/dL (79–256 µmol/L). However, as renal function usually does not stop abruptly, the increase is often much slower, and becomes manifest

Box 17.1 Clinical measures and biomarkers for identification of acute kidney injury in critically ill patients

Recommended use in critically ill patients is indicated in **bold**.

- **Overhydration**
- **Electrolyte disturbances (hyperkalaemia)**
- **↑Serum creatinine and serum urea N**
- **Oliguria/anuria/polyuria**
- **Urinalysis (protein +; glucose +; sediment: leucocytes, red blood cell, cylinders**
- Creatinine clearance [14, 15]
- Calculation of eGFR [12, 13]
- GFR by clearance of inulin, ^{99m}DTPA, or iohexol
- RBF by selective arteriography, Doppler ultrasonography, or radionuclide scanning
- RIFLE criteria [2]: → risk → injury → failure → loss (RRT >4 weeks) → endstage disease (RRT >3 months)
- **AKIN criteria** (see Table 17.1)
- Serum cystatin C
- Urine or plasma NGAL

eGFR, estimated glomerular filtration rate; GFR, glomerular filtration rate; NGAL, neutrophil gelatinase associated lipocalin; RBF, renal blood flow; RRT, renal replacement therapy.

Table 17.1 AKIN classification/staging system for acute kidney injury[a]

Stage	Serum creatinine criteria (changes within 48 h)	Urine output criteria
1	Increase ≥0.3 mg/dL (≥ 26.4 µmol/L) or increase ≥1.5–2-fold from baseline[c]	<0.5 ml kg^{-1} h^{-1} for >6 and ≤12 h
2	Increase >2–3-fold from baseline[c]	<0.5 ml kg^{-1} h^{-1} for >12 h
3[b]	Increase >3-fold from baseline[c] or ≥ 4.0 mg/dL (≥354 µmol/L), with an acute increase of at least 0.5 mg/dL (44 µmol/L])	<0.3 ml kg^{-1} h^{-1} for 24 h or anuria for 12 h

RRT, renal replacement therapy.

[a] Only one criterion—either creatinine or urine output—has to be fulfilled to qualify for a stage.

[b] Given wide variation in indications and timing of initiation of RRT, patients who receive RRT are considered to have met the criterion for stage 3 irrespective of the stage they are in at the time of RRT.

[c] If the baseline creatinine value is unknown and no chronic kidney disease is found in the history, a normal baseline serum creatinine value can be assumed and calculated from the MDRD formula (estimated GFR before acute disease: 75 mL min $^{-1}$1.73 m^{-2}).

Adapted from Mehta RL, Kellum JA, Shah SV, *et al.* Acute Kidney Injury Network: report of an initiative to improve outcomes in acute kidney injury. *Critical Care* 2007;**11**:R31. BioMed Central.

only 24–48 h after the renal insult. In addition, in patients with initially normal renal function a GFR loss of less than 50% cannot be detected by the relatively insensitive increase in creatinine.

Reduction in urine output also varies considerably in AKI, being dependent on severity of damage, hydration state, blood pressure, and medication. Urine output should be evaluated only after exclusion of dehydration and not earlier than 6–24 h after an acute renal insult.

Evaluation of the changes of serum creatinine and urine output over time allows more sensitive detection and graduation of AKI than single measurements do. Monitoring and detection of the 'pre-failure' stages is of utmost importance, since causal treatment of AKI is rarely successful. Even relatively mild renal injury—best described by the AKIN criteria (⮕Box 17.1 and ⮕Table 17.1)—drastically impairs the prognosis of the patient.

The RIFLE classification (<u>r</u>isk of renal dysfunction, <u>i</u>njury to the kidney, <u>f</u>ailure of kidney function, <u>l</u>oss of kidney function, <u>e</u>ndstage kidney disease) [2] is based on serial measurements of serum creatinine and urine output

over up to 7 days and describes three severity levels of renal impairment—'risk', 'injury' and 'failure'—in combination with the consequences of 'loss of function' and 'endstage disease'. The RIFLE classification was recently refined and published as the Acute Kidney Injury Network (AKIN) classification with stages AKIN-1 to AKIN-3 (⮕ Table 17.1; [3]). Stages AKIN-1–AKIN-3 are defined by specified increases in serum creatinine or decreases in spontaneous urine output within 48 h of an acute insult. Ensuring the patient is in a balanced fluid state is a prerequisite for calculation of the AKIN stage, however, as severe dehydration can mimic a 'pseudo-increase' of serum creatinine. The AKIN classification is more manageable in daily practice than the RIFLE classification and should be the classification of choice for monitoring acute kidney dysfunction in the critically ill patient. However, the criteria for AKIN stages do not allow early diagnosis of renal injury.

Patients who need renal replacement therapy (RRT) are classified as AKIN-3. The AKIN criteria can also be applied to patients with 'acute on chronic' renal failure if serum creatinine or GFR before the renal insult is known; the diagnosis can be difficult if this information is missing.

Akin stages correlate with mortality [4]: 18.5% in AKIN 1, 28.1% in AKIN 2, and 32.6% in AKIN 3.

Cystatin C is exclusively excreted by the kidneys through free glomerular filtration. Under physiological conditions cystatin C is not found in the urine because it is completely metabolized in the renal tubule. Its serum concentration has been suggested as a more sensitive marker for renal excretory impairment than creatinine, for both chronic [5] and acute renal disease. The serum concentration of cystatin C rises on average 1.5 days earlier after kidney injury than that of creatinine [6]. Nevertheless, serum cystatin C is not an early marker of AKI since GFR has to be impaired for several hours before the marker begins to rise.

Whether urinary cystatin C is also a true early marker of kidney injury is still an open question [7], and the search for earlier biomarkers continues. Under investigation are neutrophil gelatinase associated lipocalin (NGAL), kidney injury molecule 1 (KIM-1), and liver-type fatty acid binding protein (LFABP) [8, 9]. A steep increase of NGAL in the urine detects kidney injury as early as 2–3 h after an insult, also after cardiopulmonary bypass [10, 11]. It is likely that this new parameter will become established in the intensive care unit (ICU) soon.

Creatinine clearance or glomerular filtration rate?

Stable kidney function is a prerequisite for the estimation of GFR [12, 13]. Creatinine clearance monitoring is preferable in patients with AKI, and can easily be done by a 2-h clearance [14].

Monitoring of renal blood flow

Direct quantification of renal blood flow [15] is rarely indicated. Selective arteriography, Doppler ultrasonography, or radionuclide scanning can be used [15]; the gold standard method of para-aminohippurate (PAH) clearance is not applicable in clinical practice.

Monitoring of ischaemic versus toxic kidney injury

Ischaemic (shock), toxic (contrast media), and probably also hyperaemic (sepsis) injuries are assumed to represent the main mechanisms leading to AKI. Unfortunately, the kidneys' response to these injuries is relatively uniform so that a distinction between them can be made only from the patient's history and the underlying disease.

Only primary renal disease would be an indication for renal biopsy in AKI.

Monitoring of kidney function in cardiac disease

Patients in the critical care unit or intensive care unit

Every third critically ill patient (37.1%) has one of the AKIN 1–3 stages (AKIN 1 18.1%, AKIN 2 10.1%, AKIN 3 8.9%) [4], with about 5% of CCU patients [16], 15.4–19.2% of

cardiac surgery patients. and 51.8–67.2% of unselected ICU patients [17].

Acute heart failure with cardiorenal syndrome I

Patients with severe heart failure often have renal impairment [18], with its degree, as measured by GFR, being an independent and potent predictor of cardiorenovascular outcome [19]. Cardiorenal syndrome (CRS) I—acute heart failure, which induces rapid deterioration of renal function—mainly occurs in patients with severe impairment of systolic left ventricular dysfunction and often indicates the transition to terminal heart failure [20]. In cardiogenic shock, CRS I is present in about 70% of patients [21]. As detection of CRS I has therapeutic consequences [20], monitoring of evolving AKI is of the utmost importance.

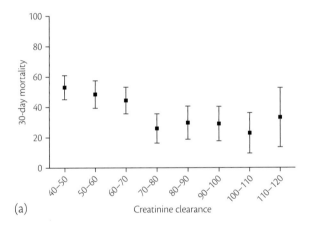

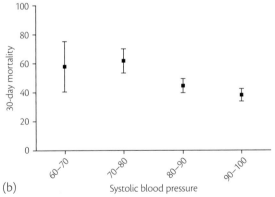

Figure 17.1 Prognostic relevance of creatinine clearance and of systolic blood pressure on vasopressor support in patients with refractory cardiogenic shock following acute myocardial infarction despite a patent infarct artery. (a) Rates of 30-day mortality among intervals of calculated creatine clearance. Creatinine clearance was estimated at baseline using the Cockroft–Gault formula [12]. (b) Rates of 30-day mortality among intervals of systolic blood pressure. Systolic blood pressure was measured on vasopressor support at shock confirmation, at least 1 h after established infarct artery patency. Reproduced from Katz JN, Stebbins AL, Alexander JH, *et al.* for the TRIUMPH Investigators. Predictors of 30-day mortality in patients with refractory cardiogenic shock following acute myocardial infarction despite a patent infarct artery. *Am Heart J* 2009;**158**:680–687, with permission from Elsevier.

Cardiogenic shock complicating myocardial infarction

AKI—defined by a rise in creatinine of more than 25% from baseline—occurs within the first 3 days in 55% of shock patients [22]. AKI risk factors are age over 75 years, left ventricular ejection fraction (LVEF) 40% or less, and use of mechanical ventilation. Patients developing AKI have a longer hospital stay, a more complicated clinical course, and a significantly higher mortality rate (50% vs 2.2%; relative risk 12.3).

In these shock patients [23], a reduced creatinine clearance is one of the three most important predictors of mortality (❯ Fig. 17.1a), besides reduced systolic blood pressure and vasopressor support [24]: for every 10 mL/h increase of the reduced creatinine clearance, 30-day mortality is lowered by 23%. In comparison, a 10 mmHg increase of systolic blood pressure at shock confirmation reduces 30-day mortality risk by 35% (❯ Fig. 17.1b).

Advanced heart failure supported by left ventricular assist device

Serum creatinine and blood urea nitrogen can be used to monitor improvement of renal organ function [25].

Liver

Monitoring of liver function

An elevated serum bilirubin concentration of more than 2 mg/dL within 48 h of admission, without a history of liver disease, occurs in 11% of critically ill patients and is an independent risk factor for poor prognosis [26], with a longer median ICU stay and an increased hospital mortality (30.4% vs 16.4%; p <0.001).

Biomarkers of liver dysfunction

When looking for the 'ideal' marker one has to bear in mind which of the specific liver organ functions should be monitored (❯ Table 17.2). Although laboratory markers are routine practice in the ICU, the functional tests described here are seldom used.

- The measurement of the plasma disappearance rate of indocyanine green (PDR$_{ICG}$) [27, 28] reflects the functional reserve of intact hepatocytes that participate in maintained nutritional perfusion [29]. ICG is almost exclusively eliminated by the liver without biotransformation and does not undergo enterohepatic recirculation. A plasma disappearance rate of less than 16–8%/min is assumed to be pathological [30].

- The MEGX test consists of intravenous injection of lidocaine hydrochloride, 1 mg/kg, and measurement of

Table 17.2 Monitoring of hepatic function

Measure	Organ function/dysfunction
AST ↑, ALT ↑	Hepatocellular injury
Cholinesterase ↓, prothrombin ratio↓	Impaired synthetic function
C-reactive protein ↑, albumin ↓	Acute phase response
Bilirubin ↑, PDR$_{ICG}$* ↓	Impaired excretory function

ALT, alanine aminotransferase; AST, aspartate aminotransferase; *PDG$_{ICG}$, plasma disappearance rate of indocyanine green.

monoethylglycinexylidide (MEGX), the oxidative degradation product via cytochrome P450, in blood after 15 and 30 min. In patients prior to liver resection, the MEGX test is of prognostic help [31]. In critically ill patients without pre-existing liver disease the MEGX test can be used to show a deterioration of splanchnic oxygenation [32].

Liver biopsy

In the case of acute liver failure, histological data (endstage liver disease; viral infections) will rarely change therapy [33]. In addition, percutaneous biopsy in an unstable, coagulopathic patient may be deemed too risky; if biopsy is really necessary, a retrograde biopsy technique via the inferior vena cava is preferable.

Monitoring of liver function in severe sepsis

Depending on the marker used, the incidence of liver dysfunction in severe sepsis is found to be 42% (bilirubin >1.2 mg/dL), 11% (bilirubin >2 mg/dL) [34], 31% (bilirubin >2 mg/dL) [35], or 74% (PDG$_{ICG}$ <16%/min) and the incidence of severe liver dysfunction—as defined as a SOFA subscore for the liver item of 3 or more (bilirubin ≥6 mg%)—is 8% [30].

Conventional markers for liver injury (ALT: AUC = 0.48, p = 0.084); bilirubin: AUC 0.43, p = 0.412) fail to predict outcome, whereas PDG$_{ICG}$ of less than 8%/min (AUC 0.81, p = 0.006) as a complex estimate of perfusion, energy metabolism, and transporter function predicts death with a sensitivity of 81% and specificity of 70% [30] (🏥 17.1).

Monitoring of hepatic blood flow

See 'Monitoring of splanchnic perfusion', below.

Monitoring of liver function in cardiac disease

Though liver dysfunction and—in the extreme—'shock liver' can tremendously complicate severe heart failure and cardiogenic shock, monitoring in most cases is limited to the determination of laboratory markers, and therapeutic consequences result mostly from an impairment of the synthesis of coagulation factors. Prognostic data, as shown in 🖳 17.1 for severe sepsis, do not exist for cardiac patients. As long as no better data are available, cardiologists should use the rise of bilirubin as a marker of hepatic organ dysfunction, as with this marker—as part of the SOFA score (see ➲ Monitoring of multiorgan dysfunction syndrome; [36]—most information is available with respect to liver dysfunction in critically ill patients [34].

In patients with advanced heart failure supported by a left ventricular assist device, serum alanine aminotransferase (ALT), aspartate aminotransferase (AST), and bilirubin can be used to monitor improvement of hepatic organ function [25].

Gastrointestinal tract

Clinical monitoring

In the critically ill cardiac patient clinical monitoring of gastrointestinal function is mandatory as several life-threatening complications (➲ Table 17.3) can occur.

- Hypotension-induced ischaemic damage of the liver without pre-existing liver disease can be prevented for a long time by a compensatory increase in hepatic artery blood flow, when portal vein flow is reduced ('hepatic arterial buffer response'). The final consequence is the 'shock liver', with a rapid increase in transaminases (especially AST), followed 3–5 days later by a rise in bilirubin. If haemodynamics can be restored, recovery can be complete, with a long-lasting hyperbilirubinaemia due to albumin-bound bilirubin.

- Ventilation associated liver dysfunction may occur during ventilation with PEEP values greater than 20 mmHg [37], as high PEEP reduces thoracic blood volume and thereby decreases cardiac output and splanchnic perfusion [38].

- Gastrointestinal haemorrhage is one of the three most prominent prognostically relevant gastrointestinal failures [39]. It occurs in 1.5% of critically ill ICU patients, and its presence increases mortality fivefold.

- ICU-related pancreatitis can be triggered—without pre-existing pancreatic disease—by ischaemia, organ hypoperfusion, and mechanical ventilation [40], with the main trigger probably being the splanchnic hypoperfusion [41]. It can be diagnosed by two of the following three criteria [40]: (1) acute abdominal pain and tenderness in the upper abdomen; (2) elevated levels of lipase and/or amylase in blood, urine, or ascitic fluid; and (3) abnormal imaging findings for the pancreas associated with acute pancreatitis.

- Splanchnic perfusion disturbances are often overlooked, because the underlying shock state dominates the clinical picture. Usually, the bowel arteries are only partially occluded, with a relatively good flow in the proximal part of the vessel, but a rather limited flow at the periphery (➲ Fig. 17.2). Initially the clinical signs of the evolving paralytic ileus may be masked and not very prominent. The increase in serum lactate and the development of metabolic acidosis are indirect measures of splanchnic hypoperfusion [42]. Ischaemia is further aggravated by long-standing catecholamine treatment.

- Ileus is defined as intestinal obstruction due to inhibition of bowel motility [39]. Sedation with opiate analogues as well as mechanical ventilation may induce motility defects which seriously interfere with enteral nutrition, most often because of atony of the stomach. In the colon, acute pseudo-obstruction—Ogilvie's syndrome—is the most prominent diagnosis which can be identified by radiography (air-filled transverse caecum).

- Intolerance of food—the impossibility of enteral feeding—is an indicator of bad prognosis (see ➲ Monitoring of gut dysfunction in cardiac patients).

Table 17.3 Monitoring of gastrointestinal dysfunctions in critically ill patients

Type of organ dysfunction	Comments
Liver dysfunction	11%[a]
Cholestasis	Impairs bactericidal activity of neutrophils[b]
Ischaemic, due to hypotension	ASAT ↑↑, 3–5 days later: bilirubin ↑↑
Ischaemic, due to abdominal compartment syndrome	Disturbed flow in liver veins due to increased intra-abdominal pressure[c]
Ventilation associated	Be careful with high PEEP
Acalculous cholecystitis	Can be a septic focus; check by sonography[d]
Gastrointestinal haemorrhage	Identify cardiac patients for stress ulcer prophylaxis[e]
ICU-related pancreatitis	Avoid low Pa_{O_2}/Fi_{O_2} values[f]
Bowel ischaemia	Increased lactate is a late phenomenon
Ileus	Diagnosis supported by radiography

[a] [34]; see also ➲ Liver.
[b] [121].
[c] [113]; furthermore, in recent studies, intra-abdominal hypertension has been associated with worse outcome in mixed critically ill patients [122]. Still, it needs to be clarified whether the measurement of intra-abdominal pressure alone is sufficient for complex assessment of gastrointestinal function [123].
[d] [124].
[e] See ➲ Monitoring of gastrointestinal failure.
[f] [40, 45].

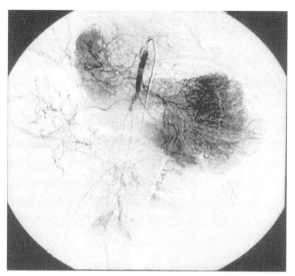

Figure 17.2 Angiography of mesenterial arteries in a patient with bowel ischaemia. Considerable rarefactions are seen in the peripheral branches of the arteries, but no complete occlusions ('nonocclusive disease'). From Winkler M, Lange B, Lemm H. [The ventilated patient with gastro-intestinal complications—if gastro-intestinal organs fail, the mortality risk increases. *klinikarzt* 2008;**37**(5):250–254. With permission from Georg Thieme Verlag KG.

◆ An increase in lactate levels (>2 mEq/L) may indicate tissue hypoxia with a switch from aerobic to anaerobic metabolism [43, 44] which—among many other reasons—can be triggered by splanchnic hypoperfusion or mesenteric infarction. However, this rise in lactate may also represent the result of an exaggerated aerobic glycolysis through Na^+,K^+-ATPase stimulation within the muscles, as shown at least for septic shock [45].

Monitoring of gastrointestinal failure

Increased mortality (43.7% vs 5.3%) as well as a longer ICU stay (10 days vs 2 days) and longer duration of mechanical ventilation (8 days vs 1 day) accompany gastrointestinal failure (GIF) [39].

Definition of gastrointestinal failure

In a retrospective analysis of 2588 adult medical and surgical ICU patients [39], about 10% had GIF, defined as at least one of the following gastrointestinal problems:

◆ Food intolerance: inability to feed the patient via nasogastric tube due to vomiting or nasogastric aspirate volumes larger than those previously given.

◆ Gastrointestinal haemorrhage: visual evidence of blood in nasogastric tube aspirates or in stool. The following patient groups are prone to gastrointestinal haemorrhage and should receive stress ulcer prophylaxis:

  · patients on mechanical ventilation for more than 4 days (15-fold risk).

  · patients with coagulopathy (platelets <50 000/μL; spontaneous PTT more than twice normal) (fourfold risk)

  · patients with arterial hypotension

  · patients with portal hypertension

  · patients with severe sepsis [46].

◆ Ileus: intestinal obstruction due to inhibition of bowel motility.

Most patients develop GIF during the first week of ICU stay. Patient's profile (emergency surgical or medical), APACHE II and SOFA scores, and the use of catecholamines (OR 4.16) on admission are risk factors for the development of GIF.

Daily monitoring of GIF is strongly recommended.

Monitoring of splanchnic perfusion

Splanchnic blood flow

In heart failure and shock, nonocclusive mesenteric ischaemia is the result of the low flow states as well as the overwhelming splanchnic vasoconstriction due to sympathetic overdrive shifting blood flow to vital organs (❥ Figure 17.2) [47]. The clinical picture varies from mild transient colitis to the development of extensive gangrene. The blood flow to the liver is usually less impaired [48–50]. Further impairment of mucosal microcirculation and disruption of the intestinal barrier results from venous congestion due to right heart failure with elevated venous pressure, splanchnic congestion, and mucosal oedema [51].

Splanchnic blood flow under therapeutic measures

◆ Enteral feeding increases blood flow in the superior mesenteric artery, and parenteral feeding decreases it [52].

◆ Reversible bowel ischaemia (up to 40%) is induced by hypothermic cardiopulmonary bypass [53, 54].

◆ PEEP values of 10–20 cmH_2O do not affect splanchnic perfusion [37].

◆ In patients with vasodilatory shock after cardiac surgery, even low to moderate doses of vasopressin induce intestinal and gastric mucosal vasoconstriction [55].

◆ In pigs with endotoxaemic shock, the combination of dobutamine plus norepinephrine but not levosimendan maintains portal blood flow [56, 57].

◆ During abdominal surgery, hydroxyethyl starch (HES) provides better protection of splanchnic microcirculation than gelatine [58].

◆ Routine nursing procedures in ventilated ICU patients may also impair splanchnic perfusion [59].

Assessment of splanchnic perfusion

Several methods for the assessment of splanchnic perfusion are used in clinical research [51], but at present none of them is really helpful in daily clinical practice in the CCU and ICU.

These direct and indirect methods [60] of measuring blood flow in splanchnic vessels such as the superior mesenteric artery and hepatic vein include laser endoscopy [126]; colour Doppler flow imaging (CDFI)/duplex ultrasound [52, 61, 62, 63]; angiography (⊃ Fig. 17.2); hepatic vein catheterization [55, 59, 64, 65]; laser Doppler flow measurement [55, 66]; near-infrared spectroscopy [66]; MRI [67, 68]; intestinal endoluminal microdialysis for the large bowel with continuous measurement of lactate, glycerol, glucose, and pyruvate [69]; plasma clearance of D-sorbitol/galactose [70]; scintigraphic methods [71]; and gastric/intestinal tonometry [37, 55, 72–76]. Gastric/intestinal tonometry is a method in which intramucosal carbon dioxide partial pressure (pCO_2) and the respective calculated pH represents a surrogate marker of splanchnic perfusion, oxygenation, and cellular energy balance. However, positive results [77] could not be reproduced in a subsequent prospective clinical trial [78].

Monitoring of gut dysfunction in cardiac patients

In general, GIF monitoring, i.e. monitoring for food intolerance, gastrointestinal haemorrhage, and ileus, should be carried out routinely every day in all critically ill cardiac patients.

The incidence of GIF is 19.1% in medical emergency patients and 5.7% in cardiosurgical patients. Development of GIF increases the risk of death markedly in medical emergency patients (OR 13.64) as well as in elective cardiac surgery patients (OR 31.82) [39].

Enteral dysfunction in chronic heart failure

Enteral dysfunction plays an important role in patients with chronic as well as with acute heart failure. The reduced tissue perfusion in congestive heart failure results in nonocclusive mesenterial ischaemia and impaired intestinal microcirculation, with the consequence of a disturbed intestinal mucosa with increased permeability to endotoxin. Then, endotoxin can enter the bloodstream, with higher lipopolysaccharide (LPS) levels found in the hepatic veins than in the left ventricle [79]. This endotoxin translocation in turn triggers a local as well as a systemic inflammatory response [51].

Coagulation

Monitoring with disseminated intravascular coagulation scores

Coagulation disturbances in cardiac patients

Coagulation disturbances of different degrees (🎦 17.2) may become relevant for those critically ill cardiac patients who develop severe inflammation, sepsis, or MODS, as seen for instance in one patient in six during the course of cardiogenic shock [80]. Coagulation monitoring is important, because early treatment can clear this coagulation dysfunction [81, 46, 82].

Monitoring of humoral and cellular coagulation and fibrinolysis

In specific coagulation disorders or therapeutic anticoagulation with coumarins or heparin, monitoring of specific coagulation parameters such as prothrombin time and INR may be sufficient. When coagulation dysfunction is considered as part of sepsis-induced organ dysfunction, platelet counts have been chosen as integral part of the SOFA score (see ⊃ Multiorgan dysfunction syndrome and sepsis).

In manifest or evolving disseminated intravascular coagulation (DIC), monitoring a single coagulation parameter usually is not enough. Hence, several scores have been recommended and validated instead [83, 84].

- The overt DIC score (⊃ Table 17.4) should be used in critically ill patients when the underlying disease is known to be associated with DIC. The maximum score is 8 points; a value of 5 or more defines DIC. However, a score value of less than 5 does not exclude evolving DIC. Scoring should be done daily.

- The nonovert DIC score (⊃ Table 17.5) should be used in critically ill patients when the underlying disease can be associated with DIC. As coagulation markers this score uses platelet counts, prothrombin time, and a fibrin-related marker (D-dimers), but not fibrinogen, as the overt DIC score does. Optional markers are the antithrombin and protein C levels which fall relatively early in evolving DIC, but seem not to be of great prognostic relevance. A score value of 5 or more for the actual state is indicative of nonovert DIC. If the score value is less than 5 then the dynamic change of the values—usually within 24 h—can also be taken into account. Scoring should be done daily.

Overt and nonovert DIC scores in critically ill patients

The overt DIC score should be used only when the underlying disease is known to predispose to DIC [84].

Table 17.4 Overt ISTH DIC score

Measure	Range	Points
Platelets (× 10^9/L)	<50	2
	50–100	1
	>100	0
Prothrombin index/INR[a]	<40%/>2.3	2
	40–70%/≤2.3	1
	>70%/≤1.4	0
Fibrinogen (mg/dL)	≤100	1
	>100	0
D-dimer (μg/L)	>5.0	3
	1.0–5.0	2
	≤1.0	0
Assuming an underlying disease associated with DIC:		
⇒ Definition of DIC		≥5

Maximum achievable points are 8. A DIC value <5 does not exclude evolving DIC.
[a] [125]; for further information see text and [83–85].

Table 17.5 Dynamic nonovert ISTH DIC score

Measure	Actual situation		Dynamic situation[b]	
	Range	Points	Range	Points
Platelets (× 10^9/L)	<100	1	+ Rising	−1
	>100	0	Stable	0
			Falling	1
Prothrombin time (s)/INR[a]	>3 s/>1.4	1	+ Rising	−1
	<3 s/≤1.4	0	Stable	0
			Falling	1
D-dimer[b]	>1-fold	1	+ Rising	−1
	<1-fold	0	Stable	0
			Falling	1
Underlying disease associated with DIC	Yes	2		
	No	0		
Optional				
Antithrombin/ protein C level	<70%	1		
	>70%	−1		
⇒ Definition of nonovert DIC		≥5		

[a] [125].
[b] The dynamic range is usually judged within 24 h. For further information see text and [83, 84].
[c] Several D-dimer tests are in use, with different normal ranges and not validated for absolute comparison. Therefore, the DIC points for D-dimers are given as x-fold of upper normal range [125]; see also ➲ Table 17.4.

However, critically ill patients without DIC predisposition, e.g. cardiac patients, may also have well-known coagulation abnormalities. In these patients, the same score can be used to calculate the severity of coagulation disturbances, but it is then called a 'coagulation score' [85].

In ICU patients, overt DIC score values vary widely, with a large and overlapping range between different patient groups [85]. Both the nonovert DIC score and, even more, so the overt DIC score correlate quantitatively with the severity of disease and mortality [84, 85].

Monitoring of coagulation dysfunction/ disseminated intravascular coagulation in cardiac patients

In ICU patients with cardiac diseases, the coagulation/overt DIC score was measured as 1.6 ±0.1, and in patients with either thrombosis or pulmonary embolism as 2.2 ±0.3 and 3.0 ±0.1 respectively [85], with scores of 5 or more in 5.9%, 3.6%, and 4.8%. There was a clear-cut correlation between the coagulation score and the severity of the disease—as measured by the initial APACHE II score—as well as with mortality (🎥 17.3).

Although critically ill cardiac patients are not uniformly susceptible to DIC, one patient in 20 is a high risk patient because of existing coagulation abnormalities. These high risk patients can be identified by serial (daily) monitoring with the overt DIC score (➲ Table 17.4).

Microcirculation

Microcirculation as final target of haemodynamic compromise

Haemodynamic compromise (acute heart failure, shock), systemic inflammation (systemic inflammatory response syndrome [SIRS], sepsis) and MODS impair microcirculation (➲ Fig. 17.3) [86] and thereby tissue oxygenation (🎥 17.4). Microcirculatory dysfunction is of prognostic relevance, independent of global haemodynamics [87].

Monitoring of microcirculation in critically ill patients

Microcirculation of the sublingual mucosa can be monitored in patients noninvasively with either orthogonal polarization spectroscopy (OPS) or sidestream dark field (SDF) technology [88–92] (🎥 17.5–17.7). In practice, both methods need training and experience, and measurements are subject to some variability. However, reliable data can

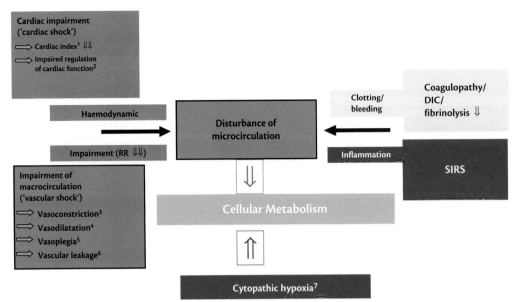

Figure 17.3 Determinants of blood flow at the microcirculatory level. Cell metabolism and particularly cellular energy metabolism depend on adequate microcirculatory support and functioning cell metabolism, especially of the mitochondria. In acute heart failure, cardiogenic and other forms of shock, multiorgan dysfunction syndrome (MODS), and sepsis, disturbances in microcirculatory flow can result from impaired cardiac function, impaired vascular function, coagulation/fibrinolysis abnormalities, and the development of a systemic inflammatory response syndrome (SIRS) [86]. A reduction in cardiac index[1] occurs not only in acute heart failure and cardiogenic shock, but also in septic shock due to septic cardiomyopathy [114].[2] Impaired regulation of cardiac function by autonomic dysfunction with dominance of the sympathetic tone indicates a worse prognosis in patients with heart failure, after MI, shock, and MODS [97]. Vasoconstriction[3] is a characteristic compensatory mechanism in cardiogenic and hypovolaemic shock to stabilize blood pressure, while vasdilatation,[4] vasoplegia to catecholamines,[5] and vascular leakage[6] (see 🖥 17.2) are typical for septic shock. An impairment of oxygen utilization at the cellular level can result from 'cytopathic hypoxia',[7] a disturbance of the mitochondrial respiratory chain induced by inflammatory trigger substances such as nitric oxide and TNF-α [117–119].

be obtained with respect to the proportion of perfused large and small vessels as well as the proportion of small vessels with absent or intermittent perfusion (➲ Table 17.6, 🖥 17.8) and other circulatory parameters [93–95]. The correlation with microcirculation of vital organs is unproven, but animal data show a good correlation with gut microcirculation [94].

Monitoring of microcirculation in cardiac patients

In acute heart failure and cardiogenic shock the proportion of perfused sublingual small vessels is reduced, more in nonsurvivors than in survivors (🖥 17.8). The topical application of acetylcholine completely restores mucosal

perfusion [96], documenting the functional character of vasoconstricted vessels, in agreement with the strongly attenuated parasympathetic tone in patients with shock and MODS [97]. In contrast to sublingual microcirculation, cerebral microcirculation is much lesser reduced in cardiogenic shock, documenting the autoregulation of this regional perfusion area [98].

Mechanical cardiopulmonary support

In patients with cardiogenic shock, an improvement of sublingual microcirculation was shown by extracorporeal membrane oxygenation [89] and cardiac assist systems [89] such as IABP [99, 17], Impella pump [99, 100], and a portable heart–lung machine (Lifebridge) [101].

Table 17.6 Semi-quantitative markers of sublingual microcirculation of patients as measured with the sidestream dark field technique

Per visual field:	
Proportion of	**Proportion of small vessels**
Perfused large vessels	With absent perfusion
Perfused small vessels	With intermittent perfusion

For further details see e.g. [93–96].

Multiorgan dysfunction syndrome and sepsis

Monitoring of multiorgan dysfunction syndrome

The prognosis of critically ill cardiac patients often depends more on the development of MODS than on the underlying (cardiac) disease. Monitoring of patients with MODS can best be done by specific scores [102]:

* APACHE II score ('acute physiology and chronic health evaluation score' II [103]

* SAPS II score ('simplified acute and physiology score' II [104]

* MOD score ('multiple organ dysfunction score' [105]

* SOFA score ('sepsis-related organ failure assessment score' [36]

Details of calculation of the scores are found in the original publications and in [102]. For many scores, computer-based software, also included in patient data management systems, is available for easy calculation. The higher the score values, the worse is the prognosis of the patient.

Initial and serial scoring

Score-based judgement of prognosis is validated only for specific patient groups, not for the individual patient. Nevertheless, according to our experience, even in the individual patient daily scoring can be helpful to identify a stable trend for improvement or deterioration.

Most of the scores have been initially validated as a single measurement within the first 24 h when the patient is admitted to the ICU [102]. Meanwhile, serial scoring is also used to give prognostic information: within the first days of MODS survivors will show a fall in score values, while the scores of nonsurvivors remain high or even rise further. This 'serial scoring' has been validated prospectively for more than 600 patients with severe sepsis and septic shock in the SBITS study [106]: in survivors the mean APACHE II score fell from day 0 to day 4 by 5.9 points, while in nonsurvivors it rose by a further 0.4 points. Detailed information regarding scoring and handling of missing values is given in [107].

Monitoring of multiorgan dysfunction syndrome in cardiac patients

The APACHE II and SAPS II scores (📇 17.9) can be used not only for patients in the ICU, but also to those in the CCU [108, 109], including patients with myocardial infarction (MI) [58].

The high mortality of these patients with MI complicated by cardiogenic shock despite early successful coronary revascularization is not only due to haemodynamic compromise, but also to the developing MODS (📇 17.10) [110]. The APACHE II score, as indicator of the severity of disease and MODS, discriminates better between survivors and nonsurvivors than either haemodynamic parameters such as cardiac index or B-type natriuretic peptide. The initial

APACHE II score values are significantly lower in survivors than in nonsurvivors, and within the next 96 h they fall in survivors, while in nonsurvivors they remain high or even further rise. The APACHE II score data point to the prognostic relevance of MODS in these patients. Monitoring the APACHE II score therefore allows us to assess the mortality risk in these patients, and treatment strategies should focus on reversing the MODS.

In cardiac patients with MODS, heart rate variability (HRV) is much more reduced than in patients with heart failure or MI, indicating a severe impairment of regulation of cardiac function by the autonomic nervous system [97]. HRV attenuation, as well as high heart rate, correlates with unfavourable prognosis [97].

Monitoring of sepsis

MODS and sepsis develop in 15–20% of patients with MI complicated by cardiogenic shock [80].

Biomarker monitoring of sepsis: procalcitonin

The biomarker of choice is procalcitonin (PCT) [46, 111], with a half-life of about 24 h. Under normal conditions, plasma PCT is below 0.1 ng/mL, but in severe sepsis levels can rise, starting within 2 h. The classification of PCT ranges in ⟩ Box 17.2 may be helpful.

Initial median PCT values have been described as 0.6 ng/mL in case of noninfectious SIRS, 3.5 ng/mL in sepsis, 6.2 ng/mL in sepsis with organ failure (severe sepsis), and 21.3 ng/mL in septic shock [111]. For a PCT cut-off value of 1.1 ng/mL the sensitivity for discrimination of sepsis and noninfectious SIRS is 97%, with a specificity of 78% [111]. PCT monitoring every 4–5 days in manifest severe sepsis and septic shock may help to see a response to therapy in the individual patient.

Increased PCT of nonseptic origin

Conditions with haemodynamic impairment and endotoxin translocation from the gut, such as cardiogenic shock [46, 112], polytrauma, and large surgical procedures, may also trigger an increase of PCT.

Box 17.2 Procalcitonin ranges in the monitoring of sepsis

* PCT <0.5 ng/mL: Severe sepsis very unlikely

* PCT >1.0–2.0 ng/mL: High risk of sepsis

* PCT >2.0 ng/mL: Diagnosis of sepsis highly probable

* PCT >10.0 ng/mL: Manifest severe sepsis or septic shock highly probable

Monitoring of septic cardiomyopathy

One patient in seven with MI complicated by cardiogenic shock develops culture-proven sepsis, thereby doubling their mortality risk [80]. On the other hand, cardiologists should also be aware that 'septic shock' has not only a vascular, but also a cardiac component ('septic cardiomyopathy' [114]).

The haemodynamics of septic shock (🖭 17.11) is characterized by a massive toxic vasoplegia with consecutive drop in blood pressure. For stabilization of blood pressure, cardiac output has to increase to very high values (up to 18 L/min). The reasons why such high cardiac output values are only rarely seen is the fact that also the heart is often severely impaired in sepsis ('septic cardiomyopathy'; [114]).

As afterload is often very low in septic patients due to vasoplegia, the impairment of cardiac function is best unmasked by correlating cardiac output with systemic vascular resistance (SVR) (🖭 17.12). The extent of sepsis-induced impairment of the heart can thereby be determined. Septic cardiomyopathy is—in principle—reversible (🖭 17.13) [114].

Evolving septic shock in a critically ill cardiac patient can be recognized by the fall in SVR [80] in combination with a further decrease of SVR-related cardiac output (🖭 17.12). This recognition is of therapeutic relevance for the treatment of sepsis.

Personal perspective

Many patients with cardiac disease in the CCU or ICU have not only 'cardiac' but also 'noncardiac' problems: reduced blood flow in vital organs impairs organ functions. This becomes evident either from the organ-to-organ crosstalk, as seen by the CRS of patients with acute heart failure, or as MODS in patients with cardiogenic shock. Consequently, cardiologists should implement noncardiac organ monitoring tools and validate their relevance for our cardiac patients. Tools such as the AKIN criteria, PDR$_{ICG}$, GIF score, and DIC score are available to monitor kidney, liver, gut and coagulation function better than we usually do, but we also have to apply them in our cardiac patients.

It is also necessary, as a critical care cardiologist, to rethink the concept of haemodynamic monitoring. Macrohaemodynamic monitoring alone is not enough and has not helped us to improve our patients' prognosis in recent years. We now have tools available to monitor microcirculation. These techniques are admittedly still experimental and not standard practice in the ICU, but they open up a new field of understanding about the detrimental consequences of cardiac failure on the tissue level of vital organs.

And finally, we have to accept that in cardiogenic shock patients an evolving MODS or sepsis can threaten the patient's life even more than the underlying cardiac disease. Consequently, cardiologists should implement MODS and sepsis monitoring in their routine ICU/CCU programmes.

Further reading

Bagshaw SM, George C, Bellomo R. A comparison of the RIFLE and AKIN criteria for acute kidney injury in critically ill patients. *Nephrol Dial Transplant* 2008;**23**:1569–1574.

De Backer D, Hollenberg S, Boerma C, *et al.* How to evaluate the microcirculation: report of a round table conference. *Crit Care* 2007;**11**:R101.

Kramer L, Jordan B, Druml W, *et al.* Austrian Epidemiologic Study on Intensive Care, ASDI Study Group. Incidence and prognosis of early hepatic dysfunction in critically ill patients—a prospective multicentre study. *Crit Care Med* 2007;**35**:1099–1104.

Reintam A, Parm P, Redlich U, *et al.* Gastrointestinal failure in intensive care: a retrospective clinical study in three different intensive care units in Germany and Estonia. *BMC Gastroenterology* 2006;**6**:29.

Schoolwerth AC, Gehr TWB. Clinical Assessment of renal function. In: Shoemaker WC, Ayres SM, Grenvik A, Holbrook PR (Eds)

Textbook of Critcial Care, 4th edition, pp. 1637–1643. W.B. Saunders, Philadelphia, 2000.

Toh CH, Hoots WK; SSC on Disseminated Intravascular Coagulation of the ISTH. The scoring system of the Scientific and Standardisation Committee on Disseminated Intravascular Coagulation of the International Society on Thrombosis and Haemostasis: a 5-year overview. *J Thromb Haemost* 2007;**5**:604–606.

Additional online material

🖭 17.1 Hepatic parameters in patients with severe sepsis

🖭 17.2 Clinical aspects of DIC and purpura fulminans

🖭 17.3 Prognostic relevance of coagulation abnormalities in ICU patients with cardiovascular diseases

🖭 17.4 Skeletal muscle partial pressure of oxygen in healthy volunteers and in patients with severe sepsis, cardiogenic shock, and limited infection

17.5 Monitoring of blood flow of sublingual microcirculation in critically ill patients with the sidestream dark field (SDF) technique

17.6 Sublingual microcirculation in a patient with stable haemodynamics, as measured by the SDF technique

17.7 Sublingual microcirculation in a patient with vasopressor-treated cardiogenic shock, as measured by the SDF technique

17.8 Sublingual microcirculation of 9 patients with acute heart failure and 31 patients with cardiogenic shock in comparison to that of 15 noncompromised controls

17.9 Predictability of mortality by SAPS II score in critically ill patients in the CCU and ICU

17.10 What determines prognosis in patients with myocardial infarction complicated by cardiogenic shock?

17.11 Cardiovascular changes in a patient with *Pseudomonas* septic shock

17.12 Correlation of CO and SVR in patients with severe sepsis and septic shock

17.13 Case report: patient with pneumococcal sepsis—reversibility of septic cardiomypathy

➔ For additional multimedia materials please visit the online version of the book (ℬ http://www.esciacc.oxfordmedicine.com).

CHAPTER 18

Blood gas analysis: acid–base and fluid–electrolyte disorders

Pavlos M. Myrianthefs and
George J. Baltopoulos

Introduction

Management of the acid–base balance and of water and electrolytes is crucial in critically ill patients. As most acid–base derangements cannot be treated by correction of the abnormal pH, treatment should be based on the diagnosis and treatment of the underlying disease/condition. Recognition of the pathophysiological mechanism underlying the acid–base abnormality is therefore essential to take the appropriate therapeutic measures; based upon the clinical context and the blood gas analysis, metabolic disorders should be distinguished from respiratory disorders, and in the latter the chronic or acute nature of the disorder should be recognized. Only then can it be assessed whether compensation of the acid–base disorder is truly appropriate.

Water and electrolytes are present in the cells, between the cells, and in the blood. They transport gases and nutrients and generate electrical activity of cells for body functions. There are two fundamentally different water disorders, dehydration and overhydration, which can be further distinguished as hypotonic, isotonic, and hypertonic according to extracellular sodium concentration. Hydration status can be clinically evaluated and confirmed by measuring serum sodium and tonicity. Management includes water restriction or administration according to need. There are at least five types of electrolyte disorders, relating to sodium, potassium, calcium, phosphate, and magnesium, each of them requiring specific therapeutic management.

CHAPTER 18A

Blood gas analysis and acid–base disorders

Contents

Summary

The combination of clinical history and physical examination along with the availability of arterial blood gas analysis can provide useful information for the management of critically ill patients. Acid–base homeostasis key to maintaining normal tissue and organ function. Acid–base disturbances, i.e. acidosis and alkalosis, can have harmful effects on the body and, when severe, can be life threatening. Patient prognosis is determined by the nature of the underlying causes of acid–base disturbance rather than the extent of pH value deviation. Correction of acid–base disturbances should be based on the diagnosis and treatment of the underlying disease/condition since most acid–base derangements are not corrected by adjustment of the abnormal pH.

The basics

Acids and bases in human blood

Although the human body produces acids we are designed to be alkaline creatures. Acids can be defined as a proton (H^+) donors and include molecules that dissociate to H^+ in solution, such as plasma. Physiologically important acids include carbonic (H_2CO_3), phosphoric (H_3PO_4), pyruvic, and lactic acids. A base is defined as a proton (H^+) acceptor, e.g. serum molecules capable of accepting H^+ ions. Physiologically important bases include bicarbonate (HCO_3^-) and biphosphate (HPO_4^{2-}).

Human body is 100 000-fold more sensitive to changes in hydrogen ion concentration ($[H^+]$) than to changes in $[K^+]$. In extracorporeal cardiopulmonary support (ECS), $[HCO_3^-]$ is 600 000-fold higher than $[H^+]$ (24 000 000/40 nEq/L). When CO_2 reacts with water it produces equal amounts of H^+ and HCO_3^- ions which, added to the existing ones, affect the $[H^+]$ more than the $[HCO_3^-]$. Human plasma ion concentration is shown in 🖳 18a.1.

The body is a continuous source of $[H^+]$ due to metabolic processes which include aerobic (carbonic acid) and anaerobic metabolism of glucose (pyruvic and lactic acid), oxidation of sulfur-containing amino acids (sulfuric acid), incomplete oxidation of fatty acids (ketone bodies), and hydrolysis of phosphoproteins and nucleoproteins (phosphoric acid).

The total amount of H^+ coming from nonvolatile acids is 561 500 mEq/24 h (lactic acid 1500 mEq/24 h, ADP 80 000 mEq/24 h, ATP 120 000 mEq/24 h, mitochondria 360 000 mEq/24 h). Most of this amount is reused for several biochemical reactions and therefore does not need to be excreted. Only the small amount of 70 mmol of nonvolatile acids per day coming from food, medication, and metabolic intermediates (lactic acid, pyruvic acid, acetoacetic acid) has to be excreted through the kidneys.

The total of H^+ coming from volatile carbonic acid equals the amount coming from the reaction of 15 moles of CO_2 produced per day with water according to the equation:

$$CO_2 + H_2O \leftrightarrow H_2CO_3 \leftrightarrow H^+ + HCO_3^- \qquad (1)$$

Hydrogen ion concentration and pH

We are very interested in $[H^+]$ because it affects normal enzyme activity as well as oxygenation (oxyhemoglobin dissociation curve), muscle, nerve, and metabolic functions. $[H^+]$ in the extracellular fluid (nEq/L) is determined by the balance between bicarbonate $[HCO_3^-]$ (mmol/L) and CO_2 ($Paco_2$ in mmHg):

$$[H^+] = 24 \times (Paco_2/HCO_3^-) \quad (2)$$

Considering that the normal values are 40 mmHg for $Paco_2$ and 24 mEq/L for $[HCO_3^-]$, from Equation 2 the normal blood $[H^+]$ is 40 nEq/L. This small concentration is usually expressed in pH units, and under normal conditions 40 nEq/L $[H^+]$ corresponds to a pH of 7.40. As $[H^+]$ increases, pH falls and as $[H^+]$ decreases, pH increases.

From the Henderson–Hasselbalch equation (📷 18a.2) we conclude that acidaemia results from conditions that increase $Paco_2$ or decrease $[HCO_3^-]$. Conversely, alkalaemia results from decreased $Paco_2$ or increased $[HCO_3^-]$. Normal values for a healthy person are shown in 📷 18a.3.

Generation of acid–base disorders

According to Equation (2), $[H^+]$ and accordingly pH depends on the values of $Paco_2$ and $[HCO_3^-]$. Changes in $Paco_2$ determine the respiratory component of acid–base balance and generate respiratory acid–base disorders including respiratory acidosis (increase in $Paco_2$) and respiratory alkalosis (decrease in $Paco_2$). Changes in $Paco_2$ are caused by hypoventilation and hyperventilation.

Changes in $[HCO_3^-]$ determine the metabolic component of acid–base balance including metabolic acidosis (decrease in $[HCO_3^-]$) and respiratory alkalosis (increase in $[HCO_3^-]$). Changes in $[HCO_3^-]$ are caused by production and accumulation of acids or acid loss.

Acid–base compensation and control

According to Equation (1), normal hydrogen concentration $[H^+]$ and thus pH is determined by a constant ratio ($Paco_2/[HCO_3^-] = 20$) which means that deviation in one of the two components (respiratory or metabolic) must be accompanied by a proportional change in the other component to keep the ratio and thus the pH constant.

This operation of the respiratory and renal systems to keep the pH constant is called the control system of acid–base balance and is activated when a primary acid–base disorder occurs. When a primary respiratory disorder (changes in $Paco_2$) occurs, a complementary metabolic response is activated (changes in $[HCO_3^-]$), and vice versa. The response to primary change is called compensatory or secondary acid–base disorder.

Acid–base disturbances and compensation

Acidaemia is defined as the condition in which pH is below normal (<7.35) and alkalaemia is defined as the condition in which pH is greater than normal (>7.45). Accordingly, acidosis is the condition leading to pH <7.35 due to acid accumulation or base loss and alkalosis is the condition leading to pH >7.45 due to base accumulation or acid loss.

There are four primary acid–base disorders which are accompanied by compensatory responses that tend to return the pH to normal.

◆ Respiratory acidosis: increase in $Paco_2$ (hypoventilation), accompanied by compensatory increase in $[HCO_3^-]$ via renal excretion of H^+ which occurs slowly over days. Pulmonary oedema, exacerbation of chronic obstructive pulmonary disease (COPD), pneumonia, chest bellows dysfunction, and opiate overdose (central nervoous system depression) are common causes of respiratory acidosis (respiratory failure).

◆ Respiratory alkalosis: decrease in $Paco_2$ (hyperventilation), accompanied by compensatory decrease in $[HCO_3^-]$ via renal function. Rapid breathing due to hypoxaemia, pain, anxiety and fear but also salicylate intoxication, liver failure, pulmonary embolism, and sepsis are common causes.

♦ Metabolic acidosis: decrease in plasma $[HCO_3^-]$ through loss of HCO_3^- or accumulation of H^+, accompanied by compensatory fall in $Paco_2$ through hyperventilation. Common causes include cardiac arrest, shock, diabetic coma, lactic acid production, renal tubular necrosis, and diarrhoea.

♦ Metabolic alkalosis: increase in plasma $[HCO_3^-]$ through H^+ loss or HCO_3^- gain, accompanied by compensatory rise in $Paco_2$ through hypoventilation. Chloride-responsive metabolic alkalosis is caused by vomiting (also gastric suctioning) with loss of gastric acid, diuretic therapy, and post-hypercapnia; chloride-unresponsive metabolic alkalosis by any hyperaldosterone state (Cushing's syndrome, Bartter's syndrome, Conn's syndrome, exogenous steroids), excess alkali, or severe hypokalaemia.

A synopsis of acid–base disorders and compensation mechanisms is shown in ⊃ Table 18a.1.

Acid–base disturbances can be defined as simple if there is one primary derangement for which compensation is adequate for pH correction. However, if there is more than one acid–base disorder in the same patient at the same time, acid–base disorder is characterized as mixed. If compensation is not achieved as anticipated, then a mixed acid–base disturbance might exists.

We need to remember that respiratory compensation occurs immediately (within minutes) but complete respiratory compensation occurs within 24 h after a metabolic disturbance. Adequate renal (metabolic) compensation starts within 6 h, but full compensation occurs within days of the initial respiratory disturbance. Also, compensation cannot restore pH to normal, but near to normal.

For consequences of acid–base disorders, see 🖳 18a.4.

Arterial blood gas analysis

Requirements for an accurate approach

Accurate interpretation of acid–base balance requires the availability of the following:

♦ Arterial blood gases (ABG) report: pH, Pao_2, $Paco_2$, HCO_3^- and the fraction of inspired oxygen (Fio_2).

♦ Serum electrolytes including Na^+, K^+, Cl^-

♦ Anion gap (AG) value, i.e. serum cations – anions: $[(Na^+ + K^+) - (HCO_3^- + Cl^-)]$ or $[Na^+ - (HCO_3^- + Cl^-)]$, assuming that K^+ values are constant and negligible. The second version is the one most often used in a clinical setting. Normal AG values are 12 ± 2. In case of severe hypoalbuminaemia a correction should be applied for AG estimation: adjusted AG = observed AG + 2.5 × [4.5 – measured albumins].

♦ Calculation of excess AG $^+$ HCO_3^- = (measured AG – normal AG) + measured HCO_3^- = (measured AG – 12) + measured HCO_3^-

For evaluation of oxygenation and oxygen uptake, see 🖳 18a.5.

Table 18a.1 (a) Acid–base disorders: pathophysiology and compensation

Disturbance	Pathophysiology	Compensation	$Paco_2$/$[HCO_3^-]$
Respiratory acidosis	CO_2 retention	Production of HCO_3^-	↑$Paco_2$/↑$[HCO_3^-]$
Respiratory alkalosis	CO_2 removal	Increased HCO_3^- removal (decreased H^+ excretion)	↓$Paco_2$/↓$[HCO_3^-]$
Metabolic acidosis	HCO_3^- removal	Hyperventilation CO_2 removal	↓$[HCO_3^-]$/↓$Paco_2$
Metabolic alkalosis	HCO_3^- retention	Hypoventilation CO_2 retention	↑$[HCO_3^-]$/↑$Paco_2$

(b) Expected changes in pCO_2 and $[HCO_3^-]$ in acid–base disorders (ΔpCO_2 and $\Delta[HCO_3^-]$ from normal 40 mmHg and 25 mmol/L respectively)

Acute respiratory acidosis	$\Delta[HCO_3^-] = 0.1\ \Delta pCO_2$
Chronic respiratory acidosis	$\Delta[HCO_3^-] = 0.35\ \Delta pCO_2$
Acute respiratory alkalosis	$\Delta[HCO_3^-] = 0.2\ \Delta pCO_2$
Chronic respiratory alkalosis	$\Delta[HCO_3^-] = 0.5\ \Delta pCO_2$
Metabolic acidosis	$\Delta pCO_2 = 1.2\ \Delta[HCO_3^-]$
Metabolic alkalosis	$\Delta pCO_2 = 0.9\ \Delta[HCO_3^-]$

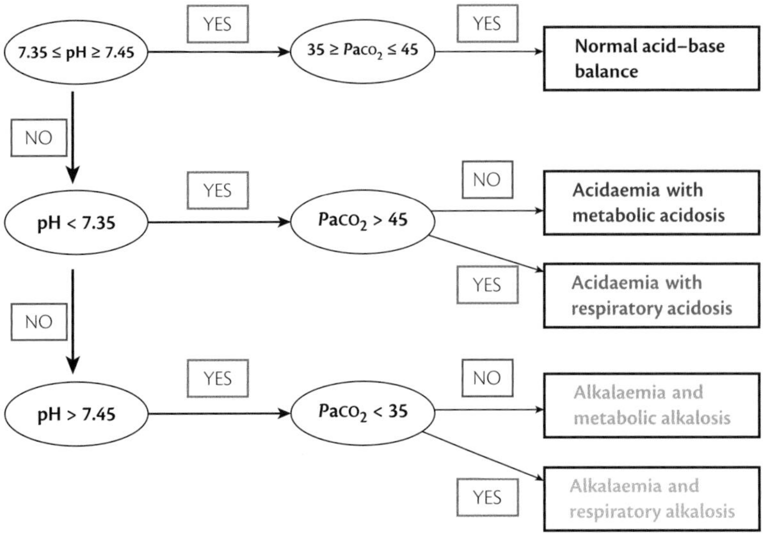

Figure 18a.1 Algorithm for initial acid–base balance interpretation.

Evaluation of acid–base balance

In general, an acid–base abnormality is present if the pH or the $Paco_2$ is out of the normal range. However, if either pH or $Paco_2$ is normal, a mixed metabolic and respiratory acid–base disorder might exist. A simple algorithm for blood gas analysis is shown in ➲ Fig. 18a.1, taking into account the pH value and $Paco_2$. However, we suggest the following six-step analysis for accurate diagnosis (see algorithm in ➲ Fig. 18a.1).

Step 1. Check ABG numbers and internal consistency, and define the acid–base status

For a pH of 7.40, [H$^+$] is 40 nmol/L. Since the pH scale is logarithmic, every increase or decrease by 0.30 (log$_2$) in the pH scale represents a 50% decrease or increase in [H$^+$]. Taking in account that the pH 8 and pH 7 represents a [H$^+$] of 10 and 100 respectively, and any change in pH by 0.01 represents a change in [H$^+$] of 1 nmol/L (approximately) we can calculate the [H$^+$] for any given pH.

When we evaluate ABGs, from the pH we estimate the [H$^+$] concentration and in addition we calculate it from Equation (2). The numbers we obtain have to be very close: otherwise there is an ABG measurement problem and the measurement must be repeated. Another approach is to calculate the nmol/L of H$^+$, using Equation (2). Subtracting the calculated [H$^+$] from 80, we have to obtain the last two digits of a pH beginning with 7 (see ➲ 18a.6 for example calculations).

Having establishing internal consistency, we now look at the pH. If it is within normal range, a normal or compensated or mixed state exists. If it is outside normal limits, assess whether acidosis or alkalosis is present. The body does not fully compensate for primary acid–base disorders

and never overcompensates; whichever state exists on the pH scale is the primary abnormality.

◆ If pH <7.36 this is acidaemia and acidosis

◆ If pH >7.45 that is alkalemia and alkalosis.

The primary disturbance (respiratory or metabolic) is determined by the pH value. Whichever side of 7.40 the pH is, the process that caused it to shift to that side is primary. See also ➲ Fig. 18a.1.

Step 2. Which is the primary disturbance (respiratory or metabolic)?

Look at the $Paco_2$ and the [HCO$_3^-$]:

◆ If $Paco_2$ is related to the change in pH, then the primary disturbance is respiratory: it needs to be elevated in acidosis and decreased in alkalosis.

◆ If [HCO$_3^-$] is related to the change in pH then the primary disturbance is metabolic: it needs to be decreased in acidosis and elevated in alkalosis.

Another way is to look at pH and $Paco_2$. If both are abnormal, compare the directional change. See also the algorithm in ➲ Fig. 18a.1.

◆ If they both change in the same direction (increase or decrease) the primary disorder is metabolic.

◆ If they change in opposite directions, the primary abnormality is respiratory.

Step 3. If the primary disturbance is respiratory, is it acute or chronic?

Look at the changes in [HCO$_3^-$] compared to the changes in $Paco_2$. Define the condition according to the rules in ➲ Table 18a.4.

Step 4. Calculate the AG to check for AG metabolic acidosis

$$AG = [[Na^+] - ([HCO_3^-] + [Cl^-])]$$

The AG is an estimate of unmeasured anions and cations (🔖18a.7) that helps to identify if there is an AG metabolic acidosis. AG maybe elevated (>12), normal, or low (<6).

An AG metabolic acidosis is probably present, regardless of pH or serum [HCO_3^-], if the AG is 20 mmol/L or more, because this value is more than four standard deviations from the mean. Metabolic or respiratory alkalosis elevates AG to a modest degree because of an increase in the negative charge of serum proteins.

Causes of elevated AG include:

♦ Metabolic acidosis: uraemia–endstage renal failure, diabetic or alcoholic ketoacidosis, lactic acidosis, methanol or ethylene glycol ingestion, salicylate intoxication, rhabdomyolisis. However, not all causes of metabolic acidosis have an increased AG.

♦ Dehydration.

♦ Carbenicillin or penicillin therapy.

♦ Alkalosis (increases the negative charge of serum proteins).

Some people use the acronym MUDPILES to remember: methanol, uraemia (renal failure), DKA (ketoacidosis), paraldahyde, inborn errors of metabolism & idiopathic & isoniazid, lactic acidosis & alcoholic ketoacidosis (i.e. sepsis, etc.), ethanol toxicity, salicylate intoxication.

Causes of low AG include:

♦ Decreased unmeasured anion: hypoalbuminaemia: AG falls 2.5 mEq/L for every 1 g/L decrease in plasma albumin.

♦ Increased unmeasured cations: lithium intoxication; hyperkalaemia, hypercalcaemia, hypermagnesaemia; myeloma cationic paraprotein (negative AG).

♦ Drugs: bromide (negative AG), iodide (negative AG), polymyxin B, tromethane.

Normal AG metabolic acidosis is the result of net increase in [Cl^-] (chloride gain) due to the loss of bicarbonates in the extracellular fluid. This metabolic acidosis is also called hyperchloraemic metabolic acidosis. Conditions usually associated with normal AG metabolic acidosis include gastrointestinal bicarbonate losses (diarrhoea, rectosigmoidostomy, pancreatic fistula ureteral diversions–ureteroenterostomy), renal bicarbonate losses (renal tubular acidosis, early renal failure, and carbonic anhydrase and aldosterone inhibitors consumption), post hypocapnia, isotonic saline infusion.

To differentiate gastrointestinal from renal bicarbonate losses the urinary anion gap ($UAG = [Na^+] + [K^+] - [Cl^-]$) has to be measured. UAG is negative in diarrhoea (–20 ±5.7 mmol/L) and positive in renal tubular acidosis (23 ±4.1 mmol/L), in hyperkalaemic distal renal tubular acidosis (30 ±4.2 mmol/L), and in selective aldosterone deficiency (39 ±4.2 mmol/L).

Step 5. Is the compensation of the primary disturbance adequate?

This can be worked out according to the following rules of compensation.

1 Metabolic acidosis: The ventilatory response (tachypnea) will reduce the $Paco_2$ for compensation. $Paco_2$ should fall from its normal value by 1.2 mmHg × $\Delta[HCO_3^-]$:

$$\Delta[HCO_3^-] \times 1.2 = \Delta Paco_2$$

If the measured value of $Paco_2$ is equivalent to the expected value then the respiratory compensation is adequate and the condition is called compensated metabolic acidosis. If the measured $Paco_2$ is higher than expected, then either the compensation time is short or the respiratory system fails to appropriately respond to the acidic stimulus. In the latter case an additional respiratory acidosis is superimposed on the existing metabolic acidosis. If the measured $Paco_2$ is lower than expected an additional respiratory alkalosis is superimposed on the existing metabolic acidosis.

2 Metabolic alkalosis: The ventilatory response (hypoventilation) will increase $Paco_2$ for compensation. The value of $Paco_2$ should rise from the normal value by 0.9 mmHg × $\Delta[HCO_3^-]$:

$$\Delta[HCO_3^-] \times 0.9 = \Delta Paco_2$$

If the measured value $Paco_2$ is equivalent to the expected value, then the respiratory compensation is adequate and the condition is called compensated metabolic alkalosis. If the measured $Paco_2$ is higher than expected, an additional

Table 18a.2 Acute vs chronic respiratory acidosis/alkalosis

Acute respiratory acidosis	$\Delta[HCO_3^-] = 0.1\, \Delta Paco_2$
Chronic respiratory acidosis	$\Delta[HCO_3^-] = 0.35\, \Delta Paco_2$
Acute respiratory alkalosis	$\Delta[HCO_3^-] = 0.2\, \Delta Paco_2$
Chronic respiratory alkalosis	$\Delta[HCO_3^-] = 0.5\, \Delta Paco_2$

respiratory acidosis has occurred. If the measured $Paco_2$ is lower than expected, then either the compensation time is short or the respiratory system has failed to respond appropriately to the alkali stimulus. In the latter case an additional respiratory alkalosis is superimposed on the existing metabolic alkalosis.

Because of the delayed renal compensation in respiratory disturbances, the respiratory acid–base disorders are classified as acute (before full renal compensation occurs) and chronic (after full renal compensation has developed).

3 Acute respiratory acidosis: The renal response (increased HCO_3^- reabsorption in proximal tubules) will increase serum $[HCO_3^-]$ levels for compensation. Plasma $[HCO_3^-]$ should rise from the normal level by 0.1 mmHg × the rise in plasma $\Delta Paco_2$:

$$\Delta Paco_2 \times 0.1 = \Delta[HCO_3^-] \text{ (max } HCO_3^- \text{ increase } 28 \text{ mmol/L)}$$

4 Chronic respiratory acidosis (compensated):

$$\Delta Paco_2 \times 0.35 = \Delta[HCO_3^-] \text{ (max } Paco_2 \text{ increase } 45 \text{ mmol/L)}$$

5 Acute respiratory alkalosis: The renal response (decreased HCO_3^- reabsorption in proximal tubules) will decrease serum $[HCO_3^-]$ levels for compensation. Plasma $[HCO_3^-]$ should decrease from the normal level by 0.2 mmHg × the rise in plasma $\Delta Paco_2$:

$$\Delta Paco_2 \times 0.2 = \Delta[HCO_3^-] \text{ (usually not less than } 18 \text{ mmol/L)}$$

6 Chronic respiratory alkalosis (compensated):

$$\Delta Paco_2 \times 0.5 = \Delta[HCO_3^-] \text{ (usually not less than } 14 \text{ mmol/L)}$$

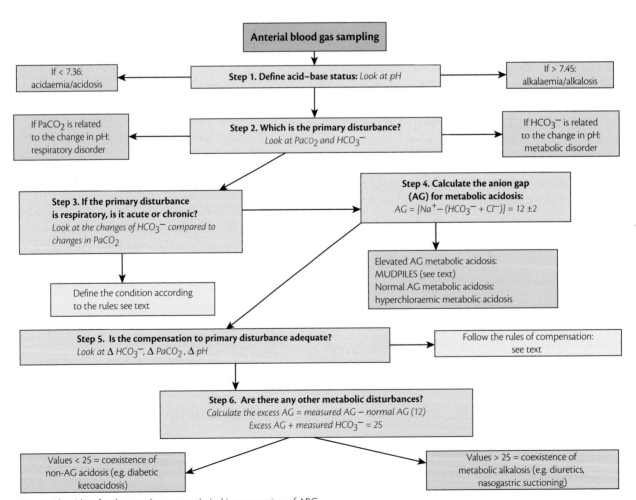

Figure 18a.2 Algorithm for the step-by-step analytical interpretation of ABGs.

Box 18a.1 Additional useful rules for interpretation of ABGs

1 Acute CO_2 rise of 10 mmHg will decrease pH by 0.05 units.

2 Acute CO_2 reduction of 10 mmHg will increase pH by 0.10 units

3 Acute CO_2 rise of 10 mmHg will be compensated by $[HCO_3^-]$ increase of 1.0 mmol/L (maximum $[HCO_3^-]$ level 28 mol/L).

4 Acute CO_2 reduction of 10 mmHg will be compensated by $[HCO_3^-]$ decrease of 2.5 mmol/L (minimum $[HCO_3^-]$ level 18 mmol/L).

5 Chronic CO_2 rise of 10 mmHg will be compensated by $[HCO_3^-]$ increase of 2.5–3.5 mmol/L (maximum $[HCO_3^-]$ level 45 mmol/L).

6 Chronic CO_2 reduction of 10 mmHg will be compensated by $[HCO_3^-]$ decrease of 5 mmol/L.

7 In metabolic acidosis the expected $Paco_2 = 1.5 \times [HCO_3^-] + (8 \pm 2)$, or equals the last two digits of pH.

8 In metabolic alkalosis an increase of 10 mmol/L in $[HCO_3^-]$ will increase $Paco_2$ by 6 mmHg (maximum 55 mmHg).

9 Derangement of pH by 0.1 is equal to 6–7 mmol/L change of $[HCO_3^-]$.

An algorithm providing a step-by-step approach to the interpretation of ABGs is shown in ➲ Fig. 18a.2.

In applying the above rules we must remember that if expected values are not achieved either the compensation time is short or an additional disturbance has occurred, resulting in mixed acid–base disorder, and should be investigated.

In order to evaluate whether compensation mechanisms are adequate, several additional rules can be applied: these are listed in ➲ Box 18a.1.

Step 6. Are there any other metabolic disturbances?

In metabolic acidosis with high AG, another metabolic disorder may be identified (normal AG metabolic acidosis or metabolic alkalosis):

1 Calculate the excess AG = measured AG – normal AG (=12).

2 Add this value to the measured $[HCO_3^-]$.

3 Excess AG $^+$ measured $[HCO_3^-]$ = 25 (normal).

The result is interpreted as follows:
◆ Values greater than 25: coexistence of metabolic alkalosis (e.g. diuretics, nasogastric suctioning)
◆ Values less than 25: coexistence of non-AG acidosis (e.g. diabetic ketoacidosis).

Conclusion

We have the necessary tools for the diagnosis of acid–base disorders. For the accurate diagnosis of these disorders, and especially for mixed disorders, the following are needed: good medical history, careful physical examination, an ABG report (pH, $Paco_2$, HCO_3^-) and electrolyte values (Na^+, K^+, Cl^-), AG and excess AG plus $[HCO_3^-]$.

Simple acid–base disorders are not followed by normal pH (it is slightly more or less than normal). Normal pH and abnormal $[HCO_3^-]$ or $Paco_2$ indicate two or more acid–base disorders. Changes of pH and $[HCO_3^-]$ greater or less than predicted from the changes of CO_2 indicate that there is an additional metabolic acid–base disorder. We should always remember that we are treating the patient and not the ABGs. We correct the underlying cause of the acid–base disorder and not the ABG abnormality. Under specific circumstances a pH of more than 7.55 or less than 7.20 should be corrected until management of the underlying condition is achieved. Every patient is a special case.

Personal perspective

ABG analysis is one of the most frequently ordered laboratory tests in the clinical setting. Almost all patients requiring admission to a critical care unit (CCU) need at least one ABG analysis for the evaluation of gas exchange and acid–base status.

The ABG report provides useful information regarding gas exchange and acid–base disorders commonly seen in patients with cardiac diseases, to guide therapy and adequate management. Thus, an ABG analyser seems to be mandatory in the CCU for the prompt evaluation and management of potentially life-threatening but also reversible conditions including respiratory failure, metabolic acidosis, and respiratory acidosis. Learning to use an ABG analyser is easy and the investment is cost effective. Interpretation of ABGs involves simple and easy-to-learn steps that enable cardiologists to manage simple as well as mixed acid–base disorders.

Further reading

Gilfix BM, Bique M, Magder S. A physical chemical approach to the analysis of acid–base balance in the clinical setting. *J Crit Care* 1993;**8**(4):187–197.

Gluck SL. Acid–base. *Lancet* 1998;**352**:474–479.

Harber RJ. A practical approach to acid–base disorders. *West J Med* 1991;**155**:146–151.

Kellum JA. Determinants of plasma acid–base balance. *Crit Care Clin* 2005;**21**:329–346.

Kellum JS. Determinants of blood pH in health and disease. *Crit Care* 2000;**4**:6–14.

Narins RG, Emmett M. Simple and mixed acid–base disorders: a practical approach. *Medicine (Baltimore)* 1980;**59**(3):161–187.

Narins RG, Gardner LB. Simple acid–base disturbances. *Med Clin North Am* 1981;**65**(2):321–346.

Online resource

℘ Acid–base calculator. http://health.adelaide.edu.au/paed-anaes/javaman/Respiratory/a-b/AcidBase.html

℘ Acid-base pHysiology. http://www.anaesthesiamcq.com/AcidBaseBook/

℘ Acid–base tutorial. http://www.acid–base.com/

℘ Arterial blood gas demonstration. http://www.youtube.com/watch?v=0Rr6vpFMKPE

Additional online material

▦ 18a.1 Normal plasma ion concentrations

▦ 18a.2 Henderson–Hasselbalch equation

▦ 18a.3 Normal arterial blood gas values at sea level, breathing ambient air

▦ 18a.4 Consequences of acid–base disorders

▦ 18a.5 Evaluation of oxygenation and oxygen uptake

▦ 18a.6 Example ABG calculations

▦ 18a.7 Unmeasured anions and cations contributing to the anion gap

➲ For additional multimedia materials please visit the online version of the book (℘ http://www.esciacc.oxfordmedicine.com).

CHAPTER 18B

Fluid and electrolyte disorders

Contents

Summary

The recognition and management of fluid and electrolyte problems are common challenges for the patient in the coronary care unit and particularly in patients with acute or chronic heart failure (CHF). In this chapter we discuss common water and electrolyte disorders and their treatment strategies.

The basics

The body's water content (total body water, TBW) is dependent on sex and age: it declines throughout life with changes in muscle mass and fat. In adult males it is approximately 60% of the body weight and in females 50%.

Water occupies two main compartments:

◆ Intracellular fluid (ICF): approximately two-thirds of total water

◆ Extracellular fluid (ECF): approximately one-third of total water; plasma (20%), interstitial fluid (80%)

Water balance is regulated by intake (meals, drinks, and oxidation of food) and water losses (urine, stools, and insensible losses). Normal water balance is shown in ♣ 18b.1). Daily water requirements maybe increased according to clinical conditions of the body (♣ 18b.2).

Fluid requirements for adults (including food water) are 30–35 mL/kg per day or 1–2 mL/kg per hour. Normal serum electrolyte values and daily requirements are shown in ♣ 18b.3.

All hospital patients are provided with sodium, potassium, and chloride solutions on a daily basis. Calcium, magnesium, and phosphorus are administered not on a day-to-day basis but according to their measured level, aiming to bring the level to normal.

Water disorders

There are two fundamentally different water disorders: dehydration and overhydration, which can be further differentiated into hypotonic, isotonic, and hypertonic according to the extracellular Na^+ concentration.

Hypotonic dehydration

There is a fluid deficit which is associated with Na^+ deficiency. Extracellular space osmolality (mosm/kg) due to Na^+ (effective osmolality or tonicity—see 📷18b.4 for definitions) is decreased, leading to intracellular water transport because of the effective osmolality difference (intracellular osmolality is higher) and therefore to a reduction of extracellular volume and an increase of intracellular volume.

Isotonic dehydration

There is a deficiency both of water and of Na^+. The extracellular volume is decreased but osmolality is normal and thus there is no water transport between extra- and intracellular spaces.

Hypertonic dehydration

There is a water deficiency with elevated osmolality and decreased extracellular volume. Water is diffused from intracellular to extracellular space to balance the osmotic (tonicity) differences, leading to decreased intracellular volume and increased osmolality.

Hypotonic overhydration

There is an excess of water with increased extracellular volume. Water is diffused from extracellular to intracellular space to balance the osmotic (tonicity) differences.

Isotonic overhydration

There is an excess of water and Na^+. The extracellular volume is increased but extracellular and intracellular osmolality is normal, so there is no water transport between extra- and intracellular spaces.

Hypertonic overhydration

There is excess of water and Na^+. Water is diffused from intracellular to extracellular space to balance the osmotic (tonicity) differences, leading to decreased intracellular volume and increased osmolality.

Sodium disorders

Sodium disorders are usually caused by excess free water (hyponatraemia) or free water loss (hypernatraemia). Changes in Na^+ concentration usually affect serum osmolality because Na^+ is the major contributor to ECF osmolality (normal range 275–299 mOsm/kg).

Hyponatraemia (serum Na^+ <135 mEq/L or mmol/L)

Common causes and therapeutic interventions are shown in 📷18b.5. Most patients become symptomatic at an Na^+ level of 120 mEq/L. Seizures are likely at a Na^+ level of 113 mEq/L or less. Gradually developing hyponatraemia is better tolerated. Hyponatraemia may be associated with high, normal, or low tonicity. Laboratory findings include decreased serum osmolality and dilution of haematocrit, and blood urea nitrogen (BUN).

Symptoms and signs vary depending on the rapidity of development, the severity of hyponatraemia and the hydration status. They include anorexia, nausea, vomiting, abdominal cramps, diarrhoea, fingerprint oedema, muscle cramps, weakness, headache, personality changes, lethargy, seizures, stupor, coma, and death.

Treatment

♦ In general, treatment of hyponatraemia with water excess is focused on the underlying cause.

♦ Hyponatraemia due to water intoxication: limitation of water intake or discontinuing medications that contributes to the syndrome of inappropriate antidiuretic hormone hypersecretion (SIADH).

♦ Hyponatraemia due to Na^+ deficiency: administration of a saline solution orally or intravenously.

♦ Symptomatic hyponatraemia (neurological symptoms): combination of hypertonic saline solution (3%) and a loop diuretic (furosemide). In chronic symptomatic hyponatraemia, the rate of serum Na^+ increase should be no more than 0.5 meq/L per hour (risk of osmotic demyelination of brain cells). If serum Na^+ is less than 100 meq/L, an initial rapid correction is required until symptoms resolve or a safer level is reached (c.120 mEq/L). The goal is to correct the serum Na^+ at a rate of 0.5–1 meq/L per hour using 3% (513 meq/L) hypertonic saline. For patients with severe symptoms, the initial correction rate is 1–2 meq/L per hour, but with a maximum correction of 25 meq/L achieved over 48 h.

- Hypovolaemic hyponatraemia: calculation of Na^+ deficit and replacement with 0.9% normal saline is needed:

$$Na^+ \text{ deficit} = [0.6 \times \text{ideal body weight} \times (140 - \text{measured } Na^+)].$$

For women, multiply this figure by 0.85.

- Hypervolaemic hyponatraemia: Na^+ and water restriction (<1 L/day), haemodialysis.
- SIADH: free water restriction. If chronic, demeclocycline.
- Remember that daily Na^+ needs are 10 g and that each bottle of 0.9% normal saline contains 4.5 g of Na^+.

Hypernatremia (plasma Na^+ >145 mEq/L or mmol/L)

Hypernatraemia is a problem of excessive water loss, decreased water intake or increased Na^+ intake. Common causes and therapeutic interventions are shown in ⚏ 18b.6. Laboratory findings include increased haematocrit and BUN.

Symptoms and signs vary depending on the rapidity of development, the severity of hypernatraemia, and the hydration status. They include polydipsia, high urine specific gravity, oliguria or anuria, dry skin and mucous membranes, decreased tissue turgor, rough and fissured tongue, decreased salivation and lacrimation, tachycardia, weak and thready pulse, decreased blood pressure, vascular collapse, headache, agitation and restlessness, decreased reflexes, seizures, and coma.

Treatment

- This is focused on the underlying disorder and fluid replacement therapy to treat the accompanying dehydration.
- Replacement fluids can be given orally or intravenously. The oral route is preferable. Oral rehydration solution contains glucose (2.0 g/L), Na^+ (90 mEq/L), K^+ (20 mEq/L), Cl^- (80 mEq/L), and $HCO3^-$ (30 mEq/L).
- Hypovolaemic hypernatraemia: volume replacement until clinically judged euvolaemic (0.45% saline until urine output at least 0.5 mL/kg per hour) and then free water replacement using the free water deficit (FWD) equation:

$$FWD = [\text{ideal body weight} \times 0.6 \times (\text{measured } Na^+/140 - 1)]$$

In women, multiply this figure by 0.85.

- Hypervolaemic hypernatraemia: loop diuretics + 5% dextrose in water.

- Central diabetes insipidus: desmopressin (dDAVP) can be used.
- Nephrogenic diabetes insipidus: treatment of the underlying cause in combination with salt restriction and thiazide diuretic is used.
- The rate of serum Na^+ correction should not exceed 0.5 meq/L per hour (risk of brain oedema). Reduction in serum Na^+ should not exceed 10–15 meq/L per day.

Potassium disorders

K^+ is the major cation in the ICF compartment (98% is within cells, intracellular concentration is 140–150 mEq/L). Total body stores of K^+ are related to body size and muscle mass. In adults, total body K^+ ranges from 50 to 55 mmol/kg body weight. Approximately 65–75% of K^+ is in muscle. Thus, K^+ content declines with age, mainly as a result of a decrease in muscle mass.

The distribution of K^+ between the ICF and ECF regulates electrical membrane potentials controlling the excitability of nerve and muscle cells as well as contractility of skeletal, cardiac, and smooth muscle tissue.

Hypokalaemia (plasma K^+ <3.5 mEq/L)

Hypokalaemia is a problem of excessive K^+ loss, decreased K^+ intake, or a drug side effect. Potassium requirement is 3–4.5 g/day. Common causes, signs, and symptoms are shown in ⚏ 18b.7.

Treatment

- Replacement of K^+ deficit intravenously when the oral route (meats, dried fruits, fruit juices (orange), and bananas) is not tolerated or when rapid replacement is needed. Rapid infusion of a concentrated K^+ solution can cause cardiac arrest and death.
- In severe hypokalaemia (K^+ <2.0 mEq/L) rapid intravenous infusion: maximum correction rate of 40 mEq/h (or 0.3 mEq/kg per hour). ECG monitoring is needed.
- If K^+ is more than 2.0 meq/L and there are no ECG changes: 10 meq/h.
- Treat any coexisting hypomagnesaemia, because Mg^{2+} deficiency may impair K^+ correction.
- Administration of K^+ solutions of more than 20 mEq/L require a central line. Administration of 20 mEq will increase serum K^+ by approximately 0.25 meq/L.
- Remember that 1 g of KCl contains 13.4 mEq K^+.

- Beware of K^+ concentrations over 4 g/L in intravenous fluid.

- In a 70-kg adult a serum K^+ level of 2.0 mEq/L represents a deficit of at least 200 mEq. To increase serum K^+ from 3.0 mEq/L to 4.0 mEq/L requires about 100 mEq of K^+.

- Intravenous aldactone (200 mg) may increase serum K^+ levels (0.20 mEq/L) and produce a dramatic diuretic response, especially in patients with secondary aldosteronism.

Hyperkalaemia (plasma K^+ >5.0 mEq/L)

Hyperkalaemia is a problem of decreased K^+ elimination, excessive K^+ intake, or K^+ release from tissues. Common causes, signs, and symptoms of hyperkalaemia are shown in 🎥18b.8.

Potassium levels of 7.0–8.0 mEq/L leads to ventricular fibrillation in 5% of cases and levels of 10 mEq/L in 90% of cases.

Treatment

- Correction of the underlying disorder and restricting dietary sources of K^+.

- Administration of sodium polystyrene sulfonate (Kayexalate), oral or rectal; 20–60 g given orally with 100–200 mL of sorbitol, or 40 g sodium polystyrene sulfonate with 40 g sorbitol in 100 mL water given as an enema. Each gram of sodium polystyrene sulfonate eliminates 1 meq K^+.

- Diuretics (furosemide 40 mg IV), haemodialysis, or peritoneal dialysis as a definitive measure.

- Administration of insulin (shifting K^+ to intracellular space, 50 mL 50% dextrose in water, IV push, with 10–15 units regular insulin).

- Administration of bicarbonates ($NaHCO_3$, 50–100 mEq IV over 2 min) for alkalization (increase of pH). Nebulized salbutamol (albuterol) may be given at a dose of 10–20 mg. It shifts K^+ intracellularly.

- To avoid arrhythmias: calcium gluconate intravenously (10mL of a 10% solution over a period of 2–3 min). It should be used in patients in whom the P wave is absent or the QRS is widened.

Other electrolytes: calcium, phosphate, and magnesium

Calcium, phosphate, and magnesium are consumed in food, absorbed from the intestine, and eliminated in the urine.

Approximately 99% of Ca^{2+}, 85% of P^{3-}, and 50–60% of Mg^{2+} is found in bone and the remaining Ca^{2+} (1%), P^{3-} (14%), and Mg^{2+} (40% to 50%) is located inside cells. A small amount of these three ions is present in ECF but is vital for the function of the body.

Calcium disorders

In the ECF Ca^{2+} is found as free (ionized), complexed, and protein-bound. Only the ionized Ca^{2+} plays an essential role in neuromuscular and cardiac excitability. Serum Ca^{2+} levels are regulated by parathyroid hormone and by renal function.

Hypocalcaemia (serum Ca^{2+} level <8.5 mg/dL)

Total Ca^{2+} levels must be interpreted relative to the plasma albumin levels. For every 1.0 mg/dL that the albumin is below 4.0, the Ca^{2+} is lowered by about 0.6 mg/dL. Alkalaemia causes more Ca^{2+} to bind to albumin and will further drop ionized Ca^{2+}. Causes, signs, and symptoms of hypocalcaemia are shown in 🎥 18b.9.

Treatment

- Always treat the underlying disorder.

- Check Mg^{2+} levels and replace if low.

- Acute symptomatic hypocalcaemia (tetany): intravenous infusion containing Ca^{2+} (e.g. Ca^{2+} gluconate, Ca^{2+} gluceptate, Ca^{2+} chloride). Usual dose is 100–200 mg of elemental calcium IV over 10 min in 50–100 mL of 5% dextrose in water followed by an infusion containing 1–2 mg/kg per hour over 6–12 h (10% Ca^{2+} gluconate contains 93 mg of elemental Ca^{2+}, 10% $CaCl_2$ contains 272mg of elemental Ca^{2+}).

- Chronic hypocalcaemia: oral intake of Ca^{2+} (one glass of milk contains 300 mg of Ca^{2+}).

- Vitamin D preparations may be required.

Hypercalcemia (serum Ca^{2+} level >10.5 mg/dL)

For causes, signs, and symptoms of hypercalcaemia, see 🎥18b.10.

Treatment

- Rehydration: normal saline 0.9% at a rate of 250–500 mL/h and loop diuretics (furosemide 20–80 mg).

- Inhibition of bone reabsorption: drugs that are used to inhibit Ca^{2+} mobilization include bisphosphonates (e.g. etidronate, pamidronate 60 mg IV over 24 h—one dose only, zoledronate, alendronate, risedronate), calcitonin (2–8 IU/kg IV or SQ every 6–12 h if diuresis has not worked after 2–3 h), mithramycin, glucocorticosteroids (hydrocortisone 50–75 mg IV every 6 h), and gallium nitrate (200 mg/m² IV infusion over 24 h for 5 days).

◆ Dialysis can be applied in hypercalcaemic patients with renal failure and in heart failure patients with fluid overload.

◆ Plicamycin is given at a dose of 25 μg/kg intravenously over 2–3 h (use as last resort).

Phosphorus disorders

Approximately 85% of the body's phosphorus is found in bones and the remainder is incorporated into organic compounds such as nucleic acids, high-energy compounds (e.g. ATP), and coenzymes that are critically important for cell function. Serum levels of Ca^{2+} and P^{3-} are reciprocally regulated to prevent the deposition of calcium phosphate crystals in the soft tissues.

Hypophosphatemia (adults: serum levels of P^{3-} <2.5 mg/dL)

Many of the manifestations of hypophosphataemia are related to a decrease in cell energy due to ATP depletion. Causes, signs and symptoms of hypophosphataemia are shown in ♟18b.11.

Treatment

◆ Oral replacement therapy unless severe (<1.0 mg/dL) in which case intravenous replacement solutions are indicated (sodium or potassium phosphate). Initial dose: 0.1 mmol/kg every 6 h intravenously (32 mmol/day). Aggressive intravenous replacement: 0.2–0.3 mmol/kg over 6 h.

◆ One glass of milk contains approximately 250 mg of phosphate.

◆ Phosphate supplements usually are contraindicated in hypercalcaemia and renal failure because of the increased risk of extracellular calcifications.

Hyperphosphataemia (adults: serum levels of P^{3-} >4.5 mg/dL)

Many of the manifestations of hyperphosphataemia reflect a decrease in serum Ca^{2+} levels. Causes, signs, and symptoms of hyperphosphataemia are shown in ♟18b.12.

Treatment

◆ This is directed at the underlying disorder and dietary restriction of foods that are high in phosphate.

◆ Calcium-based phosphate binders are useful in chronic hyperphosphataemia. Sevelamer, a calcium- and aluminium-free phosphate binder, is as effective as a calcium-based binder but without its adverse manifestations, such as elevation of the calcium × phosphate product, hypercalcaemia, and vascular and cardiac calcifications.

◆ Saline hydration or acetazolamide may help those without renal failure.

◆ Haemodialysis can be used in renal failure or endstage renal disease.

Magnesium disorders

Most of the body's Mg^{2+} is found within cells; it functions in the regulation of enzyme activity, generation of ATP, and Ca^{2+} transport. Hypomagnesaemia is a common cause of hypocalcaemia. There is also interdependency between Mg^{2+} and K^+ concentrations such that a decrease in one is accompanied by a decrease in the other. Magnesium deficiency contributes to cardiac dysrhythmias due to hypokalaemia.

Hypomagnesemia (serum Mg^{2+} level <1.8 mg/dL)

Causes, signs, and symptoms of hypomagnesaemia are shown in ♟18b.13.

Treatment

◆ Mg^{2+} replacement, which may require large doses.

◆ Symptomatic moderate to severe Mg^{2+} deficiency: intravenous administration for several days to replace stored and plasma levels.

◆ Common dose of Mg^{2+} is 2 g magnesium sulfate in 5% dextrose in water infused over 10–20 min, followed with magnesium sulfate 1–2 g/h for 3–4 h. (1 g $MgSO_4$ contains 8.3 mmol Mg^{2+}).

◆ Magnesium is often used to treat arrhythmias, and pregnancy complicated by pre-eclampsia or eclampsia. Caution to prevent hypermagnesaemia is essential especially in renal failure.

◆ In chronic intestinal or renal Mg^{2+} loss, maintenance support with oral Mg^{2+} may be required although it is poorly tolerated.

Hypermagnesaemia (serum Mg^{2+} level >2.7 mg/dL)

Causes, signs, and symptoms of hypermagnaesemia are shown in ♟18b.14.

Treatment

◆ Cessation of Mg^{2+} administration.

◆ Hydration with loop or thiazide diuretic if patient urinates.

◆ Peritoneal dialysis or haemodialysis if the patient is anuric.

◆ Intravenous administration of calcium gluconate (antagonist of Mg^{2+}) may be used for cardiac conduction abnormalities. 10 mL of 10% solution (93 mg elemental calcium) over 10–20 min in 50–100 mL 5% dextrose in water, given intravenously (useful in patients being treated for eclampsia).

Conclusion

Water and electrolyte disorders are common in coronary care unit patients and may have detrimental effects. Early identification and prompt management is required to prevent/treat fatal complications, including severe arrhythmias, cardiac arrest, and pulmonary oedema, and to improve survival.

Personal perspective

The ability to diagnose water and electrolyte disorders requires a combination of clinical skills and the availability of an ABG analyser for the measurement of serum K^+, Na^+, Ca^{2+}, and osmolality. Most therapeutic strategies for water and electrolyte disorders require easily applied measures including water restriction or administration and substitution or removal of electrolytes. Only in extreme cases is the use of invasive techniques including haemodyalysis required as a definitive measure.

Further reading

Ackrill P, France MW. Common electrolyte problems. *Clin Med* 2002;**2**:205–208.

Bushinsky DA, Monk RD. Calcium. *Lancet* 1998;**352**(9124):306–311.

Halperin ML, Kamel KS. Potassium. *Lancet* 1998;**352**(9122):135–140.

Kumar S, Berl T. Sodium. *Lancet* 1998;**352**(9123):220–228.

Moore K, Thompson C, Trainer P. Disorders of water balance. *Clin Med* 2003;**3**(1):28–33.

Weisinger JR, Bellorín-Font E. Magnesium and phosphorus. *Lancet* 1998;**352**(9125):391–396.

Online resources

- Fluid physiology. http://www.anaesthesiamcq.com/FluidBook/index.php
- Virtual anaesthesia textbook: water, electrolytes, renal and acid–base. http://www.virtual-anaesthesia-textbook.com/vat/acidbase.html

Additional online material

- 18b.1 Daily water balance in healthy adults
- 18b.2 Additional water requirements according to clinical conditions
- 18b.3 Electrolytes: serum values and daily requirements
- 18b.4 Definitions
- 18b.5 Hyponatraemia: causes, diagnosis, and management. Reproduced from Berl T, Anderson RJ, Mcdonald KM, et al. Clinical disorders of water metabolism. *Kidney Int* 1976; **10**:117–132, with permission from Nature Publishing Group.
- 18b.6 Hypernatraemia: causes, diagnosis, and management. Reproduced from Berl T, Anderson RJ, Mcdonald KM, et al. Clinical disorders of water metabolism. *Kidney Int* 1976; **10**:117–132, with permission from Nature Publishing Group.
- 18b.7 Hypokalaemia: causes, signs, and symptoms
- 18b.8 Hyperkalaemia: causes, signs, and symptoms
- 18b.9 Hypocalcaemia: causes, signs, and symptoms
- 18b.10 Hypercalcaemia: causes, signs, and symptoms
- 18b.11 Hyperphosphataemia: causes, signs, and symptoms
- 18b.12 Hyperphosphataemia: causes, signs, and symptoms
- 18b.13 Hypomagnesaemia: causes, signs, and symptoms
- 18b.14 Hypermagnesaemia: causes, signs, and symptoms

⇥ For additional multimedia materials please visit the online version of the book (⌘ http://www.esciacc.oxfordmedicine.com).

CHAPTER 19

Clinical assessment and monitoring with chest radiographs

Alexander Parkhomenko and Olga Gurjeva

Contents

Summary

Chest radiography remains the most readily available radiological imaging technique in patients in the intensive cardiac care unit (ICCU). It still provides extremely valuable diagnostic information, including presence of pulmonary overload, such as pulmonary oedema, or pulmonary infection. In addition, a chest radiograph is needed after many procedures, to check the absence of possible iatrogenic complications or inadequate placement of tubes or catheters.

Interpretation of radiographic images is often challenging due to lack of time and the need for fast clinical decisions and because of the rapidly changing spectrum of symptoms and conditions in patients with acute or severely decompensated cardiovascular disease. An understanding of the radiographic features of major findings on the chest radiograph is therefore crucial. This chapter will review several clinical conditions (water-retention and air-related problems) and radiographic features of abnormalities (e.g. line and tube malpositioning), which can be helpful for timely diagnosis.

Introduction

Despite the availability of a variety of imaging modalities, chest radiography remains an easy-to-use and informative diagnostic tool which should be obtained on patients in the intensive cardiac care unit (ICCU). Although it may reveal nonspecific signs, the chest radiograph gives diagnostic clues and sometimes makes it possible to diagnose unexpected clinically relevant conditions that may prompt changes in treatment plan [1–2]. Daily chest radiographs are not always needed.

Chest radiography in the intensive cardiac care unit

In most ICCU patients, obtaining an optimal postero-anterior (PA) radiograph is not possible. Chest radiographs are therefore usually taken in antero-posterior (AP) or decubitus projection. It is critical to have uniform approach to chest radiography in terms of distance to the plate: 72 inches (183 cm) in the upright position and 40 inches (102 cm) in the supine position). Although an upright or sitting position is desirable, in the ICCU it is sometimes impossible to achieve this because of the severity of the patient's illness. It is therefore important to remember that in the supine position lung physiology changes as a result of intra- and extravascular fluid redistribution, and this should be taken into account in interpreting a suboptimal supine AP chest radiograph. The appearance of a chest radiograph also depends on the inspiratory effort made by a patient. Excessive inspiration can complicate the diagnosis of pulmonary congestion, oedema, and small lung atelectases in the lower lobes. On the other hand, a chest radiograph from a patient with poor inspiratory effect may reveal false basilar clouding or opacities and mediastinal widening. All of these signs resolve completely if the chest radiograph is repeated on deeper inspiration.

Placement of central venous catheters, pacemaker leads, intra-aortic ballon pump (IABP), endotracheal tubes (ETT), feeding tubes, chest tubes, and drains is of critical importance for the patient's management and therefore needs to be assessed using radiographic signs of misplacement along with other typical features. It should be noted that sometimes all this equipment may distract physician's attention from other abnormalities.

The position of tubes, lines, and other indwelling devices in place should be identified and monitored. For example, although an IABP is often placed under fluoroscopy control, a chest radiograph should be obtained to verify correct positioning of the IABP balloon.

Water-retention related problems

Pleural effusion

Fluid collections are not uncommon findings on chest radiograph in ICCU patients [3]. Pleural effusions may result from thoracic surgery, fluid overload, decompensation of congestive heart failure, infection, pulmonary embolism, neoplasms, and other causes [4–5]. The content of pleural cavity may be transudate, exudate, or blood; less frequently, it may be pus or chyme. On the chest film obtained in upright position, pleural fluid usually accumulates at the basilar spaces and appears as a blunting of the costophrenic angle. Lower lobe vessels may also not be clearly visible if an effusion is present. These findings are frequent after cardiac surgery and usually resolve completely. With larger effusions, density is homogenous, diaphragm contour is not clearly seen, and the costophrenic angle is obliterated (➲ Fig. 19.1).

In most ICCU patients it is difficult to obtain a chest radiograph while standing, so physician will encounter challenges in identifying water-retention related abnormalities. Water redistributes and accumulates posteriorly to the lung in basal spaces. Loculated effusions may be difficult to differentiate from atelectases and pneumonia. Atelectases may have inhomogenous density while interlobar effusions are usually homogenous and do not cause obliteration of minor fissures. These should be better seen in a lateral chest radiograph. Smaller effusions are more easily diagnosed using ultrasound examination, which is more sensitive than the chest radiograph in detecting small to moderate amounts of fluid in pleural cavities [6]. Assessment of a better access site for placement of pleural drainage in moderate-to-large effusions may be done under ultrasound guidance as well.

Pericardial effusion

Fluid may accumulate in pericardium as a result of postoperative bleeding, or from infection, obstruction of drainage by tumour, or in patients with renal failure. Pericardial effusions are difficult to diagnose on the chest radiograph [7].

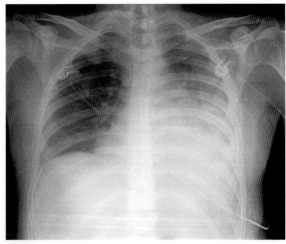

Figure 19.1 Massive left-sided pleural effusion (homogenous density, obliteration of left costophrenic angle, vessels not clearly seen).

Echocardiography is better modality to diagnose pericardial effusions and determine whether restriction is present [8], but if a chest radiograph is taken, small effusions usually appear like heart enlargement without specific features. Larger effusions may be seen in the chest radiograph as 'water bottle' or heart-shaped features.

Air-related problems

Extralveolar air collection is a quite frequent finding on the chest film in ICCU patients and could result from surgery, percutaneous interventions, mechanical ventilation, or placement of lines, drains, and devices. Intrathoracic air collection (pneumothorax, pneumomediastinum, pneumopericardium) and subcutaneous emphysema can be appreciated on chest radiographs.

Subcutaneous emphysema

This may follow catheterization of the subclavian vein or placement of mediastinal and pleural drains, and may resolve completely without serious clinical impact. Extensive subcutaneous emphysema can make it difficult to discern other abnormalities (e.g. pneumothorax). In some cases air may dissect muscle bundles extending from pleural cavities (pneumothorax) or mediastinum (pneumomediastinum). In this case lucent bubbles or gas streaks are seen along the sheaths.

Pneumothorax

Air collection within the pleural cavity may occur either spontaneously or as a result of lung injury during procedures (subclavian vein catheterization, placement of drains).

The diagnosis of pneumothorax and appearance of air on the chest radiograph largely depends on the patient's position. In most ICCU patients the radiograph is taken in the supine position, so air would be appreciated anteromedially and better seen as increased lucency on a lateral chest radiograph. If air appears on an AP chest radiograph in apical regions in a supine patient, this indicates a large pneumothorax. Increased lucency of the costophrenic sulcus with anterolateral air collections is described as deep sulcus sign. In an upright patient, air most frequently collects in an apicolateral location and appears on the chest film as a thin white pleural line ⊃ Fig. 19.2). Air sometimes collects below the lung, between the lung and the diaphragm surface, and may be seen as a basal lucency in the supine patient.

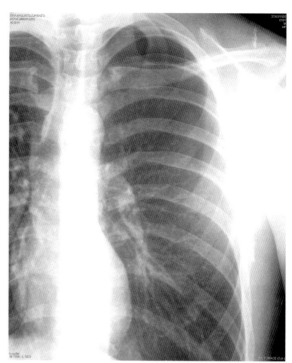

Figure 19.2 Pneumothorax.

In case of postoperative diaphragm perforation, air can be seen above and below the diaphragm, above the liver shadow. Small air collections resolve without special treatment.

The diagnosis of tension pneumothorax is usually made clinically. Sometimes lung atelectases or collapse are not seen on the chest radiograph because of reduced lung compliance resulting from chronic obstructive pulmonary disease (COPD), lung fibrosis, acute respiratory distress syndrome (ARDS), etc. Shift of the mediastinum, heart border, and cava veins may or may not be present if the patient is on positive end-expiratory pressure (PEEP) mechanical ventilation. Depression of the hemidiaphragm is one of radiographic signs that should be also kept in mind when tension pneumothorax is suspected.

Sometimes skin folds can have similar appearance and might occasionally be described as pneumothorax.

Pneumomediastinum

Pneumomediastinum occurs when alveolar rupture is present. Alveolar rupture may develop in patients with acidosis (Kussmaul respiration), after vomiting, airway obstruction, aspiration, on PEEP mechanical ventilation, and in some other conditions (ARDS, emphysema, infection). It results in interstitial emphysema with gas dissection medially to the mediastinum. Gas collecting in the mediastinum can be also a consequence of manipulations or recent surgery (upper airway, oesophagus injury) or air extending to the chest cavity from the pneumoperitoneum.

There are several typical radiographic findings, including lucent gas bubbles or streaks outlining mediastinal structures. These are sometimes better seen on a lateral chest radiograph than on AP projection, especially if located anteriorly to the heart [9].

Typically, gas collects between the visceral pleura of the lung and the parietal pleura of the mediastinum and forms the pleural line above the heart on the left, outlining the aortic arch and the main pulmonary artery on an AP chest radiograph. Ring-around-the-artery sign occurs when gas wraps round the extrapericardial portion of the right pulmonary artery. Gas may collect around the superior vena cava and azygos vein or brachiocephalic veins (V sign—gas outlining brachyocephalic veins superiorly). The continuous left hemidiaphragm sign often helps to differentiate between pneumomediastinum and pneumopericardium [10] ➲ Fig. 19.3). It is seen as a line separating the diaphragm from the heart. The superior margin of the left hemidiaphragm is not normally seen as it is obscured by contact with the heart structures. Gas separating the pericardium from the diaphragm forms a continuous left hemidiaphragm sign. Another V sign is known as Naclerio's V sign and is seen when oesophageal rupture is present, although it is not always specific. This sign consists of a lucent band of gas outlining the lateral margin of the descending aorta and seen between the medial left hemidiaphragm and the parietal pleura. Sometimes gas separates the parietal and visceral pleura from the apical chest wall and simulate pneumothorax. If air extents further it may result in pneumothorax, although pneumonediastinum and pneumothotax may be present simultaneously.

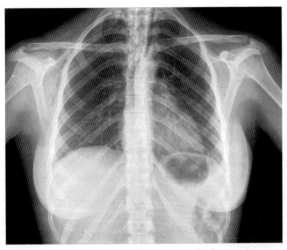

Figure 19.3 Pneumomediastinum (continuous diaphragm sign, air around heart and vessels and extending to the neck).

Pneumopericardium

Pneumopericardium is a less common condition than pneumomediastinum, found in patients postoperatively and rarely as an extension of a pneumothorax. Gas collected in the pericardium often forms a broad band, which wraps round the left ventricle and right atrium and, if large, creates the halo sign. As the gas is confined to the pericardial sac it does not extend along the trachea and bronchi to the neck. It should be noted that gas around the main and right pulmonary arteries, the ascending aorta (to the level of brachiocephalic artery), and the superior vena cava (below the azygos vein) must be inside the pericardium, whereas gas seen around the aortic arch, superior vena cava above the azygos, and distal pulmonary artery must be outside the pericardium.

Another distinguishing feature of the location of gas collection is that with changing position (upright to supine or decubitus position) gas does not shift if it is located in mediastinum, but easily redistributes within the pericardium.

Lung-related problems

Pneumonia

Community-acquired as well as nosocomial (3 days after admission) pneumonias complicate the course of cardiac disease in the ICCU and are associated with high mortality [11]. Predisposing factors to pneumonias include congestive heart failure, immune compromise, and mechanical ventilation. On the chest radiograph it is sometimes difficult to discern between pneumonic consolidation and small atelectases, pulmonary embolism associated lung infarction shadowing, early stages of ARDS and loculated pleural effusions. Consolidation can look focal or patchy and, further, may be bilateral and multifocal. Signs of an air bronchogram may be apparent. Pneumonia could be accompanied by pleural effusions (including empyema), lung atelectases, and coexisting congestion or oedema, which makes differential diagnosis difficult. Chest radiographs in changing positions (upright, decubitus) may help to differentiate between congestion, fluid collections, and pneumonic opacification, with the lung consolidation and filling of alveoli with fluid air-filled bronchi clearly seen as an air bronchogram.

Pulmonary embolism

Pulmonary embolism (PE) is caused by emboli originating from the deep veins of the legs and less frequently of the arms, right heart chambers, pelvis, and kidney. Prolonged immobilization, venous thromboembolism, tumours, and endocarditis are often responsible for development of this clinical condition. In some cases the source of emboli is not identified, which may suggest idiopathic thromboembolism. Factor V Leiden mutation, antithrombin-III deficiency, and excessive concentrations of factor VIII are responsible for most 'idiopathic' PE. Although most patients with PE have abnormalities on chest radiograph, those are quite nonspecific and the chest film aims more at assessment for underlying and concomitant disorders rather than confirmation of the PE diagnosis. Radiographic signs believed to be suggestive of PE include elevation of hemidiaphragm, lung discoid atelectases, signs of pulmonary infarction (triangular shadow or consolidation), and an enlargement of the pulmonary artery which has been described as a 'knuckle' (Palla's sign) or 'sausage'. It should be noted that there is no association between enlargement of the pulmonary artery and right ventricle hypokinesis. Beyond the occlusion, oligaemia of the pulmonary vessels could be present (Westermark's sign) [12, 13]. Pulmonary infarction occurs only with massive embolism and could be misdiagnosed with pneumonia. A Hamptom's hump is a late radiographic feature which is considered to be associated with pulmonary infarction; it is described as a rounded pleural based opacity without air bronchogram which may later convert into a thick-walled cavity.

Although the above features may suggest PE to a certain extent, they have very low sensitivity and specificity and are poor predictors of PE. It must also be noted that 12–14% of patients with a confirmed diagnosis of PE had their admission chest radiograph interpreted as normal [14, 15].

Pulmonary oedema

There are several scenarios for the development of pulmonary oedema [16]. An increased hydrostatic pressure mechanism is observed in a majority of patients, implying cardiac oedema [16, 17]. About one-third of patients have noncardiac pulmonary oedema secondary to increased permeability of the pulmonary capillary endothelium resulting from infection, aspiration of acid gastric contents, or other causes. The chest radiograph is an easily accessible assessment method for pulmonary oedema.

Radiographic features characteristic of pulmonary oedema are long (5–10 cm) septal lines which occur with fluid collection in deep septae, called Kerley's A lines. These lines run from the lung hilum laterally to the periphery. Shorter lines, Kerley's B lines (c.2 cm), appear on the

periphery and run to the pleura. Interstitial oedema progresses to alveolar oedema when bilateral opacities are seen laterally to the hilum. This syndrome is described as 'batwing' opacity. An air bronchogram is a radiographic sign which is recognized when lung consolidation due to alveolar fluid collection is present in patients with oedema or pneumonia [18]. With increased density of surrounding lung tissue, air-filled bronchi have more distinct inner contours. Increased opacification towards the bases and air bronchogram in the upper right lobe may be present in patients with congestive heart failure. In patients with pulmonary oedema of cardiac origin, pleural effusion, cardiomegaly, redistribution of pulmonary blood flow (upper lobe blood diversion) are common, although in patients with acute coronary syndrome these signs may not be present. Pulmonary oedema limited to lower lobes or one lobe may develop in patients with pre-existing COPD.

In some cases the features of pulmonary oedema on the chest radiograph are not 'classical' and may pose a challenge for interpretation. Unilateral and lobar pulmonary oedema may develop. Miliary oedema is usually observed during the transition from interstitial oedema into alveolar oedema with further generalized bilateral 'clouding'. The transformation of opacification into a homogenous appearance implies worsening of oedema and is difficult to differentiate from ARDS.

Acute respiratory distress syndrome

ARDS is associated with poor survival and results from pulmonary infection, sepsis, aspiration, or other causes leading to alveolar capillary endothelium damage and development of interstitial and further alveolar pulmonary oedema [19, 20]. Although a variety of radiographic criteria for ARDS have been described, the chest radiograph remains an important mode of diagnosis of ARDS along with confirmation of the acute onset of severe hypoxaemia (Pao_2/Fio_2 ≤300) and absence of pulmonary hypertension (pulmonary capillary wedge pressure ≤18 mmHg). The diagnosis of ARDS is more clinical, but quite distinct if bilateral infiltrates consistent with pulmonary oedema ➲ Fig. 19.4) or dense alveolar consolidation are present in all lung quadrants [21, 22]. Reduction in pulmonary longitudinal diameter has also been described in the literature [23]. Sometimes infiltrates limited to lower lobes attributable to ARDS may be mistaken for atelectases. Increased interstitial markings, indistinct vessels, and blurring of hilar structures characteristic of mild pulmonary oedema are problematic for interpretation as interstitial and alveolar pulmonary oedema may be a stages of ARDS. In addition,

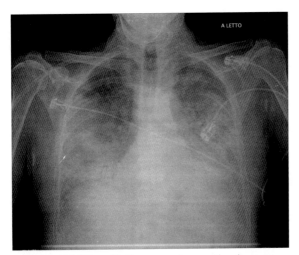

Figure 19.4 ARDS (bilateral infiltrates consistent with pulmonary oedema).

patients with ARDS may have pre-existing chronic heart failure, so basilar opacifications and upper lobe blood diversion which is usually not characteristic of ARDS still could coexist [24].

Aspiration

In ICCU patients, especially those who are unconscious, aspiration of gastric contents may occur and cause serious consequences. The acid gastric content causes not only irritation of the upper airway and bronchospasm but also release of inflammatory factors and increase in membrane permeability. Patients rapidly progress from dyspnoea and pneumonitis (Mendelson's syndrome) to chemical pulmonary oedema. Further aspiration pneumonias secondary to infection may develop. On chest radiograph, bilateral symmetric opacities can be seen in most patients, but in some cases a postaspiration chest film may show unilateral opacities [25]. These opacities may be asymmetric and located around the hilum. Signs of pulmonary consolidation may either resolve completely or persist and progress to other complications such as abscesses.

Atelectasis

Total or partial lung collapse may develop due to obstruction of the airway (by tumour, mucus, compression of left lower lobe bronchus by heart in supine position), poor ventilation (misplacement of endotracheal tube during mechanical ventilation, failure to breath deeply after surgery, general anaesthesia), pneumothorax, or pneumonia [26]. Small atelectases may occur quite frequently postoperatively due to incomplete mucus suction and may be not apparent on the chest radiograph [27]. Also, sudden mucus plugging of larger bronchus may cause hypoxia and should be differentiated from PE. Lung consolidations which occur with small or moderate atelectases may be mistaken for pneumonia; they may also be caused by pneumonia, or coexist with it. Lung collapses in most cases follow certain radiographic patterns which are helpful in diagnostics.

Radiographic features of atelectases include crowded vessels in the collapsed lobe or segment, displacement of hilum and/or trachea with upper lobe collapse and heart displacement, and elevated hemidiaphragm on side of atelectasis with lower lobe atelectases [28, 29] (↪ Fig. 19.5).

Minor subsegmental atelectases in basal lobes do not impair ventilation and appear as linear streaks on the chest radiograph. Displacement of interlobar fissures also may be appreciated on the chest film. If the collapse is extensive, compensatory hyperinflation of the remaining lung may be seen.

Lines, tubes, and temporary pacemakers

Endotracheal tube

Adequate maintenance of the airway depends on the proper positioning of the endotracheal tube (ETT), which can migrate with head movement or may not initially have been placed correctly. Misplacement of ETTs is not uncommon and has been reported in about 10% of patients [30]. Even when breath movements are present on the both

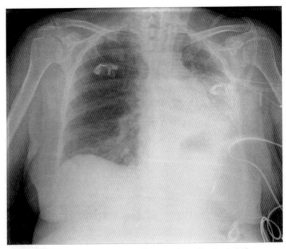

Figure 19.5 Left lung lower lobe atelectasis (mediastinal shift, elevated left hemidiaphragm).

sides and respiration is heard on auscultation bilaterally, ETT may still have been placed in proximal right bronchus [31]. Radiographic control is therefore desirable. The tip of the ETT, if placed correctly, should be found at a level of 2–7 cm cephalad to the carina on a sufficiently exposed chest radiograph. If the position of the carina is not obvious, the level of another anatomical landmark such as T4–T5 should be noted. The level of T4–T5 corresponds to the carina, and insertion of the ETT with the tip advanced to this level would be correct ➲ Fig. 19.6). Another approach was described by Dee: (1) identifying the aortic arch; (2) drawing a line through the middle of the aortic arch at 45° to the midline; (3) identifying the point of intersection of the midline and the diagonal line, which in most cases will accurately correspond to the carina. Alternatively, data exists that in a majority of patients placement of the ETT may be suggested using length marks on the tube [32, 33]: in 97.6% of patients the position of the ETT would be correct if adjusted at the corner of the mouth to 21 cm for women and 23 cm for men. If the ETT is misplaced, collapse of the left lung, aspiration, tracheal damage, haematoma, abscess, cord paralysis, and mediastinal or cervical emphysema may occur. To diagnose these serious complications a lateral chest radiograph should be taken also and the space between the trachea and vertebral column should be assessed for abnormalities suggestive of the collection of air or fluid (haematoma, pus) posteriorly to the trachea.

Chest tubes

The efficacious drainage of pleural cavities should be ensured by checking the position of the thorastomy tube. The tube position is seen as the site of interruption of

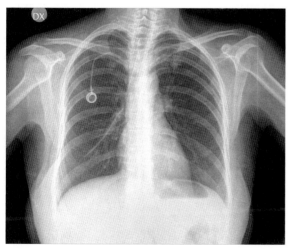

Figure 19.6 Fractured central venous catheter.

a radio-opaque line which should lie within the thoracic cavity. The presence of subcutaneous air, incompletely drained fluid in pleural cavities, etc. should be checked [34].

Nasogastric tubes

Generally a chest film is seldom needed to ensure the correct positioning of a nasogastric (NG) tube; abdominal auscultation is used to check the placement of NG tubes. If there is uncertainty about the proper advancement of the NG tube it is necessary to order abdominal rather than chest radiograph, as the tip of the NG tube should normally lie in the upper small bowel (duodenum) [35, 36].

Central venous catheters

Central venous catheters (CVCs) are quite frequently misplaced [37]. The tip of the central line should be positioned between the right atrium and the proximal valves of the subclavian or jugular veins. To check CVC placement, ultrasonography and/or chest radiography should be used. Complications associated with incorrect line placement are pneumothorax, haematomas, venous injury, thrombosis (with difficult venipuncture) as well as arrhythmias, and right atrium or right ventricular perforation (with too distal tip advancement). If a CVC breaks, a chest radiograph may help to locate the parts of the catheter ➲ Fig. 19.6).

Pulmonary capillary wedge pressure catheters

Pulmonary capillary wedge pressure (PCWP) catheters are usually introduced via the right jugular vein and placed into the distal pulmonary artery or interlobar pulmonary artery and wedged with balloon inflation ➲ Fig.19.7). Less frequently, the subclavian or right femoral vein is used as the access site. After the PCWP is taken the balloon should be deflated and the catheter should be pulled back to the main pulmonary artery. Malpositioning of the Swan–Ganz catheter or failure to deflate the balloon fully may cause serious consequences such as pulmonary artery perforation, lung infarction, and arrhythmias. Caution is required during manipulations with PA catheters [38].

Intra-aortic balloon pump

The IABP may be used in haemodynamically unstable patients or in high-risk patients before emergent percutaneous revascularization or coronary artery bypass graft (CABG) [39]. The device is usually introduced via the right femoral vein and the tip of the IABP should be

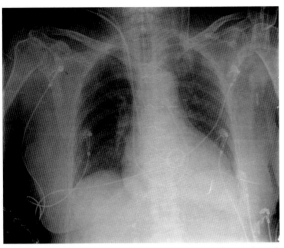

Figure 19.7 Correctly placed endotracheal tube, overadvanced jugular catheter, deflated PCWP catheter in proximal pulmonary artery.

localized using fluoscopic guidance 2 cm below the carina and 1 cm below the left subclavian artery. It can be visualized in the region of the aortic isthmus or left main bronchus. The central lumen of the catheter should be flushed, and it should be ensured by fluoroscopy that IABP balloon is out of its sheath. If the balloon is kinked or not fully inflated, it should be repositioned by pulling the sheath back. Although the IABP is usually placed under fluoroscopic control, a chest film should be obtained after pump insertion. Daily chest radiographs are recommended to secure proper position of balloon catheter. During diastole, the inflated balloon can be easily seen; during systole, the deflated balloon is fusiform in shape.

Pacemaker leads

Temporary pacing in ICCU patients is required when bradycardia with haemodynamic compromise is present. Preferred sites for pacemaker insertion are the internal jugular and subclavian veins; sometimes a femoral approach is used. Although temporary pacers are placed under ECG and echocardiographic guidance, a chest radiograph should be obtained to check lead position when a pacemaker is in place. Right atrial pacing is easiest to achieve, but the position of the catheter there is not stable. Advancing the catheter, under fluoroscopic control, to the atrial appendage anteriorly above the annulus of the tricuspid valve increases stability. In this case the catheter appears L-shaped in right

anterior projection and J-shaped in left anterior projection. Both the right atrium and the right ventricale are paced if the catheter is placed in the coronary sinus. To check the catheter position, a lateral chest radiograph is helpful [39]. For ventricular pacing the ideal catheter placement is on the diaphragmatic surface of the right ventricle between midpoint and apex. A position in the right ventricle outflow tract is not stable and leads could be easily displaced. AP and lateral chest films reveal the tip of the catheter located within the cardiac trabeculae and 3–4 mm beneath the epicardial fat. If the tip of the pacemaker lead has advanced further and is apparent beyond the epicardial fat stripe, this is suggestive of right ventricle perforation. On the chest radiograph the appearance of pacemaker wires should be assessed for continuity, presence of buckling, and sharp angulations [40]. Some extent of buckling is acceptable but excessive buckling is associated with the risk of right heart perforation.

Conclusion

Although the quality of chest radiography is not always ideal, it is still a time-saving and essential tool for clinical decision-making. In obtaining images, efforts should therefore be made to ensure optimal patient position and relevant inspiration, which is also important for interpretation of chest films. Despite the growing availability of different sophisticated imaging techniques, portable chest radiography remains one of the first line diagnostic options. It should be noted that in some cases other methods (e.g. ultrasonography in diagnosis of pleural or pericardial effusions) may give additional information but still would not completely replace radiography. In ICCU settings this simple and cheap tool is helpful for differential diagnosis of important clinical conditions, some of which may not be suspected on initial examination. Timely performance of a chest radiograph also allows monitoring of proper placement of lines, tubes, and other devices, and may also rule out procedure-associated complications. Hence, initial chest radiography is suggested for all ICCU patients, with the decision to obtain further chest radiographs based on the patient's condition and the need to check placement of devices and central lines.

Personal perspective

Our clinical experience suggests that in ICCU patients it is rarely possible to obtain good-quality chest radiographs in the ideal PA position. Despite this, AP films and those taken in decubitus or supine position are essential for monitoring of proper position of chest tubes, central lines, IABP balloon, pacemaker leads, etc. Radiographs should be taken after placement of devices and in cases when malposition is likely to occur. Portable chest radiography is an easy-to-use and informative diagnostic tool, and in critically ill patients with underlying cardiopulmonary problems quite often may reveal unsuspected clinical conditions. In addition to the initial film, chest radiographs should be taken daily in patients on mechanical ventilation and those with IABP-assisted circulation. Otherwise, daily chest radiography need not be performed routinely in ICCU patients.

Acknowledgement

All images in this chapter are courtesy of Dr Marco Tubaro MD FESC, Intensive Cardiac Care Unit, Cardiovascular Department, San Filippo Neri Hospital, Rome, Italy.

Further reading

Collins J, Stern EJ. *Chest radiology: the essentials.* 2nd edition. Lippincott Williams & Wilkins, Philadelphia, 2007, p. 432.

Moskowitz H. *ICU chest radiology: principles and case studies.* Wiley-Blackwell, Chichester, 2010, p. 183.

Planner A, Uthappa M, Misra R. *A–Z of chest radiology.* Cambridge University Press, Cambridge, 2007, p. 224.

◆ For additional multimedia materials please visit the online version of the book (http://www.esciacc.oxfordmedicine. com).

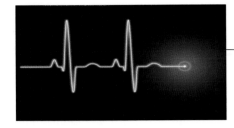

CHAPTER 20

Echocardiography in cardiac intensive care

Ruxandra Beyer and Frank A. Flachskampf

Contents

Summary

For the emergency management of cardiovascular disorders, echocardiography is the indispensable imaging technique at the bedside. In the intensive care environment, crucial questions such as left and right ventricular function, valvular heart disease, volume status, aortic disease, cardiac infection, and many others can be sufficiently and reliably answered by using echo techniques; in fact, it is near to impossible to manage patients with acute severe haemodynamic impairment reasonably without prompt and repeated access to echo. This is confirmed by the prominent place that echo has in the guideline-based diagnosis and treatment of all major cardiovascular emergencies, from acute heart failure to acute coronary syndrome, pulmonary embolism, etc. Moreover, it is the ideal tool to follow the patient, since repeat examinations pose no risk to the patient and demand relatively little in the way of logistics and resources. To benefit from the wealth of information that echo can provide, reasonably modern equipment (including a transoesophageal probe) and systematic training of echocardiographers must be ensured. Ensuring prompt and experienced echocardiography services at all times is therefore fundamental for sound contemporary cardiovascular intensive care.

Introduction

The intensive care environment poses specific and rigorous demands on availability, speed, versatility, and accuracy of cardiac imaging. Echocardiography is by far the technique which best matches these demands in the vast majority of cases and thus is clearly—as in cardiology in general—the 'first line' imaging technique in intensive care. Prompt availability of echocardiography is indispensable to any intensive care unit (ICU), and of course central to cardiac care units (CCU). In the following, a basic knowledge of echo techniques and examination procedures is assumed: the strengths, weaknesses, pitfalls and particularities of echo in specific situations are discussed. New techniques are briefly presented, but the main emphasis is on the most appropriate use of standard armamentarium, corresponding to the typical needs of intensive care management. The chapter has been organized according to clinical scenarios.

Technical considerations and equipment

Echo has always been relatively small, portable, and deployable at the bedside in contrast to other imaging modalities, but technical progress in recent years has led to further reduction in size even of state-of-the-art machines, making them well suited for use in an intensive care setting. In addition, miniaturized echo machines have begun to differentiate into two main lines. One consists of laptop-type devices which essentially have all capabilities of larger machines, including full digital storage and transoesophagal imaging. These devices typically still need a power supply or additional battery package and, although eminently mobile, they require a table or similar support platform. The other type of product is further miniaturized to allow effortless portability ('ultrasound stethoscope'), with minimal weight less than a kilogram; they can be carried in a coat pocket or around the physician's neck (📷 20.1). These devices have quite limited options, if any, e.g. for Doppler interrogation and storage, and cannot be used for transoesophageal imaging. They still provide reasonable two-dimensional (2D) quality, sufficient to identify e.g. impaired left ventricular function or a pericardial effusion.

The selection of an ultrasound machine for an ICU should consider the following fundamental issues:

- 2D image quality remains the cornerstone of echocardiographic diagnosis.

- Reasonably good colour Doppler, and, often neglected, continuous-wave Doppler are very important (e.g. to assess aortic stenosis or pulmonary systolic pressure via the tricuspid regurgitation profile).

- Transoesophageal echo is an essential option.

- Newer techniques are of limited importance; basic tissue Doppler is useful to assess left ventricular diastolic pressures, but more sophisticated techniques are rarely necessary to deal with emergencies.

- Digital storage, including long-term storage, is mandatory, ideally via a digital network. Technically, even wireless options are already available today, although still rare. It is very important to be able to promptly recall previous examinations to monitor changes, e.g. in wall motion, and given the life-and-death character of daily decisions in the intensive care environment, full documentation is vital to protect patients and physicians.

In the intensive care setting, echocardiography equipment maintenance issues are a constant headache, often because there are no clear responsibilities. This relates to equipment maintenance, cleaning, proper disinfection of transoesophageal probes, housekeeping of reports and other documentation, management of digital storage including protection against loss of data, regular software updates, providing sufficient space, and other issues.

Training

The ICU is often the first place where a cardiology or internal medicine fellow in training operates an echo machine, usually under the informal supervision of a more experienced colleague. Because of the frequent direct impact of the echo diagnosis on management, this is a particularly impressive and enlightening situation in which to learn echocardiography. However, this experience must be accompanied or followed by systematic training, in particular because the time pressures of the intensive care setting often lead to incomplete and hurried examinations. Also, crucial competencies such as eyeballing left ventricular pump function or assessing valvular regurgitation are not sufficiently well acquired without systematic training and comparison with other techniques. In a study of the diagnostic accuracy of 'point-of-care' echocardiography with portable devices, the diagnosis of impaired left ventricular function agreed in only 75% of cases between fellows with limited training and fully trained echocardiographers [1]. Therefore, the training recommendations of the European Association of Echocardiography ([2]; 📷 20.2) or national societies should be followed and it should be ensured that definitive reports are reviewed beforehand by a trained echocardiographer. For a fully trained cardiologist subspecializing in intensive cardiac care, the curriculum of the Working Group on Acute Cardiac Care requests the ability to fully and independently perform transthoracic cardiography (TTE) and transoesophageal echocardiography (TOE) (level III competence, including performance of at least 350 transthoracic and 50 transoesophageal studies).

Data storage, preferably digital, and written reporting of echo findings are of critical importance in the intensive care setting, not only for patient management, but also for medico-legal reasons. Understandably, there is a tendency to neglect these tasks in the context of life-threatening scenarios, but this temptation should nevertheless be resisted.

Echocardigraphy in specific scenarios

Acute coronary syndrome and its complications

Echocardiography is extremely valuable in the acute coronary syndrome (ACS), and therefore an echo examination should be performed at the earliest possible moment. The echocardiographic hallmark of the ACS is the wall motion abnormality as a marker of ongoing or recent myocardial ischaemia 📹 20.3). Wall motion abnormalities result from impaired systolic wall thickening and reduced systolic endocardial inward motion. They range in degree from hypokinesia (reduced thickening and inward motion) through akinesia to dyskinesia (systolic outward movement and thinning) and aneurysm (systolic and diastolic outward bulging and thinning), and in extent by the number of wall segments affected, which are most conveniently described by the standard 16- or 17-segment schemes [3]. The wall motion score is a semiquantitative way to express this: each segment receives a score from 1 (normokinetic) to 4 (dyskinetic), and the sum of all scores divided by the number of segments, called the 'wall motion score index', is a dimensionless semiquantitative parameter of wall motion impairment, being 1 for a normal ventricle and increasing in value with increasing wall motion abnormalities. The pattern of affected segments may indicate which coronary artery is affected. Degree and extent of wall motion abnormalities depend on the severity of ischaemia, which in turn depend mainly on the location of occlusive thrombus and the duration of ischaemia. However, it is frequently not possible to decide whether a wall motion abnormality is new or old, although myocardial thinning or increased echogenicity implying fibrosis are signs of an older scar. Also, it is not immediately possible to decide whether a new wall motion abnormality is reversible by an acute intervention (myocardial stunning), although some newer techniques such as left heart contrast echo or deformation imaging may be helpful. Although echo is quite good at detecting acute myocardial ischaemia, wall motion abnormalities may be missed depending on the image quality, and therefore echo is not 100% sensitive for the ACS. However, a good quality echo without any wall motion abnormalities makes acute myocardial ischaemia highly unlikely. On the other hand, the extent and severity of a detected and presumably wall motion abnormality is important for global left ventricular function and also predicts prognosis and the likelihood of postinfarction remodelling.

A second crucial piece of information is global left ventricular pump function, usually expressed as ejection fraction, with well-known prognostic and management implications (➲ Fig 20.1). Ejection fraction can be eyeballed by sufficiently experienced observers and can be measured by 2D and 3D methods with adequate image quality. A useful surrogate parameter for ejection fraction in patients who are difficult to image is the excursion of the mitral annulus or the peak systolic longitudinal (apicobasal) tissue velocity at the base of the left ventricle, e.g. the basal septal

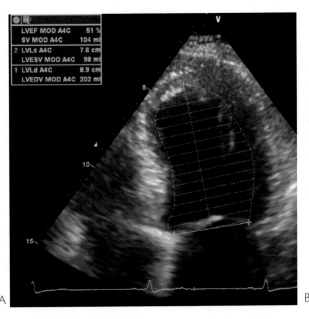

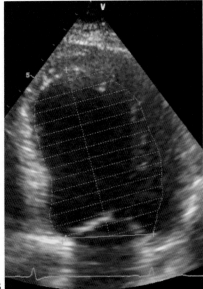

Figure 20.1 Calculation of ejection fraction (EF) by monoplane modified Simpson's rule (summation of discs) in a patient with mildly impaired left ventricular pump function. Apical four-chamber view. (a) End-systolic frame, yielding a volume of 104 mL. (b) End-diastolic frame, yielding a volume of 202 mL. The EF is (202−104)/202 = 51%. Note that the papillary muscle is included in the volume.

A   B segment in the four-chamber view. Beside this information, echo can provide evidence for increased filling pressures, e.g. the restrictive transmitral filling pattern, which carries considerable prognostic weight independently from ejection fraction [4]; for more detail the reader is referred to the literature [5, 6].

Finally, complications of acute myocardial infarction can be quickly detected in the acute phase of an ACS:

- Thrombus formation. This is quite frequent in patients with large wall motion abnormalities, especially anterior aneurysms (➲ Fig. 20.2). Thrombi are often accompanied by spontaneous echo contrast or 'smoke', a marker of thrombogenic flow conditions caused by red blood cell aggregation. To detect apical thrombi, they should be systematically sought especially in two-chamber views to minimize apical foreshortening, which is usually present to some degree in four-chamber views. Left heart contrast application can help in delineating thrombi. Fresh left ventricular thrombi are potential sources of systemic embolism and require anticoagulation.

- Aneurysm formation. Aneurysms are large wall motion abnormalities due to myocardial scar with an outward bulging shape that does not change during the cardiac cycle. They most frequently occur at the left ventricular apex and are prone to thrombus formation.

- Mitral regurgitation. Acute ischaemic mitral regurgitation may develop due to several mechanisms. Most frequently, left ventricular global dilatation and remodelling lead to functional regurgitation (➲ Fig. 20.3). In rarer cases, the subvalvular apparatus of the mitral valve may be directly

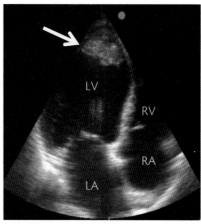

Figure 20.2 Anterior myocardial infarction, apical aneurysm and large apical thrombus (arrow). Inverted apical four-chamber view.

damaged by ischaemia, most dramatically in papillary (head) muscle rupture, which sudden onset of torrential regurgitation (see ➲ Endocarditis, acute valvular regurgitation, and prosthetic valve dysfunction). Chordal rupture may also occur, leading to less dramatic presentations. In any case, new ischaemic mitral regurgitation is a recognized negative prognostic sign and typically leads to pulmonary congestion or oedema. Mitral regurgitation is detected easily by colour Doppler, and the underlying mechanism should always be sought. In papillary muscle rupture, hypermobile mitral leaflets flapping back and forth from left ventricle to left atrium with an attached solid structure representing the ruptured distal papillary structure are seen, together with signs of severe mitral regurgitation.

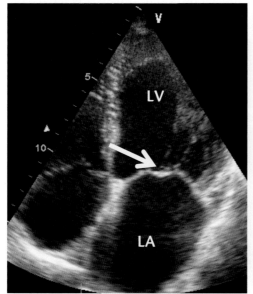 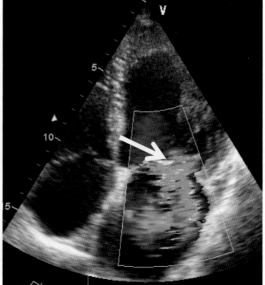

Figure 20.3 Ischemic cardiomyopathy. All heart chambers are dilated, particularlay the left ventricle and atrium. Note typical configuration of the closed mitral valve on the left, with closure line of leaflets (arrow) pulled into the left ventricle by eccentric tug of the papillary muscles. Right, color Doppler of functional, or "ischemic", mitral regurgitation (arrow).

- Right ventricular infarction: This complication of inferior infarcts manifests as an enlarged, hypokinetic right ventricle with new onset of tricuspid regurgitation. Its recognition is important because fluid restriction in this scenario is deleterious.

- Ischaemic ventricular septal defect (➲ Fig. 20.4): Rupture of the ventricular septum occurs in the muscular part of the interventricular septum, and the murmur is often taken for mitral regurgitation. Colour Doppler shows the jet in the right ventricle, and the rupture site can often be seen directly on 2D images, but sometimes the course of the rupture line is tortuous and not directly visualizable. Subcostal images are very useful to detect ventricular septal defects, since the echo beam is almost coaxial to the shunt jet. Ventricular septal defects are easily overlooked if the colour Doppler sector is not positioned in the appropriate region, which is the apical and mid right ventricle.

- Ventricular free wall rupture and pseudoaneurysm formation (➲ Fig. 20.5): Complete rupture of the left ventricular myocardium leads either to rapidly lethal tamponade, detectable as pericardial fluid and (usually) asystole, or, if the rupture is contained by the parietal pericardium, to pseudoaneurysm formation. Typical signs of a pseudoaneurysm are an abrupt decrease of myocardial thickness, an abrupt outward course (as if around a sharp corner) of the endocardial contour, and often a 'neck' that is narrower than the maximal diameter of the body of the pseudoaneurysm. There may be paradoxical systolic inflow into the pseudoaneurysm and diastolic outflow. Distinction between true aneurysm and pseudoaneurysm is important because the latter is in

principle an urgent indication for surgery; the situation is not always clear and additional imaging modalities may be necessary.

In the subacute phase and before discharge from hospital, it is important to provide a baseline study of wall motion and ventricular function for later follow-up. Regional and global function may still undergo changes in this phase, both in the direction of improvement if there is still myocardial stunning, or deterioration due to left ventricular postinfarction remodelling. Other concerns are the presence of inducible ischaemia from coronary territories other than the culprit one and the question of myocardial viability in areas of wall motion abnormality; these questions can also be addressed by (stress) echocardiography.

Shock and hypotension

Severe hypotension, shock, and cardiac arrest all call for immediate echocardiographic support. When performing such an emergency echo, it is useful to have a list of the most important echo features in mind to search for (➲ Table 20.1). The imaging conditions are almost always suboptimal, with many people surrounding the patient, frequently in the cramped conditions of an invasive laboratory, with simultaneous procedures such as creating intravenous access or even resuscitation going on in parallel. Obviously, portable echo machines are beneficial in these circumstances. Unlike the typical protocol of echo that begins with parasternal imaging, here often only apical or subcostal windows are usable and should be quickly sought. In the ventilated patient TOE, if quickly available, is very helpful. In the patient in cardiac arrest undergoing resuscitation or shortly thereafter it is typical to see diffusely

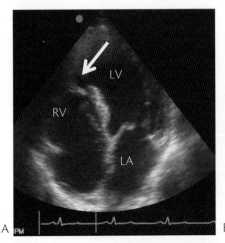
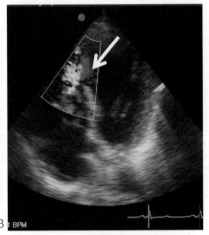

Figure 20.4 Postinfarction, ischaemic ventricular septal defect. (a) Apical four-chamber view. The discontinuity in the muscular ventricular septum is visible (arrow). (b) There is a colour Doppler jet towards the right ventricle, indicating left to right shunting. Note that this jet is easily missed if the septum is not interrogated by colour Doppler.

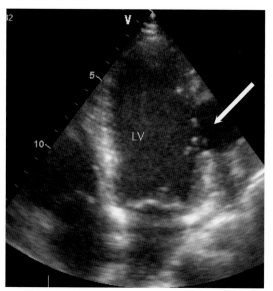

Figure 20.5 Postinfarction pseudoaneurysm arising from the lateral wall (arrow). Four-chamber view. The discontinuity of the left ventricular free wall is quite evident.

hypokinetic, dilated ventricles. This in itself does not establish a cause for the cardiac arrest. However, the presence of a pericardial effusion or of a disproportionately large right ventricle points to tamponade or pulmonary embolism as the most likely causes of arrest, and these two conditions can be detected or excluded by echo within seconds even in very unfavourable circumstances, which may lead to life-saving treatment.

Most aetiologies of an acute drop in blood pressure are discussed in more detail in the pertinent sections of this chapter. Volume depletion, which is a frequent cause of hypotension, does not have specific echocardiographic signs; typically, the right ventricle is relatively small (underfilled), and the inferior caval vein collapses with inspiration. The value of echo in this scenario lies mainly in the exclusion of cardiac pathology. See ➲ Assessment of cardiac output and volume status for more detail.

Table 20.1 Typical echocardiographic features of shock and hypotension of different aetiologies

Aetiology	Key echo signs	Remarks
Left ventricular pump failure	Enlarged, hypokinetic, spheroid left ventricle, functional mitral regurgitation	
Pulmonary embolism	Enlarged, right ventricular apex reaching cardiac apex, hypokinetic right ventricle, tricuspid regurgitation, elevated pulmonary pressure (degree varies with pre-existing pulmonary hypertension, right ventricular function, and extent of embolism)	
Pericardial tamponade	Pericardial fluid compressing the right ventricle and/or right atrium; exaggerated respiratory variation in left and right ventricular inflow	Look for signs of aortic dissection, myocardial infarction, trauma or other thoracic disease, e.g. tumours
Acute left sided valvular regurgitation	Structural damage of aortic or mitral valve, e.g., papillary muscle rupture; Doppler signs of severe aortic or mitral regurgitation; hyperkinetic left ventricle, often of normal size	Look for signs of inferior myocardial infarction in papillary muscle rupture, and for signs of aortic dissection in aortic regurgitation
Acute right heart failure	Enlarged, hypokinetic right ventricle, may occur with pulmonary embolism, chronic pulmonary hypertension, or as right ventricular infarction complicating inferior myocardial infarction	
Aortic dissection or rupture	Aortic enlargement, aortic valvular regurgitation, dissection flap in the aorta, pericardial tamponade	The typical site of aortic rupture, e.g. after deceleration trauma, is the proximal descending aorta, which is visualizable by TOE
Sepsis	Endocarditic vegetation on valve or pacemaker electrode, abscess, or destruction of valves	In sepsis due to noncardiac causes, the discrepancy between systemic hypotension in the presence of a often hyperkinetic heart is typical
Prosthetic valve obstruction	'Frozen' occluder position in mitral prostheses, often with clear thrombus; in the aortic position, difficult to see even by TOE. Massive transvalvular gradient elevation by Doppler	Always use TOE; compare to earlier transprosthetic gradients, if possible
Prosthetic valve regurgitation or dehiscence	Abnormal mobility ('rocking') of prosthesis, (colour) Doppler signs of severe regurgitation, premature mitral valve closure in aortic regurgitation	
Aortic stenosis	Severe aortic stenosis, typically with a severely depressed left ventricle	Continuity equation must be used to evaluate stenosis severity; gradients may be deceptively low

Heart failure

Assessment of systolic left ventricular function

Echocardiography provides crucial information on mechanisms, severity, and therapeutic options in congestive heart failure. Global left ventricular function is typically categorized into systolic or pump function, which assesses the ability of the left ventricle to create an adequate stroke volume, and diastolic function, which relates to the ability of the left ventricle to fill adequately at low diastolic pressures. Evaluation of global left ventricular systolic function consists of:

* Ejection fraction (EF), calculated from end-diastolic and end-systolic left ventricular volumes (➲ Fig. 20.1): This may be visually estimated from several cross-sections, or preferentially measured by tracing the left ventricle in end-diastole and end-systole in the four-chamber view (monoplane EF) or additionally in the two-chamber view (biplane EF), enabling the calculation of left ventricular volumes and EF by the modified Simpson's rule method. If 3D echo is available, volumes can be calculated from the full 'volume data set' without any geometric assumptions.

* End-systolic (LVESD) and end-diastolic (LVDD) left ventricular short axis diameters (by M-mode or by 2D echo measured from a parasternal long-axis view) and the shortening fraction (LVEDD – LVESD)/LVEDD are the oldest quantitative parameters of global left ventricular function. However, they only take into account wall motion at the base of the left ventricle.

* The systolic excursion (normally >12 mm) of the atrioventricular plane of the left ventricular, i.e. the apical displacement of the mitral annulus during systole, can serve as a measure of global systolic function.

* On tissue Doppler recordings from the mitral annular region of the septal and lateral wall in the apical four-chamber view, peak systolic longitudinal velocities are normally greater than 5 cm/s (➲ Fig. 20.6). Strain values averaged over all left ventricular segments ('global strain') may also be used to evaluate left ventricular function.

See 🔒 20.4 for normal values.

Assessment of diastolic left ventricular function

Almost all patients with impaired global systolic function also have elevated left ventricular filling pressures and hence impaired diastolic function. Echo provides an estimate of elevated filling pressures and is able to detect markers of impaired prognosis, such as the restrictive transmitral filling pressure [4, 6]. On the other hand, there is a large group of patients suffering from symptoms of heart failure, although EF is preserved, especially in the presence of hypertension and left ventricular hypertrophy. This has been termed 'heart failure with normal EF' or 'diastolic heart failure'. The following signs and parameters should be systematically used to evaluate diastolic left ventricular filling pressures:

* Impaired systolic function (EF) invariably leads to elevated filling pressures.

* Presence of left ventricular hypertrophy, independent of cause, indicates impaired relaxation and often also reduced chamber compliance, which in advanced hypertrophy requires higher than normal filling pressures.

* The size of the left atrium, measured as left atrial volume from the apical four-chamber view or in both apical four-chamber and long-axis view (🔒 20.5). Normal size ($\leq$34 ml/m^2) excludes chronic elevation of left ventricular filling pressures. However, the left atrium may also enlarge in other conditions, e.g., atrial fibrillation.

* The ratio E/e' (E, the peak transmitral early diastolic flow velocity, divided by e', peak early diastolic mitral annular tissue velocities averaged from the septal and lateral mitral annular region) (➲ Fig. 20.6). A ratio less than 8 largely excludes elevated filling pressures, while a ratio greater than 15 largely proves substantially elevated filling pressures. Between these values, other parameters have to be used to evaluate filling pressures [6]. These include a longer duration of the retrograde pulmonary atrial wave than of the transmitral A wave, an increase in the peak velocity of the retrograde pulmonary atrial wave to more than 35 cm/s, a reduction in pulmonary venous systolic forward flow (🔒 20.5), and a delay in the onset of e' in relation to the onset of E.

* Pulmonary artery systolic pressure, measured by the maximal tricuspid regurgitation velocity (see section on pulmonary embolism), is elevated in diastolic heart failure and is a measure of severity of heart failure.

* A restrictive transmitral flow pattern (peak E > 2 × peak A wave velocity and E wave deceleration time <150 ms) indicates severely impaired prognosis (➲ Fig. 20.6); however, this is usually accompanied by systolic dysfunction. Isovolumic relaxation time, a highly preload-dependent time interval measured from cessation of aortic flow

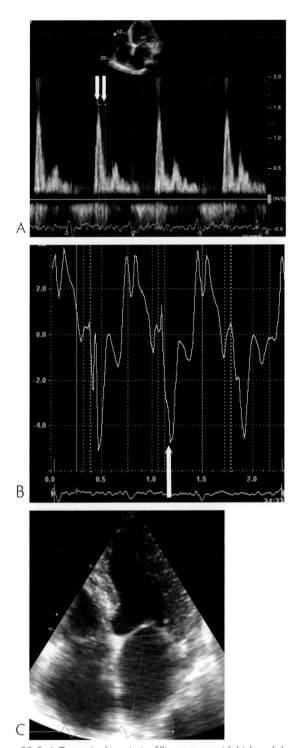

Figure 20.6 A. Transmitral restrictive filling pattern with high and short E wave and small A wave; peak E wave is more than double as high a peak A wave. The E wave deceleration (time interval between arrows) is 103 ms. B. In the same patient, basal myocardial velocities by tissue Doppler. Reduced early diastolic peak velocity e' (5 cm/s, arrow) and also low peak systolic velocities (4 cm/s). E/e' in this patient was 29, indicating massively elevated left ventricular filling pressures. C. Left atrial volume calculation from the four-chamber view by summation of disks (different patient from A and B). The left atrium is mildly enlarged at 36 ml/m2.

to onset of transmitral inflow, is severely shortened (<60 ms). A pseudo-restrictive pattern may be observed in young, perfectly healthy individuals due to very vigorous relaxation.

♦ A transmitral flow pattern with E<A peak velocities is very frequent, with isovolumic relaxation prolonged (>100 ms). This is normal in patients over 60 years of age. The pattern excludes substantially elevated filling pressures, since these would increase peak E wave.

Other aspects of heart failure

Further important information in patients with heart failure gleaned from echo includes:

♦ Presence and degree of mitral regurgitation.

♦ Signs of coronary artery disease (e.g., regional wall motion abnormalities), cardiomyopathy (especially the dilated form), myocarditis, or constrictive pericarditis causing heart failure.

♦ Signs of right ventricular dysfunction. Isolated right ventricular dysfunction is most frequently due to chronic pulmonary hypertension or acute pulmonary pressure elevation following pulmonary embolism (see ➲ Pulmonary embolism). Hallmarks are an enlarged and globally hypokinetic right ventricle, with tricuspid regurgitation and elevated peak tricuspid velocity, which enables an estimate of peak systolic right ventricular and, thus, pulmonary pressure. Importantly, in severe right heart failure after pulmonary embolism, the right ventricle may not be able to generate high pressures, leading to deceptively low peak transtricuspid regurgitant velocities and right ventricular pressure estimates. The ventricular septum is shifted to the left side, giving the cross-section of the left ventricle a D shape instead of a circular appearance ('D sign'). Right ventricular size and function are usually eyeballed, due to unreliability of M-mode or 2D measurements. A useful practical measure of right ventricular is the systolic excursion of the tricuspid annulus, with values of less than 15 mm indicating impairment of right ventricular function. Right ventricular end-diastolic free wall thickness greater than 5 mm indicates chronic pulmonary hypertension. Right ventricular infarction, a complication of inferior left ventricular infarction, is discussed in the section on ➲ Acute coronary syndrome and its complications. Rarely, advanced cardiomyopathy, e.g. right ventricular arrhythmogenic cardiomyopathy, may be the cause of right heart failure.

Echo also plays a critical role in identifying candidates for therapies and procedures which may improve heart failure or its prognosis [7]. The most important issues are:

- Measurement of EF to identify candidates for implantable defibrillator therapy (EF <35%).

- Diagnosis of hibernating myocardium with the potential to improve function after revascularization. Hibernating, i.e., dysfunctional but viable, myocardial regions can be identified by dobutamine stress echo. The identification of hibernating myocardium predicts improvement of EF and overall prognosis after revascularization.

- Identification of candidates for cardiac resynchronization therapy (CRT). Although so far the selection of CRT candidates by echo criteria has not been proved to discriminate well between potential responders and non-responders, and criteria for identifying CRT-responsive left ventricular dyssynchrony continue to evolve, several parameters seem to have at least moderate predictive value [8]:

  - The interventricular delay, measured as the delay of onset of left ventricular ejection versus the onset of right ventricular ejection (measured from pulsed-wave Doppler of pulmonary and aortic flow), considered to be significant if greater than 40 ms.

  - The differences in the time that it takes myocardial longitudinal systolic velocities to reach their systolic maximum ('time to peak') in the basal or mid segments of the left ventricle, in particular comparing septal to lateral wall segments (with a delay >65 ms considered predictive).

  - Differences in timing of onset or peak of longitudinal, radial, or circumferential systolic strain of opposing wall segments.

Assessment of cardiac output and volume status

Knowledge of cardiac output and of intravascular volume status is crucial in intensive care. These parameters can be estimated—to a degree—from echocardiography. Cardiac output is easiest calculated by measuring left ventricular outflow tract diameter (D) and the time velocity integral of left ventricular outflow tract flow by pulsed-wave Doppler (VTI), taking care to align the Doppler beam as well as possible with the long axis of the outflow tract (⊃ Fig. 20.7). Systemic stroke volume (SV) is then approximately (assuming a circular outflow tract cross-section)

$$SV = \pi \times D^2 \times VTI/4$$

provided that there is no aortic regurgitation. A similar calculation can be made at the pulmonary valve level to calculate pulmonary SV. The product of SV and heart rate is cardiac output. The calculation is far from precise, but will give a reasonable estimate of cardiac output.

The estimation of intravascular volume status, specifically of central venous pressure and of pulmonary capillary pressure, relies on indirect signs and is more complex.

- Central venous pressure may be estimated by assessing the respiratory variation of the diameter of the inferior vena cava from a subcostal echo window (🎥 20.6). Exact measurements are rather difficult since the vena cava inferior itself moves in and out of the cross-section

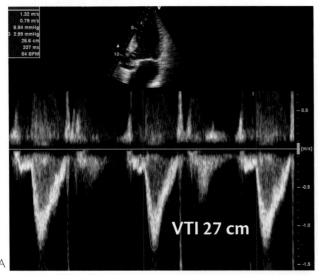
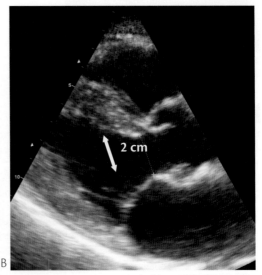

Figure 20.7 Stroke volume calculation from left ventricular outflow tract diameter (2 cm) and velocity-time-integral of the systolic flow profile in the left ventricular outflow tract, measured by pulsed-wave Doppler (27 cm), yielding a stroke volume of 85 ml.

during respiration, but a total obliteration of the vena cava during inspiration ('sniff') is usually associated with mean right atrial pressures of 5 mmHg or less. A less than 50% inspiratory decrease in caval diameter is associated with mean right atrial pressure above 10 mmHg, and no diameter change at all with severely elevated mean right atrial pressure of 20 mmHg or more. Furthermore, the systolic portion of hepatic venous flow, which usually shows a systolic and a diastolic forward wave towards the right atrium, decreases with increasing right atrial pressures. This is accentuated if there is substantial tricuspid regurgitation, which will lead to backward systolic flow in the hepatic veins. The hepatic veins can easily be sampled by pulsed-wave Doppler in held respiration from the subcostal window. Positive end-expiratory pressure (PEEP) elevates right atrial pressures and makes it difficult to use them to assess volume status.

♦ Pulmonary arterial pressure: Systolic pulmonary pressure is assumed to be equal to peak right ventricular pressure, which can be estimated using the tricuspid regurgitation Doppler signal (see section ➲ Pulmonary embolism). In the absence of a usable tricuspid regurgitation signal, the acceleration time (time from onset of pulmonary ejection to peak velocity) of the transpulmonary pulsed-wave Doppler flow profile may be used as a very rough estimate of pulmonary pressure; acceleration times greater than 100 ms make substantial pulmonary hypertension unlikely.

♦ Assessment of elevated left ventricular filling pressures and thus, elevated pulmonary capillary pressures (see ➲ Assessment of diastolic left ventricular function). Elevated pulmonary capillary pressures due to left ventricular dysfunction usually are associated with E/e′

ratios greater than 15 [6]. Further, high pulmonary capillary pressures and high left ventricular filling pressures will generate a tall, short transmitral E wave; a transmitral E/A wave ratio of less than 1 makes high filling pressures unlikely and may be normal for age or caused by hypovolaemia or slowed left ventricular relaxation.

♦ Pleural effusions are easily diagnosed and semiquantitated by applying the echo transducer to the intercostal spaces over the lungs, preferentially with the patient sitting (📷 20.10).

Endocarditis, acute valvular regurgitation, and prosthetic valve dysfunction

Infective endocarditis

Infective endocarditis may necessitate intensive care for several reasons: sepsis, acute valvular regurgitation, and central or peripheral systemic embolism. The echocardiographic hallmark of infective endocarditis is new mobile mass lesions (vegetations; ➲ Fig. 20.8, 20.9) attached to valvular structures, and valvular destruction leading to regurgitation; in fact, echo evidence of infective endocarditis is a major diagnostic criterion. Mitral and aortic valves are affected with similar frequency. Tricuspid endocarditis occurs mainly in drug addicts and patients with long-standing disease necessitating the insertion of indwelling central catheters and ports. Vegetations may also be attached to cardiac foreign bodies such as pacemaker electrodes and in rare cases directly to the endocardium, e.g. in the proximity of a ventricular septal defect. Abscess formation in the perivalvular tissue may be observed, especially in aortic valve endocarditis and in prosthetic valves. Further sequelae of endocarditis are fistulae, perforations, or the formation of a mitral pseudoaneurysm. Valve endocarditis may

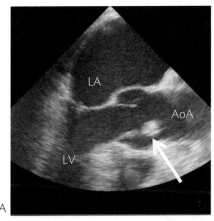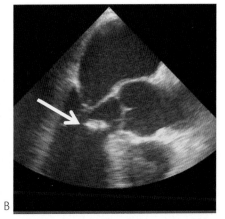

Figure 20.8 Infective endocarditis of the aortic valve with vegetation attached to the right coronary cusp. Transoesophageal long axis view at 120°. Note vegetation (arrow) changing position during the cardiac cycle. The vegetation is echo-dense, suggesting chronic or healed endocarditis. Panel A: diastole; Panel B: systole.

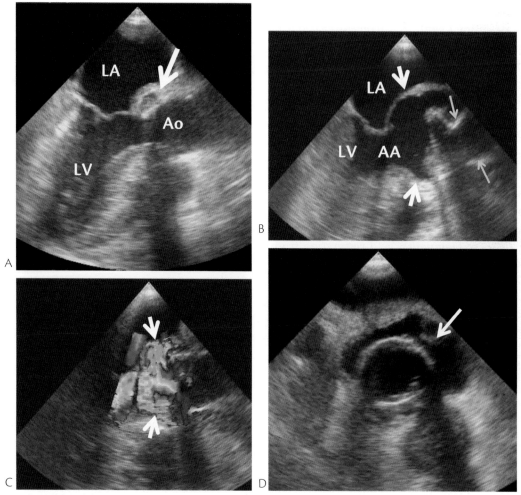

Figure 20.9 (A) Infective endocarditis. Abscess of the posterior aortic ring (arrow) in a patient with a mechanical aortic prosthesis. Transoesophageal long-axis view.
Prosthetic infective endocarditis after Bentall operation. TEE long axis view at 120°. Systolic image (B) shows ring dehiscence and migration of the entire valved conduit (yellow arrows) above the plane of aortic annulus (AA). The native aorta (white arrows) developed a pseudoaneurysm. Color Doppler in diastole (C) shows circular paraprosthetic leak (arrows). (D) TEE short axis view of conduit replacing of the ascending aorta showing a periprosthetic abscess (arrow) in the proximal remnant aorta.

induce regurgitation of all degrees by perforation or rupture of valvular structures. TOE is superior to TTE because of its higher spatial resolution and better image quality and should always be used if there is a substantial suspicion of infective endocarditis (e.g. positive blood cultures) and no definite diagnosis can be established by TTE. In the presence of prosthetic valves, use of TOE is mandatory [9], since infective endocarditis is then frequent, difficult to detect, and more prone to complications, especially ring abscesses.

Acute mitral or aortic regurgitation

◆ Acute severe mitral regurgitation occurs in several scenarios (⏏ 20.9). Due to systolic regurgitation into the left atrium, there is acute volume overload, and, consequently, pressure overload of the left atrium, leading to increases in pulmonary capillary pressure and pulmonary oedema. Forward SV is low, causing hypotension and ultimately cardiogenic shock. Key echo findings are [10]:

◆ A clear structural abnormality of the mitral valve with excessive mobility of a part of the valvular apparatus, such as a flail leaflet, or papillary muscle or chordal rupture (➲ Fig. 20.10, ⏏ 20.10).

◆ A large, consistently imaged proximal acceleration zone (>1 cm² at aliasing velocities ≥50 cm/s) on the ventricular side of the mitral valve; the regurgitant jet in the left atrium is often hard to interpret because of tachycardia, low systemic pressure, and other factors.

◆ Systolic pulmonary venous flow reversal.

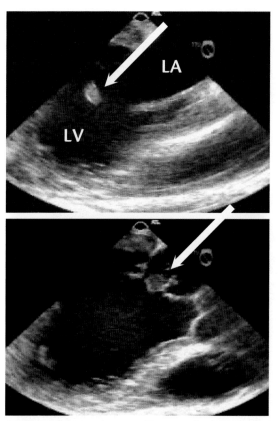

Figure 20.10 Papillary muscle rupture. Transoesophageal transgastric two-chamber view. The ruptured head of the papillary muscle (arrow) is seen in the left ventricle in diastole (top) and in the left atrium in systole (bottom).

- In extreme cases, the typically symmetric bell-shaped continuous-wave Doppler profile of mitral regurgitation becomes triangular due to dramatic late systolic pressure increase in the left atrium.

- The left ventricle is often hyperkinetic due to massive volume overload. The left atrium may be of normal size due to the acuteness of regurgitation.

Acute severe aortic regurgitation causes sudden left ventricular volume overload, increased diastolic pressures leading ultimately to pulmonary oedema, and with reduced forward SV also leads to cardiogenic shock. Key echo findings are:

- A clear structural abnormality such as endocarditic destruction, rupture of a leaflet, or an aortic dissection membrane prolapsing into the outflow tract and precluding diastolic closure of the valve.

- Doppler and colour Doppler signs of severe aortic regurgitation, including marked holodiastolic backward flow in the descending aorta and, if present, a large proximal acceleration zone (>1 cm^2 at aliasing velocities ≥ 50 cm/s) on the aortic side of the valve.

- Premature closure of the mitral valve on a mitral M-mode recording or the transmitral Doppler profile.

Prosthetic mitral or aortic valves may develop sudden severe regurgitation due to ring dehiscence, e.g. in the course of infective endocarditis, endocarditic destruction, or degenerative rupture of bioprosthetic leaflets, or thrombotic fixation or embolization of a mechanical occluder (e.g. after strut fracture of a tilting disc prosthesis).

Prosthetic valve thrombosis

Prosthetic valve thrombosis (➲ Fig. 20.11) occurs almost exclusively in mechanical valves, leading to predominant stenosis with or without regurgitation depending on the dynamic of the prosthetic leaflet(s). Symptoms and clinical findings depend on how rapidly the prosthetic obstruction develops and on the severity of obstruction [11, 12]. The incidence of prosthetic valve thrombosis is twice as high in the mitral as in the aortic position, and even higher in the tricuspid position, independently of the prosthesis type. Echo signs are increased transprosthetic Doppler gradients and, especially in mitral prostheses, absent motion of one or both occluders. Transoesophageal echocardiography is mandatory and sometimes can distinguish obstruction by thrombus or by pannus. Fluoroscopy is very helpful and indispensable in aortic prosthetic thrombosis.

Pericardial disease and trauma

The two main pericardial pathologies important for cardiac intensive care are pericardial effusion, including tamponade, and constrictive pericarditis. Pericardial effusions occur in many circumstances, including infectious, immunological, and malignant diseases, as well as perforation or rupture of coronary vessels or cardiac chambers and traumatic damage.

Cardiac tamponade is a life-threatening complication of pericardial effusion and can occur even with small, but acutely developing effusions, e.g. after coronary artery perforation or rupture due to percutaneous coronary intervention (📷 20.11). Due to the limited intrapericardial space and low compliance of the pericardium, compression of cardiac chambers ensues, typically the right atrium (in late diastole and early systole) and the right ventricle (in early diastole) because of their relatively low internal pressures. This 'collapse', along with the effusion, can be seen directly on 2D echo, especially in the four-chamber view and the subcostal view (➲ Fig 20.6, 📷 20.12). The duration of collapse during the cardiac cycle parallels the severity of haemodynamic compromise. While temporary inward displacement of the right atrial wall during the

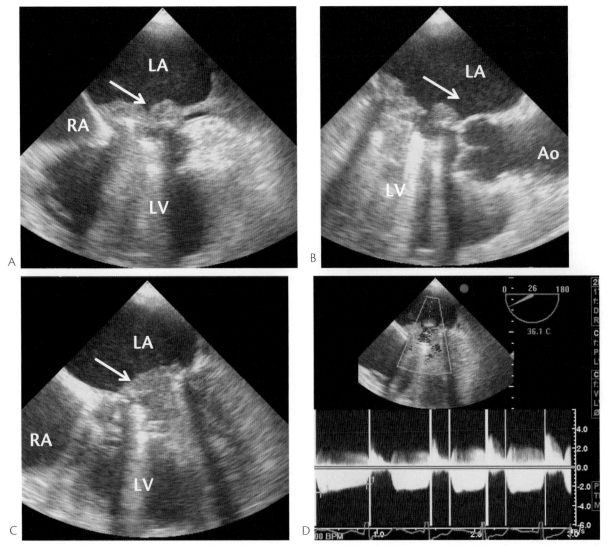

Figure 20.11 A-C. Extensive obstructive thrombosis of a mechanical mitral prosthesis (arrow) in different transoesophageal views. D. Transoesophageal continuous wave Doppler profile across the mitral prosthesis, demonstrating obstruction (note very slow deceleration slope and a mean gradient of approximately 15 mmHg).

cardiac cycle is an early and sensitive sign of haemodynamic significance of pericardial effusion, its specificity for tamponade is low; on the other hand, right ventricular collapse has lower sensitivity, but higher specificity for haemodynamic compromise. In rare cases of localized pericardial effusions (e.g. postoperatively) the left atrium or ventricle may be primarily compressed; these localized effusions may be difficult to detect and may necessitate TOE, especially in the postoperative patient. The compression of the heart chambers leads to an exaggeration of respiratory variation of inflow and outflow patterns of the ventricles: mitral inflow and aortic SV decrease with inspiration, while tricuspid inflow increases. A decrease of more than 25% in peak transmitral E wave velocity with inspiration is considered a sign of haemodynamic compromise. A 'paradoxical' septal shift to the left in early diastole,

created by the increase in transtricuspid flow, is also observed. In expiration, these changes are reversed. Furthermore, the inferior vena cava is usually distended and does not collapse with inspiration.

To prepare for pericardial puncture, the subcostal view is useful to determine the location, angle, and depth of the puncture. If the subcostal approach is not feasible, echo helps to select alternative sites for puncture, i.e. sites where the distance between skin and pericardial fluid is minimal, e.g. the apex. After puncture, the location of the tip of the needle or of a catheter introduced into the pericardial space may be confirmed by injecting an agitated infusion solution, which will create a bright contrast echo in the pericardial space.

In constrictive pericarditis, thickened (>5 mm) or calcified pericardium may be apparent, but often is not.

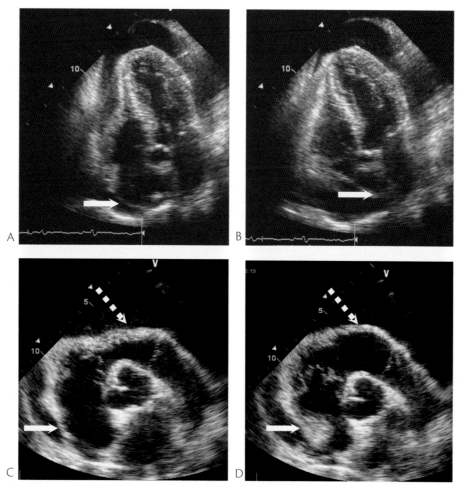

Figure 20.12 Circular pericardial effusion with beginning haemodynamic compromise (tamponade). (A) Apical four-chamber view in diastole, with normal convex contour of right atrial free wall, and (B) systole, with compression of the right atrium (arrows). (C) Parasternal short axis view in diastole, with compression of right ventricle (dotted arrows) and no compression of right atrium (continuous arrow), and (D) systole, with compression of right atrium and no compression of the pressurized right ventricle.

The ventricles are of normal size, while the atria are enlarged. Global left and right ventricular systolic function are normal, but paradoxical septal motion is present. In clearcut cases, there is an inspiratory decrease in transmitral flow and increase in transtricuspid flow, with opposite changes in expiration. Sometimes, however, this sign is blunted by massive diuretic therapy. The transmitral flow in the typical case is characterized by tall, short E waves with short deceleration time ('restrictive transmitral pattern').

Traumatic cardiac and aortic injury

Virtually all cardiac structures may be damaged by blunt trauma (📷 20.13). The ventricles may develop intramyocardial haematoma, myocardial necrosis, or frank rupture, leading to usually lethal tamponade if a free wall is affected, or else to ventricular septal defect. The right ventricular free wall is most often affected due to its anterior localization in the chest. The atria may also rupture. Coronary vessels may be lacerated, leading to haematopericardium and tamponade. Valvular structures may also be damaged, including leaflets and the support apparatus, most prominently papillary muscles or chordae. Tears of the pericardium, with or without other cardiac injury, may lead to herniation of other organs into the pericardial sac (e.g. intestinal herniation through a ruptured diaphragm) or displacement of cardiac structures outside the pericardial sac.

The thoracic aorta is affected especially by deceleration trauma (e.g. traffic accidents or falls). Traffic accidents typically cause aortic damage at the aortic isthmus, the junction of the aortic arch and descending aorta. Falls may lead to aortic damage at the level of the innominate artery. The damage to the aorta ranges from intramural haematoma to complete transection of the vessel.

Echocardiography, especially TOE, is very helpful after blunt chest trauma. In a study, more than half of

117 patients with blunt chest trauma showed clearly pathologic findings on TOE, ranging from right ventricular wall motion abnormalities to pericardial effusions; the ECG was often normal in these patients [13]. Penetrating trauma of the heart or large vessels is typically rapidly fatal, precluding echocardiographic examination.

Pulmonary embolism

A dilated and hypokinetic right ventricle is the typical echo finding in severe pulmonary embolism (PE). Additionally, there is a variable increase in right ventricular systolic pressure as estimated by measuring peak tricuspid regurgitant velocity (➲ Fig. 20.13). This is done by measuring peak tricuspid regurgitant velocity by continuous-wave Doppler, calculating the peak pressure difference between right ventricle and right atrium from the Bernoulli equation ($\Delta p = 4v^2$) and adding an estimate of mean right atrial pressure, e.g. 10 mmHg (for more detail on right atrial pressure estimation, see ➲ Heart failure). Note, however, that in the acutely failing right ventricle associated with fulminant PE, this pressure may be deceptively normal or only minimally elevated. Very high peak pulmonary pressures (e.g. >80 mmHg) cannot be generated by a previously normally loaded right ventricle and do not occur in response to an acute embolism, unless there is previous pulmonary hypertension. A shift of the ventricular septum to the left, flattening the cross-section of the left ventricle into a D shape instead of the normal circular shape in short axis views, and paradoxical septal motion are important signs of acute right ventricular pressure overload. Tricuspid regurgitation is invariably present, and the inferior vena cava may be distended and lack inspiratory collapse. Thrombi may sometimes by seen directly in the pulmonary artery imaged in parasternal or subcostal views. If TOE is performed, the right pulmonary artery can also be evaluated quite well, and thrombotic material may be seen there. The acute pressure increase in the right atrium leads to a shift of the position of the atrial septum to the left side and may create continuous right-to-left shunt through a patent foramen ovale. In the presence of severe PE, paradoxical embolism of thrombotic material through a patent foramen ovale is a recognized and devastating complication. On the other hand, small pulmonary emboli are not detectable on echo. The role of echo therefore is not the definitive exclusion of (small) PE, but assessment of whether a haemodynamically significant embolism has taken place and whether right ventricular compromise warrants thrombolytic therapy.

The echocardiographic differentiation of chronic and acute pulmonary pressure elevation is difficult. Right ventricular hypertrophy with an end-diastolic free wall thickness greater than 5 mm supports chronic pulmonary hypertension, but does not exclude an additional acute pressure increase. Several signs that have been described as relatively specific (but not sensitive) for acute PE [14] are:

◆ McConnell's sign: a hypokinetic right ventricular free wall together with a hyperkinetic or normokinetic right ventricular apex.

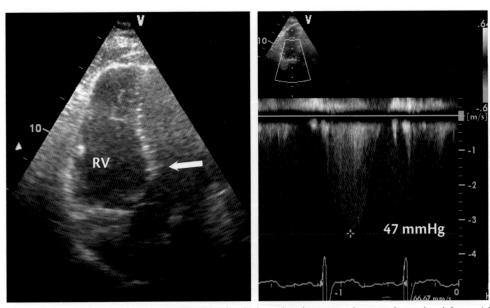

Figure 20.13 Pulmonary embolism. A. Dilated, hypokinetic right ventricle which reaches the apex and appears larger than left ventricle. Note shift of basal septum to the left (arrow) B. Continuous-wave Doppler of tricuspid regurgitation shows elevated peak right ventricular pressure (peak tricuspid regurgitant velocity 47 mmHg)

- The transpulmonary pulsed-wave Doppler flow profile may show shortened acceleration time (<100 ms) and notching, which is believed to result from reflected pressure waves created by central pulmonary thrombus.

- The '60/60' sign: a pulmonary systolic pressure of less than 60 mmHg by tricuspid regurgitation, and a pulmonary acceleration time of less 60 ms.

It should be clear, though, that these signs are far from being ideally predictive for acute PE.

Aortic emergencies

The ascending aorta can be seen to varying extents from the left and right parasternal echo windows, and the aortic arch is seen from the suprasternal window, which, however, is often obstructed in elderly or emphysematous individuals. A much better evaluation of the thoracic aorta is afforded by TOE, where almost the entire course is visible except for a 'blind spot' created by tracheal and left bronchial interposition at the distal ascending aorta and proximal arch. Dilatation and aneurysms, atheromatous disease, plaque-adherent thrombi, aortic dissection (➲ Box 20.1) or intramural haematoma, and traumatic damage (see ➲ Traumatic cardiac and aortic injury) can be diagnosed by TOE (📹 20.14). The following are important pathological features of the aorta [15]:

- Enlarged aortic diameters: These are important since the risk of rupture and also of dissection depends on aortic diameters. Diameters greater than 55 mm in general are an indication for surgery even in asymptomatic patients, and in patients with Marfan's syndrome or bicuspid aortic valve lower values (>45 mm) have been recommended for replacement [11].

- Atheromatosis is mainly observed in the descending aorta and the arch. Sometimes, mobile thrombi may be noted, which may embolize (➲ Fig. 20.14).

- Aortic dissection is diagnosed by identifying the pathognomonic dissection membrane, a thin, undulating membrane ('intimal flap') separating true and false lumen (➲ Fig. 20.15, 📹 20.15). Reverberations of the posterior wall of the ascending aorta or the posterior wall of the right pulmonary artery may create aortic intraluminal linear horizontal lines and need to be differentiated from true flaps, which are usually very well delineated and crisp [16]. Entry and re-entry sites may be identified by 2D echo and colour flow Doppler. The false lumen is typically larger, has slower flow (often spontaneous contrast

Box 20.1 Classification of aortic dissection

- Stanford A: dissection involves ascending aorta, and may also involve aortic arch and descending aorta

- Stanford B: dissection involves only descending aorta

A more recent classification of acute aortic syndromes [17] distinguishes:

- Class I: classic dissection of all types

- Class II: intramural hematoma

- Class III: subtle circumscript dissection representing a localized tear without clear-cut haematoma

- Class IV: plaque ulceration (mostly in the descending aorta, and often in the abdominal aorta)

- Class V: traumatic or iatrogenic (mostly catheter-induced, retrograde) dissection

or even thrombosis is present), and is convex towards the more highly pressurized, but smaller, true lumen. The site of the intimal rupture and the extent of the dissection are crucial for identification of the type of dissection and its management. Type A dissection is typically accompanied by some amount of aortic regurgitation and pericardial haemorrhage, which may progress abruptly to lethal tamponade. These two signs are easily recognized on TTE and should raise the 'red flag' of possible aortic dissection in the context of chest pain or other clinical presentations, like sudden hypotension or shock. When a patient with suspected aortic dissection is examined by TOE, blood pressure must be controlled tightly, since death due to progressive rupture during TOE has been reported.

- Intramural haematoma of the aorta is a variant or precursor of dissection, which often coexists with areas of classic dissection. It is characterized by a thickened aortic wall (>7 mm) with echolucent areas, a smooth intimal surface, and sometimes displacement of superficial calcifications towards the lumen. Differentiation from (1) severe atherosclerotic wall thickening, or (2) the thrombosed false lumen of a classic dissection, can be difficult.

Dissection and intramural haematoma are life-threatening diseases which require emergency surgery if they affect the ascending aorta [17]. The questions that echocardiographic examination should quickly and decisively address

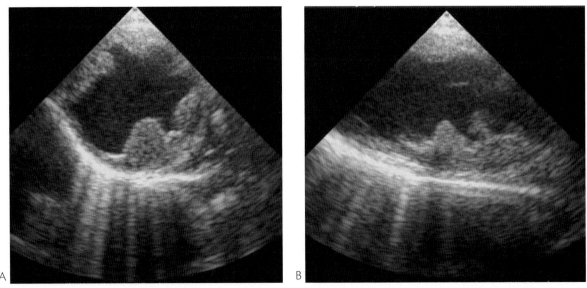

Figure 20.14 Thrombi in a non-aneurysmatic descending aorta. After a few weeks of anticoagulation, the thrombi dissolved and only atherosclerosis of the aortic wall was seen. A. Transoesophageal short axis view.B. Transoesophageal long-axis view.

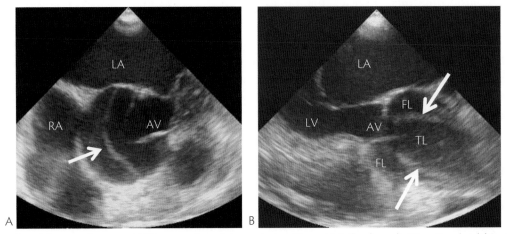

Figure 20.15 Dissection of the ascending aorta: (A) Transoesophageal short axis view. Note mobile flap (arrow). AV: aortic valve. (B) Transoesophageal long-axis view at 120°. Note circular flap (arrows). FL, false lumen; TL, true lumen.

are summarized in 📺 20.14. Importantly, nonclassical forms of the acute aortic syndrome, such as intramural haematoma or penetrating ulcer, are often difficult to detect by echo. CT or MRI should be liberally used in any cases of doubt.

Systemic embolism

Echocardiography is the method of choice if a cardiovascular source of embolism is suspected [18]. TOE has a higher

yield than TTE in identifying such sources and should be used if results may lead to a change in management. TOE is particularly valuable in assessing left atrial thrombi, endocarditic vegetations, tumours, and aortic atheromas. The presence of the following potential sources of embolism should be systematically sought:

♦ Atrial thrombi, in particular thrombi of the left atrial appendage, which frequently occur in atrial fibrillation and in some instances (e.g. aortic stenosis) also in sinus rhythm. However, in atrial fibrillation, which is by far the most frequent cardiac source of embolism, a negative TOE does not exclude that a left atrial or appendage thrombus was present before the embolism; therefore, independent from TOE findings, anticoagulation usually is indicated.

- Infective endocarditis (see ⊃ Infective endocarditis).
- Left ventricular thrombi from regions with severe wall motion abnormalities, e.g. apical aneurysm. TOE has no advantage in detecting left ventricular thrombi, but left heart contrast echocardiography may be helpful.
- Tumours, e.g. myxoma or fibroelastoma, best diagnosed or excluded by TOE.
- Atrial septal defect or patent foramen ovale as the gate for paradoxical embolism.
- Aortic atheromatosis with superimposed thrombi (TOE).

Personal perspective

Every intensive care patient with a cardiovascular disorder needs echocardiography, and the sooner the better. Especially in the cardiac intensive care environment, there is simply no other imaging method even remotely as valuable as echocardiography. The challenge today and in the future is to ensure adequate training and to use the method, which is so conveniently available at the bedside, to the full extent of its diagnostic possibilities.

This requires proper and dedicated training, which is not acquired 'on the fly'. There is no doubt that further echocardiographic refinements in haemodynamic assessment, diagnosis of myocardial ischaemia and viability, myocardial perfusion, coronary flow reserve, and others will arrive and further improve our diagnostic capabilities. The limitation, however, is often the 'human factor', which requires sufficient experience and expertise to harness the abundant imaging data for better patient care and outcomes.

Further reading

Erbel R, Alfonso F, Boileau C, et al. Diagnosis and management of aortic dissection. Recommendations of the Task Force on Aortic Dissection, European Society of Cardiology. Eur Heart J 2001;**22**:1642–1681.

Evangelista A, Avegliano G, Aguilar R, et al. Impact of contrast-enhanced echocardiography on the diagnostic algorithm of acute aortic dissection. Eur J Echocardiogr 2010;**31**(4):472–479.

Flachskampf FA, Voigt JU, Daniel WG. Cardiovascular ultrasound. In: The ESC Textbook of Cardiovascular Medicine, 2nd edition, Oxford University Press, Oxford, 2009.

Lang R, Bierig M, Devereux R, Flachskampf FA, et al. Recommendations for Chamber Quantification. A report from the American Society of Echocardiography's Nomenclature and Standards Committee, the Task Force on Chamber Quantification, and the European Association of Echocardiography. Eur J Echocardiogr 2006;**7**:79–108.

Task Force on the Prevention, Diagnosis, and Treatment of Infective Endocarditis of the European Society of Cardiology et al. Guidelines on the prevention, diagnosis, and treatment of infective endocarditis (new version 2009): the Task Force on the Prevention, Diagnosis, and Treatment of Infective Endocarditis of the European Society of Cardiology (ESC). Eur Heart J 2009;**30**:2369–2413.

Torbicki A, Perrier A, Konstantinides S, et al. Guidelines on the diagnosis and management of acute pulmonary embolism: the Task Force for the Diagnosis and Management of Acute Pulmonary Embolism of the European Society of Cardiology (ESC). Eur Heart J 2008;**29**:2276–2315.

Vahanian A, Baumgartner H, Bax J, et al. ESC guidelines on the management of valvular heart disease. Eur Heart J 2007;**28**:230–268.

Zoghbi WA, MD, Enriquez-Sarano M, Foster E, et al. Recommendations for evaluation of the severity of native valvular regurgitation with two-dimensional and Doppler echocardiography. Eur J Echocardiogr 2003;**4**:237–261.

Zoghbi WA, Chambers JB, Dumesnil JG, et al. Recommendations for evaluation of prosthetic valves with echocardiography and Doppler ultrasound. J Am Soc Echocardiogr 2009;**22**:975–1014.

Additional online material

- 20.1 Modern mobile echo devices
- 20.2 Training requirements in echocardiography
- 20.3 Wall motion abnormality in the anteroseptum (LAD territory)
- 20.4 Reference normal and abnormal values of left ventricular size
- 20.5 Reduction in pulmonary venous systolic forward flow
- 20.6 Respiratory variability of the diameter of the inferior vena cava
- 20.7 Pleural effusions

⮕ For additional multimedia materials please visit the online version of the book (✎ http://www.esciacc.oxfordmedicine.com).

CHAPTER 21

Cardiac magnetic resonance imaging

J. Schwitter and J. Bremerich

Contents

Summary

Current applications of cardiac magnetic resonance (CMR) imaging offer a wide spectrum of indications in the setting of acute cardiac care. In particular, CMR is helpful for the differential diagnosis of chest pain by detection of myocarditis and pericarditis. Also, takotsubo cardiomyopathy and acute aortic diseases can be evaluated by CMR and are important differential diagnoses in patients with acute chest pain. In patients with restricted windows for echocardiography, CMR is the method of choice to evaluate complications of acute myocardial infarction (AMI).

In AMI, CMR allows for a unique characterization of myocardial damage by quantifying necrosis, microvascular obstruction, oedema (=area at risk), and haemorrhage. These capabilities will help us to understand better the pathophysiological events during infarction and will also allow to assess new treatment strategies in AMI. To what extent the information on tissue damage will guide patient management is not yet clear and further research in this field is warranted.

In the near future, CMR will certainly become more routine in acute cardiac care units, as manufacturers are now focusing strongly on this aspect of user-friendliness. Finally, in the next decade or so, MRI of other nuclei such as fluorine and carbon might become a clinical reality, which would allow for metabolic and targeted molecular imaging with excellent sensitivity and specificity.

Introduction

In recent years, cardiac MR imaging (CMR) has emerged as a very powerful tool in the evaluation of a variety of cardiac diseases [1, 2]. CMR is now established as a useful clinical technique in the work-up of patients with heart failure [3, 4], in particular after myocardial infarction (MI), of patients with known or suspected coronary artery disease [5–10], in cardiomyopathies [11, 12], in suspected myocarditis [13, 14], and also in congenital heart disease [15] (◑ Box 21.1). However, CMR is less frequently used in the cardiac care unit

---

Box 21.1 Applications of CMR in the acute cardiac care setting

Myocardial function (without contrast medium)

- Video acquisitions: steady-state free precession (SSFP) pulse sequence

- Tagging acquisitions (apply grid pattern on to tissue)

Tissue characterization

Without contrast medium

- Oedema: T_2-weighted imaging

- Haemorrhage: T_2-weighted imaging—dark core surrounded by bright oedematous tissue

With contrast medium

- Necrosis: late gadolinium enhancement—bright area

- Microvascular obstruction: late gadolinium enhancement—dark core surrounded by bright necrotic tissue

- Ischaemia: perfusion–CMR: low signal (delayed wash-in during first-pass) in viable tissue (with vasodilator stress)

- Scar: late gadolinium enhancement—bright area

(CCU) setting. One major reason for this is most likely the still limited availability of CMR. Nevertheless, for a broad spectrum of acute cardiovascular diseases, CMR can yield crucial or at least complementary information relevant for the management of critically ill patients.

Acute myocardial infarction and acute coronary syndrome

Acute coronary artery occlusions with consequent ST-elevation MI (STEMI) represent a generally accepted indication for acute percutaneous coronary intervention (PCI) in order to reopen the culprit artery. As ischaemic time is a strong predictor of salvaged myocardium, there is no indication for these patients to undergo pre-interventional noninvasive imaging. However, in patients with unspecific ECG changes and little or no troponin elevation, noninvasive imaging may add relevant information for risk assessment and consequently, for further patient work-up and treatment decisions. In such a patient population with at least 30 min of chest pain compatible with MI but an inconclusive ECG, Kwong and coworkers [16] studied the effect of noninvasive CMR examinations on

patient management and outcome. In this setting, where persistent or transient repetitive episodes of myocardial ischaemia occur, the investigators assessed global and regional left ventricular function parameters, viability, and resting perfusion by CMR. This CMR protocol detected an underlying acute coronary syndrome with a sensitivity and specificity of 84% and 85%, respectively. Multivariate logistic regression analysis showed CMR as the strongest predictor of acute coronary syndrome (ACS) and it added diagnostic value over clinical parameters such as ECG or troponin measurements. These results indicate that stunning is a particularly important and sensitive finding in detecting ACS as the cause of chest pain. In this situation, functional imaging is advantageous, as it is able to detect stunning as a consequence of ischaemia before any necrosis, and thus enzyme leak, may occur. Perfusion–CMR during adenosine-induced hyperaemia was also shown to be highly predictive for future cardiac events in patients presenting with acute chest pain in the emergency department [17]. In patients with more than 30 min of chest pain, negative troponins, and a nondiagnostic resting ECG, a CMR examination negative for ischaemia had a 100% sensitivity and 93% specificity in predicting the future diagnosis of coronary artery disease (CAD). CAD was defined as more than 50% diameter stenosis in coronary angiography, abnormal stress test, MI, or death occurring in the first year after the CMR examination. A high sensitivity and specificity of 96% and 83%, respectively, were also reported by Plein *et al.* in patients with non-STEMI ACS for the detection of 70% or more coronary stenoses [18]. Miller and coworkers explored the utility of CMR to detect or exclude ischaemia in patients referred with acute chest pain [19]. In their study patients were either randomized to hospital admission with routine work-up, or to be evaluated in an observation unit by CMR. CMR detected ischaemia in 4% of patients, who were then successfully treated. As a result, 79% of patients could be discharged safely and a cost reduction of approximately 25% was achieved [19]. These data, although sparse, indicate the potential for significant cost reductions, when new CMR-based algorithms are implemented. CMR findings of an acute left anterior descending artery (LAD) occlusion in a patient with a history of LAD stenting are shown in 21.1.

Viability imaging by cardiac magnetic resonance: quantification of necrotic tissue

In acute plaque rupture, thrombogenic material of the plaque core may cause thombosis and acute occlusion of the epicardial coronary vessel. Alternatively, this material may also embolize into the vessel periphery to cause micro-infarctions. Viability imaging by CMR is sensitive enough to detect necrosis affecting less than 1 g of tissue [20]. Accordingly, this CMR technique was able to detect micro-infarctions after PCI in patients. Viability imaging by CMR is performed after injection of conventional MR contrast media, i.e. gadolinium chelates, which are excluded from the intracellular space by intact cell membranes. In case of acute damage of cell membranes, such as during prolonged ischaemia and ischaemia/reperfusion, these contrast media also distribute into the intracellular space, which increases the contrast media content per volume of tissue [21–23]. This increase in contrast concentration is visualized as bright area of myocardium. This approach is called late gadolinium enhancement (LGE). The images are acquired during a short breath-hold whereby the imaging parameters are selected to set the signal of viable intact myocardium to zero. This approach results in a superbe contrast-to-noise ratio between viable and necrotic tissue [21]. This unique feature, together with the excellent spatial resolution of the technique, results in an unbeatable sensitivity and repro-ducibility in detecting and quantifying myocardial necrosis noninvasively [4, 24, 25]. The amount of necrosis as meas-ured by LGE–CMR has been shown to be a strong predictor of future recovery of segmental function in patients after AMI [26, 27]. ➲Figure 21.1 shows an example of a patient with a large AMI, imaged by CMR at day 5, demonstrating akinesia of the anterior wall, necrosis with microvascular obstruction, and oedema with central haemorrhage.

As the LGE technique can quantify necrosis mass with high precision and reproducibility, this technique was recently used in a large multicenter European trial to assess the efficacy of a new fibrin-derived compound to reduce ischaemia–reperfusion induced injury in patients with STEMI [28]. This fibrin derivative reduces leucocyte pen-etration into reperfused ischaemic tissue in animals and the clinical proof-of-concept trial was positive by showing a reduced necrosis mass in the treatment arm [28]. Necrosis quantification by CMR is also increasingly utilized to assess the effect of stem cell strategies in AMI patients [29]. LGE–CMR was also used to compare treatments of AMI by pre-hospital combination fibrinolysis (reteplase and abciximab) versus prehospital combination fibrinolysis with facilitated PCI. Facilitated PCI resulted in a significantly reduced infarct size in this study [30].

Microvascular obstruction

When performing viability imaging by CMR in AMI and subacute MI, another phenomenon in addition to necro-sis formation was observed, the so-called microvascular obstruction (MVO). The LGE technique probes cell mem-brane integrity by measuring contrast medium concentra-tions, i.e. distribution volumes of contrast medium in the steady-state condition that occurs typically 10–15 minutes after injection of contrast medium. In severe myocardial damage, however, equilibrium distribution of contrast medium may not yet be achieved at this time point. This is encountered when the microvasculature of the core region of the infarct is disrupted and/or plugged with blood cells, preventing the contrast medium from reaching the infarct core. Under these circumstances, the core of the infarct region accumulates less contrast medium and it appears as a dark core region, called the MVO zone (➲Fig. 21.1). A large body of evidence demonstrates that the occurrence of such a MVO zone goes along with a particularly bad prognosis [31, 32]. The mechnism(s) responsible for this

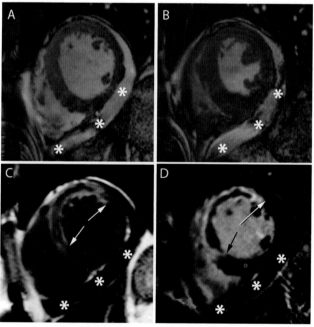

Figure 21.1 In this patient with recanalization of a proximal LAD occlusion by PCI, the CMR study at day 5 demonstrates an akinetic anteroseptal wall in the short-axis video acquisitions (A, end-diastolic phase; B, end-systolic phase). In C, a T_2-weighted acquisition in the same short-axis orientation is shown. The bright area (arrows) delineates myocardial oedema, which corresponds to the area at risk, supplied by the LAD. In the central regions, a dark core is identified, which corresponds to haemorrhage in this patient. In D, the late gadolinium enhancement (LGE) CMR technique demonstrates the necrotic tissue in the anteroseptal wall (same short-axis orientation as in A–C). In this patient, the area at risk (1C) and the necrosis extension are similar indicating that myocardial salvage by PCI in this patient was minimal. In the LGE–CMR aquisition, a dark central core in the necrosis territory is visualized which corresponds to tissue with microvascular obstruction. * identify pericardial effusion.

impaired prognosis of MVO, however, remains unclear. One may speculate that disruption of the microcirculation may negatively affect the healing processes in these infarcts.

Oedema and haemorrhage

Recently an attractive CMR application evolved to assess the myocardium at risk in the setting of reperfusion AMI. T_2-weighted MR pulse sequences are sensitive to water content and thus are able to visualize tissue oedema ($\supset$ Fig. 21.1). Accordingly, T_2-weighted CMR was shown in animal models of AMI to delineate tissue oedema and thus, to allow for accurate quantification of the area at risk [33]. While viability imaging by LGE–CMR yields excellent signal from necrosis, 5–10 times higher than in normal myocardium, T_2-weighted imaging yields signals in oedema that are only about twice as high as in normal myocardium [34]. Therefore, oedema imaging based on T_2-weighted CMR pulse sequences is still challenging and expertise is needed for correct interpretation. Oedematous regions are often located in stunned myocardium. The low contractility in these areas causes stagnant blood to appear as high signal area near the endocardial surface, sometimes making its discrimination from the high-signal edema territory difficult. To circumvent this particular problem, newer 'bright blood' T_2-weighted sequences are increasingly used for this purpose. In 70 patients with STEMI and PCI treatment, this area-at-risk assessment by CMR demonstrated a salvage of up to 90%, when interventions were performed within 90 min of coronary occlusion [35]. In the era of PCI of AMI, intramyocardial haemorrhage can develop as a complication of reperfusion. This intramyocardial haemorrhage can be readily visualized on the T_2-weighted images as dark regions in the high-signal oedema territory ($\supset$ Fig. 21.1). Hemorrhage was visualized in up to 25% of PCI-treated AMI and was shown to predict adverse remodelling 4 months after AMI [36].

Assessment of complications of acute mycardial infarction

A rare complication of AMI, necrosis of the interventricular septum and consequent ventricular septum defect (VSD), can be easily visualized by video imaging using SSFP sequences. Undergoing CMR for this indication might be relevant for patients with an inappropriate acustic window. In addition, CMR offers also a highly accurate technique, the phase contrast pulse sequence, to quantify fluxes in the aorta and pulmonary artery to quantify shunting in this condition. Phase contrast CMR yields velocity information in each pixel covering the cross-sectional area of a vessel.

This approach therefore is not limited by assumptions on the flow profile in the vessel and yields highly reproducible and accurate measurements of flow. This phase contrast or velocity CMR technique can also be used to visualize pseudo-aneurysms that might form in the setting of AMI. Necrosis of the papillary muscles is easily detected by LGE–CMR and, in case of rupture, quantification of mitral regurgitation is also possible by phase contrast CMR [37]. However, it should be mentioned, that echocardiography is certainly the method of choice in the emergency situation of an acute papillary muscle rupture.

Intracavitary thrombus formation, a frequent complication of AMI, is easily detected by LGE–CMR, which visualizes thrombi as dark, nonenhancing masses adherent to necrotic, bright tissue ($\supset$ Fig. 21.2). The sensitivity of LGE–CMR in identifying thrombi is excellent and was shown to be superior to transthoracic echocardiography [38].

Differential diagnoses in acute chest pain and acute coronary syndrome

Myocarditis and perimyocarditis

Chest pain accompanied by ST-segment alterations in the resting ECG and elevated troponins is highly suspicious for an acute coronary syndrome. However, a fraction of these patients do not exhibit relevant coronary stenoses on X-ray coronary angiography. Patients with the characteristics given above should certainly undergo invasive coronary angiography as the first-line examination in order to treat immediately in the case of a coronary artery occlusion. Nevertheless, in cases without significant coronary stenosis and/or occlusions, CMR can add relevant information. One major differential diagnosis in this setting is myocarditis. CMR, particularly its LGE application, is ideal to detect inflammatory foci, visualized as high-signal tissue, typically located in the subepicardial layers of the left ventricular myocardium [11, 13, 14, 39]. Most often, the inferolateral wall is affected, but any other region of the left or right ventricle may be involved ($\textcircled{\tiny\textbf{m}}$ 21.2). The depiction of inflammatory foci may guide endomyocardial biopsy, e.g. in patients with an unstable course of myocarditis [40].

In pericarditis, tamponade can be assessed by CMR, however, echocardiography is clearly the method of choice for these emergency situations. In acute pericarditis or perimyocarditis, CMR yields detailed information on thickened pericardium and after contrast medium administration, enhancing pericardium is indicative of an active form of the disease. For both myocarditis and pericarditis, CMR is an ideal tool to monitor disease activity over time and to assess the effect of treatment [2].

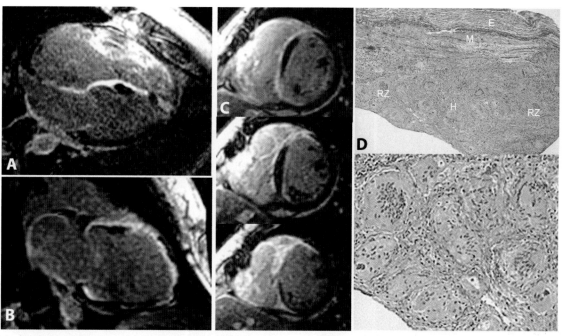

Figure 21.2 In this 43-year old woman with dyspnoea progressing to NYHA class IV, a CMR study demonstrates a massive enhancement by the LGE–CMR technique predominantly involving the right ventricle in the horizontal long axis (A) and short axis (C). Only a small region of the basal right ventricle free wall is not affected. Also large portions of the interventricular septum and anterior wall of the left ventricle are involved (B, vertical long axis). Ejection fractions of the right and left ventricle were 18% and 19%, respectively. The next day the patient developed an atrioventricular block 3. Histology confirmed a giant cell myocarditis. The patient was stabilized with immunosuppressive therapy and remained in NYHA III for 3 years.

Takotsubo cardiomyopathy

With improved access to invasive X-ray coronary angiography, Takotsubo's cardiomyopathy is now more often observed. Although its aetiology and pathophysiology are not yet fully elucidated, the typical findings are major ECG changes going along with severe regional hypo- or akinesia of left ventricular walls, most often involving the left ventricular apex, and nonstenosed coronary arteries. In this situation, CMR can demonstrate preserved viability in the hypo-akinetic regions, which predicts full recovery of function and a good outcome (➲ Fig. 21.3). Thus, this information is useful for patient management and differentiates this disease from others with a mixed prognosis such as myocarditis or AMI [11].

Aortic dissection, aortic ulcer, and intramural haematoma

Aortic dissection, intramural haematoma, and penetrating ulcer are acute aortic disorders that can present similarly with severe chest pain radiating to the back. Moreover, there is also overlap in pathophysiology between these entities which is also reflected by corresponding imaging findings [41].

Dissection is the most common of these disorders, with an incidence of up to 0.8%, and also carries the highest mortality [42]. Aortic dissection is a typical complication

in Marfan's disease and thus regular controls to monitor vessel diameters are recommended to be performed, ideally by MRI as it does not use ionizing radiation and thus allows for repetitive studies (📷 21.3). In case of dissection, an intimal tear of an abnormal vessel wall enables blood to enter the wall with subsequent propagation in the media both proximally and distally, displacing the intima inward. The Stanford classification distinguishes type A, which involves the ascending aorta or aortic arch with or without involvement of the descending aorta, from type B, with involvement of the descending aorta only. Type A dissection is a surgical emergency whereas type B is generally treated conservatively. Major risk factors are systemic hypertension, cystic media necrosis, bicuspid aortic valve, coarctation, pregnancy, trauma, and arteritis. Clinically suspected aortic dissection requires urgent imaging with CT or MRI to confirm or exclude the diagnosis [42]. Both CT and MRI enable imaging of the entire aorta and its major branches with excellent reproducibility. MRI does not required ionizing radiation and can be acquired without contrast material in case of renal failure. ECG-gated steady-state free precession images show blood with high signal intensity and allow clear delineation of the intimal flap with low signal intensity (📷 21.4). Moreover, cardiac function and the aortic valve are readily assessed with MRI. Typical complications such as pericardial tamponade and occlusion of major

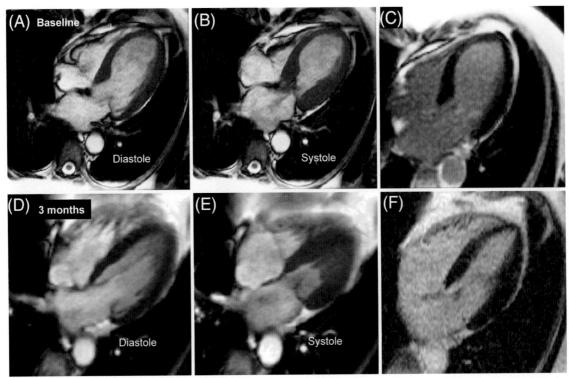

Figure 21.3 Serial LGE–CMR studies in takotsubo cardiomyopathy. Images acquired at baseline (A–C) demonstrate vigorous basal systolic function with apical hypokinesia (A and B) in the absence of LGE (C). A repeat study 3 months later shows complete normalization of ventricular function (D and E), with no LGE detectable (F).
With kind permission of the European Society of Cardiology.

side branches are readily identified. Contrast enhanced MR angiography may be helpful to visualize the whole aorta and to semiquantitatively assess organ perfusion. The convexity of the intimal flap is usually toward the false lumen that surrounds the true lumen. The false lumen usually has a larger diameter and a slower flow. Thus spin-echo images show higher signal intensity from blood in the false lumen than in the true lumen. The false lumen tends to enlarge over time because of intraluminal pressure and wall stress, with risk of aneurysm formation and rupture.

Intramural haematoma is defined as bleeding in the medial layer of the aorta, with no blood flow within the media. The most frequent source of intramural haematoma is in the media itself, representing spontaneous hemorrhage from the vasa vasorum. Other potential causes include trauma or penetrating aortic ulcer bleeding into the aortic wall [42]. Intramural haematoma is considered as an early stage or variant of dissection; systemic hypertension is the leading risk factor. Intramural hemorrhage is classified as Stanford A or B, similarly to aortic dissection. On nonenhanced CT intramural haematoma can be appreciated as thickended aortic wall with high attenuation extending longitudinally. In contrast to dissection, the lumen is rarely compromised. MRI shows the same but can provide additional information, because it may allow determination of

the age of a haematoma based on the signal characteristics of hemoglobin degradation products. On T_1-weighted images haematoma appears with intermediate signal intensity in the acute stage because of the presence of oxyhemoglobin and with high signal intensity in the subacute stage caused by the presence of methemoglobin.

Penetrating aortic ulcers occur when atherosclerotic plaques disrupt the intima with subsequent hemorrhage into the media, as shown in ➲ Fig. 21.4. Thus penetrating ulcer may progress to intramural haematoma, dissection, or rupture of the aorta through the adventitia. A potential complication is embolization of thrombi from within the ulcer. Penetrating aortic ulcers most frequently occur in elderly hypertensive patients and most frequently in the mid descending thoracic aorta [42]. CT and MRI show a localized ulcer penetrating through the aortic intima into the aortic wall and adjacent intramural haematoma. An important disadvantage of MRI as compared to CT is its inability to reveal intimal calcification and its dislodgement which is a frequent finding in aortic ulcer.

Both MRI and CT are robust tools for evaluation of aortic dissection, intramural haematoma, and penetrating ulcer. Advantages of CT are (1) availability, particularly in emergencies, (2) short imaging time, and (3) the sensitivity to calcification. Advantages of MRI are (1) the absence of

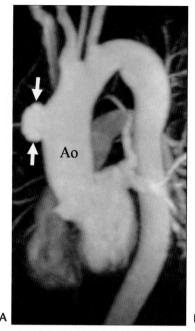

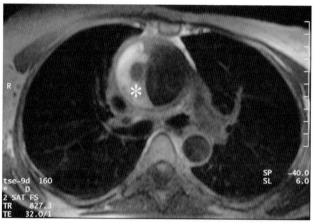

Figure 21.4 Penetrating ulcer with intramural haematoma of the ascending aorta (Ao) on contrast-enhanced 3D MR angiography (A) and axial T_1-weighted turbo spin echo with fat-suppression prepulse (B). Angiography shows outpouching of the lumen (arrows) whereas tomographic MR acquisition also shows intramural haematoma (*).

ionizing radiation and (2) the possibility to image without contrast material when renal function is impaired.

Pulmonary embolism and pulmonary diseases

Pulmonary embolism (PE) is problematic to diagnose in critically ill patients who are commonly immobile and may have decreased ability to communicate. Moreover, diagnostic testing in such patients may be hampered by mechanical ventilation or impaired renal function, precluding intravenous contrast enhanced imaging such as CT [43]. Today, MRI is not established in routine work-up of critically ill patients with suspected PE, but it can be used in suspected PE as shown by Kluge *et al.* [44]. These investigators compared a three-component MR protocol with (1) steady-state-free precession, (2) contrast enhanced perfusion imaging and (3) MR angiography with parallel imaging with multidetector CT as standard of reference. Sensitivities/specificities for the three components were 85%/98%, 77%/100%, and 100%/91%, respectively. Most interestingly, the sensitivity of MR angiography for subsegmental clot was only 55% compared to 93% for perfusion MR. Perfusion MR is sensitive but not specific, whereas angiography is specific but not as sensitive. Thus the combination of angiography with perfusion imaging appears to be attractive for detection of central and peripheral emboli.

The spatial resolution of MR was 1.2 mm × 1.5 mm which is similar to that of multidetector CT. The total average examination time was less than 10 min. This comprehensive assessment of pulmonary angiography and perfusion may be combined with venography of the lower limbs. A stepping table technique with parallel imaging allows for assessment of the entire venous system from the ankles to the inferior vena cava in less than 10 min and without additional contrast material [45]. These data show that MRI may play an important role in imaging of suspected PE in the future.

Limitations and contraindications

Probably the most important limitation of CMR today is the restricted availability of the technique. As cardiologists and radiologists are expected to obtain more experience with the technique, its use and thus its availability will most likely improve in the near future.

From an imaging point of view, small and irregularly moving structures such as valvular vegetations are difficult to detect by CMR and echocardiography is certainly the method of choice in patients with suspected endocarditis. Frequent extrasystoles (more than 20/min or atrial fibrillation) limit the accuracy of volume and function measurements by CMR, whereas viability and inflammation imaging is not compromised by arrhythmias, if the acquisition window is set to occur in mid to late systole.

Absolute contraindications to CMR are electronic devices such as pacemakers, implantable cardioverter–defibrillators (ICDs), insulin pumps, or cochlear implants [2, 46]. The device industry is very active in this field, however, and the first pacemaker approved for MR examinations is now available and it is also approved in Europe for cardiac MR applications. Some older cerebral clips post neurosurgery are contraindictions for CMR, as well as ferromagnetic bodies in the eyes. Shrapnel is another type of foreign ferromagnetic body to consider. Most other surgical metallic implants are CMR-compatible. In particular, valvular heart prostheses are MR compatible (the old ball-type Edwards prosthesis is a rare exception). For each implant, detailed information on MR compatibility can be obtained from specific literature or from the web.

For CMR, conventional contrast media, i.e. gadolinium chelates, are used. These contrast media are very safe, with a minimal risk of allergic reactions. In recent years, another complication of contrast medium administration was observed. Insufficient elimination of contrast medium in patients with severe renal failure can induce systemic nephrogenic fibrosis (SNF) [2]. This complication is so far linked to linear contrast medium only; the next generation of macrocyclic gadolinium chelates appears to be free of this complication, as so far no 'nonconfounded' cases with macrocyclic contrast medium are reported. The incidence of SNF with linear contrast medium is low, ranging from 1 in 1–1.5 million injections.

Personal perspective

Currently, considerable efforts are being undertaken to increase the user friendliness of MR machines. The next generation of CMR machines will be able to run many applications automatically. Functional imaging and localization of long-axis and short-axis acquisitions through the left ventricle will likely be achieved fully automatically. This will make the utilization of CMR much easier, faster, and even more reproducible. The device industry is very active in developing new pacemakers and ICDs with the long-term goal of offering MR compatibility for the entire spectrum of devices.

In experimental models, a fascinating new field of CMR is currently explored. This is based on imaging of nuclei other than protons. Fluorine is amenable for MRI, because of its favorable magnetic properties which are similar to those of protons. However, fluorine offers the advantage of being virtually absent in the human body. Thus, theoretically any fluorine-labelled contrast medium will yield an excellent signal to noise ratio, as no background signal from body tissue can alter the signal behavior of the contrast medium. Fluorine-labeled contrast media are available which are selectively taken up by macrophages. After intravenous injection of these contrast media, active macrophages can be detected with high sensitivity and specificity, even before any macroscopic lesions occur. This approach visualized macrophage activity during infarct healing and also during orthotopic heart transplant rejection [47, 48].

Another nucleus of interest is carbon-13. Compounds containing this isotope can undergo a process of hyperpolarization. This technique yields a contrast medium that produces signals up to 10 000 times higher than in conventional proton imaging. This enormous signal is typically available for 2–3 min and allows for spectroscopic imaging with high spatial and temporal resolution. With this technique, severe metabolic alterations in myocardium were identified in an animal model several hours after an ischaemic episode. This technique could directly demonstrate the cause for chest pain based on the detection of metabolic changes rather than on functional (stunning) or anatomical alterations (coronary artery stenosis/occlusion) [49].

Further reading

Assomull R, Lyne J, Keenan N, *et al*. The role of cardiovascular magnetic resonance in patients presenting with chest pain, raised troponin, and unobstructed coronary arteries. *Eur Heart J* 2007;**28**:1241–1249.

Giang T, Nanz D, Coulden R, *et al*. Detection of coronary artery disease by magnetic resonance myocardial perfusion imaging with various contrast medium doses: first European multicenter experienc. *Eur Heart J* 2004;**25**:1657–1665.

Ingkanisorn W, Kwong R, Bohme N, *et al*. Prognosis of negative adenosine stress magnetic resonance in patients presenting to an emergency department with chest pain. *J Am Coll Cardiol* 2006;**47**:1427–1432.

Kilner P, Geva T, Kaemmerer H, *et al*. Recommendations for cardiovascular magnetic resonance in adults with congenital heart disease. *Eur Heart J* 2010; doi: 10.1093/eurheartj/ehp586.

Kim RJ, Wu E, Rafael A, *et al*. The use of contrast-enhanced magnetic resonance imaging to identify reversible myocardial dysfunction. *N Engl J Med* 2000;**343**:1445–1453.

Mahrholdt H, Wagner A, Deluigi CC, *et al*. Presentation, patterns of myocardial damage, and clinical course of viral myocarditis. *Circulation* 2006;**114**:1581–1590.

Schwitter J. MRI and MRA of the thoracic aorta. *Appl Radiol* 2006;Suppl. May: 6–13.

Schwitter J. Myocardial perfusion imaging by cardiac magnetic resonance. *J Nucl Cardiol* 2006;**13**:841–854.

Schwitter J, Nanz D, Kneifel S, *et al*. Assessment of myocardial perfusion in coronary artery disease by magnetic resonance: a comparison with positron emission tomography and coronary angiography. *Circulation* 2001;**103**:2230–2235.

Schwitter J, Wacker C, van Rossum A, *et al*. MR-IMPACT: comparison of perfusion-cardiac magnetic resonance with single-photon emission computed tomography for the detection of coronary artery disease in a multicentre, multivendor, randomized trial. *Eur Heart J* 2008;**29**:480–489.

Wagner A, Mahrholdt H, Holly TA, *et al*. Contrast-enhanced MRI and routine single photon emission computed tomography (SPECT) perfusion imaging for detection of subendocardial myocardial infarcts: an imaging study. *Lancet* 2003;**361**:374–379.

Wu KC, Zerhouni EA, Judd RM, *et al*. Prognostic significance of microvascular obstruction by magnetic resonance imaging in patients with acute myocardial infarction. *Circulation* 1998;**97**:765–772.

Online resource

Schwitter J, *CMR update*. http://www.herz-mri.ch

Additional online material

- 21.1 CMR findings in a patient with a history of LAD stenting
- 21.2 Detection of inflammatory foci
- 21.3 Marfan's syndrome
- 21.4 Suspected aortic dissection

→ For additional multimedia materials please visit the online version of the book (http://www.esciacc.oxfordmedicine.com).

CHAPTER 22

CT angiography and other applications of CT

Joëlla E. van Velzen, Joanne D. Schuijf, Lucia J. Kroft, and Jeroen J. Bax

Contents

Summary

Patients presenting with acute chest pain constitute a common and important diagnostic challenge. Therefore, there is increased interest in using CT for non-invasive visualization of coronary artery disease in patients presenting with acute chest pain. As a result of rapid developments in coronary CT angiography technology, high diagnostic accuracies for detecting coronary stenosis can be obtained. Additionally, CT is an excellent modality in patients whose symptoms suggest other noncoronary causes of acute chest pain such as aortic aneurysms, aortic dissection, or pulmonary embolism. Furthermore, acquisition of the coronary arteries, thoracic aorta, and pulmonary arteries in a single CT examination is feasible, allowing 'triple rule-out'. Finally, other applications such as the evaluation of plaque composition, myocardial function, and perfusion are currently under investigation and may also become valuable in the setting of acute chest pain. However, although CT shows great potential in evaluating patients with acute chest pain, more randomized clinical trials are needed to determine the value of this technique in this challenging patient population.

Introduction

Since the introduction of CT in the early 1970s the technique has evolved into an essential imaging tool in general medicine. With this technique, noninvasive high resolution cross-sectional imaging of internal structures such as the brain, thorax and abdomen was permitted, thereby gradually replacing the more invasive radiographic techniques [1]. Moreover, CT angiography has evolved as a very accurate tool for the visualization of the aorta and pulmonary arteries. However, high-quality imaging of the coronary arteries remained challenging because of their small vessel size, movement, and tortuous anatomy requiring high temporal, spatial and contrast resolution. In the late 1990s, the first 4-slice spiral CT scanner was developed with sufficient resolution to allow visualization of

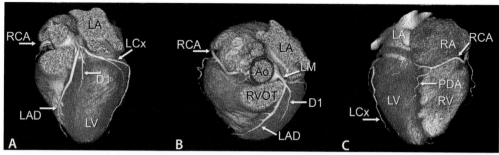

Figure 22.1 Surface-rendered volumetric 3D images of the coronary arteries and side branches, providing a 3D overview of the coronary artery tree and their relative position to the underlying cardiac structures, including the left ventricle (LV) and right ventricle (RV). A. Anterior view of the left circulation demonstrating the left anterior descending coronary artery (LAD) with first diagonal branch (D1). In addition, the left circumflex coronary artery (LCx) can be identified. B. Cranial view demonstrating a volume-rendered image of right coronary artery (RCA) and left main coronary artery (LM) and their main branches originating from the right and left coronary cusp, respectively. C. Posterior view of the RCA and the posterior descending coronary artery (PDA).

the coronary arteries, establishing the potential of multislice CT for detecting significant coronary stenosis in comparison to conventional coronary angiography (CCA) [2–4]. Since then, coronary multislice CT angiography has developed into a promising noninvasive alternative to invasive CCA. With each successive generation of scanners from 4-slice to the present 64-slice and even 320-slice scanners, temporal and spatial resolution improved markedly due to faster gantry rotation times, thinner detectors, and volumetric coverage. These new developments currently allow motion-free visualization of the entire coronary artery tree with high diagnostic accuracy for detecting coronary stenosis (⊃ Fig. 22.1) [5, 6].

Thanks to these rapid developments, interest has been raised in using CT for the evaluation of patients presenting with acute chest pain. In the intensive coronary care unit (ICCU), acute chest pain is the most common clinical presentation of coronary artery disease (CAD). The diagnosis of acute coronary syndrome (ACS) is straightforward in high risk patients with typical chest pain, typical ECG changes, and elevation of serum cardiac markers, whereas it is difficult in patients presenting with atypical chest pain, nondiagnostic or normal ECG, and normal initial markers. Indeed, up to 8% of patients with ACS are misdiagnosed and inappropriately discharged home [7]. Conversely, only a minority of 'low risk' patients (i.e. those with initially normal ECGs and cardiac enzymes) actually suffer from myocardial ischaemia [8]. Therefore, the conventional approach for patients with acute chest pain leads to many unnecessary hospital admissions and is both time-consuming and expensive and thus, resource-intensive. Therefore, a noninvasive and rapid examination to establish or exclude CAD as the underlying cause of symptoms could substantially improve the clinical care of patients admitted to the ICCU, reducing hospital admissions and costs.

This chapter focuses on the evolving role of coronary CT angiography (including coronary calcium scoring) in the diagnosis of patients with acute chest pain. An overview of a wide range of other CT applications is also provided, including triple rule-out, evaluation of plaque composition, myocardial function, and perfusion.

Coronary CT angiography: technique, acquisition, and postprocessing

CT is an imaging modality which has an X-ray source (tube) and detectors on opposite sides of a gantry that continuously rotates around the patient. During the CT scan the patient is moved through the gantry. Subsequently, the X-ray source emits photons collimated into a fan beam which are, after partial absorption and dispersion, reabsorbed by the detectors. Computer systems process these data into three-dimensional (3D) volumetric information, which can be transferred to CT workstations and evaluated using multiple postprocessing techniques. Fast image acquisition is essential for the acquirement of motion-free images and as multiple factors influence CT quality, proper patient preparation and appropriate CT acquisition techniques are critical in guaranteeing diagnostic image quality.

Patient preparation

Proper patient preparation is important for obtaining diagnostic image quality. Therefore, before referring a patient for coronary CT angiography, a short patient history should be taken. Overall, a history of a severe allergic reaction to contrast agents, impaired renal function (glomerular filtration rate <30 mL/min), presence of atrial fibrillation, and pregnancy are considered contraindications. The patient should refrain from food and liquids preferably 3 h before the examination, to prevent nausea as a reaction to the contrast agent. Moreover, a low and stable heart rate in the range of approximately 50–60 beats/min is preferred during image acquisition. To achieve a low and stable heart rate, a β-blocker is frequently administered prior to the examination, unless contraindicated. Lastly, to ensure rapid delivery of the contrast agent bolus for coronary CT angiography, an intravenous catheter should be present for delivery of the contrast agent, preferably in the right antecubital vein (18–20 gauge).

ECG triggering and image acquisition

The range of the current 64-slice scanners is not large enough to cover the entire heart in one rotation and therefore several heart cycles are needed to image the entire heart. To compensate for cardiac motion and synchronize the start of the systole, ECG gating is needed to obtain phase-compatible images. Currently, there are two approaches to scanning the beating heart; with retrospective gating and prospective triggering (🎥 22.1). First, retrospective ECG gating collects data during the whole R–R interval in several heart beats with 64-slice scanners. Afterwards, the optimal phase in which the coronary arteries have the fewest motion artefacts can be selected. As data acquisition is throughout the cardiac cycle, ventricular function can be analysed as well. A newer scanning technique is prospective triggering, in which the start of scanning is triggered by the R-wave and the scanning is performed only during diastole or another pre-specified part of the cardiac cycle. An advantage is that the patient is exposed to less radiation [9]. A disadvantage is that, afterwards, there is limited ability to correct any motion artefacts that occurred due to changes in heart rate or arrhythmias. Prospective triggering with dose modulation can be used for coronary artery imaging (full dose at the mid diastole of the cardiac cycle) in combination with ventricular function analysis (low dose throughout the other parts of the cardiac cycle).

Depending on the scanner type, imaging can be performed in helical ('spiral') mode with continuous table movement and continuous or modulated acquisition, or in step-and-shoot mode with multiple volumetric acquisitions reconstructed into a single data set. A wide-volume detector allows full cardiac acquisition in a single gantry rotation, e.g. a 320-detector-row scanner that allows a maximum of 16 cm scan range in a single rotation [10].

The patient should be placed in a supine position with both arms above the head. The ECG leads are best positioned above and below the level of the scan surface to prevent streak artefacts. Importantly, to make sure that the entire heart is imaged, the CT examination must start from approximately 1–2 cm below the carina to 2 cm below the apex. Note that if other structures (e.g. pulmonary arteries, aorta, bypass grafts) need to be visualized, a larger scan length should be selected.

For coronary calcium scoring, a low-dose ECG triggered non-contrast-enhanced scan is performed before the contrast-enhanced CT examination and reconstructed to 3-mm slices. Additionally, this scan can be used to determine the proper location and scan range for coronary CT imaging. For a regular 64-slice scanner, a rapid infusion of 60–100 mL of contrast material with a flow rate of 5 mL/s is used, followed by a saline flush. Typical scan parameters are a pitch of 0.375, rotation time of 333–500 ms, tube voltage of 120 kV and tube current of 300 mA. When using a bolus-triggered start of the CT scan, the start is automatically initiated if the preset contrast-enhancement threshold level in the descending aorta is reached. Alternatively, a test bolus injection can be used to determine the contrast transit time. Subsequently, data acquisition is performed at half-inspiratory breath hold of approximately 10 s.

Postprocessing and evaluation

After data acquisition, images are reconstructed and sent to a dedicated workstation for postprocessing. If a non-contrast-enhanced data set is acquired, the coronary calcium score can be quantified according to the Agatston method on a vessel and patient basis [11]. Commonly, coronary CT angiography data sets are reconstructed with continuous images using thin increments (typically 0.5–0.6 mm slice thickness). Retrospectively gated axial images can be reconstructed in any phase of the cardiac cycle. However, when prospective triggering was used, images can only be reconstructed in the pre-specified R–R acquisition interval. Most often reconstructions are performed in the relatively motion-free phase of mid diastole (70–80% of the R–R interval) which is generally least affected by motion artefacts.

For postprocessing, various types of algorithms are available. The thin axial slices are considered the source information of CT imaging (➲ Fig. 22.2). Accordingly, the cardiac structures and coronary arteries can easily be evaluated by scrolling through the images in axial direction (🎥 22.2). Additionally, curved multiplanar reconstructions (MPR) allow visualization of the entire coronary artery in a single image which is useful for depicting the entire coronary lumen and evaluating degree of stenosis. Furthermore, maximum intensity projections (MIP) can be reconstructed which represent a series of contiguous CT slices stacked into

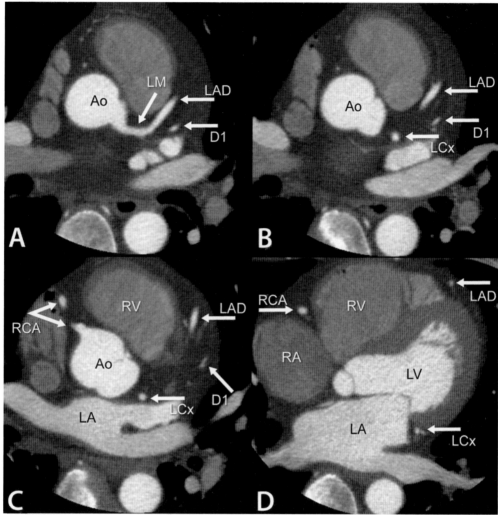

Figure 22.2 Typical example of axial contrast-enhanced images (0.5-mm slice thickness), which can be used to evaluate cardiac structures (such as the left ventricle (LV), left atrium (LA), right ventricle (RV), and aorta (Ao)) and coronary arteries by scrolling through the slices in the cranio-caudal direction. Four images have been selected to demonstrate the anatomy of the heart. A. Axial image showing the left main (LM) coronary artery at the level of the ostium which arises from the left coronary cusp and bifurcates first into the left anterior descending coronary artery (LAD). B. Slightly more distal axial image showing the left circumflex coronary artery (LCx) and the first diagonal branch (D1) which has originated from the LAD. C. Axial image demonstrating the origin of the right coronary artery (RCA) from the right coronary cusp and the mid segments of the LCx, LAD, and D1. (D) Axial image at midventricular level which shows the mid segment of the right coronary artery (RCA) and distal segments of the LAD and LCx (the latter is seen in the left atrioventricular groove).

a single image ('slab'). Moreover, MIPs are very suitable for assessment of longer length of vessel segments and may facilitate in evaluating the degree of stenosis. Lastly, 3D volume rendering provides a 3D image of the heart and vessels (📷 22.3). An excellent overview of the coronary anatomy is provided, although 3D volume rendering is generally not used for assessing the degree of stenosis.

A systematic approach is important when evaluating a coronary CT angiogram. If coronary calcium scoring has been performed, the Agatston score is reported on a patient and vessel basis (see ➲ Coronary calcium score). With regard to the coronary CT angiogram, the quality of the scan should be mentioned as this influences the diagnostic certainty of the study. Findings are commonly reported similar to the traditional CCA report. Typically, the coronary segments are described as normal, mild (<30% wall irregularities), nonsignificant (30–50% stenosis), significant (>50% stenosis), severe stenosis (>70%), and occlusion. Presence and patency of stents and bypasses are reported, if evaluable. Segments effected by severe calcifications, motion, and breathing artefacts should also be mentioned in the report.

Coronary calcium score

It has been widely verified that presence of coronary calcifications only occurs in the presence of coronary atherosclerosis [12]. Both electron beam CT (EBCT) and multislice CT have been used over the past years for the noninvasive evaluation of coronary calcifications, each demonstrating high sensitivities for the detection of CAD. An example of coronary calcium scoring is provided in 22.4 [13, 14]. For quantification of the coronary calcifications, the Agatston method (a method that multiplies the calcified area by a density factor based on the highest Hounsfield values within this area) has traditionally been used [11]. Total coronary calcium scores are generally divided into normal (zero calcium), mild (1–100), moderate (100–400), and severe (>400) [15]. Although newer quantification methods have been introduced (calcified volume (mm^3) and mass (mg) measurements), no clinical studies have provided data using these methods.

Coronary calcium score in the general population

Several population based studies have demonstrated that the calcium score increases with higher age, thereby reflecting the natural progression of atherosclerosis. In addition, men tend to have higher coronary calcium scores than women of similar age. Therefore, the coronary calcium score should be ranked in percentiles according to the distribution within age and sex [13, 16]. Moreover, the relation between the presence of obstructive CAD and presence and extent of coronary calcium has been extensively studied [17]. The coronary calcium score has a high sensitivity and negative predictive value for the presence of obstructive disease, but its specificity is rather poor [17, 18]. Indeed, extensive calcifications can be present even in the absence of significant luminal narrowing. Therefore, the technique may be more suited to provide an estimate of total plaque burden rather than stenosis severity. Interestingly, numerous investigations have shown that the extent of coronary calcium burden translates into prognostic information. Coronary calcium scoring has therefore been proposed as a tool for stratifying cardiac risk. In fact, several large trials have reported that elevated coronary calcium scores have predictive value for cardiovascular events, both independently and incrementally to cardiovascular risk factors [19, 20].

Coronary calcium score in acute coronary syndrome

In the specific clinical setting of acute chest pain, a few initial investigations with EBCT have been conducted to assess the value of coronary calcium scoring; however, the number of patients in these studies was relatively limited [21–23].

Georgiou et al. performed a prospective observational study of 192 patients with acute chest pain and demonstrated that the presence of coronary calcium was a strong predictor of future cardiac events [21]. In addition, these authors elegantly demonstrated that the absence of coronary calcifications had a very low risk for future cardiac events (<1%). Moreover, McLaughlin et al. performed coronary calcium scoring in 134 patients with suspected ACS and a normal or nondiagnostic ECG. The authors found that the absence of calcium had a high negative predictive value (98%) for ruling out the presence of ACS [23].

Nevertheless, when comparing coronary calcium scores of patients with stable angina to patients with acute myocardial infarction (AMI), significant differences have been observed [24]. Extensive calcium was more often present in the coronary arteries of patients with chronic stable angina, whereas patients with AMI demonstrated only mildly calcified or noncalcified culprit arteries. Similar results were shown in a study by Henneman et al. who showed that in 40 patients suspected of ACS, coronary calcium was absent in 13 patients (33%) [25]. Importantly, in 5 (39%) of the 13 patients without coronary calcium, significant CAD was identified on CCA (example shown in ᐅ Fig. 22.3). Thus, particularly in the acute setting, the absence of coronary calcification may not invariably imply the absence of atherosclerotic plaque. Moreover, the presence of coronary calcification does not by definition explain the actual cause of chest pain. Evidently, there is a need for more research to define the role of coronary calcium scoring in patients with acute chest pain. The current guidelines therefore do not recommend coronary calcium scoring as a screening method for patients suspected of ACS [26].

CT angiography in the evaluation of coronary artery disease

General population

With the current generation 64-slice scanners with improved temporal and spatial resolution a good diagnostic accuracy for detection of obstructive CAD both in proximal coronary vessels and smaller distal vessels has been observed. Indeed, a high sensitivity (85–99%) and specificity (83–90%) of 64-slice CT angiography for the detection of obstructive lesions as compared to CCA has been demonstrated [5, 6, 27]. More importantly, due to the high negative predictive value, coronary CT angiography has an excellent ability to exclude significant CAD (᎒ 22.5). Accordingly, if patients show normal coronary arteries on coronary CT angiography

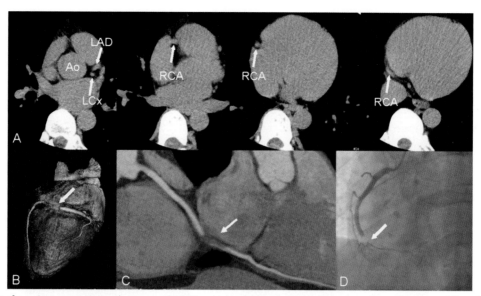

Figure 22.3 Example of a patient presenting with suspected ACS in which calcium scoring and contrast-enhanced coronary CT angiography was performed to exclude CAD. Although no calcium was demonstrated by the calcium score (A), an obstructive noncalcified plaque with a superimposed thrombus in the right coronary artery (RCA) was detected on coronary CT angiography (B, C). The volume-rendered 3D reconstruction (B) and curved multiplanar reconstruction (C) show an occlusion in the mid segment of the RCA (white arrows). (D) This finding was confirmed on invasive conventional coronary angiography (white arrow). Ao, aorta; LAD, left anterior descending coronary artery; LCx, left circumflex coronary artery. Reproduced from Henneman MM, Schuijf JD, Pundziute G, *et al.* Noninvasive evaluation with multislice computed tomography in suspected acute coronary syndrome: plaque morphology on multislice computed tomography versus coronary calcium score. *J Am Coll Cardiol* 2008;**52**(3):216–222, with permission from Elsevier.

no further testing is required and patients can be reassured. However, a significant limitation of CT angiography remains the relatively low positive predictive value (64–93%). As a result, atherosclerotic lesions are still frequently being over-estimated on CT which occasionally may lead to unnecessary referral for invasive CCA. Moreover, it should be noted that the diagnostic performance of CT coronary angiography is influenced by the pretest likelihood of significant CAD (➲ Table 22.1). Indeed, a recent study showed that the benefit from this noninvasive modality is highest in patients with a low to intermediate pretest likelihood for CAD because of its excellent ability to rule out obstructive CAD [28]. Similar results were recently published by Henneman *et al.* demonstrating that coronary CT was able to rule out coronary atherosclerosis in 58% of patients with low pretest likelihood [29]. However, in patients with a high pretest likelihood, CT was often abnormal and CAD

was ruled out in only 17% of patients. Consequently, the remaining 83% of patients with a high pretest likelihood and abnormalities on coronary CT angiography still required further functional and/or invasive testing. Therefore, to avoid layered testing and delayed diagnosis, these patients should be directly referred for either functional testing or invasive CCA. Accordingly, current guidelines state that if the pretest likelihood of CAD is high, invasive CCA remains the test of first choice and the additional value of noninvasive coronary angiography may be limited.

Suspected acute coronary syndrome

A major advantage of coronary CT angiography is that it is a noninvasive, fast, and accurate modality for ruling out the presence of CAD and severe stenosis, features that are particularly useful in the emergency department. Several investigations have assessed the value of coronary CT

Table 22.1 Diagnostic accuracy of 64-slice CT angiography for detection for significant stenosis (≥50%) according to pretest probability. As can be derived from the table, patients with a low to intermediate likelihood benefit the most from noninvasive coronary CT angiography as the sensitivity and specificity (and negative predictive value to rule out CAD) is higher in these patients

Pretest probability	N	Sensitivity (%)	Specificity (%)	PPV (%)	NPV (%)
Low	66	100	93	78	100
Intermediate	83	100	84	80	100
High	105	98	74	93	89

NPV, negative predictive value; PPV, positive predictive value.

Data adapted from Meijboom WB, van Mieghem CA, Mollet NR, *et al.* 64-slice computed tomography coronary angiography in patients with high, intermediate, or low pretest probability of significant coronary artery disease. *J Am Coll Cardiol* 2007;**50**(15):1469–1475.

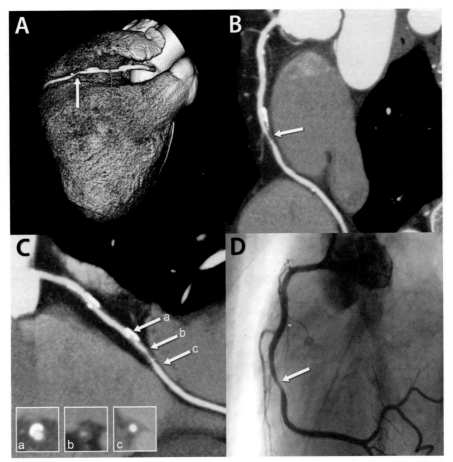

Figure 22.4 Example of noninvasive coronary angiography with CT in a patient presenting with suspected ACS. In (A), a 3D volume-rendered reconstruction is provided, showing a large dominant right coronary artery (RCA) with signs of luminal narrowing (white arrow). B. A curved multiplanar reconstruction (MPR) of the RCA is shown demonstrating the presence of significant luminal narrowing in the mid segment (arrow). C. Another curved MPR in a different view, revealing the presence of significant stenosis (arrows). Cross-sectional CT images (inlays) show the presence of calcified plaque proximal to the stenosis (a), exclusively noncalcified plaque within the stenosis (b), and no coronary plaque distal from the stenosis (c). D. Conventional coronary angiography confirming the presence of significant luminal narrowing of the RCA (arrow).

angiography in patients presenting with ACS (an example is shown in ➲ Fig. 22.4). Preliminary studies investigating the efficacy of CT in the diagnosis of ACS were performed with 4- and 16-slice systems [30, 31]. Ghersin *et al.* studied 62 patients hospitalized with suspected ACS and found a moderate sensitivity (80%) and specificity (89%) for the detection of significant CAD (defined as ≥ 50% luminal narrowing) [30]. Subsequent studies have been performed using 64-slice systems (➲ Table 22.2), with higher spatial and temporal resolution, evaluating coronary plaque and stenosis in patients presenting with ACS [32–36]. For instance, Rubinshtein and colleagues evaluated the efficacy of coronary CT angiography for initial triage in 58 patients with suspected ACS and assessed clinical outcomes during a follow-up of 15 months [36]. During the follow-up period, no deaths or myocardial infarctions occurred in

Table 22.2 Studies assessing the diagnostic accuracy of dedicated coronary 64-slice CT angiography in patients presenting with acute chest pain in the emergency department

	N	Pretest probability	ACS (%)	Sensitivity (%)	Specificity (%)	PPV (%)	NPV (%)
Hoffman *et al.* [33]	103	Low	14	100	82	47	100
Gallagher *et al.* [39]	85	Low	8	86	92	50	99
Rubinshtein *et al.* [36]	58	Intermediate	34	100	92	87	100
Goldstein *et al.* [32]	99	Low	8	100	74	25	100
Hoffman *et al.* [34]	368	Low	8	100	84	35	100

ACS, acute coronary syndrome; NPV, negative predictive value; PPV, positive predictive value.

the 35 patients discharged from the emergency department after initial triage and with normal CT findings. Most recently, the ROMICAT (Rule Out Myocardial Infarction using Computed Assisted Tomography) trial evaluated 368 patients suspected of ACS and demonstrated that 50% of patients with acute chest pain with a low to intermediate likelihood of ACS were free of CAD by coronary CT angiography and had no ACS. The authors concluded that given the large number of such patients, initial evaluation with coronary CT angiography may significantly improve patient management in the emergency department. These results are in line with most studies signifying that coronary CT angiography is useful and safe in ruling out CAD and facilitates early and accurate release of patients with acute chest pain [32–36]. Additionally, CT evaluation reduced diagnostic time, lowered costs, and required fewer repeat investigations when compared to standard of care [32]. Of note, the majority of patients included in the above-mentioned studies were classified as having a low to intermediate risk for ACS (normal or nondiagnostic ECG and normal first cardiac enzymes). In addition, the presence of a significant stenosis on coronary CT does not by definition confirm the presence of ACS. Importantly, there is no additional role for coronary CT angiography in patients with evident myocardial infarction (MI). Naturally, high risk patients should immediately be referred for invasive CCA and coronary CT angiography would only cause significant delay. At present there are no formal guidelines for the use of CT in patients with acute chest pain, although appropriateness criteria and consensus documents have recently been published [37, 38]. Currently, more large randomized clinical trials should be performed to determine the accuracy and benefits of coronary CT angiography for triage of patients with acute chest pain. However, in the future, initial evaluation with coronary CT angiography may play an important role, especially in a population with low to intermediate risk for ACS in whom the incremental value of noninvasive imaging may have a significant impact on patient management.

CT angiography of aorta and pulmonary arteries

Noncardiac causes of acute chest pain concerning vascular structures in the thorax such as aortic aneurysms, dissection, pulmonary emboli, and pathology of the chest wall can be easily visualized by CT angiography. CT angiography of other vascular beds than the heart is less complex if non-ECG gating techniques are used. ECG gating may be used to improve image quality. In addition, contrast enhancement in the blood pool is required to visualize the vascular structures, so intravenous contrast is still needed. Several common principles should be applied to all imaging protocols to provide optimal diagnostic image quality such as bolus timing for optimization of contrast delivery in the vessel, fast high resolution acquisition, and administration of approximately 60–120 mL of contrast material (dependent on patient size, contrast agent used, and scanner type) injected at rapid infusion rates (4–5 mL/s).

Thoracic aortic aneurysm

In general, an ascending aortic diameter equal to or greater than 4 cm (in an individual less than 60 years old) is considered an aneurysm (🖮 22.6). Atherosclerosis is, as expected, the most frequent cause of thoracic aneurysms (70%). Two different types of thoracic aortic aneurysms can be identified according to their pathological features. First, a true aneurysm, in which all three layers of the vessel wall are involved (intima, media, and adventitia) and which is characterized by a fusiform shape (🖮 22.6). Secondly, a false aneurysm (or pseudo-aneurysm), in which the intima is disrupted and the blood is contained by the adventitia. CT angiography is the most robust tool for evaluating aortic aneurysms and some key features should be evaluated when using CT such as maximal aortic diameter, presence of thrombus, shape and extent of the aneurysm, involvement of aortic branches, relationship to adjacent structures, and presence of aortic calcifications. In 23% of cases a thoracic aneurysm coexists with an abdominal aortic aneurysm, so evaluation of the whole aorta should be performed. Most importantly, CT shows excellent accuracy for characterizing important features of aneurysms [40].

Aortic dissection

Aortic dissection is the most common disorder of the acute aortic syndromes and also has the highest mortality rate. Aortic dissection occurs when a tear in the media layer allows blood to enter within and along the vessel wall and results in separation of the layers of the aorta. In most patients, an intima disruption is present that leads to the development of a true and false lumen, separated by a 'flap'. There are currently two classification systems: the De Bakey classification and the Stanford classification. The De Bakey type I dissection involves both the ascending and descending thoracic aorta, De Bakey type II involves only the ascending aorta, and De Bakey type III involves only the descending aorta. The Stanford system is more clinically useful. In Stanford type A the dissection is located in the ascending aorta and aortic

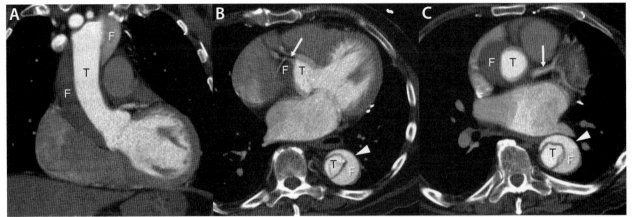

Figure 22.5 Thoracic CT angiography showing a type A aortic dissection (A). The right coronary artery is contrast enhanced and has its origin from the true lumen (arrow, B). The right coronary artery has double appearance due to motion artefacts in this non-ECG gated scan. The left main coronary artery stem (arrow, C) is also contrast enhanced and had its origin from the true lumen. Carotid and subclavian arteries as well as the visceral arteries all had their origin from the true lumen. Note the almost complete disruption between the true and false lumen of the descending aorta (arrowheads B, C). F, false lumen; T, true lumen.

arch, either with or without involvement of the descending aorta, while Stanford type B dissections are limited to the descending aorta alone. Type A acute aortic dissection has the worst prognosis and generally should be immediately surgically repaired to avoid fatal complications.

When aortic dissection is suspected, urgent high resolution imaging is required to confirm the diagnosis. For this purpose; CT angiography, MRI and transoesophageal echocardiography (TOE) have been shown to be equally accurate for confirming or excluding the diagnosis of thoracic aortic dissection [41]. Currently, CT angiography is the most commonly used technology for the assessment of patients suspected of aortic dissection (⟴ Fig. 22.5). It has an excellent sensitivity and specificity of almost 100% for the detection of aortic dissection [42, 43]. CT scanning protocols for patients suspected of thoracic aortic dissection should include unenhanced (for depicting intramural haematoma) and contrast-enhanced image acquisition with visualization of the entire aorta. The key features of dissection on contrast-enhanced images are a 'flap' separating two lumens (usually the convexity of the intimal flap is towards the false lumen), contrast arriving in the true lumen first followed by the false lumen, slower flow in the false lumen, and presence of pleural and/or pericardial effusion. CT should also be used to accurately locate the position of the intimal tear site, as this is important for the surgical approach.

Pulmonary embolism

The well-known Wells' clinical decision rule is used to risk stratify patients suspected of pulmonary embolism [44].

This is a scoring method based on various clinical risk factors and stratifies patients as low, intermediate, or high risk. If a patient has a score of 4 or more, further testing is required. CT pulmonary angiography has been demonstrated to provide high diagnostic accuracy for the detection of pulmonary embolism, and patients with a high-quality negative CT examination do not require further examination [45, 46]. On CT, pulmonary emboli are shown as filling defects in the contrast-enhanced central or (sub)segmental pulmonary arteries (⟴ Fig. 22.6). Currently, contrast-enhanced CT pulmonary angiography is the imaging method of choice for the detection of pulmonary emboli and thus replacing ventilation–perfusion imaging.

Triple rule-out CT

The concept of the 'triple rule-out' protocol is to simultaneously exclude all three potentially life-threatening causes of acute chest pain—ACS or MI, acute aortic dissection, and pulmonary embolism—in one single CT examination. A triple rule-out scan protocol includes coverage of the entire thorax cavity including the aortic arch. State-of-the-art 64-slice scanners with wide anatomical coverage are able to scan the entire thorax including the pulmonary arteries, thoracic aorta, and coronary arteries in a single breath hold of approximately 15–20 s. However, an important technical challenge of a triple rule-out scan protocol is to ensure that high contrast enhancement is present simultaneously in both the right and left circulation to evaluate the pulmonary and aorta including the coronary arteries. Recent data reporting the implementation of

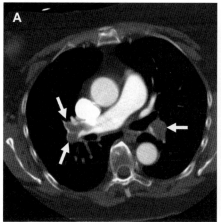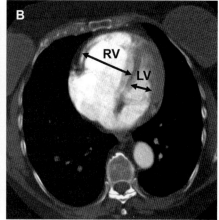

Figure 22.6 Patient with acute pulmonary embolism and high embolus load. Massive emboli in the left and right pulmonary arteries can be observed (arrows, A). Note severe dilatation of the right ventricle (RV, B) with interventricular septum shift to the left and compression of the left ventricle (LV) due to high embolus load. Normally the RV diameter does not exceed that of the LV.

a triphasic contrast injection protocol (first bolus of 100 mL at 5 mL/s, followed by a second bolus of 30 mL contrast at 3 mL/s, followed by a saline flush) showed promising results with satisfactory contrast enhancement of coronary, aortic, and pulmonary vasculature in a single breath hold [47]. Potentially, this new approach may improve the triage of patients presenting to the emergency department with acute chest pain, and provide a faster algorithm to make a diagnosis. However, it is crucial that patients should be carefully selected to ensure the appropriate use of a triple rule-out CT protocol. However, as the triple rule-out protocol may involve retrospective gating of the entire thorax, radiation dose is high, even more than the radiation dose observed in dedicated coronary CT angiography [48, 49]. Prospective gating techniques may reduce radiation dose, but cannot be applied effectively in patients with high heart rates. Therefore, patients with symptoms highly suggestive for either ACS, acute pulmonary embolism, or acute aortic dissection, should be referred for a work-up specifically designed for this purpose (such as invasive CCA if a patient has a high risk for ACS). Notably, presence of a significant stenosis on CT angiography does not automatically confirm the presence of ACS. In the remaining patients with uncertain cause of chest pain, a triple rule-out protocol can be considered. Initial studies suggest that a triple rule-out CT angiography protocol for evaluation of patients with acute chest pain is feasible and that quantitative parameters of image quality may be comparable to the conventional, dedicated coronary and pulmonary CT angiography protocols [50, 51]. A study evaluating the diagnostic value of triple rule-out with 64-slice CT in 55 patients admitted to the

emergency department demonstrated that this technique facilitated the differential diagnosis of chest pain [50]. Furthermore, the triple rule-out protocol could potentially identify a subset of patients with acute chest pain who can safely be discharged from the emergency department without adverse events during a 30-day follow-up [52]. Indeed, more randomized control trials are needed to determine whether this protocol is safe, cost-effective, and improves clinical decision making before routine use of such a technique can be justified.

Other applications of CT

Evaluation of plaque composition

An important advantage of coronary CT angiography is that not only luminal narrowing can be visualized but also atherosclerotic plaque composition. Three different plaques types can be distinguished by coronary CT; non-calcified plaque, mixed plaque, and calcified plaque. More interestingly, plaque composition on coronary CT angiography has been linked to clinical presentation. Indeed, noncalcified and mixed plaques have been shown to be more prevalent in patients with ACS whereas extensively calcified plaques have been associated with stable CAD [53]. In addition, it has been suggested that certain plaque features have prognostic value. In prospective studies, noncalcified plaques with low attenuation values, positive remodelling, and spotty calcifications have been associated with subsequent development of ACS (🎥 22.7) [54, 55].

Although further characterization of noncalcified plaque remains challenging, more improvements are expected, possibly allowing for improved identification of patients at risk [56].

Evaluation of myocardial function

Another particular advantage of CT angiography is that it allows assessment of cardiac function. If data have been collected during the whole cardiac cycle, images can be retrospectively reconstructed in several phases to derive left ventricular ejection fraction from left ventricular volumes. Indeed, numerous studies have shown that global left ventricular function by CT correlates well with echocardiography and MRI, although a slight tendency of CT to overestimate end-systolic volumes and thus slightly underestimate left ventricular ejection fraction has been reported [57, 58]. In addition, regional wall motion abnormalities can be reliably evaluated as compared to MRI [59]. However, as images should be acquired throughout the cardiac cycle, left ventricular function protocols are associated with increased radiation exposure. Accordingly the necessity of function measurements with CT should be carefully determined in each patient.

Evaluation of myocardial infarction

Over recent years, MRI has been successfully employed to image the presence of infarcted myocardium with delayed enhancement imaging. However, several studies have demonstrated that the presence of MI can be also identified on CT [60]. Because of the pharmokinetics of the contrast material, a difference between the accumulation of contrast in infarcted and normal myocardium can be visualized. Accordingly, early hypoenhancement can be observed on the CT images during the first pass of contrast medium at the area of infarcted myocardium. In addition, delayed hyperenhancement of infarcted tissue can be detected similarly to MRI. Interestingly, a good correlation between infarct imaging with CT and other imaging modalities such as MRI and nuclear imaging has been demonstrated [60–62]. Moreover, a good correlation between enhancement patterns (both early hypoenhancement and late hyperenhancement) and recovery of myocardial function at a follow-up of 3 months was found, suggesting that CT may be useful to predict myocardial functional recovery after infarction [63]. However, it is important to realize that in general, delayed enhancement imaging with CT requires additional imaging and thus involves additional radiation exposure. Also, a larger amount of contrast agent is required for delayed enhancement imaging as compared to imaging the coronary arteries alone.

Evaluation of myocardial perfusion

A major limitation of coronary CT angiography is that the haemodynamic significance of atherosclerotic lesions cannot be assessed. Indeed, functional information is of particular importance in regard to lesions with borderline luminal narrowing. Interestingly, thanks to recent developments in scanner technology, it has become possible to image myocardial perfusion and to determine the presence of ischaemia through perfusion imaging during stress [64]. The technique is based on myocardial tissue attenuation changes during the infusion of contrast medium. Consequently, CT perfusion imaging can detect the presence of myocardial perfusion defects during stress that resolve during rest, indicating the presence of ischaemia. Recent studies have been published demonstrating the feasibility of stress–rest myocardial perfusion imaging with CT in humans [65–67]. Importantly, the combination of both anatomical and functional data may improve the diagnostic accuracy of CT and optimize patient management. However, before CT perfusion imaging can be implemented in daily clinical practice, its accuracy should be confirmed in additional, larger prospective studies.

Extracardiac findings

Beyond evaluating the coronary arteries, other cardiac findings and/or extracardiac findings may be identified during coronary CT angiography. Interestingly, extracardiac findings provide an explanation for chest pain complaints in 4–8% of patients[68, 69] (🎥 22.8) or may be incidental findings not related to chest complaints. Several studies have shown that extracardiac findings are present in a large proportion of patients (~ 50%) [68, 70–72]. However, many of these findings are not significant and do not require follow-up or treatment, such as an incidental small calcified pulmonary nodule or calcified lymph nodes. However, 2–5% of patients do have significant findings requiring immediate further diagnostic action, such as a suspected malignancy which may necessitate immediate therapeutic actions, or the presence of acute pulmonary embolism or pneumonia [68, 73–75]. Other findings, e.g. pulmonary nodules with low suspicion for malignancy, may require nonurgent further investigation or follow-up [76]. It is estimated that the patient population requiring further follow-up includes approximately 15% of patients undergoing coronary CT angiography [68, 73, 77–80].

For coronary artery assessment, a zoomed-in small field of view focused on the heart is reconstructed to obtain maximal spatial resolution for evaluation. However, this focused view reveals only 36% of the total chest volume, whereas 70% of the total chest volume has been exposed to radiation [75]. Substantially more significant extracardiac pathology is found on maximum full-field reconstructions than on small-field reconstructions [73]. Therefore the maximum full-field reconstructions should be reviewed for optimal identification of extracardiac pathology [68, 73, 78, 85].

Limitations and future developments

Limitations

Coronary CT angiography has several major limiting factors that affect its usefulness in patients admitted to the emergency department and the ICCU. The technique is particularly limited in patients with an irregular heart rhythm, elevated heart rate, and a high body mass index. Indeed, the heart rate and regularity of the rhythm is closely related to image quality and accuracy of coronary stenosis assessment. Therefore, it is essential to provide adequate premedication with β-blockers (orally or intravenously) to reduce the heart rate below 65 beats/min for optimal image quality. Moreover, coronary CT angiography has particularly been criticized to be an important source of ionizing radiation in the population. The effective radiation dose with retrospective 64-slice CT coronary angiography is estimated to range approximately from 7 to 23 mSv [81]. However, with the use of ECG dose modulation, a method that reduces tube current during systole, a radiation dose reduction of 30–50% can be achieved [49]. Moreover, prospective ECG-triggered CT angiography has been shown to reduce radiation dose by 80%, often resulting in effective radiation doses of less than 3 mSv [82]. Notably, the triple rule-out CT angiography protocol is associated with an even higher radiation dose than with dedicated coronary CT and mean radiation doses of 18 mSv have been reported. However, when implementing ECG dose modulation, the mean radiation dose can be reduced to less than 10 mSv [52]. In addition, contrast administration is associated with nephrotoxicity and adverse reactions. Therefore it is essential to verify that renal function is not impaired before referring patients for contrast-enhanced CT angiography studies.

Future developments

CT technology is evolving quickly. Most recently, 256- and 320-detector-row scanners have been introduced, which have higher volume coverage and improved temporal and spatial resolution [10, 83]. Complete volume coverage of the heart in a single heartbeat is possible, thereby reducing the motion artefacts in patients with irregular heart rates. Furthermore, additional radiation dose reduction has been achieved with the implementation of prospective ECG triggering by scanning only during a small predefined phase of the R–R interval. Moreover, dual-source CT systems with 2×128 detector rows have been introduced demonstrating a high temporal resolution of 75 ms (approximately half of the temporal resolution of the fastest 64-slice CT) making it possible to freeze cardiac motion and obtain diagnostic quality images of the coronary arteries regardless of heart rate. Initial studies with dual-source coronary CT in patients presenting with chest pain have reported high negative predictive values of almost 100% for detecting coronary artery stenoses, even in patients with higher heart rates [84]. Most recently, high-pitch ECG triggered ('Flash Spiral') dual-source CT scanners have shown promising results. The novelty of this technique lies in the very high pitch which results in fast image acquisition without cardiac motion artefacts and a very low radiation exposure (mean estimated effective radiation dose of 1.0 ±0.3 mSv) [85]. Nevertheless, as these techniques are relatively new, only limited data are currently available. Prospective studies are needed to validate these novel applications of CT for use in standard clinical practice.

Conclusion

Coronary CT angiography is a feasible technique for non-invasive, fast, and accurate diagnosis of significant CAD in patients presenting with acute chest pain. In particular, a normal CT angiogram has been shown to allow safe discharge with good short-term prognosis. In addition, CT can evaluate other noncoronary causes of acute chest pain such as aortic aneurysms, aortic dissection, or pulmonary embolism. However, although CT shows great potential in evaluating patients with acute chest pain, more randomized clinical trials are needed to confirm its value in this challenging patient population.

Personal perspective

Preliminary data suggest that coronary CT angiography has the potential to evaluate patients with acute chest pain and possibly improve diagnosis and management strategies. Improvements in technology (faster gantry rotation times, thinner detectors, volumetric coverage) and consequential improvement in image quality have resulted in a high diagnostic accuracy for detecting obstructive CAD in stable patients with low to intermediate likelihood. However, despite the excellent negative predictive value for ruling out CAD, there is still a considerable number of false-positive studies. Moreover, another drawback is that at present the haemodynamic significance of a lesion cannot be evaluated. Nevertheless, there are some features distinctive for coronary CT angiography which renders this technique very suitable for use in the diagnostic work-up of patients presenting with acute chest pain. The technique is noninvasive, relatively fast and simple to use, and generally widely available. Furthermore, contrast-enhanced CT angiography is the imaging modality of choice regarding the detection of noncoronary causes of acute chest pain such as aortic aneurysms, aortic dissection, or pulmonary embolism. Notably, radiation exposure is a major concern which needs to be carefully considered when referring patients for coronary CT angiography. However, newer CT systems are available with dose saving innovations such a prospective triggering and dose modulation, allowing substantial radiation dose reduction. Overall, large randomized controlled trials are needed to assess the safety, efficacy, and cost-effectiveness of the use of coronary CT angiography in patients with acute chest pain, before an evidence based recommendation can be made.

Further reading

Bertrand ME, Simoons ML, Fox KA, *et al*. Management of acute coronary syndromes in patients presenting without persistent ST-segment elevation. *Eur Heart J* 2002;**23**(23):1809–1840.

Budoff MJ, Dowe D, Jollis JG, *et al*. Diagnostic performance of 64-multidetector row coronary computed tomographic angiography for evaluation of coronary artery stenosis in individuals without known coronary artery disease: results from the prospective multicenter ACCURACY (Assessment by Coronary Computed Tomographic Angiography of Individuals Undergoing Invasive Coronary Angiography) trial. *J Am Coll Cardiol* 2008;**52**(21):1724–1732.

Greenland P. ACCF/AHA 2007 clinical expert consensus document on coronary artery calcium scoring by computed tomography in global cardiovascular risk assessment and in evaluation of patients with chest pain: a report of the American College of Cardiology Foundation Clinical Expert Consensus Task Force (ACCF/AHA Writing Committee to Update the 2000 Expert Consensus Document on Electron Beam Computed Tomography) developed in collaboration with the Society of Atherosclerosis Imaging and Prevention and the Society of Cardiovascular Computed Tomography. *J Am Coll Cardiol* 2007;**49**(3):378–402.

Hausleiter J, Meyer T, Hadamitzky M, *et al*. Radiation dose estimates from cardiac multislice computed tomography in daily practice: impact of different scanning protocols on effective dose estimates. *Circulation* 2006;**113**(10):1305–1310.

Hoffmann U, Bamberg F, Chae CU, *et al*. Coronary computed tomography angiography for early triage of patients with acute chest pain: the ROMICAT (Rule Out Myocardial Infarction using Computer Assisted Tomography) trial. *J Am Coll Cardiol* 2009;**53**(18):1642–1650.

Hendel RC, Patel MR, Kramer CM, *et al*. ACCF/ACR/SCCT/SCMR/ASNC/NASCI/SCAI/SIR 2006 appropriateness criteria for cardiac computed tomography and cardiac magnetic resonance imaging. *J Am Coll Cardiol* 2006;**48**(7):1475–1497.

Stillman AE, Oudkerk M, Ackerman M, *et al*. Use of multidetector computed tomography for the assessment of acute chest pain: a consensus statement of the North American Society of Cardiac Imaging and the European Society of Cardiac Radiology. *Eur Radiol* 2007;**17**(8):2196–2207.

Additional online material

- 22.1 Mechanism of retrospective ECG gating versus prospective ECG triggering
- 22.2 Axial slices when scrolling from cranial to caudal
- 22.3 Volume reconstruction
- 22.4 Coronary calcium scoring with non-contrast-enhanced CT
- 22.5 Coronary CT angiography to rule out ACS
- 22.6 Aortic aneurysm
- 22.7 Cumulative event-free rate for development of ACS. Reproduced from Motoyama S, Sarai M, Harigaya H, et al. Computed tomographic angiography characteristics of atherosclerotic plaques subsequently resulting in acute coronary syndrome. *J Am Coll Cardiol* 2009; **54**(1):49–57, with permission from Elsevier Science.
- 22.8 Diaphragmatic hernia

➔ For additional multimedia materials please visit the online version of the book (⌗ http://www.esciacc.oxfordmedicine.com).

SECTION V

Procedures in the intensive cardiac care unit

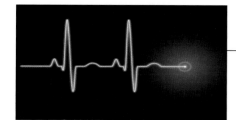

CHAPTER 23

Noninvasive ventilation

Josep Masip and Kenneth Planas

Contents

Summary

During the last 20 years the use of noninvasive ventilation (NIV) has grown substantially. NIV refers to the delivery of positive pressure to the lungs without endotracheal intubation, and has a significant role in the management of acute respiratory failure in acute care areas or general wards. The primary aim of NIV is to avoid intubation and it is mainly used in patients with chronic obstructive pulmonary disease (COPD) exacerbations, acute cardiogenic pulmonary oedema (ACPE) or in the context of weaning, situations in which a reduction in mortality has been demonstrated. The principal techniques are continuous positive airway pressure (CPAP) and pressure support ventilation (NIPSV). Whereas NIPSV requires a ventilator, CPAP is a simpler technique that can be used in unequipped areas such as the prehospital setting. The success of NIV is related to the adequate timing and selection of patients, as well as the appropriate use of interfaces and the fine-tuning of the ventilator.

Introduction

Noninvasive ventilation (NIV) started in the 1930s, when continuous negative extrathoracic pressure was applied (iron lung, chest shell, rocking bed, pneumobelt) in the treatment of epidemic poliomyelitis [1]. In the late 1950s, mechanical ventilation through endotracheal intubation provoked a dramatic decrease in the use of NIV. However, after the introduction of pressure support ventilation in the late 1980s, NIV began to be used again in patients with acute respiratory failure as an alternative to endotracheal intubation in critical care settings [2, 3]. Currently, the rate of NIV in European intensive care units (ICU) is 12–25% [4, 5] and more than 50% of all patients with respiratory failure without intubation at ICU admission will end up with NIV [3]. This rate increases to over 90% in patients with chronic obstructive pulmonary disease (COPD) or acute pulmonary oedema (APE) [5]. NIV is now a first line therapy in emergency departments [6], regular hospital wards [7], palliative [8] or paediatric [9] care units, and even for out-of-hospital patients [10, 11].

Principles of noninvasive ventilation

NIV refers to the delivery of ventilatory support or positive pressure into the lungs without an invasive endotracheal airway [12, 13]. It has several advantages over invasive mechanical ventilation [9]. NIV techniques leave the upper airway intact and may avoid complications that might occur during the endotracheal intubation procedure (upper airway trauma, laryngeal swelling), throughout mechanical ventilation (sedation, infections, tracheal granuloma) and at the time of extubation (vocal cord dysfunction). The most relevant difference with intubated patients is the reduced incidence of infections, especially ventilator-acquired pneumonia [14, 15], because the natural defence mechanism of the upper airway is preserved. By avoiding intubation and its inherent consequences, the length of stay and mortality in the ICU may be reduced, decreasing costs [16]. Furthermore, patients do not need sedation, allowing for nourishment and communication.

Besides all these benefits, there are some disadvantages. One of them is the increased demand for nursing attention in case of functional respiratory impairment due to uncoupling. Moreover, NIV has its own complications such as aerophagia, subjective sensation of air trapping, and in some cases, hypotension, bronchoaspiration, or pneumothorax [17]. However, complications are normally mild and localized, like ocular irritation, nasal congestion, skin lacerations or nasal bridge ulcers (⊃ Fig. 23.1).

Modes of noninvasive ventilation

Two major modes of NIV are used in clinical practice: continuous positive airway pressure (CPAP) and noninvasive pressure support ventilation (NIPSV).

Continuous positive airway pressure

Although it was introduced earlier, CPAP is not essentially a 'true' ventilation mode because it does not provide any inspiratory support [18]. CPAP can be generated with a simple oxygen source through a hermetic mask with a positive end-expiratory pressure (PEEP) valve or a Boussignac mask that holds a quantity of air in the lungs on expiration (⊃ Fig. 23.2). The continuous positive intrathoracic pressure recruits collapsed alveolar units and increases functional residual capacity and lung compliance, improving oxygenation and the work of breathing. However, the control of Fio_2 can be difficult unless a mixer or a ventilator is used. CPAP is currently used in hypoxaemic patients, particularly in those with atelectasis or acute pulmonary oedema.

Noninvasive pressure support ventilation

NIPSV is the foundation of NIV. Unlike CPAP, it requires a ventilator. It is usually programmed with two levels of pressure: expiratory pressure (EPAP) (similar to CPAP) and inspiratory pressure (IPAP) (⊃ Fig. 23.3). When the patient starts the inspiratory effort, the ventilator delivers inspiratory assistance or pressure support using a decelerated flow, which keeps the prefixed inspiratory pressure constant (IPAP). When the inspiratory flow descends below 25% of its maximum value, the ventilator assistance is discontinued and the pressure drops down to the predetermined EPAP (⊃ Fig. 23.4).

Other modalities

- Volume ventilation is reserved for obnubilated patients.

- Proportional assist ventilation (PAV): the inspiratory support is regulated by analysing the elasticity and resistance of the patient, delivering assisted ventilation proportional to the patient's effort. Although this modality has demonstrated a better patient–ventilator synchrony [19] this

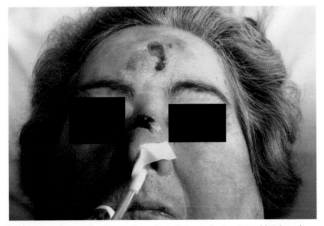

Figure 23.1 Complications of noninvasive ventilation. Nasal bridge ulcers secondary to face mask.

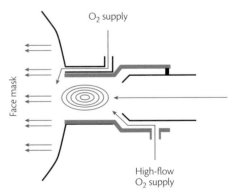

Figure 23.2 Continuous positive airway pressure system without ventilator: the Boussignac mask.

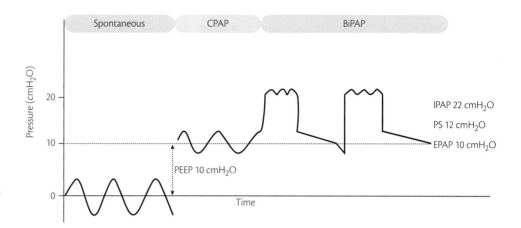

Figure 23.3 Pressure–time curves. Spontaneous breathing, CPAP (10 cmH$_2$O) and bilevel pressure support (IPAP 22 cmH$_2$O, EPAP 10 cmH$_2$O) with pressure support (PS) 12 cmH$_2$O.

advantage has not been translated into clinical outcomes [20–22].

♦ Transtracheal open ventilation: in this recently introduced modality, ventilatory support is delivered through an uncuffed minitracheostomy tube [23], which may be almost as effective as conventional ventilation in maintaining adequate gas exchange and reducing complications, duration of mechanical ventilation and ICU length of stay in COPD patients.

♦ Intrapulmonary percussive ventilation (IPV) has shown to be useful in secretion mobilization. It has been tested in paediatrics and cystic fibrosis patients, and more recently, in COPD exacerbations, improving gas exchange, reducing duration of ventilation and length of stay in ICU [24, 25].

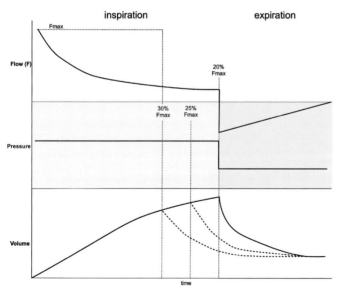

Figure 23.4 Flow–time, pressure–time, and volume–time curves in pressure ventilation modalities with the inspiration cycle set at 20% of the maximal flow achieved at the onset of inspiration. Note the differences in volume (dashed lines) when the inspiration time is limited to different percentages (30%, 25%) of maximum flow.

♦ Negative pressure ventilation: there are few groups still using this modality.

Interface

Whatever NIV technique used, an interface is needed to connect the patient to a ventilator or air/oxygen source (ᗒ Fig. 23.5). That interface is the component that really defines NIV, and it is crucial for the success of the treatment. In order to avoid leaks, a tight seal between the patient's face and the device is essential, but often difficult to obtain. There are different types of interfaces [26].

Nasal interface

This has proved useful in chronic patients or those with sleep apnoea disorders. Although nasal masks can be better tolerated [27], they are less useful in critical situations, generating more resistance than facial masks [28], and therefore are not recommended in acute respiratory distress. There are two different types:

♦ Nasal mask: covers the nose exclusively, offers the possibility of speaking and drinking, allows coughing, reducing the risk of vomiting. Disadvantages: massive air leakage through the mouth when opened, as well as nasal skin injuries.

♦ Nasal pillow: inserted into nostrils. No skin damage. Disadvantages: low flow, frequent air leaks, nasal irritation and unreliable volume monitoring.

Face mask

The most used in clinical practice, in over 70% of all patients requiring NIV [29]. There are three different types:

♦ Full face mask or oronasal mask: covers mouth and nose. It increases minute volume ventilation and reduces Pa_{CO_2} more effectively than nasal masks [27, 30]. Indicated specifically in mouth-breathing patients with dyspnoea. Different sizes and models are necessary for

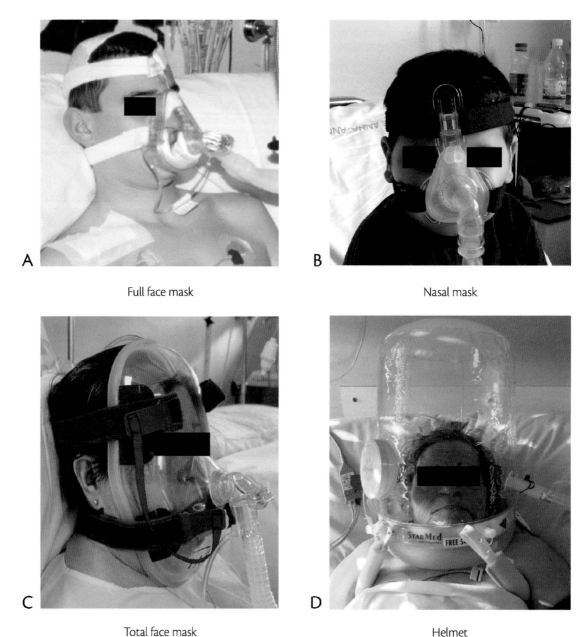

Figure 23.5 Interfaces for noninvasive ventilation. (A) Full face mask; (B) Nasal mask; (C) Total face mask; (D) Helmet.

correct adaptation. Disadvantages: unprotected from vomiting, nasal skin injuries, speaking difficulty, and possible claustrophobia.

• Total face mask: covers mouth, nose, and eyes. Little cooperation is required to achieve a correct adaptation, with an easy fitting and application, provoking fewer skin injuries than full face masks [31]. Disadvantages: higher cost, unprotected from vomiting, difficult of speaking, and claustrophobia.

• Boussignac mask: used for CPAP only. The oxygen flows through small-diameter channels in cylinder walls and is injected at high speed into the cylinder through angled side channels. The resulting turbulence, together with air

friction, creates pressure on the patient's side cylinder opening, acting as virtual PEEP valve [32] (see ➲ Fig. 23.3). This is a very simple technique that may be used in poorly equipped areas. Disadvantages: unprotected from vomiting, difficult of speaking, and claustrophobia.

Helmet

Covers the whole head and part of the neck, without contact with patient's face. Very useful when anticipating prolonged NIV treatment. It can be attached to the patient's axillae, to the abdomen, or even to the bed. Although it allows more patient autonomy (speaking and eating), its noise may be uncomfortable [33, 34]. It is not recommended with traditional ventilators, as a fresh gas flow high enough to minimize rebreathing is necessary [35]. A physiological study performed in patients with stable COPD showed that the helmet was associated with less inspiratory muscle loading but with greater patient–ventilator asynchrony [36]. A recent study certified that when used with specific settings, helmet NIPSV provided similar results to face mask NIPSV, with improvement in the triggering-on delay, and not in the cycling-off delay, leading to worse patient–ventilator synchrony compared to a face mask [37]. Disadvantages: rebreathing, noise, asynchrony, discomfort of axillae, and vomiting.

Other

Mouthpieces placed between lips and held in place by lip seal are less effective due to higher rate of leaks and asynchronies, and greater patient discomfort [38, 39]. Laryngeal masks with control volume may be useful for comatose patients.

The most important reason for patient–ventilator asynchrony is air leakage. In these cases it is recommendable to adjust the interface manually, reduce pressure support, and help the patient gain confidence with the technique.

Indications for noninvasive ventilation in acute care patients

One important point of NIV is the appropriate selection of patients that may benefit from treatment (➲ Box 23.1). NIV can be used in a wide range of disorders that may lead to acute respiratory failure [26]. NIV is currently recommended for COPD exacerbations, cardiogenic pulmonary oedema, facilitation of weaning/extubation of COPD patients, and in immunosupressed patients. It is also indicated for do-not-intubate patients, palliative treatment in endstage patients, community-acquired pneumonia (especially in COPD patients), postoperative respiratory failure, extubation failure in COPD or congestive heart failure patients, and severe asthma. It can be used with weaker evidence in neuromuscular diseases, partial upper airway obstruction, thoracic trauma, severe asthma, cystic fibrosis, and hypoventilation in obese patients.

Exacerbation of chronic obstructive pulmonary disease

Many randomized trials have compared the efficacy of NIPSV with conventional oxygen therapy in patients with exacerbation of COPD, showing NIPSV to be significantly better in improving gas exchange and symptoms [46–51]. The first significant trial was a multicentre randomized study (n = 85) performed in the ICU by Brochard et al. [47] and published in 1995. In that study, a reduction in endotracheal intubation rate (74% vs 26%), length of hospital stay (35 days vs 17 days) and mortality (31% vs 19%) was observed in patients treated with NIPSV in comparison to conventional treatment. A larger study carried out in general wards by Plant et al. [50] (n = 236) also reported a reduction in endotracheal intubation rate (27% vs 15%) and mortality (20% vs 10%) with NIPSV. Only one study (n = 24), performed in patients with mild COPD, found no significant differences [52]. In a recent systematic review by Keenan et al. [53], there was little to support the benefit of NIPSV in milder exacerbations of COPD. Further meta-analysis confirmed that appropriate candidates for NIV are COPD patients with severe acute exacerbation and hypercapnia [54], showing lower intubation rate, ICU or hospital length of stay, and mortality [41, 55–58]. These results make NIPSV the first line treatment for decompensated COPD patients [59–61] in the emergency room, ICU, and even general wards, although the latter is recommended for less severe cases (pH 7.30) [59].

Although a favourable response to NIPSV would be anticipated in acute asthma, little evidence supports this application. While some studies [60–65] suggest that NIPSV may be effective in improving airflow, correcting gas exchange abnormalities, avoiding intubation, and reducing the need for hospitalization, recent reviews concluded there is not enough evidence to use NIPSV in acute asthma [66] and medical treatment alone may be effective [67].

Box 23.1 Acute pulmonary diseases that may benefit from noninvasive ventilation

Noninvasive ventilation recommended

- Chronic obstructive pulmonary disease exacerbation
- Acute cardiogenic pulmonary oedema
- Weaning from mechanical ventilation
- Acute respiratory failure in immunocompromised patients

Noninvasive ventilation suggested

- Asthma
- Pneumonia
- Initial phases of acute respiratory distress syndrome
- Postoperative respiratory failure
- Postoperative recovery
- Do-not-intubate patients

Acute cardiogenic pulmonary oedema

Several surveys have demonstrated that COPD exacerbations and ACPE are the most frequent indications for NIV in acute care settings [4, 5, 68]. The main mode used in patients with ACPE is CPAP and NIPSV.

The use of CPAP in patients with cardiac failure has a physiological basis. In addition to previously mentioned effects on oxygenation, positive intrathoracic pressure reduces venous return and left ventricular transmural pressure (systolic wall stress) [69–72]. In patients with normal cardiac function, this may produce a mild decrease in blood pressure and cardiac output. Conversely, in patients with decompensated heart failure with hypervolaemia and elevated preload, it may decrease pulmonary congestion and increase cardiac output [72, 73].

Since 1985, numerous studies have proved the superiority of CPAP over standard oxygen therapy in patients with ACPE, improving gas exchange and symptoms [71, 74–81], and reducing the endotracheal intubation rate. The most frequent pressure used in these trials was 10 cmH_2O.

The first trial with NIPSV appeared in the year 2000 [82]. Although a study carried out in Israel with extremely low pressure support showed worse outcomes with NIPSV [83], several trials [80, 82, 84] showed a reduction in the intubation rate compared to standard therapy, especially in hypercapnic patients [85].

However, several meta-analyses including up to 19 trials and almost 900 patients were concordant: CPAP and NIPSV reduce nearly to half the risk of endotracheal intubation when compared with standard therapy [86–90]. In addition, both techniques reduced mortality by nearly 40%, although only CPAP reached statistical significance. When compared, neither technique (CPAP vs NIPSV and some cases PAV), clinical trials [80, 91–96], nor meta-analyses [86–90, 97] have been shown to be superior concerning the main outcomes. However, NIPSV tended to show a faster improvement in respiratory failure, and PAV was better tolerated.

In the latest European Society of Cardiology (ESC) guidelines for the diagnosis and treatment of acute and chronic heart failure [98], NIV was considered a class IIa recommendation, but the evidence level moved from A in the previous version [99] to B, because of the publication of the 3CPO study [100]. This multicentre randomized clinical trial, the largest trial on NIV carried out to date, analysed 1069 patients distributed into three groups: standard oxygen therapy, CPAP, and NIPSV. The results showed NIV (both CPAP and NIPSV) improved respiratory distress and metabolic disturbance more rapidly, but no effect was observed on short-term mortality. Patients were not hypoxaemic at study entry (average Pao_2 was 100 mmHg) and the intubation rate was extremely low (<3%), suggesting that patients might not be sufficiently unwell to benefit from these techniques. In addition, there was a high crossover rate (nearly 15%) of patients who did not respond to standard therapy yet were successfully treated with rescue NIV. The design of the trial, which ethically could not restrict the use of NIV, would possibly result in a considerable bias against NIV. The selection of patients, the crossover rate, the prehospital treatment, the possible delay in treatment start (abnormal chest radiograph was mandatory for inclusion), and the teams' expertise (there was a significant rate of NIV intolerance) could also have a role in these results [101, 102]. In spite of this, a recent meta-analysis [103] including the 3CPO trial, still reported a significant reduction of mortality with NIV in ACPE over standard oxygen therapy (RR = 0.75 [0.61–0.92]). Further studies are necessary to define which patients are most likely to benefit from NIV in terms of mortality. The ideal target population may be those patients with high risk for intubation [104], severe acidosis (pH<7.25), hypercapnia, and less hypertension.

In conclusion, NIV is indicated as a first line therapy in ACPE, since it improves acute respiratory failure more rapidly and may reduce the intubation rate and mortality when compared with standard therapy. CPAP may certainly be the technique of choice for its low cost and simplicity, easily implemented at home or in the ambulance. NIPSV may be used with the most severe patients (hypercapnia or respiratory fatigue) and should be performed by experienced personnel with the appropriate equipment.

Community-acquired pneumonia

Several randomized clinical trials have compared the efficacy of NIV with that of conventional oxygen therapy in patients with community-acquired pneumonia (CAP) [105]. Confalonieri et al. [106] enrolled 56 patients with severe CAP and found a significant reduction in endotracheal intubation rate (21% vs 50%), shorter ICU stay, and a reduction in mortality. However, those effects were observed entirely in the subgroup of patients with COPD. Ferrer et al. [107] found that NIV was associated with significantly lower ICU mortality, intubation rate (26% vs 76%), and ICU stay, in patients with severe CAP and hypoxaemic respiratory failure. In another study where COPD patients were excluded [108], patients with NIV had better clinical improvement, but the intubation rate was rather high (60%). However, a more recent trial [109] comparing NIV to invasive ventilation in acute respiratory failure with different aetiologies showed that patients with CAP had the worst clinical outcomes. Hence, NIPSV may be used in patients with acute respiratory failure due to severe CAP, especially if they have COPD.

Finally, it has been widely proved that the use of NIV may reduce the risk of nosocomial pneumonia [15], which may be an additional benefit in these patients.

Acute lung injury/acute respiratory distress syndrome

Studies on NIV to treat acute lung injury/acute respiratory distress syndrome (ALI/ARDS) have reported negative results, although no randomized clinical trials have focused on ALI/ARDS exclusively [105]. In a recent meta-analysis [110] that selected studies with patients with acute respiratory failure due to different aetiologies, NIV had no effect over intubation rate or mortality in patients with ARDS. The delay in endotracheal intubation may be associated with major complications. Risk factors for NIV failure in these patients include severe hypoxaemia, shock, and metabolic acidosis [111]. In a recent prospective survey [112], patients with initial ALI/ARDS (no multiple organ failure or haemodynamic instability) who were treated with NIV had excellent outcomes, avoiding intubation in 54% of the cases. Therefore, NIV can be used with caution in a selected subgroup of patients with ALI/ARDS without high oxygen requirements, multiple organ failure, or haemodynamic instability, but not in those who need invasive ventilation.

Weaning and postextubation

Several randomized trials, different studies, and two recent meta-analyses have explored the role of NIV in weaning. Ferrer et al. [113] assessed the efficacy of NIV in patients with persistent weaning failure and found shorter mechanical ventilation and length of stay, lower incidence of complications (pneumonia and septic shock), less need for tracheotomy, and better survival. However, 60% of their patients had COPD. Although these results were not observed in other trials [114], in recent meta-analyses [114–122] the application of NIV during weaning had positive effects on mortality and ventilator-acquired pneumonia, mainly in COPD patients.

On the other hand, because of the high rate of complications in patients that need reintubation (c.15% of the cases) [115], NIV has been used to prevent acute respiratory failure in high-risk patients. In the first study focused on this issue, by Jiang et al. [116], NIV was of no benefit.

However, in two recent studies [117, 118]the use of NIV was more effective than standard therapy in preventing postextubation respiratory failure, and reintubation rate, without impact on mortality, except for hypercapnic patients [118]. Recently, Ferrer et al. [119] confirmed the advantages of early NIV in patients with chronic respiratory disorders and hypercapnia to diminish the risk of respiratory failure after extubation, with a reduction in 90-day mortality.

On the other hand, Keenan et al. [120] assessed NIV in established acute respiratory failure after extubation and reported no benefits. Esteban et al. [121], in a multicentre trial with 221 patients, found similar results with different approaches, but with an increase in mortality in patients with NIV. This was attributed to delayed reintubation in the NIV group (12h vs 2.5 h). It is important to point out that only 8–12% of these patients had COPD. The authors concluded that NIV was not effective in averting the need for reintubation in unselected patients with respiratory failure after extubation [121].

In conclusion, it seems reasonable that NIV may be used as an alternative to traditional weaning and in the prevention of postextubation acute respiratory failure, especially in COPD or hypercapnic patients, but should not be used in the treatment of postextubation acute respiratory failure, since reintubation delay may be hazardous.

Immunocompromised patients

The use of NIV is well supported for immunocompromised patients with acute respiratory failure of different aetiologies, although the maximal benefit has been observed to be secondary to ACPE [123]. After a solid-organ transplant, NIV may reduce the intubation rate (20%), improve oxygenation, reduce mortality, and shorten ICU stay [124]. In patients with haematological malignancy and acute respiratory failure, the use of NIV may avert the need for endotracheal intubation and its complications, and those patients responding to NIV therapy have a better prognosis [125]. The in-hospital mortality rate for haematological patients is very high (up to 80%) and it is desirable to avoid the complications associated to endotracheal intubation.

Postoperative respiratory failure

In pulmonary postoperative patients, preventive NIV reduced the development of acute respiratory failure and improved recovery [126]. In patients who develop postoperative respiratory distress NIV has shown to reduce the intubation rate (20.8% vs 50%) and hospital mortality

(12.5% vs 37.5%) when compared with conventional therapy [127]. Some authors have reported beneficial effects with postoperative prophylactic nasal CPAP in patients undergoing thoracoabdominal aortic surgery, reducing complications and hospital stay [128]. However, Altmay et al. [129], assessed the use of CPAP in postoperative cardiac surgery and did not find advantages over standard therapy. Gaszynski et al. [130] reported the same results in patients undergoing gastric surgery, with only an improvement in oxygenation.

In conclusion, NIV may be useful in the treatment and prophylaxis of acute respiratory failure of some postoperative states, such as surgery of the lung or aortic aneurysm. To date, there have been no studies demonstrating that NIV can improve the clinical outcome for cardiac surgery patients [131].

Do-not-intubate patients

The use of NIV in patients with acute respiratory failure but a do-not-intubate status has been well described and has had positive effects [132, 133]. This has aroused debate in endstage terminal patients, since mask discomfort outweighs any palliative effect and has complications. Recovery possibilities mainly depend on the characteristics of the patient and the aetiology of the acute respiratory failure; the best results are in COPD and heart failure [30, 134].

Miscellaneous

⊃ Table 23.1 summarizes several randomized trials where NIV was used in series of patients with acute respiratory failure of different aetiologies. Most of them showed the superiority of NIV to conventional oxygen therapy regarding oxygenation, intubation rate, length of stay, and mortality, being especially conclusive in those with COPD and/or hypercapnia [49, 106, 136–139]. However, the results in a series of patients treated in the emergency department [140] and those with hypoxaemic nonhypercapnic respiratory failure were unclear [133]. Studies comparing NIV with conventional mechanical ventilation (through endotracheal intubation) reported a lower incidence of infections [141] and complications [109]. When comparing NIPSV to CPAP or PAV, no significant differences were observed [20–22, 142].

Table 23.1 Randomized trials assessing noninvasive ventilation in acute respiratory failure of different etiologies.

	Year	n	Location	ETI (%)		Mortality (%)		Characteristics
				NIV	Control	NIV	Control	
Hypoxeamic–hypercapnic acute respiratory failure (NIV vs standard)								
Wysocki [134]	1995	40	ICU	62	70	33	50	In hypercapnia ↓ETI/mortality**
Kramer [135]	1995	31	ICU	31	73*	6	13*	NIPSV ↓ ETI (74% were COPD)
Celikel [44]	1998	30	ED[a]	7	40*	0	7	Hypercapnic NIPSV ↓ ETI
Wood [140]	1998	27	ED	43.8	49.5	25	0	NIPSV Nasal NIPSV delayed ETI
Martin [136]	2000	32	ICU	28	59*	2.39	4.27	NIPSV ↓ ETI
Thys [137]	2001	20	ED[b]	0	30–100*	10	20	COPD, ACPE: NIPSV ↓ ETI
Hypoxaemic acute respiratory failure (NIV vs standard)								
Delclaux [133]	2000	123	ICU	34	39	31	30	Multicentre: CPAP vs ST (improvement in 1 h)
Ferrer [104]	2003	105	ICU	13	25*	9.1	21.3*	NIPSV vs ST. Maximum benefit in CAP
Comparison between techniques								
Antonelli [138]	1998	64	ICU	31	100	28	47	NIPSV vs ETI. ETI ↑ infections
Honrubia [106]	2005	64	ICU	58	100	23	39	NIPSV vs ETI. NIPSV ↓ complications
Gay [21]	2001	42	ICU	26	24	30	19	NIPSV vs PAV. PAV ↑ tolerance
Fernandez [20]	2003	117	ICU	37	34	29	28	NIPSV vs PAV. PAV ↑ tolerance
Cross [139]	2005	101	ED	4.7	11.5	12	16	NIPSV vs CPAP No differences

* Significant difference **Mortality at 90 days (p = 0.02)
[a] Six patients (40%) from control group were treated with rescue NIV and two needed ETI. Shorter hospital stay with NIV.
[b] Control group was treated with a placebo ventilator without NIPSV. All the patients required NIPSV due to bad evolution (ETI 30%).
ACPE, acute cardiogenic pulmonary oedema; COPD, chronic obstructive pulmonary disease; CPAP, continuous positive airway pressure; ED, emergency department; ETI, endotracheal intubation; ICU, intensive care unit; n, sample; NIPSV, noninvasive pressure support ventilation; NIV, noninvasive ventilation; PAV, proportional assist ventilation; CAP, community acquired pneumonia; ST, standard therapy.

Patient selection for noninvasive ventilation

Before starting NIV it is crucial to identify if the patient is a good candidate [62] (⊖ Box 23.2) considering the predictors of failure (⊖ Table 23.2) and possible complications of NIV (⊖ Box 23.3). Intubation may be preferred if the likelihood of NIV failure is too high [62]: high SAPS-APACHE scores, very low pH, low Glasgow Coma Score or ARDS patients) [41, 42]. Patients with no improvement after 60 min of NIV or excessive secretions may also fail [18, 68, 143–146].

In our experience, there are three levels that may influence the success of NIV (⊖ Fig. 23.6): the patient (severity of disease, adaptation, mental status), the physician (concomitant therapy, experience, team attitude) and the device (incorrect adjustment, inadequate interface, excessive leakage).

Table 23.2 Predictors of failure of noninvasive ventilation therapy in acute respiratory failure

General	After 60min
Breathing asynchrony with ventilator	No reduction in respiratory rate
Excessive air leakage	No improvement in pH
Copious secretions	No improvement in oxygenation
Extremely high respiratory rate	No reduction in carbon dioxide
Bad subjective tolerance	
Neurological impairment	
ALI/ARDS	
Metabolic acidosis	
Severe hypoxaemia with oxygen therapy	
Shock	
High severity scores	

ALI, acute lung injury; ARDS, acute respiratory distress syndrome.

How to apply noninvasive ventilation

Continuous positive airway pressure

The technique is very simple and no special training is required. However, it is important to use appropriate masks adjusted with head straps and monitoring, when

---

Box 23.2 Indications and contraindications for noninvasive ventilation

Indications

- Physical examination
  - Moderate to severe dyspnoea
  - Tachypnea
  - Increased work of breathing, accessory muscle use, abdominal paradoxic respiration
- Gas exchange
  - Ventilatory failure: hypercapnia, acidosis
- Hypoxaemia

Contraindications

Absolute

- Cardiac or respiratory arrest
- Facial anatomical abnormality (unable to fit the mask)
- Refractory hypoxaemia
- Shock established

Relative

- Mild hypotension
- Agitated or uncooperative patient
- Unable to protect airway
- Excessive secretions
- Multiple organ failure
- Recent upper airway or upper gastrointestinal surgery

Box 23.3 Complications of noninvasive ventilation

Related to interface

- Discomfort
- Facial erythema
- Claustrophobia
- Skin ulcers

Related to air flow

- Nasal congestion
- Sinusitis
- Oral and nasal dryness
- Ocular irritation
- Gastric hyperinsufflation

Major complications

- Aspiration pneumonia
- Hypotension
- Pneumothorax

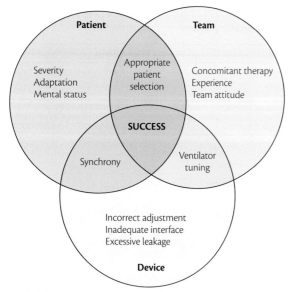

Figure 23.6 The success puzzle for noninvasive pressure support ventilation.

possible, the resulted FiO_2. Initial CPAP may be 5 cmH$_2$O. If the patient is correctly adapted, CPAP may be increased to 10 cmH$_2$O, the most common level of pressure applied in the majority of trials.

Noninvasive pressure support ventilation

This technique requires more experience. There are several factors to keep in mind when preparing to start NIPSV therapy, as mentioned previously (➲ Fig. 23.7).

Ventilator settings

It is advisable to start with low levels of pressure (IPAP 8–10 cmH$_2$O/EPAP 3–4 cmH$_2$O), increasing pressure support progressively according to patient adaptation, ensuring expired tidal volume is more than 4–6 mL/kg (it can be lower in COPD patients). If there is no control display of the expired volume, pressure support must be increased until tolerated. Normally, with a pressure support of 12–18 cmH$_2$O above PEEP, a tidal volume of 400–500 mL is reached. Elevated pressures may cause excessive air leakage, lack of coordination (when the patient is tachypnoeic) and discomfort. On the other hand, a PEEP over 4 cmH$_2$O is useful to avoid rebreathing when using portable ventilators, which may not include an expiratory valve or double inspiratory-expiratory circuit [147]. To ensure the success of NIV, close monitoring is necessary (➲ Box 23.4), especially patients' oxygen saturation (to adjust FiO_2), $PaCO_2$ (to assess efficacy) and face mask fitting (visually, air leakage volume), principally at the onset of the procedure.

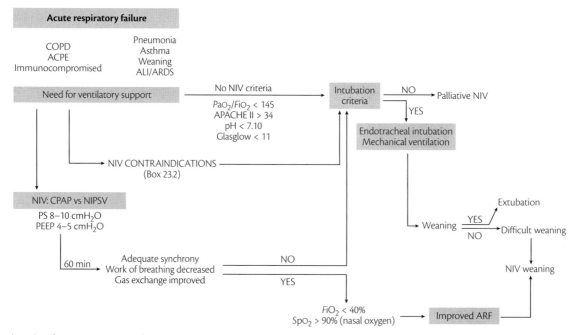

Figure 23.7 Algorithm for patient selection for noninvasive ventilation. ACPE, acute cardiogenic pulmonary oedema; ALI, acute lung injury; ARDS, acute respiratory distress syndrome; ARF, acute respiratory failure; COPD, chronic obstructive pulmonary disease; CPAP, continuous positive airway pressure; FiO_2, fraction of inspired oxygen; GCS, Glasgow Coma Scale; NIPSV, noninvasive pressure support ventilation; NIV, noninvasive ventilation; PEEP, positive end-expiratory pressure; PS, pressure support; SpO_2, pulse oximetry.

Bo x 23.4 Monitoring noninvasive ventilation in acute respiratory failure

Patient

- Respiratory rate
- Vital signs
- Dyspnoea/accessory muscle use/abdominal paradoxical breathing
- Consciousness level
- Mask comfort
- Collaboration

Ventilator parameters

- Tidal volume (6–7 mL/kg) and minute ventilation
- Air leakage volume

- Pressure support and PEEP setting
- Synchrony/ineffective efforts
- Trigger/slope/inspiration time/expiration setting
- Auto-PEEP
- Alarms (maximal peak pressure, minimal minute ventilation)

Gas exchange

- Continuous pulse oximetry
- Arterial blood gas sample (baseline and after 60 min NIV for Pao_2/Fio_2, pH, $Paco_2$)
- Venous blood gas sample (for pH)

Fio_2, fraction of inspired oxygen; $Paco_2$, arterial partial carbon dioxide pressure; Pao_2, arterial partial oxygen pressure; PEEP, positive end-expiratory pressure;

Staffing, costs, and resources

Optimal staffing and location are needed for NIV therapy. After connecting a patient to NIV, close attention from the therapeutic team is required. Several trials reported that patients with NIV may need more attention than intubated patients [137, 148]. When comparing costs, NIV seems to have a better cost–benefit ratio [149] than invasive ventilation.

Conclusion

NIV plays an important role in the management of acute respiratory failure in acute care areas (ICU, cardiac care unit, emergency department) and in general wards. It is indicated in patients with acute exacerbations of COPD and acute cardiogenic pulmonary oedema, where it must be considered as a first line treatment. It can be useful, depending on the adequate selection of patients, in cases of pneumonia, asthma, difficult weaning, in immunocompromised patients, as a palliative treatment and in the prevention of postextubation or postoperative respiratory failure. Caregivers must develop skills in the technique, paying special attention to face mask fitting and patient–ventilator synchrony. Many other potential applications are undergoing further investigation, and additional studies are necessary to confirm all the benefits of NIV extending its indications in the future.

Personal perspective

Although in developed countries NIV has shown a sustained growth for two decades, it seems to have stabilized in the last years. There are several reasons to explain this. First, familiarity with the technique has reached extensive areas of the health care system. Second, the number of trials analysing NIV has decreased since they usually repeat previous data, resulting in a low acceptance rate in relevant medical journals. Third, no significant technological discoveries have been presented in the last few years.

Finally, the real weight of NIV therapy has become more evident since it cannot be considered a substitute for mechanical ventilation through intubation for all patients. In this context, new improvements in the devices, either ventilators or interfaces, as well as new scenarios of where to apply the technique (prehospital, developing countries) would expect to improve patient's comfort and adaptation, further spreading the use of the technique. However, additional large, well-designed studies are necessary to definitively establish the role of NIV in mortality, especially in critically ill cardiac patients.

Further reading

Antonelli M, Conti G, Rocco M, *et al.* A comparison of noninvasive positive-pressure ventilation and conventional mechanical ventilation in patients with acute respiratory failure. *N Engl J Med* 1998;**339**:429–435.

Bersten AD, Holt AW, Vedig AE, *et al.* Treatment of severe cardiogenic pulmonary edema with continuous positive airway pressure delivered by face mask. *N Engl J Med* 1991;**325**:1825–1830.

Brochard L, Mancebo J, Wysocki M, *et al.* Noninvasive ventilation for acute exacerbations of pulmonary disease. *N Engl J Med* 1995;**333**:817–822.

Gray A, Goodacre S, Newby DE, *et al.* Noninvasive ventilation in acute cardiogenic pulmonary edema. *N Engl J Med* 2008;**359**:142–151.

Liesching T, Kwok H, Hill NS. Acute applications of noninvasive positive pressure ventilation. *Chest* 2003;**124**:669–713.

Masip J, Betbesé AJ, Páez J, *et al.* Non-invasive pressure support ventilation versus conventional oxygen therapy in acute cardiogenic pulmonary oedema: a randomized trial. *Lancet* 2000;**356**:2126–2132.

Masip J, Roque M, Sánchez B, *et al.* Noninvasive ventilation in acute cardiogenic pulmonary edema. Systematic review and meta-analysis. *JAMA* 2005;**294**:3124–3130.

Pañuelas O, Frutos-Vivar F, Esteban A. Noninvasive positive-pressure ventilation in acute respiratory failure. *CMAJ* 2007;**177**:1211–1218.

Potts JM. Noninvasive positive pressure ventilation. Effect on mortality in acute cardiogenic pulmonary edema: a pragmatic meta-analysis. *Pol Arch Med Wewn* 2009;**119**:349–353.

Ram FS, Picot J, Lightower J, Wedzicha JA. Non-invasive positive pressure ventilation for treatment of respiratory failure due to exacerbations of chronic obstructive pulmonary disease. *Cochrane Database Syst Rev* 2004;**3**:CD004104.

Additional online material

- Video 1. Patient NIV asynchrony.
- Video 2. Patient NIV synchrony.

➲ For additional multimedia materials please visit the online version of the book (http://www.esciacc.oxfordmedicine.com).

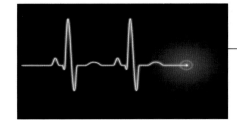

CHAPTER 24

Mechanical ventilation

Gihan Abuella and Andrew Rhodes

Contents

Summary

Mechanical ventilation is used to assist or replace spontaneous respiration. Gas flow can be generated by negative pressure techniques, but it is positive pressure ventilation that is most efficacious in intensive care. There are numerous pulmonary and extrapulmonary indications for mechanical ventilation and it is the underlying pathology that will determine the duration of ventilation required. Ventilation modes can broadly be classified as volume or pressure controlled, but modern ventilators combine the characteristics of both in order to complement the diverse requirements of individual patients. To avoid confusion it is important to appreciate that there is no international consensus on the classification of ventilation modes. Ventilator manufacturers can use terms that are similar to those used by others that describe very different modes, or have completely different names for similar modes. It is well established that ventilation in itself can cause or exacerbate lung injury, so the evidence-based lung protective strategies should be adhered to.

Introduction

Mechanical ventilation is a machine-driven method of assisting or replacing spontaneous breathing. In order for gas to flow into the lungs, a pressure difference between the atmosphere and the alveoli is required. In spontaneous respiration the respiratory muscles expand the chest wall, generating negative intrapleural pressure that draws air in. Mechanical ventilation is classified into negative pressure ventilation (NPV) and positive pressure ventilation (PPV).

In PPV gas flow is achieved by applying positive pressure at the upper airway, either externally through a face mask as described in ◑ Chapter 23 on noninvasive ventilation (NIV) or internally through a tracheal tube. NPV requires the use of a rigid external chest wall device such as the cuirass, a modern version of the iron lung, which generates negative pressure inside the shell that helps to expand the chest wall. NPV is rarely used in intensive care because of its many

Box 24.1 Oxygen delivery

Oxygen delivery (Do_2) = cardiac output (CO) × arterial oxygen content (Cao_2)

$$Cao_2 = [O_2 \text{saturation}(\%) \times Hb(g/dL) \times 1.34m(mL/g)] + [Pao_2 (kPa) \times 0.023 (mL\ kPa^{-1}\ dL^{-1})]$$

practical limitations, thus the ventilation modes described in this chapter refer to PPV only.

Mechanical ventilation is indicated for any cause of type I and/or type II respiratory failure; where the airway is compromised; in nonrespiratory disorders where oxygen delivery (◉ Box 24.1) is impaired and shock ensues; and postoperatively for 'warming, weaning, and waking' (◉ Table 24.1).

Respiratory physiology

This section provides a brief overview of the respiratory physiology relevant to mechanical ventilation, to define and place in context terms that are used subsequently in this chapter.

Functional anatomy

The respiratory system is composed of the upper and lower respiratory tracks. The nose, mouth, pharynx, and larynx form the upper respiratory track which accounts for two-thirds of the resistance to airflow. The lower respiratory track is subdivided according to Weibel's classification into 23 generations.

Table 24.1 Indications for mechanical ventilation

Respiratory	Nonrespiratory
Pneumonia	Airway obstruction, e.g. Ludwig's angina
Cardiogenic pulmonary oedema	Airway protection for obtunded GCS
ALI	Severe sepsis/septic shock
ARDS	Postoperative hypothermia or acidosis
PE	Cardiogenic shock
Acute severe asthma	Therapeutic hypothermia post VF arrest
Acute exacerbation of COPD	Neuromuscular disorders, e.g. GBS
Impaired respiratory drive causing apnoea or hypoventilation due any cause e.g. drug overdose	Severe anaemia where transfusion is contraindicated i.e. Jehovah's Witness after major blood loss

ALI, acute lung injury; ARDS, acute respiratory distress syndrome; COPD, chronic obstructive pulmonary disease; GBS, Guillain–Barré syndrome; GCS, Glasgow Coma Scale; PE, pulmonary embolus; VF, ventricular fibrillation.

◆ The conducting airways start at the trachea and bifurcate for 16 generations from major bronchi to the bronchioles. These do not take part in gas exchange. The larger airways are held open by cartilaginous half-rings, while lower airway patency relies on the elastic recoil of the lung parenchyma; collapse of these smaller airways is therefore more likely at low lung volumes.

◆ The gas exchange units are the respiratory bronchioles (generations 17–19) and the alveolar ducts and sacs (generations 20–23). Alveoli consist of three types of cells. Type I cells provide a very thin layer of cytoplasm that forms the alveolar epithelium; type II cells have several metabolic functions including surfactant production; type III cells are macrophages that contain proteolytic enzymes and form part of the lung's defence system.

Each lung is partitioned by connective tissue into 10 bronchopulmonary segments, each with its own artery, vein, and bronchus. The pulmonary arteries feed the respiratory units, but the bronchi receive their blood supply directly from the aorta. A rich network of lymphatics drains fluid from the interstitium into the thoracic duct. Nerve supply comes from the sympathetic and vagal plexuses.

Gas exchange

Alveoli are the fundamental units of gas exchange. An adult has 300 million alveoli, giving a total surface area in excess of 50 m². Pulmonary capillaries line the alveoli in densely packed sheets to match this large area of ventilated lung. Gas exchange occurs between the alveolar-capillary membrane which is 0.3 μm thick in healthy lung tissue. The rate of oxygen diffusion depends on the oxygen partial pressure (Po_2) gradient between the alveolus and pulmonary capillary; and the thickness of the endothelium between them. The Po_2 gradient is largely determined by the inspired oxygen concentration, however alveolar $Paco_2$ will also affect Pao_2. The sum of the partial pressures of all the alveolar gases cannot exceed atmospheric pressure, therefore the higher the $Paco_2$, the lower the Pao_2 will be. Oxygen diffusion will be impeded by any accumulation of fluid between the alveolar-capillary membrane (pulmonary oedema) or other material such as collagen (pulmonary fibrosis).

Oxygenation is also affected by the contact time between the red blood cells and alveoli, which is inversely related to the cardiac output. Cooperative bonding of oxygen by haemoglobin allows alveolar and RBC Po_2 to equilibrate by the time the RBC has traversed one-third of the capillary. This only takes a quarter of a second, so a very high cardiac output can contribute to desaturation if the contact time is less than this.

CO_2 diffuses rapidly from pulmonary capillaries into the alveoli down its concentration gradient, therefore elimination relies on alveolar ventilation. The tidal volume needs to match CO_2 production which is 200 mL/min in an average 70-kg man; and account for physiological and equipment dead space. In conventional mechanical ventilation (as described in ventilation modes), increasing minute volume enhances CO_2 clearance as long as tidal volume exceeds the total dead space.

Ventilation–perfusion mismatch

Ventilation (V) needs to match perfusion (Q) in order to optimize gas exchange ($V/Q = 1$). Dead space ($V/Q > 1$) describes areas that are ventilated but not perfused, whereas shunt ($V/Q < 1$) refers to areas of lung that are perfused but not ventilated or the dilution of arterial blood with venous blood. V/Q mismatch represents a spectrum with dead space at one end and shunt at the other.

Anatomical dead space is the part of the respiratory tract that does not take park in gas exchange, from the mouth and nose down to the 16th-generation bronchioles. This is normally 2–3 mL/kg and is generally taken to be approximately 150 mL. Anatomical shunt is the dilution of arterial blood by deoxygenated blood from the bronchial veins that drain into the left atrium and the endocardium of the left ventricle that drains into the left heart chambers via the thebesian veins. This right to left shunt only causes a slight drop in Pao_2. In pathological shunting, increasing the Fio_2 does not fully reverse the hypoxia; the supplementary oxygen increases dissolved oxygen which has a minor role in oxygen delivery. Haemoglobin passing through the ventilated areas becomes fully saturated early and cannot compensate for the deoxygenated haemoglobin with which it subsequently mixes. Hypoxic pulmonary vasoconstriction (HPV) diverts blood away from under ventilated areas thereby provides physiological compensation to minimize the effects of V/Q mismatching.

Even in normal healthy lungs alveolar V/Q varies from apex to base. This arises as a result of a natural gradient in intrapleural pressure which gradually increases vertically regardless of the patient's position. The lung is divided into three functional zones (West zones) (⮑ Fig. 24.1). Lower intrapleural pressure at the apex allows alveoli to distend; therefore alveolar pressure is highest and perfusion is reduced. Alveolar dead space (D_A) is normally negligible but if alveolar pressure is increased significantly with PPV or PEEP, or capillary artery pressure is reduced

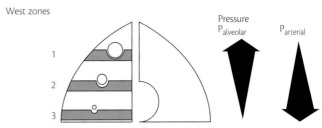

Figure 24.1 Functional zones of the lung (upright position).

due to hypovolaemia or shock, D_A will increase. At the lung bases, pulmonary capillary pressure is higher and alveoli have smaller volumes. Physiological dead space is the sum of anatomical and alveolar dead space. Pathological causes of increased dead space and shunt are listed in ⮑ Table 24.2.

Respiratory mechanics

The thoracic cage, formed of ribs and intercostal muscles along with the diaphragm, represents the chest wall. The thoracic cage has a tendency to spring outwards whereas the lungs, being elastic, tend to collapse: these opposing forces generate negative intrapleural pressure. Inspiration occurs mainly through diaphragmatic contraction and augments the negative intrapleural pressure. This decrease in transpulmonary (alveolar minus pleural) pressure draws air in. The volume of gas that remains in the lungs at the end of normal expiration and holds the lung open is the functional residual capacity (FRC) and represents a point of equilibrium between the opposing recoil of the lungs and thoracic cage. Lung volumes vary with age, gender, and height; in an adult tidal volume is approximately 7 mL/kg (500 mL) and FRC is 2500 mL.

The ease with which the lungs inflate in response to a change in transpulmonary pressure is the lung compliance. The more distended alveoli at the lung apex and the more collapsed alveoli at the base have a lower compliance compared to those in the mid zones. Surfactant has a crucial role in maximizing lung compliance by reducing the surface tension within the alveoli. Pressure in the alveoli is related to tension and radius: $P_A = 2T/r$. In the absence of surfactant, alveoli with the smallest radii would have the

Table 24.2 Pathological causes of increased dead space and shunt

Dead space	Shunt
PPV	Atelectasis
Pulmonary embolus	Pneumonia
Haemorrhage	PFO and septal defects, especially Eisenmenger's
Hypotension	Hepatopulmonary syndrome in cirrhosis

PFO, patent foramen ovale; PPV, positive pressure ventilation.

greatest pressure, therefore would tend to collapse and empty into larger alveoli. Total respiratory compliance combines lung and chest wall compliance; any alveolar or interstitial infiltrate such as pulmonary oedema or fibrosis will decrease lung compliance, whereas chest wall compliance is increased by conditions such as generalised oedema and obesity. At FRC the respiratory compliance is optimum; the lung sits on the steepest part of the pressure/volume curve subsequently a small change in pressure results the largest change in volume (◘ Fig. 24.2).

Note that during spontaneous respiration, the basal alveoli sit on a more favourable part of the *P/V* curve and therefore are more compliant than apical alveoli. Greater expansion of these alveoli gives preferential ventilation to the lung bases, matching the greater basal blood flow. In situations where FRC is reduced (supine position, mechanical ventilation) the lungs shift down the *P/V* curve and compliance, therefore the distribution of ventilation changes and will be greater at the apices thereby increasing *V*/*Q* mismatch.

Gas flow into the lungs is proportional to pressure change but inversely related to airways resistance. In the larger airways (generations 1–5) flow is predominantly turbulent and accounts for the higher resistance whereas resistance in the more distal airways is lower due to laminar flow. High velocity flow increases turbulence and therefore airways resistance. During deep inspiration flow rates as high as 60 L/min can be reached. The energy required to overcome airways resistance and elastance (reciprocal of compliance) amounts to the work of breathing.

Ventilation modes

Ventilation modes are classified according to (1) the type of breath delivered in terms of cycling (phase variables) and (2) how the gas flow is driven (control variables).

Phase variables

The terminology used to describe ventilator breaths revolves around the two phases of the natural respiratory cycle: inspiration and expiration. Like normal respiration, ventilators provide active inspiration and passive expiration. The inspiratory time (T_I) and expiratory time (T_E) represent the duration of inspiration and expiration respectively, while the transition from one phase to another is known as cycling. Inspiratory cycling marks the beginning of inspiration and expiratory cycling marks the beginning of expiration. These four variables are referred to as the phase variables as they can be manipulated to suit the patient's respiratory mechanics and gas exchange requirements. The inspiratory phase itself can have two components: an active or flow phase followed by a pause. Inspiration is said to have ended at the end of the flow phase, whereas the inspiratory phase ends after the pause (◘ Fig. 24.3).

Cycle time is the sum of T_I and T_E expressed in seconds and the respiratory rate or frequency is the number of cycles per minute. The usual ratio of T_I to T_E is 1:2. These variables are interconnected so that setting any two parameters determines the third.

An intubated patient who is breathing spontaneously controls every aspect of the breathing cycle: continuous positive airway pressure (CPAP) is usually delivered to keep the alveoli open, but the breath is not supported.

If the ventilator determines both inspiratory and expiratory cycling, so that the patient has no control over ventilation, the mode is described as mandatory. This is the mode used intraoperatively as patients are often paralysed or their respiratory drive is abolished by deep anaesthesia. Terms that describe this mode are intermittent positive pressure ventilation (IPPV), continuous mandatory ventilation (CMV),or, if the patient is allowed to take other breaths in between, intermittent mandatory ventilation (IMV).

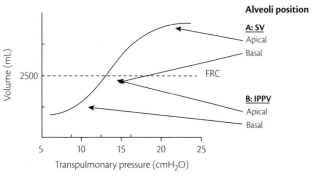

Figure 24.2 Total respiratory system compliance curve during (A) spontaneous ventilation; (B) mechanical ventilation.

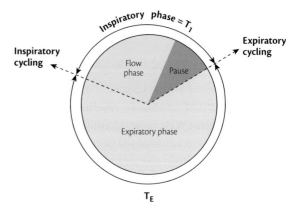

Figure 24.3 Respiratory phases and cycling.

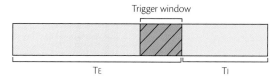

Figure 24.4 Illustration of trigger window.

When a patient takes breaths during ventilation on a mandatory mode, the ventilator may allow the patient to draw in gas, in which case these breaths are accommodated. If not, the circuit pressure falls and the ventilator alarm sounds.

Unlike in theatre, on intensive care units the sedation dose used is the lowest that will keep the patient comfortable. It is preferable to allow the patient to make some respiratory effort to minimize respiratory muscle weakness and facilitate weaning off the ventilator. If the patient's respiratory effort determines inspiratory cycling, then the breath is said to be triggered and the ventilator is on a demand, assist, or support mode.

A hybrid mode is combination of mandatory and triggered ventilation. Synchronized intermittent mandatory ventilation (SIMV) is a hybrid mode where mandatory breaths are set at a certain frequency. If the patient makes an inspiratory effort, this triggers the ventilator to give a breath instead of the mandatory breath (this breath will have the same control characteristics as the mandatory breath in terms of pressure or volume). This will not happen every time an inspiratory effort is made, but only when that inspiratory effort falls within a 'trigger window' (➲ Fig. 24.4) in the time interval before the mandatory breath was due. Inspiratory effort outside this trigger window may be accommodated or supported with different control variables than the mandatory breath.

When inspiratory cycling depends completely on triggering, an apnoea interval is employed so that if the patient stops breathing for a set period of time, the ventilator alarm sounds and it changes to a mandatory mode.

Phase variable are summarized in ➲ Table 24.3.

Control variables

The control variables that determine how gas flow is delivered by the ventilator are pressure and volume, and those that determine inspiratory and expiratory cycling are flow and time.

In volume controlled ventilation (VCV), a target tidal volume is set on the ventilator. Flow is constant for a fixed time period. Inspiration and expiration are determined by the time allocated for each respiratory cycle (frequency) and the $T_I{:}T_E$. Ventilation is said to be time cycled. The ventilator will deliver the tidal volume to the patient and the pressure generated will be determined by the patient's compliance (➲ Fig. 24.5). Larger tidal volumes or a shorter inspiratory time produce higher peak pressures. The consistency of minute volume with VCV results in more predictable CO_2 elimination. Theoretical disadvantages of VCV include a risk of barotrauma (see ➲ Ventilator-associated lung injury') and increased incidence of patient–ventilator asynchrony.

With pressure control ventilation (PCV), the inflating pressure is set on the ventilator and the breath is delivered using a decelerating flow pattern. Initially both airway pressure and flow rise briskly to a peak; the pressure is maintained at this level for the remainder of inspiration, whereas flow decreases exponentially (➲ Fig. 24.6). The tidal volume delivered depends on the patient's compliance and airway resistance. Cycling is flow dependent and expiration occurs when flow drops below a predetermined level which is usually 25% of the peak flow. Patient comfort is improved because an increase in inspiratory effort is matched with an increase in gas flow however changes in compliance will increase or decrease tidal volume proportionately and risk volutrauma (see ➲ Ventilator-associated lung injury').

While each mode of ventilation has theoretical advantages and disadvantages, clinical trials have failed to show any difference in complication rates, length of intensive care unit (ICU) stay, or mortality.

The above descriptions of VCV and PCV are simplified schemes to illustrate the basic principles behind the control variables. Modern ventilators have sophisticated sensors and controls that allow multiple ventilation parameters to be adjusted in order to fine tune the breath characteristics. The beneficial features of VCV and PCV can be combined.

In dual modes the variable that drives the gas flow is labelled as 'control' while the limiting variable is labelled

Table 24.3 Summary of mode phase variables

Ventilation mode	Inspiratory cycling	Expiratory cycling	Ventilator delivers breath
Spontaneous	Patient	Patient	No
Mandatory	Ventilator	Ventilator	Yes
Assist/support/demand	Patient	Ventilator	Yes
Accommodated	Patient	Patient	No

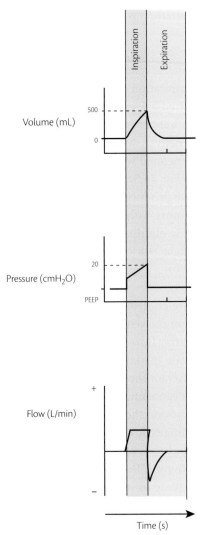

Figure 24.5 Volume, pressure, and flow waveforms for volume controlled ventilation.

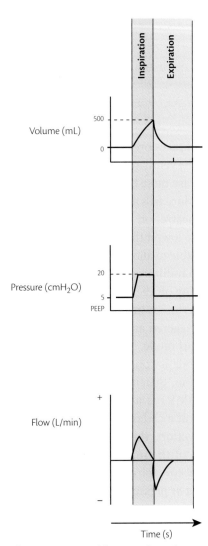

Figure 24.6 Volume, pressure, and flow waveforms for pressure controlled ventilation.

'limit' or 'target' or 'regulated', e.g. pressure-regulated volume control (PRVC). In this mode the desired volume and a pressure limit are set. The full tidal volume will only be delivered so long as the pressure remains below the pressure limit. If the pressure limit is reached then the ventilator cycles to expiration and sounds an alarm. An additional feature of modern ventilators is the automatic (auto) mode which can sense the patient's respiratory effort and switch between mandatory and triggered modes accordingly. The ventilator responds to a gradual change in the patient's compliance by increasing or decreasing the pressure support given in small increments. Theoretically these multi-faceted ventilation modes will encourage weaning as the patient improves, and shorten the duration of mechanical ventilation; however, this hypothesis needs to be validated by clinical trials.

There are several dual ventilation modes which can be pressure controlled and volume targeted or, as described above, volume controlled and pressure limited. They can be mandatory or triggered, or hybrids of these phase variables. Confusion occurs because of the numerous combinations of control and phase variables. There is no universally agreed classification or terminology for ventilation modes; manufacturers have different names for similar ventilation modes, or may use the same name to describe very different modes.

Patient–ventilator asynchrony

Asynchrony, also known as 'fighting the ventilator', arises out of mismatching of the patient's intrinsic respiratory rhythm and the ventilator settings. The patient's inspiratory drive, timing, and respiratory mechanics influence the interaction with the ventilator. If the ventilator does not accommodate or trigger when a patient tries to inspire, considerable discomfort will be felt. Equally if the patient's peak inspiratory flow rate is not

Table 24.4 Cardiovascular effects of mechanical ventilation and PEEP

Effect	Explanation
RV preload decreases	Increased intrathoracic pressure reduces venous return, decreases RV volume but increase RV pressure
RV afterload increases	Due to increased PVR
RV contractility unchanged	No evidence of impaired contractility
LV preload decreases (2 hypotheses)	1. Reduced filling due to increased PVR: may respond to volume replacement 2. Reduced compliance due to bulging of interventricular septum with very high PEEP as RV pressure increases: does not respond to volume replacement
LV afterload decreases	Circulatory reflexes reduce SVR and improve LV emptying
LV contractility unchanged	May be impaired in IHD due to altered coronary blood flow (unproven hypothesis)
HR unchanged or decreased	Impaired baroreceptor reflexes
CO decreases	Reduced preload and HR reduces CO by up to 26%

CO, cardiac output; HR, heart rate; IHD, ischaemic heart disease; PVR, pulmonary vascular resistance; LV, left ventricle; PEEP, positive end-expiratory pressure; RV, right ventricle; SVR, systemic vascular resistance.

matched by the ventilator's, flow restriction will occur. This problem tends to occur with VCV with a constant flow rate. The patient will respond by making a greater inspiratory effort, which generates a large negative pressure in the airway. In PCV the pressure rise time, support level, and flow threshold for expiratory cycling affect patient–ventilator asynchrony. Patients with high airways resistance require a higher flow threshold for expiratory cycling than the preset 25%, and those with poor compliance may need a lower threshold.

It is by understanding the patient's mechanics that complementary ventilator modes and settings can be established. In difficult cases, the patient's respiratory drive can be abolished by deepening of sedation or muscle paralysis.

Ventilator-associated lung injury

Mechanical ventilation itself is associated with lung damage, ventilator-associated lung injury (VALI), which resembles acute lung injury (ALI). ALI is a term that covers a wide spectrum of disease characterized by (1) hypoxaemia where the Pao_2/Fio_2 is below 40 kPa or 300 mmHg, (2) low lung compliance, (3) widespread infiltrates on chest radiograph and (4) normal left atrial pressure (pulmonary capillary wedge pressure) <18 cmH$_2$O). Acute respiratory distress syndrome (ARDS) is at the severe end of the spectrum, requiring Pao_2/Fio_2 less than 27 kPa (200 mmHg) for diagnosis. Four mechanisms underlie VALI: volutrauma, atelectrauma, barotrauma, and biotrauma.

Volutrauma

Overdistension of alveoli leads to direct damage to the alveolar-capillary membrane as a result of excessive wall stress (ratio of alveolar wall tension to thickness). This leads to a rapid increase in permeability with leakage of protein-rich fluid into the alveoli and interstitium. The action of surfactant is severely impaired, leading to alveolar collapse and a reduction in lung compliance. The increase in extravascular lung water occurs more readily in animal models with established lung injury. Animal studies have also clearly demonstrated that this form of pulmonary oedema is directly related to the high volumes and not the increase in pressure that is usually associated with the delivery of a high tidal volume.

Atelectrauma

The repeated cyclical opening and closing of small airways and alveoli that occurs with ventilation at low lung volumes. Ventilation associated with supine positioning and reduced FRC, particularly in the absence of PEEP, results in an atelectatic (collapsed) lung where the air–liquid interface is more proximal at the terminal conducting bronchioles instead of in the alveoli. The high shearing forces required to open these airways are associated with surfactant depletion and physical disruption of the alveolar epithelium.

Barotrauma

The use of excessive pressures leads to epithelial damage and air leakage causing pneumothoraces, subcutaneous emphysema, or less commonly pneumomediastinum or pneumopericardium. Studies suggest that high transpulmonary pressures are more relevant than airway pressure as such; however, it is not easy to measure transpulmonary pressures clinically, so plateau and mean pressures are used as surrogate markers.

Biotrauma

The release of proinflammatory cytokines such tumour necrosis factor alpha (TNFα) and interleukins 1 and 6 (IL-1, IL-6) contributes to lung injury and they enter the systemic circulation to cause systemic inflammation and multiple organ dysfunction syndrome (MODS).

Lung protective ventilation strategies

Positive end-expiratory pressure

Positive end-expiratory pressure (PEEP) is synonymous with CPAP but applies to the continuous airway pressure applied during ventilation with a mandatory or assisted mode. It maintains the small airways and alveoli open, and helps return the FRC towards the normal physiological range. Preventing derecruitment reduces atelectrauma and allows adequate oxygenation to be achieved using lower tidal volumes. PEEP therefore reduces shearing stress and cytokine release and curtails surfactant depletion. Chest CT imaging of patients with ARDS showed a more homogenous distribution of tidal volume at PEEP of 20 cmH_2O than at lower levels of 0, 5, 10, and 15. There is no easy method of establishing optimal PEEP for each individual patient. Some studies suggest that the patient's pressure/volume curve should be used to determine the lower inflection point ($\Rightarrow$ Fig. 24.7) and set PEEP slightly above that level, but this is time consuming and is subject to considerable observer variability. In reality the level of PEEP used is based on clinical judgement, depending on the patient's body habitus and underlying pathology with the aim of minimizing the Fio_2, and is usually no more than 10 cmH_2O except in patients with ARDS. Clinical trials have failed to show a mortality benefit between low or high PEEP, although there may be a reduction in ventilator days which was greatest in those with more severe lung oedema.

Low tidal volumes

It is now accepted that ventilation with traditional tidal volumes of 10–15 mL/kg is harmful, particularly in patients with pre-existing lung injury. These high tidal volumes often lead to high peak and plateau pressures and significantly increase the risk of both volutrauma and barotrauma. A number of early small studies using lower tidal volumes did not consistently demonstrate any benefit. However, a landmark study by the ARDS network compared a traditional ventilation strategy with tidal volumes of 12 mL/kg and plateau pressures up to 50 cmH_2O with a protective strategy using tidal volumes of 6 mL/kg and plateau pressures less than 30 cmH_2O. PEEP was set according to the Fio_2 and ranged from 4 to 15 cmH_2O. The PEEP and Fio_2 required to maintain oxygenation in the lower tidal volume group was significantly higher. This large multicentre trial was stopped early because interim analysis showed a significantly lower mortality in the protective strategy group. The number of ventilator-free days and nonpulmonary organ failure was also lower in this group.

Most studies of protective ventilation strategies involved patients with established lung injury however large tidal volumes have also been associated with acute lung injury within 5 days of mechanical ventilation in other patient groups without ALI.

Permissive hypercapnia

The use of low tidal volumes often leads to hypercapnia and acidosis. Carbon dioxide causes pulmonary hypertension, vasodilation, reduction in systemic vascular resistance, and tachycardia resulting in an increase in cardiac output. These effects are transient and do not cause myocardial depression in patients without cardiac disease. Hypercapnia increases both end-diastolic and end-systolic volume and can impair left ventricular contractility particularly in conjunction with acidaemia. The vasodilation which normally increases coronary blood flow can decrease perfusion of ischaemic areas. Profound hypercapnia is therefore not recommended in the ischaemic or failing heart.

Oxygenation strategies

Oxygen toxicity

Hyperoxia increases production of oxygen-derived free radicals and causes neutrophil recruitment and the release of inflammatory mediators. Surfactant production is impaired, pulmonary interstitial oedema occurs followed by fibrosis. An increase in intrapulmonary shunting occurs as a result of collapse of unstable alveolar units. High inspired oxygen concentrations (Fio_2) should therefore be avoided if possible, to minimize this risk of dose-related cellular toxicity and reabsorption atelectasis. There is no

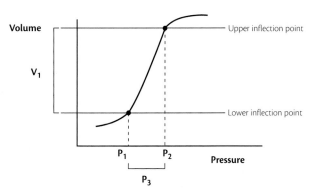

Figure 24.7 Pressure/volume curve to illustrate the lower inflection point. V_1, tidal volume, P_1, PEEP, P_2, maximal desired inflation pressure; P_3, pressure range for ventilation.

evidence-based threshold for Fio_2; recommendations are to take aggressive measures to reduce Fio_2 below 0.65, but limiting airway pressure takes precedence. Lower Sao_2 and Pao_2 should be accepted unless contraindicated.

Recruitment

Recruitment refers to the reinflation of atelectic lung to decrease intrapulmonary shunting and improve oxygenation. The principle is to apply sustained high airway and therefore transpulmonary pressure to open up the collapsed airways and alveoli. CPAP at 10 cmH_2O above plateau pressure is applied for 30–60 s. An alternative protocol is to increase CPAP in a stepwise fashion in increments of 5 cmH_2O for 40 s up to 20 cmH_2O above plateau pressure. Recruitment manoeuvres can be employed by hand using a separate circuit (usually Mapleson C circuit) or through the ventilator if it has an inspiratory hold function. Caution is required because high CPAP reduces venous return, cardiac output and blood pressure inevitably drop and can precipitate a period of cardiovascular instability in susceptible patients.

Inverse ratio ventilation

Increasing inspiratory time in relation to expiratory time so that the I:E ratio is greater than 1 can provide more uniform inflation of alveoli with varying time constants. This can be achieved by increasing the inspiratory time during PCV or by adding an inspiratory pause during VCV (modern ventilators simply allow the I:E to be altered and will adjust the mode settings accordingly). Prolonging inspiratory time can maintain tidal volume and mean airway pressure at lower peak alveolar pressure, and reduces dead space. However, reduced expiratory time can lead to air trapping, barotrauma, and cardiovascular instability.

Prone ventilation

Lung perfusion that favours dependent areas in the supine position becomes more uniformly distributed in the prone position. The normal ventral to dorsal transpulmonary pressure gradient is reversed, resulting in more homogenous ventilation. Patients with any form of ALI exhibit an exaggerated transpulmonary pressure gradient and are more susceptible to atelectasis. Proning significantly improves V/Q matching and improves oxygenation in the majority of patients. The process of turning a patient to the prone position requires much staff input and risks cardiovascular instability as well as dislodgement of tracheal tubes, lines, and chest drains. The main complications are pressure sores and facial and periorbital oedema. Prone ventilation is usually reserved for those with the most severe impairment

in oxygenation, although studies have failed to show a significant mortality benefit. Several contraindications exist, including patients with unstable cardiac rhythms requiring defibrillation or cardiopulmonary resuscitation and those with abdominal or thoracic wounds at risk of dehiscence.

High-frequency oscillatory ventilation

This alternative to conventional ventilation uses sustained lung inflation set as mean airway pressure and extremely high respiratory frequencies of 4–5 Hz (300 breaths/min). An oscillating diaphragm produces a sinusoidal air flow pattern whereby both inspiration and expiration are active. The amplitude required for air flow is proportional to the patient's compliance. Tidal volumes generated are very small, typically less than anatomical dead space, therefore gas transport does not occur by the usual physiological process. A combination of seven potential mechanisms accounts for alveolar ventilation including augmented diffusion, turbulence, and coaxial flow patterns. Minute volume is maintained and hypercapnia does not necessarily occur.

High-frequency oscillatory ventilation (HFOV) improves V/Q mismatch and increases mean airway pressure, thereby improving oxygenation. The lungs are held open and tidal volumes are minimized. In theory this is the ultimate in protective ventilation; however, breath stacking can occur, causing barotrauma. There is no evidence to date that HFOV improves ICU length of stay or survival in adults.

Practical tips

When a patient desaturates, particularly if this occurs rapidly or unexpectedly; there is a sequence of events that should ensue to exclude some common causes. These should only take a few minutes and are not a substitute for full respiratory examination and appropriate investigations.

- 100% oxygen may be required immediately.
- Visual check of patient and ventilator for signs of asynchrony or any other clues.
- Breathing circuit check for disconnection, from endotracheal tube (ETT) to ventilator. Most ICU ventilators sound an alarm if there is a leak, but most portable ventilators do not.
- ETT length check, as endobronchial displacement can occur when the patient is repositioned or the ETT tie

Table 24.5 Complications associated with prolonged mechanical ventilation

Directly associated with MV	Indirectly associated with MV
Upper airway: trauma, oedema, sinusitis	ICU delirium
Tracheal stenosis	GI stress ulceration
Endobronchial tube displacement	Critical illness neuropathy
Atelectasis and *V/Q* mismatch	Critical illness myopathy
VALI	Pressure sores
VAP	Deep venous thrombosis
Reduced CO and hypotension	Reduced splanchnic and renal perfusion

CO, cardiac output; GI, gastrointestinal; MV, mechanical ventilation; VALI, ventilator-associated lung injury; VAP, ventilator-associated pneumonia.

Conclusion

Mechanical ventilation is a important component of the management of many postoperative and critically ill patients. Positive pressure techniques are used in most cases, but there is a role for negative pressure ventilation, e.g. on the paediatric cardiac ICU following complex surgery for congenital heart disease.

A basic comprehension of respiratory physiology and mechanics is essential in order to understand mechanical ventilation. There are numerous ventilation modes and terminology is inconsistent; nevertheless, these can be simplified by classification into their basic elements of phase and control variables. Ventilation itself can induce or exacerbate pre-existing lung injury and lead to multiple organ dysfunction: recommendations for protective lung ventilation therefore aim to minimize this effect. In view of this and improvements in technology, in recent years there has been a resurgence of interest in extracorporeal support in adults for both oxygenation and CO_2 removal.

is replaced. The length at the incisors should be up to 21 cm for women and up to 23 cm for men.

- The suction catheter should be inserted through the whole length of the ETT to check tube patency and to aspirate any secretions or mucus plugs.
- It is useful and often necessary to disconnect the ventilator and 'bag' the patient by hand through a Water's circuit to assess compliance.
- Recruitment manoeuvres should be performed either on the ventilator or manually.
- Following manual recruitment, the ETT can be clamped before reconnection to the ventilator to prevent decruitment.

Personal perspective

The role of cardiac intensive care has expanded rapidly in light of advances in diagnostic and therapeutic strategies in clinical cardiology and cardiac surgery. The increasing availability of sophisticated support mechanisms such as the intra-aortic balloon pump (IABP) and ventricular assist device (VAD) along with developments in cardiac transplantation provide hope for patients with previously irreversible complex and severe cardiac disease. Mechanical ventilation is a crucial component of the care of these patients, but prolonged mechanical ventilation is associated with complications (⮫ Table 24.5) as well as increased morbidity and mortality. Ventilator technology has evolved in line with better understanding of patient–ventilator interactions and the pathophysiology of VALI. HFOV provides protective lung ventilation, better oxygenation, and potentially less cardiovascular instability, but evidence for its efficacy has been lacking. The OSCAR trial comparing conventional PPV with HFOV is currently underway. The use of extracorporeal membrane oxygenation (ECMO) abolishes the need for both ventilation and the cardiac component of oxygen delivery, thereby temporarily 'resting' the cardiorespiratory system and potentially providing time for recovery. The recently published CESAR trial that compared conventional ventilation with extracorporeal membrane oxygenation (ECMO) showed a significant improvement in survival without disability in the ECMO group. Like the majority of adult ventilation studies, these trials are in populations with ALI/ARDS; however, any benefit demonstrated will inevitability generate interest in other patient groups that may be susceptible to lung injury. (Note that all the published trials mentioned in this chapter have attracted criticisms that the reader should be aware of.)

Further reading

Acute Respiratory Distress Syndrome Network (ARDSNet). Ventilation with lower tidal volumes as compared with traditional tidal volumes for acute lung injury and the acute respiratory distress syndrome. *New Engl J Med* 2000;**342**:1301–1308.

Malarkkan N, Snook NJ, Lumb AB. Review article. New aspects of ventilation in acute lung injury. *Anaesthesia* 2003;**58**:647–667.

Mackenzie I. *Core topics in mechanical ventilation.* Cambridge University Press, Cambridge, 2008.

West JB. *Respiratory physiology: the essentials*, 8th edition. Lippincott Williams & Wilkins, Philadelphia, 2008.

Luce, JM. The cardiovascular effects of mechanical ventilation and positive pressure ventilation. *JAMA* 1984; **252**(6):807–811.

Shekerdemian L, Bohn D. Cardiovascular effects of mechanical ventilation. *Arch Dis Child* 1999;**80**:475–480.

Patel P, Clague J, Cordingley J. Case report. Successful use of biventricular pacing to facilitate weaning from mechanical ventilation in a patient with severe left ventricular failure. *Br J Cardiol* 2006;**13**(1):26–28.

Online resources

🔗 Critical Care Tutorials. http://www.ccmtutorials.com

🔗 Standards of Managing Patients after Cardiac Arrest. http://www.ics.ac.uk

➲ For additional multimedia materials please visit the online version of the book (🔗 http://www.esciacc.oxfordmedicine. com).

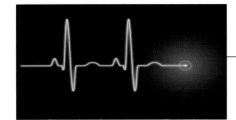

CHAPTER 25

Temporary pacing

Bulent Gorenek

Contents

Summary

Temporary pacing is a life-saving procedure for patients in the intensive cardiac care unit (ICCU). As symptomatic bradycardias and severe conduction disturbances may occur in many acute cardiac care settings, temporary pacing can be necessary to treat acute myocardial infarction patients, patients undergoing percutaneous coronary intervention, and patients with sinus node dysfunction. This type of pacing can also be considered useful to terminate or suppress some supraventricular and ventricular arrhythmias in the ICCU. Single chamber, dual chamber, and biventricular pacing are available. When haemodynamic support is required, physiological pacing is preferred.

Typically, temporary pacing can be easily carried out in most acute cardiac care cases; however, occasionally transvenous pacing electrodes may need to be placed. Optimally, this procedure is performed under fluoroscopy, but electrode catheters can also be inserted without fluoroscopy, using ECG monitoring.

Methods of temporary pacing include transvenous pacing, external pacing, and transoesophageal pacing. Transvenous pacing is the most common method. Although this method is safe and easy, some complications may occur either during or after the operation related to venous access, implanted electrode catheters, and the electrical performance of the device.

Introduction

Conduction disturbances are notable problems for many intensive cardiac care unit (ICCU) patients. These include partial and complete bundle branch blocks, various degrees of atrioventricular (AV) block, and sinus node dysfunction.

All of these events are particularly well recognized complications of acute myocardial infarction (MI). Sinus bradycardia is common in the first hours, especially in inferior infarction. It is estimated that approximately 20% of patients with an acute MI develop AV block [1–3], which can be induced either by ischaemia and necrosis of the conduction system or by autonomic imbalance. Patients with peri-infarction AV block have a higher in-hospital and late mortality than those with preserved AV conduction. The increased mortality is related to the extensive myocardial damage that is required to develop heart block, rather than to the heart block itself.

The management of patients with conduction disturbances after an MI depends in part on the location of the infarct. High degree AV block that is associated with inferior wall MI is located above the bundle of His in 90% of patients [4, 5]. As a result, third degree AV block often results in only a modest and usually transient bradycardia, with escape rhythm rates above 40 beats/min. However, high degree AV block that is associated with anterior MI is more often located below the AV node [4], is usually symptomatic, and has been associated with a higher mortality rate.

Patients at high risk of developing advanced degrees of conduction block or cardiac arrest are candidates for temporary pacing, and this is considered to be a necessary skill for every cardiologist. Temporary pacing was first accomplished transcutaneously by Zoll in 1952 [6] and transvenously by Furman in 1958 [7]. Pacing techniques have since been refined and new pacing modalities have been developed. The goal of temporary cardiac pacing in the ICCU is to restore effective cardiac depolarization and myocardial contraction, resulting in the delivery of adequate cardiac output.

In this chapter, we review the indications and methods of temporary pacing in the ICCU.

Indications

The indications for temporary pacing are less certain than those for permanent pacing. Indeed, there is no clear consensus on many of the indications for temporary pacing, with most recommendations coming from clinical experience rather than from clinical trials. Various authorities differ slightly when defining the indications.

Patients with acute myocardial infarction

Temporary pacing is necessary for patients with symptomatic bradycardias, but should also be considered for those at high risk of developing third degree AV block as a consequence of acute MI. Most physicians think that patients with third degree AV block and a wide QRS complex escape rhythm require a temporary pacemaker, even though symptoms are absent. The same is true of new onset

type 2 second degree AV block. Temporary pacing is also indicated in trifascicular block. However, there is no common consensus for the use of temporary pacing in patients with bifascicular block, which carries a 15–31% risk of progression to second or third degree AV block in acute MI [8, 9]. First degree AV block requires no treatment. A new left bundle branch block usually indicates extensive anterior infarction, with a high likelihood of developing complete AV block and pump failure. The preventive placement of a temporary pacing electrode may be warranted.

Temporary pacing may also need to be considered if the patient with acute MI experiences episodes of asystole, or develops ventricular tachycardia or fibrillation in response to bradycardia. Bradycardia-induced sustained ventricular arrhythmias can be prevented by rapid pacing in acute MI patients. One example is torsades des pointes (TdP) that is associated with a long QT interval. Atrial or ventricular pacing at higher rates can prevent the initiation of TdP by shortening the QT interval and by preventing ventricular ectopic beats that might initiate the tachycardia.

The administration of thrombolytic therapy is a priority in acute MI, and it should not be delayed by the need to insert a temporary pacing electrode catheter. If necessary in the bradycardic patient, temporary transcutaneous pacing can be instituted while thrombolytic therapy is being given.

Although pacing has not been shown to increase long-term survival, it may still be indicated in symptomatic bradyarrhythmias that are associated with acute MI. Recommendations regarding temporary transvenous pacing in the setting of acute MI were included in the 1996 ACC/AHA guidelines for the management of patients with ST-elevation MI (⊃ Table 25.1) [10]. No changes in the recommendations were made in the new version of the guidelines. The recommendations for temporary pacing are clearer and briefer in the 2008 ESC Guidelines for the Management of Acute MI in patients presenting with persistent ST-segment elevation (⊃ Box 25.1) [11].

Patients undergoing percutaneous coronary intervention

New conduction defects occur in approximately 1% of the patients that undergo percutaneous coronary intervention (PCI) [12]. Right bundle branch blocks are the most common conduction disturbances in these patients, and this is followed by first degree AV block. Although these defects almost always disappear without treatment before the time of hospital discharge, they occasionally require the elimination of the drugs that depress cardiac activity [13].

Table 25.1 Recommendations for temporary transvenous pacing in acute MI

Class I	1. Asystole
	2. Symptomatic bradycardia (includes sinus bradycardia with hypotension and type I second degree AV block with hypotension not responsive to atropine)
	3. Bilateral BBB (alternating BBB or RBBB with alternating LAFB/LPFB) (any age)
	4. New or indeterminate age bifascicular block (RBBB with LAFB or LPFB, or LBBB) with first degree AV block
	5. Mobitz type II second degree AV block
Class IIa	1. RBBB and LAFB or LPFB (new or indeterminate)
	2. RBBB with first degree AV block
	3. LBBB, new or indeterminate
	4. Incessant VT, for atrial or ventricular overdrive pacing
	5. Recurrent sinus pauses (>3 s) not responsive to atropine
Class IIb	1. Bifascicular block of indeterminate age
	2. New or age-indeterminate isolated RBBB
Class III	1. First degree heart block
	2. Type I second degree AV block with normal haemodynamics
	3. Accelerated idioventricular rhythm
	4. Bundle branch block or fascieular block known to exist before acute MI

AV, atrioventricular; BBB, bundle branch block; LAFB, left anterior fascicular block; LBBB: left bundle branch block, LPFB, left posterior fascicular block; MI, myocardial infarction; RBBB, right bundle branch block; VT, ventricular tachycardia.
ACC/AHA Classification:
Class I: Conditions for which there is evidence and/or general agreement that a given procedure or treatment is useful and effective.
Class II: Conditions for which there is conflicting evidence and/or a divergence of opinion about the usefulness/efficacy of a procedure or treatment.
Class IIa: Weight of evidence/opinion is in favour of usefulness/efficacy.
Class IIb: Usefulness/efficacy less well established by evidence/opinion.
Class III: Conditions for which there is evidence and/or general agreement that the procedure/treatment is not useful and in some cases may be harmful.
Data from *J Am Coll Cardiol*. 1996;**28**:1328–1428.

Box 25.1 Recommendations for temporary pacing in acute phase of ST-segment elevation

Class I

- Sinus bradycardia associated with hypotension, if failed response to atropine
- AV block II (Mobitz 2) or AV block III with bradycardia that causes hypotension or heart failure, if atropine fails

ESC Classification: Class I: Evidence and/or general agreement that a given treatment or procedure is beneficial, useful, effective.
Adapted from *Eur Heart J* 2008;**29**:2909–2945.

Conduction disturbances are more common in acute MI patients undergoing primary PCI. In a study published a few years ago, 6.3% of acute MI patients developed third degree AV block. In 86.3% of these cases, the block occurred before or during PCI, and in 94.5% of the patients resolution of the block occurred in the catheterization laboratory [14].

When third degree AV block develops, atropine (though rarely helpful in the setting of inadequate escape and deterioration) should be given. Coughing may help support the circulation and maintain consciousness while a temporary pacing catheter is inserted.

Sinus node dysfunction

In sinus node dysfunction, when there are signs or symptoms of haemodynamic compromise, temporary pacing may be necessary if intravenous atropine administration fail to stabilize the patient. Patients with compromised sinus node function may develop sinus nodal depression following drug therapy with antiarrhythmic drugs in the ICCU. Therapy with these agents can be carried out more safely if a temporary pacemaker is inserted to prevent drug-induced bradycardia and circulatory decompensation; permanent pacing is frequently required, and its early use in selected patients can avoid the need for the additional invasive procedure of temporary pacing [15].

In a tachycardia–bradycardia syndrome, there is often an oscillation between rapid rates that are due to atrial fibrillation and slow rates that are caused by sinus bradycardia. The slow sinus rates can result in atrial fibrillation as an escape arrhythmia; maintenance of a faster heart rate with pacing may prevent this.

Prevention, diagnosis, and termination of tachycardias

Temporary pacemakers can be used for the prevention of pause-dependent ventricular tachycardias, which may occur in some patients with long QT syndrome, with the use of antiarrhythmic drugs, and also in acute MI.

Pacing may also be used for the differential diagnosis of tachycardias. In patients with wide complex tachycardia, an atrial recording may differentiate between ventricular tachycardia and supraventricular tachycardia with aberrancy. The atrial recording may be either transvenous or transoesophageal.

Overdrive antitachycardia pacing is a method that is used to terminate a tachycardia by pacing at a rate faster than the tachycardia. It may be helpful for the acute management of patients with frequent recurrent episodes, particularly when drug therapy is ineffective. Although this method is not effective in converting atrial fibrillation to the sinus rhythm, many supraventricular re-entrant tachycardias can be terminated by pacing techniques if the pathway is susceptible to penetration by exogenous electrical stimuli, a phenomenon known as entrainment [16–18]. Re-entrant arrhythmias that can be interrupted following entrainment include sinus node re-entrant tachycardia, AV nodal re-entrant tachycardia, atrial tachycardia, atrial flutter, and AV re-entrant tachycardia [15, 19–23]. Re-entrant monomorphic ventricular tachycardia can also be ended by antitachycardia pacing. However, ventricular tachycardia rates that exceed 200 beats/min might be more likely to be accelerated by antitachycardia pacing, and subsequently deteriorate into ventricular fibrillation.

There are no known contraindications to the use of temporary pacing as a therapeutic or prophylactic modality. Nevertheless, certain relative contraindications may exist in any given patient. Among others, the application of asynchronous pacing in competition with an intrinsic rhythm may provoke arrhythmias in electrically unstable individuals.

Methods of temporary pacing

Methods of temporary pacing include transvenous (endocardial) pacing, external (transcutaneous) pacing, and transoesophageal pacing.

Transvenous (endocardial) pacing

Although transvenous pacing is the most reliable pacing method available, its effective use requires an invasive procedure as well as an experienced operator [23, 24].

Modes of pacing

A number of pacing modes are available for temporary use; pacing can be single chamber (atrial or ventricular), or dual chamber.

Single chamber pacing

In a single chamber temporary pacing, only one electrode catheter is placed into a chamber of the heart. Usually it is placed into a ventricle, but occasionally an atrium is used.

Ventricular pacing is the most commonly used pacing mode in the ICCU. The advantages of ventricular pacing include the requirement for only a single electrode catheter and the ability to protect the patient from dangerous bradycardias. However, ventricular pacing cannot maintain AV synchrony, and a lack of AV synchrony can result

in 'pacemaker syndrome', which can be defined as a loss of AV synchrony, retrograde ventriculoatrial conduction, and absence of a rate response to physiological need. Atrial pacing is appropriate for patients with sinus node dysfunction who have intact AV nodal function or for termination of some of supraventricular tachycardias.

Dual chamber pacing

In dual chamber pacing, electrode catheters are placed in two chambers of the heart. One paces the atrium and the other paces the ventricle. This approach more closely matches the natural pacing of the heart, and this type of pacing can coordinate function between the atria and ventricles.

This was demonstrated by Murphy and colleagues in 1992; temporary ventricular pacing at 80 beats/min was found to be no better than spontaneous bradycardia, whereas dual chamber pacing resulted in improved cardiac output, blood pressure, and falls in pulmonary wedge pressure and right atrial pressure [25]. This would suggest that temporary pacing should generally be AV synchronous in the presence of normal sinus node activity; however, despite these findings, the more complex procedure associated with temporary transvenous dual chamber has led to the continued routine use of ventricular pacing in the temporary setting [26].

Biventricular pacing

Temporary biventricular pacing may improve cardiac performance in patients with major intraventricular conduction block and severe heart failure that is related to left ventricular dysfunction [27]. A transvenous pacing catheter placed in a coronary vein via the coronary sinus may improve heart failure symptoms in these patients. It was demonstrated that this mode of pacing may provide short-term benefit to selected patients in cardiogenic shock [28]. Moreover, responses to this therapy may also help to determine the benefit of a permanent biventricular pacing. However, clinical experience on the use of temporary biventricular pacing is limited, and this method does not change the mortality rate within the ICCU.

Electrode catheters (leads)

The tip of a bipolar temporary pacing electrode catheter has a distal tip electrode and a proximal ring electrode. As cathodal pacing has a lower threshold, it is customary to give negative polarity to the tip and positive polarity to the ring electrode. The proximal connectors of the electrode catheter are connected to an external pacemaker.

Temporary pacing electrode catheters are classified as flexible, semifloating, or nonfloating catheters. The last group carries a higher risk of cardiac perforation, and thus they are generally used only under fluoroscopic guidance, where their stiffness yields the benefit of easier manipulation [29]. In emergency situations, a semifloating catheter with or without a balloon tip is used most commonly [29–31]. In patients who are experiencing cardiac arrest, inflating the balloon carries no benefit; this is because there is no forward flow of blood to guide an inflated balloon through the venous system into the right side of the heart [32].

Most manufacturers misguidedly pack their temporary ventricular electrodes with a near 90° bend fashioned at the tip, often with a stiff former to keep this shape. This does not aid placement of the electrode. Ideally there should be a 20–30° curve at the tip, and it may be necessary to straighten some of the bend out of the electrode before insertion [33].

The external generator

The external pacing generator is used to deliver the electrical current through the pacing catheter. The various available generators share the same basic features; these allow adjustment of the pacing output, pacing rate, pacing mode, and sensitivity to intrinsic activity. Dual chamber generators will allow greater flexibility in pacing mode and will enable adjustment of atrioventricular delay and refractory periods [26].

Generators can either be small enough to allow the patient to be ambulant, or require to be placed at the bedside. Batteries must be checked at least daily and the generator sited so that it cannot fall and exert traction on the pacing electrode catheter. Spare batteries should be kept available at all times. It is recommended that new batteries be used with each patient. Low battery condition is usually signalled by a flashing red light during sensing or pacing. When this occurs, the batteries should be replaced without delay. Some generators may also offer high rate pacing to allow overdrive pacing of tachyarrhythmias [26].

Implantation procedure

The implantation can be done at the bedside in the ICCU or in a specially equipped room near the ICCU. The equipment needed for implantation includes an introducer sheath, electrode catheter, and external generator. An ECG machine and a cardiac monitor should also be available. Once all the equipment has been assembled, the patient is prepared in the usual sterile fashion. A wide area should be cleaned, and the patient should be generously draped to ensure that all the equipment remains in a sterile field [32].

Venous access may be achieved via the internal jugular, external jugular, subclavian, antecubital, or femoral veins.

The choice of venous access site may depend on physician preference or experience, and on the urgency of the clinical situation. The subclavian route should be avoided following fibrinolysis or in the presence of antithrombin therapy. If a permanent pacemaker is anticipated, the left subclavian site should generally be reserved, and a different site should be used for temporary pacing. The right internal jugular and left subclavian veins may be accessed quickly in an emergency, and they may afford direct passage of the pacing catheter to the right ventricular apex without requiring fluoroscopic imaging [24].

For electrode catheter placement, fluoroscopy can be used. However, many physicians prefer the blind technique in the ICCU because it is faster and technically less complex. To perform the blind procedure, the catheter electrodes are connected directly to the pacing generator. The catheter is then inserted and the generator turned on.

Temporary atrial pacing electrode catheters have a pre-shaped J curve to enable positioning in the right atrial appendage. This necessitates an approach from a superior vein, and positioning is greatly assisted by a lateral screening facility on fluoroscopy. The tip of the electrode catheter should point forward, with the J shape slightly opened out when slight traction is applied; unless this is achieved, it is unlikely that the electrode catheter will be stable [26].

After positioning the electrode catheter, the chamber must be paced 10 beats/min above the patient's rate, and then the amplitude of the voltage delivered is slowly turned down until capture is lost. Capture is the depolarization and resultant contraction of the atria or ventricles in response to a pacemaker stimulus. Threshold is the minimum voltage needed for capturing the chamber paced. Ideally, the ventricular capture threshold should be lower than 1 mA. The output should be set at 3–5 times the capture threshold [24].

Sensing is the ability of the pacemaker to sense an intrinsic electrical signal, which depends upon the amplitude, slew rate, and frequency of the signal. The sensing threshold should also be measured if intrinsic ventricular activity is present. Following the positioning of either or both of the electrode catheters, they must be secured to the skin to prevent displacement by movement or traction [26].

Complications

Complications occur in over 20% of patients treated with temporary pacemakers [34]. These are related to venous access, electrode catheters, and the electrical performance of the device.

Venous access-related complications include pneumothorax, haemothorax, and air embolism. The risk of pneumothorax is related to the experience of the implanter, and the number and difficulty of subclavian punctures. Pneumothorax is often small, asymptomatic, and noted incidentally on follow-up chest radiography. However, tension pneumothorax should always be part of the differential diagnosis when hypotension or pulseless electrical activity ensues during an implantation. Haemothorax results from trauma to the great vessels [35]. Special care with regard to catheter insertion and manipulation should be taken in order to prevent air embolism, especially in patients with coexisting pulmonary disease, in whom coughing may increase the likelihood of venous air embolism. Massive air embolism, which is very rare, is potentially fatal and should be recognized and treated promptly.

Electrode catheter-related complications include perforation, dislodgement, diaphragmatic stimulation, malpositioning [36], and catheter-induced arrhythmias. Perforation, which is very rare, can involve the great vessels, right atrium, or right ventricle. It usually occurs without serious sequelae. However, a most devastating manifestation is cardiac tamponade, which requires prompt diagnosis and pericardiocentesis. An initial suspicion should be evaluated by fluoroscopy of the heart border, which is an immediately available diagnostic method. Confirmation of the diagnosis is obtained by emergent bedside echocardiography. Electrode catheter dislodgement takes place in 2–5% of implants, usually in the first 24–48 h postimplant. Intermittent undersensing or loss of capture on postimplant telemetry should prompt consideration of this complication. Definitive correction needs electrode catheter repositioning or replacement. Diaphragmatic stimulation results from phrenic nerve stimulation. Screening for this complication by pacing at maximum outputs is a requisite part of correct implantation procedure. Malpositioning is diagnosed by unacceptable implant pacing, sensing, or defibrillation thresholds. The presence of an atrial or ventricular septal defect can allow the passage of an electrode catheter to the left heart, which is one of the most common causes of malpositioning. Passage into the left heart is more common with ventricular electrode catheters [35]. The operator must be alert to the resultant-paced ECG–QRS complex morphology. If a right bundle is involved, a left-sided ventricular lead position should be excluded. Various arrhythmias, including ventricular tachycardia and ventricular fibrillation, may also occur in some patients as an electrode catheter-related complication which requires repositioning of the electrode catheter. Rarely, such arrhythmias (when they are frequent) do not allow the electrode catheter to be placed [35].

Some complications may be related to the electrical performance of the pacemaker electrode catheter and generator (➲Boxes 25.2–25.4). If pacing suddenly fails, the connections to the external generator, generator batteries, and the possibility of oversensing must be checked. If pacing spikes can be seen but no capture occurs, the output should be increased and consideration should be given to repositioning or replacing the electrode [26].

External (transcutaneous) pacing

Chest wall electrodes with a high impedance interface are required for external pacing. Although these can be used during an asystolic cardiac arrest, there is little evidence that external pacing is successful in this setting. Most hospital and prehospital studies report no long-term survivors from asystole when using external pacing.

Another possible indication is use as a standby therapy for patients at high risk of developing a symptomatic bradycardia. The available external pacemaker systems are suitable for providing standby pacing in acute MI, especially for those not requiring immediate pacing and at only moderate

---

Box 25.2 Causes of loss of capture[a]

- Perforation
- Electrode catheter dislodgement
- Electrode catheter fracture
- Generator malfunction or battery depletion
- Generator-lead connection problems
- Poor endocardial contact
- Local myocardial necrosis or inflammation
- Hypoxia—acidosis
- Electrolyte disturbances

[a] Depolarization and resultant contraction of the atria or ventricles in response to a pacemaker stimulus.

Box 25.3 Causes of undersensing[a]

- Perforation
- Inadequate cardiac signal
- Exit block
- Electrode catheter dislodgement
- Electrode catheter fracture
- Generator malfunction or battery depletion
- Local myocardial necrosis or inflammation

[a] Failure of the pacemaker circuitry to sense intrinsic P- or R-waves.

Box 25.4 Causes of oversensing[a]

- Myopotentials
- Electromagnetic interference
- Extrasystoles
- Electrode catheter dislodgement
- Electrode catheter fracture
- Generator malfunction

[a] The sensing of events other than P- or R-waves by the pacemaker circuitry.

---

risk of progression to AV block. These do not entail the difficulty in application and risk of complications of intravenous systems. External pacing technology is also well suited to patients receiving thrombolytic therapy, as it reduces the need for vascular interventions. Recommendations regarding temporary transcutaneous pacing in the setting of acute MI were included in the 1996 ACC/AHA guidelines for the management of patients with ST-elevation MI (➲Table 25.2) [10].

This method can also be used to terminate some sustained tachycardias. Single and multiple beat pacing stimulation have been described as a useful treatment for these arrhythmias.

Despite some advantages, external pacing is not a preferred pacing technique for many physicians. In addition to causing significant discomfort, sedation or a state of unconsciousness is required to use this approach effectively for more than back-up or emergency pacing.

Transoesophageal pacing

A transoesophageal pacemaker electrode catheter can be used for atrial and ventricular pacing. Depending on the type of catheter used, it can be inserted through the mouth or the nose. This technique has been used to convert supraventricular tachycardias, such as atrial flutter. It results in the immediate restoration of the sinus rhythm in 15–50% of patients with atrial flutter. Moreover, an additional 40% convert to sinus rhythm after a transient period of atrial fibrillation. Oesophageal ventricular pacing has also been well described. However, the use of transoesophageal pacing is not common in daily practice as the catheter is uncomfortable to place, pacing is usually unreliable, and pain is common because it requires a high current for capture.

Table 25.2 Recommendations for placement of transcutaneous patches[a] and active (demand) transcutaneous pacing[b] in acute MI

Class I	1. Sinus bradycardia (rate <50 beats/min) with symptoms of hypotension (systolic blood pressure less than 80mm Hg) unresponsive to drug therapy[b]
	2. Mobitz type II second degree AV block[b]
	3. Third degree heart block[b]
	4. Bilateral BBB (alternating BBB, or RBBB and alternating LAFB, LPFB (irrespective of time of onset)[a]
	5. Newly acquired or age-indeterminate LBBB, LBBB and LAFB, RBBB, and LPFB[a]
	6. RBBB or LBBB and first degree AV block[a]
Class IIa	1. Stable bradycardia (systolic blood pressure >90 mmHg, no haemodynamic compromise, or compromise responsive to initial drug therapy)[a]
	2. Newly acquired or age-indeterminate RBBB[a]
Class IIb	1. Newly acquired or age-indeterminate first degree AV block[a]
Class III	1. Uncomplicated acute MI without evidence of conduction system disease

AV, atrioventricular; BBB, bundle branch block; LAFB, left anterior fascicular block; LBBB, left bundle branch block; LPFB, left posterior fascicular block; MI, myocardial infarction; RBBB, right bundle branch block.
For ACC/AHA Classification, see ➲ Table 25.1.
[a] Apply patches and attach system; system is in either active or standby mode to allow immediate use on demand as required. If transvenous pacing or expertise are not available to place an IV system, consideration should be given to transporting the patient to a facility equipped and competent in placing transvenous systems.
[b] Transcutaneous patches applied; system may be attached and activated within a brief time if needed. Transcutaneous pacing may be very helpful as an urgent expedient. Because it is associated with significant pain, high-risk patients likely to require pacing should receive a temporary pacemaker.
Data from *J Am Coll Cardiol* 1996;**28**:1328–1428.

Conclusion

Temporary pacing is a potentially life-saving intervention that is used primarily to correct profound bradycardia and conduction disturbances. Any patient with acute haemodynamic compromise that is caused by bradycardia or episodes of asystole should be considered for temporary cardiac pacing in the ICCU. The procedure needs the appropriate instruments, a sterile environment, trained support staff, and good quality fluoroscopy equipment. However, the blind technique is preferred in the ICCU by many physicians, because it is faster and technically less complex. Despite the advances in techniques, the complication rates remain high, and operators should do their best to minimize the risk of complications.

Personal perspective

The benefits of temporary pacing in patients with severe conduction disturbances are well known. Although the techniques of cardiac pacing have been developed since 1958, there are still some problems with temporary pacing. In the future, I believe that easier and faster electrode catheter placement methods will be developed, in particular for use in the ICCU. More steerable electrode catheters will be used routinely. Noninvasive pacing methods will become more comfortable and more effective. Furthermore, physiological pacing modes will be preferred to ventricular pacing. The use of temporary biventricular pacing in patients with severely reduced left ventricular function is a new therapeutic measure. The results obtained from small studies provide hope for the use of biventricular pacing, which appears to be haemodynamically beneficial in selected patients.

Further reading

Echt DS, Cowan MW, Riley RE, Brisken AF. Feasibility and safety of a novel technology for pacing without leads. *Heart Rhythm* 2006;**3**:1202–1206.

Fitzpatrick A, Sutton R. A guide to temporary pacing. *BMJ* 1992;**304**:365–369.

Gammage MD. Temporary cardiac pacing. *Heart* 2000;**83**:715–720.

Ganz LI. Temporary cardiac pacing. *Card Electrophysiol Rev* 1999;**2**:389–392.

Hamad MA, van Gelder BM, Bracke FA, *et al*. Acute hemodynamic effects of cardiac resynchronisation therapy in patients with poor left ventricular function during cardiac surgery. *J Card Surg* 2009;**24**:585–590.

Harrigan RA, Chan TC, Moonblatt S, *et al*. Temporary transvenous pacemaker placement in the Emergency Department. *J Emerg Med* 2007;**32**:105–111.

Lee KL, Tse HF, Echt DS, Lau CP. Temporary leadless pacing in heart failure patients with ultrasound-mediated stimulation energy and effects on the acoustic window. *Heart Rhythm* 2009;**6**:742–748.

Ryan TJ, Anderson JL, Antman EM, *et al*. ACC/AHA guidelines for the management of patients with acute myocardial infarction. A report of the American College of Cardiology/ American Heart Association Task Force on Practice Guidelines (Committee on Management of Acute Myocardial Infarction). *J Am Coll Cardiol* 1996;**28**:1328–1428.

Silver MD, N Goldschlager. Temporary transvenous cardiac pacing in the critical care setting. *Chest* 1988;**93**:607–613.

Van de Werf F, Bax J, Betriu A, *et al*. Management of acute myocardial infarction in patients presenting with persistent ST-segment elevation: the Task Force on the Management of ST-Segment Elevation Acute Myocardial Infarction of the European Society of Cardiology. *Eur Heart J* 2008; **29**:2909–2945.

Online resource

∽ UpToDate in Pulmonary, Critical Care, and Sleep Medicine. http://www.uptodate.com/home/clinicians/specialties/ pulmonary.html

↪ For additional multimedia materials please visit the online version of the book (∽ http://www.esciacc.oxfordmedicine. com).

CHAPTER 26

Pericardiocentesis

Bernhard Maisch, Arsen Ristic,
and Konstatinos Karatolios

Contents

Summary

Pericardiocentesis guided either by fluoroscopy or by echocardiography, and subsequent drainage, is a live-saving measure in patients with acute or chronic tamponade of different pericardial syndromes. Subsequent evacuation avoids lethal cardiac compression. It has to be carried out most frequently for effusions of neoplastic origin, followed by infective or autoreactive aetiology, rarely but then acutely in pericardial haemorrhage following cardiac interventions. Subsequent pericardial fluid analysis by histochemistry, cytology, and microbiology, and additional epi- and pericardial biopsy for (immuno)histology and microbiology (polymerase chain reaction for infective agents) guided by pericardioscopy add important information to the underlying aetiology of the effusion and may permit causative intrapericardial treatment in addition to systemic therapy.

Introduction: anatomy and function of the pericardium

The normal pericardium as a double-layered membrane consists of an outer fibrous cover and an inner serous sac, which is invaginated by the heart. The serous pericardium has a visceral layer, the epicardium which covers the heart and the great vessels, and a parietal layer at the inner side of the fibrous pericardium. The pericardium fixes the heart in its proper anatomical place; prevents excessive motion with changes in body position; prevents sudden dilatation of the cardiac chambers during exercise and hypervolaemia; facilitates atrial filling during ventricular systole; and minimizes friction between the heart and surrounding structures. In addition, it serves as a barrier against the extension of infection and malignancy. It also distributes hydrostatic forces and enforces the diastolic coupling of the ventricles [1].

The capacity of the normal pericardial cavity, a virtual space with a superior, transverse, and oblique sinus and several small recesses, is limited by the size and extensibility of the pericardial sac and the rate of fluid accumulation over time. Fat can be found either outside the pericardial sac as pericardial fat or underneath the visceral layer of the epicardium as epicardial fat. In effusion it can be visualized as a 'halo phenomenon' and serves as hallmark for pericardial puncture [2]. Pericardial innervation functions over the phrenic nerves: vagal fibres are supplied from the oesophageal plexus. Only a small portion of the pericardial surface responds to painful stimuli, e.g. in acute pericarditis. Lymphatic drainage occurs mainly to the anterior mediastinal, tracheobronchial, lateropericardial, and posterior mediastinal lymph nodes and not to the hilar nodes [3, 4].

The normal pericardial fluid is a serous ultrafiltrate of plasma with a lower protein concentration but a relatively higher albumin level than plasma. Its osmolarity is less than that of plasma. In healthy individuals, 15–50 mL of this fluid may be present in the pericardial space [4].

Pericardiocentesis in patients with an effusion gives access to the space between the epicardium and the parietal serous layer of the fibrous pericardium.

Pericardial syndromes

Although idiopathic pericarditis/pericardial effusion is the diagnosis most frequently made in pericardial disorders, it only demonstrates our ignorance or inability to make an aetiologically correct diagnosis. Pericardiocentesis is the chance to make a correct aetiological diagnosis and to start effective intrapericardial treatment based on the correct individual diagnoses. ⊃ Table 26.1 gives an overview of the aetiology, pathogenesis, and pathophysiology of the pericardial syndromes at a tertiary referral centre, which is able to combine different diagnostic measures for a correct diagnosis. In general practice the diagnosis of 'idiopathic' pericarditis still prevails.

Assessment of pericarditis and pericardial effusion

The diagnostic pathway in acute pericarditis according to the European Society of Cardiology (ESC) guidelines [5] follows the sequence of diagnostic tests in ⊃ Table 26.2 and ⊃ Fig 26.1.

Indications for pericardiocentesis and drainage

Indications for pericardiocentesis and drainage according to the ESC guidelines [5] are listed in ⊃ Box 26.1. In principle

each cardiac tamponade, except in aortic dissection, has to undergo timely pericardiocentesis, also every suspected bacterial or purulent pericardial effusion (class I). In aortic dissection the cardiac surgeon has to treat both the dissection and the haemopericardium. In purulent pericardial effusion, extensive saline rinsing by large lumen catheters is advisable. In these cases the cardiac surgeon should be involved as well.

In suspected neoplastic pericardial effusion, pericardiocentesis will also establish the underlying tumour by cytology. It is possible to differentiate neoplastic from radiation-induced effusions in patients with breast or bronchial cancer. Pericardiocentesis is also advisable in large effusions of unknown origin (class IIa) without tamponade [4, 7], although this is not undisputed [8]. In patients with smaller pericardial effusions of unknown origin, the rationale for pericardiocentesis lies in the possibility to clarify the underlying aetiology. It may permit intrapericardial therapy.

Diagnosis of cardiac tamponade

The diagnosis of cardiac tamponade is based on the algorithm described in ⊃ Table 26.3 and ⊃ Fig 26.2. In pregnancy special conditions apply (🔬 26.1), since many pregnant women develop a minimal to moderate clinically silent hydropericardium by the third trimester, but cardiac compression and therefore pericardiocentesis is rare. In these rare cases echocardiographically-guided pericardial puncture should be preferred. Note that caution is necessary in medical therapy; high-dose aspirin may prematurely close the ductus arteriosus. Colchicine is contraindicated in pregnancy.

Standard techniques

Pericardiocentesis should be guided either by fluoroscopy or by echocardiography. In Europe, guidance by fluoroscopy is much more frequent. Echocardiography is carried out immediately before the procedure. It is essential that the operator performing the pericardiocentesis should see the echocardiogram [5].

Strict aseptic conditions, ECG and blood pressure monitoring, and local anaesthesia must be provided. Under sedation with midazolam or diazepam (5–10 mg IV) and under pain management with morphine preceded by metoclopramid the blood pressure has to be monitored closely. Direct ECG monitoring from the puncturing needle is insufficient,

Table 26.1 Aetiology, incidence, and pathogenesis of pericardial syndromes with effusion undergoing pericardiocentesis (n = 300) in the Marburg Registry and from the ESC guidelines or literature

Aetiology	Incidence of pericardiocentesis[a] (%)	Incidence of pericarditis ± effusion[b] (%)
Infectious	All 21	Pericarditis in myocarditis:
-viral (CVB A9, B1–4, Echo B, CMV, EBV, parvo B19, HIV, other	14	~25 in viral myocarditis
Bacterial	7	~10 in endocarditis
Fungal	0	Unknown
Parasitic	0	Unknown
Systemic autoimmune disorders	All 1.5	
Systemic lupus erythematosus	0.5	~30
Rheumatoid arthritis	0.5	~30
Systemic sclerosis	0.5	~50
Type 2 (auto)immune process	all 24	
Rheumatic fever	0	20–50
Postcardiotomy syndrome	1	<20 after operation
Postmyocardial infarction syndrome	0.5	<5 after infarction
Autoreactive pericarditis (or idiopathic)	22.5	~25 in autoreactive myocarditis
Pericardial effusion in diseases of surrounding organs		**Tamponade is rare**
Myocarditis	14.5 (see Infectious aetiology)	~25
Aortic aneurysm	Contraindicated	~5
Lung infarction	0	<1
Hydropericardium in CHF	4	Rare in heart failure and pulmonary hypertension
Paraneoplastic/malignant	43	~5–10
Pericarditis in metabolic disorders		Rare
Uraemia/renal failure	1	Frequent in uraemia
Myxoedema	0.3	~30
Addison's disease	0	Rare
Diabetic ketoacidosis	0.3	Rare
Cholesterol pericarditis	0.3	No data available
Pregnancy	0	Rare. mostly hydropericardium
Traumatic pericarditis		
Direct penetrating injury	0.15	No data available
Indirect injury (by mediastinal irradiation)	5	No data available
Neoplastic pericardial disease		
Primary tumours	0.5	41.5
Secondary metastatic tumours	41	40
Lung carcinoma	25	22
Breast carcinoma	15	15
Leukaemia and lymphoma	0.5	Rare
Other tumours	0.5	No data available
Idiopathic pericarditis	4.0; in other publications often >50%	

CHF, chronic heart failure; DCM, dilated cardiomyopathy; my, myocarditis.

[a] Incidence of pericardiocentesis (n = 300) from the Marburg Registry (in %) [4].

[b] Incidence of pericarditis ± effusion in respective aetiological syndrome or disease (%) from the ESC guidelines [5] or literature (*).

Table 26.2 Diagnostic pathway and sequence of performance in acute pericarditis (level of evidence B for all procedures)

Technique	Characteristic findings
Obligatory (indication class I)	
Auscultation	Pericardial rub (mono-, bi-, or triphasic)
ECG[a]	Stage I: anterior and inferior concave ST-segment elevation. PR segment deviations opposite to P polarity
	Early stage II: ST junctions return to the baseline, PR deviated
	Late stage II: T waves progressively flatten and invert
	Stage III: generalized T wave inversions
	Stage IV: ECG returns to prepericarditis state
Echocardiography	Effusion types B–D (Horowitz [6]) Signs of tamponade
Blood analyses	1. ESR, CRP, LDH, leucocytes (inflammation markers) 2. cTnI, CK-MB (markers of myocardial lesion)[b]
Chest radiograph	Ranging from normal to 'water bottle' heart shadow. Revealing additional pulmonary/mediastinal pathology
Mandatory in tamponade (indication class I), optional in large/recurrent effusions or if previous tests inconclusive (indication class IIa) in small effusions (indication class IIb)	
Pericardiocentesis and drainage	Pericardial fluid cytology, and cultures, PCRs and histochemistry for determination of infection or neoplasia
Optional or if previous tests inconclusive (indication class IIa)	
CT	Effusions, peri-, and epicardium
MRI	Effusions, peri-, and epicardium, myocarditis MRI criteria
Pericardioscopy, pericardial biopsy	Establishing the specific aetiology

[a] Typical lead involvement: I, II, aVL, aVF, and V3–V6. The ST segment is always depressed in aVR, frequently in V1, and occasionally in V2. Occasionally, stage IV does not occur and there are permanent T wave inversions and flattenings. If ECG is first recorded in stage III, pericarditis cannot be differentiated by ECG from diffuse myocardial injury, 'biventricular strain,' or myocarditis. ECG in early repolarization is very similar to stage I. Unlike stage I, this ECG does not acutely evolve and J-point elevations are usually accompanied by a slur, oscillation, or notch at the end of the QRS just before and including the J point (best seen with tall R and T waves - large in early repolarization pattern). Pericarditis is likely if in lead V6 the J point is >25% of the height of the T wave apex (using the PR segment as a baseline).

[b] cTnI (cardiac troponin) is detectable in 32.2–49%, more frequently in younger, male patients, with ST-segment elevation, and pericardial effusion at presentation. An increase beyond 1.5 ng/ml is rare (7.6–22%), and associated with CK-MB elevation. cTnI increase is not a negative prognostic marker regarding the incidence of recurrences, constrictive pericarditis, cardiac tamponade or residual LV dysfunction.

Data from Maisch B, Ristic AD, Seferovic PM, Tsang TSM. *Interventional pericardiology, pericardiocentesis, pericardioscopy, pericardial biopsy, balloon pericardiotomy, and intrapericardial therapy*, Springer, Heidelberg, 2010 and Maisch B, Seferovic PM, Ristic A, *et al*. ESC Guidelines—Guidelines on the diagnosis and management of pericardial diseases. Executive summary. *Eur Heart J* 2004;**25**:587–610.

and without an imaging modality it is also not an adequate safeguard. Right-heart catheterization can be performed simultaneously, not only to monitor the improvement after drainage but also to allow the exclusion of constriction.

Pericardiocentesis guided by fluoroscopy

Pericardiocentesis guided by fluoroscopy is performed in the cardiac catheterization laboratory under local anaesthesia and sedation. The patient should lie in supine position, with the thorax elevated to 45% to increase accumulation of the fluid in lower and frontal portions of the pericardium. However, in patients with large pericardial effusions, pericardiocentesis is also successful without this elevation of the thorax. The subxiphoid approach has been most commonly used, with a long needle directed towards the left shoulder at a 30° angle to the skin (➲ Fig. 26.3). We use a long Touhy needle with a rounded tip. During the puncturing procedure its sharp side is turned to the sternum. It can be twisted by 180° immediately after entry into the pericardial sac. The needle approaches the pericardium slowly and under steady manual aspiration (negative pressure). It is stopped as soon as the effusion is aspirated. During the puncturing process it is helpful to locate the position of the puncturing needle in relation to the diaphragm and the pericardial sac with a small amount of contrast medium. The orientation of the puncturing needle is best when both the lateral and the anterior–posterior view are available. In the lateral view the halo phenomenon clearly marks the epicardial fat pad, which is best seen when the effusion is fairly large (insert in ➲ Fig. 26.3). After the first aspiration of pericardial fluid a soft J-tip guide wire is introduced into the pericardial space. Dilatation of the entry with a 5 or 7 French introducer set follows, then a multi-holed pigtail catheter is advanced. We recommend inserting a second wire as a safety guide wire; it can easily be introduced via a common 7 French introducer sheath when pericardioscopy and epi- or pericardial biopsy is carried out later. In large effusions it is prudent to drain no more than 1 L at the beginning, to avoid acute right ventricular dilatation. The procedural success of pericardiocentesis is high (>90%) in patients with an anterior effusion and an echocardiographically measured pericardial free space of 10 mm or more in diastole [9]. The Marburg Registry reports an overall procedural success of more than 98% in 587 patients with effusions of different sizes, including small effusions [4]. We had no fatal complications, only 6 chamber lacerations out of the 587 procedures, which required a second (successful) puncture of the then somewhat larger pericardial space. In these cases of haemopericardium with no suspicion of

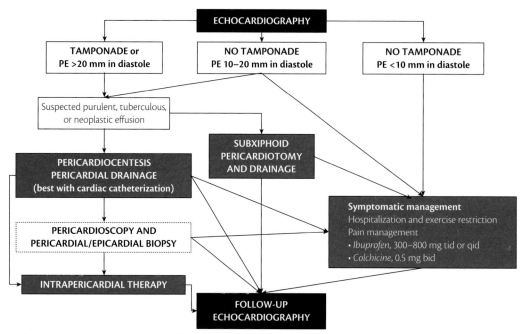

Figure 26.1 Diagnosis and management in acute pericarditis with effusion.
From Maisch *et al* 2004, Guidelines on the diagnosis and management of pericardial diseases. *Eur Heart J* 2004; **25**:587-610.

neoplastic origin we perform concomitant autotransfusion [2, 10, 11] as described later.

Pericardiocentesis guided by echocardiography

Pericardiocentesis guided by echocardiography was introduced into routine clinical practice in the late 1970s, with the Mayo Clinic spearheading this technique [4, 12]. Echo-guided pericardiocentesis was successful in withdrawing pericardial fluid and/or relieving tamponade in 97% of the procedures. It can be performed in the intensive care unit or in operating theatre. Echocardiography should identify the shortest route where the pericardium can be entered intercostally. This is usually in the sixth or seventh intercostal space in the anterior axillary line, from which a straight needle trajectory avoids vital structures. Since ultrasound does not penetrate air, lung injury can be avoided and intercostal arteries remain untouched. Aseptic conditions, adequate local anaesthesia and sedation are mandatory. From the 'ideal' entry side a polytef (PTFE)-sheathed Deseret needle ('intracath', 16–18 gauge, 5.1–3.3 cm length) is advanced in a straight line with an attached saline-filled syringe. The position of the polytef sheath during the procedure can be confirmed at any time from a remote window while agitated saline is injected as echo contrast. After insertion, pericardial pressure can be measured as well. On entering the pericardial fluid, the needle is moved about 2 mm further. The polytef sheath is then advanced over the needle and the steel core is withdrawn. Thus only the

polytef sheath remains in the fluid space. A pigtail catheter is introduced into the pericardial sac via a guide wire.

In the Mayo experience [12] there were a total of 14 major (1.2%) and 40 minor complications (3.5%), including one lethal complication due to haemorrhagic tamponade. Nonfatal complications included chamber lacerations requiring surgery (5), injury to an intercostal vessel necessitating surgery (1), pneumothoraces requiring chest tube placement (5), ventricular tachycardia (1), and bacteraemia possibly related to pericardial catheter placement (1). Minor complications did not require specific treatment. The contraindications to echo-guided pericardiocentesis are similar to those mentioned in ⭢ Table 26.2 for any pericardiocentesis.

Emergency pericardiocentesis

If a cardiac chamber is perforated occurs during pericardial puncture, the perforating catheter should be kept in place. Percutaneous puncture can then be attempted again. If it is successful the perforating catheter can be withdrawn and surgery can be avoided by prompt drainage and autotransfusion of pericardial blood into the femoral vein [13]. Autotransfusion should not be carried out in malignant pericardial effusions after perforation of a ventricle.

Prolonged pericardial drainage

Prolonged pericardial drainage is performed until the volume of effusion obtained by intermittent pericardial

Box 26.1 Indications and contraindications for pericardiocentesis independent of access site or method

Indications

Class I

- Cardiac tamponade
- Effusions >20 mm in echocardiography (diastole)
- Suspected purulent or tuberculous pericardial effusion

Class IIa

- Effusions 10–20 mm in echocardiography in diastole for diagnostic purposes other than purulent pericarditis or tuberculosis (pericardial fluid and tissue analyses, pericardioscopy, and epicardial/pericardial biopsy)
- Suspected neoplastic pericardial effusion

Class IIb

- Effusions <10 mm in echocardiography in diastole for diagnostic purposes other than purulent; neoplastic, or tuberculous pericarditis (pericardial fluid and tissue analyses, pericardioscopy, and epicardial/pericardial biopsy)

Contraindications (Class III)

Absolute contraindication

- Aortic dissection, myocardial rupture (e.g. in transmural infarction)

Relative contraindications

- These contraindications include uncorrected coagulopathy; anticoagulant therapy; thrombocytopenia <50 000/mm^3; small, posterior, and loculated effusions

Adapted from the ESC guidelines [5].

aspiration (every 4–6 h) falls to less than 25 mL/day. This can last several days. Under these circumstances intravenous antibiotic prophylaxis (e.g. cefalosporin or ampicillin) must be continued at least as long as the intrapericardial pigtail catheter is in place.

Surgical drainage of the pericardium

If the heart cannot be reached by a needle, surgical drainage is required. Usually a subcostal incision will do. In aortic dissection or rupture of a ventricle in transmural infarction, surgical drainage is unavoidable. In loculated pericardial effusion the surgeon can break up adhesions with a finger or a suction device, which is particularly important in purulent pericardial effusion. McDonald *et al.* [14] compared outcomes in a single-institution study with 96 patients undergoing pericardial catheter drainage and 150 patients with subxiphoid surgical drainage. Although no procedural mortality occurred in either condition the in-hospital mortality was significantly higher in the percutaneous group (22.9%) than in the surgical patients (10.7%). Also recurrence rates were seen more frequently (16.5%) in the percutaneous group than in the surgical group (4.6%). It must be borne in mind, however, that in both groups no intrapericardial therapy and no balloon pericardiotomy was applied. The advantage of surgical drainage in this study and the one by Allen *et al.* [15] is that larger samples of tissue were available for diagnosis and that a larger pleuropericardial or abdominopericardial window could be created. The disadvantage is the need for general anaesthesia. The diagnostic advantages described in the surgical studies are nowadays compensated by pericardial and epicardial biopsy sampling under pericardioscopical control. Furthermore, both intrapericardial instillation and balloon pericardiocentesis are now available for the interventional pericardiologist.

Alternative techniques

A small effusion or even a dry pericardium can be entered in specialized centres with devices that are still experimental, such as the Touhy needle, the Perducer or the Marburg PeriAttacher [4]. This can be of particular interest in cases where intrapericardial therapy with few or no systemic side effects is preferable, e.g. in severe forms of fulminant virus-negative myocarditis, eosinophilic myocarditis, or in giant cell myocarditis. In these patients intrapericardial triamcinolone instillation can cure the disease [4]. In patients with severe dysrhythmias, pericardial access to ablation therapy may also be helpful.

Pericardioscopy

Pericardioscopy was first introduced by Maisch *et al.* in 1994 from the subxiphoid access site [10]. Further experience followed, both from cardiologists [7] and from cardiac surgeons [16]. The limited view of the first-generation rigid endoscopes (e.g. rigid 'urethroscopes') has nowadays been expanded by the flexible fibroscopic devices to the entire pericardial space [4]. By use of a flexible 16 French fibroscope the peri- and epicardial surfaces as well as the pericardial space can be visualized (➲ Fig. 26.4) and the targeted sampling of pericardial and epicardial tissue under the control of the naked eye is possible. To avoid any

Table 26.3 Diagnosis of cardiac tamponade

Clinical presentation	Elevated systemic venous pressure[a], hypotension[b], pulsus paradoxus[c], tachycardia[d], dyspnoea, or tachypnoea with clear lungs
Precipitating factors	Drugs (ciclosporin, anticoagulants, thrombolytics, etc.), recent cardiac surgery, indwelling instrumentation, blunt chest trauma, malignancies, connective tissue disease, renal failure, septicaemia[e]
ECG	Can be normal or nonspecifically changed (ST-T wave), electrical alternans (QRS, rarely T), bradycardia (endstage), electromechanical dissociation (agonal phase)
Chest radiograph	Enlarged cardiac silhouette with clear lungs
M mode/2D echocardiogram	Diastolic collapse of the anterior RV free wall[f], RA collapse, LA and very rarely LV collapse, increased LV diastolic wall thickness 'pseudohypertrophy', IVC dilatation (no collapse in inspiration), 'swinging heart'
Doppler	Tricuspid flow increases and mitral flow decreases during inspiration (reverse in expiration)
	Systolic and diastolic flows are reduced in systemic veins in expiration and reverse flow with atrial contraction is increased
M-mode colour Doppler	Large respiratory fluctuations in mitral/tricuspid flows
Cardiac catheterization	1. Confirmation of the diagnosis and quantification of the haemodynamic compromise:
	RA pressure is elevated (preserved systolic x descent and absent or diminished diastolic y descent)
	Intrapericardial pressure is also elevated and virtually identical to RA pressure (both pressures fall in inspiration)
	RV mid-diastolic pressure elevated and equal to the RA and pericardial pressures (no dip-and-plateau configuration)
	Pulmonary artery diastolic pressure is slightly elevated and may correspond to the RV pressure
	Pulmonary capillary wedge pressure is also elevated and nearly equal to intrapericardial and right atrial pressure
	LV systolic and aortic pressures may be normal or reduced
	2. Documenting that pericardial aspiration is followed by haemodynamic improvement
	3. Detection of the coexisting haemodynamic abnormalities (LV failure, constriction, pulmonary hypertension)
	4. Detection of associated cardiovascular diseases (cardiomyopathy, coronary artery disease)
RV/LV angiography	Atrial collapse and small hyperactive ventricular chambers
Coronary angiography	Coronary compression in diastole
CT	No visualization of subepicardial fat along both ventricles, which show tube-like configuration and anteriorly drawn atria

IVC, inferior vena cava; LA, left atrium; LV, left ventricle; RA, right atrium; RV, right ventricle.

[a] Jugular venous distension is less notable in hypovolemic patients or in 'surgical tamponade'. An inspiratory increase or lack of fall of the pressure in the neck veins (Kussmaul sign), when verified with tamponade, or after pericardial drainage, indicates effusive-constrictive disease.

[b] Heart rate is usually >100 beats/min, but may be lower in hypothyroidism and in uraemic patients.

[c] The blood pressure cuff is inflated above the patient's systolic pressure. During slow deflation, the first Korotkoff sound is intermittent. Correlation with the patient's respiratory cycle identifies a point at which the sound is audible during expiration, but disappears when the patient breathes in. As the cuff pressure drops further, another point is reached when the first Korotkoff sound is audible throughout the respiratory cycle. The difference of >10 mmHg in systolic pressure between these two points is accepted as positive pulsus paradoxus. For quick clinical orientation the sign can be also investigated by simply feeling the pulse, which diminishes significantly during inspiration, when the patient is breathing normally. Pulsus paradoxus is absent in tamponade complicating atrial septal defect and in patients with significant aortic regurgitation. Caution: the patient should breathe normally—no deep inspirations.

[d] Occasional patients are hypertensive especially if they have pre-existing hypertension.

[e] Febrile tamponade may be misdiagnosed as septic shock.

[f] Right ventricular collapse can be absent in elevated right ventricular pressure and right ventricular hypertrophy or in right ventricular infarction.

[g] If after drainage of pericardial effusion intrapericardial pressure does not fall below atrial pressure, the effusive-constrictive disease should be considered.

From Maisch B, Seferovic PM, Ristic A, *et al.* ESC Guidelines—Guidelines on the diagnosis and management of pericardial diseases. Executive summary. *Eur Heart J* 2004;**25**:587–610, with permission.

perforation, the fibroscope is moved along a first guide wire, which runs through the endoscope itself. The bioptome is handled via a second working channel. The biopsy can be controlled both by the fibreoptics and by X-ray. In the rare case of a perforation during an epicardial biopsy, a second guide wire positioned outside the fibroscope can be helpful in order to immediately introduce a pigtail catheter to perform the evacuation of blood and to permit autotransfusion from the pericardial space into the femoral vein [5, 13].

Pericardial fluid analysis

Pericardial fluid analysis should be carried out whenever fluid is available. Possible analyses comprise cytology, bacteriology, possibly virology, and immunology as well as simple analysis of the protein content, haemoglobin, electrolytes, cardiac enzymes, and biomarkers or mediators. Specific tests should be ordered according to the clinical presentation and suspicion for the underlying disease [17].

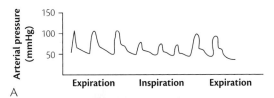

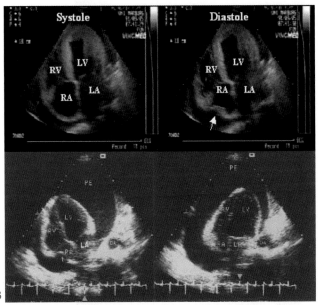

Figure 26.2 Clinical criteria, echocardiography, and pathophysiology of tamponade.
Reproduced from Maisch B, Ristic AD, Seferovic PM, Tsang TSM. *International Pericardiology, Pericardiocentesism Pericardioscopy, Pericardial biopsy, ballon Pericardiotomy, intrapericardial therapy,* Springer, Heidelberg, 2010. With kind permission of Springer Science + Business Media.

The indications for tests in the ESC guidelines [5] have recently been updated, as follows [4].

Class I indication

◆ In suspected malignant disease cytology can ascertain or disprove the neoplastic disease.

◆ In suspected tuberculosis, acid-fast bacilli staining, mycobacterium culture, and polymerase chain reaction (PCR) are obligatory. Adenosine deaminase (ADA; >40 IU/L) [18]), γ-interferon (≥200 pg/L), pericardial lysozyme levels (≥6.5 µg/dL) provide additional diagnostic information [5].

◆ In suspected bacterial infection, at least three cultures of pericardial fluid for aerobes and anaerobes as well as three blood cultures are mandatory. Positive cultures should be followed by sensitivity tests for antibiotics [4, 5].

Class IIa indication

◆ PCR analyses for the RNA or DNA of cardiotropic viruses discriminates viral from autoreactive pericarditis or hydropericardium.

◆ Tumour markers (e.g. carcinoembryonic antigen (CEA), alpha-fetoprotein (AFP), carbohydrate antigens CA 125, CA 72–4, CA 15–3, CA 19–9, CD30, CD25, etc.) give additional information on suspected neoplastic pericarditiseven when cytology for neoplastic cells is unequivocal. Sensitivity and specificity of the intrapericardial values have to be established for each test and compared with serum values.

◆ The combination of epithelial membrane antigen, CEA, and vimentin immunocytochemical staining can be useful to distinguish reactive mesothelial and adenocarcinoma cells.

Class IIb indication

◆ Analyses of the pericardial fluid specific gravity (>1.015), protein level (>3.0 g/dL; fluid/serum ratio >0.5), LDH (>200 mg/dL; serum/fluid >0.6), and glucose (exudates vs transudates = 77.9±41.9 vs. 96.1±50.7 mg/dL) can separate exudates from transudates but are not directly diagnostic [17].

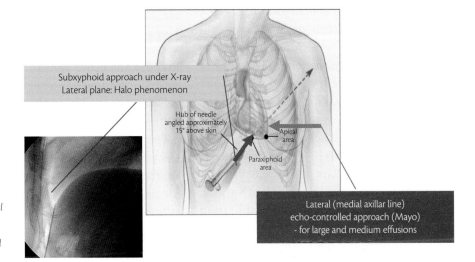

Figure 26.3 Pericardiocentesis and halo phenomenon.
Adapted from Maisch B, Ristic AD, Seferovic PM, Tsang TSM. *Interventional pericardiology, pericardiocentesis, pericardioscopy, pericardial biopsy, balloon pericardiotomy, intrapericardial therapy,* Springer, Heidelberg, 2010.

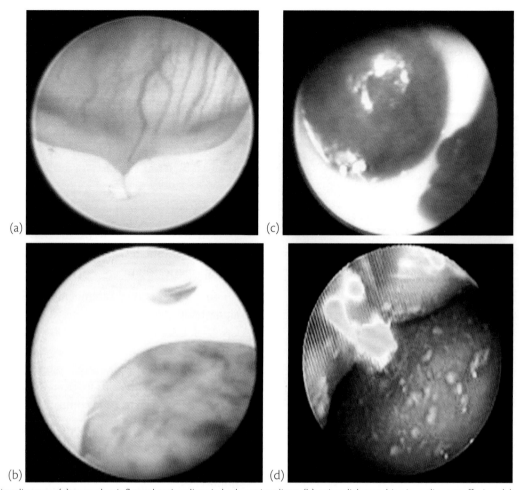

Figure 26.4 Pericardioscopy: (a) normal uninflamed pericardium in hydropericardium; (b) epicardial petechiae in malignant effusion; (c) calcification in tuberculous (epi-) and pericarditis; (d) epicardial biopsy in fibrinous pericarditis.
Reproduced from Maisch B, Ristic AD, Seferovic PM, Tsang TSM. *International Pericardiology, Pericardiocentesism Pericardioscopy, Pericardial biopsy, ballon Pericardiotomy, intrapericardial therapy*, Springer, Heidelberg, 2010. With kind permission of Springer Science + Business Media.

Pericardial and epicardial biopsy

Pericardial [19] and epicardial biopsy [4, 11,20] add relevant information for the aetiology and pathogenesis of the underlying disease, similar to endomyocardial biopsy in inflammatory heart muscle disease or (peri)myocarditis. Since in perimyocarditis the pericardial effusion is in itself already diagnostic for inflammation, the analysis of the biopsy tissue should target the specific aetiology either by specific staining for bacteria (Gram, acid fast) or fungi (fungal staining), or by PCR for cardiotropic agents (e.g. enterovirus, Coxsackie A9 in particular, echo-, adeno-, influenza-, hepatitis C, HIV, parvo B19, human herpesvirus 6, herpes simplex, Epstein–Barr, cytomegalovirus or xenotropic murine leukaemia virus related virus (XMRV), *Borrelia burgdorferi*, *Rickettsia burnetii*), the infiltration of malignant cells, or specific forms of inflammation (e.g. eosinophilic heart disease, Churg–Strauss syndrome,

giant cells, granuloma forming cells, immune complex binding to cardiac structures, etc). For detailed descriptions of these methods, see ➲ Chapter 56 and [4].

Intrapericardial therapy

Evacuation of the pericardial fluid is essential, followed by saline rinsing. Subsequent intrapericardial therapy can be sclerosing and/or causative, thus directly targeting the pathogenetic process.

For sclerosing treatment we introduce 80 mg gentamycin into the pericardial space. Unlike tetracyclines, gentamycin neither causes any pain nor does it increase cardiac enzymes. It has additional local bactericidal effects.

Specific intrapericardial and systemic treatment is summarized in ➲ Table 26.4.

Table 26.4 Specific intrapericardial and systemic treatment of pericardial effusions

Disease/effusion	Intrapericardial treatment	Systemic treatment	Comment
Bronchus carcinoma PE	Cisplatin 50 mg/m² or Thiothepa	Antineoplastic Tx	Prevents recurrence in 85% of cases [21, 11, 4, 5]
Breast cancer PE	Cisplatin 50 mg/m² or Thiothepa	Antineoplastic Tx	Prevent recurrence in 80-85% of cases [21, 11, 4, 5]
Autoreactive PE	Triamcinolone 500 mg/m²	NSAIDs for symptomatic Tx or colchicine 0.5mg three times daily	Prevents recurrence in 85% cases [20]
Giant cell PE, sarcoid PE	Triamcinolone 500 mg/m² or systemic therapy	Azathioprine 50–100mg/m² initial dose, tapering of to 50 mg for 6 m or more	Corticoid treatment is life saving [4]
Bacterial PE	Intensive rinsing with saline, repeated intrapericardial gentamycin	Systemic IV antibiotics (e.g. vancomycin 1 g twice daily, ceftriaxone 1–2 g twice daily, and ciprofloxacin 400 mg/day)	Surgical drainage is advisable [5]
Tuberculous PE	Intensive rinsing with saline, repeated intrapericardial gentamycin or surgery	Systemic tuberculostatic antibiotics (e.g. isoniazid 300 mg/day, rifampicin 600 mg/day, pyrazin-amide 15–30 mg/kg/day, and ethambutol 15–25 mg/kg/day. After 2 months most patients can be switched to two-drug regimen (isoniazid and rifampicin) for a total of 6 months	Check for accompanying HIV infection. In this case add systemic antiretroviral therapy, consider corticoid treatment [22]
Uremic PE	Extensive rinsing, triamcinolone 500 mg/m²		
Fibrotic PE	Urokinase 250–500 U, repeatedly		Only case report available [4, 5]

PE: pericardial effusions; Tx, therapy.

Systemic treatment options

In addition to the specific intrapericardial treatments listed in ➲ Table 26.4, systemic antineoplastic treatment should accompany malignant pericarditis according to current protocols. However, care should be taken to avoid drugs or dosages of drugs with negative effects on cardiac function or arrhythmogenic potential. In tuberculous pericarditis, adequate long-term antituberculostatic treatment possibly accompanied by corticosteroids in double infections with HIV [5, 22], is required. In bacterial pericardial effusion, systemic antibiotic treatment of at least 3–4 weeks is recommended [4, 5].

The mainstay of symptomatic treatment of precordial pain in acute pericarditis are nonsteroidal anti-inflammatory drugs (NSAIDs) [5]. Indomethacine should be avoided in elderly patients because it causes flow reduction in the coronaries. Ibuprofen (300–800 mg three time daily) is preferred for its few side effects, favourable impact on the coronary flow, and large dose range. Colchicine (0.5 mg twice daily) added to an NSAID or as monotherapy also appears to be effective for the initial attack and the prevention of recurrences [23], as shown in the COPE trial [24]. It is well tolerated, with fewer side effects than long-term NSAIDs. Systemic corticosteroids should be restricted to connective tissue diseases, autoreactive or uraemic pericarditis [5]. Intrapericardial application of triamcinolone is effective and avoids systemic side effects [4, 5, 20].

Systemic corticosteroids should be used only in patients in whom viral or bacterial pericardial effusions have been excluded. A common mistake is to use a dose too low to be effective, or to taper the dose too rapidly. The regimen recommended in the guideline is prednisone 1–1.5 mg/kg, for at least 1 month. If patients do not respond adequately, azathioprine (75–100 mg/day) or cyclophosphamide can be added. Corticosteroids should be tapered over a 3-month period. Towards the end of the taper, introduce anti-inflammatory treatment with colchicine (0.5 mg twice or three times daily) or an NSAID [4]. In chronic or recurrent pericarditis, apart from the intrapericardial treatment outlined above, balloon pericardiotomy or pericardiectomy may be considered [4]. In all other cases, particularly in those in whom the aetiology was not established ('idiopathic'), long-term colchicine is recommended. In the patients with 'idiopathic' pericarditis who have been treated with oral corticosteroid therapy, recurrences appear to be more frequent. In these aetiologically poorly characterized patients, low-dose oral cortisone prevents recurrences more effectively than a high dose [25].

Personal perspective

Apart from life-saving emergency pericardiocentesis in patients with tamponade, pericardial access to the heart opens a new diagnostic window for intraperi- and epicardial inspection by pericardioscopy, targeted biopsy, and molecular and immunohistochemical diagnosis. Pericardiocentesis is already becoming the key to pericardial and myocardial treatment by instillation of drugs in a restricted compartment, avoiding systemic side effects, and to ablation or pacemaker therapy.

Further reading

Chamoun A, Cenz R, Mager A, *et al.* Acute left ventricular failure after large volume pericardiocentesis. *Clin Cardiol* 2003;**26**(12):588–590.

Maisch B, Ristic AD, Seferovic PM, Tsang TSM. *Interventional pericardiology, pericardiocentesis, pericardioscopy, pericardial biopsy, balloon pericardiotomy, and intrapericardial therapy,* Springer, Heidelberg, 2010.

Maisch B, Seferovic PM, Ristic A, *et al.* ESC Guidelines—Guidelines on the diagnosis and management of pericardial diseases. Executive summary. *Eur Heart J* 2004;**25**:587–610.

Palacios IF. Pericardial effusion and tamponade. *Curr Treat Options Cardiovasc Med* 1999;**1**:79–89.

Seferović PM, Ristić AD, Maksimović R, Mitrović V. Therapeutic pericardiocentesis: Up-to-date review of indications, efficacy, and risks. In: Seferović PM, Spodick DH, Maisch B (eds.) *Pericardiology: contemporary answers to continuing challenges, Science,* Belgrade, 2000, pp. 417–426.

⟳ For additional multimedia materials please visit the online version of the book (⬙ http://www.esciacc.oxfordmedicine.com).

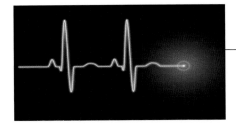

CHAPTER 27

Chest tubes

Karim Tazarourte, Christian Laplace,
and Arthur Atchabahian

Contents

Summary

Percutaneous insertion of chest tubes is routinely performed in surgical wards, in the intensive care unit, in the emergency department, and in pulmonary medicine. Although it has been shown that trained physicians can safely insert chest tubes, severe complications have been described, associated with lack of proper training and/or incorrect insertion or management of chest tubes. The proper technique of thoracic drainage is key for safety and effectiveness. Chest tube insertion is well described, step by step, in the British Thoracic Society (BTS) guidelines. The level of scientific proof of these recommendations ranges from a high level of evidence (level A) to an expert opinion (level C).

Introduction

Despite a long history of clinical use, the role and management of chest tubes and pleural drainage devices remain incompletely defined [1]. The many types of chest tube and the host of clinical indications for their use account for wide variations in the use of these devices. The purpose of pleural drainage is to restore the vacuum of the pleural space: appropriate chest tube size selection depending on the clinical situation is crucial, especially in the case of a tension pneumothorax, a massive haemothorax, or a malignant pleural effusion. The appropriate pleural drainage unit and the timing of chest tube removal are equally important, but remain controversial as well.

Indications and equipment for chest tube insertion

Chest tubes can be used in many clinical situations. The main indications are listed in ➲ Box 27.1. All the equipment required to safely insert a chest tube (listed in ➲ Box 27.2) must be available prior to performing the procedure.

Box 27.1   Indications for chest tube insertion

- Pneumothorax:
  - In all patients mechanically ventilated regardless of the size of the pneumothorax
  - Tension pneumothorax after initial needle aspiration
  - Persistent or recurrent spontaneous pneumothorax after simple aspiration
  - Iatrogenic pneumothorax
  - Traumatic haemopneumothorax regardless of its size
- Malignant pleural effusion
- Postoperative, after cardiac or thoracic surgery

Reproduced with permission from Laws D, Neville E, Duffy J, *et al.* BTS guidelines for the insertion of a chest drain. *Thorax* 2003;**58**:ii53–ii59.

Aseptic technique is essential to avoid wound site infection or empyema and must be used during chest tube insertion (level C evidence; see ➲ Table 27.1).

Predrainage risk assessment

There is no published evidence that abnormal coagulation or platelet count affects bleeding complications of chest tube insertion [1]. However, it is preferable to correct any coagulopathy or platelet defect before chest tube insertion (level C).

Box 27.2   Equipment used for chest tube insertion

- Surgical cap and mask, sterile gloves and gown
- Antiseptic solution for skin disinfection: iodine or chlorhexidine alcohol solution
- Sterile drapes
- Syringes (10 and 20 mL) and intramuscular needles
- Lidocaine 1 or 2%
- Scalpel and blade
- Curved clamp for blunt dissection
- Suture material
- Chest tube, possibly trocar
- Connecting tube
- Closed drainage system (pleural drainage unit or bottle water seal system)
- Sterile dressing

From Laws D, Neville E, Duffy J, *et al.* BTS guidelines for the insertion of a chest drain. *Thorax* 2003;**58**:ii53–ii59.

Table 27.1   Scientific proof level of British Thoracic Society recommendations

A	One or more randomized controlled trial
B	One or more studies with good scientific quality but no randomized controlled trials
C	No studies: expert advice

Reproduced with permission from Laws D, Neville E, Duffy J, *et al.* BTS guidelines for the insertion of a chest drain. *Thorax* 2003;**58**:ii53–ii59.

Analgesia

If the patient is conscious, premedication must be administered. Chest tube insertion has been reported to be a painful procedure, with 50% of patients experiencing pain levels of 9–10 on a 10-point visual analogue pain scale [2]. Premedication with an opioid and a benzodiazepine to achieve adequate analgesia and sedation is recommended. The usefulness of atropine to prevent vasovagal reactions has not been demonstrated [1]. Local anaesthetic should be infiltrated before insertion of the chest tube (level C).

Technique of chest tube insertion

Whenever possible, ultrasound guidance must be used to identify and localize a pleural effusion and to guide chest tube insertion.

Patient position and insertion site

The tube for drainage of a pneumothorax should be placed in the second intercostal space on the midclavicular line. An insertion site that is too medial may injure the internal mammary artery, which is located about 2 cm lateral to the lateral border of the sternum. The disadvantages of this insertion point are the transfixion of the pectoralis major and the highly unsightly scar it causes. However, it is possible to perform the drainage without mobilizing the upper extremity, and the chest tube insertion is far away from the diaphragm. It is imperative to remember that the diaphragm reaches the fifth intercostal space during expiration.

The drainage for fluid or mixed effusions is performed at the fourth intercostal space on the anterior axillary line just lateral to the lateral edge of the pectoralis major muscle. The main risk is to place the chest tube too low and to injure the diaphragm and the underlying abdominal organs (liver, spleen) (➲ Fig. 27.1) [1]. The preferred patient's position is supine, with the operative side propped up and with the ipsilateral arm behind the patient's head to expose the axillary area. A chest tube should never be inserted more caudad or more medial than the nipple, or through the

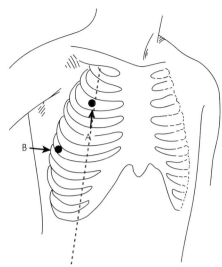

Figure 27.1 Insertion site: A, anterior; B, lateral.

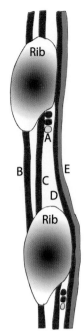

Figure 27.2 Schematic representation of the intercostal space, demonstrating the position of the neurovascular bundle (A) under the lower aspect of the upper rib of the space. The tube should therefore be inserted as close as possible to the upper aspect of the lower rib of the space. B, external intercostal muscle; C, internal intercostal muscle; D, innermost intercostal muscle; E, parietal pleura.

track of a previous surgical drain, or through a traumatic wound. Drawing a vertical line through the midpoint of the clavicle and the nipple and a horizontal line through the nipple defines four quadrants on the anterior thorax of the patient; the entry point for chest drainage should always be in the upper lateral quadrant [1].

Regardless of the insertion site, it must be remembered that the intercostal neurovascular bundle is located on the inferior aspect of the rib, overlying the intercostal space. Therefore, chest tube insertion should always be done as close as possible to the upper aspect of the lower rib of the intercostal space chosen (➲ Fig. 27.2).

Needle decompression

Needle decompression is a salvage procedure. It is performed in cases of gas tamponade associated with a tension pneumothorax or a compressive haemothorax. The indication for decompression is limited to pneumothorax or haemothorax compression that induces respiratory distress and/or circulatory instability [3]. In this situation, the procedure to perform is not drainage, but rather immediate needle decompression. This will confirm the diagnosis and vent the excessive intrapleural pressure. The technique is extremely simple and fast and has no contraindications. After skin disinfection, the puncture is made in the area of resonance at the second intercostal space in the midclavicular line. A trocar-type short 14 gauge venous catheter is mounted on a syringe and the operator inserts the needle perpendicular to the skin. To prevent damage to the neurovascular bundle, the puncture must always be done as close as possible to the cephalad edge of the lower rib of the space. The entry of air under pressure into the syringe

confirms the diagnosis. The air then escapes through the catheter disconnected from the syringe (➲ Fig. 27.3). The pleural space pressure is thus restored to atmospheric pressure and clinical improvement should be immediate. One potential problem with this technique is when the length of the selected trocar is insufficient, especially in an obese patient [3]. The aspiration of the effusion is a procedure that allows salvage decompression of the tamponade but does not drain the effusion completely. It does not bring the lung back to the chest wall. However, by equalizing pleural and atmospheric pressure, it allows adequate ventilation, and performance of the chest drainage in better haemodynamic conditions. Drainage is necessary after the decompression.

Blunt dissection and chest tube insertion

A 1.5–2 cm skin incision is made, and the subcutaneous plane is then bluntly dissected with a curved clamp such as a Kelly clamp (➲ Fig. 27.4). The parietal pleura should be opened by a gloved finger, in order to avoid injuring the underlying lung. Furthermore, when inserting the finger into the pleural cavity it is possible to verify the absence of adhesions around the entry point by rotating the finger 360° around the hole. The key is then to insert the chest tube while avoiding advancement of the trocar beyond the

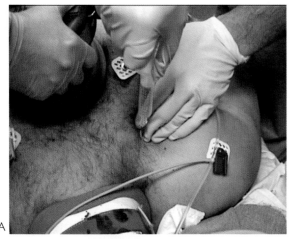
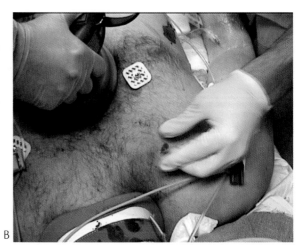

A B

Figure 27.3 Needle decompression for tension pneumothorax.

parietal pleura (◐ Fig. 27.5). Flexible perforated silicone drains introduced through a Monod-type trocar have the lowest likelihood of causing pulmonary lesions. Internal trocar-type drains, with a sharp tip sticking out of the tube, carry a higher risk of endothoracic injury if the trocar is not held in place after passing the parietal pleura. Their use is therefore best avoided because it can result in injury to the lung or the mediastinum. The chest tube is introduced under the control of a finger. It should penetrate into the pleural cavity without resistance. The direction of insertion of the chest tube should be chosen accordingly to the

gravity-induced distribution of air and fluid effusions. For an isolated air effusion, the chest tube should be directed cephalad and anteriorly. In contrast, for a fluid effusion, the preferred insertion point is lateral rather than anterior, and the chest tube will be inserted caudad and posteriorly. Chest tube insertion should be performed without using substantial force [1].

Type and size of chest tube

There are three types of drains, according to size and insertion method [4] (◐ Fig. 27.6).

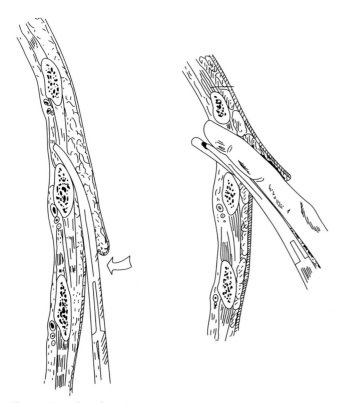

Figure 27.4 Blunt dissection.

◆ Drains with short trocar (Monod) or long trocar (Mallinckrodt): the diameter of these drains is often large (>24 French). After blunt dissection and after removal of the intrathoracic finger, a blunt-tipped guide, surrounded by a trocar 10 cm in length, is introduced 1–2 cm into the pleural cavity. Care should be taken to prevent the trocar from sliding on the intercostal muscles. One may erroneously believe that the trocar has entered the pleural cavity, and insert the chest tube between the intercostal muscles and the chest wall. Once the tip is inside the pleural cavity by 1–2 cm, the guide and trocar are directed anteriorly or posteriorly, depending on the nature of the effusion. The guide is then removed, leaving the trocar in place. The chest tube, whose diameter is adapted to the internal diameter of the trocar and whose outer end is occluded by a clamp, is then inserted through the trocar. Once the chest tube is in place, the trocar is removed along the tube until reaching the clamp. A second clamp is then placed on the tube between the trocar and the skin incision. The first clamp is removed, allowing the complete removal of the trocar while the tube is continuously clamped. For the Mallinckrodt drain, the equipment used is a large chest tube (maximum 28 French), pack-

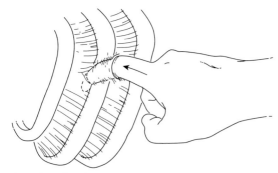

Figure 27.5 Insertion site.

aged with a disposable trocar within the tube. The blunt dissection is performed as described above. It is especially important to control the insertion of the tube and guide while going through the intercostal space. Uncontrolled insertion of the trocar can cause serious intrathoracic injuries. The insertion phase of the chest tube, however, is simplified, as there are fewer manipulations. Drain and guide are introduced into the pleural cavity by 1–2 cm, then directed anteriorly or posteriorly depending on the nature of the effusion. The guide is removed at half the length of the tube, leaving the tube in place. A clamp is placed on the tube between the guide and the skin incision. The guide is then completely withdrawn.

◆ Chest tubes without trocar but with a sharp needle (e.g. 'Pleurocath'): the tube is a small calibre (8 French) fairly rigid, multiperforated, blunt catheter about 8 cm long. It is packaged in a long plastic sheath ending in a needle

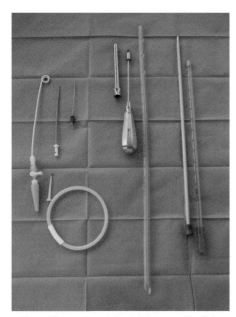

Figure 27.6 Chest tubes. Left to right: Seldinger method drain, Monod drain, Mallinckrodt drain.

tip bevel and a long handle. The insertion is performed by puncturing the intercostal space with the needle, with the chest tube partially engaged on the needle. As with any pleural puncture, the needle should be kept as close as possible to the superior edge of the lower rib to avoid injury to the intercostal neurovascular bundle. Once the tip enters the pleural cavity, air or pleural fluid will pass between the tube and the internal wall of the needle and appear at the base. The needle is then redirected and the tube is pushed through the needle by manipulating the tube through the plastic sheath. When the tube is in place, the needle is withdrawn. Clamping these small chest tubes is not recommended (risk of crushing). A three-way stopcock system (supplied with the chest tube) is attached to the end of the tube to connect to the continuous suction system. These chest tubes are rarely used nowadays because of the risk of injuring intrathoracic structures with the sharp needle.

◆ Chest tubes using the Seldinger technique: this type of drainage is the gold standard in radiology. Kits contain a disposable needle, syringe, guide wire with a flexible tip, a dilator and a small- or medium-bore (9–14 French) multiperforated tube with a distal hole. This technique has several advantages: it is less painful for the patient and does not require blunt dissection. However, there are few data on its effectiveness: in a recent study including 52 small-bore Seldinger-type chest tube, the overall drain failure rate was 37%. This was especially true for empyemas. These small chest tubes, however, have a failure rate in pneumothorax and uncomplicated fluid effusion comparable to that of large-bore tubes [5].

The main criterion for selecting chest tube size is the flow of either air or fluid that can be accommodated by the tube [4]. Internal diameter and length are the critical flow determinants. Chest tube selection must take into account not only the nature of the material being drained but also its rate of formation. For a constant level of suction at least 20 cmH$_2$O, the air flow will vary from 5 L/min for an 8-French chest tube to 28 L/min for a 28-French chest tube [4]. Clinical experience indicates that large leaks, such as may occur in a mechanically ventilated patient with a persistent bronchopleural fistula, can be in excess of 20 L/min [6]. Appropriate chest tube size is therefore key to prevent the occurrence of a tension pneumothorax.

It also seems logical that viscous fluids such as blood or pus would require a larger-bore tube. However, data from the literature are few and contradictory. A retrospective review including 59 patients with malignant pleural effusion was unable to detect any major difference in the efficacy of chest drainage between small-bore and large-bore chest tubes [7].

The quality of the initial drainage is an important factor in preventing the subsequent onset of pulmonary complications. An incompletely drained haemothorax has been shown to be associated with a higher incidence of early complications such as empyema, and late complications such as fibrosis and atelectasis [8].

Indications for large-bore chest tubes (>24 French)

These chest tubes are inserted by blunt dissection and usually have a trocar. Pneumothorax ranks second to rib fracture as the most common complication of traumatic chest injury, and justifies a large-bore chest tube [3]. Mechanically ventilated patients sustaining a spontaneous or iatrogenic pneumothorax may develop a tension pneumothorax and require a larger-bore chest tube [1,3]. The same applies if these patients develop a bronchopleural fistula or an empyema.

Indications for medium-bore chest tubes (16–24 French)

Medium-size chest tubes may be inserted by a Seldinger technique or by blunt dissection. However, it is not possible to insert a finger to explore the pleura when inserting a tube of this size. The indications are not clearly defined; the diameter is too small for mechanically ventilated patients with a pneumothorax, and too large for a primary spontaneous pneumothorax [9, 10]. However, these tubes can be used in case of haemothorax secondary to rib fracture. There is indeed a slow seepage of blood from the various fractures with pleural fibrinolysis and absence of clot, in contrast to immediate massive haemothorax [11]. Reactive effusions and transudates may be evacuated using a medium-bore chest tube. In contrast, exudates, and especially empyemas, require large-bore chest tubes (28 French) because of the high viscosity of the fluid. For these indications there are also double-lumen tubes, used to irrigate the pleura and/or instil streptokinase; the usefulness of streptokinase instillation is still being debated [12].

Indications for small-bore chest tubes (8–14 French)

Small-bore chest tubes are usually inserted without blunt dissection. They have been successfully used for recurrent pneumothorax in spontaneously breathing patients, and for uncomplicated fluid effusions [13]. However, for the management of primary spontaneous pneumothorax, despite the lack of randomized control trials, there was no difference in the immediate rate of success and requirement for

pleurodesis at 1 year between simple percutaneous aspiration and chest tube drainage [9, 10]. It therefore appears preferable, in these cases, to perform a simple aspiration [1].

Securing the chest tube

Immediately after the insertion of the chest tube, it must be connected to a drainage device or to a one-way valve such as a Heimlich valve. For large- and medium-bore chest tubes, the incision should be closed by a suture appropriate for a linear incision. The chest tube should be secured after insertion to prevent it from falling out. A suture is not usually required for the small-bore tube. Large amounts of tape and padding to dress the site are not necessary. A transparent dressing allows the wound site to be inspected by the nurse for leakage or infection [1]. A chest radiograph should always be performed after insertion of a chest tube to assess tube position and to determine the volume of residual fluid or pneumothorax (level C).

Drainage of a massive haemothorax

In cases of initial massive haemorrhage (>1 L of blood upon chest tube insertion) or in cases of persistent bleeding (>150 mL/h), a vascular lesion must be suspected and an exploratory thoracotomy for surgical haemostasis is warranted without delay. Classically, the chest tube should not be placed on suction in cases of massive bleeding; it only vents the fluid and avoids tamponade. However, this dogma is questionable and the use of suction does not appear to influence prognosis. In remote locations, when rapid access to banked blood is unlikely, a rudimentary autotransfusion device can be set up on the chest tube to retransfuse some of the fresh blood [14]. This allows immediate availability of compatible red cells for hemodynamically unstable patients. However, this technique has been criticized as the retransfusion of incoagulable blood can trigger coagulation disorders and increase bleeding [15].

Experimentally, the study by Napoli et al. [16] using this technique showed that reinfusion of a volume equivalent to 25% of blood volume results in a 25–30% reduction of coagulation factors without significantly altering coagulation. We therefore reserve this technique for the initial management of polytrauma patients (or thoracic vascular emergencies) with extreme instability and an immediate need for red blood cells, while limiting it to the immediate reinfusion of up to one-quarter of the patient's blood volume. Special devices exist (e.g. Pleur-Evac retransfusion bag, Teleflex Medical) that are inserted between the pleural drain and the Pleur-Evac device itself. Once the bag is filled, blood product infusion tubing with a filter can be connected and the collected blood transfused (◆ Fig. 27.7) [16].

Management of the drainage system

Once a chest tube is placed, depending on the clinical indication, a pleural drainage device (PDD) will be connected to provide suction, or a water seal to prevent the backflow of air into the pleural space. Spontaneous pneumothorax and free-flowing fluid will generally drain without need for suction [1, 4]. The chest tube is attached with a closed underwater seal bottle in which a tube is placed under water at a depth of 3 cm. The disadvantages of the system include mandatory inpatient management and the difficulty of patient mobilization. The use of Heimlich flutter valves has been advocated in these patients, especially as they permit ambulatory management with a high success rate [17]. If the quantity of pleural air or liquid is large or that drainage is incomplete with gravity and water seal, suction must be applied. Many types of PDDs are available: they consist of a three-compartment system, including a compartment to trap fluids from the patient's pleural space and to allow pleural air to pass through to the next compartments, a compartment to prevent air flow back into the pleural space and to detect an air leak, and a compartment to regulate the amount of negative pressure transmitted back to the patient from the wall suction device [6]. All models are not equal in terms of maximum suction flow. This may have important clinical consequences in cases of bronchopleural fistula with a throughput greater than the maximum flow allowed by the device: The development of a tension pneumothorax is then inevitable. Of eight models tested, three posed this risk if they were set at –10 cmH$_2$O and one if set at –20 cmH$_2$O. At this pressure, the suction flow rates ranged from 10 to 40 L/min depending on the model [6].

Clamping a chest tube in the presence of a ongoing air leak may lead to a tension pneumothorax with fatal outcome. A bubbling chest tube must never be clamped.

Drainage of a large pleural effusion should be performed in a stepwise, controlled fashion to prevent the potential complication of re-expansion pulmonary oedema (level C).

Monitoring pleural drainage

Chest tube drainage should be checked at each nursing shift, and every time the patient is examined. The correct installation and seal of individual connections must be given special attention. The absence of inflammation or discharge from the insertion site and the tightness of the dressing should be checked. The level of suction (or the absence of suction) must be confirmed regularly. Loops of the tubing between the chest tube and the drainage device, especially common with an excessive length of tubing, must be avoided in order to avoid siphoning. The tubing should be milked regularly only in the presence of clots. The purpose of milking is to briefly create a very deep depression, to fragment the clots, and to maintain the patency of the chest tube. The volume of collected secretions, the persistence of bubbling, and the oscillations of the water column will be evaluated each time vital signs are taken. In case of persistent bubbling, if the patient is mechanically ventilated, the amount of leakage should be evaluated by comparing the set tidal volume and the expired volume measured by the respirator. It is standard practice to monitor the daily chest radiograph: the correct positioning of the chest tube, the absence of any hole excluded from the pleural cavity, and the quality of lung re-expansion are checked.

Chest tube complications

Chest tube complications are categorized as related to insertion, position, or infection. With trained physicians, early and late complications appeared in respectively 3% and 8% [1]. Recently, more severe complications have been described, including empyema and chest tube malposition associated with thoracic or abdominal injuries [18]. Two recent prospective studies have shown that malposition

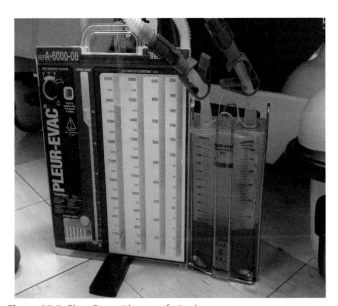

Figure 27.7 Pleur-Evac with retransfusion bag.

was detected by thoracic CT in 30% of percutaneous inserted chest tube [18, 19]. In these studies, avoiding the use of a trocar and an appropriate training of operators significantly reduced the incidence of chest tube complications [20]. Chest radiography failed to identify half of the malpositions [19, 20].

The malposition risk is not influenced by the insertion site: in a study comparing 101 chest tubes placed in 68 major trauma patients (20% anterior site, 80% lateral site), 22 (20%) were malpositioned, but only 6 out of these 22 were ineffective [21]. The risk of malposition was not related to a particular insertion site [21].

Learning how to perform the procedure correctly is key to avoiding complications. An audit survey of junior doctors working in a teaching hospital showed that 45% of doctors would have placed a chest tube outside the insertion site recommended. The most common error was the selection of too low an insertion site [22].

A brief teaching module using a simulation model is effective in building confidence and skill in chest tube insertion [23].

Antibiotic use

Despite the absence of broad consensus, the BTS guidelines suggest that prophylactic antibiotics should be given only when a chest tube is inserted after chest trauma (level A) [1]. The available data (five randomized controlled trials) suggest a significant reduction in the incidence of pneumonia and post-traumatic empyema [24]. A first-generation cephalosporin should be used for no longer than 24 h [25].

When to remove a chest tube

The most significant complication after chest tube removal is the recurrence of the pleural effusion. The timing of removal is dependent on the original indication for insertion and the clinical evolution. In the case of a pneumothorax, the chest tube should not be removed until bubbling has ceased for several hours and a chest radiograph demonstrates lung reinflation [1,4].

Clamping of the chest tube before removal is not necessary and not recommended: in one study, the removal of chest tube was performed while on continuous suction or following disconnection from suction to a underwater seal. No significant difference in outcome was observed between these two methods. In each group, 2 out of 80 patients (2.5%) required reinsertion of a chest tube [26].

In cases of fluid effusion, the timing for removing the chest tube is empirically established, with wide variations among centres. The minimum daily chest tube fluid output before tube removal is not clearly established. Younes *et al.* prospectively studied 139 randomized post-thoracotomy patients and found no difference in hospital stay, reaccumulation rates, or thoracentesis rate among those patients whose tubes were removed when the daily output rate was 100 mL/day or less, 150 mL/day or less, or 200 mL/day or less (thoracentesis rate was 2.3%) [27]. Even a threshold as high as 400 mL/day did not adversely affect drainage and fluid reaccumulation in postsurgical patients: a retrospective cohort study included, in one centre, all patients who underwent elective pulmonary resection (n = 2077) and found no difference when the chest tubes were removed with fluid output rate 450 mL/day or less [28]. In this study, only 0.5% patients had to be readmitted because of recurrent symptomatic effusion and were treated with video-assisted thoracoscopy.

Whether one should remove a chest tube at the end of inspiration or the end of expiration remains a subject of controversy. It is essential to understand the relationship between the respiratory cycle and the risk of recurrence of a pneumothorax. At the end of inspiration, the lung is maximally expanded and the parietal and visceral pleura are most closely opposed; at the end of expiration, the pressure difference between the atmospheric and the intrapleural space is minimized, thus the risk of inadvertent airflow into the chest cavity during tube removal is limited. The BTS guidelines advocate that the chest tube should be removed when the patient performs a Valsalva manoeuvre or during expiration [1]. One prospective randomized study that compared these two methods has demonstrated that removal of a chest tube at the end of inspiration or at the end of expiration is equally safe regarding complications such as recurrent pneumothorax (7% in each group) and the need for reinsertion a new chest tube (3% in each group) [29].

The chest tube should be removed with a brisk motion while an assistant ties the previously placed closure suture [1].

Controversy persists regarding the best time to perform a chest radiograph to rule out the presence of a recurrent pneumothorax after chest tube removal. The BTS guidelines do not address that topic [1]. Traditionally, chest radiography has been suggested between 12 and 24 h after tube removal, but data are sparse and radiographic protocols have not been validated. Recently, a small study regarding mechanically ventilated patients showed that performing a chest radiograph within 1–3 h after chest tube removal identified all recurrent pneumothoraces [30].

Ultrasound guidance

The diagnosis and assessment of pleural effusions using ultrasound is well documented [31, 32].

In a recent study, the ultrasonographic appearance of the pleural effusion (anechoic, heterogeneous nonseptated, or heterogeneous septated) before the procedure was a predictor of drainage success. Moreover, the ultrasound-guided percutaneous catheter drainage of empyemas ensures accurate catheter placement with a high success and a low complication rate, especially in the case of unsuccessful initial chest drainage [33].

Whenever possible, ultrasound guidance should be used to identify and localize a pleural effusion and to guide chest tube insertion.

Conclusion

Chest drainage can be performed using several techniques. Ultrasound diagnosis of the effusion and drainage guidance should be used whenever possible. Poorly tolerated tension pneumothorax or haemothorax requires immediate needle decompression. Large-bore chest tubes (24 French or larger) inserted by blunt dissection technique should be used in case of haemothorax, empyema, post-traumatic pneumothorax or large bronchopleural fistula. Other types of pleural effusions, especially well-tolerated pneumothoraces in awake patients, should be drained by small-bore tubes inserted using the Seldinger technique. The lateral insertion site is the most common. Particular attention should be paid to the suction devices. Training and well-defined policies and protocols for procedure performance and for subsequent management ensure quality care and minimize complications.

Personal perspective

Percutaneous pleural drainage is widely used. Yet, indications and management are not evidence-based and vary considerably between countries or even between institutions. Several studies have shown chest tube complications to be significantly underestimated, sometimes severe, and often related to lack of skill and practice. At the same time, the development of ultrasonography in the intensive care unit has profoundly changed the detection, localization, and evaluation of effusions. Chest tube insertion under ultrasound guidance, once the province of radiologists, is now being performed by other specialists.

Further reading

Baumann MH. What size chest tube? What drainage system is ideal? And other chest tube management questions. *Curr Opin Pulm Med* 2003;**9**:276–281.

Baumann MH, Patel PB, Roney CW, Petrini MF. Comparison of function of commercially available pleural drainage unit and catheter. *Chest* 2003;**123**:1878–1886.

Horsley A, Jones L, White J, Henry M. Efficacy and complications of small-bore, wire-guided chest drains. *Chest* 2006;**130**:1857–1863.

Hutton A, Kenealy H, Wong C. Using simulation models to teach junior doctors how to insert chest tubes: a brief and effective teaching module. *Intern Med J* 2008;**38**:887–891.

Laws D, Neville E, Duffy J *et al*. BTS guidelines for the insertion of a chest drain. *Thorax* 2003;**58**:ii53–ii59.

Remérand F, Luce V, Badachi Y, *et al*. Incidence of chest tube malposition in the critically ill. *Anesthesiology* 2007;**106**:1112–1119.

Younes RN, Gross JL, Aguiar S, *et al*. When to remove a chest tube? A randomized study with subsequent prospective consecutive validation. *J Am Coll Surg* 2002;**195**:658–662.

⮑ For additional multimedia materials please visit the online version of the book (⌦ http://www.esciacc.oxfordmedicine.com).

CHAPTER 28

Renal support therapy

Piotr Rozentryt, Paweł Siwołowski,
Marian Zembala, and Piotr Ponikowski

Contents

Summary

In everyday clinical practice, the term 'renal replacement therapy' is used to in the context of therapies designed to modify the size and composition of fluid compartments. Usually such procedures can be carried out using extracorporeal circulation and various membranes, or with peritoneal dialysis. In an appropriately designed system, blood connects with a specifically composed fluid through a semipermeable membrane in order to replace the kidney as an excretion organ.

Different methods of renal support therapy are used, including haemodialysis (intermittent, continuous venovenous), haemofiltration (intermittent, continuous venovenous, arteriovenous), and peritoneal dialysis. These methods differ in complexity, efficiency, cost, and risk of complications.

Indications for renal support therapies include numerous clinical conditions, among which acute kidney injury is most common. Once this form of therapy has been decided on, it must be remembered that it also carries a risk of complications at different stages. In cardiology, with the progress of knowledge on pathophysiology of acute decompensated heart failure it become evident that different forms of renal support therapy may be more effective in managing volume overload in selected patients. In future, systems with living renal tubule epithelial cells attached to the semipermeable membranes ('bio-artificial kidney') are likely to replace the function of the kidneys.

History

The phenomenon of haemodialysis through a semipermeable membrane was described in 1889 by the English scientist B. R. Richardson. It was first used in the treatment of intoxication in a human patient in Giessen, Germany in October 1924. In September 1944 a haemodialysis device built by Willem Kolff in the Netherlands enabled the survival of a woman with acute renal failure [1]. Since then there have been rapid technical developments, providing treatment of chronic uraemia [2], acute renal failure [3], and other pathologies not directly associated with impaired renal function [4].

Terminology

The term 'renal replacement therapy' may be misleading and does not reflect the possibilities of modern treatment. Therapy can partially replace the excretion function of the kidneys, but not their endocrine, metabolic, and immune functions which all contribute to maintain the body's homeostasis. Thus, it is more appropriate to use the term 'renal support therapy', designed to modify the size and the composition of the fluid compartments. Such procedures can be carried out using extracorporeal circulation and different sorts of filters or with peritoneal dialysis. Another procedure used in nephrology, therapeutic apheresis, can modify concentrations of substances in the blood (proteins, cytokines, antibodies, and lipoproteins) and also affects the function of blood cells. In the future, systems with living renal tubule epithelial cells attached to the semipermeable membranes ('bioartificial kidney') are most likely to replace the function of the kidneys [5–7].

The whole spectrum of procedures intended to replace or support the excretory function of the kidneys and to provide possible interventions in the composition and the volume of the body fluids can be called 'blood purification procedures'.

For a review of the biophysics of renal replacement therapy and derived techniques, see 28.1–28.4.

Review of selected procedures used in extracorporeal purification

The clinical consequences of changes in osmolarity, electrolyte concentrations, and fluid compartment volumes induced by the procedures listed in Table 28.1 are an important issue. The rapid reduction of urate concentration in the extracellular fluid causes a decrease in plasma osmolarity and encourages osmotic transport of water to the cells, resulting in oedema; neurological signs and symptoms, known as disequilibrium syndrome, occur as a consequence. The removal by means of ultrafiltration of several litres of fluid in 4–5 h of intermittent haemodialysis causes a drop in blood pressure, ischaemia of organs, and secondary activation of the blood pressure regulating systems, with all the subsequent consequences. Continuous therapies were introduced, in an attempt to overcome these difficulties by avoiding significant hypotension and tuning rapid changes in electrolyte concentrations and osmolarity to reduce water imbalance between fluid compartments and the risk of disequilibrium syndrome.

The continuous procedure introduced in the 1980s [8], taking blood from an artery and returning it to a vein, using an arteriovenous pressure gradient, is very rarely carried out nowadays.

Slow continuous ultrafiltration

In slow continuous ultrafiltration (SCUF) no dialysate is used, there is no substitution flow and a reduction of only the extracellular compartment during the procedure. It can be done from peripheral access, with a duration of up to several hours depending on patient's needs and haemodynamic parameters. Such procedures can be applied in patients with acute decompensated heart failure (ADHF) and volume overload (see Volume overload in acute heart failure). A diagram of the process is shown in Fig. 28.1.

Intermittent haemodialysis

The duration of intermittent haemodialysis (IHD) is usually 4–5 h. The dialysis fluid flow generally reaches 400–500 mL/min, with a high clearance of the small molecules.

Table 28.1 Methods of renal support therapy

Modality	Use in haemodynamically unstable patients	Solute clearance	Volume control	Anti-coagulatiion
PD	Yes	++	++	No
IHD	Possible	++++	+++	Yes/no
IHF	Possible	+++	+++	Yes/no
Intermittent IHF	Possible	++++	+++	Yes/no
Hybrid techniques	Possible	++++	++++	Yes/no
CVVH	Yes	+++/++++	++++	Yes/no
CVVHD	Yes	+++/++++	++++	Yes/no
CVVHDF	Yes	++++	++++	Yes/no

HDF, haemodiafiltrations; CVVH, continuous veno-venous haemofiltration; CVVHD, continuous veno-venous haemodialysis; CVVHDF, continuous veno-venous haemodiafiltration; IHD, intermittent hemodialysis; IHF, intermittent hemofiltration, PD, peritoneal dialysis;

Reproduced with permission from Cerda J, Ronco C. Modalities of continuous renal replacement therapy: technical and clinical considerations. *Semin Dial* 2009;**22**:114–122.

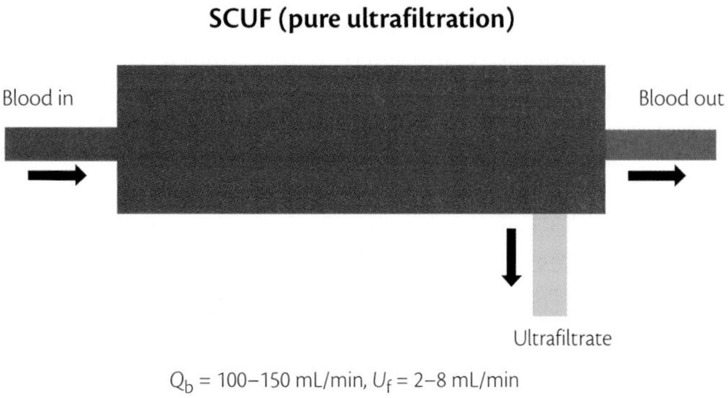

SCUF (pure ultrafiltration)

Blood in → Blood out →

Ultrafiltrate ↓

Q_b = 100–150 mL/min, U_f = 2–8 mL/min

Figure 28.1 Slow continuous ultrafiltration (SCUF).

In everyday practice haemodialysis procedures are often merged with ultrafiltration. Unlike in SCUF this effect is obtained by lowering the pressure on the dialysate side. No replacement fluid is used, so no convection contributes to the global clearance. These procedures are efficient only in eliminating small molecules from the circulation. The speed of fluid resorption from the extracellular compartment to vessels (refilling) limits the ultrafiltration rate during IHD procedures. There are several IHD-related procedures (e.g. sodium concentration programming, individual ultrafiltration programming), which are used to minimize the consequences of fast changes in osmolarity and extracellular fluid volume. Currently IHD remains the most accessible and cheapest method, and therefore a very valuable form of renal replacement therapy. A diagram of the process is shown in ➔ Fig. 28.2.

Continuous venovenous haemodialysis

The next step was continuous venovenous haemodialysis (CVVHD), which limits some disadvantages of IHD while preserving its high potential to eliminate small molecules. CVVHD makes it possible to spread ultrafiltration over a longer period (theoretically up to 24 h) and to avoid the

clinical consequences of fast changes in osmolarity and extracellular fluid volume; the clearance of small molecules remains at a level comparable to IHD. A diagram of the process is shown in ➔ Fig. 28.3.

Sustained low-efficiency dialysis

Sustained low-efficiency dialysis (SLED) is carried out daily for at least 12 h, which leaves some time for diagnostics and other procedures.

Haemofiltration

This is the model procedure using convective transport. No dialysate is needed. During the procedure a high-flux membrane is used that allows removal and continuous replacement of as much as 60–100 L of fluid within 24 h. Additionally, removal of the medium-sized and larger molecules (up to 12 kDa) is possible [9]. The haemofiltration procedure requires a precisely calibrated system to balance the amount of removed fluid with the speed of infusion of the replacement fluid, which needs to be ultra-pure.

Convective transport demands considerable ultrafiltration. The amount of replacement fluid administered must therefore equal the ultrafiltration volume minus the fluid volume that we aim to remove as a part of the therapy. This offers unique possibilities of controlling the intracellular compartment and leaves some space for the fluid regimen and nutrition. The replacement fluid can be administered before the filter (pre-dilution) or after the filter (post-dilution). With pre-dilution, the efficacy of the clearance is decreased, but the filter has a longer life; with post-dilution, the clearance is increased, but there is faster filter blockage.

Continuous venovenous haemofiltration

A continuous venovenous haemofiltration procedure (CVVHDF) combines continuous haemofiltration and

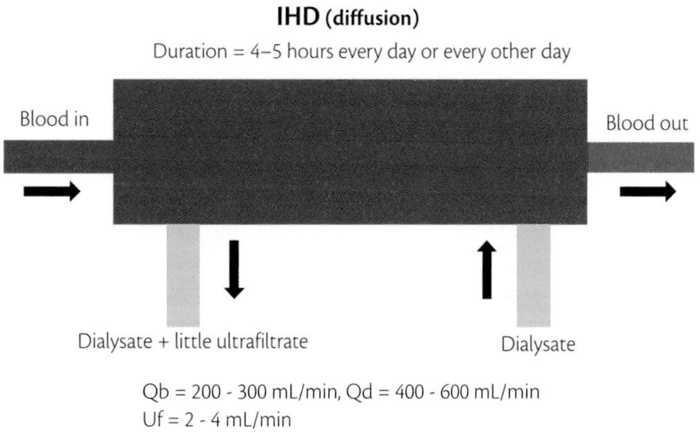

IHD (diffusion)

Duration = 4–5 hours every day or every other day

Blood in → Blood out →

Dialysate + little ultrafiltrate ↓   Dialysate ↑

Qb = 200 - 300 mL/min, Qd = 400 - 600 mL/min
Uf = 2 - 4 mL/min

Figure 28.2 Intermittent haemodialysis (IHD).

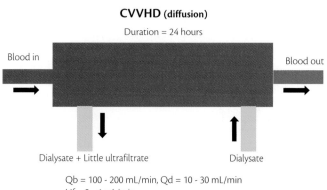

CVVHD (diffusion)

Duration = 24 hours

Blood in → Blood out →

Dialysate + Little ultrafiltrate ↓   Dialysate ↑

Qb = 100 - 200 mL/min, Qd = 10 - 30 mL/min
Uf = 2 - 4 mL/min

Figure 28.3 Continuous venovenous haemodialysis (CVVHD).

haemodialysis and is sometimes called hybrid therapy. A high-flux membrane and a large volume of replacement fluid are needed (➲ Fig 28.4).

Plasmapheresis

This requires a special filter, with permeability as much as 3×10^6 kDa, which can separate blood cells from plasma. Replacement fluid administration is needed to replace the removed plasma. The fluid consists of fresh plasma, possibly enriched in albumins. During a single procedure 40–50 mL plasma/kg body mass is replaced and it should not take longer than 3 h. To shorten the plasmapheresis time two filters can be connected, or cascade plasmapheresis is used. Plasmapheresis can be merged with other procedures such as CVHF or CVVHDF. A diagram of the process is shown in ➲ Fig. 28.5.

Continuous haemoperfusion

Continuous haemoperfusion (CHP) comes in several variants depending on the therapeutic goal (➲ Fig. 28.6). The simplest example is low-density lipoprotein (LDL) apheresis; more complex haemoperfusion systems are used in the treatment of drug intoxication and liver failure. CHP procedures can be merged with procedures such as CVVHF, CVVHDF, and plasmapheresis.

Peritoneal dialysis

The peritoneum serves as a semipermeable membrane. Unlike in other methods transport through the peritoneum takes place in both directions: from blood to peritoneal fluid and back. Therefore molecules from the peritoneal fluid (e.g. glucose) are transported through the lymphatic system to the circulation. The peritoneal dialysis technique involves diffusion, convection, ultrafiltration, and adsorption.

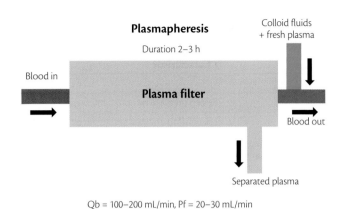

Qb = 100–200 mL/min, Pf = 20–30 mL/min

Figure 28.5 Simple plasmapheresis.

Many methods of peritoneal dialysis have been described, from the intermittent dialysis to automatic dialysis with the use of special device called a cycler.

Major indications for renal replacement therapies

Deterioration in renal function is common in hospitalized patients. It is related to poor outcome, and in some cases renal replacement therapy is needed [10–17]. Acute kidney injury (AKI) is the major clinical problem requiring treatment with the use of blood purification methods. The consequences of AKI can vary and there is no single recommendation regarding its management. Indications for starting renal replacement therapy were introduced in 2000 by the Working Group Acute Dialysis Quality Initiative (ADQI) [18, 19]. ➲ Table 28.2 summarizes the indications for renal replacement therapy in critically ill patients. As the dynamics of AKI are different from the dynamics of chronic renal failure, especially if AKI is a part of another condition, the decision to start therapy should be individualized. AKI and its consequent homeostasis disturbances are not the only indications for a clinician to use blood purification techniques in intensive care setting. ➲ Table 28.3 summa-

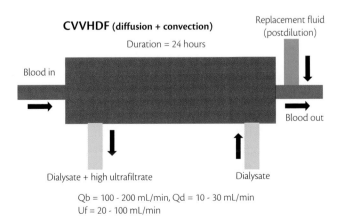

Qb = 100 - 200 mL/min, Qd = 10 - 30 mL/min
Uf = 20 - 100 mL/min

Figure 28.4 Continuous venovenous haemofiltration (CVVHDF).

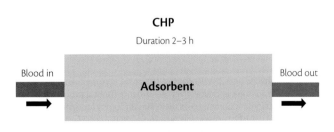

Qb = 100–200 mL/min

Figure 28.6 Continuous haemoperfusion (CHP).

Table 28.2 A summary of absolute or 'rescue therapy' indications for initiation of renal support therapy in critically ill patients

Category	Characteristic
Metabolic	
Uraemia	Serum urea ≥36 mmol/L (100 mg/dL)
Uraemic complications	Encephalopathy, pericarditis, bleeding
Hyperkalaemia	K^+ ≥6 mmol/L and/or ECG abnormalities
Hypermagnesaemia	Mg^{2+} ≥4 mmol/L and/or anuria/absent deep tendon reflexes
Acidosis	Serum pH ≤7.5
Oligo/anuria	Urine output <200 mL/12 h or anuria
Fluid overload	Diuretic-resistant organ oedema (i.e. pulmonary oedema) in the presence of acute kidney injury

Table 28.3 Indications for blood purification therapy regardless of diagnosis of acute kidney injury

Indication	Type of procedure
Familial hypercholesterolaemia	LDL apheresis, PL
Tumour lysis syndrome	IHD, CVVHF
Selected poisoning or overdose	IHD, CVVHF, PL
Periprocedural after contrast administration in patients with impaired glomerular filtration	CVVH
Presence of graft-versus-host antibodies after renal, cardiac or pulmonary transplant	PL
Acute liver failure	PL, MARS, SPAD
ANCA-associated acute glomerulonephritis	PL
Catastrophic antiphospholipid syndrome	PL
Heart transplant rejection	ECP, PL
Thrombotic angiopathy, haemolitic–uraemic syndrome	PL
Hypertriglyceridaemic pancreatitis	PL
Hyperviscosity syndromes	PL
Sepsis	PL
Systemic lupus erythematosus	PL
Thyrotoxicosis	PL
Dilated cardiomyopathy	IA

ECP, extracorporeal photopheresis; IA, immunoadsoption; MARS, molecular adsorbents recirculation system; PL, plasmapheresis; SPAD, single pass albumin dialysis.

Data from Szczepiorkowski ZM, Bandarenko N, Kim HC et al. Guidelines on the use of therapeutic apheresis in clinical practice—evidence-based approach from the Apheresis Applications Committee of the American Society for Apheresis. *J Clin Apheresis* 2007;**22**:1–70 and Joannidis M, Druml W, Forni LG, et al. Prevention of acute kidney injury and protection of renal function in the intensive care unit. Expert opinion of the working group for nephrology, ESICM. *Intensive Care Med* 2010;**36**:392–411.

rizes indications for blood purification therapy regardless of an AKI diagnosis [4, 20].

Continuous versus intermittent treatment

Despite numerous studies, the superiority of continuous over intermittent therapy has not been proved [21–27]. None of the meta-analyses, including randomized and restrospective studies in varying proportions, have provided any new information [24, 25]. A Cochrane review [26] did not demonstrate any difference in mortality, percentage of renal function recovery, or frequency of hypotension episodes between continuous and intermittent methods of renal replacement therapy. The study showed only higher mean blood pressure in patients on continuous therapy [26]. Higher blood pressure should indicate an earlier renal function recovery, so the lack of this effect makes the conclusions less reliable. As the current evidence is inconclusive [27], everyday clinical practice should be guided by personal experience and experts opinion. A prevalent current view limits the use of intermittent therapies to patients who are haemodynamically stable, as continuous therapy provides better stabilization of the cardiovascular system.

Dose and timing of therapy

Since the introduction of the concept of a dose in dialysis more than 30 years ago [28] there has been no doubt that more intense dialysis is related to better prognosis in chronic renal failure [29–30]. Whether dose of dialysis affects prognosis in AKI remains unknown. Ronco *et al.* [11] demonstrated a reduction in mortality in patients treated more intensively, which was confirmed in another study [15]. However, more recently, large multicentre studies [13, 17] have failed to show a reduction in mortality with the higher dialysis doses. The concept of a point of inflection, according to which an increase in the dialysis dose improves prognosis only to a certain level (📷 28.5) above which there would be no further benefit, is an attempt to summarize all these results. Further improvement may be dependent on the time when therapy was started, the choice of the method, and other yet unknown factors [31].

Apart from the dose of dialysis, the optimal timing of therapy initiation plays an important role. Although it is commonly accepted that therapy should be initiated as early as possible, there are no definitive studies to prove it [32,

33]. The Acute Kidney Injury Network (AKIN) has begun intensive work on the standardization of AKI criteria and its management. As a result a multilayered classification of acute injury called the RIFLE classification (risk, injury, failure, loss of function, and endstage renal disease) has been proposed [34] with a modification known as AKIN classification [35]. The RIFLE classification (➲ Fig. 28.7) is a useful starting point for a qualitative description of a role of early and late start of renal replacement therapy.

No clear conclusions can be drawn from the studies that have used the RIFLE classification [36, 37] and a recent meta-analysis [38]. Since there is no reliable evidence for the early start of therapy, it seems reasonable to rely on several individual premises. Such an approach forms the basis for the working scheme of renal replacement therapy initiation which was recently presented for discussion in the AKIN experts group [39] (➲ Fig. 28.8). The scheme follows the idea of many variables that should be taken into consideration while deciding on therapy initiation, methods used, and dose of dialysis, as well as on the moment when the therapy is completed. According to these authors there are three groups of factors influencing the decision to initiate renal replacement therapy in critically ill patients (▣ 28.6).

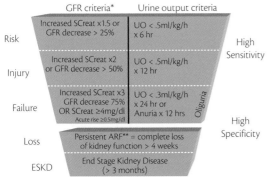

Figure 28.7 The RIFLE classification: a proposed classification scheme for acute renal failure (ARF). The classification system includes separate criteria for creatinine and urine output (UO). A patient can fulfil the criteria through changes in serum creatinine (SCreat) or changes in UO, or both. The criteria that lead to the worst possible classification should be used. Note that the F component of RIFLE (failure of kidney function) is present even if the increase in SCreat is less than threefold, as long as the new SCreat is greater than 4.0 mg/dL (350 μmol/L) in the setting of an acute increase of at least 0.5 mg/dL (44 μmol/L). The designation RIFLE-F$_O$ should be used in this case to denote 'acute-on-chronic' disease. Similarly, when the RIFLE-F classification is achieved by UO criteria, a designation of RIFLE-F$_O$ should be used to denote oliguria. The shape of the figure denotes the fact that more patients (high sensitivity) will be included in the mild category, including some who do not actually having renal failure (less specificity). In contrast, at the bottom of the figure the criteria are strict and therefore specific, but some patients will be missed.
From Bellomo R, Ronco C, Kellum JA, et al. Acute renal failure-definition, outcome measures, animal models, fluid therapy and information technology needs: the Second International Consensus Conference of the Acute Dialysis Quality Initiative (ADQI) Group. Crit Care 2004;**8**: R204–R212. Copyright 2004 Bellimo et al; licensee BioMed Central Ltd.

Vascular access

The efficacy of all procedures depends on the appropriate vascular or peritoneal access. In the acute setting arteriovenous fistulas and PET (Dacron) grafts are not used because of a high risk of bleeding and vessel injury. Silicon or polyurethane double lumen catheters (11–14 French), especially soft, are commonly used. Catheters 15–16 cm long are used to cannulate the internal jugular vein (or another location in smaller patients), 19–20-cm catheters are used for the subclavian vein, and 24-cm catheters are usually used for the femoral vein. If therapy for longer than 3 weeks is in prospect, tunnelled cuffed catheters should be used [40]. Catheter insertion is performed in a fully sterile manner using a modified Seldinger technique. The National Kidney Outcome Quality Initiative (KDOQI) recommends ultrasound support for catheter insertion [40, 41].

The site of catheter placement plays a significant role. The right internal jugular vein is preferable because of easy access and almost straight course of the catheter, keeping the tip of the catheter 2–3 cm above the right atrium. Left-sided access is also possible, but more tortuous course of the vessel can obstruct sufficient flow. Catheter insertion in the femoral vein should be a second choice; it provides good blood flow but has a higher risk of infection. Subclavian vein access incurs a high risk of vein thrombosis, further stenosis, and periprocedural risk. According to the KDOQI recommendations, radiographic verification of the catheter location should be performed after insertion in the internal jugular or subclavian vein [40].

Peritoneal dialysis requires peritoneal catheter insertion. The most commonly used Tenkhof catheter is made of silicon. It can be inserted into peritoneal cavity by means of modified Seldinger, laparoscopic, or surgical techniques. Antibiotic prophylaxis is needed each time.

Anticoagulation

Despite the lack of unified anticoagulation guidelines, it appears that most of the renal replacement procedures require anticoagulation in order to avoid filter thrombosis. Choice of anticoagulation agent and the administration method should depend on the clinical circumstances, the team's experience, and the agents available (▣ 28.7) [42].

The main factors to consider in deciding on the anticoagulation method are history of heparin-induced thrombocytopenia (HIT), active bleeding, impaired liver function, and history of recent surgical procedures especially within the central nervous system.

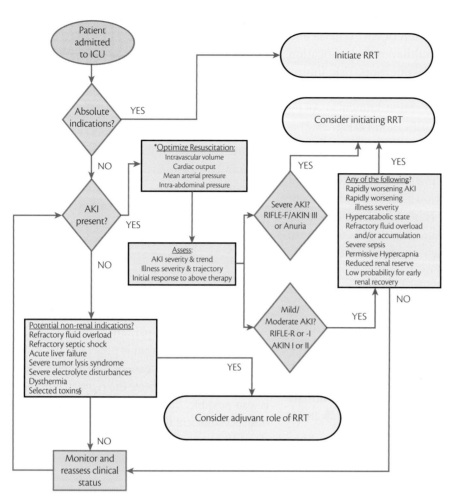

Figure 28.8 Algorithm for initiation of renal replacement therapy.
Reproduced with permission from Bagshaw SM, Cruz DN, Gibney N, Ronco C. A proposed algorithm for initiation of renal replacement therapy in adult critically ill patients. *Crit Care* 2009;**13**:317–325.

Unfractionated heparin (UFH) is the most commonly used anticoagulation agent. Renal replacement therapy has an unpredictable impact on its pharmacokineticsdepending on the method used, membrane type, and the amount of the blood flow through the filter. It is necessary to monitor activity of anti-factor IIa by measuring the activated partial thromboplastin time (APTT). When unfractionated heparin is used the filter usage time is proportional to APTT but not to the heparin dose [43]. Additionally, HIT or bleeding with an incidence risk of up to 50% [43] can occur while using unfractionated heparin.

To avoid complications, methods limiting anticoagulation to the filter region only have been developed. Regional heparinization is one of them [44, 45], but this method is reserved for teams with much experience in performing this procedure.

Low-molecular-weight heparin (LMWH) is another option, with more predictable pharmacokinetics despite being excreted by kidneys. There is a lower risk of developing HIT, equal effectiveness in preventing filter thrombosis [46, 47], and greater safety [47, 48].

Alternatively to protamine sulfate, an infusion of sodium citrate to the arterial line of the filter can be used in regional anticoagulation. Citrate ions chelate calcium ions and if the ionized calcium concentration is below 0.35 mmol/L they provide anticoagulation in the filter. The advantages are no risk of developing HIT, good anticoagulation control in the filter if there is an appropriate calcium concentration there, and acidosis control. Many [49, 50] but not all [51] of the studies show the superiority of citrate anticoagulation over heparin administration with regard to filter life and the risks of bleeding.

Limited experience is available with heparinoids. Dosing information and the methods of controlling basic agents are shown in 📹 28.7 [52].

Complications

Renal replacement therapy carries a risk of complications at various stages [53] (➲ Table 28.4).

Table 28.4 Complications of renal support therapy

Vascular access	Haemodynamic instability
Bleeding	**Electrolyte disturbances**
Thrombosis	Hypophosphataemia
Arteriovenous fistula formation	Hypomagnesaemia
Haematoma	Hypocalcaemia
Aneurysm formation	Hypokalaemia
Haemothorax	Hyponatraemia
Pneumothorax	Hypernatraemia
Pericardial tamponade	**Acid–base disturbances**
Arrhythmias	Metabolic acidosis
Air embolism	Metabolic alkalosis
Infection	Citrate-induced alkalosis and acidosis
Extracorporeal circuit	**Nutritional losses**
Reduced filter life	Amino acids and proteins
Reduced dialysis dose	Poor glycaemic control
Hypothermia	Vitamin deficiencies
Bioincompatibility	Trace minerals
Immunological activation	**Volume management errors**
Anaphylaxis	**Altered drug removal**
Haematologic complications	**Delayed renal recovery**
Need for anticoagulation	
Metabolic alkalosis	
Hypernatraemia	
Citrate intoxication	
Bleeding	
Thrombocytopenia	
Bleeding	
Haemolysis	
Heparin-induced thrombocytopenia	

Reproduced with permission from Finkel KW, Podoll AS. Complications of continuous renal replacement therapy. *Semin Dial* 2009;**22**: 155–159.

The expected duration of therapy must be considered before the vascular access is placed. The NF/KDOQI guidelines recommend insertion of tunnelled cuffed catheters within 5 days for femoral access and within 3 weeks for jugular access [40]. If catheters that are inappropriately short or too long are used, the therapy may be less efficacious or may even have to be discontinued. A catheter placed close to the vessel wall can damage the vessel and may need to be repositioned. There is a risk of infection if catheters are kept too long.

The risk of electrolyte abnormalities, especially hypokalaemia and hypophosphataemia, is increased in therapy with high ultrafiltration and with a large volume of replacement fluid [54]. Alterations in acid–base and electrolyte balance may be caused by citrate or lactate use.

Hypotension is an important complication leading to multisystem hypoperfusion (including kidneys) and can impede renal function recovery. In haemodynamically unstable patients, continuous therapy should be used.

Medication dosing

All renal replacement therapies influence the concentration of protein-unbound medication fractions, especially for medications that are not tightly bound to proteins. An additional dosing problem is nonphysiological pharmacokinetics of medications administered in patients with AKI. Changes in volumes of medication distribution can be especially important. It is difficult, if not impossible, to assess the distribution volume. It must be noted that the influence of intermittent therapy, e.g. IHD, and continuous treatment is not the same. Continuous therapies with differing proportions of diffusion and convective transport in global clearance have differing effects on drug concentrations. For a given proportion of dialysate flow/ultrafiltration, the order is CVVH > CVVHDF > CVVHD.

From the practical point of view, another fact should be noted. The influence of continuous therapy on drug excretion through the filter varies over time, since in the course of dialysis proteins are gradually adsorbed on the filter so that the dynamics of the semipermeable membrane's filtration and diffusion change. As a result there can be significant differences in the serum levels of a medication after administration of the same dose at the beginning or at the end of the life of the filter. When the filter is new the drug concentration tends to be subtherapeutic, but when the dynamics of the semipermeable membrane become limited drug toxicity can occur.

As there are no studies on the pharmacokinetics of more than 80% of medications described in the basic handbooks on drug dosage in renal disease [55], it seems to be reasonable to manage patients depending, if possible, on the monitoring of plasma levels of medications.

Special clinical circumstances: renal replacement therapy in acute decompensated heart failure

Renal dysfunction is one of the most common comorbidities in heart failure patients, proven to be an independent factor in unfavourable outcome [56]. Most of the patients admitted to hospital as a result of ADHF suffer from renal dysfunction *de novo* or from an exacerbation of previously diagnosed chronic renal disease [57] With the progress of knowledge on volume overload physiology in ADHF (➡ Box 28.1), cardiologists have become more interested in renal replacement therapy techniques, use of which has traditionally been reserved for nephrologists.

Volume overload in acute heart failure

Volume overload symptoms and pulmonary congestion are the most common causes for hospital admission in patients with ADHF. Prolonged overload leads to neurohormonal activation, subendocardial ischaemia causing cell damage and necrosis, structural disturbances of the left ventricle, impaired drainage of cardiac veins, progression of myocardial dysfunction, and, consequent irreversible remodelling [58]. On the basis of these pathophysiological concepts ADHF can be classified as:

+ Acute vascular failure, which is common in women, older people, and patients with a previous history of hypertension and relatively preserved left ventricle ejection fraction, and is more often a clinical manifestation of the patient's first episode of acute heart failure syndrome.

+ Acute decompensated cardiac failure with normal or mildly decreased blood pressure, common in young male patients or in patients with a previous history of heart failure.

In acute vascular failure the volume overload in the pulmonary circulation is a consequence of its redistribution rather than retention. The mechanisms of fluid redistribution in ADHF include [58–60]:

+ Increase in vascular resistance (peripheral and renal).

Box 28.1   Renal replacement therapy in ADHF: some important dates

+ 1949: Schneierson proposed intermittent peritoneal dialysis for refractory ADHF

+ 1954: Kolff noted that ultrafiltration could be used for a 'reduction of intractable oedema'

+ 1977: Haemofiltration was first described as a means of removing extracellular fluid from patients with oedema refractory to diuretic agents

+ 1979: Paganini *et al.* reported the practical application of ultrafiltration in a volume-overloaded patient

---

+ Neurohormonal activation (renin–angiotensin–aldosterone system activation, natriuretic peptide resistance, inadequated nonosmotic vasopressin secretion).

+ Proinflamatory activation (iNOS, COX-2, IL-1β, TNF-α).

+ Progressing renal dysfunction with sodium and water retention (vasomotor nephropathy).

+ Inappropriate use of some medications (NSAIDs, derivatives of thiazolidinedione).

Cardiorenal syndrome in acute heart failure

According to the definition proposed by Ronco *et al.*, cardiorenal syndrome (CRS) can be defined as a pathophysiological disorder of the heart and kidneys whereby acute or chronic dysfunction of one organ may induce acute or chronic dysfunction of the other [56].

Among the haemodynamic factors underlying CRS and renal function deterioration in the course of ADHF, the following can be mentioned: (1) adequacy of arterial filling and renal perfusion; (2) degree of venous congestion; (3) the presence of raised intra-abdominal pressure [61] (👥 28.8).

The decrease in stroke volume in the course of ADHF activates neurohormonal compensatory mechanisms to maintain systemic and renal perfusion pressure. It leads to systemic and renal vasoconstriction, which, together with decreased cardiac output, results in the deterioration in renal perfusion and glomerular filtration rate (GFR) [62]. As a consequence of activation of the autonomic system and renin–angiotensin–aldosterone system and an increase in nonosmotic vasopressin secretion, sodium and water retention in the kidneys, further overload, an increase in afterload, and subsequent decrease in the stroke volume occur. An increase of sodium concentration in the distal tubule and in the area of the macula densa induces secretion of adenosine (by the juxtaglomerular apparatus), which stimulates adenosine A_1 receptors causing constriction of afferent arterioles and a further drop in eGFR. This phenomenon, known as tubuloglomerular feedback, also explains the unfavourable impact of loop diuretics on renal function and constitutes one of the proposed mechanisms for the development of diuretic resistance [63]. It has also been shown that furosemide has a direct toxic impact on renal tubules which is mediated by prostaglandins and is not related to the renal flow alterations [64].

Refractory heart failure: the place of renal replacement therapy

According to the recent European Society of Cardiology (ESC) guidelines, the use of diuretics is always a first line treatment to correct the body fluid volume (class of recommendation I, level of evidence B) [65]. According to data from multicentre registries, 87–93% of patients with AHFS are treated with diuretics [66]. However, some patients tend to inadequately respond to diuretic therapy and develop diuretic resistance. The causes of diuretic resistance are:

◆ Decreased renal perfusion (small cardiac output)

◆ Neurohormonal activation

◆ Decreased intravascular volume

◆ Elevated uptake of Na^+ in distal tubule

◆ Distal tubule epithelial hypertrophy

◆ Decreased tubular secretion (renal failure, NSAIDs)

◆ Impaired absorption of diuretics

◆ Abnormal distribution of loop diuretics

◆ Lack of patient's cooperation.

The recognition of a high incidence of diuretic resistance in ADHF has aroused an interest in alternative treatment methods that can protect kidney function. One of these is renal replacement therapy. Currently, three types of renal replacement therapy are used in the treatment of patients with ADHF: (1) intermittent isolated ultrafiltration (IUF), (2) SCUF, and (3) CVVH.

Ultrafiltration has been shown to improve the symptoms of congestion and lower right atrial and pulmonary arterial wedge pressure, improve cardiac output, decrease neurohormone levels, correct hyponatraemia, restore diuresis and reduce requirements for diuretics [67]. Recent studies have also demonstrated that early ultrafiltration in patients with signs of volume overload and diuretic resistance is an efficient alternative form of treatment and is associated with shorter hospital stay, fewer hospital readmissions, faster fluid removal with earlier clinical recovery as compared with the standard diuretics regime [67, 68]. According to the ESC guidelines [65] ultrafiltration should be considered in selected patients with signs of overload (pulmonary congestion or peripheral oedema) and in order to correct hyponatraemia in symptomatic patients with diuretic resistance (class of recommendation IIa, level of evidence B).

Potential limitations of ultrafiltration

Ultrafiltration can remove fluid from the blood at the same rate that fluid can be naturally recruited from the tissue. The transient removal of blood triggers compensatory mechanisms, termed plasma or intravascular refill, to minimize this reduction [69]. The plasma refill response is a compensatory response by the circulation in response to

---

Box 28.2 Potential complications of ultrafiltration

◆ Bleeding

◆ Haematomas

◆ Thrombosis

◆ Membrane bioincompatibility

◆ Infection and sepsis

◆ Allergic reactions to the extracorporeal circuit

◆ Hypotension

---

volume loss. If the rate of ultrafiltration is too fast, intravascular volume may significantly decrease because the rate of refill from the interstitial to the intravascular space is not sufficient. This in turn may lead to haemodynamic instability and renal dysfunction. There have been studies that document an increase in creatinine and haemodynamic instability when ultrafiltration rates are too aggressive in a high-risk subset of patients with advanced heart failure [67, 69] and thus the clinician should be aware of this risk.

For potential complications of ultrafiltration and advantages of SCUF over diuretics, see ➲ Boxes 28.2 and 28.3.

Box 28.3 Proposed advantages of SCUF compared with diuretics

◆ More rapid removal of fluid and improvement in symptoms

◆ Higher clearance of sodium

◆ Decreased risk of electrolyte abnormality (e.g. hypokalaemia)

◆ Lack of neurohormonal activation

◆ Removal of proinflammatory cytokines (with potential restoration of responsiveness to diuretics)

◆ Shortened length of stay for heart failure-related hospitalizations

◆ Decreased rate of readmission for heart failure -related hospitalizations

◆ Decreased risk of worsening renal function

Data from Kazory A, Ross EA. Contemporary trends in the pharmacological and extracorporeal management of heart failure: a nephrologic perspective. *Circulation.* 2008;117:975–983.

Personal perspective

More than 60 years have passed since the first clinical application of haemodialysis, and during this period there has been rapid development and technological progress in renal support therapies. This term is now used in the broad context of all therapies designed to modify the size and composition of fluid compartments. In general, this type of therapy makes use of appropriately designed systems connecting blood with specially formulated fluid through a semipermeable membrane in order to replace the kidney as an excretory organ. Indications for renal support therapies include numerous clinical conditions among which AKI, regardless of underlying cause, is the most common. Quite recently, it has become evident that this method can also be used in cardiology to effectively manage volume overload in patients with ADHF. In the near future, systems with living renal tubule epithelial cells attached to the semipermeable membranes ('bioartificial kidney') are likely to be used as genuine renal replacement therapies.

Further reading

Bagshaw SM, Cruz DN, Gibney N, Ronco C. A proposed algorithm for initiation of renal replacement therapy in adult critically ill patients. *Crit Care* 2009;**13**:317–325.

Bellomo R, Ronco C, Kellum JA, *et al.* Acute renal failure-definition, outcome measures, Animals models, fluid therapy and information technology needs: the Second International Consensus Conference of the Acute Dialysis Quality Initiative (ADQI) Group. *Crit Care* 2004;**8**:R204–R212.

Finkel KW, Podoll AS. Complications of continuous renal replacement therapy. *Semin Dial* 2009;**22**:155–159.

Gheorghiade M, Pang PS. Acute heart failure syndromes. *J Am Coll Cardiol* 2009;**53**:557–573.

Pannu N, Klarenbach S, Wiebe N, *et al.* Renal replacement therapy in patients with acute renal failure: a systematic review. *JAMA* 2008;**299**:793–805.

Ronco C, Anker S, McCullough P, *et al.* Cardio-renal syndromes: report from the consensus conference of the Acute Dialysis Quality Initiative. *Eur Heart J* 2010; **31**:703–711.

Ronco C, Bellomo R, Homel P, *et al.* Effects of different doses in continuous veno-venous hemofiltration on outcomes of acute renal failure: a prospective randomised trial. *Lancet* 2000;**356**:26–30.

Song JH, Humes HD. The bioartificial kidney in the treatment of acute kidney injury. *Curr Drug Target s* 2009;**10**:1227–1234.

The RENAL Replacement Therapy Study Investigators. Intensity of continuous renal-replacement therapy in critically ill patients. *N Engl J Med* 2009;**361**:1627–38.

Thorsgard M, Bart BA. Ultrafiltration for congestive heart failure. *Congest Heart Fail* 2009;**15**:136–143.

Additional online material

📺 28.1 Biophysics of renal replacement therapy and derived techniques

📺 28.2 Membrane permeability for different molecules in comparison to the permeability of the filtering membrane of the renal glomerulus

📺 28.3 A diagrammatic representation of diffusion

📺 28.4 A diagrammatic representation of convection

📺 28.5 The concept of a point of inflection

📺 28.6 Factors that may influence the decision to initiate renal replacement therapy in critically ill patients

📺 28.7 Comparison of anticoagulants used in renal replacement therapies. Reproduced with permission from Davenport A, Bouman C, Kirpalani A, *et al.* Delivery of renal replacement therapy in acute kidney injury: what are the key issues? *Clin J Am Soc Nephrol* 2008;**3**:869–75. Copyright American Society of Nephrology.

📺 28.8 Pathophysiology of cardiorenal syndrome

⮊ For additional multimedia materials please visit the online version of the book (🔗 http://www.esciacc.oxfordmedicine.com).

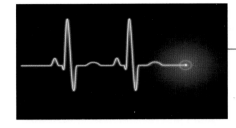

CHAPTER 29

The intra-aortic balloon pump

K. Werdan, M. Ruß, and M. Buerke

Contents

Summary

The intra-aortic balloon pump (IABP) is widely used in patients with cardiogenic shock, with high-risk percutaneous coronary interventions (PCIs), and in cardiac surgery patients. IABP support improves coronary perfusion, heart function, and thereby macro- and microcirculation. The conversion of these cardiovascular effects into prognostic relevance in the critically ill cardiac patient is, however, not well established. This is especially the case for acute myocardial infarction (AMI) patients with cardiogenic shock and early revascularization by PCI, although this indication is a class I recommendation of the European and American guidelines.

Introduction

An IABP benchmark registry [1] presents 'real life' information on intra-aortic balloon pump (IABP) applications, complications, and results in 5495 patients with acute myocardial infarction (AMI) in 250 institutions worldwide between June 1996 and August 2001. Indications were cardiogenic shock (27.3%), haemodynamic support (27.2%) during percutaneous coronary intervention (PCI), high-risk cardiac surgery (11.2%), mechanical infarct complications (11.7%), and refractory postinfarction angina (10%). Mortality was 20%, and in cardiogenic shock 30.7%. Severe complications were seen in 2.7%, during a mean duration of IABP support of 3 days. Premature termination was necessary in 2.1%.

The concept of the intra-aortic balloon pump

Some IABP milestones are the description of the concept by Kantrowitz in 1953 [2], the first clinical use in 1968 [3–5], and percutaneous insertion in the 1980s [6, 7]. Further developments took the form of smaller balloons and sheathless insertion techniques [8–10], miniaturization [11], mathematical modelling [12, 13], continuous versus pulsatile augmentation [14], and a stroke volume blood chamber [15].

The conventional indication for IABP is 'manifest or impending acute heart failure/cardiogenic shock of ischaemic aetiology'. With the IABP in place in the descending thoracic aorta, inflation of the balloon in diastole and active deflation in systole induce higher diastolic perfusion pressures in the coronary arteries and unload the diseased heart by reducing left ventricular afterload in systole [16]. Volume shifting of about 40 mL/beat by the IABP increases left ventricular ejection fraction and thereby cardiac output (CO) by up to 1 L/min. IABP improves oxygen supply, decreases oxygen demand and may improve arterial functional capability [17]. However, the effects vary widely from patient to patient due to a number of clinical and technical factors, as described below [18–20].

Effects on coronary blood flow

♦ Normal blood pressure and patent coronary arteries: In this condition balloon pumping decreases myocardial oxygen demand, but has no effect—probably because of autoregulation—on total coronary blood flow [19, 21–23], nor on blood flow through saphenous vein or internal mammary artery bypass grafts [24].

♦ Severe hypotension and patent coronary arteries: IABP-induced rise in systemic blood pressure can increase coronary blood flow.

♦ Severe coronary artery stenosis or acute coronary syndrome (ACS): Despite an increase in coronary perfusion pressure, IABP pumping does not increase coronary blood flow beyond a very narrowed or occluded vessel [5, 25–30]. Some results argue for a favourable influence of IABP pumping on the distribution of global coronary blood flow in myocardial ischaemia, especially in hypotension [18, 23, 31–34].

♦ Thrombolysis treatment of ST-segment elevation myocardial infarction (STEMI): IABP pumping may support systemic thrombolysis therapy to achieve successful reperfusion of the reopened infarct-related coronary artery [35, 36] and may reduce risk of reocclusion [37–40], most likely by the increase of diastolic flow velocity by 100% or even more [21, 22, 41].

Effects on heart function

♦ Reduction in ventricular afterload and improvement in ventriculoarterial coupling [42, 43] produces an increase in stroke volume and cardiac index (CI) of 15–30%, with the largest increases in CO seen in patients with reduced CO [30, 43–46].

♦ Heart rate remains stable or decreases slightly [30, 45, 46].

♦ Ventricular preload, left ventricular end diastolic pressure, and pulmonary capillary wedge pressure are often found to be reduced [28, 23, 45].

♦ In patients with myocardial ischaemia, a decrease in left ventricular wall stress and of myocardial oxygen supply has been described, thereby improving the myocardial oxygen supply/demand ratio [18, 30, 43–45, 47]. The fall in levels of N-terminal pro-brain natriuretic peptide (NT-proBNP) [48] and brain natriuretic peptide (BNP) [49] is in agreement with this positive effect.

♦ The reduction of left ventricular afterload is especially helpful in patients with acute mitral insufficiency or ventricular septal defect [50, 51].

♦ Right ventricular afterload: IABP may reduce pulmonary artery pressure and limit deleterious ventricular interdependence, thereby improving right ventricular ejection fraction [46, 52, 53].

Effects on systemic macro- and microcirculation

♦ Blood pressure: Mean blood pressure generally does not change in patients with normal baseline pressures but does increase in shock [30, 44, 46]. Systolic pressure in haemodynamically stable patients tends to decrease by 5–20%, while in shock an increase may be observed [5, 23, 28, 30, 43, 45, 47]. A marked increase in diastolic pressure, from 10% to 90% or even more, can be seen; this is due to diastolic augmentation [5, 23, 28, 30, 43, 45, 47].

♦ Regional blood flow: IABP pumping may improve renal blood flow and correct metabolic acidosis in patients with severe heart failure and cardiogenic shock [45, 54], but without improvement of kidney function [54]. Interestingly, blood flow in the carotid artery is not increased [55].

♦ Microcirculation: With the sidestream dark field technique, sublingual microcirculation in humans can be monitored online (see ◗ Chapter 17). IABP findings were described as positive [56], as well as neutral, despite clear-cut positive effects on macrocirculation (mean arterial pressure increased by 6 mmHg; CI 0.5 L min^{-1} m^{-2}; cardiac power index (CPI) increased by 0.1 W m^{-2} [57].

♦ Haemodynamic IABP effects in a randomized trial with patients with AMI complicated by cardiogenic shock: BNP levels are lower in the IABP group, indicating some unloading of the left ventricle. However, no significant difference is observed with respect to CI [49]. Furthermore, no relevant effects of IABP support are seen with respect to CO, systemic vascular resistance (SVR), pulmonary vascular resistance (PVR), pulmonary artery pressure (PAP), pulmonary artery occlusion pressure (PAOP), left ventricular stroke work index (LVSWI), or cardiac power output (CPO) (unpublished results), with the CPO being a good prognostic indicator in this patient group [58].

Practical approach

Equipment

The equipment consists of the balloon catheter, an insertion set for femoral access (sheath, guide wire, puncture cannula), the console, and the control panel with monitor screen [16].

The balloon catheter has two lumens. The central lumen allows insertion into the artery over a guide wire and subsequent continuous arterial pressure monitoring, while helium gas exchange to and from the balloon is enabled by the outer lumen. The shaft sizes range from 7 to 8 French, with the 7-French catheter being small enough to be inserted through a 7-French arterial sheath. Sheathless insertion is also possible.

For adults, the balloon is positioned in the descending aorta, distal to the left subclavian artery and proximal to the renal arterial. The inflated balloon should ideally occupy 80–90% of the diameter of the aorta. Too small a balloon will provide ineffective counterpulsation, whereas one that is too large may result in either balloon rupture or aortic damage.

Triggered by blood pressure tracing or ECG, low-viscosity helium is rapidly injected into the balloon during cardiac diastole and withdrawn during systole. The frequency with which the balloon inflates can be timed to each, every other, or every third/fourth cardiac cycle.

Insertion technique

For a depiction of the technique, see 📷 29.1.

Insertion before or after percutaneous coronary intervention?

Inserting the IABP before PCI provides all possible advantages of IABP support for PCI, i.e. increase of mean arterial pressure and coronary perfusion pressure [16]. However, difficulties in positioning the balloon catheter can sometimes prolong the time to reperfusion. Furthermore, as well as the femoral artery access for the IABP another access for coronary angiography has to be established and takes up 'reperfusion time'. When the IABP is placed first and the lack of a second arterial access becomes evident, the IABP catheter must be removed. Many centres therefore prefer to perform PCI first and insert IABP by the same access route afterwards.

Femoral approach

◆ The IABP is usually placed by the percutaneous femoral artery approach over a guide wire, under fluoroscopic guidance, although it can also be placed at the bedside without fluoroscopy, if necessary. In latter case, the correct position must be checked by chest radiograph or transoesophageal echocardiography. Strict aseptic technique is followed throughout the complete insertion procedure.

◆ Before insertion the pulses in both lower extremities should be assessed, and the balloon catheter should be placed through the femoral artery with the stronger pulse, if necessary with the help of a pocket Doppler.

◆ Arterial access is obtained in the common femoral artery using the Seldinger technique with the patient under local anaesthesia. The puncture site should be below the inguinal ligament to avoid a noncompressible injury to the artery, but the puncture should be above the femoral bifurcation; placing the IABP through the smaller profunda or superficial femoral branches will result in limb ischaemia.

◆ A guide wire is then advanced into the descending thoracic aorta. If the standard J-tip wire cannot be passed smoothly, alternative wires (e.g. a large J or steerable wires) may be tried. If these manoeuvres are unsuccessful, a small contrast injection under fluoroscopy may reveal the problem, such as a tight atherosclerotic narrowing in the iliac artery. Placement of the balloon via an alternative site, such as the contralateral femoral artery, may then be necessary. Alternatively, peripheral balloon angioplasty may be performed to permit successful balloon insertion [59].

◆ After the wire is passed, an appropriately sized sheath (usually 8 French) is placed over the guide wire; if sheathless insertion is planned, predilation with an 8-French dilator is performed [9, 60]. Sheathless insertion is not recommended in patients with groin scarring, very tortuous iliac vessels, or severe obesity.

◆ The balloon catheter is prepared for insertion by application of negative pressure to the gas lumen, using the supplied syringe and one-way valve, and flushing of the guide-wire lumen with heparinized saline. The catheter is then advanced over the wire until the radiopaque marker at its tip lies just distal to the take-off of the left subclavian artery. If fluoroscopy is not used, how far to insert the balloon may be estimated by placing the tip of the catheter at the sternal notch, laying it flat on the patient to the umbilicus, and then angling the catheter from the umbilicus to the femoral puncture site.

• The wire is removed, and the central lumen is flushed and connected via a pressure transducer to the pump console. The one-way valve is removed from the gas lumen and connected via the supplied tubing to the helium tank. The balloon is purged and filled, correct positioning of the catheter tip is verified by fluoroscopy, and pumping is initiated. If adjustment of the balloon position is needed at any time, it must be placed in standby mode while it is repositioned; if a sheath is used, the balloon may be moved into the sheath, but the sheath itself must not be advanced because this may damage the artery.

• The left radial pulse is palpated to ensure that the balloon tip is not obstructing the left subclavian artery, and the pulses distal to the balloon pump site are assessed and recorded.

• Unless there has been a breach of aseptic precautions, prophylactic antibiotic administration is not necessary, because it has not been shown to reduce infection risk or to improve overall outcomes [61].

• A chest radiograph must be taken immediately after the procedure, particularly if fluoroscopy was not used.

Alternative insertion techniques

These are seldom necessary. They include interventional or surgical axillary, brachial, subclavian, iliac, or retroperitoneal approaches [62–68].

Care of the patient

• Comfort of the patient: Most patients tolerate IABP well, even in the conscious, nonventilated state. Sedation and analgesia are usually unnecessary.

• Heparin anticoagulation: In many centres, the patient is fully anticoagulated with heparin to reduce the risk of balloon-related thrombosis [69], though the advantage over low-dose heparin is unproven [70].

• Nursing: Nursing care recommendations are given in [71].

• In experienced hands, IABP can be safely carried out in the intensive care unit (ICU) as well as in the emergency department [72].

• Transfer of patients dependent on IABP support: These patients can be safely transported by helicopter or aeroplane, by personnel trained in IABP care [73].

Removal technique

Before removal of the IABP it is preferable to provide a margin of safety for reinstituting therapy without requiring reinsertion of the IABP. Ideally, mechanical ventilation should be discontinued and vasopressor and inotropic support adjusted. Patients are usually weaned by gradual reduction of the pump mode from 1:1 to 1:2 to 1:3 (on some consoles, even 1:8). If the patient tolerates the reduction in pumping without clinical deterioration, anticoagulation is stopped; counterpulsation is continued to decrease the risk of thrombosis. When the anticoagulation decreases to a safe level, the IABP may be removed.

The technique of removal of the IABP differs in several respects from the removal of most other intravascular devices. In the stop mode, the balloon is deflated completely. Then it is withdrawn to (not into) the sheath, if one is present. It is important to remember that a used balloon cannot be withdrawn into the sheath because it will not fold back to its original size; attempts to pull a balloon into a sheath may result in rupture and possibly embolization of the balloon membrane.

Firm manual pressure is applied distal to the insertion site, and balloon and sheath are removed as a unit. Distal pressure is maintained for two to three heartbeats, which permits free bleeding from the site and allows thrombus and other debris to clear from the vessel. Then pressure is applied proximal to the insertion site, usually for 20–40 min, until haemostasis is secure.

If significant limb ischaemia or another vascular complication is present, or if the balloon was placed by means of an open surgical approach, surgical removal is usually indicated. Haemostasis may be difficult to obtain with manual compression in patients with high puncture sites (above the inguinal ligament), morbid obesity, or prolonged periods of IABP support, and these patients may also benefit from surgical removal [74].

Timing

Proper timing of balloon inflation and deflation is critical for optimal IABP support (⊃ Fig. 29.1) [16, 75]. Errors in the timing of IABP inflation and deflation may be harmful. There are four potential errors of IABP timing:

• Inflation too early. Inflation of the balloon before aortic valve closure (pressure rise before dicrotic notch) may result in diastolic augmentation encroaching into systole.

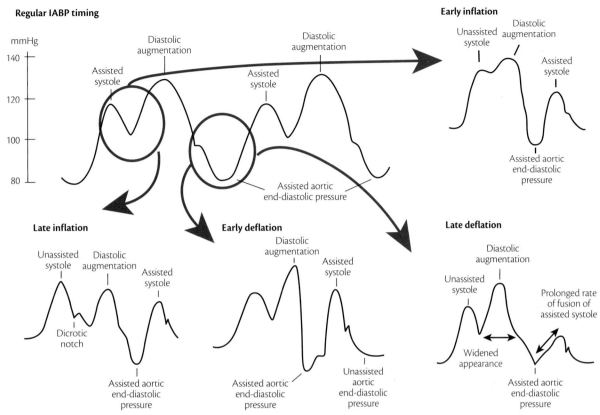

Figure 29.1 Correct timing and pitfalls in timing of inflation and deflation of the IABP balloon.

This then results in potential premature closure of the aortic valve or aortic insufficiency, increased left ventricular wall stress, increase in left ventricular end diastolic pressure, and finally increased myocardial oxygen demand.

- Inflation too late. The inflation of the balloon late after closure of the aortic valve, characterized by the absence of a sharp V in the pressure curve, leads to suboptimal diastolic augmentation and thereby suboptimal augmentation of coronary artery perfusion.

- Deflation too early. Premature deflation of the balloon during the diastolic phase is recognized as a sharp drop following diastolic augmentation, leading to suboptimal diastolic augmentation, suboptimal coronary perfusion, and possibly retrograde coronary and carotid blood flow. As a result, angina may occur and there is inefficient afterload reduction and increased cardiac oxygen demand.

- Deflation too late. With prolonged pressure support lasting till the next systole, assisted aortic end diastolic pressure may be equal to the unassisted aortic end diastolic pressure, which prolongs the rate of rise of assisted systole, and the diastolic augmentation may appear widened. In this case, afterload reduction is essentially absent, with

increased cardiac oxygen consumption due to the left ventricle ejecting against a greater resistance (increased afterload) and a prolonged isovolumetric contraction phase.

The newer IABP models with advanced algorithms allow automatic triggering even in difficult conditions such as tachyarrhythmias; nevertheless, IABP timing should be checked regularly (at least every 8 h).

Contraindications and complications

- Limb ischaemia—which in our opinion is less frequent nowadays—usually necessitates discontinuation of the IABP; it generally resolves when the balloon is removed [76–78], but in up to 14% of cases surgical intervention seems necessary [76].

- Vascular complications are also associated with worse overall outcome, including higher mortality [79, 80]; chronic ischaemia with pain and diminished or absent pulse may be evident in 2–18% [76, 81].

- The incidence of complications is strikingly increased in patients with peripheral arterial disease; further risk factors for vascular complications include female gender, diabetes, smoking, shock, an ankle/brachial index less than 0.8, and atherosclerotic debris in the aorta [16, 78, 82].

◆ Not unexpectedly, large catheter size [8, 10, 83] and long duration of IABP support [10, 74] also contribute to the risk of complications.

⮕ Box 29.1 summarizes the contraindications and complications of IABP use.

Adjunctive intra-aortic balloon pump treatment

Commonly accepted criteria under optimal medical therapy for implementation of an IABP are [84]:

◆ CI <2.0 L m^2 min^{-1}

◆ Mean arterial pressure <65 mmHg

Box 29.1 Contraindications and complications of IABP use

Contraindications

Absolute contraindications

◆ Moderate to severe aortic valvular incompetence: increase in diastolic pressure may exacerbate valvular regurgitation

◆ Aortic aneurysm and aortic dissection: risk of rupture; risk of IABP insertion and inflation into the false lumen

◆ Patent ductus arteriosus: increase in left-to-right shunting

Relative contraindications

◆ Severe bilateral peripheral arterial disease and bilateral femoral–popliteal bypass grafts: increased risk of severe vascular complications

◆ Major bleeding disorders: risk of haemorrhagic complications at the insertion site

◆ Hypertrophic cardiomyopathy with dynamic left ventricular outflow obstruction: IABP-triggered afterload reduction may worsen degree of obstruction[a]

Complications

Total complications

◆ Registry data:[b] 2.7%

◆ Review data:[c]
  • major complications 15.0%
  • minor complications 42.0%

Mortality

◆ 30-day mortality during AMI treatment:[c,d] 1%

◆ 30-day mortality during treatment of AMI with shock and early PCI:[d] 6%

◆ 30-day mortality during treatment of AMI with shock and early PCI:[e] 0%

◆ Mortality due to vascular complications in open heart surgery:[f] 8.49%

Stroke during AMI treatment:[d] 2%

Bleeding

◆ Major bleeding during AMI treatment:[d] 6%

◆ Increase in major bleeding during PCI:[g] 3.5-fold

◆ PCI in the presence of glycoprotein IIb/IIIa antagonists:[h]
  • major bleeding 9%
  • minor bleeding 15%

Vascular complications

◆ In patients undergoing open heart surgery:[f] 9.4% (leg ischaemia, leg ischaemia with compartment syndrome, groin haematoma needing wound exploration)

◆ Limb ischaemia—acute or chronic[i]

◆ Thrombosis, embolism (e.g. into bowel vessels[j])

◆ Haematoma, bleeding, pseudoaneurysm[k]

◆ Arterial perforation, laceration, or dissection (risk of paraplegia)[l]

◆ Cholesterol embolism

Infection—superficial or deep

Haemolysis[m]

Renal and visceral ischaemia[n]

◆ (due to juxtarenal and juxtamesenteric-artery balloon positioning)

Thrombocytopenia[o]

Balloon rupture[c]

Specific complications with an IABP inserted thoracically[p]

---

[a] [148]; [b] [1]; [c] [16]; [d] [90]; [e] [49]; [f] [149]; p for mortality = <0.005; [g] [150]; OR 3.5, 95% confidence interval 1.0–12.1; p = 0.47); [h] [151]; [i] [76, 77, 79, 78, 81, 80]; [j] [152]; [k] [152, 153]; [l] [154]; [m] haemolysis is generally mild; [n] [155, 156]; [o] usually mild and reversible; [157];[p] [158]; may occur in up to 5%; appearance of blood in the gas lumen tubing; prompt removal of the catheter is necessary, even if the balloon had been functioning properly, to prevent helium embolism or balloon entrapment.

◆ Left or right atrial or PAOP > 20 mmHg

◆ Urine output <20 mL/h

◆ SVR >2100 dyne s cm^{-5}

Type of ventricular dysfunction

Most data on the beneficial effect of IABP are available for left ventricular systolic dysfunction and to a lesser extent for right ventricular systolic failure (see ➲ Cardiac surgery). Disease-specific indications are listed in ➲ Table 29.1. However, most of the indications for IABP are not validated by randomized trials.

Table 29.1 Indications for implementation of IABP

Indications	Guidelines		
	ESC	AHA	German/Austrian
In selected patients with myocardial infarction (STEMI)			
Complicated by cardiogenic shock	I/C	I/B	
Treatment with PCI			⇔/3/4
Treatment with fibrinolysis/with no perfusion strategy			⇑/3/4
Before transport to an interventional centre for PCI			⇑/3/4
With mechanical complications (acute mitral insufficiency due to papillary muscle rupture, ventricular septal rupture) for preoperative haemodynamic stabilization	+	+	⇑/3/4
With hypotension (RRsyst <90 mmHg or 30 mmHg below baseline RR, who do not respond to other interventions)		I/B	
With low output states		I/B	
As stabilizing measure for angiography and prompt revascularization when cardiogenic shock is not quickly reversed with pharmacological therapy		I/B	
In addition to medical therapy in case of recurrent ischaemic-type chest discomfort and signs of haemodynamic instability, poor left ventricular function, or a large area of myocardium at risk, as additional support to the urgently needed revascularization procedure		I/C	
With refractory polymorphic ventricular tachycardia to reduce myocardial ischaemia		IIa/B	
With refractory pulmonary congestion		IIb/C	
In selected patients without complications after reperfusion therapy			

Table 29.1 (Cont'd) Indications for implementation of IABP

Indications	Guidelines		
	ESC	AHA	German/Austrian
In selected non-STEMI patients with identical indications as in STEMI patients[a]			
In selected patients with unstable angina			
With ischaemia refractory to medical management till PCI/ACB intervention[b]			
With haemodynamic instability			
In selected patients with severe systolic heart failure			
Caused by reversible myocardial depression			
Acute myocarditis			
Drug-induced myocardial dysfunction[c]			
Myocardial contusion			
Post-cardiac arrest syndrome[d]			
Anorexia nervosa[e]			
With haemodynamic instability			
In selected patients during PCI[f]			
With haemodynamic instability			
With severely depressed left ventricular function			
With left main or three-vessel disease			
In selected cardiac surgery patients			
Preoperative			
With unstable clinical syndromes			
With poor left ventricular function			
With high-risk coronary anatomy			
With acute mitral insufficiency			
Intraoperative or postoperative			
With haemodynamic instability			
With difficulty in weaning from CBP			
Bridge to transplantation/permanent LVAD			
In selected patients with high-risk cardiac disease during urgent or emergency surgery			
(?) In selected patients with septic shock and severe septic cardiomyopathy			

[a] For IABP-treated non-STEMI patients a higher mortality rate has been reported than with STEMI patients [159].
[b] [111].
[c] [160].
[d] Therapeutic hypothermia after cardiac arrest can be safely carried out with inserted IABP [161].
[e] [162].
[f] 104, 101, 105, 153, 19, 5, 26, 28, 163].
The recommendations and evidence levels of the following guidelines are given: ESC [99], AHA/ACC [100], German/Austrian [89].

Myocardial infarction, especially if complicated by cardiogenic shock

80% of AMI patients with cardiogenic shock suffer from systolic pump failure [85].

What do meta-analyses tell us?

Although there are several registries [18, 6] and uncontrolled trials [87–89] the number of controlled trials with mortality as an endpoint is very small. Recent meta-analyses [90] have summarized the available data:

- High-risk STEMI patients (➲ Fig. 29.2): This meta-analysis included 7 randomized trials with 1009 patients. IABP did not reduce 30-day mortality or improve left ventricular ejection fraction, but strokes (+2%) and bleeding (+ 6%) were increased.

- STEMI patients with cardiogenic shock (➲ Fig. 29.3): 9 cohorts with 10 529 patients were analysed. In those

patients treated with systemic thrombolysis, IABP support was associated with an 18% decrease in 30-day mortality (*p* <0.001), albeit with significantly higher revascularization rates compared to patients without support. These data go along with those from the SHOCK Trial Registry, where mortality in patients with thrombolysis plus IABP was nonsignificantly lower (47%) than in those without IABP (63%) [91]. In patients treated with primary PCI, however, IABP was associated with a 6% increase in 30-day mortality (p <0.0008). Why IABP could work as adjunctive therapy together with thrombolysis but not with PCI remains a subject for speculation [89, 90].

Effects on haemodynamics, systemic inflammation, and multiorgan dysfunction syndrome

Prognostic factors in cardiogenic shock complicating AMI are not only impaired cardiac function, but also the development of systemic inflammatory response syndrome (SIRS), measured by interleukin-6 (IL-6), and multiorgan

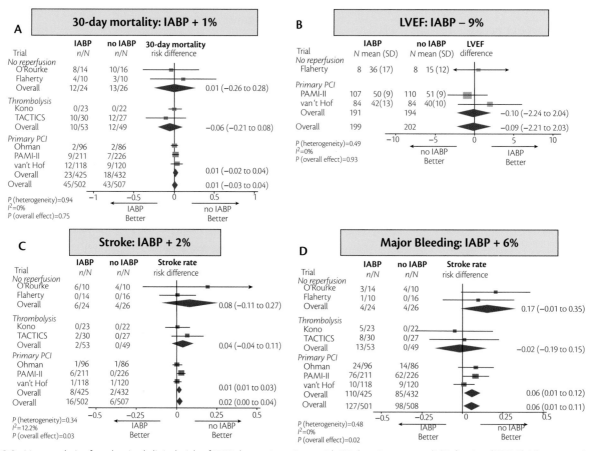

Figure 29.2 Meta-analysis of randomized clinical trials of IABP therapy in patients with ST-elevation myocardial infarction (STEMI). All meta-analyses show effect estimates for the individual trials, for each type of reperfusion therapy and for the overall analysis. The size of each square is proportional to the weight of the individual trial. In (A), the risk difference in 30-day- mortality is shown, in (B) the mean difference in left ventricular ejection fraction, in (C) the risk difference in stroke, and in (D) the risk difference in major bleeding rate. IABP, intraaortic balloon counterpulsation; LVEF, left ventricular ejection fraction; PCI, percutaneous coronary intervention.
Modified from Sjauw KD, Engstrom AE, Vis MM, *et al.* A systematic review and meta-analysis of intra-aortic balloon pump therapy in ST-elevation myocardial infarction: should we change the guidelines? *Eur Heart J* 2009;**30**:459–468. Editorial: 389–390. With permission from Oxford University Press.

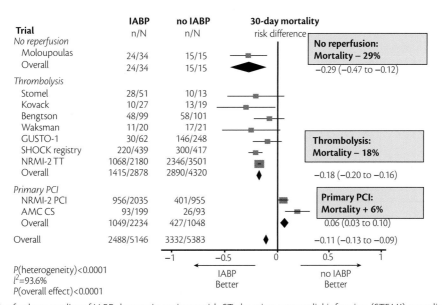

Figure 29.3 Meta-analysis of cohort studies of IABP therapy in patients with ST-elevation myocardial infarction (STEMI) complicated by cardiogenic shock. The risk differences in 30-day mortality for the individual studies, for each type of reperfusion therapy, and for the overall analysis are given. The size of each square is proportional to the weight of the individual study. PCI, percutaneous coronary intervention.
Modified from Sjauw KD, Engstrom AE, Vis MM, *et al.* A systematic review and meta-analysis of intra-aortic balloon pump therapy in ST-elevation myocardial infarction: should we change the guidelines? *Eur Heart J* 2009;**30**:459–468. Editorial: 389–390. With permission from Oxford University Press.

dysfunction syndrome (MODS), measured by serial APACHE II scoring—a fall indicates better survival in septic shock [92] (see ⮞ Chapter 17). In a prospective randomized trial (⮞ Fig. 29.4) [49] no effect of IABP on these measures was seen: neither serial APACHE II score over the first 96 h, nor CI, nor IL-6 was significantly different. Only plasma BNP levels at 48 and 72 h were significantly (p <0.05) lower in the IABP patients, though this biomarker was of no prognostic relevance in this study [49]. If effective medical inotropic therapy, including levosimendan [93, 94] is employed, adjunctive IABP support seemingly has only, at best, few additional beneficial effects in these patients.

Transfer for percutaneous coronary intervention

In hospitals where PCI is not available, adjunctive IABP with or without thrombolysis might be a helpful option before the patient is transferred to a cardiological intervention centre [95]) or cardiac surgery unit [96] (uncontrolled studies).

Mechanical complications of myocardial infarction

Especially in ventricular septal defect [97], an IABP should be implemented as short-term support in advance of surgical or interventional repair, as many of these patients develop cardiogenic shock, thereby increasing mortality risk sevenfold [98]. IABP support increases CI, decreases left-to-right shunt, improves metabolic acidosis, and reduces lactate levels [51].

Conclusions to be drawn from the evidence

In view of the level 1 recommendations of the European [99] and American [100] guidelines for the use of IABP in patients with complicated myocardial infarction (⮞ Table 29.1), the reported meta-analyses [90] yielded surprising and disappointing results (⮞ Figs. 29.2, 29.3). In consequence, a rethinking of IABP recommendations is required:

◆ In high-risk patients with myocardial infarction without cardiogenic shock, the use of IABP cannot be recommended.

◆ In STEMI/non-STEMI patients with cardiogenic shock, analysis is hampered by bias and confounding [90]. Hence, a randomized controlled trial (IABP Shock II trial; ClinicalTrials.gov identifier NCT00491036; see ⮞ Online resource) has recently been initiated that will address the potential benefit of IABP counterpulsation adjunctive to medical treatment and primary PCI in 600 patients.

A German–Austrian guideline for AMI patients with cardiogenic shock [89] took these meta-analyses [90] into account and gives the following recommendations (⮞ Table 29.1):

◆ In primary systemic thrombolysis, adjunctive IABP therapy is recommended (low recommendation and evidence level).

◆ In primary PCI, IABP use may be considered. Whether this might be helpful is unclear.

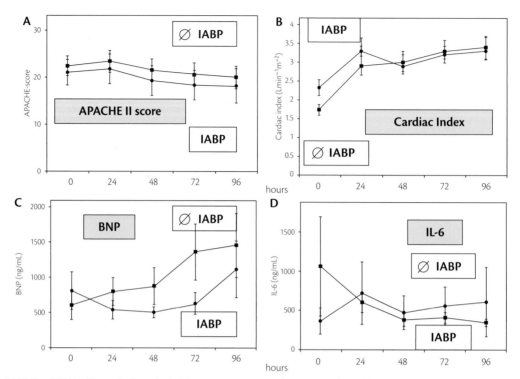

Figure 29.4 The 'IABP Shock' Trial: effects of adjunctive IABP support. Patients with AMI complicated by cardiogenic shock and treated by primary PCI have randomly been adjunctively supported by IABP (n = 19; 'IABP') or not (n = 21; 'ø IABP'). Serial biomarker monitoring is presented during the first 96 h after starting treatment. APACHE II score represents severity of disease and MODS, CI represents heart function, BNP represents pump failure, and IL-6 represents systemic inflammation. Only BNP plasma levels at 48 h and at 72 h were significantly different between the groups ($p < 0.05$).
Adapted with permission from Prondzinsky R, Lemm H, Swyter M, *et al.* Intra-aortic balloon counterpulsation in patients with acute myocardial infarction complicated by cardiogenic shock—the prospective, randomized IABP SHOCK trial for attenuation of multi-organ dysfunction syndrome. *Crit Care Med* 2010;**38**:152–160.

♦ When transferring a patient to a PCI centre, an IABP should be inserted for haemodynamic stabilization (low recommendation and evidence level).

♦ If there are mechanical AMI complications, especially a ventricular septal defect, an IABP should be inserted for haemodynamic stabilization before the patient is transferred for cardiac surgery (low recommendation and evidence level).

High-risk percutaneous coronary intervention

27% of IABP insertions in patients with AMI are to support high-risk catheterizations and angioplasty procedures [1, 90,101, 102]. The combination of IABP plus levosimendan has also been reported [103].

Recent evidence from nonrandomized trials

Registry data and retrospective study analysis describe beneficial effects of prophylactic IABP use during 'high-risk PCI', especially in those patients with severe left ventricular dysfunction, cardiogenic shock, large amount of myocardium at risk [104–106], and advanced age [107]: the results showed

an increased freedom from adverse events, fewer cardiac and cerebral events, lower hospital rates of major adverse cardiac events, and better in-hospital and 6-month survival.

Rationale of the BCIS-1 study

Because high-level evidence is still missing, the Balloon pump-assisted Coronary Intervention Study (BCIS-1) has been designed [108] (http://www.clinicaltrials.gov, trial ID NCT00910481 and http://www.controlled-trials.com, ISRCTN 40553718).

Cardiac surgery

About 2–8% of cardiac surgical procedures, mostly aortocoronary bypass (ACB), are carried out with IABP support [109–112]; the tendency is decreasing [112].

Choosing the right patient

There are two indications:

♦ The emergency indication, in case of the development of low cardiac output syndrome during surgery, or during weaning from the cardiopulmonary bypass, or postoperative haemodynamic instability in the ICU.

◆ The prophylactic/preemptive indication, with IABP implementation in high-risk cardiac surgery patients, characterized by two or more of the following criteria [113, 114]:

  · refractory unstable angina despite intravenous administration of heparin and nitroglycerine

  · left ventricular ejection fraction ≤40%

  · coronary left main stenosis ≥70%

  · previous coronary artery bypass grafting (CABG)

  · diffuse coronary artery disease (four or more distal anastomoses to achieve complete revascularization).

◆ Slightly changed 'high-risk' criteria in cardiac surgery patients are also used.

◆ Another approach for prophylactic IABP support is to select high-risk patients with a high EuroSCORE (≥12) [115]: prophylactic use of IABP starting preoperatively appears to shift high-risk patients undergoing ACB into a lower risk category.

Aortocoronary bypass risk patients

◆ For on-pump ACB surgery the evidence of retrospective, nonrandomized trials can be summarized as follows:

  · In high-risk patients, prophylactic use seems favourable [112, 116–120].

  · In low-risk patients, the results of one study [120] argue that early IABP implementation should be established whenever cardiac complications are suspected, because of its beneficial impact on enzymatic leakage, myocardial recovery as seen by echocardiography, hospital outcome, mid-term follow-up survival, and freedom from cardiovascular events.

◆ For off-pump coronary artery bypass surgery, convincing data are available favouring prophylactic use of IABP in high-risk patients with severe left ventricular dysfunction [121], especially in those with left main coronary artery disease [122]. Perioperative morbidity and mortality are considerably reduced by prophylactic IABP.

Cardiac surgery patients with right ventricular systolic failure

In patients with right ventricular low CO syndrome, IABP support of cardiac surgery increases mean CI and mean arterial pressure within 1 h after IABP insertion, while central venous pressure and PAOP decrease; 75% of these patients can be weaned from IABP [110].

When an intra-aortic balloon pump is not enough

In patients with postoperative low CO syndrome despite adjunctive IABP therapy, several indicators measured 1 h after IABP insertion document a worse prognosis: adrenaline dose >0.05 µg kg^{-1} min^{-1}; oliguria <100 mL/h, Svo_2 <60–65%; left atrial pressure >15–17 mmHg. In these patients, the addition of levosimendan [123] or implantation of a ventricular assist device should be considered [110, 124].

Pulsatile or nonpulsatile perfusion during cardiopulmonary bypass

The negative effects of cardiopulmonary bypass during cardiac surgery may be partly counteracted by inducing a pulsatile flow with IABP, especially in elderly patients [125–127], with improving coronary bypass graft flows during nonpulsatile peripheral extracorporeal membrane oxygenation [38].

Bridge to cardiac transplantation

IABP can be used for short-term support in advance of cardiac transplantation in patients with both ischaemic and nonischaemic cardiomyopathy [41, 128–132], although IABP is not ideal for this indication because it is designed for brief temporary support, usually no longer than 2 weeks. However, for at least one-third of these patients, IABP support is insufficient [133, 132].

Patients with cardiogenic shock and sepsis

13–18% of AMI patients with cardiogenic shock develop severe inflammation and sepsis [134, 135], as shown by sepsis criteria and a fall in SVR (see ⊃ Chapter 17). IABP is used in these patients too, with higher median duration, but still with no more complications reported [134, 135]. Nevertheless, in septic patients a device such as an IABP could trigger further infectious events and might be harmful. In view of this the use of IABP would be better avoided.

To better judge this situation, cardiologists should know that septic cardiomyopathy contributes considerably to septic shock (⊃ Chapter 17; [136–140]) and there is controversial experimental evidence [141–143] and some (not convincing) clinical evidence [144–146] that IABP support of patients with septic shock could be of benefit.

Other means of haemodynamic support

In comparing IABP and percutaneous left ventricular assist devices (Impella, Tandem Heart) in cardiogenic shock it is necessary to distinguish haemodynamic from prognostic effects [147]. A higher CI ($+0.35$ L min^{-1} m^{-2}) and mean arterial pressure ($+12.8$ mmHg) as well as a greater decrease in PAOP (-5.3 mmHg) in the group with a left ventricular assist device did not result in better survival. In terms of side effects, limb ischaemia was no more frequent, but bleeding episodes occurred 2.35-fold more often in the left ventricular assist device group.

Personal perspective

Experimental and clinical studies have documented the effects of IABP on coronary circulation, heart function, and circulation, but almost none have considered its prognostic relevance. Also, most of this work was carried out decades ago, before effective measures like PCI were available. It is really questionable whether the results obtained can usefully be transferred to current practice.

Nevertheless, the use of IABP in the adjunctive treatment of cardiogenic shock is widely accepted, even on the guideline level. Nevertheless, the promise of IABP use as an evidence-based standard procedure is by no means fulfilled. This is especially the case when we

Conclusion

The use of IABP can help to improve haemodynamics in cardiogenic shock and also to support high-risk PCIs and ACBs. For patients with cardiogenic shock complicating myocardial infarction, the European STEMI guidelines give a class I recommendation for IABP use. This recommendation, however, needs further evidence-based support.

consider the use of IABP in the large group of patients with myocardial infarction complicated by cardiogenic shock: the available low-quality study evidence may favour IABP use when patients are treated with systemic thrombolysis, but patients treated with primary PCI might even be harmed. Unfortunately, percutaneous left ventricular assist devices—though haemodynamically more efficient than IABP—have not shown superiority over IABP in terms of prognosis. Nevertheless, the STEMI guidelines should critically discuss the evidence for IABP support in AMI patients complicated by cardiogenic shock, and more high-quality study evidence should be sought, in interventional cardiology as well as in cardiac surgery.

Further reading

Kelly RF. Intraaortic balloon counterpulsation. In: Parrillo JE, Dellinger RP (eds) *Critical care medicine—principles of diagnosis and management in the adult*, 2nd edition, Mosby, St. Louis, 2001, pp. 91–106.

Sjauw KD, Engstrom AE, Vis MM, *et al*. A systematic review and meta-analysis of intra-aortic balloon pump therapy in ST-elevation myocardial infarction: should we change the guidelines? *Eur Heart J* 2009;**30**:459–468. Editorial: 389–390.

Van de Werf F, Bax J, Betriu A, *et al*. Management of acute myocardial infarction in patients presenting with persistent ST-segment elevation: the task force on the management of ST-segment elevation acute myocardial infarction of the European Society of Cardiology. *Eur Heart J* 2008;**29**:2909–2945.

Online resource

ClinicalTrials.gov. http://www.clinical trials.gov

Additional online material

29.1 IABP insertion technique

➔ For additional multimedia materials please visit the online version of the book (http://www.esciacc.oxfordmedicine.com).

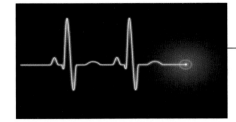

CHAPTER 30

Left ventricular assist devices in acute heart failure

Susanna Price, Martin Strueber, and
Pascal Vranckx

Contents

Summary

Medical therapy remains the mainstay of treatment for the majority of heart failure patients. In recent years, however, advanced mechanical support of the circulation has been developed to provide an additional therapeutic option. Initially designed as a temporary solution for the failing heart to allow ventricular recovery, or as a bridge for patients to cardiac transplantation, in more recent times, with demand for cardiac transplantation outstripping organ supply, these devices have been used as destination therapy for highly selected patients in whom transplantation is not an option. The available devices are generally classified by their mechanism of action (centrifugal, volume displacement) and the intended duration of support (short- or long-term). Each is limited by the invasive nature of the procedure, the requirement for central cannulation, the risks of bleeding, thromboembolism, and infection. In all cases, the key requirements for success are appropriate patient selection, and care in a cardiothoracic centre of excellence. This chapter concentrates on the application of advanced mechanical assistance relevant to the interventional cardiologist.

Introduction

Mechanical cardiac support became a potential therapeutic option with the successful implementation of cardiopulmonary bypass (CPB) in 1953 [1]. Subsequent development of more long-term support over the decades since then has resulted in a number of devices, each with their own indications and limitations. Treatment with mechanical circulatory support must be tailored to each patient in order to optimize the benefits and minimize the risk of complications.

Portable (percutaneous) cardiac assist devices

Concept

Management of the ischaemic patient with significant acute hemodynamic compromise undergoing percutaneous intervention is a challenge for myocardial intervention centres. Although the intra-aortic ballon pump (IABP) provides an important method of mechanical circulatory support, where it is inadequate, immediate triage to more advanced percutaneous (or implantable) circulatory support may be warranted in specific settings. In some circumstances, transfer to a centre with an active cardiac assist programme may be the most appropriate course of action.

Portable (short-term) mechanical circulatory support (PMCS) may be indicated for three reasons:

♦ to resuscitate patients

♦ as a stabilizing measure for angiography and (prompt) revascularization

♦ to buy time until more definite measures can be taken.

In addition, there is experimental evidence that ventricular unloading of the left ventricle can significantly reduce infarct size and influence myocardial remodelling after myocardial infarction (MI). Left ventricular (LV) remodelling after MI is complex, dynamic, and time dependent and results in a number of topographic and functional changes in the left ventricle in response to the abrupt loss of myocytes [2–5]. Mechanical offloading of the myocardium during ischaemia and reperfusion has been shown to reduce LV work and myocardial oxygen consumption [6–10]. Indeed, the reduction in infarct size has been shown to be related to the degree of offloading of the left ventricle [11]. During mechanical support

and subsequent weaning, pharmacological support should be titrated according to the patient's clinical condition.

Design, performance requirements, and safety issues

PMCS can be provided by a variety of devices and modalities designed to increase forward blood flow and reduce filling pressures. A minimal flow rate of 70 mL/kg body weight per minute, representing a cardiac index of at least 2.5 L/m^2, is generally required to provide adequate organ perfusion. This flow is the sum of the PMCS output and the remaining function of the heart The main considerations when choosing PMCS include patient safety, deliverable flow rate, durability, device and cannula size, and ease of handling. The safety of the patient is the pre-eminent concern, with main considerations shown below, and contraindications listed in ⊃ Table 30.1.

Peripheral vascular disease

Generally access is percutaneously via the transfemoral route, with a cannula size of 10 Fr. However, PMCS pump flow is limited by the size of the arterial cannula. Therefore in cardiogenic shock larger cannula sizes (13–17 Fr) are required to achieve adequate organ perfusion. To solve the problem of possible limb ischaemia many centres use a second (5 Fr) cannula inserted percutaneously in the distal femoral artery, connected to a side port of the arterial line of the PMCS. Before insertion, abdominal and iliofemoral angiography should be performed in order to size vessels, assess the extent and severity of atherosclerotic disease, and select the most appropriate insertion site. In case of emergency in patients with severe atherosclerotic disease, angioplasty (PTA) of the femoral artery or direct surgical cutdown may be performed.

Table 30.1 Different methods of renal support therapy

Modality	Use in hemodynamically unstable patients	Solute clearance	Volume control	Anti-coagulation
PD	Yes	++	++	No
IHD	Possible	++++	+++	Yes/no
IHF	Possible	+++	+++	Yes/no
Intermittent IHF	Possible	++++	+++	Yes/no
Hybrid Techniques	Possible	++++	++++	Yes/no
CVVH	Yes	+++/++++	++++	Yes/no
CVVHD	Yes	+++/++++	++++	Yes/no
CVVHDF	Yes	++++	++++	Yes/no

HDF, hemodiafiltration; CVVH, continuous veno-venous hemofiltration; CVVHD, continuous veno-venous hemodialysis; CVVHDF, continuous veno-venous hemodiafiltration; IHD, intermittent hemodialysis, IHF, intermittent hemofiltration, PD, peritoneal dialysis.

From Cerda J, Ronco C. Modalities of Continuous Renal Replacement Therapy: Technical and Clinical Considerations. *Seminars In Dialysis* 2009;**22**:114–122.

Thromboembolism and bleeding

The occurrence of thromboembolic events depends on a number of factors including the type of device, duration of support, location and number of cannulation sites. Numerous physical factors must also be considered, including mechanical trauma, blood temperature, and blood flow. Embolization may occur during device insertion, function, and removal. The rate of thromboembolic events is relatively low with a heparin anticoagulation regimen. Heparin therapy remains the mainstay of anticoagulation during PMCS, monitored using the ACT or aPTT or by measurement of heparin levels. An ACT of 160–200 s is usually recommended. There is no evidence for the benefit of additional antiplatelet therapy in PMCS.

In long-term mechanical circulatory support a combination of anticoagulation (coumadin) and platelet inhibition is used. As with all anticoagulation, where there is a significant discrepancy between results, or excessive bleeding/unexpected thrombosis occurs, expert haematological advice must be sought. Regional anticoagulation (within the device) may reduce the systemic anticoagulation and reduce the risk of bleeding, although systemic anticoagulation is the norm.

Valvular heart disease

Valvular dysfunction can have a significant impact in patients being considered for PMCS, depending on device selection and site of cannulation. In cases where LV assistance is initiated with left atrial to aortic cannulation, aortic insufficiency may result in left ventricular ballooning in the presence of significant left ventricular dysfunction. In the presence of severe mitral valve stenosis, left atrial to aortic cannulation may be the access route of choice.

Right-sided circulatory failure

Adequate right heart function is required to maintain LVAD filling and therefore flow. Right-sided circulatory failure may result from stunning due to myocardial ischaemia, MI, or volume loading, and from alteration of right ventricular septal geometry induced by LV unloading. Concomitant pulmonary hypertension in this setting may be catastrophic. In selected patients where it is felt that there is prospect for recovery and survival, either bypass should be instigated (see below) or surgical implantation of biventricular support should be considered.

Devices for percutaneous mechanical support

In this section we focus on devices and modalities of percutaneous mechanical support. Understanding the interaction of the patient–device circuit is the cornerstone of proper monitoring, troubleshooting, and assessment of device performance.

Intra-aortic balloon pump

See ➲ Chapter 29.

Percutaneous cardiopulmonary support (short-term, centrifugal): extracorporeal life support (ECLS)

Rapid percutaneous institution of CPB remains the most potent means of haemodynamic support in patients with cardiogenic shock, cardiac arrest, refractory arrhythmias, and high-risk or complicated coronary angioplasty [12, 13].

The percutaneous technique for initiation of femorofemoral CPB support (PCPS) using the Bard portable percutaneous cardiopulmonary support system was described as far back as 1990 [14, 15]. Here, blood is aspirated by a Biomedicus vortex-centrifugal pump from the right atrium through a 18- to 20-Fr bypass cannula positioned in the femoral vein, and returned by means of a membrane oxygenator to a femoral artery cannula. Flows of up to 6 L/min may be obtained, providing almost complete circulatory support, independent of intrinsic cardiac rhythm or cardiac function. In the early days (P)CPS use beyond 6 h was limited by severe haematological and pulmonary complications [16]. Because of the oxygenator in the circuit, PCPS has an extensive artificial area for blood contact, leading to haemostatic disorders (activation of the intrinsic coagulation system, thrombocytopenia, and platelet dysfunction). With the use of modern pump technology and more biocompatible oxygenators full heparinization is no longer required, avoiding the problems of bleeding from the cannulation. However, significant complications related to anticoagulation and infection, in addition to insufficient unloading of the left ventricle, still remain major problems.

Percutaneous, left atrial-to-femoral artery left ventricular support device (short-term, centrifugal)

Closed chest left heart bypass, with left atrial-to-femoral artery cannulae, has shown promise in the high-risk PCI setting [17–19]. As opposed to the PCPS, the recently introduced Tandemheart system (Cardiac Assist Technologies, Inc, Pittsburgh USA) uses the patient's lungs as their own ventilator, avoiding the need for the highly procoagulant/prothrombotic oxygenator, and may be used to support the patient for relatively prolonged periods of time (up to 18 days). The Tandemheart PTVA (➲ Fig. 30.1a) incorporates arterial perfusion cannula configurations ranging from 9 to 17 Fr, a 21 Fr venous trans-septal cannula, and a centrifugal blood pump (➲ Fig. 30.1b). Oxygenated blood from the patient's left atrium is supplied to the pump via

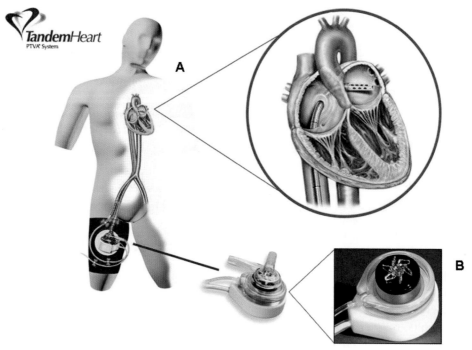

Figure 30.1 The Tandemheart pVAD is a percutaneous, left atrial-to-femoral artery Left Ventricular Support device. Oxygenated blood from the patient's left atrium is supplied to a small centrifugal pump by a 21 French transseptal cannula and then returned to the patient by femoral route.

the trans-septal cannula and then returned to the patient's systemic circulation via the femoral artery.

Successful deployment of this device requires a team of trained operators, including an operator familiar with transeptal puncture [20]. In experienced hands, LV assist can be instituted in under 30 min. The system is can deliver up to 4.5–5 L of blood flow per minute, depending on the size of the arterial cannulation and the filling conditions of the left atrium, while operating at a relatively low speed (7500 rev/min). As with any left-sided assist device, preload to the pump, and therefore flow, is dependent on adequate right heart function. With adequate flows, organ dysfunction in may potentially be avoided, and possibly reversed in cardiogenic shock patients [21].

Intracardiac axial flow pumps: the Impella Platform (short-term, axial)

Intracardiac axial flow pumps incorporate a rotor driven by an electrical motor, and a cannula implanted across the aortic valve aspirating blood from the LV cavity and expelling it into the ascending aorta. The device has a pigtail catheter at its tip to ensure a stable position in the LV and to prevent adherence to the myocardium. The Impella acute pump (diameter 12 Fr) (Aachen, Germany) is a recently introduced catheter-mounted intravascular axial flow pump for short-term use (up to 5 days). This device operates in a way similar to a previous device (Hemopump,14 Fr), which was shown to reduce the risk of cardiac arrest during high-risk

PCI, and provide superior unloading compared with intra-aortic counterpulsation [20, 22]. As with all axial pumps, the performance of this pump (up to 2.5 L/min) depends on the rotary speed (maximal at 32 000 rotations/min) and the pressure head (aortic pressure minus LV pressure, continuously monitored, ⮕ Fig. 30.2). As the flow maximum in catheter-mounted axial flow pumps is limited (2.5–3.5 L/min) this may be inadequate to reverse the features of acute shock [23]. So far, there is only limited clinical experience, with the Impella acute, in particular in stable patients with high-risk PCI [24, 25].

The Impella Recover LP 5.0 (XX) is a microaxial flow pump capable of delivering a continuous flow of up to 5 L/min, which can also be implanted surgically. In a sheep infarction model the Impella Recover was shown to reduce oxygen and reduce infarct size [26].

Limitations of axial support devices are related to the position across the aortic valve, with the presence of a mechanical aortic prosthesis or aortic stenosis, and the presence of significant aortic regurgitation is a contraindication for implantation.

(Implantable) left ventricular assist devices

Even with optimal management many patients with severe heart failure reach a stage at which medical therapy

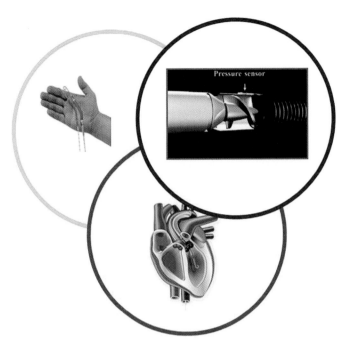

Figure 30.2 The Impella-acute® microaxial blood pump A differential pressure sensor (upper panel) continuously measures the pressure difference between the inflow and outflow of the pump (pressure head) and allows the calculation of the produced pump flow.

is insufficient to sustain an acceptable quality of life (see ⊃Chapter 23). Until recently the only additional treatment option 49, ESC Textbook of cardiovascular medicine 2nd edition for patients with advanced heart failure was transplantation. However, with the lack of suitable donors there is increased impetus to develop safe mechanical cardiac support as an alternative, or as a bridge to buy time before a suitable organ is available. Although the totally implantable heart is not currently a therapeutic option, medium and longer-term cardiac assistance of the left and/or right heart is increasingly performed. Thus far, the clinical experience with LVADs has consistently shown dramatic improvements in cardiac output and (New York Heart Association) functional class. Importantly, these clinical changes have been attended by concomitant decreases in levels of neurohormones and cytokines, suggesting that LVAD support may alter the heart failure milieu. Ventricular assist device therapy is available, effective, and safe for well-selected patients [27, 28]. Although there are no consensus guidelines for VAD implantation, criteria have been developed to help optimize patient selection and outcomes. Patients who may benefit from a mechanical assist device include those who cannot be weaned from inotropic therapy (including postcardiac surgery), who develop intolerance to angiotensin converting enzyme (ACE) inhibitors because of progressive cardiorenal dysfunction, have a peak oxygen consumption of 12 mL kg^{-1} min^{-1} or less, and/or cannot be restored to NYHA class III symptoms despite optimization of medical therapy [29–31].

A key to selection of patients for implantable ventricular assist devices, as for any available therapy, is the expected benefit that is defined as the improvement in predicted outcomes with the device. Benefit can be dominated by either survival or quality of life, as long as the other factor is sufficient to render the improvement meaningful. Outcomes are improving with device modifications being 50% for first-generation devices [32, 33] and improving to more than 70% with more recent devices [28]. Yet, (disabling) stroke remains a major challenge.

In addition to screening for cardiac transplantation eligibility, there are additional cardiovascular clinical considerations in the selection of a patient for mechanical circulatory support [34]:

◆ Aortic valve competency. An LVAD is generally contraindicated if there is moderate to severe aortic regurgitation, for this will simply distend the left ventricle, generating haemodynamically compromising volume overload of the VAD and inadequate forward flow. Concomitant aortic valve closure or replacement with a biological valve may be required. The presence of a mechanical aortic valve is a relative contraindication to LVAD implantation, because of the high risk of valve thrombosis.

◆ Preload to the VAD, mitral valve function, and intracardiac shunts: under optimal VAD function, the left ventricle is a passive, offloaded conduit to the VAD pumping chamber and must have unimpaired filling. Significant mitral stenosis must be considered when selecting the optimal cannulation sites. Right ventricular function is a major determinant of early postimplantation outcomes, and concomitant RVAD implantation should also be considered.

◆ Ischaemic heart disease. Myocardial ischaemia resulting from coronary artery disease should be corrected; preservation or maximization of right ventricular function now becomes paramount.

◆ Arrhythmias. Where an LVAD only is implanted, the patient will not tolerate significant arrhythmias, as adequate cardiac output from the right heart supplies preload to the LVAD. ICD placement may be required when not already present.

Type of devices

Volume displacement pump

This consists of a chamber that fills (either passively, or by suction applied during chamber expansion), and empties cyclically. The motor drives a pusher plate, expanding and compressing the volume displacement chamber, and the direction of blood flow is maintained by inflow and outflow valves. The pump is generally placed in the abdomen with the inflow cannula is inserted into the LV apex, and the outflow cannula inserted into the ascending aorta. These first-generation devices are currently no longer used in Europe.

Axial flow pump

Examples include the Jarvik 2000 (Jarvik Heart), the MicroMed DeBakey device (MicroMed), the HeartMate II (Thoratec), and the INCOR (Berlin Heart). Much like the Impella device, these contain an impeller, a rotor with helical blades that curve around a central shaft. An external drive line provides electrical power to a motor that drives the rotation of the impeller by electromagnetic induction. Blood is drawn by the spinning impeller from the inflow cannula to the outflow cannula. Blood flow is nonpulsatile. These second-generation devices represent the backbone of current LVAD technology used in Europe.

Centrifugal pump

This uses centrifugal force to drive nonpulsatile blood flow and contains magnetically levitated rotors in a plastic or metal housing. It is more effective in power consumption than axial flow pumps and there is no mechanical wear on the rotating parts. Blood enters at the centre of the spinning rotor, gains kinetic energy by centrifugal force, and exits at the outside of the rotor. It generates a constant, nonpulsatile flow. The Levitronix Centrimag pump has provided an option for short and intermediate temporary cardiac support of one or both ventricles in the management of postcardiac surgery heart failure or bridge to transplantation. The Hearteware HVAD is an example of a long-term device used as an alternative to axial flow devices. Details of their indications and use are beyond the scope of this chapter.

Personal perspective

As the general population continues to age and assist devices continue to evolve, these pumps will become increasingly prevalent in our society. LVADs have already evolved into small, unobtrusive devices that run on small, portable, long-lasting battery supplies. This, in turn, will allow LVADs to serve as a very reliable alternative to transplantation for many patients with advanced heart failure who cannot receive transplants or who cannot be weaned from LVAD support. Adverse events have decreased with newer devices, but still remain substantial. The issues of infection, bleeding, thromboembolism, and limited mobility have not been resolved by the advent of more sophisticated devices, although each pump has its own approach to reducing the likelihood of complications. Further refinements of this technology are already in the pipeline, but full implantability without percutanous lines, or a complete artificial heart for long-term support, will not be seen in the near future.

Further reading

Meyns B, Stolinski J, Leunens V, Verbeken E, Flameng W. Left ventricular support by catheter-mounted axial flow pump reduces infarct size. *J Am Coll Cardiol.* 2003 Apr 2;**41**(7): 1087–95.

Ronan JA, Shawl FA. Echocardiographic and hemodynamic changes during percutaneous cardiopulmonary bypass. In: shawl FA, ed. Supported complex and high risk coronary angioplasty. Kluwer Academic, Boston, 1991, 57–63.

Vranckx P, Schultz CJ, Valgimigli M. Assisted Circulation using the Tandemheart® during very high-risk PCI for Unprotected Left Main Coronary Artery disease in patients declined for CABG. *Catheter Cardiovasc Interv* 2009, **74**: 302–310.

Thiele H, Lauer B, Hambrecht R et al. Reversal of cardiogenic shock by percutaneous left atrial to femoral arterial bypass assistance. *Circulation* 2001; **104**: 2917–22.

Stevenson LW, Couper G. On the fledgling field of mechanical circulatory support. *J Am Coll Cardiol.* 2007; **50**: 748–751.

Lietz K, Long JW, Kfoury AG, et al. Outcomes of left ventricular assist device implantation as destination therapy in the post-REMATCH era: Implications for patient selection. *Circulation* 2007; **116**:497–505.

➲ For additional multimedia materials please visit the online version of the book (𝄢 http://www.esciacc.oxfordmedicine.com).

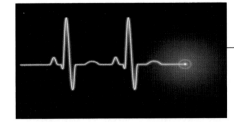

CHAPTER 31

Nutrition support in acute cardiac care

Pierre Singer and Ilya Kagan

Contents

Summary

Cardiovascular disease is a common pre-existing condition in many hospitalized patients. Acute myocardial infarction, cardiac surgery, and cardiomyopathy are three of the most common reasons for admission to the intensive care unit (ICU). Some patients are malnourished and have to be recognized and treated immediately, preventing refeeding syndrome. Others are well nourished but may have a prolonged stay in the ICU and will require appropriate nutritional assessment and nutritional therapy including the adequate nutrients. The route of feeding should be chosen in accordance to the haemodynamic condition of the patient. Glycaemic control should be targeted to avoid hypoglycaemia and prevent significant hyperglycaemia. Use of specific nutrients such as fish oil, glutamine, or antioxidants has been demonstrated to improve outcome. In addition, the new technologies introduced in the field have metabolic implications and nutritional therapy should take these changes into account. Metabolic control of the acute cardiac patient has become one of the cornerstones in the better care of these patients.

Introduction

In critical patients, artificial nutritional support is now considered to be the standard care, as it reduces complication rate and improves clinical outcomes. Most of guidelines that discuss metabolic support in general intensive care (ICU) do not differentiate between the types of intensive care. Patients in the intensive cardiac care unit (ICCU) are not a homogenous population. Acute coronary syndrome (ACS), acute exacerbation of congestive heart failure (CHF), and life-threatening arrhythmias are some of the most common ICCU admissions and are associated with considerable morbidity and mortality. Usually, ICCU patients are characterized by a short time stay while patients hospitalized in a general ICU will stay around 5–7 days on average. In addition, most patients who have had cardiovascular surgery leave the postoperation unit within 72 h after the procedure. For them, the nutrition goal is to prevent hospital complications and preventable cardiac pathology. Other patients, such as those with severe heart failure with cardiac cachexia, or with severe complications after cardiac surgery, or patients after cardiac transplantation, will remain in the ICCU or cardiothoracic unit for a longer period of time. The final group of patients are those suffering from cardiovascular complications, e.g. pulmonary oedema, ACS, and arrhythmias due to severe stress, aggressive fluid therapy, and inotropic support. These patients need also metabolic and nutritional support.

Nutrition support in acute cardiac care

Nutritional assessment

Patients with heart failure often experience malnutrition characterized by a depletion of fat and muscle. This malnutrition contributes to longer hospitalization, perioperative complications, and increased mortality [1]. To maintain body cell mass and function, daily energy intake should be maintained in equilibrium with expenditure. Body weight and body mass index (BMI) are easy and cost-effective markers of nutritional status, and an unintentional 10% loss in body weight is a sign of malnutrition. The high prevalence of oedema makes body weight and BMI a poor indicator for patients with heart failure [1, 2]. Lean body mass determinations by anthropometric measurements (skin fold thickness, arm-muscle circumference) are probably slightly more reliable. Nonspecific plasma proteins such as C-reactive protein, albumin, and prealbumin may also be indicative of a patient's nutritional status. Indirect calorimetry is the gold standard tool to measure resting energy expenditure, which is the major constituent of total daily energy expenditure. This measurement may target the individual's nutritional requirements.

Nutritional and metabolic support of heart failure in the intensive care unit

Berger and Mustafa reported that acute myocardial infarction (MI), cardiac surgery, and acute cardiomyopathy were the most common causes of admission to the ICU in Western countries [2]. Most patients could be discharged within a few days, but some do not follow the standard course after cardiac surgery or treatment for acute coronary disease, and will require prolonged ICU stay.

Patients with congestive heart failure can be admitted to ICCU after CHF exacerbation, MI, or surgery. In a patient who is already critically ill, cardiac failure is an ominous sign deserving aggressive treatment [1]. Catabolism shifts with heart failure. The anabolic–catabolic imbalance is evinced as increased plasma catecholamine, cortisol, aldosterone and renin levels, and the activation of heat shock proteins [3]. Additionally, proinflammatory cytokines such as TNF-α, IL-1, and IL-6 are unregulated [4–6]. Cardiac cachexia has been recognized as an independent predictor of higher mortality rates in patients with chronic heart failure [7], whereas moderate obesity appears to be protective. Cardiac cachexia is also associated with poor outcome after cardiac transplantation, with an increase in the 30-day mortality in cachectic recipients (13% versus 7% in normal weight recipients) and a doubling of the 5-year mortality [8]. CHF patients often suffer from anorexia, early satiety, and nausea; this alone does not explain their level of malnutrition. Nutritional depletion is complex and results from decreased nutrient intake and fat absorption, protein wasting secondary to activated inflammatory cascade, immunologic changes, and neurohormonal imbalance [9]. Patients with cardiac cachexia have an increased resting energy expenditure (REE) [10], but, due to decreased physical activity, total energy expenditure is reduced by 10–20% compare to patients without cachexia [11].

Current recommendations suggest that 25 kcal kg^{-1} day^{-1} is a reasonable target for most ICU patients. Carbohydrates should not exceed 6 g kg^{-1} day^{-1} and lipids should not exceed 2.0 g kg^{-1} day^{-1}. Evidence suggests that 1.2–1.5g kg^{-1} day^{-1} of protein is needed [12]. In the absence of a good level of evidence there is an urgent need for controlled studies of nutritional treatment with enteral feeding in cardiac cachexia [13–16], with the aim of improving function through increased supply of nutrients and energy. A further aim of such treatment might also be to complement other therapies, e.g. to supply extra protein during treatment with anabolic steroids, growth factors, or exercise training. There are no specific contraindications to enteral nutrition in CHF patients, but fluid overload should be avoided [7] and fluid balance carefully handled.

Micronutrients are essential dietary components present in small amounts [17]. They enable the body to produce antioxidants, enzymes, hormones, and other essential substances. Tiny though the amounts are, the consequences of their absence are severe. Lack of micronutrients such as selenium and thiamine (vitamin B$_1$) are reported causes of heart failure and micronutrient support may aid the failing heart in the ICU [18]. Many patients with heart failure are thiamine deficient, particularly older people and those with severe heart failure, malnutrition, or maintained on diuretic therapy [19]. In a prospective study of 100 hospitalized heart failure patients [20], 33% were found to be thiamine deficient. Vitamin supplementation seemed to be moderately efficacious in the prevention of thiamine deficiency. Patients with thiamine deficiency may have volume retention with oedema, weakness, vasodilation, and a reduction in ejection fraction, and thiamine supplementation should be considered for heart failure patients in the ICU [21]. In addition to thiamine, it appears that many patients hospitalized with heart failure have deficiencies in riboflavin (vitamin B_2) and pyridoxine (vitamin B_6) [19]. Ascorbic acid (vitamin C) is a water-soluble vitamin with antioxidant properties. It is still currently unknown if the administration of vitamins changes outcome. The benefit of combined antioxidant supplementation containing thiamine, selenium, and ascorboic acid among other things has not been suggested in patients with sepsis, systemic inflammatory response syndrome (SIRS), burns, trauma, and ischaemic stroke. Combined antioxidant supplementation has not been evaluated in critically ill heart failure patients. This subject was reviewed several years ago [22, 23].

Glucose control and insulin therapy in intensive care

An association between hyperglycaemia and adverse outcome during hospitalization has been demonstrated [24, 25]. Glucose is proinflammatory and induces increased intranuclear NF-κB, activator protein 1, and early growth response-1 (EGR1) binding [26]. Under high glucose conditions, increased reactive oxygen species (ROS) production is observed with subsequent damage to cellular components like liver mitochondria [27] and development of insulin resistance [28]. Several mechanisms are involved, such as glucose autoxidation and superoxide production, glycation and formation of advanced glycation end products, and increased sorbitol production by the polyol pathway [28, 29]. The signal transduction networks activate lipid peroxidation, protein oxidation, and DNA oxidation [30]. Enough evidence exists to conclude that high concentrations of glucose induce increased production of oxygen free radicals.

The association of hyperglycaemia with increased in-hospital mortality has been demonstrated in the last 15 years, and this association was stronger in nondiabetic patients [31]. The association persisted in patients receiving thrombolytic therapy and primary percutaneous coronary intervention (PCI). An increase of 1 mmol/L in admission glucose concentration was associated with a 4% increased mortality after acute MI and 4.3% increased mortality in ACS. Moreover, in a study of 16 871 ACS patients, there was a significant association between in-hospital death and increased levels of admission blood glucose but also mean glucose during hospitalization and persistent hyperglycaemia [32]. The hypothesis of reaching euglycaemia was proposed, with treatments using insulin and potassium [32]. Many treatments have been proposed, including the DIGAMI [33], HI-5 [34], and CREATE-ECLA studies [35]. Intervention using insulin therapy was problematic in many studies since there was a delay in starting the infusion, a paucity of nondiabetic patients, and mainly a lack of difference in blood glucose between comparator groups. The conclusion was that insulin in the absence of significant lowering of blood glucose appears to have no effect on outcome. The European Association for the Study of Diabetes and the European Society of Cardiology recommend strict glucose control with insulin therapy in patients in critical illness (grade IB) rather than those with ACS [36]. The American Heart Association [37] suggests that patients with glycaemia greater than 9.9 mmol/L should be treated intensively with insulin.

Glucose control (80–110 mg/dL) using intensive insulin therapy was proposed in a large prospective randomized study in the ICU. In this landmark study [38], van den Berghe included 1548 ICU patients, 63% of them having undergone cardiac surgery, and found a significant decrease in ICU and hospital morbidity and mortality. These results have not been duplicated successfully, and two studies [39, 40] had to be stopped for concern about hypoglycaemia and no clear advantages; a recent study [41] even showed an increased 6-month mortality in the study group. However, the patients included in these studies were largely underfed, while those in the van den Berghe study were reaching protein-calorie goals.

Specifically, Gandhi et al. [42] compared intraoperative tight glucose control to conventional therapy. Patients were treated with intensive insulin therapy management when admitted to the ICU. Morbidity and mortality were not affected by the insulin management. In addition, the study group had an increased incidence in stroke and death. The Portland diabetic project [43] is an ongoing 18-year prospective interventional trial studying the relationship between glycaemia and outcome of diabetic cardiac surgery patients. Clinical improvement was observed with target between 100 and 150 mg/dL in terms of risk of death (57% decrease) and incidence of deep sternum wound infection (66% decrease).

Fish oil in acute coronary care

Prevention of myocardial infarction

Polyunsaturated fatty acids (PUFAs) are subdivided into ω-3 (linolenic) and ω-6 (linoleic) fatty acids and are also termed essential fatty acids because they can only be obtained from the diet. Fish oil is rich in ω-3. A number of epidemiologic studies [44–48] and randomized clinical trials [49–53] have shown that dietary changes to increase ω-3 intake result in reduced cardiovascular mortality and risk in sudden death, without a consistent change in risk of MI [54]. In the Diet and Reinfarction Trial (DART) [51], Burr *et al.* checked the effects of dietary intervention in the secondary prevention of MI compare with increase in the ratio of polyunsaturated to saturated fat and an increase in cereal fibre intake. The subjects advised to eat fish had a 29% reduction in 2-year all-cause mortality compared with those not so advised. Gruppo Italiano per lo Studio della Sopravvivenza nell'Infarto miocardico (GISSI) [52] study checked dietary supplementation with ω-3 polyunsaturated fatty acids and vitamin E after MI. The primary combined efficacy endpoint was death, nonfatal MI, and stroke. Treatment with ω-3 PUFA, but not vitamin E, significantly lowered the risk of the primary endpoint (relative risk decrease 10% by two-way analysis, 15% by four-way analysis). Benefit was attributable to a decrease in the risk of death (14% two-way, 20% four-way) and cardiovascular death (17% two-way, 30% four-way).

Many studies have checked the effect of ω-3 PUFAs on arrhythmia. Some animal and *in vitro* studies have suggested a propensity for arrhythmia; more recent studies [54, 55] investigating the effect of fish oil supplementation on ventricular tachyarrhythmia in patients with implantable defibrillators did not find protective effects of PUFAs. The outcome measures of a randomized, double-blind, placebo-controlled trial performed at six United States medical centres [55] were time to first episode of implantable defibrillator (ICD) treatment for ventricular tachycardia (VT) or ventricular fibrillation (VF), changes in red blood cell concentrations of ω-3 PUFAs and frequency of recurrent VT/VF events. Two hundred patients with an ICD and a recent episode of sustained VT or VF were randomly assigned to receive fish oil or placebo and were followed up for a median of 718 days. Among patients with a recent episode of sustained ventricular arrhythmia and an ICD, fish oil supplementation did not reduce the risk of VT/VF and in some patients was pro-arrhythmic. Brouwer *et al.* [54] have published a meta-analysis to determine the effects of ω-3 PUFAs from fish on the incidence of recurrent ventricular arrhythmia in ICD patients. The main outcome was time to first confirmed VF or VT combined with death for the meta-analysis, and time to first spontaneous confirmed VF or VT for the pooled analysis. The findings do not support a protective effect of ω-3 PUFAs from fish oil on cardiac arrhythmia in all patients with an ICD. The current data neither prove nor disprove either a beneficial or a detrimental effect for subgroups of patients with specific underlying pathologies.

Treatment

Fish oil-based nutrition is protective in severe critical care conditions. Fatty acids from fish oil are emerging as powerful yet safe disease-modifying nutrients, as evident in the results of three clinical trials published in 2006 [56–58]. Two randomized controlled studies compared an enteral nutrition formula based on fish oil, borage oil, and antioxidants to a standard high-fat, low-carbohydrate formula in patients with acute respiratory distress syndrome (ARDS) [56] and severe sepsis or septic shock [57] and one in patients with acute lung injury (ALI) [58]. Clinical outcomes were superior in patients receiving fish oil-based nutrition. Marik and Zaloga in a recently published systemic review [59] found that immunomodulating diets (IMD) supplemented with fish oil improved the outcome of medical ICU patients (with SIRS/sepsis/ARDS). In 2006 the authors, in a single-centre, unblinded prospective randomized controlled study [58] checked the effects of an enteral diet enriched with eicosapentaenoic acid (EPA), γ-linolenic acid (GLA), and antioxidants on the respiratory profile and outcome of patients with acute lung injury. Primary outcome parameters were oxygenation and respiratory mechanics, and secondary outcomes included length of ventilation (LOV), length of stay (LOS), and mortality. Oxygenation was significantly higher in the EPA + GLA group on day 4 and on day 7; the advantage was lost by day 14 or at discharge. Tidal volumes and positive end-expiratory pressure (PEEP) values used during the trial were not significantly different between groups. Patients receiving a diet enriched in EPA + GLA had a significantly shorter LOV expressed in hours free from ventilation (40 patients were still ventilated in the control group and only 34 in the study group). LOS did not reach significance. Length of hospital stay was similar in the two groups. Overall survival was similar in the two groups. The conclusion of another recent review [60] is that enteral administration of fish oil, GLA, and antioxidants may improve oxygenation and clinical outcomes in ICU patients with impaired oxygenation.

There are several mechanisms of action of EPA and GLA. The prostaglandins and leukotrienes that are formed from EPA by cyclo-oxygenases (COXs) and lipoxygenases (LOXs) are less proinflammatory than their counterparts derived from amino acids (AA). Increasing the (DHA + EPA)/AA ratio in membrane phospholipids, thereby skewing the production of lipid inflammatory mediators towards less powerful agents, is a well-characterized form of protection conferred by ω-3 consumption in inflammatory states [61, 62]. The ω-3 fatty acids are also known to inhibit the activity of the pivotal proinflammatory transcription factor NF-jB, which induces the expression of many proinflammatory genes that encode adhesion molecules, cytokines, chemokines, and other effectors of the innate immune response. There is now evidence that ω-3 fatty acids block each of the three stages of LPS-induced NF-κB activity independently. Finally, in 2006 the ESPEN guidelines on enteral nutrition in ICU [63] recommended immunomodulating formulae (formulae enriched with arginine, nucleotides and ω-3 fatty acids) for several categories of patients:

- elective upper gastrointestinal surgical patients (level of evidence A)

- patients with mild sepsis (APACHE II <15) (level of evidence B)

- patients with severe sepsis; however, immunomodulating formulae may be harmful and are therefore not recommended (level of evidence B)

- patients with trauma (level of evidence A)

- patients with ARDS (formulae containing ω-3 fatty acids and antioxidants) (level of evidence B)

Tight energy balance control for prevention of complications

Increasing knowledge has been accumulated in the recent years regarding the importance of energy balance. Protein-calorie malnutrition is frequent in patients suffering from cardiopulmonary diseases. Malnutrition adversely affects cardiopulmonary and immune functions, creating a vicious circle. The combination of poor food intake as well as the extra energy costs of the metabolic disturbances associated with acute illness can lead to a state of negative nitrogen balance and significant loss of lean body mass [64]. In a recent study, 57 ischaemic heart disease patients and 34 heart failure patients were followed and compared to elderly patients with chronic obstructive pulmonary disease (COPD) and chest infection. Patients with heart failure and COPD were found to have poor anthropometric measures compared to the rest of the patients. Nutrition status deteriorated between admission and 6 weeks in heart failure, and over 6 months 39% of heart failure patients were readmitted to hospital compared to 35% of all the population [65].

Nutritional therapy is an indispensable part of therapy in these patients. If a cardiac patient is not following a standard course after acute coronary event or cardiac surgery and will require prolonged critical therapy, nutrition will be an integral part in the treatment of this acutely ill patient. Enteral nutrition (EN) is the preferred route of providing this support according to the European, American, and Canadian guidelines [63, 65, 67]. It follows the physiological route of feeding, preserves the gut from atrophy, and prevents bacterial translocation. It has been demonstrated in critically ill patients, mainly after open heart surgery, that negative cumulative energy balance was correlated with complication rate, length of ventilation, and length of ICU stay [68]. Therefore, EN should reach the calorie target as soon as possible in the course of the ICU stay. Unfortunately, this is difficult to achieve, mainly because of lack of protocols, poor gastric emptying and larger gastric residuals, use of noradrenaline and sedation, and inadequate consideration of energy balance [69]. The ASPEN/SCCM guidelines [67] recommend waiting 7–10 days to administer complementary parenteral nutrition to these poorly fed patients, whereas ESPEN [70] recommends not waiting more than 48 h to administer complementary parenteral nutrition. Recent studies have observed that the patients reaching the protein–energy target had a better survival, but more prospective studies are required to demonstrate the theory of protein–energy goal-oriented therapy [71].

Enteral feeding can be effectively administered to critically patients after a few days. However, at an earlier stage, cardiac patients often suffer from haemodynamic instability and from splanchnic hypoperfusion. The controversy about the possibility of feeding the hypoperfused gut is still open. The Lausanne group, in several studies, demonstrated [1] that enteral feeding increased cardiac index, and decreased mean arterial pressure and systemic vascular resistance. This response was appropriate, according to the authors [72]. Berger studied the absorptive capacity of the intestine in cardiac surgery patients undergoing cardiopulmonary bypass using the paracetamol test, and showed that the postpyloric absorption capability remained intact in stable as well as unstable patients [73], In another study [74], EN delivery was observed in unstable patients and was initiated at 20 mL/h and increased slowly every 12–24 h to reach an energy goal of 25 kcal/kg. Of the 70 patients included in this study, 18 were dependent on an intra-aortic balloon pump. A mean energy delivery of 70% was achieved within the first 2 weeks. If no gastrointestinal complications were observed, patients requiring elevated levels of norepinephrine or dopamine were more difficult to feed enterally. In these patients, complementary parenteral nutrition should be prescribed. In very unstable patients, caution is warranted. To our opinion, when mean arterial pressure (MAP) reaches 60–70 mmHg and haemodynamic stability is achieved even with high doses of vasopressors, enteral nutrition is safe.

Impact of new technologies

In recent decades many patients in the ICU or ICCU have been treated by new technologies such as continuous renal replacement therapy (CRRT) or vascular assist devices (VAD). CRRT has become the modality of choice in most ICUs for the treatment of severe cases of acute kidney injury (AKI) [75]. Patients with AKI have a high prevalence of malnutrition, a condition that is associated with morbidity and mortality [76]. AKI develops mostly in the context of critical illness and multiple organ failure, which are associated with major changes in substrate metabolism and body composition, overwhelming the alterations induced by AKI itself. Key effectors of these changes are inflammatory mediators and neuroendocrine alterations. The development of AKI further adds fluid overload, uraemia, acidosis, and electrolyte disturbances. In addition, AKI is associated with increased inflammation and oxidative stress [77]. Although active solute transport in a functioning kidney is an energy-consuming process, the presence of AKI in itself (in the absence of critical illness) does not seem to affect REE [78]. Energy expenditure in AKI patients is therefore determined mainly by the underlying condition. Consequently, when acute renal failure (ARF) occurs in the setting of hypercatabolic illness in the ICU, an increased REE must be taken into account [79]. Additionally, extracorporeal treatments facilitating nutritional support may induce derangements of nutrient balance [80]. As a result, a daily caloric intake of 25–35 kcal/kg has been advocated for patients in the ICU with ARF [81], although energy requirements should be individualized based on comorbidities and heat losses from extracorporeal blood circulation [82]. There are also increased protein losses in ARF patients, especially with continuous forms of dialysis and use of high-flux dialysate. Hence, protein requirements can vary from 1.0 to 2.0 g kg^{-1} day^{-1}, depending on the degree of hypercatabolism present and type of renal replacement therapy used [83] (see ➲ Chapter 28). Alterations in serum concentration of amino acid are predictable in different forms of AKI. Glutamine clearance rates correspond with plasma glutamine levels and effluent flow rates during CRRT [79]. Consistent with this, Wernerman [84] recommends 25–35 g/24 h of intravenous glutamine for those patients undergoing CRRT. A recent meta-analysis [85] on the use of CRRT described improved control of uraemia with a high amino acid intake. There was also an improvement in nitrogen balance with high amino acid doses, up to 2.5 g kg^{-1} day^{-1} on CRRT. Glucose losses in the effluent in continuous venovenous hemofiltration (CVVH) can range up to 60 g/day [86]. Increasing the glucose concentration and rate of administration of replacement solutions can help minimize this glucose loss. Water-soluble vitamins and trace elements, e.g. selenium, zinc, and thiamine, may also be lost during dialysis, particularly with CVVH. The ESPEN guidelines state that micronutrient losses should be supplemented, with careful monitoring to prevent toxicity [87].

VADs are used in patients requiring cardiovascular support in severe, acute or chronic, class IV heart failure. They have significant complications including infection, bleeding, and individual organ dysfunction. Not infrequently, VAD patients progress to multiple organ dysfunction syndrome (MODS). As this technology continues to advance, it will be even more important for the nutrition support team to work hand-in-hand with the cardiologist, cardiac surgeon, and intensive care specialist in the care of these complex patients. VAD patients face multiple barriers that may result in inadequate nutrition. Some of these difficulties, such as nausea, delayed gastric emptying, and anorexia may be secondary to anatomical problems created by the placement of the device. Moreover, there is a multifactorial metabolic process in patients with chronic heart failure that results in cardiac cachexia [79].

Conclusion

Our understanding of the nutritional and metabolic management of the acutely ill cardiovascular patient has changed over the past decade. Metabolic support may play a role in decompensated heart failure. Micronutrient and antioxidant therapy has been prescribed in the chronically critically ill. Further studies elucidating its role in the acute setting are needed. Hyperglycaemia has emerged as a marker of outcome in patients with cardiovascular disease. Intensive insulin therapy in the critically ill may play a role, particularly in patients who are in the ICU for several days. At this time, the clinical benefit of glucose–insulin–potassium (GIK) therapy remains uncertain. In addition to haemodynamic and respiratory support, nutritional and metabolic therapy needs to be considered in our critically ill patients.

Personal perspective

Year after year, more severely ill patients are admitted to acute coronary units, ICCUs post cardiac surgery, and medical or surgical ICUs. The patients are older, sicker, suffering more from comorbidities, and requiring longer and more sophisticated therapies. Better understanding of the requirements of the acutely ill patient is mandatory to better avoid deficiencies and to allow adequate administration of calories, nutrients, minerals, vitamins, and trace elements. New tools able to assess insulin resistance, closed-loop systems preventing severe disturbances in term of glucose control or electrolytes, are intensively tested and will be available in the near future. The intelligent use of specific nutrients at specific dosage and with precise timing will also allow the practitioner to manipulate cellular processes and improve clinical outcomes.

Further reading

Ankera SD, John M, Pedersenc PU, *et al.* ESPEN guidelines on enteral nutrition: cardiology and pulmonology. *Clin Nutr* 2006;**25**:311–318.

Scurlock C, Raikhelkar J, Mechanick JI. Impact of new technologies on metabolic care in the intensive care unit. *Curr Opin Clin Nutr Metab Care* 2009;**12**:196–200.

Singer P, Berger MM, van den Berghe G, *et al.* ESPEN guidelines for parenteral nutrition: intensive care. *Clin Nutr* 2009; **28**:387–400.

Singer P, Shapiro H. Enteral omega-3 in acute respiratory distress syndrome. *Curr Opin Clin Nutr Metab Care* 2009;**12**:123–128.

Van den Berghe G, Wouters P, *et al.* Intensive insulin therapy in critically ill patients. *N Engl J Med* 2001;**345**:1359–1367.

➲ For additional multimedia materials please visit the online version of the book (🔗 http://www.esciacc.oxfordmedicine.com).

CHAPTER 32

Physiotherapy in critically ill patients

R. Gosselink and J. Roeseler

Contents

Summary

Physiotherapists are involved in the management of patients with critical illness. Physiotherapy assessment of critically ill patients is less driven by medical diagnosis; instead, there is a strong focus on deficiencies at a pathophysiological and functional level.

Accurate and valid assessment of respiratory conditions (retained airway secretions, atelectasis, and respiratory muscle weakness), physical deconditioning, and related problems (muscle weakness, joint stiffness, impaired functional exercise capacity, physical inactivity, and emotional function) makes it possible to identify targets for physiotherapy.

Evidence-based targets for physiotherapy are deconditioning, impaired airway clearance, atelectasis, avoidance of (re-)intubation, and weaning failure. Early physical activity and mobility are key in the prevention, attenuation, or reversion of physical deconditioning related to critical illness. A variety of modalities for exercise training and early mobility are evidence based and are implemented depending on the stage of critical illness, comorbid conditions, and cooperation of the patient.

The physiotherapist should be responsible for implementing mobilization plans and exercise prescription and make recommendation for progression for progression of these jointly with medical and nursing staff.

Introduction

The progress of intensive care medicine has dramatically improved survival of critically ill patients, especially in patients with acute respiratory distress syndrome (ARDS) [1]. This improved survival is, however, often associated with general deconditioning, muscle weakness, dyspnoea, depression and anxiety, and reduced health-related quality of life after intensive care unit (ICU) discharge [2, 3]. Deconditioning and specifically muscle weakness, but not pulmonary function, are suggested to have a key role in impaired functional status after ICU stay [2].

Optimal physiological functioning depends on the upright position [4], so bed rest and limited mobility during critical illness result in profound physical deconditioning and dysfunction of the respiratory, cardiovascular, musculoskeletal, neurological, renal, and endocrine systems. These effects can be exacerbated by inflammation and pharmacological agents, such as corticosteroids, neuromuscular blockers and antibiotics. Skeletal muscle weakness is observed in 25% of ICU patients who were ventilated for more than 7 days [5]. Development of neuropathy or myopathy also contributes to weaning failure [6]. Finally, muscle weakness has been linked with increased mortality [8].

Respiratory dysfunction is one of the most common causes of critical illness necessitating ICU admission. Failure of either of the two primary components of the respiratory system (i.e. the gas exchange membrane and the ventilatory pump (⊃ Fig. 32.1), can result in a need for mechanical ventilation. Respiratory dysfunction includes impaired global and/or regional ventilation and lung compliance, increased airway resistance, and work of breathing. Although most patients under mechanical ventilation are extubated in less than 3 days, approximately 20% require prolonged ventilatory support [7]. Chronic ventilator dependence is a major medical problem, but it is also an extremely uncomfortable state for a patient, carrying important psychosocial implications.

Physiotherapists are involved in the prevention and treatment of deconditioning and in the treatment of respiratory conditions in critically ill patients. Their role varies across units, hospitals, and countries [9] and is appreciated by medical directors as well as patients. Physiotherapy assessment of critically ill patients is driven less by the medical diagnosis than by deficiencies at a physiological and functional level [10]. Accurate and valid assessment of respiratory conditions, deconditioning, and related problems is of paramount importance for physiotherapists. In addition, physiotherapists can contribute to the patient's overall well-being by providing emotional support and enhancing communication.

Respiratory conditions

The aims of physiotherapy in respiratory dysfunction are to improve lung inflation, clear airway secretions, reduce the work of breathing, and enhance inspiratory muscle function [11]. In the following sections the physiotherapy treatment is discussed in relation to different clinical conditions.

Prevention of pulmonary complications after abdominal and thoracic surgery

Most patients undergoing major thoracic or abdominal surgery recover without complications. Preoperative physiotherapy, including inspiratory muscle training, in cardiac surgery patients with an increased risk profile for postoperative pulmonary complications reduced the development of these complications [12].

After routine cardiac surgery, optimal postoperative management includes early mobilization and body positioning [13]. Further prophylactic physiotherapy interventions are not required in patients without complications [14] or during intubation and mechanical ventilation [15]. Early mobilization and upright body positioning after major surgery is of primary importance to increase lung volume and to prevent pulmonary complications. Routine breathing exercises should not be used following uncomplicated coronary artery bypass surgery. Perioperative physiotherapy should be instituted if warranted, e.g. in high risk patients, rather than administered routinely. Two randomized controlled studies have provided strong evidence that supports the role of prophylactic physiotherapy in preventing pulmonary complications after upper abdominal surgery [16, 17]. However, in contrast, a meta-analysis showed no added value of physiotherapy to the effectiveness of early mobilization in high risk patients after abdominal surgery [18].

Incentive spirometry and noninvasive ventilation (continuous positive airway pressure, CPAP) are frequently used in the postoperative setting:

◆ Incentive spirometry (IS) is used in the management of nonintubated patients to encourage lung volume recruitment. IS has not been shown to be of added benefit (beyond physiotherapy, early mobilization, and

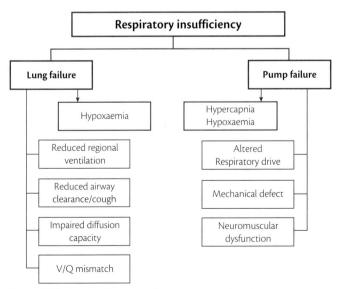

Figure 32.1 Model of causes and consequences of respiratory insufficiency.

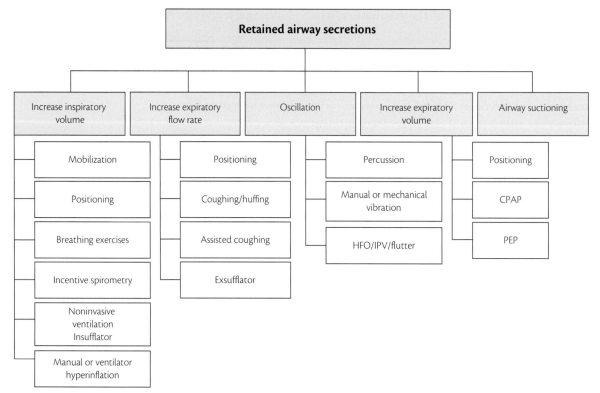

Figure 32.2 Pathways and treatment modalities for increasing airway clearance. CPAP, continuous positive airway pressure; HFO, high frequency oscillation; IPPB, intermittent positive pressure breathing; IPV, intrapulmonary percussive ventilation; NIV, noninvasive ventilation; PEP, positive expiratory pressure.
Reproduced with permission from Gosselink R, Bott J, Johnson M, *et al.* Physiotherapy for adult patients with critical illness: recommendations of the European Respiratory Society and European Society of Intensive Care Medicine Task Force on Physiotherapy for Critically Ill Patients. *Intensive Care Med* 2008;**34**:1188–1199.

body position) in the routine management of postoperative patients [19].

◆ Noninvasive ventilation (NIV) has been used successfully to support patients following thoracotomy [20]. CPAP is effective in the treatment of atelectasis, since it increases functional residual capacity (FRC) and improves compliance, minimizing postoperative airways collapse. NIV has been shown to be superior to CPAP in the treatment of atelectasis in patients after cardiac surgery [21].

Retained airway secretions and atelectasis

⮕ Figure 32.2 provides an overview of pathways and treatment modalities for increasing airway clearance. Interventions aimed at increasing inspiratory volume (deep breathing exercises, mobilization, and body positioning) may affect lung expansion, increase regional ventilation, reduce airway resistance, and optimize pulmonary compliance. Interventions aimed at increasing expiratory flow include forced expirations (huffing and coughing). Manually assisted cough, using thoracic or abdominal compression, may be indicated for patients with expiratory muscle weakness or fatigue [22]. The mechanical in- and exsufflator can be used to deliver an inspiratory pressure

followed by a high negative expiratory force, via a mouthpiece or face mask. It has been successfully applied in the management of neuromuscular patients with retained secretions secondary to respiratory muscle weakness [23]. Airway suctioning is used solely to clear central secretions that are considered a primary problem when other techniques are ineffective.

Treatment of acute lobar atelectasis and airway clearance should incorporate body positioning and techniques to increase inspiratory volume and enhance forced expiration. The effectiveness of physiotherapy has been confirmed in several studies [24, 25]. Chest wall vibration provided no additional benefit. CPAP has been shown to be effective in the treatment of atelectasis [26].

Mechanically ventilated patients

In intubated and ventilated patients manual hyperinflation (MHI) or ventilator hyperinflation, positive end-expiratory pressure (PEEP) ventilation, postural drainage, chest wall compression, and airway suctioning may assist in secretion clearance. The aims of MHI are to prevent pulmonary atelectasis, re-expand collapsed alveoli, improve oxygenation, improve lung compliance, and facilitate movement of airway secretions towards the central airways [27, 28]. MHI involves a slow, deep inspiration with manual resuscitator bag, an inspiratory hold of 2–3 s [29], followed by a quick release of the bag to enhance expiratory flow and mimic a forced expiration. MHI may have important negative side effects:

- It can precipitate marked haemodynamic changes associated with a decreased cardiac output, which result from large fluctuations in intrathoracic pressure [30].

- It can also increase intracranial pressure, which might have implications for patients with brain injury. This increase is usually limited, however, such that cerebral perfusion pressure remains stable [31]. A pressure of 40 cmH$_2$O has been recommended as an upper limit.

Two studies in ventilated patients reported that bronchoscopy offered no additional benefit over physiotherapy (postural drainage, percussion, manual hyperinflation, and suctioning) in the management of acute lobar atelectasis [32, 33].

Airway suctioning may have detrimental side effects (bronchial lesions, hypoxaemia), but reassurance, sedation, and pre-oxygenation of the patient may minimize these effects [34]. Suctioning can be performed via an in-line closed suctioning system or an open system. The in-line system does not appear to decrease the incidence of ventilator-associated pneumonia (VAP) [35], nor the duration of mechanical ventilation, length of ICU stay, or mortality [35], but it increases costs. Closed suctioning may be less effective than open suctioning for secretion clearance during pressure support ventilation [36]. The routine instillation of normal saline during airway suctioning has potential adverse effects on oxygen saturation and cardiovascular stability, and variable results in terms of increasing sputum yield [37]. Chest wall compression prior to endotracheal suctioning did not improve airway secretion removal, oxygenation, or ventilation after endotracheal suctioning in an unselected population of mechanically ventilated patients [38].

VAP is a common complication in mechanically ventilated patients and is associated with higher mortality rates, prolonged hospitalization, and high medical costs [39]. Studies have shown that avoidance of intubation with NIV reduces the incidence of nosocomial pneumonia [40, 41]. Physiotherapy including MHI and positioning plus suctioning showed no differences in VAP versus suctioning alone [42]. Yet, in contrast, another reported a significantly lower incidence of VAP (8% vs 39%) in the group receiving physiotherapy [43]. However, the duration of mechanical ventilation, length of ICU stay, and mortality were not significantly different between the groups. The addition of physiotherapy in a population of ventilated patients for various reasons of respiratory insufficiency was associated with prolongation of mechanical ventilation [44].

Weaning failure

Only a small proportion of patients fail to wean from mechanical ventilation, but they require a disproportionate amount of resources. A therapist-driven weaning protocol was shown to reduce the duration of mechanical ventilation and ICU cost [45]. However, a recent study showed that protocol-directed weaning may be unnecessary in an ICU with generous physician staffing and structured rounds [46].

A spontaneous breathing trial can be used to assess readiness for extubation with the performance of serial measurements, such as tidal volume, respiratory rate, maximal inspiratory airway pressure, and the rapid shallow breathing index [47]. Early detection of worsening clinical signs such as distress, airway obstruction, and paradoxical chest wall motion ensures that serious problems are prevented (➲ Box 32.1). Airway patency and protection (i.e. an effective cough mechanism) should be assessed before the commencement of weaning. Peak cough flow is a useful parameter to predict successful weaning in patients with neuromuscular disease or spinal cord injury when extubation is anticipated [48]. An 'airway care score' has been developed based on quality of the patient's cough during airway suctioning, the absence of 'excessive' secretions, and the frequency of airway suctioning [45]. NIV can facilitate weaning [49], reduces ICU costs [50], and is effective in preventing postextubation failure in patients at risk [51].

Inspiratory muscle training may be beneficial in patients with weaning failure. There is accumulating evidence that weaning problems are associated with failure of the respiratory muscles to resume ventilation [52]. Uncontrolled trials of inspiratory muscle training (threshold loading; see ➲ Fig. 32.3) observed an improvement in inspiratory

---

Box 32.1 Criteria for weaning

- Maximal inspiratory pressure >20 cmH$_2$O
- Minute ventilation <15 L/min
- Respiratory frequency <25/min
- Rapid shallow breathing index (f/VT) <105
- Pao$_2$/Fio$_2$ >200

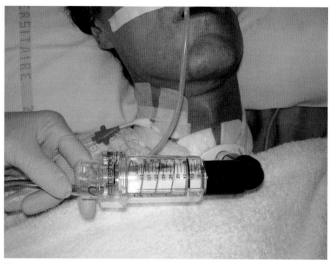

Figure 32.3 Respiratory muscle resistive training with threshold loading in a patient weaning from mechanical ventilation.

muscle function and a reduction in duration of mechanical ventilation and weaning time [53]. Interim analysis of a randomized controlled trial comparing inspiratory muscle training at moderate intensity (~50% PI_{max}) versus sham training in patients with weaning failure showed that a statistical significant larger proportion of the training group (76%) could be weaned compared to the sham group (35%) [54]. Biofeedback to display the breathing pattern has been shown to enhance weaning [55]. Voice and touch may be used to augment weaning success, either by stimulation to improve ventilatory drive, or by reducing anxiety [56]. Environmental influences, such as ambulating with a portable ventilator, have been shown to benefit attitudes and outlooks in long-term ventilator-dependent patients [57].

Physical deconditioning and related complications

The progress of intensive care medicine has dramatically improved survival of critically ill patients, especially in patients with ARDS. This improved survival is, however, often associated with general physical deconditioning, muscle weakness, dyspnoea, depression, and anxiety reduced health-related quality of life after ICU discharge [2].

Physical deconditioning and specifically muscle weakness are suggested to have a key role in impaired functional status after ICU stay [2]. Optimal physiological functioning depends on the upright position [4], so bed rest and limited mobility during critical illness result in profound physical deconditioning and dysfunction of the respiratory, cardiovascular, musculoskeletal, neurological, renal,

and endocrine systems. These effects can be exacerbated by inflammation and pharmacological agents. Denervation atrophy may complicate critical illness and sepsis has been shown to be one of the most important determinants of critical illness polyneuropathy [58]. Clinically significant muscle weakness is observed in 25% of patients who were ventilated for more than 7 days [5]. Muscle wasting appears to be highest during the first 2–3 weeks of ICU stay [59].

Early mobility and physical activity

The changes in functional performance and peripheral and respiratory muscle function mentioned above indicate the need for rehabilitation following ICU stay, but also underscore the need for assessment and measures to prevent deconditioning and loss of physical function even during the ICU stay. The amount of rehabilitation performed in ICUs is often inadequate and, as a rule, rehabilitation is better organized in weaning centres or respiratory intensive care units [60, 61]. The main reason is that in rehabilitation the approach is less driven by medical diagnosis; rather, rehabilitation focuses on deficiencies in the broader scope of health problems as defined in the International Classification of Functioning, Disability and Health. This leads to identification of problems and the prescription of one or more interventions at a level of body structure and function as well as activities and participation. Members of the rehabilitation team in the ICU (doctors, physiotherapists, nurses, and occupational therapists) should be able to prioritize, and identify aims and parameters of treatments, ensuring that these are both therapeutic and safe by appropriate monitoring of vital functions [62]. This team approach has been shown to be effective [60, 63–65].

It is important to prevent or attenuate muscle deconditioning as early as possible in patients with expected prolonged bed rest [66]. Recent scientific and clinical interest and evidence provide support for a safe and early physical activity and mobilization approach to the critically ill patient by ICU team members [63–65, 67, 68].

Exercise training is considered as a cornerstone component of any rehabilitation programme, in addition to psychosocial interventions. Accurate assessment of cardiorespiratory reserve and rigorous screening for other factors that could preclude early mobilization is of paramount importance. ➲ Figure 32.4 outlines the steps involved in safe mobilization of critically ill patients [62]. In addition to assessment of the safety and readiness of the patient for exercise and physical activity, specific measures of function (e.g. muscle strength, joint mobility), functional status (Functional Independence Measure, Berg Balance

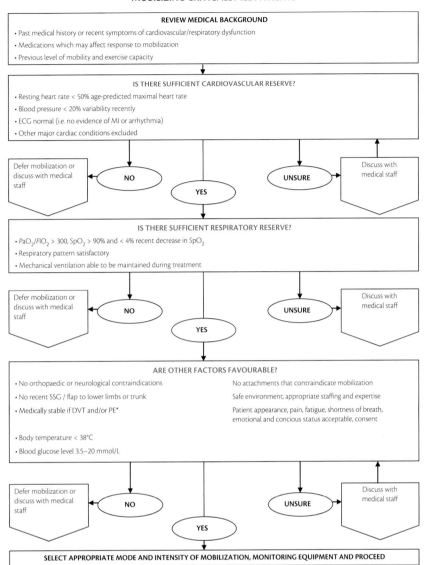

Figure 32.4 Overview of safety issues before mobilizing critically ill patients.
Reproduced from Stiller K, Phillips A. Safety aspects of mobilising acutely ill inpatients. *Physiother Theory Pract* 2003;**19**:239–257, with permission of Taylor and Francis Group..

scale, Functional Ambulation Categories) and quality of life (e.g. SF-36, disease-specific questionnaires) must be considered.

Physical activity and exercise should be targeted at the appropriate intensity and exercise modality. These will be dependent on the stability and cooperation of the patient. The risk of moving a critically ill patient is weighed against the risk of immobility and recumbency and, when employed, requires stringent monitoring to ensure the mobilization is instituted appropriately and safely [62]. Acutely ill, unco-operative patients will be treated with modalities such as passive range of motion, muscle stretching, splinting, body positioning, passive cycling with a bed cycle, or electrical muscle stimulation that do not need the patient's coopera-tion and will not put stress on the cardiorespiratory sys-tem. On the other hand, a stable cooperative patient who

is beyond the acute illness phase but still on mechanical ventilation can be mobilized on the edge of the bed, trans-fer to a chair, perform resistance muscle training or active cycling with a bed cycle or chair cycle, and walk with or without assistance. The flow diagram developed by Morris *et al.* [65] (⮕Fig. 32.5) has face validity and is an example of such a step-up approach.

The uncooperative critically ill patient

The importance of body positioning ('stirring up' patients) was reported as early as the 1940s [69]. To simulate the normal perturbations that the human body experiences in health, the patient who is critically ill needs to be positioned upright (well supported), and rotated when recumbent. These perturbations need to be scheduled frequently to avoid the adverse effects of prolonged static

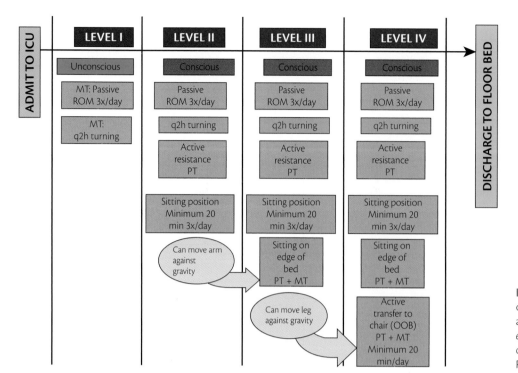

Figure 32.5 Step-up approach of progressive exercise and ambulation as suggested by Morris *et al.* [65]. MT, mobility team; OOB, out of bed; PT, physiotherapy; ROM, range of motion.

positioning on respiratory, cardiac, and circulatory function. Other indications for positioning include the management of soft tissue contracture, protection of flaccid limbs and lax joints, nerve impingement, and skin breakdown. The efficacy of two-hourly patient rotation, which is common in clinical practice, has not been verified scientifically. Bed design features in critical care should include hip and knee breaks so that patients can approximate upright sitting to the extent that they can tolerate. Heavy care patients, such as those who are sedated, heavy, or overweight may need chairs with greater support such as stretcher chairs. Hoists may be needed to change a patient's position safely.

Passive stretching or range of motion exercise may have a particularly important role in the management of patients who are unable to move spontaneously. Studies in healthy subjects have shown that passive stretching decreases stiffness and increases extensibility of the muscle. Continuous passive motion (CPM) prevents contractures and has been assessed in patients with critical illness subjected to prolonged inactivity [70]. In critically ill patients, three 3 h sessions of CPM per day reduced fibre atrophy and protein loss, compared with passive stretching for 5 min, twice daily [70]. For patients who cannot be actively mobilized and have high risk of soft tissue contracture, such as following severe burns, trauma, and some neurological conditions, splinting may be indicated.

The application of exercise training in the early phase of ICU admission is often more complicated because of lack of cooperation and the clinical status of the patient. Recent technological developments have resulted in a bedside cycle ergometer for (active or passive) leg cycling during bed rest (➲ Fig. 32.6, 📹 32.1). The bedside cycle ergometer can perform prolonged continuous mobilization allowing rigorous control of exercise intensity and duration. Furthermore, the training intensity can be continuously

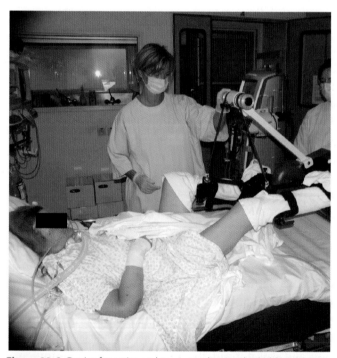

Figure 32.6 Device for active and passive cycling in a bedridden patient in the intensive care.

adjusted to the patient's health status and the physiological responses to exercise. A recent randomized controlled trial of early application of daily bedside leg cycling in critically ill patients showed improved functional status, muscle function, and exercise performance at hospital discharge compared to patients receiving standard physiotherapy without leg cycling [68].

In patients unable to perform voluntary muscle contractions, electrical muscle stimulation (EMS) has been used to prevent disuse muscle atrophy. A slower muscle protein catabolism and increase in total RNA content were also seen after EMS in patients with major abdominal surgery [71]. In patients in the ICU not able to move actively, a reduction of muscle atrophy was seen when using EMS [72], while EMS of the quadriceps, in addition to active limb mobilization, enhanced muscle strength and hastened independent transfer from bed to chair [73].

The cooperative critically ill patient

Mobilization and ambulation has been part of the physiotherapy management of acutely ill patients for several decades. Mobilization refers to physical activity sufficient to elicit acute physiological effects that enhance ventilation, central and peripheral perfusion, circulation, muscle metabolism, and alertness. Strategies—in order of intensity—include sitting on the edge of the bed, standing, stepping in place, transferring in bed and from bed to chair, and walking with or without support. Although the approach of early mobilization has face validity, the concept has only recently been studied in two randomized controlled trials [63, 65]. Morris *et al.* demonstrated that patients receiving early mobility therapy had reduced ICU stay and hospital stay, with no differences in weaning time. No differences were observed in discharge location or in hospital costs of the usual care and early mobility patients. Schweickert *et al.* observed that early physical and occupational therapy improved functional status at hospital discharge, shortened duration of delirium, and increased ventilator-free days. These findings did not result in differences in length of ICU or hospital stay [63].

The team approach (doctor, nurse, physiotherapist, and occupational therapist) is an important and strong point in establishing an early ambulation programme. The costs of this approach outweigh the benefits. The early intervention approach, although not easy, especially in patients still in need of supportive devices (mechanical ventilation, cardiac assists) or unable to stand without support of personnel or standing aids, is a worthwhile experience for the patient [65, 67]. This difference in the mentality of the team was

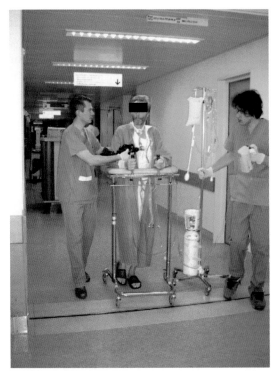

Figure 32.7 Use of a walking frame to assist a ventilator-dependent patient.

elegantly demonstrated in the study of Thomsen *et al.* [60]. Transferring a patient from the acute ICU to the respiratory ICU substantially increased the number of patients ambulating (threefold, compared with pretransfer rates). Improvements in ambulation with transfer to the respiratory ICU were allocated to the differences in the team approach towards ambulating the patients [60].

Standing and walking frames (◑ Fig. 32.7) enable the patient to mobilize safely with attachments for bags, lines, and leads that cannot be disconnected. The frame either needs to be able to accommodate a portable oxygen tank, or a portable mechanical ventilator and seat; or a suitable trolley for equipment can be used. Walking and standing aids, and tilt tables, enhance physiological responses and promote early mobilization of critically ill patients. Transfer belts facilitate heavy lifting and protect both the patient and staff. In ventilated patients, the ventilator settings may require adjustment to the patient's needs (i.e. increased minute ventilation).

Aerobic training and muscle strengthening, in addition to routine mobilization, improved walking distance more than mobilization alone in ventilated patients with chronic critical illness [61]. A randomized controlled trial showed that a 6-week upper and lower limb training programme improved limb muscle strength, ventilator-free time, and functional outcomes in patients requiring long-term mechanical ventilation compared to a control group [74]. These results are in line with a retrospective analysis of patients on long-term mechanical ventilation who participated in whole-body training and respiratory muscle training [75] In patients recently weaned from mechanical ventilation [76], the addition of upper-limb exercise enhanced the effects of general mobilization on exercise endurance performance and dyspnoea. Low-resistance multiple repetitions of resistive muscle training can augment muscle mass, force generation, and oxidative enzymes. Sets of repetitions within the patient's tolerance can be scheduled daily, commensurate with their goals. Resistive muscle training can include the use of pulleys, elastic bands, and weight belts. Patients with cardiovascular dysfunction may benefit from resistance training, although high resistance of large muscle masses may have detrimental cardiovascular effects in older patients with cardiovascular disease [77].

The chair cycle and the earlier mentioned bed cycle allow patients to perform an individualized exercise training programme. The intensity of cycling can be adjusted to the individual patient's capacity, ranging from passive cycling via assisted cycling to cycling against increasing resistance.

Conclusion

Physiotherapists are involved in the management of patients with critical illness. Physiotherapy assessment of critically ill patients is not mainly driven by medical diagnosis, focusing instead on deficiencies at a pathophysiological and functional level. Accurate and valid assessment of respiratory conditions (retained airway secretions, atelectasis, and respiratory muscle weakness) and deconditioning and related problems (muscle weakness, joint stiffness, impaired functional exercise capacity, physical inactivity, and quality of life) allows the identification of underlying problems amenable to physiotherapy. Evidence-based targets for physiotherapy are deconditioning, impaired airway clearance, atelectasis, intubation avoidance, and weaning failure. Early physical activity and mobility are key in the prevention, attenuation, or reversal of the deconditioning. A variety of modalities for exercise training and early mobility are evidence based and are applied depending on the stage of critical illness, comorbid conditions, and cooperation of the patient. The physiotherapist should be responsible for implementing mobilization plans and exercise prescription and make recommendations for progression of these jointly with medical and nursing staff.

Personal perspective

Physiotherapy practice needs to be further utilized in this highly technological, highly invasive, and costly health care setting. Evidence exists to support the use of physiotherapy in ICU patients, and, given this knowledge base, randomized controlled clinical trials with untreated controls would be unethical. The use of multicentre studies may allow ethical comparisons between differing physiotherapy strategies in different units, but differences in patient characteristics between ICUs may confound the results. In addition to traditional outcome measures of the direct effects of physiotherapy interventions on outcomes such as oxygenation, lung mechanics, rate of respiratory complications, weaning success, muscle strength, and joint mobility, quality of life outcomes and functional outcomes in all levels of care should be included.

Critical care as a whole has lagged behind compared with less acute settings with respect to the inclusion of the evaluation of these outcomes. Reducing length of ICU and hospital stay are outcomes highly consistent with the goals of physiotherapy, i.e. to exploit noninvasive interventions of care and minimize invasive care as much as possible. This should be associated with reduced health care costs, undoubtedly an important outcome. Physiotherapy might also improve functional outcome after ICU stay, which should in turn reduce health care costs.

Future studies of the efficacy of physiotherapy should include duration of ICU stay as an essential outcome, recognizing that this measure will be influenced by the care provided by other team members. Further study is required to determine which components of physiotherapy are most effective in resolving atelectasis and whether optimal lung recruitment, positioning, and mobilization are effective in both the prevention and treatment of atelectasis. The effectiveness of physiotherapy management in preventing hypoventilation in cases of chest trauma requires further investigation, as does the use of NIV in inhalation injury. Last but not least, further evaluation of physiotherapy interventions, such as respiratory muscle training and early mobilization or exercise training in the treatment of difficult to wean critically ill patients is needed.

Acknowledgement

This work is partially funded by Research Foundation—Flanders grant G0523.06.

Further reading

Burtin C, Clerckx B, Robbeets C, et al. Early exercise in critically ill patients enhances short-term functional recovery. *Crit Care Med* 2009;**37**:2499–2505.

De Jonghe B, Sharshar T, Lefaucheur JP, et al. Paresis acquired in the intensive care unit: a prospective multicenter study. *JAMA* 2002;**288**:2859–2867.

Gosselink R, Bott J, Johnson M, et al. Physiotherapy for adult patients with critical illness: recommendations of the European Respiratory Society and European Society of Intensive Care Medicine Task Force on Physiotherapy for Critically Ill Patients. *Intens Care Med* 2008;**34**:1188–1199.

Herridge MS, Cheung AM, Tansey CM, et al. One-year outcomes in survivors of the acute respiratory distress syndrome. *N Engl J Med* 2003;**348**:683–693.

Morris PE, Goad A, Thompson C, et al. Early intensive care unit mobility therapy in the treatment of acute respiratory failure. *Crit Care Med* 2008;**36**:2238–2243.

Needham DM. Mobilizing patients in the intensive care unit: improving neuromuscular weakness and physical function. *JAMA* 2008;**300**:1685–1690.

Ntoumenopoulos G, Presneill JJ, McElholum M, Cade JF. Chest physiotherapy for the prevention of ventilator-associated pneumonia. *Intens Care Med* 2002;**28**:850–856.

Pasquina P, Tramer MR, Walder B. Prophylactic respiratory physiotherapy after cardiac surgery: systematic review. *BMJ* 2003;**327**:1379.

Schweickert WD, Pohlman MC, Pohlman AS, et al. Early physical and occupational therapy in mechanically ventilated, critically ill patients: a randomised controlled trial. *Lancet* 2009;**373**:1874–1882.

Stiller K, Philips A. Safety aspects of mobilising acutely ill patients. *Physiother Theory Pract* 2003;**19**:239–257.

⮕ For additional multimedia materials please visit the online version of the book (🖰 http://www.esciacc.oxfordmedicine.com).

SECTION VI

The laboratory in intensive and acute cardiac care

CHAPTER 33

The use of biomarkers for acute cardiovascular disease

Allan S. Jaffe

Contents

Summary

Understanding the proper use of biomarkers requires clinicians to appreciate some critical preanalytic and analytic issues as well as how to use the markers properly. They must focus on learning from the peer-reviewed literature and be willing to lose prior biases and embrace the new realities. The benefits of such an approach will not only facilitate the care of patients today but will also prepare clinicians to understand and embrace the new generation of markers that is coming and that will continue to make this area transformational for cardiology.

Introduction

Cardiac biomarkers are now used extensively to help evaluate patients with acute cardiovascular disease. They facilitate the diagnosis of cardiac injury and thus acute myocardial infarction (AMI), and the diagnosis of heart failure. They are also instrumental in the risk stratification of these acutely ill patients. This was not always the case; the use of these markers has evolved over many years.

Cardiac biomarkers have been appreciated since the early 1940s, when it was first appreciated that C-reactive protein (CRP) rose in patients with AMI [1]. Their use in acute cardiovascular disease did not really begin to become extensive however, until the landmark work of Carmen and Wroblewski in the 1950s who described increases in aspartate transaminase (SGOT) [2] and lactate dehydrogenase (LDH) [3] in patients with AMI. At the time, these advances were not appreciated as important, largely because of the lack of specificity of increases for cardiac disease. This changed substantially when Rosalki in the late 1950s developed an assay for total creatine kinase (CK) [4]. At the time, intramuscular injections were being given therapeutically in patients with AMI, but even at this time, it was appreciated that a marker like CK might be useful. The use of these markers was further promulgated by the work of Sobel, Braunwald, and colleagues in San Diego who began to use CK as a surrogate for infarct size [5] and were able to show that this measure provided potent prognostic information [6].

Subsequently, the development of CK-MB assays initially by electrophoretic separation [7] and subsequently by radioimmunoassay [8] further facilitated the use of cardiac biomarkers. During roughly the same period, an appreciation of the endocrine nature of the heart itself [9] and with it the field of natriuretic peptides began to evolve with the description of atrial natriuretic peptide (ANP) by de Bold and colleagues [10]. It rapidly became appreciated that ANP had important biological effects, and that the granules containing ANP found in the atrium were associated with vasodilation and sodium excretion [11]. This led to the concept that ANP would be an important counter-regulatory hormone in hypertension, and early studies focused more on its use as a therapeutic agent, rather than as a diagnostic agent [11]. Nonetheless, it was appreciated that ANP also appeared to be helpful in diagnosing heart failure [12]. When brain natriuretic peptide (now more appropriately called B-type natriuretic peptide or BNP) was discovered, it changed the field markedly. BNP is a very different marker, requiring stimulation of its messenger RNA for synthesis rather than being mostly granularly based like ANP. It rapidly became clear that it had the potential to be a more helpful diagnostic tool [13]. By the mid-1990s, it was appreciated that from the point of view of diagnosis, BNP was probably a better marker than ANP, but nonetheless, it did not become extensively used [14] until the pivotal 2002 Breathing Not Properly trial [15].

During this same period, Dr Attilio Maseri demonstrated the usefulness of CRP in the risk stratification of patients with acute coronary syndromes [16, 17], in keeping with experimental data suggesting that inflammation was important in acute coronary artery disease [18]. The assay for CRP had been developed initially for use in infection [18]. It is perhaps not surprising it is elevated in AMI [1] since it is an acute phase reactant. Maseri and colleagues were the first to use CRP to characterize patients with unstable angina. They recognized that elevations in inflammatory markers were prognostically important [16, 17]. This group emphasized the need to correlate the CRP elevations with the clinical characteristics of the patients [17]. This is a critical issue, as it is clear that an acute necrotic event such as an infarction in itself causes substantial elevations in inflammatory markers [19]. Thus, the need to distinguish between elevations indicative of the unstable plaque and those occurring due to necrosis is critical.

The 1990s was an important time for the development of all of these efforts. Troponin assays began to be developed [20, 21], and it became clear that the problems of specificity seen with CK-MB were no longer present with troponin [22]. In addition, troponin assays were substantially more sensitive than CK-MB, leading to many of the issues that still complicate their use in patients with acute cardiovascular disease [23]. Nonetheless, the appreciation of increased specificity helped tremendously. These advances have continued as troponin assays have improved in sensitivity while not diminishing in specificity [24].

During this time, BNP was not being used extensively as a diagnostic marker although there were many publications documenting the ability to use measures of BNP in patients with valvular heart disease [25, 26] and even in patients with heart failure [14]. However, it was not until Biosite developed a easily usable point of care (POC) assay that the use of BNP became extensive. The assay was analytically not well configured, which added to the very substantial biological variability seen with BNP [27]. Nonetheless, this POC assay allowed values of BNP to be measured and evaluated rapidly. The validation work in this area focused initially on the emergency department (ED) in the evaluation of patients with acute dyspnoea [15] and to general internists and family practitioners in the outpatient setting [28, 29]. The landmark studies were done predominantly in Europe in the outpatient setting [28, 29] and in the ED in a large multicentre trial in the United States called the Breathing Not Properly (BNP) trial. This trial evaluated the ability of ED physicians to diagnose the presence of heart failure as adjudicated retrospectively by a panel of physicians including cardiologists. The data (◔ Fig. 33.1) suggested that BNP alone was superior to clinical judgement and that the combination added substantially to diagnostic accuracy (from 74% to 81.5%). Cardiologists might argue that these physician groups are less astute in the diagnosis of heart failure and thus the small incremental value documented in these studies might not be replicated if the evaluations were done by cardiologists. Nonetheless, over time, they too began to use BNP values to assist in

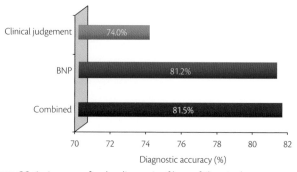

Figure 33.1 Accuracy for the diagnosis of heart failure in the emergency department based on clinical judgement, BNP, and their combined use. N = 1538; p >0.0001 from clinical judgement to combined.
From McCullough PA, Nowak RM, McCord J, et al. B-type natriuretic peptide and clinical judgment in emergency diagnosis of heart failure: analysis from Breathing Not Properly (BNP) Multinational Study. *Circulation* 2002;**106**:416–422, with permission.

the diagnosis of heart failure. This was facilitated when the prognostic value of the marker was documented [30, 31]. These trends led to the development of a large number of BNP assays based on different antibodies, and an assay for the NT-pro fragment of BNP (NT-proBNP), which under normal circumstance is also produced when the proBNP peptide cleaved after if it is released from myocytes [32].

The use of CRP in the acute setting progressed slowly after the initial landmark work of Maseri (⊃ Fig. 33.2) because (in this author's opinion) of the confounding of high levels of CRP found as a response to necrosis in patients with myocardial infarction [17]. This led some to advocate its use and some not, but very careful work was done in documenting that there is important prognostic information in CRP values taken on admission. It also became clear that the importance of those values was related to prognosis in a time course later than the elevations of troponin [33, 34]. These studies were done even with appropriate use of cut-off values of troponin—something that has been missing in a substantial proportion of the literature.

It has now become clear that biomarkers are an integral part of our diagnostic armamentarium. Troponin is the marker of choice for the evaluation of patients with any putative cardiovascular injury [35]. Its specificity has remained pristine, and assays have been improved to reduce the frequency of analytic false positives [24]. Accordingly, troponin has supplanted CK-MB as the marker of choice for the detection of cardiac injury and thus AMI. Many would argue that CK-MB no longer has any role to play in the evaluation of patients with putative cardiovascular disease [36]. BNP has also emerged as a frequently used marker [23]. Recent data suggest that using it in a bayesian

manner, i.e. in patients with an intermediate probability of disease, optimizes the cost effectiveness and benefit of testing [37]. Indeed, the data with NT-proBNP, which has always resulted in somewhat more complex algorithms, has perhaps really come closer to the mark of clinical utility by using multiple cut-offs [38]. BNP researchers originally focused predominantly on a solitary cut-off value, although it is well known that, as with NT-proBNP, there is a very substantial grey zone for BNP between values of 100 and 500 pg/mL [39]. CRP has also emerged with confirmatory data of the original trials of Maseri and colleagues, and in particular with an explanation for why the late prognostic significance may be present. In the PROVE-IT trial, it was shown that when evaluation was late (at 4–6 weeks after the acute event), continuing increases in CRP as well as inadequate treatment of LDL cholesterol were associated with more adverse events [40]. In those individuals, it appears that elevated CRP is related to comorbidities that are associated with increased inflammatory markers such as diabetes, obesity, smoking, and lack of exercise [41]. Thus, it is not totally clear whether it is most efficacious to use drugs or whether primary prevention with behavioural modification would be more appropriate.

However, the use of biomarkers in patients with acute cardiovascular disease has now become an essential part of our armamentarium and this trend is likely to accelerate in the future.

Principles guiding the use of biomarkers in acute cardiac care

Many clinicians have not been educated about to some of the important variables that can affect the accuracy of biomarker determinations. The details are not important, and are often closely monitored by those doing the assays, but a variety of principles relating to how biomarkers are collected and analysed are critical. Often little attention is paid to these issues, although if they are not understood, clinicians will have difficulty in interpreting results. Accordingly, the present chapter does not attempt to cover all of the analytic issues but rather focuses on those areas where changes might be important for analytes such as BNP, troponin, and CRP—the markers that are frequently used in critically ill cardiovascular patients.

Preanalytic factors

Although clinicians rarely consider how samples have been obtained, this is critical to the measurement of every analyte. For example, when samples are drawn through intravenous

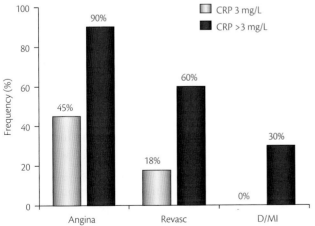

Figure 33.2 Relationship of C-reactive protein elevations at the time of admission with unstable angina and subsequent events. CRP, C-reactive protein; D/MI, death or myocardial infarction.
From Liuzzo G, Biasucci LM, Gallimore JR, *et al.* The prognostic value of C-reactive protein and serum amyloid A protein in severe unstable angina. *N Engl J Med* 1994;**331**:417–424. With permission.

or arterial lines, if contaminating fluids are not removed or if they adhere to the tubing, they can cause major alterations in values. This has recently been described in patients receiving catecholamines, where the effect markedly lowered creatinine levels [42]. The frequency of abnormal values obtained when one is drawing from indwelling lines is substantially greater than when one is doing separate venepunctures, and this has the potential to substantially delay appropriate care [43]. Major analytic issues in acute cardiology predominantly involve two of the analytes, troponin and BNP; CRP seems to be reasonably stable. Troponin can be markedly affected and may be differentially measured in heparin versus nonheparinized fluids [44, 45]. Indeed, the troponin T assay was reconfigured specifically to avoid the issues relating to heparin interference [46]. Troponin I assays have similar problems [44, 45]. In addition, there can be differences between serum and plasma independent of heparin [47]. This may not be very important in circumstances where the assays are not very sensitive, but for the newly developed highly sensitive assays for troponin, especially where there is a need to evaluate changing patterns [48], the differences could be key.

In regard to natriuretic peptides, BNP is an extremely fastidious molecule. Some have argued that it requires specific protease inhibitors to preserve activity [49], but most samples collected on EDTA and ice seem to provide adequate results if measured expeditiously [50]. However, EDTA samples that stay on ice for prolonged periods degrade to some extent as there are a variety of proteases in human blood that will affect the values [51]. This is one advantage of NT-proBNP, which is extremely stable regardless of how samples are collected [52]. These issues are even more important when considering long-term storage. Most of the samples for these assays can be stored fairly well, with the exception of BNP. The data suggest that BNP values diminish even if samples are stored at –70°C [52]. It is important for researchers to be aware of this when dealing with stored samples.

Analytic factors

There are a variety of analytic issues that clinicians need to at least consider. The first is the sensitivity of the assay. This is not a problem for CRP or even for most of the BNP assays, but it is for troponin assays [53]. This issue cannot be evaluated by looking at numbers or values for the assays, since there is no standardization in the field. At present, there is a standard material that is used by all assays that is made by the National Institute of Standards and Technology (NIST), but unfortunately it has not been capable of adequately harmonizing troponin assays [54]. Thus, numbers

do not serve us well in this regard. Accordingly, one needs to do clinical comparisons in order to know the sensitivity of one assay versus another, and companies often avoid such comparisons. This is a very complicated area and clinicians are often not aware of this issue, but it is key in understanding the troponin literature. Many articles touting the use of ancillary markers for diagnosis have used insensitive assays, and clinicians who do not work regularly in this area may not understand that these assays are so insensitive. Furthermore, the cut-off values used can have a major effect. Thus, if insensitive assays or high cut-off values are used, the data for a given marker might appear better than it really will be when used clinically [55]. This issue of cut-off values for troponin has been confusing to clinicians. The initial assays for troponin were approved at a cut-off value known as the ROC cut-off, where troponin is equivalent to CK-MB in terms of diagnostic performance [56]. Subsequently, in 2000, the European Society of Cardiology (ESC) and the American College of Cardiology (ACC) [57] suggested that troponin should be used like any other analyte, i.e. based on the distribution of normal values. Thus, what is needed is to measure a large number of normal subjects (most would suggest at least 320 subjects) and determine a 'normal' reference range. Since biomarker values are often skewed, the values may need to be normalized by logarithmic transformation to determine a cut-off value. Traditionally, this is done by taking two standard deviations from the mean so that 2.5% of all values would be elevated. With troponin, the biochemistry group of the Global Task Force of the ACC/ESC Task Force [58] suggested using three standard deviations from the mean so that there would only be 1% putative false positives. It turns out that with the present iteration of assays (not the novel high-sensitivity assays being developed which soon may be available for use), the 99% value is still substantially higher than values that are seen in normal individuals [24]. It should also be recognized that the accuracy of the 'normal' reference range depends heavily on how well the individuals used for this purpose are screened. Very few if any 'normal' value studies do more than a screening history and physical examination, and most are even less demanding.

This issue of sensitivity is often confused with issues of precision, i.e. how accurately one measures a given analyte. In the laboratory world, having good precision, so that values are reproducible, is a virtue. There are many circumstances in which lack of precision has caused confusion, and for that reason, many of the guidelines groups have advocated a low degree of imprecision near the cut-off value for troponin [35, 57]. For troponin, this has been embraced by some who have even advocating raising the cut-off value from the 99th percentile value to the 10% CV value if imprecision is even slightly greater than 10% at the 99th percentile [56]. This has never been an approach endorsed by guidelines groups [35, 57]. Some have suggested that this is why minor elevations in troponin are 'false positives'. This is not correct. In fact, if the assay is appropriately validated, imprecision should make the upper limit of the normal range higher, protecting against false positives [59]. This has been tested in at least two circumstances for diagnosis and one for prognosis with both troponin and BNP in large multicorrelate Monte Carlo simulations, with large numbers of samples predicated on real assays and based on real data from clinical trials (➲ Fig. 33.3). In both instances, modest imprecision (up to 20%) made little difference in terms of clinical diagnosis or prognosis [59, 60].

However, precision does affect the evaluation of what sort of change might be clinically important. In general, the difference between values analytically is roughly three standard deviations of the variation around those values [35]. Thus, greater imprecision would lead to a larger difference in values (delta) needing to occur in order to call the values different from one another. With very high-sensitivity assays, where one can begin to measure biological variability, one could add biological variability to this assessment. This makes the values slightly higher. Biological variation (➲ Fig. 33.4) has recently been measured by Wu and colleagues with a high-sensitivity troponin assay [61]. Biological variability cannot be measured with most of the present-day assays, because they do not measure normal values in the vast majority of patients. Direct measurements for each assay of both biological and analytic variability would be a much more potent way of developing an appropriate delta value. With troponin, there are publications suggesting that a 20% change [35] with some assays and a 30% change with others [62] is of significance. This sort of analysis needs to be done on an assay by assay basis and would be substantially assisted if there were some sort of biobank that would allow all the assays to use the same patient samples and data.

The issue of what is a significant change in values is even more complicated for natriuretic peptides. Both BNP and NT-proBNP are known to have a very large biological variability, both short term (➲ Fig. 33.5) and long term (➲ Fig. 33.6) [63]. The reference change value (RCV) is between 80% and 100%, so only very large differences can be relied on. This has led some to argue that perhaps BNP assays do not need to be quite as precise. This author would argue that imprecision is additive with biological variability, and although minor degrees of imprecision above 10% are not critical, having assays that are more precise will in the long run allow one to rely on less marked changes as significant. This is an important issue, because changing values often are relied on to monitor patients in hospital, and the question is what percentage change is significant. Based on the data that is available in regard to biological and analytic variability, one would say these changes need to be roughly 80–100% [63]. Some have argued that in critically ill patients smaller increments may still be important and have argued for 20% or 30% changes based on their clinical experience. This claim has been included in a lot of consensus documents, but there are very few data to substantiate it [64]. Indeed, there are robust data about biological variation and it is at a minimum 25%, which supports the idea that much larger RCVs are necessary to be sure

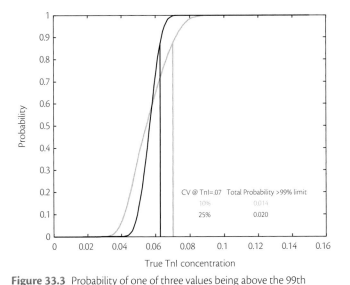

Figure 33.3 Probability of one of three values being above the 99th percentile value predicated on imprecision. The frequency of this phenomenon is clinically insignificant.
From Apple FS, Parvin CA, Buechler KF, *et al*. Validation of the 99th percentile cutoff independent of assay imprecision (CV) for cardiac troponin monitoring for ruling out myocardial infarction. *Clin Chem* 2005;**51**:2198–2200. With permission.

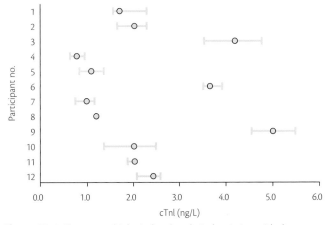

Figure 33.4 Short-term biological and analytical variation with the high-sensitivity Singulex assay.
From Wu AH, Smith A. Biological variation of the natriuretic peptides and their role in monitoring patients with heart failure. *Eur J Heart Fail* 2004;**6**:355–358. With permission.

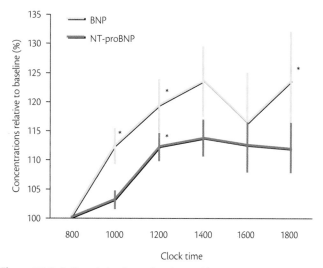

Figure 33.5 Daily variation in natriuretic peptides.
From Wu AH, Smith A, Wieczorek S, *et al*. Biological variation for N-terminal pro- and B-type natriuretic peptides and implications for therapeutic monitoring of patients with congestive heart failure. *Am J Cardiol* 2003;**92**:628–631. With permission.

a change has occurred [65]. In a recent publication, Miller *et al.* showed that, during follow-up in patients with chronic heart failure, either increases or decreases of 80% or greater were necessary to show associations with differences in outcome [66]. This may be why some of the trials using natriuretic peptides for monitoring therapy have not been positive as they have not induced sufficient increments in change in natriuretic peptide values [67].

Normal value issues

For each analyte, one needs to establish what are normal values, and their distribution; ideally this should be done across different ethnic groups, by gender, and by age. This has been

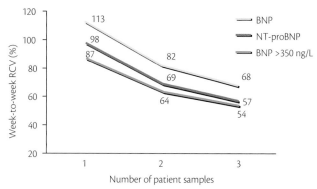

Figure 33.6 Long-term (week to week) variation in natriuretic peptides including putatively normal subjects and those with elevated values with RCVs. The RCVs for BNP (yellow), NT-proBNP (red), and BNP >350 ng/L (green) are shown separately, as derived from single, duplicate, and triplicate sampling, with each sample analysed singly, for estimating the homeostatic setpoints of the two serial results.
From Wu AH, Smith A, Wieczorek S, *et al*. Biological variation for N-terminal pro- and B-type natriuretic peptides and implications for therapeutic monitoring of patients with congestive heart failure. *Am J Cardiol* 2003;**92**:628–631. With permission.

done in part for the present analytes used in acute cardiac care, but more data are necessary and it is not clear that clinicians have an appreciation of this information. For troponin, no one has seen a gradient in values until recently, when studies with some of the high-sensitivity assays have reported a difference between men and women with the Roche [68] and Singulex [69] assays but not with the Beckman assay [70]. There are no data suggesting that there are differences between racial or ethnic groups for troponin, but that seems to be because the majority of the world has simply embraced the values generated in the United States and Europe, perhaps incorrectly. Several evaluations have tried to determine whether increases above the guideline suggested cut-off value of the 99th percentile represent subtle comorbidities or changes in values with age. At least with present-day assays, in almost each instance it has been found that these increases represent comorbidities and not increases related solely to age [71,72]. Thus, for the troponin assays in use today, correction for age and gender is not necessary. This may change with some of the high-sensitivity assays [68, 69].

For BNP, the studies have been far more extensive. Age and gender differences are clear [73, 74]. It was initially thought that the differences by gender might be related to increases in women induced by oestrogens, but recent data suggest they may be more related to testosterone, which appears to suppress values [75, 76]. Nonetheless, normal values rise with age and are much lower in younger individuals [73,74]. Women also have higher values of both BNP and NT-proBNP [73, 74]. There are sparse data in regard to normal values in different ethnic groups, but the data from large trials suggest that abnormal values do not need to be established separately [77,78] Most reports ignore these sorts of distinctions and try and generate simple paradigms for the use of these markers, which is how values of 100 pg/mL for BNP come about [15, 77]. Nonetheless, this author considers that using age- and gender-determined differences and correcting for body mass index (BMI) as well [79, 80] would lead to greater accuracy. For each analyte (BNP and NT-proBNP), substantially lower values are observed in obese individuals [78, 80]. This observation was initially hard to explain. It was known that BNP binds to the BNP clearance receptor, and it was initially thought that perhaps fat provided more clearance receptors. However, this was not thought to be an adequate explanation for the relationship of BMI and NT-proBNP values, since the NT-proBNP fragment should not bind to clearance receptors. It now appears that the majority of what is measured by both NT-proBNP assays and BNP assays is actually proBNP, [81] which does bind to the clearance receptor. Thus, the original hypothesis for this relationship between natriuretic

Table 33.1 Cut-off values with NT-proBNP. Rule-out cut-point 300 pg/mL; rule-in cut-point with renal failure 1200 pg/mL

Age strata	Optimal cut-point (pg/mL)	Sensitivity (%)	Specificity (%)	PPV (%)	NPV (%)	Accuracy (%)
All <50 years (n = 183)	450	97	93	76	99	95
All 50–75 years (n = 554)	900	90	82	82	88	85
All >75 years (n = 519)	1800	85	73	92	55	83
Overall		90	84	88	66	86

Reproduced with permission from Pascual-Figal DA, Domingo M, Casas T, *et al.* Usefulness of clinical and NT-proBNP monitoring for prognostic guidance in destabilized heart failure outpatients. *Eur Heart J* 2008;**29**:1011–1018. With permission.

peptide values and BMI may be correct. This is just one of many issues related to normal or reference values for the natriuretic peptides. There are other issues to consider as well. As one might expect, subtle comorbidities such as atrial fibrillation, even if not present at the time the patient presents, are associated with increased values [82]. In addition, renal dysfunction also increases values. This phenomenon is quantitatively more marked for NT-proBNP than for BNP. The reasons for this are not totally clear, since the renal clearance of both of these peptides does not appear to be different across a wide range of renal function [83]. Nonetheless, higher cut-off values to diagnose heart failure are needed for those with renal failure [84, 85]. For all these reasons, the use of multiple cut-off values as opposed to a solitary value seems prudent. This has been proposed for NT-proBNP (➲Table 33.1) [86].

This area is also one that is important for the use of CRP, although there is some controversy. It appears that there are differences that need to be taken into account, based on both gender and ethnicity (➲Fig. 33.7) [87, 88]. Black individuals, especially black women, have higher values than white men and white women [88]. It is also clear that oestrogens raise CRP, as do any concomitant inflammatory diseases [87]. Thus, if the patient is ill at the time the sample is obtained, a second sample must be taken when the patient has returned to their baseline health status. In addition, if the individual is on oestrogens, one should expect higher values. Similarly, obesity and diabetes are associated with higher values, likely because these comorbidities are associated with increased inflammation.

Issues of interpretation

All of the analytes discussed above (troponin, natriuretic peptides and CRP) can be elevated by a large number of processes. There is a very long list of things that cause cardiac injury, and one of the great advances troponin has provided is an appreciation of the large number of additional disease entities that can damage the heart [23]. One way to start differentiating those elevations that are acute from those that are chronic is by looking for a rising pattern of values [48], which suggests an acute change. These increases still have a broad differential diagnosis and could be due to inflammatory cytokines that damage the myocardium in patients who are septic or due to direct trauma, cardiac infections such as myocarditis, or coronary artery disease. Chronic elevations tend not to rise acutely [48]. The best-understood paradigm for these chronic elevations are the renal failure patients where elevations especially in cardiac troponin T (cTnT) are importantly prognostic and likely related to the metabolic consequences of severe renal dysfunction. However, even when baseline elevations are present, a changing pattern of values occurs during acute events [89, 90]. It is now appreciated that many patients with stable angina [91, 92], and certainly many patients with chronic heart failure, have troponin elevations [93]. In addition, they can also have intermittent acute elevations when decompensations occur [93]. Thus, sensitivity to a changing pattern is extremely important. For troponin,

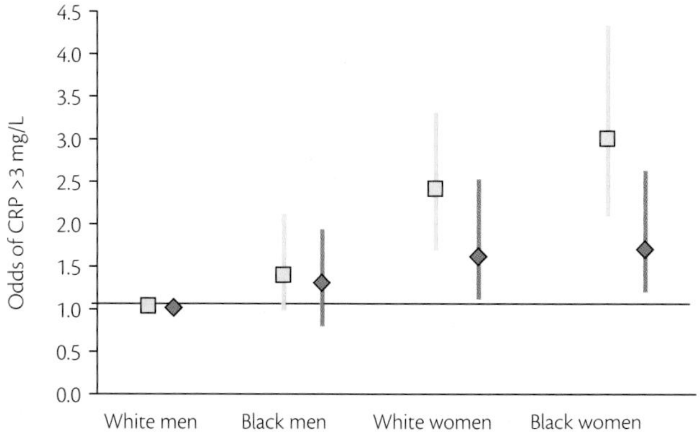

Figure 33.7 CRP values by gender and race after adjustment for relevant covariates. Yellow squares show values adjusted for weight only; red diamonds are values adjusted for age, diabetes, hypercholesterolaemia, high-density lipoprotein cholesterol, hypertension, smoking, body mass index, oestrogen use, statin use, creatinine, and sample weight.
From Chang AY, Abdullah SM, Jain T, *et al.* Associations among androgens, estrogens, and natriuretic peptides in young women: observations from the Dallas Heart Study. *J Am Coll Cardiol* 2007;**49**:109–116. With permission.

determining the appropriate RCV is related to precision, as indicated above, but in general this is the sort of issue that should be defined by the laboratories and reported as part of the results section of interpretation since it can be complex. If very high values of troponin are present without a changing pattern, one should always consider the rare circumstance of an interfering substance [94]. Interfering substances tend to cause very high values that do not change until the interfering substance is totally gone. Thus samples do not dilute linearly in this situation, which is diagnostic for an interfering substance. Many of these interfering substances are due to antibody problems and can be unmasked with the use of additional blocking antibodies, which are readily available in most high-quality laboratories.

With regard to the interpretation of BNP values, natriuretic peptides can also be elevated in many circumstances including all patients who are critically ill, those with volume increases, renal failure, Cushing's disease, and/or hyperaldosteronism [65]. Thus, one needs to interpret increases with close attention to the clinical context. One of the major differences between the presently available assays for natriuretic peptides is the difference between BNP and NT-proNBP in patients with renal failure. The aetiology for this is not understood, but increases in NT-proBNP become very high in many patients with renal failure with values that can be as high 35 000 ng/mL. It is often difficult for clinicians to know what to do with such high values, or whether a change from 35 000 to 20 000 is significant. This should not really be a problem, since the same principles in defining the change criteria are involved: the numbers are simply higher. It was initially thought that this elevation was due to renal clearance of the NT-proBNP fragment, but the renal clearance of BNP, and NT-proBNP are similar despite renal dysfunction [83]. Thus, the aetiology of this phenomenon is unclear. Nonetheless, the fact that the ratio between the two peptides changes remarkably is clear [95]. It is not clear to this author whether or not natriuretic peptides can be used diagnostically in complicated critically ill patients if renal function is below 30 mL/min, because the values are so high.

Similar issues of interpretation exist with CRP, having to do with concomitant illnesses and specifically other inflammatory processes that may confound the values. In this instance, there are few options because the CRP needs to be taken early after presentation before the acute response to necrosis occurs [19]. Thus, correction for concomitant disease may not be possible in this situation once this critical time window has passed. If the value is elevated in the absence of these confounders and it is fairly early after the onset of symptoms, it is likely that these values will persist and have long-term prognostic significance [17]. The

PROVE-IT data [40] suggesting a CRP value at 4–6 weeks post event from this perspective makes good sense. It is likely but unproven that this later group is similar to the group that has elevations at the time of presentation.

Contemporary issues with the use of acute cardiovascular biomarkers

Biomarkers are discuss in detail from the point of view of diagnostic utility in other chapters of this section. Here, we consider some generic issues concerning the contemporary use of biomarkers.

Sensitivity and detection of new disease entities

One of the issues that biomarkers pose for all clinicians—is best shown with troponin although it could occur with any of the various analytes—is that elevations will be found in circumstances where they were not expected or previously reported [24]. Such elevations pose a clinical challenge. It is easy in this situation to simply decide that the increases are spurious, and it is known that all tests can have false positives related to their analytic performance [94]. Alternatively, one could also explore the possibility that additional disease entities may participate in the development of these elevations. This principle is best demonstrated in regard to troponin elevations where we now appreciate a huge number of relatively modest increases that had not been anticipated. For example, we can now monitor doxorubicin drug toxicity with troponins, given the landmark studies of Cardinale and colleagues [96]. Not only do we now know that these troponin elevations presage reductions in ventricular performance, but it is also known that reducing troponin elevations with angiotensin converting enzyme (ACE) inhibitors also prevents short-term reductions in ventricular performance. It is very likely that many additional drug-related and toxic aetiologies for cardiac damage will become clearer as we improve the sensitivities of our assays. It is known, for example, that carbon monoxide poisoning causes troponin elevations acutely and that elevations are associated with an adverse prognosis, probably because cardiotoxicity requires significantly more marked increases in carboxyhemoglobin [98]. Thus, as opposed to ignoring or impugning these elevations, clinicians need to begin to explore the extent to which they open new pathophysiologic opportunities. This is exactly what was done by Assomull and colleagues [99] who investigated 60 patients who had elevated troponins and ECG changes that appeared acute and were thought to have AMI clinically. All of these individuals had coronary angiograms that were reassuring and therefore underwent ciné magnetic resonance (cMR) imaging. Important results (⊃Table 33.2) were elucidated in 65% of patients, including the finding that 11% of these patients had a cMR signal suggestive of AMI with delayed hyperenhancement in the subendocardium. This pattern is highly suggestive of infarction and, in this particular circumstance, one might argue it is probably diagnostic. These findings reinforce the concept that myocardial infarction can occur in the absence of overt angiographically detectable coronary disease, especially in women. There are now several series showing exactly this [100, 101]. This could be because of the timing of the angiography *per se*, to the presence of microvascular disease in smaller vessels or endothelial dysfunction in larger ones, and perhaps a to variety of yet unappreciated pathophysiological determinants. Nonetheless, AMI with normal coronary arteries is known to occur and is not new [102]. In addition, 50% of the patients in the Assomull study were found to have a cMR pattern suggestive of myocarditis, a relatively underdiagnosed and probably unappreciated disease. Indeed, cMR has begun to unmask a relatively substantial number of cases of myocarditis previously not diagnosed [103]. It had been previously reported that myocarditis could mimic AMI [104], but the frequency with which it occurred was unclear. As troponin assay sensitivity improves still further [24], it is likely that we will find still more new examples of abnormal pathophysiology manifesting as cardiac injury. In almost all instances, it is likely that the findings will be prognostically important. Thus, as opposed to immediately thinking that a given troponin value that does not correspond to acute coronary artery disease is a 'false positive,' clinicians might consider other disease entities that could potentially cause cardiac damage.

Some of this thinking may be facilitated by the designation of what has been termed 'type 2 myocardial infarction' by the most recent definition of AMI [35]. This is a circumstance where underlying coronary disease may be present but is stable until, in response to marked haemodynamic stress, increases in myocardial oxygen consumption cause cardiac injury which is then marked by the elaboration of troponin. Alternatively, in patients who are septic, it may be that the toxic cytokines are predominantly responsible [24]. Irrespective of the aetiology, the complication of having cardiac injury associated with critical illness is known to be associated with an adverse prognosis, both short and long term, and thus needs to be taken seriously [105]. One of the dilemmas in this area is that the appropriate therapeutic responses are not clear. Therefore, physicians need to think through the pathophysiology of the specific clinical entities involved as a way of attempting to craft a reasonable therapeutic response. For example, in the patient with sepsis, one possible suggestion would be to try to use the lowest possible dose of catecholamines for haemodynamic support rather than a higher dose, if one has options where both provide some degree of haemodynamic stability. This is not something that has been emphasized, but perhaps is part of what this troponin signal may be telling us in patients with sepsis. There are other possibilities as well, having to do with more specific therapies that might be targeted. However, the purpose of this chapter is not to try to define the entire range of pathophysiological circumstances clinicians should consider, but rather to help clinicians understand the principle that many of these markers are very likely to be detected in a vast array of clinical circumstances, where new disease entities will need to be considered. Indeed, if one can do that conscientiously, it is very likely to improve the diagnostic yield from the use of these markers. Similar issues are likely to evolve with natriuretic peptides as they are explored in a variety of pathophysiological situations.

Issues of organ versus clinical specificity

We would like all of our markers to be totally specific, but this is not the case and is not likely ever to become so. Troponin comes closest, but tissue specificity does not imply clinical specificity for the aetiology of the elevation [23]. This has been a disappointment from the point of view of many clinicians who viewed troponin as only being elevated as a result of ischaemic heart disease. This mindset will lead to confusion, as indicated above in the section about new diagnoses. Thus, one needs to appreciate that troponin elevations, as well as those for natriuretic peptides and CRP, are likely to be observed commonly and that these biomarkers will unmask new, previously unknown, problems.

Table 33.2 cMR findings in 60 patients who presented with chest pain, elevated troponin values, and normal or near normal coronary arteries by angiography

cMR findings	No.	%
Myocarditis	30	50
Acute	19	31.7
Nonacute	11	18.3
Myocardial infarction	7	11.6
Takatsubo cardiomyopathy	1	1.7
Dilated cardiomyopathy	1	1.7
Normal CMR findings	21	35.0

Reproduced with permission fromrom Assomull RG, Lyne JC, Keenan N, *et al*. The role of cardiovascular magnetic resonance in patients presenting with chest pain, raised troponin, and unobstructed coronary arteries. *Eur Heart J* 2007;**28**:1242–1249.

Elevations of natriuretic peptides in the absence of heart failure are probably not 'false positives' but likely to represent alternative pathophysiology such as anaemia or volume overload in the absence of heart failure. Similarly, CRP elevations are often found in obese patients, and perhaps that is a risk factor for coronary artery disease, but it should be appreciated that obesity alone is an inflammatory disorder.

Difficulties with legacies from the past

As we are educated about taking care of patients during our training, we all learn certain paradigms. Many clinicians learned about the use of CK-MB and therefore have had difficulty giving up its use, despite the fact that there is no circumstance in which it provides additional information over and above troponin [36]. Indeed, some have argued that using CK-MB actually prevents clinicians learning how to use troponin values properly and is therefore detrimental [36]. Whether this is true or not is debatable, but the concept of learning new markers—whether they are CRP, BNP, or troponin—is a critical one. In fact, many clinicians do not like using BNP because they consider that it is a substitute for clinical judgement. It is not; it should be synergistic with clinical judgement and, if used properly, can be of benefit in explaining natriuretic peptide elevations in clinical syndromes. For example, when patients have concurrent chronic obstructive pulmonary disease (COPD) and heart failure, it is often difficult to determine which of the aetiologies might be responsible for increasing shortness of breath. The use of BNP is remarkably efficacious in that circumstance, and changes in values over time once one understands biological and analytical variation can be extremely helpful. However, this can only occur if one understands the analytic and preanalytic distinctions discussed above and if one is astute to the use of the marker. Education is key. Similar caveats exist for CRP. The literature support for CRP in the acute setting is fairly robust if one looks at prognostic significance [33]. Using CRP to identify those patients who may receive closer follow-up and who then could/should be evaluated using the PROVE-IT [40] suggested paradigm (see ➲ Introduction) makes ultimate sense. However, one cannot do that unless one learns the issues related to the measurement of CRP, rather than simply reacting to negative criticism or positive hype. Neither has the interest of the clinician at heart. Advocates often believe that it is essential to provide physicians with a simple paradigm, because they believe that clinicians will have difficulty if they have to learn too much about a marker. This is often the approach of companies who make biomarker assays, rather than facilitating the most

complete understanding of a given biomarker. Indeed, critics of the use of biomarkers often refer to complexity as a detriment. Both positions are insults to clinicians. There are critical issue that clinicians need to understand; we are perfectly capable of understanding these issues and need to learn them, not from the critics or the advocates but from the experts, from textbooks, and from the peer-reviewed literature. Hopefully, this chapter is a start in this direction.

The future

Troponin assays will become much more sensitive. This increase will make an understanding of all of the analytical issues much more essential for clinicians. For example, the minor differences between values seen with plasma and serum may become important. Usually, a small difference of, say, 1–2 pg/mL (➲ Fig. 33.8) would not be important, but with a very sensitive assay it could be [24]. There also may be differences in values predicated on gender with some assays [68, 69] but not with all [70]. In addition, there are substantive clinical issues that need to be defined. It is now clear that there will be large numbers of elevations in many patients with cardiovascular disease. For example, over 50% of patients with pacemakers will have such elevations and after pacemaker implantation an additional 30% or more will manifest elevations, some with a 'rising' pattern [69]. It is also unclear whether the current treatment paradigms used in patients with acute coronary syndromes with elevations of contemporary troponin assays—aggressive anticoagulation, Gp IIb/IIIa inhibitors, and an early invasive strategy—are still appropriate with the new, more sensitive assays [106]. For that reason, many of us have recommended that such assays not be deployed for clinical use until additional information is available about how to use them [106].

Additional markers in this area are unlikely to be necessary for diagnosis. It is already clear that, when the 99th percentile cut-off value is used, so-called 'rapidly rising markers' do not add to early diagnosis [107, 108]. This has recently been confirmed yet again using one of the more sensitive contemporary assays [109]. There is still some question about additional markers for ruling out AMI, since the recent literature has not addressed how early or late one needs to monitor patients in order to be sure that they do not have cardiac injury. For that reason, there is an ongoing trial evaluating copeptin for that use [110]. When the focus turns to this issue it may be that that highly sensitive troponin assays will suffice, but time will tell. However, a marker that could help to identify those with acute coronary syndromes who are in need of urgent revascularization would be extremely

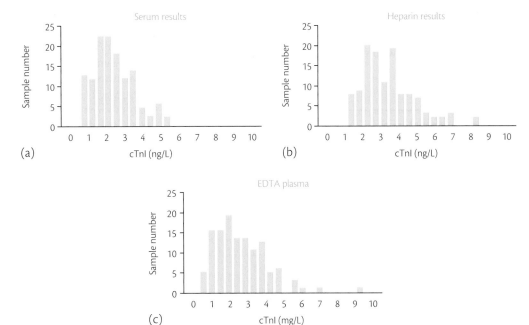

Figure 33.8 Histograms showing differences between samples collected in various ways and assayed with a novel high-sensitivity assay: (a) serum results; (b) heparin results; (c) EDTA plasma.
From Kavsak PA, MacRae AR, Yerna MJ, Jaffe AS. Analytic and clinical utility of a next generation, highly sensitive cardiac troponin I assay for early detection of myocardial injury. *Clin Chem* 2009;**55**:573–577. With permission.

valuable. Given the paradigm of aggressive anticoagulation and antiplatelet therapy, a marker of procoagulant activity as proposed previously [111] might be of benefit.

In the area of natriuretic peptides, it is now clear that the most common circulating form of BNP is proBNP [81], implying that heart failure itself is a failure of the synthesis and release of natriuretic peptides. This opens a large number of opportunities for therapeutic manipulations but also for new markers such as corin, the protease thought to be responsible for cleaving proBNP into its active form [112]. In addition, multiple new analytes such as mid-range ANP and an assay for proBNP are being developed to compete with BNP and NT-proBNP for clinical use [113, 114]. Each has theoretical advantages, but clinically so far none seem superior to the more established markers. In addition, although the natriuretic peptides predict mortality much more substantively

than recurrent events such as AMI, it appears that there may be markers that are still better at this type of prognostication, such as ST2 [115] and GDF-15 [116]. How important they will be turn out to be clinically is unclear.

New markers to assess inflammation are also present in large numbers, but very few have been evaluated systematically in the acute cardiovascular setting. Obviously, finding a marker that would improve on the specificity of CRP would be an advance. On the other hand, the value of CRP is that it amplifies the inflammatory signals from multiple inputs [117], and that may be why it has been so useful.

Ultimately, combinations of markers will be employed, but in the acute cardiac area this has not yet become a high priority [118]. Thus, for now, the need of clinicians are to understand only one marker at a time but to do that well.

Personal perspective

The principles articulated above are ones that clinicians need to embrace in order to understand how to use biomarkers in the evaluation, diagnosis, and treatment of patients with acute cardiovascular disease. There has been a lack of adequate education in this area, which leaves clinicians at the whim of lectures and special guideline documents that may sometimes represent bias rather than fact, because so often they are written by advocates. If clinicians understand some basic information about assays and how to think about them, they will be prepared for the new assays that are being developed.

Troponin assays will become much more sensitive, and that will be a challenge unless one understands how to think about the values. It is likely that new diagnostic and therapeutic approaches will develop with natriuretic peptides and inflammatory markers, built on a better understanding of the processes involved. In this area, the biomarkers have actually been developed far in advance of our understanding of the pathophysiology. As we understand more, the biases of the past will be replaced by more scientifically based information and this will likely alter which markers we use and how we use them. However, if clinicians understand the some basic principles, the transition to new markers will be much easier.

Acknowledgement

Dr Jaffe is or has been a consultant to most of the major diagnostic companies who produce assays for cardiovascular biomarkers.

Further reading

Apple FS, Parvin CA, Buechler KF, *et al*. Validation of the 99th percentile cutoff independent of assay imprecision (CV) for cardiac troponin monitoring for ruling out myocardial infarction. *Clin Chem* 2005;**51**:2198–2200.

Apple FS. A new season for cardiac troponin assays: it's time to keep a scorecard. *Clin Chem* 2009;**55**:1303–1306.

Apple FS, Jesse RL, Newby LK, *et al*. National Academy of Clinical Biochemistry. IFCC Committee for Standardization of Markers of Cardiac Damage. National Academy of Clinical Biochemistry and IFCC Committee for Standardization of Markers of Cardiac Damage Laboratory Medicine Practice Guidelines: Analytical issues for biochemical markers of acute coronary syndromes. *Circulation* 2007;**115**:e352–e355.

Apple FS, Wu AH, Jaffe AS, *et al*. NACB Committee. IFCC C-SMCD. National Academy of Clinical Biochemistry and IFCC Committee for Standardization of Markers of Cardiac Damage Laboratory Medicine Practice Guidelines: analytical issues for biomarkers of heart failure. *Clin Biochem* 2008;**41**:222–226.

Assomull RG, Lyne JC, Keenan N, *et al*. The role of cardiovascular magnetic resonance in patients presenting with chest pain, raised troponin, and unobstructed coronary arteries. *Eur Heart J* 2007;**28**:1242–1249.

Babuin L, Vasile VC, Rio Perez JA, *et al*. Elevated cardiac troponin is an independent risk factor for short- and long-term mortality in medical intensive care unit patients. *Crit Care Med* 2008;**36**:759–765.

Daniels LB, Laughlin GA, Clopton P *et al*. Minimally elevated cardiac troponin T and elevated N-terminal pro-B-type natriuretic peptide predict mortality in older adults: results from the Rancho Bernardo Study. *J Am Coll Cardiol* 2008;**52**:450–459.

Giannitsis E, Kurz K, Hallermayer K, *et al*. Analytical validation of a high-sensitivity cardiac troponin T assay. *Clin Chem* 2010;**56**:254–261.

Jaffe AS, Babuin L, Apple FS. Biomarkers in acute cardiac disease—the present and the future. *J Am Coll Cardiol* 2006;**48**:1–11.

Jaffe AS, Katus H. Acute coronary syndrome biomarkers—the need for more adequate reporting. *Circulation* 2004;**110**:104–106.

Jaffe AS. Chasing troponin. How low can you go if you can see the rise? *J Am Coll Cardiol* 2006;**48**:1763–1764.

Januzzi JL Jr, Peacock WF, Maisel AS. *et al*. Measurement of the interleukin family member ST2 in patients with acute dyspnea: results from the PRIDE (Pro-Brain Natriuretic Peptide Investigation of Dyspnea in the Emergency Department) study. *J Am Coll Cardiol* 2007;**50**:607–613.

Januzzi JL, van Kimmenade R, Lainchbury J. *et al*. NT-proBNP testing for diagnosis and short-term prognosis in acute destabilized heart failure: an international pooled analysis of 1256 patients: the International Collaborative of NT-proBNP Study. *Eur Heart J* 2006;**27**:330–337.

Katus HA, Giannitsis E, Jaffe AS, Thygesen K. Higher sensitivity troponin assays: Quo vadis? *Eur Heart J* 2009;**30**:127–128.

Kavsak PA, MacRae AR, Yerna MJ, Jaffe AS. Analytic and clinical utility of a next generation, highly sensitive cardiac troponin I assay for early detection of myocardial injury. *Clin Chem* 2009;**55**:573–577.

Kempf T, von Haehling S, Peter T, *et al*. Prognostic utility of growth differentiation factor-15 in patients with chronic heart failure. *J Am Coll Cardiol* 2007;**50**:1054–1060.

Khera A, McGuire DK, Murphy SA, *et al*. Race and gender differences in C-reactive protein levels. *J Am Coll Cardiol* 2005;**46**:464–469.

Kupchak, P, Wu AHB, Ghani F, *et al*. Influence of imprecision on ROC curve analysis for cardiac markers. *Clin Chem* 2006;**51**:752–753.

Redfield MM, Rodeheffer RJ, Jacobsen SJ, *et al*. Plasma brain natriuretic peptide concentration: impact of age and gender. *J Am Coll Cardiol* 2002;**40**:976–982.

Saenger AK, Jaffe AS. Requiem for a heavyweight: the demise of creatine kinase-MB. *Circulation* 2008;**118**:2200–2206.

Steinhart B, Thorpe KE, Bayoumi AM, *et al*. Improving the diagnosis of acute heart failure using a validated prediction model. *J Am Coll Cardiol* 2009;**54**:1515–1521.

Thygesen K, Alpert JS, White HD *et al*. Universal definition of myocardial infarction. *Eur Heart J* 2007;**28**:2525–2538; *Circulation* 2007;**116**:2634–2653; *J Am Coll Cardiol* 2007;**50**:2173–2195.

Tsimikas S. Willerson JT. Ridker PM. C-reactive protein and other emerging blood biomarkers to optimize risk stratification of vulnerable patients. *J Am Coll Cardiol* 2006;**47**(8 suppl):C19–31.

Venge P, Johnston N, Lindahl B, James S. Normal plasma levels of cardiac troponin I measured by the high-sensitivity cardiac troponin I access prototype assay and the impact on the diagnosis of myocardial ischemia. *J Am Coll Cardiol* 2009;**54**:1165–1172.

Wu AH, Jaffe AS. The clinical need for high-sensitivity cardiac troponin assays for acute coronary syndromes and the role for serial testing. *Am Heart J* 2008;**155**:208–214.

Wu AH, Smith A. Biological variation of the natriuretic peptides and their role in monitoring patients with heart failure. *Eur J Heart Fail* 2004;**6**:355–358.

Wu AH, Smith A, Wieczorek S, *et al*. Biological variation for N-terminal pro- and B-type natriuretic peptides and implications for therapeutic monitoring of patients with congestive heart failure. *J Am Coll Cardiol* 2003;**92**:628–631.

Wu AHB, Lu QA, Todd J, *et al*. Short- and long-term biological variation in cardiac troponin I measured with a high-sensitivity assay: implications for clinical practice. *Clin Chem* 2009;**55**:52–58.

Zethelius B, Johnston N, Venge P. Troponin I as a predictor of coronary heart disease and mortality in 70-year-old men: a community-based cohort study. *Circulation* 2006;**113**:1071–1078.

➲ For additional multimedia materials please visit the online version of the book (𝄐 http://www.esciacc.oxfordmedicine.com).

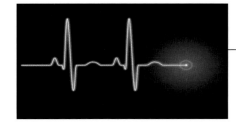

CHAPTER 34

Biomarkers in acute coronary syndromes

Evangelos Giannitsis and Hugo A. Katus

Contents

Summary

Biomarker testing in the evaluation of the patient with acute chest pain is best established for cardiac troponins (cTn) that allow diagnosis of myocardial infarction (MI), risk estimation of short- and long-term risk of death and MI, and guidance of pharmacological therapy, as well as the need and timing of invasive strategy. Newer, more sensitive troponin assays are now becoming commercially available and have the capability to detect MI earlier and more sensitively than standard assays, but are hampered by lack of clinical specificity, i.e. the ability to discriminate myocardial ischaemia from myocardial necrosis not related to ischaemia such as myocarditis, pulmonary embolism, or decompensated heart failure. Strategies to improve clinical specificity (including strict adherence to the universal MI definition and need for serial troponin measurements to detect an acute rise and/or fall of cTn) will improve the interpretation of the increasing number of positive results.

Other biomarkers of inflammation, activated coagulation/fibrinolysis, and increased ventricular stress mirror different aspects of underlying disease activity and may help to improve our understanding of pathophysiological mechanisms of acute coronary syndromes. Among the flood of new biomarkers, some appear to allow a refinement of cardiovascular risk, and some may help to identify candidates for an early invasive versus conservative strategy. A multimarker approach to biomarkers becomes more and more attractive, as increasing evidence suggests that combination of several biomarkers may help to predict individual risk and treatment benefits, particularly among troponin-negative subjects.

In the future, integration of biomarker information with biological or anatomical information obtained from sophisticated imaging modalities may open new avenues for research and clinical routine. In addition, there is increasing evidence that genotyping may help risk stratification and improve efficacy and safety of pharmacotherapy with a variety of cardiovascular drugs.

Introduction

The aetiology of acute coronary syndromes (ACS) is complex and consists of multiple interrelated mechanisms, many of which are not yet been fully understood. Our current understanding is that a plaque may rupture or erode in response to inflammation, leading to local occlusive or nonocclusive thrombosis [1]. Depending on the degree and reversibility of this dynamic obstruction, the clinical manifestations of ACS make up a continuous spectrum of risk that progresses from unstable angina (UA) to non-ST-elevation myocardial infarction (non-STEMI) to ST-elevation myocardial infarction (STEMI). Non-STEMI is distinguished from UA by ischaemia sufficiently severe in intensity and duration to cause myocyte necrosis, which is recognized by the detection of troponin, the most sensitive and specific biomarker of myocardial injury [2].

The advent of novel, sensitive biomarkers of inflammation, activation of coagulation, myocyte necrosis, vascular damage, and haemodynamic stress enables a more differentiated characterization of the individual components and their contribution at different stages of the disease (⊃ Fig. 34.1).

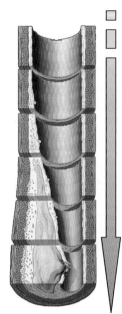

- Proinflammatory cytokines
  - IL-6
- Plaque destabilization
  - MPO
- Plaque rupture
  - sCD40L, PAPP-A, PLGF
- Acute phase reactants
  - (Hs)-CRP, fibrinogen, serum amyloid A
- Ischaemia–micronecrosis
  - Glycogen phosphorylase BB, free fatty acids, IMA, h-FABP, copeptin, hsTnT, hsTnI
- Necrosis
  - cTnT
  - cTnI
- Myocardial dysfunction
  - BNP, NT-proBNP
  - GDF-15, etc.

Figure 34.1 Panel of biomarkers allowing insights into several pathophysiological aspects of atherothrombosis at different stages.

Cardiac troponins

Cardiac troponins (cTn) are now considered to be the biomarkers of choice for the diagnosis of myocardial injury, as the cardiac isoforms of troponin T or I are expressed almost exclusively on the thin myofilament of the contractile apparatus and to a lesser degree (3–6%) as unbound protein in the cytoplasm of myocytes [2, 3]. Thus, cTn constitute the most sensitive and specific biochemical markers of myocardial damage presently available. The criterion of the universal definition of acute MI [4] is a rising and/or falling pattern of cTn values with at least one value above the 99th percentile of a reference control group in the setting of a patient with evidence of myocardial ischaemia (⊃ Box 34.1). Evidence of myocardial ischaemia is indicated by symptoms of ischaemia, typical ECG changes indicative of ischaemia, new Q-waves, or imaging evidence of the new loss of viable myocardium or new regional wall motion abnormalities. After elective coronary revascularization procedures, myocardial ischaemia may occur in a considerable proportion of cases, and a postinterventional rise of more than three times the 99th percentile value following elective percutaneous coronary intervention (PCI) and more than five times the 99th percentile value following

coronary artery bypass grafting (CABG) should be termed a postinterventional MI.

The diagnosis of MI is also made in patients who have died suddenly with signs or symptoms suggestive of myocardial ischaemia with death occurring before blood samples could be obtained, or before troponin appeared in blood [4].

Box 34.1 Joint ESC/ACCF/AHA/WHF Task Force definition of acute myocardial infarction

Myocardial infarction should be diagnosed when there is evidence of myocardial necrosis in a clinical setting consistent with myocardial ischaemia. Under these conditions the following criteria meet the diagnosis for myocardial infarction:

- ◆ Detection of rise and/or fall of cardiac biomarkers (preferably troponin) with at least one value above the 99th percentile of the upper reference limit (URL), together with evidence of myocardial ischaemia with at least one of the following:

  - Symptoms of ischaemia

  - ECG changes indicative of new ischaemia (new ST–T changes or new left bundle branch block)

  - Development of pathological Q waves in the ECG

  - Imaging evidence of new loss of viable myocardium or new regional wall motion abnormality

Elevated cTn values in patients with acute ischaemic presentations are related to more extensive coronary artery disease, procoagulant activity, and lower TIMI flow grades [5]. Angioscopic and angiographic evidence suggests a clear relationship between the presence and concentration of cTn and the presence and magnitude of intracoronary thrombus [6]. As such, an elevated troponin indicates a higher risk for acute coronary events due to the increased prothrombotic activity and the development of cardiac events during mid- and long-term follow-up due to its relation to disease severity and persistent inflammatory activity of the atherosclerotic plaque. Consistently, benefits of more aggressive antithrombotic or antiplatelet therapies with dalteparin [7], and antiplatelet therapies with abciximab [8], tirofiban [9], lamifiban [10], or triple antiplatelet therapy followed by early coronary intervention [11] were almost restricted to patients with elevated troponins.

As patients may not reliably state the time of onset of symptoms, repeated measurements are needed. According to current recommendations, cTn must be measured on presentation, and 6–9 h after admission [4, 12]. In patients with an intermediate or high clinical index of suspicion who remain troponin negative, and after recurrence of typical symptoms, a later measurement at 12–24 h should be considered for optimal rule-in or rule-out.

Clinical indicators other than cTn also provide an estimate of the acute thrombotic risk include dynamic ST-segment deviations, refractory angina, diabetes mellitus, renal failure, older age, and an intermediate or high GRACE or TIMI risk score [13]. Current guidelines therefore advocate an early invasive strategy within 72 h rather than a conservative strategy when troponin is elevated (◑ Fig. 34.2).

Using cardiac troponin: some caveats

When an increased cTn value is encountered in the absence of evidence of myocardial ischaemia, a careful search for other possible aetiologies of cardiac damage should be undertaken [14]. A variety of non-ACS related conditions including pulmonary embolism, myocarditis, endstage renal disease (ESRD), acute heart failure, or relevant valvular heart disease may cause prognostically adverse elevations of cTn in the absence of overt ischaemic heart disease (◑ Box 34.2).

Interpretation of elevated cTn is particularly difficult in the setting of severe renal failure [15, 16]. In the symptomatic patient with suspected ACS, cTn(s) retain their independent prognostic capability across all degrees of renal insufficiency [15] and represent one of several indicators of increased cardiovascular risk that advocate the need for an early invasive strategy within 72 h [13]. In asymptomatic patients with ESRD undergoing chronic haemodialysis, a persistent stable elevation of cTn may be encountered in

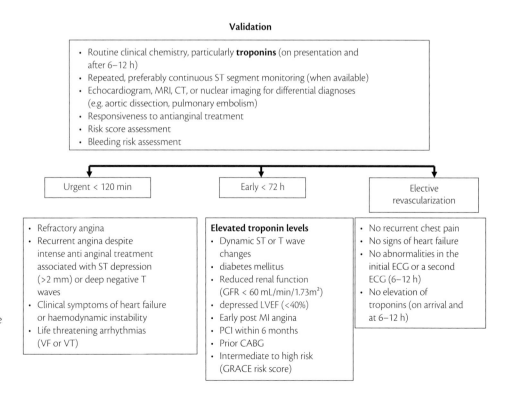

Figure 34.2 Current ESC guideline recommendations regarding selection of early invasive strategy within 72 h versus a conservative strategy according to the presence of elevated cardiac troponin.

Validation

- Routine clinical chemistry, particularly **troponins** (on presentation and after 6–12 h)
- Repeated, preferably continuous ST segment monitoring (when available)
- Echocardiogram, MRI, CT, or nuclear imaging for differential diagnoses (e.g. aortic dissection, pulmonary embolism)
- Responsiveness to antianginal treatment
- Risk score assessment
- Bleeding risk assessment

Urgent < 120 min
- Refractory angina
- Recurrent angina despite intense anti anginal treatment associated with ST depression (>2 mm) or deep negative T waves
- Clinical symptoms of heart failure or haemodynamic instability
- Life threatening arrhythmias (VF or VT)

Early < 72 h
Elevated troponin levels
- Dynamic ST or T wave changes
- diabetes mellitus
- Reduced renal function (GFR < 60 mL/min/1.73m²)
- depressed LVEF (<40%)
- Early post MI angina
- PCI within 6 months
- Prior CABG
- Intermediate to high risk (GRACE risk score)

Elective revascularization
- No recurrent chest pain
- No signs of heart failure
- No abnormalities in the initial ECG or a second ECG (6–12 h)
- No elevation of troponins (on arrival and at 6–12 h)

> **Box 34.2** Differential diagnoses of elevated cardiac troponins in the absence of an acute coronary syndrome
>
> - Cardiac contusion, including ablation, pacing, cardioversion, or endomyocardial biopsy
> - Congestive heart failure—acute and chronic
> - Aortic dissection, aortic valve disease, or hypertrophic cardiomyopathy
> - Tachy- or bradyarrhythmia, or heart block
> - Apical ballooning syndrome
> - Rhabdomyolysis with cardiac injury
> - Pulmonary embolism, severe pulmonary hypertension
> - Renal failure
> - Acute neurological disease including stroke, or subarachnoidal hemorrhage
> - Infiltrative diseases, e.g. amyloidosis, hemochromatosis, sarcoidosis, and scleroderma
> - Inflammatory diseases, e.g. myocarditis, or myocardial extension of endo/pericarditis
> - Drug toxicity, e.g.adriamycin, 5-fluorouracil, herceptin, snake venom
> - Critically ill patients, especially with respiratory failure or sepsis
> - Burns, especially if affecting >30% of body surface area

the absence of acute myocardial ischaemia [16]. For this subset of patients the National Academy of Biochemistry (NACB) guidelines [17] recommend a repeat measurement with a change of the cTn value of 20% or more in the 6–9 h after presentation as this change represents a significant (3 SD) change in cTn on the basis of a 5–7% analytical coefficient of variation.

Prevalence of positive troponin results is greater for TnT (18–75%) than for TnI (4–17%); the prevalence and magnitude of cTnT (and to a lower degree cTnI)are related to prognosis and thus may refine risk assessment by cardiologists and nephrologists [16, 18].

Other biomarkers of myocardial necrosis

A major limitation of current troponin assays is a lack of sensitivity at presentation and within the first hours due to a delayed appearance in blood after the index event. Therefore, biomarkers that appear earlier in blood have been advocated as an adjunct to cardiac troponin. Several markers, including heart-type fatty acid binding protein (h-FABP), ischaemia-modified albumin (IMA), and myoglobin have been proposed. Most experience is available for myoglobin, which is the most established marker for the rule-out of MI in patients at low risk [17].

Free fatty acids unbound to albumin, IMA, and h-FABP have been proposed as biochemical markers of cardiac ischaemia. After initial enthusiasm, recent and more thorough work indicates that IMA is specific neither for myocardial ischaemia nor for infarction. Reduced cobalt binding has also been reported after endurance exercise, such as a marathon race, after radiofrequency catheter ablation, after skeletal muscle ischaemia, or in patients with peripheral vascular disease, as well as in diseases associated with oxidative stress such as systemic sclerosis [19, 20]. In essence, IMA does not appear to fulfil the criteria for an ideal marker of myocardial ischaemia and its results must be interpreted cautiously, taking into consideration clinical circumstances and comorbidity.

h-FABP is a 15-kDa protein thought to be involved in myocardial lipid homeostasis. It is present in substantial amounts in the cytoplasm of myocardial tissue, but is also expressed in tissues outside the heart. The lack of specificity in detecting AMI is obviously a major disadvantage of using h-FABP without the concomitant measurement of cTn in this setting. Numerous studies have investigated the utility of h-FABP for assisting in the diagnosis of AMI and for prognostic stratification. A critical review of six studies using qualitative and quantitative assays analysed the performance of FABP in ACS [21]. These studies had significant weaknesses, with most studies employing now outdated gold standards for AMI diagnosis and being subject to significant verification bias. h-FABP can be detected as early as 1 h and peaks at 6–8 h after an acute coronary occlusion [22]. However, to make a meaningful difference in early detection of AMI, new cardiac biomarkers will need a higher sensitivity during the first 1–2 h after chest pain. Therefore, although there has been interest in h-FABP as an early marker of AMI for many years, it has never gained widespread acceptance for use in clinical practice.

More recently, the use of copeptin, the C-terminal part of the vasopressin prohormone, has been found effective for rapid and reliable rule-out of MI already at presentation [23]. Copeptin is secreted in response to endogenous stress and has been shown to be elevated in heart failure, in different states of shock, and very early after onset of myocardial ischaemia. However, because of the lack of cardiac specificity, copeptin and other earlier markers of ischaemia have to be measured in addition to cardiospecific troponin.

Newer troponin assays with improved sensitivity

In order to comply with the precision criteria of the European Society of Cardiology (ESC) and American College of Cardiology (ACC) [4], high-sensitivity generations of cTn assays are being developed by manufacturers. These precision criteria require the measurement of cTn at the 99th percentile value with an imprecision (coefficient of variation) of less than 10%. Strategies to improve assays performance include refinement of signal and detection antibodies of contemporary assays, or development of novel technologies such as single molecule detection systems [24]. These high-sensitivity assays allow measurement of picograms per litre rather than nanograms per litre, and are now able to detect cardiac troponin in most healthy individuals. Recent reports demonstrate that use of more sensitive cTn assays also allow a more accurate and earlier detection of MI [25], and will increase the number of cases of MI at the expense of UA [26, 27]. However, lowering the diagnostic cut-off by the implementation of more sensitive assays will also increase sensitivity at the cost of clinical specificity, as more non-ACS related acute, subacute, or chronic cardiac diseases such as heart failure or cardiomyopathies will be detected [28–31]. In order to ensure clinical specificity for MI diagnosis, adherence to the criteria of the universal definition of MI (see ⊃ Chapter 39) is paramount, as there is an emerging need for serial testing in order to distinguish an acute from a chronic elevation of hs-cTnT. The magnitude of such a rise or fall indicative of AMI in patients with ACS has not been determined. Today, only a few novel assays are used in clinical routine and there are still unresolved issues, e.g. regarding the therapeutic benefits of early invasive strategies among those with very low cTn concentrations, or the issue of biovariability which is critical in the assessment of the critical difference of serial blood samples, in order to differentiate acute from chronic myocardial damage. Whether implementation of more sensitive troponin assays may decrease the time to the second recommended blood test (6–9 h after presentation), or will obviate the need for an earlier marker of myocardial ischaemia, is still unsettled.

Other biomarkers

Biomarkers of inflammation

Inflammation represents a key pathophysiological mechanism in ACS. An exponentially rising number of publications on the prognostic role of inflammatory markers is being published every year [32].

C-reactive protein (CRP) is one of the most extensively investigated markers of inflammation. An acute elevation of CRP is believed to reflect the acute inflammatory process associated with plaque vulnerability and rupture [33]. Several studies have demonstrated unequivocally that there is a direct relationship between the presence and magnitude of elevated CRP levels and adverse prognosis, which may persist for several years [34]. As the prognostic value of CRP is independent of cTn, the combination of CRP and cTn allows a better and more than additive prognostication of future ischaemic events [35, 36]. However, the levels of CRP at the time of PCI do not provide information on who might benefit from an early invasive strategy [37].

Myeloperoxidase (MPO) is abundantly expressed in the azurophilic granules of neutrophils and monocytes, is released in a state of inflammation, and catalyses the formation of several reactive species, including hypochlorous acid [38]. Several clinical studies indicate that measurement of MPO in patients presenting with acute chest pain provides clinically relevant information in addition to and independent from cTn, and thus appears to allow a refined risk stratification [39]. However, it should be noted that comparison of the diagnostic and prognostic performance between MPO and troponin may have been influenced by inappropriate use of troponins with respect to cut-offs, sampling protocols, and outdated infarct definitions [40]. In addition, there are some preanalytical and analytical issues regarding the measurement of MPO that limit its general acceptance for clinical routine. The concentrations of MPO are sensitive to storage conditions at room temperature; depend on the type of specimen, i.e. serum or plasma; and are markedly increased by bolus injection of heparin which mobilizes MPO from vascular compartments. The comparability of trials is limited by the heterogeneous use of assay procedures (mass or activity) and differing reports of MPO concentrations on a molar or weight basis, or as MPO/protein ratios [39].

As with CRP, other inflammatory proteins, proinflammatory cytokines, and markers of vascular dysfunction have been linked to increased long-term mortality. However, these markers are also not specific for a vascular process and can be found in a variety of inflammatory conditions. This is the major reason that probably preclude their value for the acute phase of ACS.

Whether some plaque-specific biomarkers such as placental associated plasma protein A (PAPP-A) or placental-growth factor (PLGF) may indicate earlier stages of vulnerable plaque formation and anticipate the final event of plaque rupture before the occurrence of myocardial necrosis is still under investigation [41–43].

Natriuretic peptides and growth differentiation factor 15

B-type natriuretic peptides (BNP and NT-proBNP) reflect cardiac function and the release into blood may be stimulated directly or indirectly by myocardial ischaemia [44]. Across the entire spectrum of ACS, increasing levels of BNP or NT-proBNP have been shown to predict adverse clinical events during short, medium, and long-term follow-up [45–47]. In direct comparison to creatinine clearance and levels of CRP and cTn, an elevated NT-proBNP was found less predictive for death or MI within 30 days, but provided superior independent prediction of death at 1 year [45]. In this context, the combination of NT-proBNP with creatinine clearance emerged as the best predictor of 1-year mortality after ACS [45]. Although there are some data suggesting a benefit from an invasive management of patients with elevated BNP/NT-proBNP levels, particularly in patients with elevated levels of IL-6, the link to therapeutic measures could not yet be established as convincingly as for troponins [48].

On the other hand, risk of adverse events following revascularization therapy for ACS proved higher in patients with a negative cTnT (<0.01 ng/L) and a low NT-pro BNP result (<237 ng/L) highlighting the need for risk estimation in high and low risk subgroups [49].

Recent studies indicate growth differentiation factor 15 (GDF-15) as another promising marker for early risk stratification among patients with ACS [50, 51]. GDF-15 is a member of the transforming growth factor β cytokine superfamily and is induced in the myocardium after ischaemia and reperfusion injury, pressure overload, and heart failure, possibly via proinflammatory cytokine and oxidative stress-dependent signalling pathways [52]. In a retrospective analysis of the FRISC-II study, GDF-15 added independent prognostic information to ST-segment depression, renal function, NT-proBNP and troponin, and a graded relationship was found between the levels of GDF-15 and the absolute and relative benefits from an invasive strategy [50]. Although results are promising, the lack of performance data in large prospective cohorts presenting with chest pain still prohibits a general recommendation to measure GDF-15 in addition to cTn.

Renal function

Impaired renal function is associated with higher mortality in patients with ACS [53]. It is believed that creatinine clearance indicates the cumulative extent of vascular damage caused by hypertension, dyslipidaemia, and diabetes. The knowledge of renal function is important for risk assessment and for dose adjustment of anticoagulation and antiplatelet therapies, as patients with renal failure are prone to excess bleeding due to overdosing. Glomerular filtration rate (GFR) estimates based on creatinine levels can be an unreliable indicator of renal function, as creatinine serum concentrations may be affected by tubular secretion, age, sex, muscle mass, physical activity, and diet.

There is accumulating evidence that plasma cystatin C level is an accurate marker of renal function and an independent predictor of mortality in patients with coronary artery disease (CAD), but only few studies have evaluated the prognostic role of cystatin C specifically in patients with ACS [54]. In a study on 726 patients with suspected ACS, cystatin C had better discrimination power than creatinine clearance or creatinine and this suggests that its measurement can improve early risk stratification [54].

Markers of coagulation

Markers of activated thrombosis contain useful information with regard to the ongoing thrombotic process in ACS [55]. Previous studies have shown an association between the risk of MI and concentrations of fibrinogen, soluble fibrin, and markers of the fibrinolytic pathway including plasminogen activator inhibitor-1 [56, 57]. In addition, many of the novel markers are also associated with the inflammatory atherosclerotic process. However, for several reasons none of these markers appears to possess enough clinical information to be included in the present recommendations for the management of ACS [55].

Figure 34.3 256-row multislice CT of the right coronary artery showing luminal obstruction and distinction of plaque components.

Conclusion

The pathophysiology of ACS is complex and cannot be reflected by a single marker. There is growing evidence that combining a biomarker of haemodynamic stress (BNP or NT-proBNP) or a biomarker of inflammation (high-sensitivity CRP) with a biomarker of necrosis (cardiac troponin) enhances risk assessment among patients with ACS [58, 59]. It has also been shown that implementation of a biomarker of renal dysfunction adds independent prognostic information [45]. Elevated levels of CRP and BNP at presentation have been found to indicate a higher mortality risk in patients with normal troponin, thus allowing a more refined risk stratification [56] independent of troponin.

Personal perspective

New modalities including cardiac MRI, multislice CT, and new intravascular ultrasound technologies enable more detailed imaging of coronary anatomy, vessel wall and plaque composition. Today, multislice CT already allows visualization of luminal obstruction, calcium score, and distinction of plaque components, i.e. soft plaque or calcification (⊃ Fig. 34.3). Molecular imaging may also give information on specific targets such as inflammatory activity of the plaque.

Combination with biomarkers that are likely to anticipate an acute coronary event and/or mirror the actual pathophysiological process is likely to improve our understanding of the pathophysiology and may open new avenues for the noninvasive visualization and characterization of a vulnerable plaque, or at least identification of individuals at higher risk of suffering cardiovascular events in the future.

After validation using a sensitive imaging method as reference standard, a biomarker algorithm may become an easier, less expensive, and more convenient alternative for visualization and quantification of infarct size after large MIs or microvascular obstruction post-MI.

Genotyping has emerged as a new promising tool for risk stratification and guidance of therapy in patients with ACS. More recently, higher platelet reactivity and less effective platelet inhibition due to the variable response of the P2Y12 receptor to clopidogrel has been identified as a reason for future higher cardiovascular events [60–62]. CYP2C19 is one of several cytochromes that are involved in the conversion of inactive clopidogrel to its active metabolite. In a cohort of young patients post-MI it has been shown that allelic CYP2C19 variants account for more major adverse cardiac events [61]. These findings were recently confirmed by a French registry on patients with acute STEMI and non-STEMI [62], and in a randomized controlled phase III trial [63] comparing clopidogrel to prasugrel in patients with ACS undergoing PCI. In the registry [62], patients with an AMI who were receiving clopidogrel and carried the CYP2C19 loss-of-function allele had a higher rate of subsequent cardiovascular events than those who were not. This effect was particularly marked among patients undergoing PCI. In the randomized controlled trial [63], clopidogrel-treated subjects who carried this allele had a relative increase of 53% in the composite primary efficacy outcome of the risk of death from cardiovascular causes, MI, or stroke, as compared with noncarriers, and a three fold higher risk of stent thrombosis.

Another interesting finding is the interaction of substrates that compete for the same cytochrome P450 metabolism. In a double-blind placebo-controlled trial, a higher platelet P2Y12 reactivity was observed in cases where the proton-pump inhibitor omeprazol, a substrate that competes with clopidogrel for CYP2C19 metabolism, was co-administered [64]. Conversely, no CYP2C19 interaction with prasugrel has been reported in carriers versus noncarriers of a reduced-function CYP2C19 allele [65].

Thus, by analogy with current clinical practice for patient selection and customized therapy in several malignant tumours, it appears that genotyping in patients with ACS or chronic cardiovascular disease may be helpful not only for risk stratification but also for individualized therapy with clopidogrel and other drugs not yet identified.

Further reading

Armstrong EJ, Morrow DA, Sabatine MS. Inflammatory biomarkers in acute coronary syndromes: part I: introduction and cytokines. *Circulation* 2006;**113**:e72–75.

Bassand JP, Hamm CW, Ardissino D, *et al.* Guidelines for the diagnosis and treatment of non-ST-segment elevation acute coronary syndromes. The Task Force for the Diagnosis and Treatment of Non-ST-Segment Elevation Acute Coronary Syndromes of the European Society of Cardiology. *Eur Heart J* 2007;**28**:1598–1660.

Braunwald E. Unstable angina: an etiologic approach to management. *Circulation* 1998;**98**:2219–2222.

Goetze JP. Markers of activated coagulation in acute coronary syndromes. *J Am Coll Cardiol* 2008;**51**:2430–2431.

Hamm CW, Giannitsis E, Katus HA. Cardiac troponin elevations in patients without acute coronary syndrome. *Circulation* 2002;**106**:2871–2872.

Jaffe AS, Ravkilde J, Roberts R, *et al.* It's time for a change to a troponin standard. *Circulation* 2000;**102**:1216–1220.

Morrow DA, Cannon CP, Jesse RL, *et al.* National Academy of Clinical Biochemistry Laboratory Medicine Practice Guidelines: Clinical characteristics and utilization of biochemical markers in acute coronary syndromes. *Circulation* 2007;**115**:e356–375.

Thygesen K, Alpert JS, White HD, Joint ESC/ACCF/AHA/WHF Task Force for the Redefinition of Myocardial Infarction Universal definition of myocardial infarction. *J Am Coll Cardiol* 2007;**50**:2173–2195.

Thygesen K, Mair J, Katus H, *et al.* Principles for the application of troponins in acute cardiac care. *Eur Heart J* 2010 (in press).

Wu AH, Jaffe AS, Apple FS, *et al.* National Academy of Clinical Biochemistry laboratory medicine practice guidelines: use of cardiac troponin and B-type natriuretic peptide or N-terminal proB-type natriuretic peptide for etiologies other than acute coronary syndromes and heart failure. *Clin Chem* 2007;**53**:2086–2096.

➲ For additional multimedia materials please visit the online version of the book (🕮 http://www.esciacc.oxfordmedicine.com).

CHAPTER 35

Biomarkers in acute heart failure

Kevin Shah, Pam R. Taub, and Alan Maisel

Contents

Summary

Acute heart failure (AHF) continues to be a worldwide medical problem, associated with frequent readmissions, and high mortality. AHF has a profound economic impact on national health care systems with a high number of rehospitalizations and deaths. In the past decade, biomarkers have shifted the way in which AHF is managed by the cardiologist. The search for the ideal biomarker to aid in the diagnosis, prognosis, and treatment of AHF is ongoing. The natriuretic peptides (NPs) have proved extremely useful in determining whether acute dyspnoea has cardiac aetiology. In addition, recent trials have demonstrated the use of NPs in inpatient and outpatient prognosis. In the future, this could lead to titrating outpatient medications in outpatients with chronic heart failure to prevent AHF hospitalizations. In future there will be a myriad of biomarkers for AHF, such as midregional pro-adrenomedullin (MR-proADM), midregional pro-ANP (MR-proANP), troponin, ST2, and neutrophil gelatinase-associated lipocalin (NGAL), to comprehensively treat the AHF patient in multiple settings.

Introduction

Acute heart failure (AHF) is a growing epidemic, with 35% of admitted patients having heart failure related deaths or readmissions in 60 days [1]. The diagnosis of AHF is often challenging, given a patient's multiple comorbidities and the nonspecific presenting symptoms. Clinical examination findings such as rales, elevated jugular venous pressure, and oedema are specific but not sensitive for elevated cardiac filling pressures. It is important to establish the diagnosis of AHF rapidly so that treatment can be instituted promptly. Over the past decade B-type natriuretic peptide (BNP) has become the gold standard biomarker in the diagnosis or exclusion of AHF [2]. Other biomarkers such a troponin, neutrophil gelatinase-associated lipocalin (NGAL), ST2, and midregional pro-adrenomedullin (MR-proADM) are also emerging as adjuncts to BNP for prognosis and management of AHF. A multimarker guided strategy will likely become the mainstay in the management of AHF

In this chapter, we discuss the use of biomarkers in the diagnosis, prognosis, and management of patients with AHF. In addition, we discuss novel biomarkers that will likely be incorporated in to the clinical landscape in the upcoming years.

What is the ideal biomarker for acute heart failure?

When selecting a biomarker to use with respect to AHF or any other acute disease, many criteria must be considered. Morrow and de Lemos delineate three criteria that must be met in order for a biomarker to clinically useful: (1) it must be cost-effective, precise, and with a rapid measurement; (2) it must add to clinical judgement/examination; (3) it must be useful in clinical decision-making [3].

Unfortunately, no single biomarker completely fulfils all these criteria. Sensitivity and specificity are often sacrificed interchangeably, through setting different quantifiable cut-points. Some biomarkers may prove too expensive in certain settings, or do not translate to patient benefits and outcomes when analysed in clinical trials. Even BNP, which is one of the best biomarkers available, must be interpreted in the setting of multiple confounding variables such as renal function, obesity, etc. Nonetheless, understanding the limitations of biomarkers and employing a multimarker strategy will allow the clinician to manage the AHF patient effectively.

Acute heart failure

There are limitations to clinical examination, imaging, and biomarkers in diagnosing heart failure. The physical exam is often challenging in AHF as there are many clinical scenarios in which the jugular venous pressure does not reflect pulmonary capillary wedge pressure (PCWP), such as systolic heart failure with intact right heart function. Radiographic findings are often useful in detecting pulmonary vascular congestion, but often lag behind clinical findings. Biomarkers such as BNP are useful in diagnosis but the multiple patient comorbidities that can affect the levels need to be taken into consideration in interpretations. Thus the accurate diagnosis of AHF requires the synthesis of clinical, imaging, and biomarker data and understanding the limitations of each modality. Key features of the clinical history and clinical examination are listed in ⊃ Table 35.1 and ⊃ Table 35.2.

Table 35.1 Key features of the clinical history in patients with heart failure

Symptoms	Breathlessness (orthopnoea, paroxysmal nocturnal dyspnoea)
	Fatigue (tiredness, exhaustion)
	Angina, palpitations, syncope
Cardiovascular events	Coronary heart disease
	Myocardial infarction
	Intervention
	Other surgery
	Stroke or peripheral vascular disease
	Valvular disease or dysfunction
	Thrombolysis
	PCI
	CABG
Risk profile	Family history, smoking, hyperlipidaemia, hypertension, diabetes
Response to current and previous therapy	

Natriuretic peptides

The natriuretic peptides (NPs) are hormones synthesized in the heart which regulate water–electrolyte balance in the body. The first NP, atrial natriuretic peptide (ANP) was initially discovered in 1984, followed by BNP 4 years later [4] (⊃ Fig. 35.1).

Physiology

BNP is a 32-amino-acid cardiac natriuretic peptide hormone originally isolated from porcine brain tissue. The human *BNP* gene is located on chromosome 1 and encodes the prohormone proBNP. The biologically active BNP and

Table 35.2 Key feature of the clinical examination in patients with heart failure

Appearance	Alertness, nutritional status, weight
Pulse	Rate, rhythm, and character
Blood pressure	Systolic, diastolic, pulse pressure
Fluid overload	Jugular venous pressure
	Peripheral oedema (ankles and sacrum) hepatomegaly, ascites
Lungs	Respiratory rate
	Rales
	Pleural effusion
Heart	Apex displacement
	Gallop rhythm, third heart sound
	Murmurs suggesting valvular dysfunction

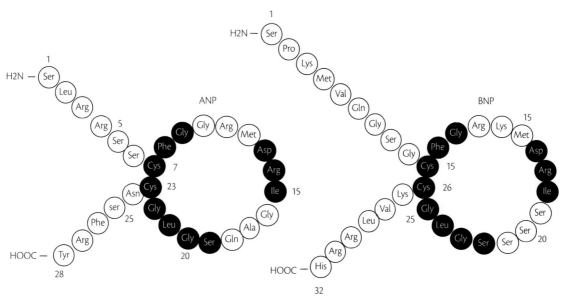

Figure 35.1 Atrial natriuretic peptide (ANP) and B-type natriuretic peptide (BNP). ANP (28 amino acids) and BNP (32 amino acids) are homologous in structure, forming a ring with a disulphide bridge. Identical amino acids are marked black.
Reproduced with permission from Hall C (2004). Essential biochemistry and physiology of (NT-pro) BNP. *Eur J Heart Fail* 2004;**6**(3):257–260; Oxford University Press.

the remaining part of the prohormone, NT-proBNP (76 amino acids) can be measured by immunoassay in human blood. Cardiac myocytes constitute the major source of BNP-related peptides. The main stimulus for peptide synthesis and secretion is myocyte stretch. In contrast to ANPs, which derive mainly from atrial tissue, BNP-related peptides are produced mainly from ventricular myocytes. In peripheral organs BNP binds to the natriuretic peptide receptor type A, causing increased intracellular cGMP production. The physiological effects include diuresis, vasodilation, inhibition of renin and aldosterone production, and inhibition of cardiac and vascular myocyte growth. BNP is cleared from plasma through binding to the natriuretic peptide clearance receptor type C [5].

Pathophysiology

Elevated levels of natriuretic peptides are a result of the body's response to a volume-overloaded state. ANP and BNP are released in response to atrial and ventricular wall stretch. They maintain sodium homeostasis by enhancing renal sodium and water excretion. BNP is a cardiac neurohormone specifically secreted from the ventricles in response to volume expansion and pressure overload [6]. These peptides also have haemodynamic effects, dilating arteries and especially, veins. They also suppress the renin–angiotensin–aldosterone system (RAAS) and, possibly, the sympathetic nervous system. Consequently, the natriuretic peptides are thought to play an important protective role in heart failure, countering the detrimental

actions of the sympathetic nervous system in heart failure. The pathophysiological interplay between the natriuretic peptides, the nervous system, the body's vasculature, the cardiac system, and the renal system is intricate (➲ Fig. 35.2). Understanding the pathogenesis of BNP production and its interaction with other organ system is important in interpreting BNP values.

Natriuretic peptides in the diagnosis of acute heart failure

NP testing has a profound effect on clinical decision-making for AHF. In the Breathing Not Properly Study of 1586 patients, a BNP cut-point of 100 pg/mL was 76% specific and 90% sensitive for the diagnosis of heart failure in patients presenting to the emergency department (ED) with dyspnoea [2]. Subsequent studies have shown that use of NPs for diagnosis of AHF is cost-effective, with a 10% reduction in admissions and decrease in the median length of hospital study by 3 days [7] (➲ Fig. 35.3).

As a quantitative marker of heart failure, NP levels are best interpreted as a continuous variable. The higher the value, the greater the likelihood that the dyspnoea is due to heart failure. When BNP is low (<100 pg/mL), it is unlikely that heart failure is primary cause of the clinical presentation. However, a high BNP (>400 pg/mL) suggests that heart failure is a contributor to the patient's symptoms with specificity exceeding 90%. The 'rule out' level (BNP <100 pg/mL) can exclude heart failure from the

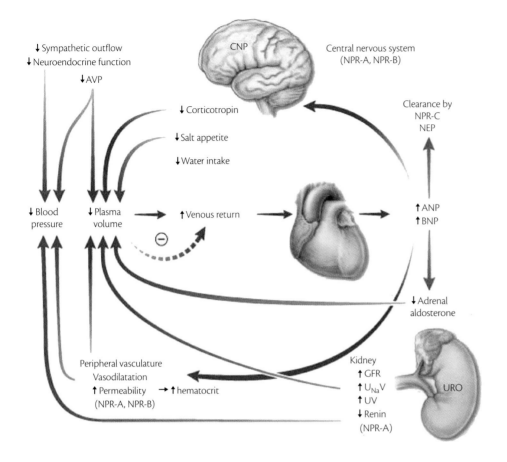

↓ Sympathetic outflow
↓ Neuroendocrine function
↓ AVP

CNP

Central nervous system
(NPR-A, NPR-B)

↓ Corticotropin

↓ Salt appetite

↓ Water intake

Clearance by
NPR-C
NEP

↓ Blood
pressure

↓ Plasma
volume

→ ↑ Venous return

↑ ANP
↑ BNP

⊖

↓ Adrenal
aldosterone

Peripheral vasculature
Vasodilatation
↑ Permeability → ↑ hematocrit
(NPR-A, NPR-B)

Kidney
↑ GFR
↑ U$_{Na}$V
↑ UV
↓ Renin
(NPR-A)

URO

Figure 35.2 Effects of natriuretic peptides released from the heart when venous return is increased. Increased secretion of the natriuretic peptides due to cardiac wall stretch reduces blood pressure and plasma volume through coordinated actions in the brain, adrenal gland, kidney, and vasculature. Overall actions of the natriuretic peptides include vasodilation and diuresis. Reproduced from Levin ER, Gardner DG, Samson WK, *et al.* Natriuretic peptides. *N Engl J Med* 1998;**339**(5):321–328. With permission from the Massachusetts Medical Society.

differential diagnosis (⊃ Fig. 35.4). However, 'ruling in' heart failure (BNP>400 pg/mL) is more complex. This requires addressing the fact that BNP may be persistently elevated in chronic heart failure and may not be representative of an acute haemodynamic change [8].

During ventricular stretch, pro-B-type natriuretic peptide is cleaved into BNP and NT-proBNP. NT-proBNP is larger, more rapidly detected, and more stable than BNP. NT-proBNP is similar to BNP in that is elevated in patients with AHF. It can be used to diagnose AHF as well, but cut-points are set by age. They have been established at 450 pg/mL, 900 pg/mL, and 1800 pg/mL for the identification of AHF in subjects aged <50, 50–75, and >75 years, respectively [9].

In addition, an increased level of NT-proBNP has been shown to be a strong independent predictor of a final diagnosis of AHF. NT-proBNP testing alone has been shown to be superior to clinical judgement alone for diagnosing AHF. NT-proBNP measurement is a valuable addition to standard clinical assessment for the identification and exclusion of acute congestive heart failure in the ED setting [10]. The decision between NT-proBNP versus BNP is usually institution-specific. However, both are invaluable tools for the diagnosis of AHF in patients presenting with acute dyspnoea.

Prognosis and risk stratification using natriuretic peptides

An ageing population and the successive prolongation of the lives of patients through the use of novel therapeutic innovations have led to an increasing incidence of heart failure; however, the mortality rate in patients with heart failure has remained quite high. There is an urgent need for simple measurements to allow better risk stratification of these patients. Chronic obstructive pulmonary disease (COPD) and heart failure produced the highest readmission rates for Europe and the United States. The nature of chronic diseases such as COPD and heart failure make it difficult to manage patients at home for extended periods of time, because of periodic deteriorations or exacerbations resulting in readmissions [11]. The NPs have proven useful as an adjunct tool to clinical intuition in the risk stratification of heart failure patients.

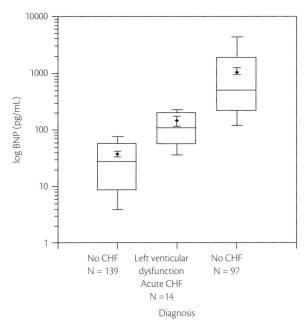

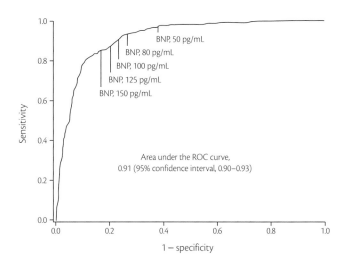

Figure 35.3 BNP levels of patients with CHF, non-CHF, and baseline ventricular dysfunction without an acute exacerbation. Patients diagnosed with CHF had the highest BNP levels, while patients not diagnosed with CHF group had the lowest BNP levels. A smaller group identified as baseline ventricular dysfunction without an acute exacerbation had intermediate BNP levels. Reproduced from Dao Q, Krishnaswamy P, *et al.* Utility of B-type natriuretic peptide in the diagnosis of congestive heart failure in an urgent-care setting. *J Am Coll Cardiol* 2001;**37**(2):379–385. With permission from Elsevier.

BNP	Sensitivity	Specificity	Positive predictive value	Negative predictive value	Accuracy
(pg/mL)		(95% confidence interval)			
50	97 (96–98)	62 (59–66)	71 (68–74)	96 (94–97)	79
80	93 (91–95)	74 (70–77)	77 (75–80)	92 (89–94)	83
100	90 (88–92)	76 (73–79)	79 (76–81)	89 (87–91)	83
125	87 (85–90)	79 (76–82)	80 (78–83)	87 (84–89)	83
150	85 (82–88)	83 (80–85)	83 (80–85)	85 (83–88)	84

Figure 35.4 Receiver operating characteristic (ROC) curve for various cut-off levels of BNP in differentiating between dyspnoea due to congestive heart failure and dyspnoea due to other causes. In patients presenting to the emergency department with acute dyspnoea, plasma BNP levels of 100 pg/mL were an effective cut-point for diagnosing heart failure. Sensitivities and specificities at other cut-points are shown below the ROC. Reproduced from Maisel AS, Krishnaswamy P, *et al.* Rapid measurement of B-type natriuretic peptide in the emergency diagnosis of heart failure. *N Engl J Med* 2002;**347**(3):161–167. With permission from the Massachusetts Medical Society.

Inpatient setting

Hospitalized patients whom are being treated for decompensated heart failure have a BNP level that can be interpreted as having a baseline and a volume-overloaded component: a 'dry' and 'wet' component, respectively [12].

It was demonstrated by Cheng *et al.* that in patients admitted with decompensated heart failure, changes in BNP levels during treatment were strong predictors for mortality and early readmission. This study suggested that BNP levels might be used to effectively guide treatment of inpatients [13]. In addition, predischarge BNP levels in decompensated heart failure patients have been shown to be useful in predicting postdischarge outcomes. An elevated predischarge BNP level (>700 pg/mL), an indication of subclinical pulmonary congestion, was an independent predictor of readmission and death. Patients with lower discharge BNP levels (<350 pg/mL), had a lower incidence of death and readmission [14]. The use of BNP levels in the inpatient setting is a valuable tool to risk-stratify heart failure patients and determine whether inpatient stay should be lengthened or more aggressive treatment administered.

Outpatient/emergency department setting

In an outpatient with chronic heart failure, the ability to use NPs to guide therapy is a long-term management strategy. Recent studies have begun to point in that direction. Dyspnoea is a common complaint in the ED, and the emerging knowledge on how NP testing can be used to make decisions in this setting has an effect on patient prognosis. In the REDHOT trial study of 464 patients, it was demonstrated that in patients presenting to the ED with heart failure symptoms, there is an apparent disconnect between the perceived severity of heart failure by ED physicians and severity as determined by BNP levels. BNP levels were shown to predict future outcomes and can aid physicians in making triage decisions about whether to admit or discharge patients. In this study, BNP levels were a stronger 90-day predictor of outcomes than an ED physician's intent to admit or discharge a patient [15].

Traditional methods of monitoring congestion through daily weights is difficult because of variability in patient food and fluid intake, as well as the time of day when measurements are taken. Thus, NP levels may prove to be useful in the outpatient setting as a surrogate for detecting and monitoring subclinical decompensation. Observations from several studies indicated that monitoring NP levels in outpatients could ultimately improve outcomes. In the Valsartan Heart Failure Trial (Val-HeFT), treatment with valsartan caused sustained reduction in BNP levels, which were consistent with clinical benefits, i.e. quality of life, clinical signs, NYHA class, and left ventricular ejection fraction.[16] In a smaller study, treatment with β-blockers in heart failure patients already taking angiotensin-converting enzyme (ACE) inhibitors also resulted in decreased BNP levels [17]. Findings like these have led to studies in which BNP levels were used to titrate drug therapy in patients who had chronic heart failure.

In the STARS-BNP Multicenter Study, the benefit of BNP-guided therapy on outcomes in outpatients with heart failure was assessed. In this study 220 patients were divided into a clinical arm and a BNP arm; the goal of the latter group was to decrease BNP levels to less than 100 pg/mL. The BNP-guided group received higher dosage of β-blocker and ACE inhibitor therapy and had fewer hospital visits and deaths at follow-up. This trial suggests that a BNP-guided strategy is better than a 'clinically guided' strategy [18].

Using NP levels to guide therapy in trials has become more and more popular in recent studies. The BATTLESCARRED trial studied 364 outpatients with heart failure with N-terminal pro-B-type natriuretic peptide (NT-proBNP) greater than 150 pmol/L (roughly 1300 pg/mL) [19]. Subjects were randomly assigned to a usual care arm or to one of two aggressive arms: NP guided or clinically guided. This study demonstrated a number of improved outcomes out to 2 years with the NT-proBNP-guided strategy among patients under 75 years of age. These included all-cause mortality, survival or heart failure readmission, and days alive and not hospitalized with heart failure. However, after 2 and 3 years of follow-up, the two intensive management treatment strategies were no longer significantly better than usual care in terms of mortality.

Studies like this demonstrate that there is a pressing need for more trials which include a number of prognostic biomarkers that pertain to chronic heart failure and renal function as well. Identifying biomarkers that truly focus on the pathophysiology of the disease mechanisms for these trials will help to identify ideal treatment strategies for heart failure patients. In the future, the use of home biomarker monitoring as a method to monitor a patient's level of congestion and to help titrate medications in the outpatient setting may prevent hospitalizations for AHF.

Systolic versus diastolic heart failure

NPs have been demonstrated to be elevated in both systolic and diastolic heart failure. A diagnosis of systolic heart failure is made through interpretations of signs and symptoms, and through the use of a handful of diagnostic tests. An algorithm for the diagnosis of heart failure is shown in ➲ Fig. 35.5.

For the diagnosis of heart failure with normal ejection fraction (HFNEF), cut-off values for NT-proBNP (220 pg/mL) and for BNP (200 pg/mL) are used. For the exclusion of HFNEF, the respective cut-off values of NT-proBNP (120 pg/mL) and of BNP (100 pg/mL) are chosen. NPs are recommended mainly for exclusion of HFNEF and not for diagnosis of HFNEF. Furthermore, when used for diagnostic purposes, NPs do not provide diagnostic stand-alone evidence of HFNEF and always need to be implemented along with other noninvasive investigations (➲ Fig. 35.6).

Diagnostic caveats and confounders

NPs are an effective tool for the diagnosis of AHF in patients presenting with acute dyspnoea. However, as stated earlier,

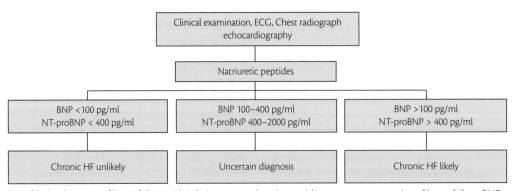

Figure 35.5 Flowchart for the diagnosis of heart failure with NPs in untreated patients with symptoms suggestive of heart failure. BNP and NT-proBNP levels can be used to rule in and rule out heart failure. There is a 'grey zone' for NPs, in which more specific investigation is necessary.
Reproduced with permission from Dickstein, K., *et al.*, ESC Guidelines for the diagnosis and treatment of acute and chronic heart failure 2008: The Task Force for the Diagnosis and Treatment of Acute and Chronic Heart Failure 2008 of the European Society of Cardiology. Developed in collaboration with the Heart Failure Association of the ESC (HFA) and endorsed by the European Society of Intensive Care Medicine (ESICM). *Eur J Heart Fail* 2008;**10**(10):933–989.

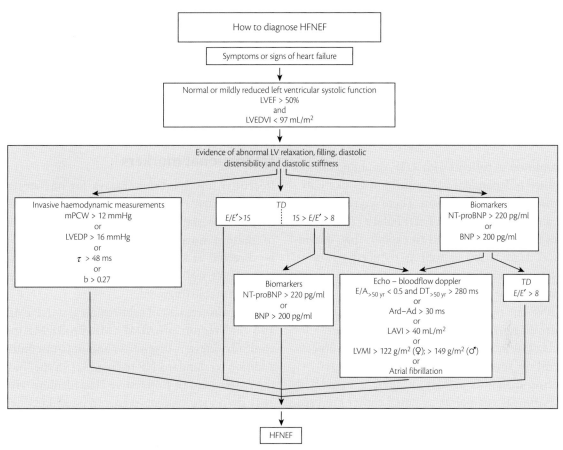

Figure 35.6 Diagnostic flowchart on how to diagnose HFNEF in a patient suspected of HFNEF. Ad, duration of mitral valve atrial wave flow; Ard, duration of reverse pulmonary vein atrial systole flow; BNP, brain natriuretic peptide; DT, deceleration time; E, early mitral valve flow velocity; E/A, ratio of early (E) to late (A) mitral valve flow velocity; E′, early TD lengthening velocity; LAVI, left atrial volume index; LVEDVI, left ventricular end-diastolic volume index; LVMI, left ventricular mass index; mPCW, mean pulmonary capillary wedge pressure; LVEDP, left ventricular end-diastolic pressure; NT-proBNP, N-terminal-pro brain natriuretic peptide; τ, time constant of left ventricular relaxation; b, constant of left ventricular chamber stiffness; TD, tissue Doppler. Reproduced with permission rom Paulus WJ, Tschope C, Sanderson JE *et al.* How to diagnose diastolic heart failure: a consensus statement on the diagnosis of heart failure with normal left ventricular ejection fraction by the Heart Failure and Echocardiography Associations of the European Society of Cardiology. *Eur Heart J* 2007;**28**(20):2539–2350.

there is no perfect diagnostic biomarker and there are caveats that must be considered when incorporating NPs into clinical practice.

The 'grey zone'

A two-cut-point method of using BNP to diagnose AHF provides higher diagnostic accuracy, but leaves a 'grey zone' of BNP values (100–400 pg/mL). In this zone, the patient is neither a definite 'rule out' nor 'rule-in' for AHF. When a patient's levels lie in this area, clinical insight and additional testing are often required to make an accurate diagnosis. If a large proportion of patients with acute breathlessness had values in the grey zone this could reduce the clinical utility of NP, but in practice 75% of patients have values above or below these cut-off values [8]. When patients have a BNP value in the 'grey zone,' conditions such as right ventricular failure from cor pulmonale, acute pulmonary embolism, and renal failure should all be considered.

Renal dysfunction

Cardiac dysfunction and renal dysfunction are intricately linked. The prevalence of congestive heart failure increases greatly as the patient's renal function deteriorates, and, in endstage renal disease, can reach 65–70%. There is evidence that chronic kidney disease itself is a major contributor to severe cardiac damage and, conversely, that heart failure is a major cause of progressive chronic kidney disease [20]. Uncontrolled heart failure is often associated with a rapid fall in renal function and adequate control of heart failure can prevent this. The opposite is also true: treatment of chronic kidney disease can prevent the onset of heart failure.

BNP and NT-proBNP concentrations are elevated in patients with renal failure. In patients with chronic kidney disease, decreased estimated GFR is associated with increased plasma BNP and even greater elevation in NT-proBNP concentrations. Because most BNP is not cleared in the renal system, the mechanism of elevated BNP levels in renal failure is likely multifactorial, representing in part a true counter-regulatory response from the heart to the kidney, and not simply decreased passive renal clearance [21]. In order to maintain optimal diagnostic performance the cut-point for detecting heart failure may need to be raised when eGFR is less than 60 mL/min [22].

Obesity

Obesity is common in patients with AHF, doubling the risk of heart failure independent of comorbidities like coronary heart disease and hypertension. There is a reduced NP level in the obese individual with heart failure [23]. Several mechanisms have been proposed to explain this, including increased degradation as well as reduced synthesis. Because BNP values are lower in obese patients, lower cut-points are needed for obese patients if sensitivity is to be preserved. BNP cut-points to maintain 90% sensitivity for a heart failure diagnosis have been shown at 170 pg/mL for lean subjects, 110 pg/mL for overweight/obese subjects, and 54 pg/mL in severely/morbidly obese patients [24]. With respect to diagnosis of AHF in obese patients with NT-proBNP, similar cut-points as stated earlier are used. Using adjusted values is important to improve diagnostic accuracy and patient management in obese individuals with AHF [25].

Age

Age has an impact on circulating NP levels, as it does with many endogenous hormones. Two studies looked at BNP levels in normal subjects without cardiovascular disease or ventricular (systolic or diastolic) dysfunction and found clear increases with age [26, 27]. Therefore, 'normal' values vary. As a general guideline, in young, healthy adults, 90% will have BNP less than 20–25 pg/mL [28]. BNP levels increase significantly with age and are higher in women than in men, leading to age-, gender-, and assay-specific reference ranges.

Lung disease

NP levels can be elevated in patients with dyspnoea due to primary lung disease, as well as dyspnoea due to AHF. The levels are, however, not as elevated in lung disease as they are in AHF [29]. BNP levels are elevated in patients with acute pulmonary embolism (PE), probably as a result of increased myocardial shear stress, mainly in the right ventricle, and depending on the degree and dynamics of embolic events [30]. Similar findings are present in patients with severe COPD and essential pulmonary hypertension [31]. Therefore, one should not assume that patients presenting

with dyspnoea and elevated NP levels have decompensated heart failure, especially if the NP levels are in the 'grey zone' (BNP 100–500 pg/mL; NT-proBNP 300–900 pg/mL for 50- to 75-year-olds).

Emerging biomarkers

Midregional markers

Recently, novel immunoassays for analytes relevant in cardiovascular regulation have been developed for detection of the stable prohormone fragment as a 'mirror' of mature hormone release. New immunoassays can be directed at stable mid-region prohormones that are stoichometrically related to synthesis of the biologically active unstable fragment.

The measurement of mid-region proANP (MR-proANP) and mid-region proADM (MR-proADM) may provide clinically relevant diagnostic and outcome information in addition to standard NP testing.[32] In the 'Biomarkers in the Assessment of Congestive Heart Failure' (BACH) trial, 1641 dyspnoeic patients were recruited and one-third were ultimately diagnosed with heart failure. Results showed that MR-proADM was prognostically more accurate than BNP or NT-proBNP at predicting outcome at 90 days. NT-proBNP did not add additional prognostic information to MR-proADM alone. The findings await confirmation, especially in lower risk populations, as most patients with a recent episode of worsening heart failure could be considered at high risk. MR-proADM could be a useful alternative to NT-proBNP for risk stratification [33].

MR-proANP itself is being examined as a diagnostic adjunct to BNP and NT-proBNP, to potentially be added to the diagnostic criteria for AHF. In addition, it has potential to assist in diagnosing AHF where BNP has caveats, such as in the 'grey zone' levels, or in renal disease.

ST2

The *ST2* gene, a member of the interleukin-1 receptor family, was recently described to be markedly up-regulated in an experimental model of heart failure [34]. The *ST2* gene is markedly up-regulated in cardiac myocytes and fibroblasts subjected to mechanical strain [34], which is important as the functional ligand of ST2 was identified to be IL-33, a cardiac fibroblast product also induced by mechanical strain [35].

Circulating ST2 concentrations might be prognostically meaningful in those with chronic severe heart failure [36] or acute myocardial infarction [37].

Results from the PRIDE study demonstrated that ST2 levels were higher among those with AHF compared to those without, but ST2 was not as useful for diagnosing heart failure as NT-proBNP. In addition, among dyspnoeic patients with and without AHF, ST2 concentrations were strongly predictive of mortality at 1 year and might be useful for prognostication when used alone or together with NT-proBNP [38].

Troponin

Cardiac troponins are regulatory proteins of the thin actin filaments of the cardiac muscle. Troponin T and troponin I are highly sensitive and specific markers of myocardial injury. Serial measurement of troponin I or troponin T has become an important tool for risk stratification of patients presenting with acute coronary syndromes [39]. Recent studies have also demonstrated that is it useful in assessing prognosis in AHF.

In a study of 84 872 patients from the ADHERE registry who were hospitalized with acute decompensated heart failure, patients who were positive for troponin had lower systolic blood pressure on admission, a lower ejection fraction, and higher in-hospital mortality than those who were negative for troponin. A positive cardiac troponin test is associated with higher in-hospital mortality, independently of other predictive variables in heart failure patients [40].

Neutrophil gelatinase-associated lipocalin

NGAL is emerging as a marker of acute kidney injury. Many of the treatments for heart failure such as diuretics and vasodilators result in renal injury and often result in the cardiorenal syndrome. If is often difficult to discern when kidney injury occurs and NGAL may be an early biomarker signal of renal dysfunction which can be used to titrate therapies for heart failure (◘ Fig. 35.7).

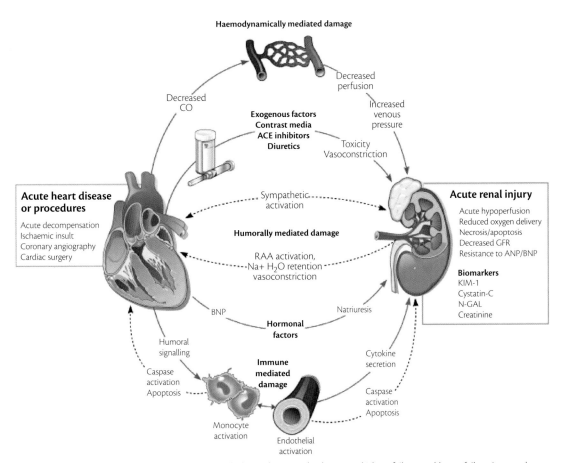

Figure 35.7 Pathophysiological interactions between heart and kidney. The interplay between kidney failure and heart failure is complex, as one failing organ often precipitates failure of the other. Decreased perfusion as well as release of NPs can eventually damage the kidney; sympathetic drive initiated by the renin–angiotensin–aldosterone system leads to increased vasoconstriction, a prothrombotic state, and potential downstream damage on the heart. ACE, angiotensin-converting enzyme; ANP, atrial natriuretic peptide; BNP, B-type natriuretic peptide; CO, cardiac output; GFR, glomerular filtration rate; KIM, kidney injury molecule; NGAL, neutrophil gelatinase-associated lipocalin; RAA, renin–angiotensin–aldosterone.
Reproduced from Ronco C, Haapio M, House AA, *et al.* Cardiorenal syndrome. *J Am Coll Cardiol* 2008;**52**(19):1527–1539. With permission from Elsevier.

NGAL is a novel cytokine involved in several systemic processes. This marker, originally identified as a 25-kDa protein associated with purified gelatinase and obtained from the supernatant of activated neutrophils, plays a role as an innate antibacterial factor. Various tissues produce and release NGAL in response to particular conditions. Diseases such as atherosclerosis and myocardial infarction, which appear to be frequently associated with age or heart failure, alter the local and systemic balance of NGAL [41].

In a study of 46 elderly patients with heart failure, NGAL levels were elevated in these patients versus healthy controls. In addition, like the NPs, NGAL levels increased with severity of heart failure (by NYHA classification). Prognostically, NGAL at a cut-point of 783 ng/mL had a higher mortality than the other subjects considered. NGAL levels may be of important prognostic value in the assessment of survival, thus extending the predictive properties of this cytokine beyond the clinical field of renal disease [42].

Conclusion

In the past decade the application of biomarkers in the diagnosis of AHF has revolutionized AHF management. In the future a more sophisticated and comprehensive multimarker biomarker strategy will aid not only in diagnosis but in prognosis and therapy titration. In addition these biomarkers are giving us insight into the pathogenesis of AHF. We anticipate that the standard of care for AHF patient will be to have a BNP taken in the ED, followed by multiple BNP levels during hospitalization to assess response to therapy. The patient will then have a discharge BNP to assess prognosis, and this 'dry' BNP level can then followed in the outpatient setting through a home BNP monitoring system to prevent future AHF hospitalizations. This patient likely also had a troponin test on admission, which will provide important prognostic information. ST2 and MR-proANP could also be used for supplemental prognostic information. NGAL might also be checked during the hospital course of this patient to assess when the patient maybe overdiuresed.

Personal perspective

NP levels can help clinicians manage patients in a great variety of settings. They are helpful in screening to identify or exclude cardiovascular disease and for the differential diagnosis of symptoms that might be due to heart failure, and are astonishingly powerful prognostic tools. As our armamentarium of biomarkers increases, it is important to have well-designed clinical trials to better understand the relevant clinical scenario in which they are useful. It is also important to understand the limitations of biomarkers. The future will also see integration of biomarkers into clinical algorithms that incorporate multiple data modalities for improved clinical decision-making and more efficient and cost-effective patient management.

Further reading

Anderson JL, Adams CD, Antman EM, *et al*. ACC/AHA 2007 guidelines for the management of patients with unstable angina/non–ST-elevation myocardial infarction. *J Am Coll Cardiol* 2007;**50**(7):e1–e157.

Apple FS, Wu AH, Mair J, *et al*. Future biomarkers for detection of ischemia and risk stratification in acute coronary syndrome. *Clin Chem* 2005;**51**(5):810–824.

Braunwald E. *Braunwald's heart disease: a textbook of cardiovascular medicine*, 3rd edition, W.B. Saunders, Philadelphia, 1997.

Christenson RH, Duh SH, Apple FS, *et al*. Standardization of cardiac troponin I assays: round robin of ten candidate reference materials. *Clin Chem* 2001;**47**(3):431–437.

Fromm RE, Roberts R. Sensitivity and specificity of new serum markers for mild cardionecrosis. *Curr Probl Cardiol* 2001;**26**(4):241–284.

Gillard JM. Bedside cardiac markers: troponin I, CK-MB, and myoglobin at the point of care. *Resid Staff Physician* 2001;**47**(14):33.

Gillard JM. Troponins: the new cardiac markers of choice. *Emerg Med* 2003;**35**(11):35.

Goetz JP. Biochemistry of pro-B-type natriuretic peptide-derived peptides: the endocrine heart revisited. *Clin Chem* 2004;**50**(9):1503–1510.

Hamm CW, Braunwald E. A classification of unstable angina revisited. *Circulation* 2000;**102**(1):118–122.

Hamm CW, Goldmann B, Heeschen C, *et al*. Emergency room triage of patients with acute chest pain by means of rapid testing for cardiac troponin T or troponin I. *N Engl J Med* 1997;**337**(23):1648–1653.

Jaffe AS, Babuin L, Apple FS. Biomarkers in acute cardiac disease: the present and the future. *J Am Coll Cardiol* 2006;**48**(1):1–11.

Labugger R, Organ L, Collier C, *et al*. Extensive troponin I and T modification detected in serum from patients with acute myocardial infarction. *Circulation* 2000;**102**(11):1221–1226.

Maisel A, Mueller C, Adams K Jr, *et al.* State of the art: using natriuretic peptide levels in clinical practice. *Eur J Heart Fail* 2008;**10**(9):824–839.

Newby LK, Storrow AB, Gibler WB, *et al.* Bedside multimarker testing for risk stratification in chest pain units: the chest pain evaluation by creatine kinase-MB, myoglobin, and troponin I (CHECKMATE) study. *Circulation* 2001;**103**(14):1832–1837.

Newman DJ, Olabiran Y, Bedzyk WD, *et al.* Impact of antibody specificity and calibration material on the measure of agreement between methods for cardiac troponin I. *Clin Chem* 1999;**45**(6 Pt 1):822–828.

Omland T, Sabatine MS, Jablonski KA, *et al.* Prognostic value of B-type natriuretic peptides in patients with stable coronary artery disease: the PEACE trial. *J Am Coll Cardiol* 2007;**50**(3):205–214.

Porela P, Pulkki K, Helenius H, *et al.* Prediction of short-term outcome in patients with suspected myocardial infarction. *Ann Emerg Med* 2000;**35**(5):413–420.

Shi Q, Ling M, Zhang X, *et al.* Degradation of cardiac troponin I in serum complicates comparisons of cardiac troponin I assays. *Clin Chem* 1999;**45**(7):1018–1025.

Solaro RJ, Rarick HM. Troponin and tropomyosin: proteins that switch on and tune in the activity of cardiac myofilaments. *Circ Res* 1998;**83**(5):471–480.

Wu AH, Feng YJ, Moore R, *et al.* Characterization of cardiac troponin subunit release into serum after acute myocardial infarction and comparison of assays for troponin T and I. *Clin Chem* 1998;**44**(6 Pt 1):1198–1208.

⮑ For additional multimedia materials please visit the online version of the book (📖 http://www.esciacc.oxfordmedicine.com).

CHAPTER 36

Coagulation and thrombosis

Anne-Mette Hvas, Erik Lerkevang Grove, and Steen Dalby Kristensen

Contents

Summary

Coagulation is evaluated by conventional analyses, often supplemented by point-of-care tests. Currently, a number of point-of-care tests for evaluation of platelet function and the efficacy of antiplatelet therapy are being investigated. Thrombophilia contributes to the risk of thrombosis, and a battery of complex assays is required to identify all thrombophilias.

Disseminated intravascular coagulation (DIC) is characterized by microthrombosis and clinical bleeding. A scoring system for overt DIC provides a five-step diagnostic algorithm. The cornerstone of DIC management is treatment of the underlying triggering condition.

Heparin-induced thrombocytopenia (HIT) is an adverse immunological effect of heparin therapy. Besides thrombocytopenia, the major clinical consequence of HIT is an enhanced risk of thrombosis. The diagnosis is based on the clinical picture and detection of platelet-activating HIT antibodies. When HIT is strongly suspected, it is recommended to stop heparin treatment, order laboratory tests for HIT antibodies, and initiate nonheparin anticoagulant treatment.

Introduction

Haemostatic dysfunction ranges from a compromised clot formation in the bleeding patient to an increased clot formation in patients with thrombotic disorders. Laboratory tests are used to detect and analyse haemostatic abnormalities and provide guidance for proper intervention. In the present chapter, strengths and limitations of standard coagulation analyses are presented, as well as point-of-care tests used for guidance in acute cardiac care and cardiac surgery. In addition, diagnosis of thrombophilias and the two acute medical complications, disseminated intravascular coagulation (DIC) and heparin-induced thrombocytopenia (HIT), are summarized.

Haemostatic disorders in acute cardiac care and cardiac surgery—point-of-care tests for diagnosis and targeted treatment

The concept of coagulation

The concept of the coagulation cascade as a series of stepwise enzymatic conversions was described as early as in 1964 under the headings of the *intrinsic* pathway and the *extrinsic* pathway culminating in the conversion of fibrinogen to fibrin [1, 2] (→ Fig. 36.1a).

Many clinicians have adopted this easily conceptualized view of haemostasis; however, the concept is not applicable to *in vivo* haemostasis, although it is a valuable scheme for diagnostic purposes. The current view of *in vivo* coagulation is that the coagulation process can be divided into three phases: initiation, amplification, and propagation (→ Fig. 36.1b) [3, 4].

In the initiation phase, exposure of subendothelial tissue factor leads to formation of a catalytic complex with factor (F) VIIa, and small amounts of FIXa, FXa and thrombin are formed. Besides being a cofactor for FVII, tissue factor serves as a receptor with signal transduction resulting in the induction of genes involved in inflammation, apoptosis,

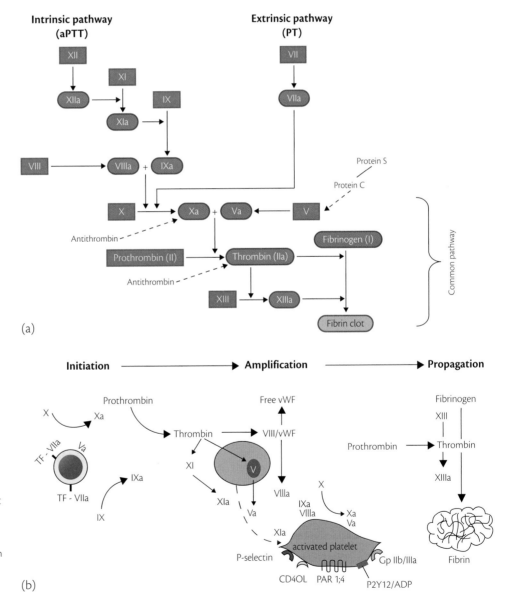

Figure 36.1 (a) The intrinsic and extrinsic pathway as described in the cascade model of coagulation reflected in the laboratory measurements of activated partial thromboplastin time (aPTT) and prothrombin time (PT). (b) Current concepts of the coagulation process.
Part (b) Reproduced with permission from De Caterina R, Husted S, Wallentin L, *et al.* Anticoagulants in heart disease: current status and perspectives. *Eur Heart J* 2007;**28**(7):880–913, Oxford University Press.

and cell migration [5]. Tissue factor is expressed by many extravascular tissues, especially perivascular tissues [6], and, importantly, tissue factor expression can also be induced on the endothelium in response to inflammatory stimuli such as sepsis. Thus, coagulation and inflammation are strongly integrated processes.

During amplification, low concentrations of thrombin activate platelets, and a positive feedback loop is initiated causing increasing amounts of thrombin to be formed. In the propagation phase, this thrombin burst results in the formation of physiologically relevant amounts of cross-linked fibrin, leading to a stable haemostatic clot. Fibrinolysis is essential for removing the clot. The principal mediator of fibrinolysis is plasmin, which cleaves fibrin, resulting in the production of fibrin degradation products.

Acute cardiac care and cardiac surgery

The frequent use of potent antithrombotic therapy in cardiac care often challenges sufficient haemostasis in these patients. Furthermore, coagulation management in patients undergoing cardiac surgery is difficult, because of the delicate balance between sufficient anticoagulation during cardiopulmonary bypass and the required haemostasis soon afterwards. During cardiopulmonary bypass activation of coagulation occurs because of contact with the nonendothelial surface of the extracorporeal circuit and because of tissue factor release in the late phase of cardiopulmonary bypass [7]. Thus, systematic anticoagulation with heparin is required during the procedure to inhibit the coagulation cascade in order to prevent thrombus formation and microvascular consumption of coagulation factors.

Characterization of the haemostatic defects responsible for bleeding is crucial for optimal clinical management of these patients [4]. Evaluation of coagulation status is performed by routine coagulation analyses, now often supplemented by point-of-care tests with the goal of assessing haemostatic function in a timely and accurate manner [8].

Strengths and limitations of standard coagulation analyses

There is no single global test available to adequately evaluate overall haemostasis. The initial formation of fibrin can easily be determined by routine laboratory tests such as prothrombin time (PT) and the activated partial thromboplastin time (aPTT) supplemented by thrombin time, fibrinogen (functional), and platelet count to assess the coagulation status of the patient (● Fig. 36.1a).

These methods have been widely used for diagnosing and monitoring patients with coagulation abnormalities.

However, the value of standard coagulation tests has been questioned because of a number of drawbacks: delays from blood sampling to obtaining the results (30–60 min); tests are determined in plasma rather than whole blood; no information is available on platelet function; and the assays are performed at a standard temperature of 37°C rather than at the patient's body temperature.

In the operating room, activated clotting time (ACT) is often used before and during cardiopulmonary bypass. ACT might be used before the procedure to assess heparin requirements, during the procedure to maintain adequate anticoagulation and, finally, after the procedure to monitor the reversal of heparin [9].

The introduction of point-of-care coagulation monitoring addresses some of the above-mentioned limitations [10] and might provide a useful supplement to standard coagulation analyses.

Thromboelastometry—a dynamic whole blood coagulation profile

Thromboelastometry (or thromboelastography) (TE) is a diagnostic point-of-care test that measures initial clotting, platelet interaction, and fibrinolysis in a sample of whole blood.

TE was introduced more than 60 years ago to assess primary and secondary haemostasis [11]. After the development of PT and aPTT, the utility of TE in clinical settings became limited. With an increasing number of complex surgical procedures such as cardiac bypass, TE has been revisited because of the need for rapid assessment of global haemostatic function.

As TE is performed using whole blood, it allows *in vivo* interaction between the coagulation system, platelets, and red blood cells. A major advantage is that the analysis has a short turnaround time (15 min) and that clot development can be visually displayed in real time. Furthermore, the use of TE provides a basis for targeted therapy and a reduced need for blood products after cardiac surgery [12, 13].

Evaluation of the response to antiplatelet therapy

Finding the optimal balance between adequate haemostasis and a beneficial degree of platelet inhibition is a growing challenge as more and more patients are receiving antiplatelet therapy.

Recent evidence suggests that not all patients respond uniformly to antiplatelet agents, with some being low responders ('resistant') [14;15]. This is the case for both aspirin and clopidogrel [14, 15]. A low response to antiplatelet therapy may be associated with an increased risk of thrombosis [16–18]. As pointed out by the Working Group on Thrombosis of the European Society of Cardiology [15], the main problem with 'resistance' is the lack of a clear definition due to lack of standardized methods of platelet function monitoring and evidence-based cut-off values for platelet function measurements to classify patients as 'responders' or 'nonresponders'.

The traditional platelet aggregation test was developed by Born [19] and O'Brien [20] and became the gold standard. This test measures platelet aggregation in response to an agonist in platelet-rich plasma by turbidometry. The basic advantage of platelet aggregometry is that it measures the aggregation of platelets with one another in a glycoprotein IIb/IIIa-dependent manner. On the other hand, this test has several drawbacks including poor reproducibility, high sample volume, requirement for sample preparation with potential loss of large and dense platelets, length of assay time, requirement for a skilled technician, and high costs [21].

Newly developed point-of-care tests have advantages including the use of anticoagulated whole blood (no need for sample preparation), usage of disposable cartridges or cups (no cleaning required), low sample volume, no requirement for a skilled technician, and rapid availability of results.

Currently, a number of point-of-care tests are under investigation, including the platelet function analyser 100 (PFA-100™), VerifyNow™, and the multiple platelet function analyser (Multiplate™) [22].

The PFA-100™ assay draws an anticoagulated blood sample through a 150-µm diameter, collagen-coated aperture in the presence of ADP or adrenaline (epinephrine), thus mimicking arterial high-shear conditions. Shear stress and platelet agonists lead to platelet plug formation, and the time until closure of the capillary is recorded [23]. The PFA-100™ could be regarded as an *in vitro* bleeding time recorder. However, this method has shown considerable variability in evaluating low responsiveness to aspirin [24, 25].

The VerifyNow™ device is based on the ability of platelets to aggregate with fibrinogen. The system measures changes in light transmission as a result of platelet aggregation [26]. Three VerifyNow™ assays are currently available: the VerifyNow IIb/IIIa Assay™ (sensitive to glycoprotein IIb/IIIa antagonists), the VerifyNow Aspirin Assay™ (sensitive to aspirin), and the VerifyNow P2Y12 Assay™ (sensitive to e.g. clopidogrel, prasugrel, and ticagrelor). The variability of the VerifyNow Aspirin Assay™ has been reported to be low [27].

The Multiplate™ analyser is based on whole blood impedance aggregometry [28]. The device has five channels with test cells for parallel testing. Each test cell contains a stirring magnet and two pairs of electrodes, on which activated platelets adhere and aggregate, resulting in an increase in electrical resistance. Several specific test reagents are available for stimulation of different platelet receptors or activation of signal transduction pathways in order to detect changes induced by drugs as well as by acquired or hereditary platelet disorders.

It is not possible to estimate the exact prevalence of 'resistance' to antiplatelet drugs because of the lack of a univocal definition [15]. As suggested by the Working Group on Thrombosis of the European Society of Cardiology, the proposed test is measurement of aggregation induced by arachidonic acid and determination of serum thromboxane B_2 for assessment of aspirin specific effects [15]. For assessment of P2Y12-specific effects, the proposed test is aggregation induced with ADP or vasodilator-stimulated phosphoprotein (VASP) phosphorylation. However, routine determination of platelet function while on antiplatelet therapy cannot yet be recommended because of the lack of evidence on how to interpret the results in a clinical setting.

Limitations of point-of-care coagulation tests

Point-of-care coagulation tests are difficult to standardize. The blood collection site, processing of the sample (e.g. native versus anticoagulated samples, time delay between collection and measurement), patient age, and gender may significantly affect test results [10]. The equipment and activators will alter the assay specificity, and currently no single point-of-care platelet function analyser has conclusively been shown to be highly reproducible and superior to other tests. Furthermore, the utility of these analysers for predicting clinical outcomes has not yet been fully established.

Thrombophilia

Thrombophilia is an inherited or acquired coagulation defect, which predisposes to thrombosis. Importantly, most individuals with thrombophilia do not develop thrombosis. When thrombophilia presents clinically, the predominant manifestation is venous thromboembolism.

Strong risk factors are deficiencies of the natural anticoagulants antithrombin, protein C, and protein S. Deficiencies of antithrombin, protein C, and its cofactor protein S are found in less than 1% of the population [29, 30], but a tenfold increased risk for thrombosis has been reported among heterozygous carriers [31].

Factor V Leiden and prothrombin 20210A are moderately strong risk factors. Among white people the prevalence of factor V Leiden is approximately 5% [32]. This variant leads to resistance to activated protein C (APC-resistance) [33], and the risk of venous thromboembolism is increased fivefold in heterozygotes, and around fiftyfold in homozygotes [34, 35].

A mutation in the prothrombin gene (prothrombin 20210A) leads to increased prothrombin levels, which are associated with a twofold increased risk of venous thrombosis [36]. The prevalence of this mutation is around 2% among whites.

Several genetic factors are known to have a weak effect on thrombosis with relative risks between 1.0 and 1.5. The variant in methylenetetrahydrofolate reductase (MTHFR) results in elevated levels of homocysteine. Around 10% of the general population are carriers, but the effect on homocysteine levels are small, and there are conflicting results on the risk of thrombosis [37, 38].

The antiphospholipid syndrome is an acquired condition defined by thrombotic and/or obstetric events together with the presence of antiphospholipid antibodies. The antiphospholipid antibodies can currently be detected by three different assays: lupus anticoagulant IgG/IgM anti-β_2 glycoprotein I antibodies, and IgG/IgM anti-cardiolipin antibodies [39, 40]. The presence of lupus anticoagulants consistently shows the highest strength of association with both arterial and venous thrombotic complications [41].

Currently, there is no single laboratory assay or simple set of assay to identify thrombophilia. Consequently, a battery of complex and expensive assays is usually required.

Disseminated intravascular coagulation

DIC is a clinical pathological syndrome characterized by systemic activation of the coagulation system leading to widespread vascular deposition of fibrin resulting in multiple organ dysfunction. The continuous activation of coagulation causes consumption of platelets and coagulation factors, which may lead to clinical bleeding (➲ Fig. 36.2).

DIC is always secondary to an underlying disorder that causes activation of the coagulation system, e.g. sepsis.

Diagnosis and laboratory tests

The diagnosis of DIC should be based on an appropriate clinical suspicion supported by laboratory tests. No single

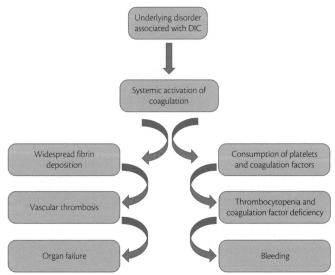

Figure 36.2 The process of disseminated intravascular dissemination (DIC).

laboratory test exists to establish or rule out DIC. A combination of tests can be used to support the diagnosis with reasonable certainty, when done in patients with a condition known to be associated with DIC [42, 43].

Screening tests for haemostatic function such as the PT, activated partial thromboplastin time (aPTT), functional plasma fibrinogen, and platelet count reflect the degree of platelet activation and consumption of coagulation factors. The extent of fibrin formation can be indirectly evaluated e.g. by measurement of fibrin D-dimers. A reduced level of the natural anticoagulant antithrombin indicates consumption of natural anticoagulants during the process of DIC.

Repeated determinations of platelet counts are essential when DIC is suspected. A clear downward trend at repeated measurements is a sensitive sign of DIC. Thrombocytopenia is seen in up to 98% of patients with DIC, and in around 50% of patients, platelet count is below 50×10^9 /L [44]. Importantly, a single determination of platelet count is not sufficient as the original platelet count may remain within the normal range of $150–400 \times 10^9$ /L. A low or decreasing platelet count is not specific for DIC, as many of the underlying conditions associated with DIC, such as sepsis, may also cause a low platelet count *per se* [45].

The PT and aPTT are prolonged in about half of the patients with DIC at some point during the course of the illness [42]. This is mainly caused by consumption of coagulation factors. However, reduced liver function, and thereby impaired synthesis of coagulation factors, may also contribute to the reduced level of coagulation factors and a prolongation of PT and aPTT [42]. Importantly, a normal PT and/or aPTT do not exclude activation of the haemostatic system and repeated measurements are required.

Sequential measurements of fibrinogen might also be useful in the diagnosis of DIC, although several limitations must be considered. Fibrinogen is an acute-phase reactant and despite an ongoing consumption, plasma levels of fibrinogen can remain within the normal range for a long period. Thus, hypofibrinogenaemia is primarily seen in very severe cases of DIC [43].

Plasma levels of antithrombin, the most important inhibitor of thrombin, are reduced during DIC, as a result of consumption, increased degradation, and impaired synthesis. A reduction of another natural anticoagulant, protein C, further compromises adequate regulation of coagulation. Accordingly, the levels of antithrombin and protein C are often reduced in DIC, and these markers have prognostic significance [46, 47]. Repeated measurements are needed, as single determinations are neither sensitive nor specific for DIC.

A definition and a diagnostic scoring system for overt DIC has been proposed by the Subcommittee of the Scientific and Standardization Committee (SSC) on DIC of the International Society on Thrombosis and Haemostasis (ISTH) [48]. These ISTH criteria suggest a five-step diagnostic algorithm to calculate a DIC score, using laboratory tests available in almost every hospital laboratory (➲ Table 36.1). Using this system, overt DIC is identified by a score of 5 or more [48, 49].

Treating the underlying triggering condition is the cornerstone of DIC management [50]. However, additional supportive treatment, specifically aimed at the coagulation and platelet abnormalities, may be required. For further information on treatment, see ➲ Chapter 69.

Heparin-induced thrombocytopenia

HIT is an immunologic adverse effect of heparin therapy associated with an increased thrombotic risk. Antibody-mediated platelet activation causes thrombin generation, resulting in the paradox that despite thrombocytopenia induced by heparin, the major clinical consequence of HIT is an enhanced risk of venous and/or arterial thrombosis. Prompt diagnosis, discontinuation of heparin, and initiation of nonheparin anticoagulants are essential to prevent further complications.

HIT typically occurs 5–14 days after start of heparin treatment [51] (➲ Fig. 36.3). In case of re-exposure to heparin within 1–2 months, HIT can occur at day 1 of heparin treatment (rapid-onset HIT). Delayed-onset HIT begins several days and up to a few weeks after heparin exposure and is caused by antibodies activating platelets independently of heparin, thus mimicking an autoimmune disease. HIT enhances the risk of both venous and arterial thrombosis, but thromboembolic complications predominantly affect the venous system.

The more unusual a new thrombotic event during heparin treatment seems, the more HIT should be considered. The risk

Table 36.1 ISTH diagnostic scoring system for disseminated intravascular coagulation

Risk assessment:			
Does the patient have an underlying disorder known to be associated with overt DIC?			
If yes: Proceed			
If no: Do not use this algorithm			
Order global coagulation tests:			
Platelet count, PT, aPTT, fibrinogen, fibrin D-dimer			
Score the test results:			
Platelet count	$>100 \times 10^9$/L = 0	$50–100 \times 10^9$/L = 1	$<50 \times 10^9$/L = 2
Prolonged PT	<3 s = 0	3–6 s = 1	>6 s = 2
Fibrinogen	>1 g/L = 0	<1 g/L = 1	
Fibrin D-dimer [a]	No increase = 0	Moderate increase = 2	Strong increase = 3
Calculate score:			
≥5 compatible with overt DIC; repeat score daily			
<5 suggestive for nonovert DIC; repeat next 1–2 days			

DIC, disseminated intravascular coagulation.

[a] In most prospective validation studies, a fibrin D-dimer assay was used as fibrin-related marker. A value above the upper limit of normal (0.4 μg/L) was considered moderately elevated, whereas a value more than 10 times the upper limit of normal (4.0 μg/L) was considered a strong increase.

Data from Taylor FB Jr, Toh CH, Hoots WK, *et al.* Towards definition, clinical and laboratory criteria, and a scoring system for disseminated intravascular coagulation. *Thromb Haemost* 2001;**86**(5):1327–1330.

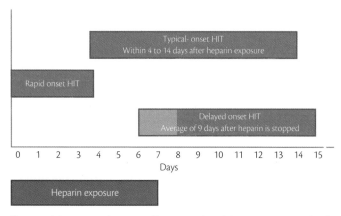

Figure 36.3 Temporal aspects of heparin-induced thrombocytopenia (HIT).

of HIT is influenced by the heparin preparation (bovine unfractionated heparin > porcine unfractionated heparin > low-molecular-weight heparin), duration of heparin exposure, patient gender (female > male), and patient population (postsurgical > medical > obstetric) [52].

Diagnosis and laboratory tests

The diagnosis should be based on both the clinical picture and detection of platelet-activating HIT antibodies, as HIT is a clinical pathologic syndrome based on clinical symptoms and detection of antibodies [53].

The '4 Ts' score is a standardized tool to assess the probability of HIT (➲Table 36.2) [54]. Combining the clinical score with a laboratory test for HIT provides the highest predictivity for HIT [55].

HIT is unlikely if (1) platelet counts decrease between days 1 and 5 of heparin treatment, (2) the patient shows overt bleeding, (3) the patient receives GP IIb/IIIa inhibitors, or (4) the patient is septic.

Laboratory tests can confirm or refute a clinical suspicion of HIT. Currently used laboratory tests fall into one of two categories: antigen assays (i.e. platelet factor 4/polyanion immunoassay) and functional (platelet activation) assays (e.g. platelet serotonin release assay [^{14}C-SRA] or heparin-induced platelet activation [HIPA] assay). Both types of tests are very good at ruling out HIT, as the negative predictive value is close to 99% [56]. However, the specificity is limited and therefore these tests only have a moderate positive predictive value. The optimal laboratory diagnostic approach is a combination of both functional and antigen assays [57].

When HIT is strongly suspected, the recommendation is to stop heparin treatment, order laboratory test for HIT antibodies, and initiate nonheparin anticoagulant treatment in therapeutic dose even in patients without thrombosis. For further information on treatment, see ➲Chapter 69.

Conclusion

Cardiac surgery and antithrombotic treatment of cardiac patients predisposes to bleeding, whereas thrombophilia and the acute medical conditions DIC and HIT mainly predispose to thromboembolic disease. Furthermore, a reduced antiplatelet effect of aspirin and/or clopidogrel ('resistance') might increase the risk of thromboembolic events in patients with coronary artery disease.

Table 36.2 Standardized clinical assessment of the probability of heparin-induced thrombocytopenia

Clinical features: the 4 T's	Probability score		
	2	1	0
Thrombocytopenia	platelet count fall >50% and platelet nadir ≥20	platelet count fall 30–50% and platelet nadir 10–19	platelet count fall <30% and platelet nadir ≤10
Timing of fall in platelet count or other sequelae	Onset day 5–10 or <1 day if heparin exposure within 30 days	>10 days, or timing unclear	Platelet count fall < 4 days, without recent heparin exposure
Thrombosis or other sequelae	New thrombosis; skin necrosis; post-heparin bolus acute systemic reaction	Progressive or recurrent thrombosis; erythematous skin lesions; suspected thrombosis—not confirmed	None
Other causes of thrombocytopenia	No other cause of platelet count fall is evident	Possible other cause is evident	Definite other cause is present

HIT, heparin-induced thrombocytopenia.
Score 0–3: HIT is very unlikely; no further testing is needed, and heparin treatment can be maintained.
Score 4–5: A minority of patients have HIT.
Score 6–8: HIT is likely, and these patients usually require substitution with a nonheparin anticoagulant.
Reproduced with permission from Lo GK, Juhl D, Warkentin TE, et al. Evaluation of pretest clinical score (4 T's) for the diagnosis of heparin-induced thrombocytopenia in two clinical settings. J Thromb Haemost 2006;**4**(4):759–765.

In acute bleeding, coagulation is evaluated by conventional coagulation analyses, often supplemented by thromboelastography. A major advantage of thromboelastography is a short turnaround time (15 min) and visual real-time display of clot development. In addition, the use of thromboelastography provides guidance for targeted haemostatic intervention.

A number of tests for evaluation of platelet function and the efficacy of antiplatelet therapy are currently being investigated. However, routine measurements of platelet function in patients on antiplatelet therapy cannot yet be recommended, because of lack of evidence on how to interpret the results in a clinical setting.

Thrombophilia is an inherited or acquired coagulation defect, which predisposes to thrombosis. Currently, there is no single laboratory assay or simple set of assays to identify thrombophilia, so a battery of complex and expensive assays is usually required.

DIC is characterized by microthrombosis and, later on, clinically overt bleeding. DIC is always secondary to an underlying disorder that causes activation of the coagulation system, e.g. sepsis. In patients with a condition known to be associated with DIC a combination of tests can be used to support the diagnosis with reasonable certainty. The cornerstone of DIC management is treatment of the underlying triggering condition.

Besides thrombocytopenia, the major clinical consequence of HIT is an enhanced risk of thrombosis. The diagnosis is based on the clinical picture and detection of platelet-activating HIT antibodies.

Personal perspective

Many new drugs now in development might be more effective in preventing ischaemic events but are also likely to increase bleeding complications. As bleeding increases cardiovascular mortality, future strategies will focus on reducing bleeding complications. By tailoring specific therapy to individual patients, such strategies may hopefully improve the benefit–risk ratio of oral antiplatelet drugs. These strategies are likely to include individual drug dosing, individual duration of therapy, and identification of risk factors and patient subgroups with a particularly increased risk of bleeding. These points are already major research areas. In particular, efforts to develop simple and reliable platelet function tests and to identify polymorphisms in key receptors and metabolic enzymes may put the concept of individually tailored therapy into practice.

Novel classes of antithrombotic drugs will be developed, including dual-function drugs inhibiting several platelet-activating pathways, or combining antiplatelet and anticoagulant activity. The safety and efficacy of these drugs will be tested in large randomized trials to select the drugs to be implemented in clinical practice to further improve the prognosis of patients with cardiovascular disease.

The scoring system for DIC will be further validated, and similar approaches for capturing coagulopathy through readily available and future assays will be developed. The potentially deleterious therapies used for treatment of DIC will be further evaluated.

Future studies performed to understand the immunobiology of HIT may help explain why host defences can result in autoimmunity. Prospective studies will be required to test the clinical utility and safety of the pretest clinical scores for HIT.

Further reading

Angiolillo DJ, Fernandez-Ortiz A, Bernardo E, *et al.* Variability in individual responsiveness to clopidogrel: clinical implications, management, and future perspectives. *J Am Coll Cardiol* 2007;**49**:1505–1516.

Grove EL, Kristensen SD. Update on oral antiplatelet therapy: principles, problems and promises. *Future Cardiol* 2009;**5**:247–258.

Hoffman M, Monroe DM. Coagulation 2006: a modern view of hemostasis. *Hematol Oncol Clin North Am* 2007;**21**:1–11.

Kuliczkowski W, Witkowski A, Polonski L, *et al.* Interindividual variability in the response to oral antiplatelet drugs: a position paper of the Working Group on antiplatelet drugs resistance appointed by the Section of Cardiovascular Interventions of the Polish Cardiac Society, endorsed by the Working Group on Thrombosis of the European Society of Cardiology. *Eur Heart J* 2009;**10**:426–435.

Levi M, Toh CH, Thachil J, Watson HG. Guidelines for the diagnosis and management of disseminated intravascular coagulation. British Committee for Standards in Haematology. *Br J Haematol* 2009;**145**:24–33.

Taylor FB, Jr., Toh CH, Hoots WK, *et al.* Towards definition, clinical and laboratory criteria, and a scoring system for disseminated intravascular coagulation. *Thromb Haemost* 2001;**86**:1327–1330.

Warkentin TE, Greinacher A, Koster A, Lincoff AM. Treatment and prevention of heparin-induced thrombocytopenia: American College of Chest Physicians Evidence-Based Clinical Practice Guidelines (8th edition). *Chest* 2008;**133**:340S–380S.

➲ For additional multimedia materials please visit the online version of the book (ℰ http://www.esciacc.oxfordmedicine.com).

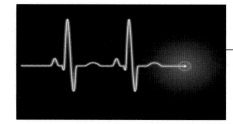

CHAPTER 37

Biomarkers for renal and hepatic failure

Martina Zaninotto, Monica Maria Mion, and Mario Plebani

Contents

Summary

In the last few years there have been major advances in the understanding of the molecular and pathophysiological mechanisms that underlie the complex interactions between the heart and the kidney, as well as between the heart and the liver, and that may explain their involvements in several diseases. According to these new insights, new biomarkers have been proposed for better evaluation and monitoring of patients affected by cardiovascular disease (CVD). In addition, some biomarkers can be considered as risk factors and offer an early identification and treatment of these severe diseases. Here we revise the most important biomarkers for evaluating the so-called cardiorenal syndrome. In particular, the measurement of serum creatinine and its use for calculating the glomerular filtration rate (eGFR) with new and more efficient equations, namely the MDRD (Modification of Diet in Renal Disease), still remains the most widely used biomarker. However, the measurement of cystatin C provides additional information, particularly in paediatric patients and in the early phase of kidney disease. Neutrophil gelatinase-associated lipocalin (NGAL) is a recently developed and very promising new biomarker for the diagnosis of acute kidney injury. The albumin/creatinine ratio has recently been re-evaluated as a simple and useful tool for the early identification of kidney disease. For liver diseases, a growing body of evidence demonstrates the usefulness of noninvasive markers of hepatic fibrosis, e.g. Fibrotest, that may avoid the need for liver biopsy in most patients. A promising field of research is represented by the role of nonalcoholic fatty liver disease (NAFLD) in the pathogenesis of CVD. C-reactive protein and fibrinogen are well-known CVD risk factors, and the role of adiponectin is under investigation.

The cardiorenal syndrome

Pathophysiological mechanisms

The term 'cardiorenal syndrome' (CRS) has increasingly been used in recent years without a clear meaning or an agreed definition [1, 2]. Actually, CRS can be generally defined as a pathophysiological disorder of the heart and kidney whereby acute or chronic dysfunction in one organ may induce acute or chronic dysfunction in the other. Although it is generally defined as a condition characterized by the initiation or progression of renal insufficiency secondary to heart failure, the term CRS is also used to describe the negative effects of reduced renal function on the heart and circulation. The absence of a clear definition, and the complexity of the heart–kidney interactions, contribute to a lack of clarity with regard to diagnosis and management. Consequently, in order to include the vast array of interrelated derangements and to stress the bidirectional nature of the heart-kidney interactions, the proposed classification now includes five subtypes whose etymology reflects the primary and secondary pathology, the time frame, and the simultaneous cardiac and renal codysfunction secondary to systemic disease [3] (see ➲ Chapter 66 for further details):

- ◆ type I: acute cardiorenal syndrome
- ◆ type II: chronic cardiorenal syndrome
- ◆ type III: acute renocardial syndrome
- ◆ type IV: chronic renocardial syndrome
- ◆ type V: secondary cardiorenal syndrome.

Biomarkers

Quantitation of overall renal function is based on the assumption that all functioning nephrons are performing normally and that a decline in renal function is due to loss of functioning nephrons quantitatively related to the loss. Thus, in nearly all types of renal disease, impaired kidney function is attributed to a reduced number of nephrons rather than to compromised function of individual nephrons. Because glomerular filtration is the initiating phase of all nephron functions, quantitative or qualitative assessment of filtration generally provides the most useful indices for physicians to assess the severity and progress of kidney damage. Several biochemical markers have proved to be the most practical and useful system for the screening and diagnosis of impaired kidney function, as well as for monitoring the course and managing the progression of the disease.

Here we review some of the most popular and widely used biochemical markers as well as new tests recently proposed.

Creatinine

The most widely used endogenous marker of glomerular filtration rate (GFR) is creatinine, expressed either as its plasma concentration or its renal clearance. In fact, creatinine (molecular mass 113 Da) is freely filtered at the glomerulus and its concentration is inversely related to GFR. As a GFR marker, it is convenient and cheap to measure but is affected by age, sex, exercise, certain drugs, muscle mass, nutritional status, and meal intake. Further, a small (but significant) and variable proportion of creatinine, typically 7–10%, is due to tubular secretion but this is increased in the presence of renal insufficiency [4]. Plasma creatinine remains within the reference interval until significant renal function has been lost, showing an unsatisfactory sensitivity in the early diagnosis of kidney insufficiency. Thus, although an elevated plasma creatinine concentration generally equates to impaired kidney function, a normal plasma creatinine does not necessarily imply normal kidney function. Because of all these limitations, it is recommended that plasma creatinine measurement alone is not used to assess kidney function [5].

Creatinine clearance and glomerular filtration rate

Because creatinine is endogenously produced and released into body fluids at a constant rate, its clearance has been measured as an indicator of GFR. Historically, creatinine clearance has been seen as more sensitive for detection of renal dysfunction than measurement of plasma creatinine, but it requires a timed urine collection which introduces its own inaccuracies. Furthermore, in adults the intraindividual day-to-day creatinine clearance variability may exceed 25%, and this further devalues the use of creatinine clearance as a measure of GFR. Creatinine clearance and GFR are not equivalent: as kidney function declines, creatinine clearance becomes significantly higher because of the preserved tubular secretion of creatinine, and may be twice the true GFR when the GFR is severely reduced. The best overall measure of kidney function is GFR, measured as the urinary or plasma clearance of an ideal filtration marker such as inulin or of alternative exogenous markers such as iothalamate or EDTA [6].

Estimated glomerular filtration rate

More than 25 different formulas have been derived that estimated GFR using plasma creatinine corrected for some or all of gender, body size, race, and age. Indeed, the National Kidney Foundation has recommended that the Cockcroft and Gault or Modification of Diet in Renal Diseases (MDRD) formula should be used in adults.

The Cockcroft–Gault formula was developed in 1976 [7] with the data from 249 men with creatinine clearance (C_{cr}) from 30 to 130 mL per minute. It systematically overestimates GFR because of the tubular secretion of creatinine. The values are not adjusted for body surface area; a comparison with normal values of creatinine clearance requires measurement of height, computation of body surface area, and adjustment to 1.73 m^2.

The MDRD study equation was developed in 1999 [8], using data from 1628 patients with chronic kidney disease (CKD), and re-expressed in 2005 for use with a standardized serum creatinine assay. This estimating equation takes into consideration some simple variables such as age, sex, and race, already available in the laboratory information system. In ⊃ Fig. 37.1, the accuracy of different proposed mathematical equations for assessing estimated GFR (eGFR) is compared: the MDRD equation seems to be the most accurate evaluation.

On the basis of eGFR values obtained with the MDRD equation, five stages of kidney disease have been defined, as shown in ⊃ Table 37.1.

The National Kidney Disease Education Program suggests that laboratories should report estimated GFR using the original four-variable MDRD study equation, recognizing less accuracy when the calibration used was not traceable to the reference method, especially at a level of less than 60 mL min^{-1} 1.73 m^{-2}. More recently, a new equation called CKD-EPI has been developed by the same authors who developed the MDRD. The CKD-EPI equation is more accurate than the MDRD and makes it possible to obtain a

Table 37.1 Stages of kidney disease and eGFR values

Stage	mL min^{-1} 1.73 m^{-2}
1 Normal GFR	>90
2 Mild impairment	60–90
3 Moderate impairment	30–59
4 Severe impairment	15–29
5 Established	<15

lower bias, especially at an estimated GFR greater than 60 mL min^{-1} 1.73 m^{-2} [9]. The improved accuracy of the CKD-EPI equation overcomes some limitations of the MDRD equation and could replace it for routine clinical use.

Cystatin C

Cystatin C is a low molecular weight protein (13 kDa) synthesized at a constant rate by virtually all nucleated cells. It is a member of a family of competitive inhibitors of lysosomal cysteine proteinase [10]. With regard to renal function, due to its free filtration at the glomerulus, complete reabsorption, and catabolism in the proximal tubule without tubular secretion, the circulating concentration of plasma cystatin C has been thought to depend almost exclusively on GFR. Several variables influence cystatin C circulating levels [11], and a cystatin C-based equation performs better when factors such as age, sex, race, and body mass index (BMI) are considered in the formula. The influence of muscle mass on cystatin C plasma concentration is far less than for creatinine [12]. The pooled diagnostic odds ratios for cystatin C and creatinine overlap, making it difficult to clarify which biomarker perform better [13].

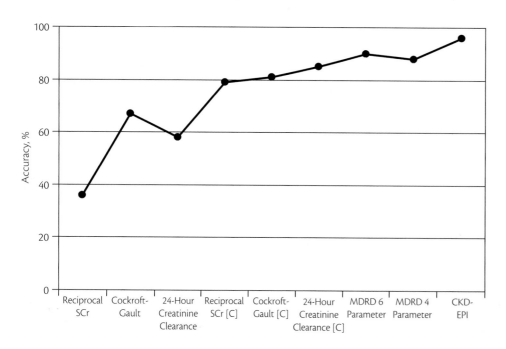

Figure 37.1 GFR estimation. See text for details of methods. SCr, serum creatinine.

Data from Myer GL, Miller WG, Coresh J, et al. Recommendations for improving serum creatinine measurement: a report from the laboratory working group of the National Kidney Disease Education Program. Clin Chem 2006;**52**:5–18; and Stevens LA, Coresh J, Schmid CH, et al. Estimating GFR using serum cystatin C alone and in combination with serum creatinine: a pooled analysis of 3,418 individuals with CKD. Am J Kidney Dis 2008;**51**:395–406.

Cystatin C and established cardiovascular risk factors

In recent years cystatin C has been proposed as a new risk marker for cardiovascular events. An independent association between high concentrations of cystatin C and established cardiovascular risk factors (age, female sex, smoking, low HDL cholesterol, BMI) has been observed in individuals without CKD or microalbuminuria, showing a risk profile similar to that of patients suffering from CKD, and interestingly, individuals with high cystatin C concentrations and no CKD showed higher prevalence of obesity and hypertension than those with low cystatin C concentrations and CKD [14]. Similarly, not only the prevalence of cardiovascular risk factors but also the prevalence of cardiovascular disease (CVD), such as myocardial infarction (MI), angina pectoris, or stroke, was higher among patients showing higher cystatin C concentrations. Furthermore, an independent association between cystatin C and hypertension has also been demonstrated in some studies [15].

Cystatin C and prediction of cardiovascular outcome

The prognostic role of cystatin C in older people (age: ≥65 years; median follow-up 7.4 years), investigated for all-cause mortality and for death from CVD, shows an adjusted hazard ratio increasing from the lowest to the highest cystatin C concentrations, as well as an independent association with the risk of developing MI and stroke for patients showing the highest cystatin C concentrations. In recent years, cystatin C has been demonstrated to be a better risk factor for the development of heart failure and peripheral arterial disease than conventional renal failure markers, also after multivariable adjustment [16]. Furthermore, in elderly patients without clinical CKD, cystatin C concentrations were also associated with cardiovascular and renal outcomes [17]. In nonhospitalized patients with coronary artery disease (previous MI, ≥50% coronary stenosis in epicardial vessels, myocardial ischaemia, previous coronary revascularization), higher cystatin C concentrations were associated with higher incidence of fatal and nonfatal events apart from renal function, while in acute coronary syndrome patients, cystatin C evidences a more accurate prognostic value for the mortality rate, in comparison to other traditional markers of renal function [18]. However the association between cystatin C concentrations and CVD mortality did not reach statistical significance after adjustment for biochemical markers of cardiac function, such as cardiac natriuretic peptide, or for chronic inflammation, such as C-reactive protein (CRP) concentrations.

Cystatin C appears to be of particular value in identifying patients at a higher risk for cardiovascular events among those classified as low risk by traditional markers (creatinine, eGFR), because it seems more sensitive than serum creatinine in detecting a small reduction in GFR (preclinical kidney dysfunction), thus revealing early GFR abnormalities potentially associated with adverse clinical outcomes [19].

Renal function is the link between cystatin C and cardiovascular outcome, even if this predictive ability has not been studied in patients with completely normal renal function. An important common limitation of these studies is that they have not measured GFR directly. Specific, well-designed trials are required to answer the important question of whether pathogenetic mechanisms other than renal dysfunction could account for a high cystatin C concentration and explain its predictive value for future cardiovascular risk.

Inflammation, associated with atherogenic changes, may be one mechanism associated with cystatin C and cardiovascular risk, and high cystatin C concentrations have been found to be associated with high concentrations of CRP: it has been suggested that high cystatin C concentrations are directly related to both inflammation and atherosclerosis (➲ Fig. 37.2). Inflammatory cytokines associated with atherosclerosis stimulate the production of lysosomal cathepsin, and consequently of cystatin C, a cathepsin inhibitor. Moreover, human cathepsin is expressed in many cells (endothelial cells, smooth muscle cells, macrophages) involved in the progression, composition, and rupture of atherosclerotic plaques [20].

Neutrophil gelatinase-associated lipocalin

NGAL (also known as lipocalin 2, siderocalin, 24p3, LCN2 or human neutrophil lipocalin) is a small molecule (25 kDa) belonging to the secreted lipocalin superfamily of cytosolic proteins with barrel-like structures carrying hydrophobic ligands [21]. It is expressed by neutrophils and various human tissues, with the loop of Henle and collecting ducts as main production sites in the kidney [22]. Recent studies suggest that NGAL may have an important role in defending against bacterial strains depending on siderophores through iron sequestration [23], in kidney development, as a growth factor, in renal regeneration and repair after ischaemic injury and in kidney protection [24]. The potential role of NGAL as a biomarker has been evaluated in many renal and nonrenal conditions, in particular in acute kidney injury (AKI), renal transplantation, CKD, and other systemic disorders.

Acute kidney injury

AKI is a serious and frequent clinical complication among hospitalized patients [25]. Serum creatinine as well as blood urea nitrogen (BUN) or urinary markers of kidney

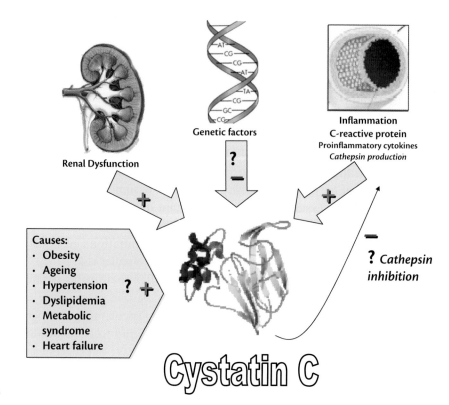

Figure 37.2 Proposed mechanisms linking renal dysfunction, inflammation, atherogenesis, and cardiovascular events.
Data from Iseki K, Ikemiya Y, Iseki C, Takishita S. Proteinuria and the risk of developing end-stage renal disease. *Kidney Int* 2003;**63**:1468–1474.

injury reflect the delayed functional alteration of the kidney, rising after cellular damage when a significant amount of renal function has been lost, thus limiting their usefulness in the early detection of AKI. An early diagnosis of AKI could allow the early institution of therapeutic measures for kidney function protection, which may result in preserved renal function and avoidance of renal replacement therapy. Rapid identification of the early phase of AKI still represents a major clinical challenge: recently, NGAL has been reported as an emerging early biomarker of AKI.

The predictive value of NGAL for AKI has been studied in various clinical settings [26] and NGAL appears to be a valuable renal biomarker in all settings of AKI, even if the predictive value seems to be lower in adults than in children. Plasma/serum and urine NGAL levels appear to perform similarly well, providing a relevant advantage in comparison to serum creatinine [27], in particular in term of sensitivity and risk stratification. In studies with standardized assay platforms, the reported cut-off value for NGAL was more than 150 ng/mL; different cut-offs have been reported

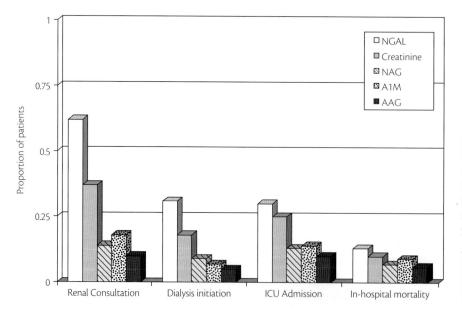

Figure 37.3 Values of different kidney injury biomarkers and clinical outcome. A1M, α1-microglobulin; AAG, α1-acid glycoprotein; NAG, *N*-acetyl-B-glucosaminidase.
Adapted with permission from Nickolas TL, O' Rourke MJ, *et al.* Sensitivity and Specificity of a Single Emergency Department Measurement of Urinary Neutrophil Gelatinase–Associated Lipocalin for Diagnosing Acute Kidney Injury. *Ann Intern Med* 2008;**148**:810–819.

for research-based assays. In patients undergoing cardiopulmonary bypass, NGAL concentration in plasma increased much more quickly than serum creatinine, in case of AKI. Furthermore, a single measurement of urinary NGAL helps to distinguish acute injury from normal function, prerenal uraemia, and CKD, and predicts poor in-hospital outcome [28, 29] (⊃ Fig. 37.3). In conclusion, NGAL seems to be an earlier and a more sensitive marker of renal injury compared with serum creatinine level: NGAL value may allow earlier and more successful renal interventions and thus serve as a useful marker of renal injury in clinical studies of renoprotective strategies and in risk stratification.

Urinary proteins and albumin/creatinine ratio

Proteinuria is the main sign of kidney disease, and testing urine samples for the measurement of total protein loss is a well established and inexpensive test for kidney injury. Urinary protein determination is indicated not only in newly diagnosed or suspected clinical conditions (kidney disease, hypertension, haematuria, diabetes mellitus, heart failure, pre-eclampsia, oedema, systemic vasculitis, and multisystem disease) to detect underlying kidney injury, but also in the monitoring of patients with CKD. Proteinuria in CKD identifies patients at increased risk of renal injury progression [30], CVD, and death [31]. Moreover, the reduction in proteinuria and the residual level of proteinuria achieved with renoprotective therapy represent useful prognostic tools [32].

There is no agreement about the level that identifies clinically significant proteinuria [33], although there is relatively good agreement on the definitions of normo-, micro- and macroalbuminuria. Normally only small quantities of albumin are lost in urine, and about 50% of the urinary total proteins is Tamm–Horsfall glycoprotein (THG) [34]. In the past, proteinuria was detected by measuring total protein or albumin in a timed collection (usually a 24-h urine collection). More recently the 'urine total protein/creatinine ratio' (PCR) or 'albumin/creatinine ratio' has been proposed and adopted as a more convenient solution, and several studies have demonstrated that PCR determined on a random urine sample represents a reliable alternative to protein measurement on a 24-h urine sample [35]. Measurement of urinary albumin is the test of choice for detection of diabetic nephropathy, while urinary total protein determination is used prevalently to investigate renal diseases. Measurement of urinary albumin as the front-line test for proteinuria detection allows a reliable and sensitive approach for an early detection and management of kidney injury [36]. Increased albuminuria is associated with onset of heart failure in various clinical settings. Mild levels of albuminuria appear to be associated with systemic endothelial dysfunction that increases the risk for hypertension, insulin resistance, diabetes, and CVD. On the other hand, high levels of albuminuria appear to reflect overt kidney injury in patients with high cardiovascular risk [37, 38]. In patients with cardiovascular risk (hypertension, left ventricular hypertrophy, diabetes, history of CVD), albuminuria represents a further risk factor at low or high concentrations. In patients with established heart failure, albuminuria is highly prevalent and appears to be associated with a worse prognosis [39]. In conclusion, albuminuria may represent a valuable tool for the physician in predicting the risk for heart failure and in evaluating the effectiveness of the established therapy.

The heart–liver connection

Chronic as well as acute heart diseases can affect the function of the liver and, vice versa, liver dysfunction affects the heart [40]. Liver injury encountered in clinical practice of CVD patients is arbitrarily divided into acute and chronic, based on the duration or persistence of liver injury.

Acute insults may arise from transient deprivation of blood flow and oxygen, and from the return of blood flow during reperfusion in acute MI and cardiogenic shock. Chronic heart disease, namely haemodynamic changes owing to right or left cardiac failure, can lead to reduced liver perfusion and, secondarily, to the impairment of liver function. In particular, liver damage in congestive heart failure may further progress to liver cirrhosis.

Acute liver diseases

Ischemia and reperfusion injury (IRI) represents a complex series of events that result in cellular and tissue damage of the liver. In particular, cardiogenic ischaemic hepatitis (CIH) is often seen in the face of acute cardiogenic shock. CIH is defined as a rapid and marked increase of serum transaminases and is diagnosed when there are extremely high levels (>1000 U/L) of alanine aminotranferease (ALT) and/or aspartate aminotransferase (AST), acute arterial hypertension is present and acute liver failure is excluded [41]. The liver enzymes fall rapidly to normal levels once the circulation is restored. Oxygen free radicals, nitric oxide, and several chemokines and cytokines may mediate and modulate this process [42].

Oxygen free radicals and scavengers

Oxygen free radicals (OFRs) are considered one of the most significant components of cell and tissue damage during ischaemia and reperfusion. Among OFRs, hydrogen peroxide, superoxide anion, and hydroxyl radical represent the main aggressive components, while among the OFRs scavengers and inhibitors, superoxide dismutase (SOD) represents an important and even measurable biomarker [43].

Leucocytes and inflammatory mediators

Leucocytes are highly involved in liver IRI and function both to amplify the molecular pathways, and to cause cellular damage directly [44, 45]. A number of mechanisms may account for leucocyte infiltration during liver IRI: P-selectin, phosphatidylserine (PS), various cytokines and chemokines (CXCL10, RANTES, MCP-1, MIP-1α, MIP-1β) and metalloproteinases (MMP), e.g. MMP-9 [46]. Moreover, nitric oxide (NO) plays a significant role in the microcirculation and organ IRI, exerting both beneficial and harmful effects [47].

However, these new insights and experimental evidence have not been translated into clinical practice and currently none of previously described mediators other than transaminases is a valuable biomarker for detecting acute liver damage in CVD.

Chronic liver diseases

The distinction between acute and chronic liver injury is a mechanistic oversimplification. Chronic liver injury reflects, in part, continuous acute liver injury extended over time; however, it leads to progressive fibrosis that can eventually result in cirrhosis, liver failure, or hepatocellular carcinoma [48]. Liver fibrosis represents a hallmark of chronic liver diseases and cirrhosis, and staging of hepatic fibrosis is of paramount clinical importance for the prognostic assessment in the individual patient. Liver biopsy still represents the gold standard for evaluating presence, type, and stage of liver fibrosis but this procedure is invasive, costly, and difficult to standardize [49]. In recent years there has been increasing interest in identifying and describing liver fibrosis by using noninvasive biochemical markers measurable in the peripheral blood.

Biochemical markers of liver fibrosis

Biochemical markers of liver fibrosis may be classified into two broad groups: direct or indirect markers of fibrogenesis.

Direct markers of fibrogenesis

These are a direct expression of either the deposition or the removal of extracellular matrix in the liver, and they include several glycoproteins (hyaluronan, laminin, YKL-40), the collagen family (procollagen III, type IV collagen), collagenases and their inhibitors, and a number of cytokines connected with the fibrogenetic process (TGF-β1, TNF-β). Some of these biochemical markers, e.g. hyaluronan

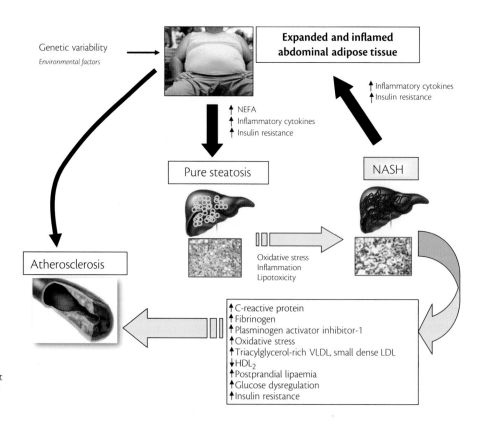

Figure 37.4 Biochemical and genetic mechanisms linking nonalcoholic fatty liver disease (NAFLD) to pathogenesis of cardiovascular disease. NASH, nonalcoholic steatohepatitis. Adapted with permission from Targher G, Marra F, Marchesini G. Increased risk of cardiovascular disease in nonalcoholic fatty liver disease: causal effect or epiphenomenon? *Diabetologia* 2008; **51**:1947–1953..

and type III procollagen, have demonstrated a good accuracy in excluding cirrhosis, but their performance in defining the stage of liver fibrosis greatly varies from one study to another, with a wide range of sensitivity and specificity [49].

Indirect markers

These are single or combined haematological or biochemical parameters that reflect the stage of liver disease. The first indirect markers of liver fibrosis are transaminases, particularly when reported as AST/ALT ratio (AAR). A further evolution of this index is the so-called APRI (AST/platelet ratio index). In the last few years many other test panels have been proposed, but the most widely investigated combination set of noninvasive markers of liver fibrosis is Fibrotest. This is a combination of five blood tests including γ-glutamyl transpeptidase (GGT), bilirubin, haptoglobin, apolipoprotein A1, and $α_2$-macroglobulin, adjusted for gender and age by using a patent algorithm [50]. Fibrotest has been extensively tested in chronic hepatitis, namely virus C hepatitis, where the area under the curve (AUC) turns out to be around 0.85 for significant fibrosis. Recently, a new combination algorithm of noninvasive markers of liver fibrosis in chronic hepatitis C was able to identify significant fibrosis with a high diagnostic accuracy (>94%), allowing a 50% reduction in the number of liver biopsies [51].

Cirrhotic cardiomyopathy

Cirrhotic cardiomyopathy is defined as 'a cardiac dysfunction in patients with cirrhosis that is characterized by impaired contractile responsiveness to stress and/or altered diastolic relaxation with electrophysiological abnormalities in the absence of other known cardiac disease' [52]. Elevations of B-type natriuretic peptide (BNP) and NT-proBNP correlate with the severity of cirrhosis and with the degree of cardiac dysfunction, as well as with the intraventricular septal and left ventricular wall thickness [53]. A possible role for adrenomedullin, a hormone involved in the regulation of vascular tone and natriuresis, was recently reported [54]: adrenomedullin may contribute to myocardial dysfunction in cirrhosis via the negative inotropic effect of NO. Serum levels of this hormone are higher in cirrhosis, more in ascitic than in nonascitic patients.

Risk of cardiovascular disease in liver disease

Recent cross-sectional and prospective studies on the association between nonalcoholic fatty liver disease (NAFLD) and intermediate markers of CVD or clinical outcomes indicate not only a link but a causal role of NAFLD in the pathogenesis of CVD [55]. Current understanding of the pathogenesis of NAFLD implies that lipids accumulate in hepatocytes in the presence of insulin resistance and that multiple factors including nonessential fatty acids (NEFA), hormones, proinflammatory cytokines and adipocytokines are involved in atherogenetic process, as shown in ⊃ Fig. 37.4.

The liver is central for the production of classical biomarkers of inflammation and endothelial dysfunction, the secretion of which depends, at least in part, on factors that are up-regulated in the presence of insulin resistance and the metabolic syndrome. Fibrinogen and CRP are increased in NAFLD patients, particularly in those with steatohepatitis (NASH). In the last few years, the importance of adiponectin has been increasingly recognized and hypoadiponectinaemia resulted to be independently associated with NASH and with more severe hepatic steatosis and necroinflammation [56]. The measurement of these biochemical markers should be suggested to allow an early diagnosis and effective treatment of these disease.

Conclusion

Noninvasive biomarkers should be useful for better evaluation and monitoring of patients affected by cardiovascular diseases and, in addition, as risk factors as well as for the early identification and treatment of these severe diseases.

Although some biomarkers, such as eGFR, albumin/creatinine ratio and natriuretic peptides (BNP and/or NT-pro-BNP) have a well-defined role in current clinical practice, for some other promising biomarkers such as NGAL, cystatin C, and noninvasive tests for liver fibrosis further studies are necessary to translate research insights into well-defined clinical guidelines. In addition to the evidence of analytical efficiency and standardization, more data on diagnostic and clinical effectiveness are necessary.

Personal perspective

The major advances in the understanding of molecular and pathophysiological mechanisms which underlie the complex interactions between the heart and the kidney, as well as between the heart and the liver, have paved the way to the development of new biomarkers aiming to better evaluate and monitor patients affected by CVD.

From our viewpoint, the most promising biomarkers in the field of kidney involvement in CVDs are cystatin C and NGAL. Cystatin C measurement may detect a small reduction in GFR (preclinical kidney dysfunction), thus revealing early GFR abnormalities potentially associated with adverse clinical outcomes in patient affected by CVD. In addition, as the rapid identification of the early phase of AKI still represents a major clinical challenge,

NGAL seems to be an effective tool for improving its diagnosis.

Regarding the association between heart and liver diseases, the most promising biomarkers seem to be related to the noninvasive diagnosis and monitoring of liver fibrosis in patients suffering from chronic conditions. The rational combination of existing panels of laboratory tests has proved to be an effective and inexpensive tool for reducing the number of inappropriate liver biopsies. Current understanding of the pathogenesis of NAFLD in the presence of insulin resistance, multiple factors including NEFA, hormones, pro-inflammatory cytokines, and adipocytokines has clarified its role in the atherogenetic process. This, in turn, may support the utilization of new biomarkers, e.g. adiponectin, in clinical practice in order to evaluate the early steps of liver disease and CVD.

Further reading

Arnlov J, Evans JC, Meigs JB, *et al*. Low-grade albuminuria and incidence of cardiovascular disease events in nonhypertensive and nondiabetic individuals: the Framingham Heart Study. *Circulation* 2005;**112**:969–975.

Cirillo M, Lanti MP, Menotti A, *et al*. Definition of kidney dysfunction as a cardiovascular risk factor: use of urinary albumin excretion and estimated glomerular filtration rate. *Arch Intern Med* 2008;**168**:617–624.

Iwao T, Oho K, Nakano R, *et al*. High plasma cardiac natriuretic peptides associated with enhanced cyclic guanosine monophosphate production in preascitic cirrhosis. *J Hepatol* 2000;**32**:426–433.

Keller T, Messow CM, Lubos E, *et al*. Cystatin C and cardiovascular mortality in patients with coronary artery disease and normal or mildly reduced kidney function: results from the AtheroGene study. *Eur Heart J* 2009;**30**:314–320.

Levey AS. Measurement of renal function in chronic renal disease. *Kidney Int* 1990;**38**:167–184.

MacDonald J, Marcova S, Jibani M, *et al*. GFR estimation using cystatin C is not independent of body composition. *Am J Kidney Dis* 2006;**48**:712–719.

Muntner P, Mann D, Winston J, *et al*. Serum cystatin C and increased coronary heart disease prevalence in US adults without chronic kidney disease. *Am J Cardiol* 2008;**102**:54–57.

National Kidney Foundation. K/DOQI clinical practice guidelines for chronic kidney disease: evaluation, classification, and stratification. Kidney Disease Outcome Quality Initiative. *Am J Kidney Dis* 2002;**39**:S1–S246.

Pan CS, Jin SJ, Cao CQ, *et al*. The myocardial response to adrenomedullin involves increased cAMP generation as well as augmented Akt phosphorylation. *Peptides* 2007;**28**:900–909.

Ronco C, House AA, Haapio M. Cardiorenal syndrome: refining the definition of a complex symbiosis gone wrong. *Intensive Care Med* 2008;**34**:957–962.

Ruggenenti P, Perna A, Mosconi L, *et al*. Urinary protein excretion rate is the best independent predictor of ESRF in non-diabetic proteinuric chronic nephropathies. 'Gruppo Italiano di Studi Epidemiologici in Nefrologia' (GISEN). *Kidney Int* 1998;**53**:1209–1216.

Uttenthal O. NGAL: a marker molecule for the distressed kidney? *Clin Lab Int* 2005;**29**:39–41.

⊃ For additional multimedia materials please visit the online version of the book (🕮 http://www.esciacc.oxfordmedicine.com).

SECTION VII

Acute coronary syndrome

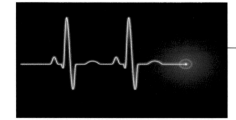

CHAPTER 38

Atherosclerosis and thrombosis

Lina Badimon, Gemma Vilahur, and Teresa Padró

Contents

Summary

Atherosclerosis is the underlying cause of nearly all causes of coronary artery disease and peripheral arterial disease and many cases of stroke. Atherosclerosis is a systemic inflammatory process characterized by the accumulation of macrophages/lymphocytes and lipids within the intima of large arteries. The deposition of these blood-borne materials and the subsequent thickening of the wall may significantly compromise the residual lumen, leading to ischaemic events distal to the arterial stenosis. However, these initial fatty streak lesions may also evolve into fibrous plaques vulnerable to rupture or erosion. Plaque disruption initiates both platelet adhesion and aggregation on the exposed vascular surface and the activation of the clotting cascade leading to the so-called atherothrombotic process. In fact, many local and systemic 'thrombogenic risk factors' at the time of plaque disruption influence the duration of thrombus deposition and hence the different pathological and clinical syndromes.

This chapter describes our current understanding of the pathophysiological mechanisms involved in atherogenesis, from fatty streaks to complex and vulnerable atheromas, and highlights the molecular machinery used by platelets and the coagulation components to initiate and accelerate the thrombotic process.

Introduction

Atherosclerosis is a systemic disease that starts early in life, asymptomatically progressing though adulthood, until clinically manifested [1]. Initial fatty streak lesions evolve into fibrous plaques, some of which develop into forms that are vulnerable to rupture or erosion, causing the so-called atherothrombotic process. This common pathophysiological process results in morbid or fatal ischaemic events with clinical manifestations such as coronary artery disease, cerebrovascular disease, and peripheral artery disease [2]. Treatments such as diet modification, exercise, and drugs that affect cardiovascular risk factors, mainly plasma lipids and hypertension, may induce changes in the clinical manifestations and in the natural pathology of plaques and arteries. Besides, the beneficial role of antiplatelet drugs in reducing the incidence of events supports a major role of platelets in the atherothrombotic process in the arterial tree.

Atherosclerosis

Atherosclerotic lesions result from a complex interplay between circulating factors and various cell types in the vessel wall, triggered by the chronic and repeated exposure to several systemic and local injurious stimuli. A high level of plasma lipids, particularly low-density lipoproteins (LDL) is a major cause of vascular damage [3]. Several risk factors may intensify or provoke atherosclerosis, including hypertension, smoking, diabetes, obesity, and genetic predisposition. Apart from epidemiological evidence for the proatherogenic role of lipoproteins, mechanistic studies suggest that they play a role in relevant features for initiation and progression of lesions, as endothelial dysfunction, intimal disorganization and thickening. In advanced atheromatous plaques, high content of extra- and intracellular lipid deposits are associated with a high risk of vulnerability to rupture, causing thrombosis and its clinical complications [4].

Initial changes in the vascular wall

The influx of LDL into the subendothelial tissue, its focal retention on extracellular matrix molecules and subsequent transformation in modified LDL (e.g. aggregated and oxidized), is accompanied by increased adhesiveness of leucocytes and platelets to the endothelium. In particular, monocytes enter the subendothelium and differentiate into macrophages. Eventually, T cells and mast cells enter the lesions, and along with macrophages contribute to the known inflammatory response. This, along with the migration of smooth muscle cells (SMC) from the media into the intima and their change into a dedifferentiated phenotype, are the major changes during initiation and progression of atherosclerotic lesions.

Lipoprotein infiltration and retention

LDL is a heterogeneous class of lipoprotein particles consisting of a hydrophobic core containing triglycerides and cholesterol esters in a hydrophilic shell of phospholipids, free cholesterol, and apolipoproteins, predominantly B-100. The entry and retention of LDL within the subendothelial space mainly depend on its sustained plasma levels [5]. However, other possible determinants such as lipoprotein

size, cholesterol enrichment, and endothelial permeability (trancytosis or intercellular transport) and endothelial cell derived biosynthetic activity (i.e. synthesis of the basement membrane and extracellular matrix) may also affect entry and retention [6].

Extracellullar proteoglycans are the most important lipoprotein-retaining molecules in the subendothelium [7]. Proteoglycans are abundant in atherosclerotic lesions, and they associate with several specific regions of the apoB-fraction of subendothelial located lipoproteins, especially LDL particles of lowest density. The main proteoglycans in the extracellular matrix (ECM) are those that contain side chains of chondroitin sulphate (CS-PG), such as versican or biglycan. In addition, LDL retention within the vessel wall may occur via lipoprotein association with other matrix molecules like lipoprotein lipase, sphingomyelinase, and phospholipase A_2 [5]. Lipoproteins retained in the subendothelial space become modified, displaying characteristics different from native LDL that make them even more atherogenic. Thus LDL can be oxidized (oxLDL) by exposure to EC, SMC, or monocytes/macrophages expressing lipooxygenases [8]. Our group demonstrated that the interaction between versican and LDL produces structural changes in the LDL particle that lead to fused LDL similar in size to aggregated LDL (agLDL) obtained by vortexing and those described in atherosclerotic lesions [9]. Other routes of LDL modification include glycation, enzymatic proteolysis, lipolysis, and incorporation in immune complexes. Collagen, considered to be the major extracellular protein in advanced lesions, has a high capacity to interact with nLDL and oxLDL by ionic interactions, and glycated collagen binds LDL covalently. Also elastin of human arterial intima has been shown to contain large amounts of 'perifibrous lipid' (small lipid droplets and vesicles), and elastin extracted from atherosclerotic intima has higher capacity to bind LDL than that extracted from normal arterial intima.

Endothelial and vascular smooth muscle cell responses

Regional phenotypes of vascular endothelial cells and SMC have significant implications in the progression of vascular disease. During early atherogenesis, the endothelium becomes activated, and SMCs undergo 'phenotypic switching. The endothelium is a crucial regulator of vascular physiology, producing in healthy conditions several substances with potent antiatherothrombotic effects. Indeed, endothelium is involved in the release of various vasodilators, including nitric oxide (NO), prostacyclin, and endothelium-derived hyperpolarizing factor, as well as vasoconstrictors such as endothelin-1. NO plays an important role in the regulation of vascular tone, inhibition of platelet aggregation, and suppression of SMC proliferation. In addition, NO blocks the expression of proinflammatory molecules such as NFκB [10], adhesion molecules (ICAM-1, VCAM-1, P-selectin), as well as leucocyte adhesion and infiltration [11]. Endothelial dysfunction is the initial step in the pathogenesis of atherosclerosis and is induced in response to local and systemic risk factors. Thus, NO release by endothelial cells can be up-regulated (i.e. estrogens, exercise, and dietary factors) and/or down-regulated (i.e. high levels of LDL, smoking, or oxidative stress). A decrease in the bioavailability of endothelial NO may derive from a reduction in the concentration and/or activation of NO synthetase as well as with an enhanced NO degradation through the formation of superoxide anions (O^{2-}) [12]. Deactivation of NO by O^{2-} gives rise to highly cytotoxic peroxynitrite radicals that in turn inhibit the expression of prostacyclin synthetase and favour its nitrosylation, a process that has recently been linked to superoxide-induced endothelial dysfunction in vascular disease. Besides NO, other vasoactive compounds such as cytochrome P450 (CYP), monooxygenases, and endothelin-1 are altered in endothelial dysfunction [1]. Cell–cell connections such as tight junctions and gap junctions are essential structures in the control of the endothelial permeability function. The formation of gap junctions is regulated by the presence and functionality of connexins, proteins whose expression is altered during the formation of atherosclerotic lesions [13]. Gap junctions, in addition to facilitate intercellular signalling, regulate NO-dependent vasodilation processes.

SMCs, the major component of the vascular wall, are characterized by their high plasticity. Under the effect of atherogenic stimuli, SMCs undergo phenotypic changes ranging from differentiation to the acquisition of a synthetic phenotype. Thus, SMCs with a nonproliferative contractile phenotype, typical in the vascular media of healthy arteries, transform into actively proliferative cells (synthetic phenotype) and migrate toward the vascular intima, attracted by chemotactic agents expressed by activated endothelial cells, monocytes, and platelets [14]. Recent data indicate, as potential source of SMCs in the intima, migrating resident SMCs from the tunica media, circulating progenitor cells from bone marrow, and progenitor cells present in the vessel adventitia [15]. SMC express a variety of receptors for cholesterol uptake, thereby participating in the early accumulation of plaque lipid. These include different members of the LDL receptor family (LDL-R, LRP, VLDL-R) and the scavenger receptor family (i.e. CD36, type I and type II scavenger receptors, CXCL16/SR-PSOX) [15]. In the presence of agLDL, the SMCs over-express receptors such as LRP-1, which not only facilitates LDL internalization and the subsequent transformation of SMC into foam cells, but also acts as a receptor for many other ligands and participates in signalling processes [9].

Effects of flow and geometry

Local haemodynamic factors are major determinants of the initiation and progression of individual atherosclerotic plaques. Atherogenesis occurs predominantly at branches and bends of the arterial tree that are exposed to relatively low or recirculating blood flow, whereas arterial regions that are exposed to relatively higher time-averaged shear stress and pulsatile laminar flow are less susceptible to plaque formation. Atheroprone regions in vivo and atheroprone shear stress on the endothelium in vitro can induce proinflammatory priming indicated by the activation and regulation of downstream inflammatory targets [16]. Using an in vitro coculture method of endothelial cells and SMC, atheroprone shear stress applied to endothelial cells modulate a proinflammatory phenotype in endothelial cells and SMCs and proatherogenic phenotypic switching in SMCs via epigenetic modifications at the chromatin level [17]. In addition, high shear stress down-regulates angiotensin type 1 receptor expression in endothelial cells and abrogates apoptosis induced by different stimuli in this vascular cell type.

Progression of vascular lesions
Immunoinflamatory response

Inflammation is central to cardiovascular disease. The infiltration of leukocytes (monocytes and T cells) into the intravascular space is an important feature during the development of atherosclerotic lesions. Atherosclerotic lesions from the early stage (fatty streak) to complicated lesions possess all the features of chronic inflammation. It has been shown that LDLs play a critical role in the proinflammatory response, whereas high density lipoproteins (HDL; antiatherogenic lipoproteins) exert anti-inflammatory functions.

Monocyte diapedesis takes place through the spaces (junctions) between endothelial cells, preferably in areas where the basal lamina is enriched with modified LDL particles [11]. Once within the arterial intima, infiltrated monocytes differentiate into macrophages and express scavenger receptors, which internalize many of the cholesterol molecules and cholesterol esters contained in modified LDL particles and become foam cells, a characteristic cell constituent of atherosclerotic lesions, that in turn secrete molecular components that facilitate plaque progression (e.g. proinflammatory cytokines, growth factors, tissue factor [18], interferon-γ). As described above for SMC, agLDL are potent inducers of massive cholesterol accumulation in macrophages [19]. Recently, it has been reported that LRP-1 is involved in macrophage internalization of LDL retained in the matrix and/or degraded by sphingomyelinase in a process regulated by SREBP1 and SREBP2, which in turn control LRP-1 expression [20].

Vascular remodelling and fibroproliferative changes

The vascular remodelling that takes place during the development and complication of atherosclerotic plaques involves modification of the composition and structure of the extracellular matrix (ECM). An imbalance between synthesis and degradation of ECM components occurs in all stages of the atherosclerotic process. In this context, deregulation of enzymes directly involved in proteolysis such as matrix metalloproteinases (MMPs) and urokinase-type plasminogen activator (UPA), or their respective inhibitors, tissue inhibitor of metalloproteinases (TIMPs) and plasminogen activator inhibitor-1 (PAI-I), as well as of lysyl oxidase (LOX), an enzyme implicated in the formation and repair of the extracellular matrix, may play a key role in lesion development.

Although endothelial cells, macrophages, and SMC may all contribute to ECM molecular composition, SMC are known to be the major producers of connective tissue both in healthy and atherosclerotic vessels. SMC synthesize and secrete collagen fibres (type I and III) that maintain the tensile strength of the fibrous plaque. As atherosclerosis progresses, the presence of LDL and atherogenic cytokines stimulate SMC to produce proteoglycans, fibronectin, and proteolytic enzymes (e.g. MMPs, UPA), that alter the ECM composition [1, 14]. Thus, MMP9 is a proteolytic enzyme of different ECM-related proteins such as collagen IV, laminin, and elastin, which is expressed by SMCs and macrophages in the vascular wall. It is latently secreted to the ECM where it is activated by plasmin in a process mediated by UPA. ECM content can in turn influence the cellularity of the lesions, when SMCs bound to healthy fibrillar collagen or laminin quickly become arrested in G_1. In contrast, when SMC are bound to fibronectin and proteoglycans, cell cycle arrest pathways are down-regulated, and SMC proliferation is promoted [14]. In addition, extracellular proteases as UPA

regulate mechanisms necessary for cell migration and proliferation either directly or through a process mediated by the generation of plasmin through pericellular proteolysis [1].

Evolution of atherosclerotic lesions: from fatty streaks to complex atheroma

Classical morphological studies in human autopsy specimens have provided valuable information on the evolution of the atherosclerotic plaques.

Fatty streaks

Diffuse intimal thickening, mainly composed of SMCs, elastin, and proteoglycans, develops from an early age in human arteries. However, the earliest stage of human atherosclerosis is the fatty streak that develops via intracellular accumulation of lipids in phagocytes, mainly monocyte-derived macrophages. As the lesion progresses, fat droplets may accumulate in the cytoplasm of SMCs. These first changes in the arterial wall occur at the branching points of arteries, where adaptive intimal thickening occurs in response to haemodynamic stress. Thus, fatty streaks are the hallmark of atherogenesis but they never obstruct the arterial lumen and are clinically silent.

Atheroma and vulnerable plaques

Fatty streaks are precursors of true atherosclerotic lesions, in which lipids also accumulate extracellularly deep in the intima, forming lipid cores and causing cell necrosis. Fibrous tissue is added to form a fibrous cap over the lipid-rich necrotic cores and just under the endothelium at the blood interface. This forms the fibrous plaque lesions that develop to become the dominant lesion (atheroma). The fibrous plaques at a few sites become thin and weakened. The predominant factors that affect the stability of atherosclerotic plaques are their cell composition and the ratio of ECM to lipid content. Unstable plaques and those with a high risk of rupture contain a substantial lipid core, rich in cholesterol esters and with little collagen, and a small number of SMCs. Inflammation within the fibrous cap, increased neovascularization, and fatigue are additional factors. Whereas SMCs account for 90–95% of the cell component in initial lesions, this proportion decreases to 50% in advanced atherosclerotic plaques. These data reflect the importance of identifying and elucidating the mechanisms that lead to loss of SMCs in advanced lesions, as this might help to define new therapeutic strategies. Atherogenic concentrations of LDL significantly reduce the migratory capacity of human vascular SMCs. Using proteomic techniques and confocal microscopy, our group has recently shown that LDL particles affect the expression and phenotypic profile of different proteins associated with the cytoskeleton of the SMCs [3]. In addition, the internalization of LDL by SMCs induces a decrease in MMP9 activity and may also potentiate the inhibitory effect of LDL on SMC migration, thereby contributing to the instability and vulnerability of plaques in advanced stages [21]. Typically, plaques with a fine fibrous layer covering the lipid core and a high tissue factor (TF) content are those with greatest potential for rupture and induction of thrombosis [22]. The proximity of TF and lipid-rich areas in advanced atherosclerotic lesions indicates that LDL particles are implicated in TF cell expression. In support of this hypothesis, it has been shown that modified lipoproteins affect the expression and activity of TF in SMCs [23]. In fact, there is evidence of an increase in circulating TF-rich microparticles in patients with acute coronary syndrome (ACS) and in patients with metabolic syndrome [24]. Our group has shown that the interaction between LRP-1 and agLDL is one of the mechanisms that induce TF expression in a process that depends on RhoA translocation to the membrane and the release of microparticles enriched in active TF to the ECM [25].

Calcification

Calcium deposits in the vascular wall occur through all these steps, initially as small aggregates, and later as large nodules. Arterial calcification is now understood to be an actively regulated process with promoters and inhibitors similar to those seen in bone remodeling. It occurs in two distinct forms involving either the atherosclerotic intima or the tunica media. After plaque rupture, calcified nodules are exposed to the lumen and become sites for thrombosis. Thus, in the tibial arteries of the lower extremity, the amount of calcification has been demonstrated to be a better predictor of amputation than atherosclerosis risk factors and the ankle brachial index. Recent studies suggest that MMPs play a critical role in the development of experimental arterial calcification in rodent models [26]. The mechanisms by which MMPs may regulate arterial calcification are not completely understood, however.

Atherosclerotic plaque burden and plaque imaging

Atherosclerosis is a systemic process with focal manifestations; therefore, once atherosclerosis has been diagnosed in a certain territory, it can be assumed that all arterial beds will be also affected, although the correlation between the degree of disease in different territories is still to be fully demonstrated with state-of-the-art imaging modalities. Indeed, conventional imaging of the vascular tree using ultrasonography, CT, contrast angiography, and MRI allows us to obtain anatomical and morphological information about localized vascular disease. Moreover, recently available imaging techniques have further provided a molecular and cellular assessment of atherothrombosis at the level of the vascular wall giving a better understanding of the pathogenesis of atherothrombosis (◯ Table 38.1) [27]. In fact, advances in noninvasive imaging have helped to identify novel approaches to plaque stabilization, with the potential to prevent plaque rupture, including lifestyle modification and dietary adjustments, as well as pharmacological interventions such as statins. Indeed, given the role of lipids in atherothrombosis, interventions affecting lipid metabolism have been studied most. Although studies addressing lipid reduction/plaque regression/reduced rate events are yet to be performed, it has been demonstrated by noninvasive MRI that an aggressive statin treatment halts atherosclerotic plaque progression at 6 months [28] and may even induce regression after a 2-year treatment period [29]. In addition, other studies using intravascular ultrasound (IVUS) have demonstrated regression of established atherosclerotic plaques with aggressive statin treatment promoting a lowering in LDL-C and a rise in HDL-C [30]. Interestingly, another study with similar dose regimens showed that the aggressive lipid lowering treatment resulted in fewer events [31]. In line with these observations, and taking into consideration that a major goal in atherothrombosis is effectively inducing plaque regression, increase of HDL-C has been regarded as an attractive approach. The first preclinical evidence of HDL-atheroprotective properties was found by our group in 1990 [32]. For the first time, we demonstrated the possibility of inducing regression in pre-existent atheroma lesions by HDL-C infusion in a rabbit model of atherosclerosis. At the clinical level, several HDL-raising interventions [30, 33] have demonstrated the ability to reduce atheroma plaque burden. Specifically, some therapies were developed taking into account that certain genetic polymorphisms are associated with high HDL-C levels such as CETP deficiency and the apoA-I mutation, apoA-I Milano. Five weekly infusions of a reconstituted version of Apo A-I Milano resulted in marked plaque regression in ACS patients, assessed by coronary IVUS [34]. Moreover, we have recently demonstrated by MRI in a rabbit model of atherosclerosis that such regression is associated with plaque stabilization resulting from an enhanced reverse cholesterol transport and decreased inflammatory milieu [27, 35]. Whether such rapid atherosclerotic plaque regression will translate into reduced cardiovascular events remains to be elucidated.

Table 38.1 Main features and limitations of the state-of-the art imaging modalities for atherosclerotic plaque assessment

Imaging modality	Features	Limitations
Contrast angiography	Depicts luminogram of the vessel (lumen size)	Invasive method X-ray fluoroscopic examination Does not detect eccentric plaque growth Unable to measure plaque changes with accuracy Not reliable in assessing the effect of different atherosclerosis-related therapies
Intravascular ultrasound (IVUS)	Measures coronary plaque volume (atheroma burden) with accuracy and may reveal signs of recent disruption Measures plaque composition (virtual histology IVUS) Reliable to assess the effect of different therapies	Invasive method Calcification creates artefacts
Magnetic resonance imaging (MRI)	Noninvasive method. Accurate tool for plaque burden analysis in aortic and peripheral artery beds Characterization of plaque composition (use of paramagnetic contrast agents and iron oxide derivatives Reliable for aortic and peripheral artery beds	Lack of studies correlating changes in atheroma volume with a reduction in events Calcification creates artefacts Cardiac and respiratory motion artefacts that limits its use in coronary arteries
Computerized tomography (CT)	Noninvasive method Accurate technique for the luminal coronary stenosis assessment Calcification assessment	Use X-rays Value in estimating the atheroma burden is controversial Requires validation from preclinical studies, and is awaiting a viable clinical application
Intima media thickening (IMT)	Noninvasive method Accurate carotid and aortic arteries wall thickness Changes in wall thickness correlates with clinical events	Examination of vessels is limited to those that are close to the skin (carotids) Not adequate for coronary atherosclerosis assessment
Scintigraphy (SPECT)	Noninvasive method Provides three-dimensional information Provides *in vivo* molecular imaging (apoptosis, activated platelets)	Uses gamma rays
Positron emission tomography (PET)	Noninvasive method Detects highly metabolic active cells (e.g., macrophages / inflammation) in the arterial wall	A radioactive tracer isotope has to be injected; uses X-rays Relatively low spatial resolution limits its use in coronary arteries

Thrombosis

Cellular and molecular mechanisms in thrombus formation

Platelets

Recent studies provide consistent evidence that platelets play a pivotal role in various phases of atherothrombosis, including the initial steps of atherogenesis, the progression of atherosclerotic lesions, and the ensuing thrombotic complications. Indeed, fissuring or rupture of an atherosclerotic plaque leads to exposure of the thrombogenic lipid core and subendothelial matrix proteins (primarily collagen) to circulating platelets, initiating platelet recruitment to the injured vessel wall in a series of events that is well coordinated in both time and place, including: (1) platelet 'arrest' on to the exposed subendothelium; (2) recruitment and activation of additional platelets through the local release of major platelet agonists; and (3) stabilization of the platelet aggregates [36].

The molecular mechanisms responsible for platelet activation in the onset of atherosclerosis are unknown. However, it has been postulated that platelet activation may be attributed to either a reduction in the mechanisms implicated in maintaining endothelial antithrombotic properties or an increase in both reactive oxygen species and prothrombotic and proinflammatory mediators generated by atherosclerotic risk factors. Thrombus formation at the site of plaque rupture initiates with platelet interactions with the ECM components exposed to blood including fibrillar collagen and/or noncollagenic adhesion proteins such as von Willebrand factor (VWF), fibronectin, thrombospondin, and laminin (➔ Fig. 38.1). The rheological conditions largely influence these adhesive interactions. Thus, while at low shear rate, platelet adhesion to the vessel wall primarily involves binding to fibrillar collagen, fibronectin, and laminin, under conditions of elevated shear stress, platelet tethering to the damaged subendothelium is critically dependent on their interaction with subendothelial bound VWF. Platelets tethered to VWF roll along the vessel

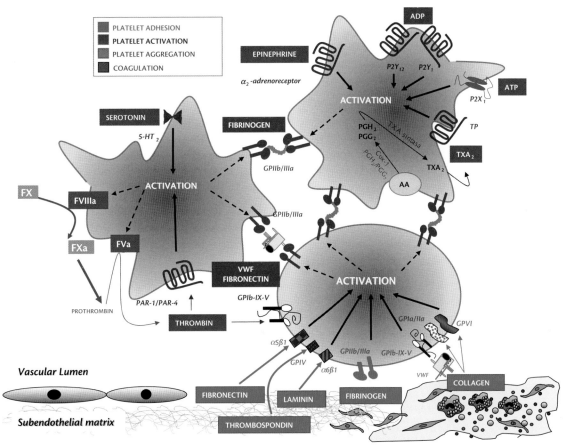

Figure 38.1 Platelet, bloodstream, and vessel-related mechanisms involved in platelet adhesion, activation, and further aggregation. AA, arachidonic acid; PG, prostaglandin; TXA$_2$, thromboxane A$_2$; VWF, Von Willebrand factor.

wall in the direction of the flow until other receptors provide stable attachment. In contrast, platelet receptor GPVI binding to collagen induces the activation of other platelet adhesion receptors, such as integrins αIIbβ$_3$ (GPIIb/IIIa) and α2β1 (GPIa/IIa) (➲ Fig. 38.1), that act in concert promoting subsequent firm, irreversible, and stable platelet adhesion to the damaged surface [37]. Firm adhesion of platelets to collagen then provides the stimulus for platelet activation, shape change, and exocytosis of granule constituents. Indeed, platelets contain three types of storage compartments—α-granules, δ-granules, and lysosomes—that are released into the circulation or translocated to the platelet surface upon activation. As such, α-granules release relevant adhesive proteins (fibrinogen, VWF, fibronectin, vitronectin, and thrombospondin), coagulation factors (FV, FIX, protein-S), fibrinolytic inhibitors (PAI-1 and α$_2$-plasmin inhibitor) whereas δ-granules liberate nucleotides (ADP, ATP), serotonin, histamine, calcium, and factor XIII. Besides delivering many thrombotic agonists into the circulation, the degranulation process also alters the composition of the platelet membrane, resulting in surface expression of P-selectin and the generation of lipid-derived mediators

such as thromboxane A$_2$ (TXA$_2$). P-selectin and other activation-dependent glycoproteins, including CD40L, mediate platelet binding to neutrophils and monocytes. In fact, leucocytes are able to roll on platelets, which are immobilized on the subendothelium, in a P-selectin-dependent manner [38]. On the other hand, TXA$_2$ released to the circulation binds to thromboxane (TP) receptors largely distributed in platelets, circulating inflammatory cells, the vascular wall, and atherosclerotic plaques, enhancing platelet activation, vasoconstriction, and promoting plaque progression. Finally, activated platelets participate in a positive feedback loop that amplifies and perpetuates the platelet response to the given original stimulus, causing a change in the conformation of both the ligand-binding extracellular region and the cytoplasmic tails of αIIbβ$_3$, expressing a high affinity binding site for fibrinogen and VWF, allowing stable bridges between platelets—a process commonly referred to as platelet aggregation (➲ Fig. 38.1). Ligand binding to αIIbβ$_3$ induces additional conformational changes which lead to phosphorylation of tyrosines of the cytoplasmatic β$_3$ chain. Disulphide changes in the αIIbβ$_3$ complex by the surface-associated protein disulphide isomerase induce high affinity binding sites for fibrinogen [39]. In addition, platelets recruit leucocytes and T cells into the growing plug. Interactions via P-selectin/PSGL1 or CD40L/CD40 mediate activation of leucocytes which trigger thrombus growth [40].

Coagulation

One of the early events after vascular disruption, and complementary to platelet activation, is the activation of the coagulation cascade. Strong evidence supports that TF [18] expressed by foam cells, is the principal nonfibrillar thrombogenic factor in the plaque's lipid-rich core, that by binding clotting factor VII/VIIa promotes local thrombin generation by initiating the extrinsic pathway of the coagulation cascade [41]. However, in addition to TF, both dysfunctional endothelium and activated platelets also play an important role in further promoting the coagulation cascade and the subsequent production of fibrin. Indeed, endothelium has switched from an anticoagulant to a procoagulant phenotype releasing tissue plasminogen inhibitor (tPA). On the other hand, activated platelets expose phospholipids in the outer surface of the plasma membrane that allow binding of several coagulation factors (➲ Fig. 38.2). Indeed, coagulation proteins usually circulate in plasma as inactive zymogens which are activated in the platelet surface. Nevertheless, either way of coagulation cascade activation leads to thrombin formation resulting in conversion of fibrinogen to fibrin monomers, which cross-link to stabilize the platelet-rich thrombus and, ultimately, form a solid clot.

Fibrinolysis

The stability of the resulting thrombus is governed by the activity of various elements with a thrombus specific lytic action including tPA and/or uPA activator. tPA, stimulated either by thrombus-bound fibrin or by ECM proteins, initiates fibrinolysis by converting plasminogen to the fibrin-degrading protease plasmin [42]. However, in stable thrombi, cross-linking of fibrin masks tPA binding sites, protects fibrin from degradation. However, these prothrombolytic actions are counterbalanced by plasminogen activator inhibitor type-1 (PAI-1), which is activated

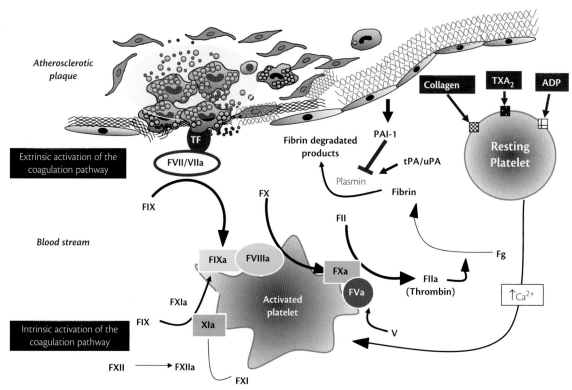

Figure 38.2 Activation of the coagulation cascade (extrinsic and intrinsic pathways) upon atherosclerotic plaque rupture and the contribution of activated platelets in catalysing coagulation factors conversion from their inactive (zymogens) to active forms on the platelet membrane surface. As seen in the figure, both coagulation cascades converge in the activation of FX (FXa) and subsequent thrombin formation (FIIa). Then, thrombin cleaves fibrinogen to fibrin. Plasmin, a key enzyme of the fibrinolytic system activated by urokinase- or tissue-plasminogen activator (uPA and tPA, respectively), may break down fibrin into fibrin degradation products fragments (polypeptides). However, these prothrombolytic actions are counterbalanced by plasminogen activator inhibitor type-1 (PAI-1), which is activated by phospholipid membrane components released at sites of vascular injury enhancing thrombus resistance to proteolysis.

by phospholipid membrane components released at sites of vascular injury and enhances thrombus resistance to proteolysis (➲ Fig. 38.2).

Local and systemic regulation of thrombus growth

A wide range of factors have been identified in prospective epidemiological studies as having a systemic effect on blood thrombogenicity. Certainly, there is increasing evidence of a close relationship between the traditional cardiovascular risk factors such as diabetes mellitus, hypertension, or hyperlipidaemia, and the increased thrombogenicity, which is characterized by hypercoagulability, hypofibrinolysis, or increased platelet reactivity [43]. Conversely, improvements of these cardiovascular risk factors have been associated with a lower prothrombic tendency [44]. In recent years several publications have suggested that the role of platelets in atherosclerosis and its thrombotic complications may be mediated, in part, by local secretion of platelet-derived microparticles (PMps; microvesicular platelets formed during the platelet activation process) [45]. Indeed, high concentrations of circulating PMps have been reported in patients with atherosclerosis, acute vascular syndromes, and/or diabetes mellitus, suggesting a potential correlation between the quantity of microparticles and the clinical severity of the atherosclerotic disease.

Platelets are probably the main source of microparticles in the vascular compartment, whereas the contribution of other vascular cells to the release of microparticles varies in accordance with the pathophysiological context and the extent of the cellular damage. Regarding the contribution of PMps to *in vivo* thrombus formation, PMps possess procoagulant properties which lead to thrombin generation. Such procoagulant activity relies on both presence of TF and the exposure of membrane anionic phospholipids that enable the assembly of coagulation complexes at the microparticle surface and on the eventual thrombin formation. Whether TF is constitutively active on the microparticle surface or needs to be de-encrypted from an inactive form to become available for factor VIIa is still an open question [46]. Additionally, PMps may also intervene in inhibition of fibrinolysis by promoting vimentin-mediated PAI-1 activation [47]. The PMp surface also presents an array of platelet-derived adhesion and chemokine receptors, such as P-selectin, $\alpha IIb\beta_3$, GPIbα, and PF4-receptor, that induce cytokine production by monocytes and endothelium, and an increase in leucocyte aggregation and recruitment via P-selectin/PSGL-1 dependent interactions [48]. PMps may also adhere to both activated subendothelium where they enhance the adhesion of leukocytes via up-regulation of the adhesion molecule ICAM-1 and enhance the inflammatory environment through the production of interleukins

Table 38.2 Antiplatelet agents currently used in the clinical setting, under clinical testing, and under development

Target	Agents	Mechanisms of action
Thromboxane inhibitors	Aspirin Triflusal	Platelet Cox-1 inhibitors
	Terutroban (S18886)	Thromboxane receptor blockade
ADP P2Y(12) receptor antagonists	Thenopyidines: Ticlopidine (1st generation) Clopidogrel (2nd generation) Prasugrel (CS-747, LY640315; 3rd generation)	Require hepatic metabolism. Irreversibly bind the ADP receptor P2Y12
	Nonthenopyridines: Ticagrelor (AZD6140) Cangrelor (AR-C69931 MX)	Do not require hepatic metabolism Reversibly block the ADP receptor P2Y12 Cangrelor is intravenously administered
GPIIb/IIIa inhibitors($\alpha IIb\beta_3$ antagonists)	Abciximab	Monoclonal antibody that irreversibly block GPIIb/IIIa receptor
	Eptifibatide Tirofiban	Synthetic molecules that competitively and reversible block GPIIb/IIIa receptor
Thrombin receptor antagonists	E5555 TRA-SCH 530348	Oral antagonists of platelet thrombin receptor PAR-1
Agents under preclinical investigation	vWF-GPIb inhibitors	Inhibit platelet adhesion by preventing vWF-GPIb interaction
	NCX-4016	Nitric-oxide donor + aspirin releaser
	Soluble CD39	ATP and ADP metabolism
	Nitric oxide donors	

(IL-1, IL-6, and IL-8). Moreover, Mause *et al.* [49] have interestingly suggested that circulating PMps may even serve as a transfer module system for the platelet-derived chemokine RANTES on activated early atherosclerotic endothelium. Thus, elevated levels of PMps may not solely reflect an epiphenomenon of platelet activation but may rather be regarded as an active transcellular delivery system for proinflammatory mediators and platelet receptors.

Therapeutic implications in atherothrombosis

Atherosclerosis prevention is mainly focused on the management of so-called 'cardiovascular risk factors'. Indeed, many studies have reported on the effect of healthy lifestyle habits such as exercise [50], control of body weight[51], Mediterranean diet [52], light to moderate alcohol consumption [53], smoking cessation[54], and stress reduction [55] on not only limiting atherosclerosis progression but also reducing blood thrombogenicity.

In terms of preventing and/or treating thrombosis-related complications, progress in understanding the processes of platelet activation/aggregation and the role of acute thrombus formation has led to a widespread use of antiplatelet therapy in cardiovascular disease (⊃ Table 38.2, and see ⊃ Chapter 42). On the other hand, taking into consideration that recurrent events in patients with unstable angina are unrelated to the initial culprit lesion but arise from complications in other segments of the coronary vasculature, there has been an increasing interest in changing plaque composition in order to reduce the propensity for plaque rupture and thrombosis. ⊃ Table 38.3 shows potential therapeutic strategies that have been shown to achieve plaque stabilization, resulting in a reduced incidence of ACS.

Conclusion

Atherosclerosis is a diffuse pathological process that involves structural changes in the intima and media of arterial vessels driven mainly by cholesterol accumulation,

Table 38.3 Potential therapeutic strategies to achieve plaque stabilization targeted towards the intrinsic and extrinsic features that promote plaque vulnerability

Therapy	Agents	Mechanisms of action
Invasive treatment	Stents	Correction of the shear stress variations
Lipid lowering agents	HMG CoA inhibitors Niacin Bile acid resins Fibrates PPAR-γ LDL apheresis Diet and exercise	Modest retardation of angiographic disease progression Endothelial function improvement Small degree of plaque regression Decrease in MMPs activity
Antithrombotic therapy	ASA/clopidogrel GPIIb/IIIa inhibitors Warfarin	Thrombus inhibition
Antioxidants	Vitamin E (α-tocopherol) Vitemin C Probucol	Inhibition of LDL oxidation Reduction of matrix degradation in the plaque
Blood-pressure control	β- blockers ACE inhibitors	Reduction of the haemodynamic forces that promote plaque rupture
Gene therapy	Transfer of the LDL receptor gene in patients with familial hypercholesterolaemia type IIb Apo A1 Bcl-2	Lipid removal Apoptosis suppression
Induction of ECM synthesis/ prevention of ECM degradation	Anti-inflammatory agents (ASA) Growth factors (IGF-1, PDGF) MMPs inhibitors	Increase collagen synthesis
Macrolide antibiotics	Azithromycin	Reduction in IgG *Chlamydia pneumoniae* antibody titres
Cannabinoids	δ-9-tetrahydrocannabinol	Pleiotropic immunomodulation effects on lymphoid and myeloid cells

ACE, angiotensin converting enzyme; ASA, aspirin; ECM, extracellular matrix; HMG CoA, 3-hydroxy-3-methylglutaryl coenzyme A; IGF-1, insulin-like growth factor-1; LDL, low density lipoproteins; MMP, matrix metalloproteinases; PDGF, platelet derived growth factor; PPAR, peroxisome proliferator-activated receptors.

inflammatory cell infiltration, and SMC migration. Although an atherosclerotic plaque may remain clinically silent, it is prone to disruption, leading to local platelet activation, aggregation, and the subsequent atherothrombotic episode. Interestingly, in recent years it has been shown that atherosclerotic plaque composition rather than the degree of arterial stenosis can be the determinant of rupture. Indeed, several anatomic non-invasive imaging modalities can currently identify several morphological features characteristic of the vulnerable plaque. There is a need for new imaging techniques/approaches that can provide information regarding molecular and cellular processes that occur within the atherosclerotic lesions, helping to classify the risk of plaque rupture.

Personal perspective

The clinical manifestations of atherothrombosis involve not only the atheroma progression but also the interplay with circulating blood. Despite the established safety and effectiveness of several antithrombotic therapies, there is still much room for improvement. Indeed, new insights at the cellular–proteomic level will help us to understand platelet pathology in the course of atherosclerosis and unveil molecular interactions prevalent in thrombosis. Undoubtedly, these advances will aid the development of more accurate, safe, and powerful strategies of pharmacological intervention for selectively inhibiting the pathways most relevant to the atherothrombotic disease process. Advances in the cellular and molecular characterization of the components and signalling pathways that contribute to the atherothrombotic process may guarantee an earlier detection of vulnerable plaques, greater predictive value of serum markers, and more specifically targeted pharmacological interventions to find and treat the vulnerable patient at risk of an acute ischaemic event.

Further reading

Badimon JJ, Ibañez B, Fuster V, Badimon L. Coronary thrombosis: local and systemic factors. Chapter 53 in: Fuster V, O'Rourke R, Walsh R, *et al.* (eds) *Hurst's the heart*, 12th edition. McGraw-Hill, New York, 2008.

Davì G, Patrono C. Platelet activation and atherothrombosis. *N Engl J Med* 2007;**357**(24):2482–2494.

Libby P, Ridker PM, Hansson GK, *et al.* Inflammation in atherosclerosis: from pathophysiology to practice. *J Am Coll Cardiol* 2009;**54**(23):2129–2138.

◑ For additional multimedia materials please visit the online version of the book (🕮 http://www.esciacc.oxfordmedicine.com).

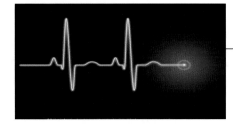

CHAPTER 39

The universal definition of myocardial infarction

Kristian Thygesen, Joseph S. Alpert,
Allan S. Jaffe, and Harvey D. White

Contents

Summary

Myocardial infarction is defined pathologically as myocyte necrosis due to prolonged ischemia. These conditions are met when there is a detection of a rise and/or fall of cardiac biomarkers, preferably troponins, with at least one value above the 99th percentile of the upper reference limit together with evidence of myocardial ischemia as recognized by at least one of the following: symptoms of ischemia, ECG changes of new ischemia, development of pathological Q waves, imaging evidence of new loss of viable myocardium or new regional wall motion abnormality is present. Myocardial infarctions are divided into 5 types and can be spontaneous, secondary, or related to sudden cardiac death, percutaneous coronary intervention, or coronary artery bypass grafting.

Introduction

In 2000, the European Society of Cardiology (ESC) and the American College of Cardiology (ACC) redefined criteria for the diagnosis of myocardial infarction (MI), changing the criteria of older MI definitions based on epidemiology to a clinical definition involving elevation of troponins in the clinical setting of myocardial ischaemia [1]. However, considerable advances in the diagnosis and management of MI have occurred since the original redefinition document was published.

Furthermore, there was a pressing need at that time for a classification of MI to be employed in various clinical settings. For example when a patient arrives at the intensive cardiac care unit (ICCU) with complex, multiorgan failure accompanied by a minor or modest elevations of cardiac troponin (cTn) values, it is unclear whether this represents an MI secondary to increased myocardial oxygen demand (related to hypoxia, tachycardia, etc.) in a patient with underlying coronary artery disease (CAD), or whether the myocardial damage is secondary to elevated levels of circulating cytokines, or endogenous or exogenous cathecholamines in a critically ill patient.

Therefore, the leadership of the ESC, the ACC and the American Heart Association convened, together with the World Heart Federation, a Global Task Force to update the 2000 consensus document. The Global Task Force was composed of a number of expert working groups (biomarkers, ECG, imaging, interventional cardiology, clinical investigation, and global perspectives) in order to refine as precisely as possible the original ESC/ACC criteria for the diagnosis of MI from various perspectives. During several Task Force meetings the recommendations of the various working groups were co-coordinated, resulting in an updated consensus document [2].

Definition of myocardial infarction

MI is defined pathologically as myocardial cell death due to prolonged ischaemia. In the clinical setting these conditions are met when the following criteria are present: detection of a rise and/or fall of cardiac biomarkers with at least one value above the 99th percentile of the upper reference limit (URL) together with evidence of myocardial ischaemia as recognized by at least one of the following: symptoms of ischaemia, ECG changes of new ischaemia or development of pathological Q waves, or imaging evidence of new loss of viable myocardium or new regional wall motion abnormality (➲ Box 39.1) [2].

Cardiac biomarkers

Cardiac troponins I and T are the preferred markers for the diagnosis of myocardial injury since these have nearly

---

Box 39.1 Definition of myocardial infarction

Acute myocardial infarction
Any one of the following criteria meets the diagnosis for MI:

1 Detection of elevated values of cardiac biomarkers (preferably troponin) above the 99th percentile of the upper reference limit (URL) together with evidence of myocardial ischaemia with at least one of the following:
   (a) Ischaemic symptoms
   (b) ECG changes indicative of new ischaemia (new ST-T changes or new left bundle branch block (LBBB))
   (c) Development of pathological Q waves in the ECG
   (d) Imaging evidence of new loss of viable myocardium or new regional wall motion abnormality.

2 Sudden unexpected cardiac death, including cardiac arrest, with symptoms suggestive of myocardial ischaemia, accompanied by new ST elevation, or new LBBB, or definite new thrombus by coronary angiography but dying before blood samples could be obtained, or in the lag phase of cardiac biomarkers in the blood.

3 For percutaneous coronary interventions (PCI) in patients with normal baseline values, elevations of cardiac biomarkers above the 99th percentile URL are indicative of periprocedural myocardial necrosis.

By convention, increases of biomarkers greater than 3 × 99th percentile URL have been designated as defining PCI-related MI.

4 For coronary artery bypass grafting (CABG) in patients with normal baseline values, elevations of cardiac biomarkers above the 99th percentile URL are indicative of periprocedural myocardial necrosis. By convention, increases of biomarkers greater than 5 × 99th percentile URL plus either new pathological Q waves or new LBBB, or angiographically documented new graft or native coronary artery occlusion, or imaging evidence of new loss of viable myocardium have been designated as defining CABG-related MI.

5 Pathological findings post-mortem of an acute myocardial infarction.

Prior myocardial infarction

1 Development of new pathological Q waves with or without symptoms.

2 Imaging evidence of a region of loss of viable myocardium that is thinned and fails to contract, in the absence of a nonischaemic cause.

3 Pathological findings post-mortem of a healed or healing myocardial infarction.

From Thygesen K, Alpert JS, White HD, *et al.* Universal definition of myocardial infarction. *Eur Heart J* 2007;**28**:2525–2538.

absolute myocardial tissue specificity, as well as high sensitivity, reflecting even microscopic zones of myocardial necrosis [3]. Optimal precision at the 99th percentile URL for each assay should be defined as a coefficient of variation of 10% or less [4, 5]. If troponin assays are not available, the best alternative is the MB fraction of creatine kinase (CK-MB) measured by mass assay. As with troponin, an increased CK-MB mass value is defined as a measurement above the 99th percentile URL using gender-appropriate normal ranges [6]. However, given its greater sensitivity and specificity, troponin is greatly preferred for the diagnosis of MI.

Assuming good assays and appropriate cut-off values, both cTnI and cTnT perform comparably in terms of their diagnostic accuracy. The one difference between these two troponin assays occurs in renal failure patients where there are greater numbers of elevations of cTnT compared with cTnI. These elevations are usually stable over time [7]. Pathology studies suggest that these elevated values denote cardiac abnormalities in these patients with renal insufficiency [8]. Moreover, they are highly prognostic [7] and thus, patients with renal insufficiency who have elevated levels of cTnT require further clinical evaluation. Although there is a relationship between cTnT elevations and CAD in these patients, not all elevations are due to coronary artery disease [9] If this group displays the characteristic rise and/ or fall of cTnT values, albeit from an abnormal baseline, these renal patients are having acute events and should be assessed as having acute MI if there are signs and/or symptoms of ischaemia [10].

Indeed, a variety of disease entities can injure myocardium (e.g. trauma, myocarditis, chemotherapeutic agents, etc.) thereby leading to elevated values of troponin. These other entities are not the result of acute ischaemic heart disease and careful clinical evaluation should be used to prevent these patients from being labelled as having had an acute MI (➲ Box 39.2).

Classification of myocardial infarction

MI can be a spontaneous event related to plaque rupture, fissuring, or dissection of an atherosclerotic plaque; or, as recently described, nodular plaque rupture, which is classified as MI type 1. Alternatively, MI can result from increased myocardial oxygen demand combined with inadequate myocardial supply of oxygen and nutrients.

Box 39.2 Elevations of troponin in the absence of overt ischaemic heart disease

- Cardiac contusion, including ablation, pacing, cardioversion, or endomyocardial biopsy
- Congestive heart failure, acute and chronic
- Aortic dissection, aortic valve disease, or hypertrophic cardiomyopathy
- Tachy- or bradyarrhythmias, or heart block
- Apical ballooning syndrome
- Rhabdomyolysis with cardiac injury
- Pulmonary embolism, severe pulmonary hypertension
- Renal failure
- Acute neurological disease, including stroke, or subarachnoid haemorrhage
- Infiltrative diseases, e.g. amyloidosis, hemochromatosis, sarcoidosis, scleroderma
- Inflammatory diseases, e.g. myocarditis, or myocardial extension of endo-/pericarditis
- Drug toxicity, e.g. adriamycin, 5-fluorouracil, herceptin, snake venoms
- Critically ill patients, especially with respiratory failure, or sepsis
- Burns, especially if affecting >30% of body surface area

From Thygesen K, Alpert JS, White HD, *et al.* Universal definition of myocardial infarction. *Eur Heart J* 2007;**28**:2525–2538.

This could be the result of anaemia, arrhythmia, and hyper- or hypotension. Vasoconstriction or arterial spasm, causing a marked reduction in myocardial blood flow can also lead to severe myocardial ischaemia and MI. This second group of entities is termed MI type 2 (➲ Box 39.3) [2].

One circumstance in which biomarkers are not of value in the diagnosis of MI is when the patient with a typical presentation for myocardial ischaemia/infarction dies before it is possible to detect blood biomarker elevation, either because blood samples for troponin determination were not obtained or the patient succumbed soon after the onset of symptoms before troponin values could be elevated. Such patients are designated as having a MI type 3 (➲ Box 39.3) [2].

Elevated troponin values (>3 × 99th percentile URL) following a percutaneous coronary intervention (PCI) is designated as an acute MI resulting from myocardial

Box 39.3 Clinical classification of different types of myocardial infarction

- Type 1: Spontaneous MI related to ischaemia due to a primary coronary event such as plaque erosion and/or rupture, fissuring, or dissection

- Type 2: MI secondary to ischaemia due to either increased oxygen demand or decreased supply, e.g. coronary artery spasm, coronary embolism, anaemia, arrhythmias, hypertension, or hypotension

- Type 3: Sudden unexpected cardiac death, including cardiac arrest, often with symptoms suggestive of myocardial ischaemia, accompanied by presumably new ST elevation, or new LBBB, or evidence of fresh thrombus in a coronary artery by angiography and/or at autopsy, but death occurring before blood samples could be obtained, or at a time before the appearance of cardiac biomarkers in the blood

- Type 4a: MI associated with PCI

- Type 4b: MI associated with stent thrombosis, as documented by angiography or at autopsy

- Type 5: Myocardial infarction associated with CABG

From Thygesen K, Alpert JS, White HD, *et al.* Universal definition of myocardial infarction. *Eur Heart J* 2007;**28**:2525–2538.

Box 39.4 ECG manifestations of acute myocardial ischaemia (in absence of LVH and LBBB)

ST elevation

- New ST elevation at the J-point in two contiguous leads with the cut-off points ≥0.2 mV in men or ≥0.15 mV in women in leads V_2–V_3 and/or ≥0.1 mV in other leads

ST depression and T wave changes

- New horizontal or down-sloping ST depression ≥0.05 mV in two contiguous leads; and/or

- T inversion ≥0.1 mV in two contiguous leads with prominent R wave or R/S ratio >1

LBBB, left bundle branch block; LVH, left ventricular hypertrophy. From Thygesen K, Alpert JS, White HD, *et al.* Universal definition of myocardial infarction. *Eur Heart J* 2007;**28**:2525–2538.

As shown in ➲ Box 39.5, Q waves or QS complexes are usually pathognomonic of a prior MI in the absence of QRS confounders [13]. ST or T wave deviations alone are nonspecific findings for myocardial necrosis. However, when these abnormalities occur in the same leads as the Q waves, the likelihood of MI is increased [2].

Imaging techniques

Imaging techniques can be useful in the diagnosis of MI because of the ability to detect wall motion abnormalities in the presence of elevated cardiac biomarkers. If for some reason biomarkers have not been measured, or may have normalized, demonstration of new loss of myocardial viability alone in the absence of nonischaemic causes meets the

ischaemia (MI type 4a). A second category of type 4 MI can be caused by stent thrombosis, and is termed MI type 4b (troponin value >99th percentile URL). Moreover, elevations of troponin measurements (>5 × 99th percentile URL) at the time of coronary artery bypass grafting (CABG) defines a type 5 MI (➲ Box 39.3). Elevations of troponin at baseline are associated with greater elevations postprocedurally. Accordingly, these guidelines require a normal baseline value [2].

ECG

The ECG criteria for the diagnosis of acute myocardial ischaemia that may lead to infarction are listed in ➲ Box 39.4 [2]. The J-point is used to determine the magnitude of the ST elevation. J-point elevation in men decreases with increasing age; however, that is not observed in women, in whom J-point elevation is less than in men [11]. The term 'posterior' to reflect the basal part of the left ventricle wall that lies on the diaphragm is no longer recommended. It is preferable to refer to this territory as inferobasal [12].

Box 39.5 ECG changes associated with prior myocardial infarction

- Any Q wave in leads V_2–V_3 ≥0.02 s or QS complex in leads V_2 and V_3

- Q wave ≥0.03 s and ≥ 0.1 mV deep or QS complex in leads I, II, aVL, aVF or V_4–V_6 in any two leads of a contiguous lead grouping (I, aVL,V6; V_4–V_6; II, III, aVF)

- R wave ≥0.04 s in V_1–V_2 and R/S ≥1 with a concordant positive T wave in the absence of a conduction defect

From Thygesen K, Alpert JS, White HD, *et al.* Universal definition of myocardial infarction. *Eur Heart J* 2007;**28**:2525–2538.

criteria for MI. However, if biomarkers have been measured at appropriate times and are normal, the determination of these takes precedence over the imaging criteria.

Echocardiography is the imaging technique of choice for detecting complications of acute infarction including myocardial free wall rupture, acute ventricular septal defect, and mitral regurgitation secondary to papillary muscle rupture or ischaemia. However, echocardiography cannot distinguish regional wall motion abnormalities due to myocardial ischaemia from infarction. An important role of acute echocardiography or radionuclide imaging is in patients with suspected MI and a nondiagnostic ECG. A normal echocardiogram or resting ECG-gated scintigram has a 95–98% negative predictive value for excluding acute infarction [14, 15]. Thus, imaging techniques are useful for early triage and discharge of patients with suspected MI [16].

Recent data suggest that the use of cardiac magnetic resonance (see ➲ Chapter 21) can help to define aetiologies for elevated troponin values in patients who present with findings suggestive of acute MI but who have normal coronary arteries angiographically. Some of these patients, especially women, still appear to have acute MI but myocarditis is a common mimicker [17].

Definition of reinfarction

Traditionally, CK-MB has been used to detect reinfarction. However, recent data suggest that troponin values provide similar information [18]. If a recurrent MI is suspected from clinical signs or symptoms following the initial infarction, an immediate measurement of the employed cardiac marker (preferably troponin) is recommended. A second sample should be obtained 3–6 h later. Recurrent infarction is diagnosed if there is a 20% or more increase of the value in the second sample. Analytic values are considered to be different if they are different by more than three standard deviations of the variance of the measures [19]. This value should also exceed the 99th percentile URL.

The ECG diagnosis of reinfarction following the initial infarction may be confounded by the initial evolutionary ECG changes. Reinfarction should be considered when ST elevation of 0.1 mV or more reoccurs in a patient having a lesser degree of ST elevation or new pathognomonic Q waves, in at least two contiguous leads, particularly when associated with ischaemic symptoms for 20 min or longer. ST depression or left bundle branch block alone should not be considered valid MI criteria [2].

Myocardial infarction associated with revascularization procedures

Periprocedural MI is different from the spontaneous infarction, because it is associated with the instrumentation that is required during mechanical revascularization procedures by either PCI or CABG [20].

In PCI, balloon inflation during a procedure almost always results in ischaemia whether or not accompanied by ST-T changes. The occurrence of procedure-related cell necrosis can be detected by measurement of cardiac biomarkers before or immediately after the procedure, and again at 6–12 and 18–24 h [21, 22]. Elevations of biomarkers above the 99th percentile URL after PCI, assuming a normal baseline troponin value, are indicative of postprocedural myocardial necrosis. If the baseline value is elevated, it is impossible to distinguish the injury associated with the procedure and that associated with the inciting event that led to the elevation. If there are chronic elevations, criteria for reinfarction can be employed [2]. There is currently no solid scientific basis for defining a biomarker threshold for the diagnosis of periprocedural MI. Pending further data, and by arbitrary convention, the suggestion is to designate increases greater than 3 × 99th percentile URL as PCI-related MI type 4a. However, in the event of stent thrombosis as documented by angiography and/or autopsy in association with a troponin value above the 99th percentile URL, the suggestion is to designate this subcategory as PCI-related MI type 4b [2].

Any increase of cardiac biomarkers after CABG indicates myocyte necrosis, implying that an increasing magnitude of biomarker is likely to be related to an impaired outcome [23, 24]. One cannot distinguish between elevations of biomarkers related to the details of anaesthesia, cardioprotection, and technical aspects of the surgery from those related to graft or native coronary abnormalities. Thus, biomarkers cannot stand alone for the diagnosis of infarction in this context. In view of the adverse impact on survival observed in patients with significant biomarker elevations, it is suggested, by arbitrary convention, that biomarker values greater than the 5 × 99th percentile URL during the first 72 h following CABG should prompt a search for other associated criteria such as appearance of new pathological Q waves or new left bundle branch block, or angiographically documented new graft or native coronary artery occlusion, or imaging evidence of new loss of viable myocardium. If such criteria are met, the patient should be considered to have suffered a CABG-related MI type 5 [2].

Myocardial infarction associated with noncardiac surgery

Studies of patients undergoing noncardiac surgery strongly support the concept that many of the infarctions diagnosed in this context are caused by prolonged imbalance between myocardial oxygen supply and demand on the background of CAD [25, 26], which together with rise and fall of cardiac markers points towards MI type 2. The fact that many such patients have type 2 infarctions should not obscure the likelihood that some of the infarctions are type 1 as well. Pathology of fatal peri- or postoperative MI shows plaque rupture and platelet aggregation leading to thrombus formation in approximately half of these events [27]. Given the differences that probably exist in the therapeutic approaches to each, close clinical scrutiny to identify this group is essential. However, some patients may not have had an MI at all. Careful clinical evaluation including a detailed history, examination, and evaluation by means of further investigations to identify and treat those with pulmonary embolism, sepsis, and/or the many other conditions associated with myocyte necrosis and troponin elevations is also strongly advocated [2, 28].

Myocardial infarction in the intensive cardiac care unit

Elevations of cardiac troponin are common in ICCU patients and associated with an adverse prognosis regardless of the underlying disease state [29–31]. Some elevations may reflect a type 2 MI due to underlying CAD and increased myocardial oxygen demand [30], but the relationship in this setting is less secure than that observed in noncardiac surgery patients [26]. Some patients may have elevations due to myocardial damage induced by catecholamines, direct toxic effects from circulating toxins, or, in some cases, even type 1 MI. Many of these patients do not need a detailed CAD evaluation once they recover from their serious illness. However, this is a case for careful clinical analysis and judgement. If the myocardial event appeared to be related to underlying CAD, either a noninvasive or an invasive evaluation of the coronary circulation may be indicated.

Myocardial infarction in clinical investigations

In clinical trials, MI may be an entry criterion or an endpoint. The definition of MI employed in these trials will thus determine the characteristics of patients entering the studies as well as the number of outcome events. In recent investigations, different infarct definitions have been employed, thereby hampering comparison and generalization among these trials. Consistency among investigators and regulatory authorities with regard to the definition of MI used in clinical investigations is essential.

The investigators should ensure that a trial provides comprehensive data for the various types of MI (e.g. spontaneous, periprocedural) and include the decision limits used for MI of the cardiac biomarkers in question. In clinical trials, as in clinical practice, measurement of cardiac troponin T or I is preferred to measurement of CK-MB or other biomarkers for the diagnosis of MI. Assessment of the quantity of myocardial damage (infarct size) is also an important trial endpoint. It is suggested that the data should be reported as multiples of the 99th percentile URL of the applied biomarker, enabling comparisons between various classes and severity of the different MI types as indicated in ⮞ Table 39.1 [2].

Table 39.1 Tabulation of MI types according to multiples of the 99th percentile URL of the applied cardiac biomarker

Multiples × 99%	MI type 1 (spontaneous)	MI type 2 (secondary)	MI type 3[a] (sudden death)	MI type 4[b] (PCI)	MI type 5[b] (CABG)	Total number
1–2 ×						
2–3 ×						
3–5 ×						
5–10 ×						
>10 ×						
Total number						

[a] Biomarkers are not available for this type of MI since the patients expired before biomarker determination could be performed.

[b] For the sake of completeness, the total distribution of biomarker values should be reported. The hatched areas represent biomarker elevations below the decision limit used for these MI types.

Conclusion

The new universal definition of myocardial infarction is based on troponin elevation together with ischemic symptoms, typical ECG changes, or imaging evidence of loss of viable myocardium. Myocardial infarctions are classified into 5 types whether spontaneous, secondary, or related to sudden cardiac death, percutaneous coronary intervention, or coronary artery bypass grafting.

Further reading

Thygesen K, Alpert JS, White HD, Joint ESC/ACCF/AHA/WHF Task Force for the Redefinition of Myocardial Infarction. Universal definition of myocardial infarction. *Eur Heart J* 2007;**28**:2525–2538; *Circulation* 2007;116:2634–2653; *J Am Coll Cardiol* 2007;50:2173–2195.

➲ For additional multimedia materials please visit the online version of the book (🔗 http://www.esciacc.oxfordmedicine.com).

CHAPTER 40

Systems of care for patients with acute coronary syndrome

Kurt Huber, Keith A. A. Fox, Patrick Goldstein, and Nicolas Danchin

Contents

Summary

Although primary percutaneous coronary intervention (PCI) is the preferred strategy for patients with ST-elevation myocardial infarction (STEMI), offering fast access to this procedure often remains difficult because of local resources and capabilities and a lack of cooperation and organization. Accordingly, for most countries worldwide primary PCI can be provided for only part of the population. Moreover, not all patients referred for primary PCI receive optimal mechanical reperfusion within the recommended time intervals with the procedure performed in an experienced centre by an experienced team. Intravenous thrombolytic therapy, preferably administered prehospital and as part of a pharmaco-invasive strategy, offers a reasonable therapeutic option in selected cases. Network organization is central to offering fast and optimal reperfusion treatment in the individual case. It has been shown repeatedly that early recognition of STEMI as well as minimizing time delays is important for the achievement of optimal clinical results. These findings should encourage the building up of regional networks according to specific local constraints, and monitoring their effectiveness by ongoing registries. Financial, regulatory, and political barriers can be resolved and prompt, guideline-recommended care becomes feasible and affordable if stakeholders and participants agree and cooperate.

Introduction

About 20 years ago the concept of primary percutaneous coronary intervention (PCI) was developed and randomized clinical trials consistently exhibited the superiority of this reperfusion technique compared with thrombolytic therapy (TT) [1], making it the reference reperfusion strategy in acute STEMI [2, 3]. The major issue in treatment of acute STEMI today is to offer reperfusion strategies and adjunctive measures to all patients as early as possible. If primary PCI or TT is offered with little delay from symptom onset, the clinical outcome is significantly improved. Potential differences between the two reperfusion strategies are modest compared with the outcomes of any reperfusion strategy versus no reperfusion.

Minimizing differences between reperfusion strategies

Primary percutaneous coronary intervention versus thrombolytic therapy

The CAPTIM trial, as well as recently published registry studies [4–7], revealed comparable mortality data between patients treated with either reperfusion strategy if patients were treated 2–3 h of onset of pain, and if TT, preferably prehospital, was followed either by rescue PCI in nonresponders or by routine angiography and PCI in initial responders to pharmacological reperfusion.

In contrast, in most trials showing a clear benefit of primary PCI over TT including the early phase of STEMI [1], TT was not administered in an optimal way: (1) at that time adjunct treatment with clopidogrel and enoxaparin, as recommended by the new guidelines [2, 3], was not yet proven; (2) the data obtained were generated with fibrin-specific agents as well as with the less efficient non-fibrin-specific thrombolytic agents; and (3) the use of coronary angiography and angioplasty in TT-treated patients was limited to a minority: in only one of all trials selected for the meta-analysis of Keeley *et al.* [3], the CAPTIM trial [8], was early angiography part of the protocol in patients randomized to pharmacological reperfusion. In this study rescue PCI was performed in 26% of the patients after prehospital TT; whereas in the DANAMI-2 trial, another important contributor to this meta-analysis, only 1.9% of patients had a rescue procedure [9]. Moreover, PCI procedures after initially successful TT during the hospital stay were offered in 34.5% and 16.4%, respectively.

The pharmaco-invasive approach

Several trials have examined the value of coronary angiography and PCI after TT. The REACT trial showed that in patients who had failed TT rescue PCI was better than a conservative approach or repeated TT [10]. The role of systematic PCI within 24 h of TT was investigated in the SIAM-III trial [11], the GRACIA-1 trial [12], the CAPITAL-AMI trial [13], and the CARESS in AMI trial [14], respectively. In all instances, a strategy of systematic PCI after intravenous TT yielded better results than conservative management. More recently, the TRANSFER-AMI trial [15] enrolled acute STEMI patients less than 12 h after symptom onset, who were randomly assigned to transfer for angioplasty within 6 h or to elective angiography in those not needing rescue angioplasty. There was no difference in mortality between the standard and invasive strategy (3.6% vs 3.7%, $p = 0.94$), but the composite endpoint of death, MI, or recurrent ischaemia was strongly in favour of the invasive strategy (11.7% vs 6.5%, $p = 0.004$). The WEST study [16] further strengthened this concept by suggesting that rapidly applied pharmacological reperfusion with follow-up PCI (rescue or routine) within 24 h produces equivalent results to primary PCI. Similar data were reported for the FAST-MI trial [7] and the Vienna STEMI registry [4], in both of which rescue PCI was offered (in up to 39% of patients) to nonresponders, while routine angiography and PCI was performed in initial responders to therapy. Both studies confirmed the concept of a pharmaco-invasive approach demonstrating comparable hard clinical endpoints for patients receiving primary PCI or TT, when treated in the early phase of acute STEMI. In favour of a pharmaco-invasive strategy are also the German PREMIER registry [17], the Haifa experience from Israel [18], and the Polish Wielkopolska registry, in which TT with tPA followed by PCI in 26% of the patients provided results that compared with those of primary PCI in patients with onset of chest pain < 4 h [19]. Recently, in the NORDISTEMI trial 266 patients with acute STEMI living in rural areas with more than 90-min transfer delay to PCI initially received tenecteplase, and were randomized to immediate transfer for PCI or conservative management in the local hospitals with early transfer for rescue PCI only in nonresponders to therapy [20]. The primary combined endpoints (death, re-infarction, stroke, or new ischemia at 12 months) showed a trend in favour of the early invasive treatment (21%) as compared to the conservatively treated group (27%; $p = 0.19$), while a composite of death, re-infarction and stroke at 12 months was significantly reduced in the early invasive versus the conservative group (6 vs 16%; $p < 0.01$), respectively.

Remaining problems in STEMI treatment

The main remaining problems in STEMI treatment are to ensure timely reperfusion therapy and to treat the approximately 35% of patients who are eligible for reperfusion therapy, but do not receive it, as documented in international registries [21, 22]. In developing countries this percentage may approach 60%. The reasons for this finding include lack of treatment resources as well as the absence of clear, systematic protocols for identifying treatment-eligible patients and offering the best reperfusion strategy based on the individual situation. Furthermore, available resources are frequently not properly used or mobilized to provide timely care 24 h per day.

The importance of time delays

The success of reperfusion in STEMI is dependent on the time of administration, and total ischaemic time (from onset of symptoms until reperfusion of the infarct-related artery) is the key to success or failure of reperfusion therapy. However, registry data show that the recommended time intervals of 30 min door-to-needle and 90–120 min first medical contact (FMC)-to-balloon are difficult to achieve. FMC-to-balloon times are often much longer than expected, as weather conditions, geographic location, initial personnel involved, or poor management strategies can lead to long delays [21]. In a real world setting it seems that only 15% of patients referred for primary PCI can be treated within 2 h of symptom onset [23]. Furthermore, the GRACE registry failed to document any meaningful improvement in time delays for reperfusion therapy between 2000 and 2005 and, surprisingly, the prehospital delay time was slightly longer in the latest time period (133 min between July 2005 and June 2006) compared with the earliest measurement (120 min between April 1999 and June 2000). However, times from hospital admission to primary PCI or TT decreased (from 99 to 80 min for primary PCI and from 40 to 34 min for TT) [21]. Organizational delays within PCI-capable hospitals are longer if personnel are not sufficiently trained to perform procedures and/or if the caseload is too low to maintain quality. There is additional time delay when patients are transferred to emergency rooms or coronary care units rather than directly to the cardiac care unit (CCU) and/or catheterization laboratory [24–26].

Time delays to primary PCI are associated with increased mortality. A recent analysis of 43 801 STEMI patients enrolled in the National Cardiovascular Data Registry (NCDR) found that as door-to-balloon time increases, there is a minute-by-minute increase in in-hospital mortality [27].

Accordingly, expected time delays are also crucial in determining the best reperfusion strategy: the superiority of primary PCI over TT exists only as far as the time to reperfusion is not too much increased by opting for PCI rather than the faster approach of intravenous TT. The balance between primary PCI and TT varies according to time from symptom onset, infarct location, and patient's age [28]. Importantly, the superiority of PCI over TT was lost when the PCI-related delay (FMC-to-balloon minus FMC-to-needle) was longer than 40 min for patients younger than 65 years of age with an anterior MI presenting within 2 h of symptom onset, demonstrating the critical importance of time to reperfusion in the early phase of STEMI [28].

Optimizing diagnosis and treatment

The current challenge is to organize care in order to optimize the implementation of early reperfusion therapy in STEMI patients, with a tailored approach based on the individual situation. In an optimized STEMI network the local emergency medical system (EMS), non-PCI-capable hospitals, and hospitals with PCI facilities cooperate closely, with the goal of treating all comers with chest pain with the most appropriate and timely reperfusion strategy for the individual situation. A well-organized network is usually able to perform timely primary PCI in the majority of patients, to administer prehospital TT, to apply in-hospital TT in non-PCI-capable hospitals, and to guarantee immediate transfer of patients to a PCI centre for angiographic diagnosis and consecutive PCI if required. The best option for patients with acute STEMI in terms of receiving the fastest available mechanical reperfusion is the direct way via the EMS into a PCI capable department (◐ Fig. 40.1).

Patient-related time delays are still responsible for about two-thirds of the total ischaemic time. Therefore, prerequisites for early activation of the EMS are a single call number for chest pain emergencies, and repeated educational efforts via the media to inform the general public about symptoms and prompt them to call for medical help as early as possible. Further factors for improving delivery of reperfusion therapy have been described in a large survey [29]:

◆ Direct activation of the catheterization laboratory by the emergency physicians

Pre-hospital Management

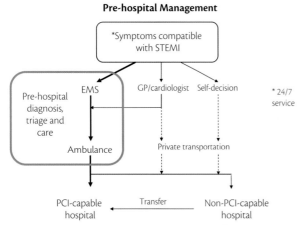

EMS: Emergency Medical System; STEMI: Acute ST-segment Elevation Myocardial Infarction; GP: General Practitioner; PCI: Percutaneous Coronary Intervention
Thick arrows: preferred patient flow; dotted line: to be avoided

Figure 40.1 Prehospital management. Thick arrows indicate preferred patient flow; dotted lines are routes to be avoided. EMS, emergency medical system; GP, general practitioner; PCI, percutaneous coronary intervention; STEMI: acute ST-segment elevation myocardial infarction. Reproduced with permission from Van de Werf F, Bax J, Betriu A, *et al.* Management of acute myocardial infarction in patients presenting with persistent ST-segment elevation: the Task Force on the Management of ST-Segment Elevation Acute Myocardial Infarction of the European Society of Cardiology. *Eur Heart J* 2008;**29**:2909–2945.

- A single call number to activate the catheterization laboratory

- Having staff arriving at the catheterization laboratory within 20 min after being paged or having an attending cardiologist on site.

➲ Box 40.1 summarizes important constituents of well-organized STEMI networks.

Prehospital triage can be made either by physicians or with specially trained paramedics [30]. ECG teletransmission, especially when the ambulance staff are paramedics,

---

Box 40.1 Network components

- One call number
- EMS (car, helicopter)
- 12-lead ECG, defibrillator
- Basic and advanced life support
- Cell phone (direct contact with catheterization laboratory)
- Trained (emergency) physicians or paramedics
- Automatic ECG diagnosis or ECG-telemetry (paramedics)
- Options for prehospital treatment (pain relief, antithrombins, antiplatelet agents, prehospital lysis)

---

or in rural areas with long transfer times, can be helpful in achieving a faster initial diagnosis and has been shown to reduce time to initiation of reperfusion therapy [24, 31]. Ambulance teams should also triage for the best reperfusion method in the individual case and transfer the patient with/ without prehospital TT directly to a PCI-capable facility, while simultaneously mobilizing the interventional team [6, 22]. When prehospital TT has been performed patients should be transferred directly to a PCI-capable hospital, even when a noninterventional hospital is closer, avoiding a time-consuming two-stage transfer for the patient. Implementing such strategies might require changes in hospital operations and changes in regulatory or legal guidance.

Experienced PCI centres (heart attack centres) are analogous to trauma centres and, as in trauma centres, patients should be transferred back to their originating hospital as soon as possible after the acute intervention. The originating hospital will handle further diagnosis and treatment, including the very important initiation of secondary prevention measures. Non-PCI-capable hospitals should therefore be included in networks and be responsible for all but the acute phase of STEMI care.

Examples of STEMI networks in practice

In practice, most networks now deliver three forms of reperfusion therapy: Primary PCI; in-hospital TT; and prehospital TT with follow-up angiography (and any required mechanical intervention).

The Vienna STEMI network

Although organized by cardiologists, in this network about 60% of patients are first seen by physicians of the Viennese ambulance systems [4]. About 40% of patients are self-presenters, and half of these present to hospitals without catheter facilities. Under these circumstances, patients are quickly transferred to a PCI-capable hospital by primary transportation (special ambulance staffed with emergency doctor and required equipment). If FMC-to-balloon time is expected to exceed 90–120 min, patients receive TT with tenecteplase (prehospital) before transfer. Under an inter-hospital rotational agreement, for a population of about 1.8 million inhabitants there are always two catheter-equipped hospitals available 24 h a day on weekdays during off-hours, and one open 24 h on weekends. The advantage

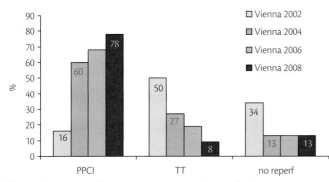

Figure 40.2 Vienna STEMI registry: changes in reperfusion strategies 2002–2008.

of this rotational system is that only highly experienced interventional cardiologists and well-trained personnel are on duty.

In the first 2 years of the Vienna STEMI network (2003–2004) the percentage of patients receiving any reperfusion therapy increased from 66% to 87% [4], while, as a consequence, in-hospital mortality of all registered STEMI patients decreased from 16% to 9.5% (*p* <0.01). Over time the percentage of patients referred for primary PCI further increased, while TT decreased to less than 10% in the sixth year of the network, with a stable 13% of patients not receiving any reperfusion therapy because of contraindications, e.g. severe comorbidities (➲ Fig. 40.2).

One-year mortality reflected a persistent beneficial effect of early TT in patients with STEMI of <2 h of symptom onset, as compared with primary PCI, or pharmacological

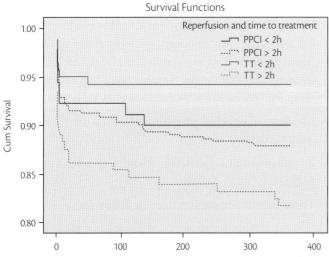

Figure 40.3 Vienna STEMI Registry: 1-year survival rate (2003–2004). From Fox KA, Huber K. A European perspective on improving acute systems of care in STEMI: we know what to do, but how can we do it? *Nat Clin Pract Cardiovasc Med* 2008;**5**:708–714. Reprinted by permission from MacMillan Publishers Ltd.

reperfusion or primary PCI in patients with infarction of more than 2 h duration [32] (➲ Fig. 40.3).

The French experience with the SAMU system

The French SAMU system (Service d'Aide Médicale Urgente; see ➲ Chapter 4) is a nationwide system with a unique nationwide call number and one SAMU medical response centre for each French administrative region, which dispatches one or several mobile intensive care units (MICUs). By French law, each MICU team is staffed by a senior emergency physician, a nurse, and a basic life support (BLS)-certified driver. Management on scene by the MICU team and precise notification to the medical centre of the patient's status allow direct admission to the most appropriate setting.

The FAST-MI registry evaluated all patients hospitalized for acute MI in an ICU in France with participation of approximately 60% of all French hospitals [7]. It was demonstrated that 21% of patients received prehospital TT, 11% in-hospital TT, 38% primary PCI, and 30% no reperfusion therapy. By use of the SAMU system median time from first call to reperfusion was 110 min versus 154 min with other routes, and more patients with SAMU received reperfusion therapy (77% vs 59%) [7].

When primary PCI cannot be performed in a timely fashion, the most widely used strategy in France is a pharmaco-invasive approach, with 96% of patients undergoing coronary angiography after TT [7]. Approximately 85% of patients undergo subsequent PCI and 58% of these patients undergo PCI within 24 h after initiation of TT. In-hospital mortality was comparable for TT and primary PCI, with 4.3% and 5.0%, respectively. In patients after TT 30-day mortality was 9.2% without and 3.9% with subsequent PCI. These results confirm that, in selected patients presenting early after symptom onset, TT followed by systematic angiography and, when needed, PCI, is a true alternative to primary PCI.

The Mayo Clinic network

This network includes 28 non-PCI hospitals and rural areas located up to 150 miles (240 km) away from the single catheter-equipped centre (St Mary's Hospital in Rochester, Minnesota) [5].

Patients presenting within the city limits of Rochester are delivered directly for primary PCI. Patients presenting to a regional hospital beyond 3 h of symptom onset receive morphine, aspirin, clopidogrel, and heparin and

---

Box 40.2 Improving systems of care

- Public information campaigns
- Cooperation and communication between EMS, PCI-capable hospitals, and non-PCI hospitals
- Involvement of health politicians
- Financial support
- Education
- Registry

Box 40.3 Barriers for building up STEMI networks

- Lack of patient awareness
- Communication problems between participating parties
- Nonavailability of 24/7 catheterization facilities
- Transfer problems
- Legal impediments
- Insufficient use of prehospital TT if indicated
- Financial barriers
- Absence of treatment protocols
- Insufficient reimbursement and insurance

---

are directly transferred to the catheterization laboratory, bypassing the emergency department there. Patients presenting to a regional hospital within 3 h of onset of pain receive TT (tenecteplase) and are immediately transferred to the catheterization laboratory or the CCU, where they receive rescue PCI in nonresponders to TT. Patients in the TT group showed the lowest mortality rates compared to both primary PCI groups, although this was not statistically significant [5]. At 6 months, this trend continued, with mortality rates of 10.5% at the PCI centre, 8.8% among transfer patients, and 6.9% with TT, respectively.

The North Carolina network

The RACE (Reperfusion of Acute Myocardial Infarction in North Carolina Emergency Departments) network in the state of North Carolina is a statewide STEMI system of more than 100 hospitals and 700 EMSs [6]. Regional, non-PCI-capable hospitals are coordinated with nearby PCI centres to maximize the number of patients undergoing timely primary PCI. EMS dispatchers are trained to recognize potential STEMI patients and to dispatch ECG-equipped ambulances. Diagnosis is performed on site by paramedics, and patients with STEMI are transported directly to the nearest PCI-capable hospital for primary PCI provided the time from FMC-to-balloon is less than 90 min. If the anticipated delay exceeds 90 min, patients receive prehospital TT and are transferred to the nearest PCI-capable hospital for follow-up.

Based on the experience of these and other examples of STEMI networks several factors have been identified, which are main determinants of the success of systems of care (◗ Box 40.2).

Barriers to building up networks

Important barriers for the organization of networks include:

- Lack of patient and public awareness of symptoms and how to react when they occur
- Communication problems between ambulance transportation systems and interventional cardiology departments
- Nonavailability of PCI facilities and staff around the clock
- Lack of agreement to transfer patients directly to PCI-capable facilities
- Restrictions imposed by national legislation on bypassing local hospitals
- Insufficient advocacy of prehospital TT
- Financial barriers to staffing and training of EMS personnel and providing modern equipment for ambulances (minimum 12-lead ECG, optimal 17-lead ECG, optimal telemedicine devices for transmittal of ECGs, reimbursement for cost of thrombolytic agents)
- Absence of treatment protocols used to prevent in-hospital delays
- Reimbursement policies, funding, and insurance policies.

These factors are summarized in ◗ Box 40.3.

Personal perspectives

The formation of networks to improve treatment of acute STEMI is one of the most important recommendations of the recent international guidelines. In many countries, however, the essential structures for building up systems of care, e.g. local diagnosis and treatment protocols, well-equipped and staffed EMS systems, well-organized ambulance transfer of STEMI patients to PCI centres, or 24/7 active catheter facilities with experienced personnel, are either totally absent or only partially available. Moreover, even in the presence of all necessary network constituents, financial, regulatory, and personal impacts not infrequently impede the formation and optimal action of STEMI networks. Cooperation and conversation between participating centres and the inclusion of health politicians on a local and national basis for financial and regulatory support are prerequisites for optimization of such systems of care. Those who have already built up successful STEMI networks need to educate and support others who are willing to do so but lack experience in order to improve clinical outcome in STEMI nation- and worldwide.

Conclusion

Geographic considerations and distribution of PPCI centers mean that for most countries and regions in Europe and North America primary PCI can be provided for the majority of the population if systems are in place to optimize its use. At present, between 20–90% of patients with STEMI undergo primary PCI, a range that reflects local resources and capabilities. Accordingly, there will be still an important role for thrombolytic therapy, especially when offered pre-hospital, in most countries. Moreover, of those patients with acute STEMI who are referred for primary PCI, not all receive optimal mechanical reperfusion within the recommended time range, i.e. first medical contact-to-balloon time of < (90-) 120 minutes with the procedure performed in an experienced center with an experienced team. The key to success begins with local organization of dedicated care-providers in each community. With the agreement of all stakeholders and participants in optimized networks, financial, regulatory, and political barriers can be resolved, and prompt, guidelines-recommended care becomes feasible, achievable, and affordable.

Further reading

Antman EM, Hand M, Armstrong PW, *et al.* 2007 focused update of the ACC/AHA 2004 guidelines for the management of patients with ST-elevation myocardial infarction. A report of the American College of Cardiology/American Heart Association Task Force on practice guidelines. *Circulation* 2008;**117**;296–329.

Danchin N, Coste P, Ferrières J, *et al.* Comparison of thrombolysis followed by broad use of percutaneous coronary intervention with primary percutaneous coronary intervention for ST-segment-elevation acute myocardial infarction: data from the French registry on acute ST-elevation myocardial infarction (FAST-MI). *Circulation* 2008;**118**:268–276.

Diercks DB, Kontos MC, Chen AY, *et al.* Utilization of paramedic transport with prehospital 12-lead electrocardiography on door-to-balloon time for patients with ST-segment elevation myocardial infarction. *J Am Coll Cardiol.* 2009;**53**:161–166.

Eagle KA, Nallamothu BK, Mehta RH, *et al.* Trends in acute reperfusion therapy for ST-segment elevation myocardial infarction from 1999 to 2006: we are getting better but we have got a long way to go. *Eur Heart J* 2008;**29**:609–617.

Fox KA, Huber K. A European perspective on improving acute systems of care in STEMI: we know what to do, but how can we do it? *Nat Clin Pract Cardiovasc Med.* 2008;**5**:708–714.

Huber K, De Caterina R, Kristensen SD, *et al.* Pre-hospital reperfusion therapy: a strategy to improve therapeutic outcome in patients with ST-elevation myocardial infarction. *Eur Heart J* 2005;**26**:2063–2074.

Kalla K, Christ G, Karnik R, *et al.* Implementation of guidelines improves the standard of care: the Viennese registry on reperfusion strategies in ST-elevation myocardial infarction (Vienna STEMI registry). *Circulation* 2006;**113**:2398–2405.

Nallamothu BK, Bates ER, Herrin J, *et al.* Times to treatment in transfer patients undergoing primary percutaneous coronary intervention in the United States: National Registry of Myocardial Infarction (NRMI)-3/4 analysis. *Circulation* 2005;**111**:761–767.

Steg PG, Cambout JP, Goldstein P, *et al.* Bypassing the emergency room reduces delays and mortality in ST-elevation myocardial infarction: the USIC 2000 registry. *Heart* 2006;**92**:1378–1383.

Ting HH, Rihal CS, Gersh BJ, *et al.* Regional systems of care to optimize timeliness of reperfusion therapy for ST-elevation myocardial infarction: the Mayo Clinic STEMI Protocol. *Circulation.* 2007;**116**:729–736.

Van de Werf F, Bax J, Betriu A, *et al.* Management of acute myocardial infarction in patients presenting with persistent ST-segment elevation: the Task Force on the Management of ST-Segment Elevation Acute Myocardial Infarction of the European Society of Cardiology. *Eur Heart J* 2008;**29**:2909–2945.

⮕ For additional multimedia materials please visit the online version of the book (🔗 http://www.esciacc.oxfordmedicine.com).

CHAPTER 41

ST-segment elevation myocardial infarction

Nicolas Danchin, Nadia Aissaoui and
Eric Durand

Contents

Summary

ST-elevation myocardial infarction (STEMI) is a true medical emergency. It is usually caused by an acute thrombotic occlusion of a coronary artery. The first therapeutic objective is to achieve reperfusion of the infarct-related artery as quickly as possible after symptom onset, in order to limit infarct size. Primary percutaneous coronary intervention (PCI) is the preferred reperfusion method; when it cannot be performed in due time, fibrinolysis followed by coronary angiography in the next few hours constitutes a valid alternative.

Beside reperfusion therapy, treatment of STEMI requires antithrombotic medications combining dual antiplatelet therapy and anticoagulants, β-blockers, and angiotensin converting enzyme (ACE) inhibitors. Statins are prescribed before hospital discharge.

The main complications are cardiac arrest and ventricular fibrillation, arrhythmias and conduction disturbances, mechanical complications and shock due to pump dysfunction. All require specific therapeutic measures.

Organization of care is crucial in the management of STEMI, and registry data show continuous improvement in outcomes over the past 15 years.

Introduction

ST-segment elevation myocardial infarction (STEMI) represents the most common form of acute coronary syndrome (ACS) [1]. It is also the form of ACS that incurs the highest early mortality, and this in spite of the fact that STEMI occurs at a younger age than non-ST-segment-elevation myocardial infarction (non-STEMI) [2–4]. The incidence of myocardial infarction in European countries parallels that of cardiovascular disease [5]. In the World Health Organization MONICA project, the incidence of major coronary events was monitored in 37 different populations in 21 countries (including 29 populations in 16 European countries). Although the data are now more than 10 years old and the populations selected for the project are not necessarily representative of the whole countries to which the MONICA centres belonged, they still represent the most recent source of data on cardiovascular morbidity across European countries. The incidence of definite or likely myocardial infarction was higher in northern, central and eastern Europe, than in western or southern Europe. The relative incidence of myocardial infarction (MI) across centres was similar in men and women, with the highest figures found in Glasgow; likewise, the geographical pattern for MI was similar to that for cardiovascular death. During the period the study was carried out (1983–1996), the incidence of MI decreased markedly in northern and western Europe, while, if present, the decrease was much less in eastern and central European countries. Case fatality rates were also higher in central and eastern European countries, compared with the other European regions. In the past 10 years, however, enormous efforts have been made in the organization of care for patients with STEMI, particularly in some countries of central and eastern Europe, and it is likely that rapid improvement in case fatality will be observed in these countries. There are also convincing data suggesting that an important part in the decline in cardiovascular mortality is attributable to improved patient care and decreased mortality in patients developing acute MI [6, 7].

Finally, there is evidence that the prevalence of STEMI is currently declining [8]. In the ARIC study [9], the incidence of STEMI decreased by 1.9% per year from 1987 to 2002. The Framingham heart study showed that ECG-documented incidence of acute MI (i.e. mostly STEMI) declined by 50% from 1960 to 1999, while the incidence of markers-documented AMI (i.e. non-STEMI) doubled [10].

Definitions

The universal definition of MI is discussed in ➲ Chapter 39. For clinicians, acute MI is defined by a combination of criteria including ischaemic symptoms, ECG abnormalities, and rise in cardiac markers [11]. From an operational standpoint, STEMI is defined by the combination of ischaemic symptoms and persistent ST-segment elevation on the ECG. ECG is therefore central for diagnosing STEMI. ST-segment elevation is considered to be present when new ST elevation is observed at the J-point in at least two contiguous leads with the following cut-off values: at least 0.2 mV in men or at least 0.15 mV in women in leads V_2–V_3 and/or at least 0.1 mV in other leads. Most patients will subsequently show a typical rise and fall of biological

markers of myocardial necrosis and many will progress to Q-wave MI.

Pathophysiology

Atherosclerosis is the leading cause of coronary artery disease. STEMI is usually caused by an occlusive intracoronary thrombus developing at the site of an atherosclerotic plaque. The trigger for the occurrence of intracoronary thrombus is plaque rupture or erosion [12, 13], but the mechanisms leading to coronary plaque rupture are yet incompletely elucidated. Increased haemodynamic stress may trigger acute MI; strenuous physical activity [14, 15], or major emotional stress, as was documented after the 1994 earthquake in Los Angeles [16], during emergency duties in firefighters [17], or during football matches [18, 19] are recognized triggering factors for STEMI. Clinical observations suggest that acute stress promotes the development of MI, but that it is not its underlying cause: thus, an important increase in the incidence of AMI was observed immediately after the Californian earthquake, but the incidence of AMI was lower in the following days, suggesting that acute stress had simply accelerated the occurrence of the acute event [16]. Other environmental factors, such as air pollution, have been incriminated as triggering factors for STEMI [20, 21]. Likewise, a circadian pattern in the timing of onset of MI exists, with a peak in the early hours, when levels of catecholamines are high and levels of coagulation factor are increased [22]. Inflammation, with monocytes, macrophages and T-cell infiltrates, together with a large lipid core and thin fibrous cap of the atheromatous plaque, plays a key role in the genesis of plaque rupture. In addition, hyperaggregability and prothrombotic states are usually observed. Finally, coronary vasoconstriction and coronary artery spasm may play an additional role. In rare instances, STEMI can be caused by pure coronary artery spasm, leading to subsequent thrombosis or by spontaneous dissection of a coronary artery.

Of note, STEMI is often caused by an occlusive thrombus which develops on mild, rather than tight, coronary plaques. In a seminal work in patients undergoing repeated coronary angiograms after fibrinolytic treatment for STEMI, Cribier et al. observed that the average stenosis of the residual plaque in the infarct-related artery was only 47% [23]. Conversely, complete occlusions occurring on tight coronary artery stenoses often do not lead to STEMI, because chronic ischaemia promotes diverse protective mechanisms including the development of collateral circulation and myocardial preconditioning [24]. The protective effect of preinfarct angina on infarct size gives evidence of the clinical reality of this protective mechanism [25]. Overall, in a word, most STEMIs are caused by complete coronary artery occlusions, but all complete coronary artery occlusions do not cause STEMI. There is no direct relationship between the degree of a coronary stenosis and the risk of developing STEMI [26].

The consequences of acute coronary thrombosis are a major decrease in epicardial flow and possibly also distal embolization of thrombus. Both lead to a myocardial necrosis wavefront beginning in the myocardial subendocardial layers and progressively reaching the subepicardium, until full transmural necrosis is constituted. Following recanalization of the culprit artery, impaired distal perfusion (no-reflow phenomenon) may occur. The no-reflow phenomenon can be observed in up to one-third of patients treated with primary PCI. Its pathophysiology is not fully elucidated; it seems largely related to reperfusion injury following prolonged ischaemia, leading to microvascular damage, caused by the effects of oxidative stress. Vasoconstriction caused by endothelial dysfunction, obstruction of the capillaries by endothelial debris and neutrophils, and compression by myocardial oedema can lead to microvascular obstruction. In addition, iatrogenic embolization of thrombus and/or plaque material during coronary intervention may aggravate this phenomenon.

Clinical presentation and ECG findings

The typical presentation of STEMI consists of a retrosternal chest pain, which does not stop spontaneously. Frequently patients report repeated brief and milder episodes of pain during the preceding hours and days. The pain is of a crushing nature, sometimes associated with a feeling of immediate death. There are usually no specific immediate triggering circumstances, and it is common that the chest pain starts when the patient is at rest. The pain is unrelieved by the use of nitroglycerine. It may radiate to all usual locations (neck and jaw, arm, upper abdomen). It is not rare, however, for the pain to be of a lesser intensity, particularly in diabetic or elderly patients. The MI pain, sometimes also epigastric in location, may be accompanied by vagal symptoms with diaphoresis and nausea or vomiting; this is particularly frequent in inferior MI. In rarer instances the initial symptom may be acute dyspnoea, pulmonary oedema, or syncope. Cardiac arrest may be the first manifestation of STEMI.

Physical examination is often normal. A degree of tachycardia is frequent. Pulmonary rales may be heard if left ventricular dysfunction is present. There are no cardiac murmurs in uncomplicated forms, but a fourth heart sound is common. A mild fever is often present at the initial stage. Arterial pressure is most often normal or mildly elevated. Low systolic blood pressure may correspond to either a vasovagal reaction, or to onset of shock. Cardiogenic shock is accompanied with signs of peripheral hypoperfusion, on top of low blood pressure unresponsive to fluid administration. Right ventricular infarction is characterized by the combination of low arterial blood pressure and signs of right heart dysfunction, particularly jugular vein distension.

The presence of left ventricular dysfunction is graded using the Killip classification [27] (◑ Box 41.1)

An ECG recording must be made as soon as possible and is essential in establishing the diagnosis. The main ECG finding is the presence of ST-segment elevation, which is usually of a greater magnitude when located inferior or inferobasal (posterior) leads. The ECG may also reveal a previously unrecognized left bundle branch block. It is not unusual to document conduction disturbances, particularly in inferior MIs, where atrio-ventricular block (up to third degree block) may occur.

In the absence of reperfusion therapy, pain usually lasts for several hours, and may even be present for more than one full day, although its intensity progressively decreases.

Differential diagnoses include aortic dissection, pericarditis (or myocarditis), Takotsubo's syndrome, and noncardiac pains such as pneumonia or pulmonary embolism, as well as gastrointestinal disorders.

Complications

Four main groups of complications may be observed: complications related to left ventricular dysfunction, complications related to rhythm disturbances, mechanical

---

Box 41.1 Killip classification

- Class I: no evidence of congestive heart failure or shock
- Class II: mild–moderate heart failure: presence of pulmonary rales in less than half of both lung fields
- Class III: severe congestive heart failure: pulmonary oedema
- Class IV: cardiogenic shock

complications, and pericardial reaction. Right ventricular infarction can also have specific complications.

Left ventricular failure and cardiogenic shock

Pump failure remains a major complication of STEMI. Left ventricular dysfunction is correlated with the extent of the necrotic area; it ranges from the simple presence of pulmonary rales, to that of cardiogenic shock. From the clinical standpoint, left ventricular dysfunction is classified according to the Killip classification (→ Box 41.1). Cardiogenic shock is defined by the presence of tissue hypoperfusion, with the association of low systemic blood pressure (<90 mmHg) unresponsive to fluid loading or atropine, with high central pressure (pulmonary wedge pressure >20 mmHg) or a cardiac index less than $1.8 \text{ L min}^{-1}\text{m}^{-2}$. It is caused by extensive myocardial damage, severe global ischaemia due to diffuse coronary artery disease, right ventricular infarction, or mechanical complications. Cardiogenic shock is also considered to be present when inotropes or intra-aortic ballon pump (IABP) are needed to maintain a blood pressure greater than 90 mmHg or a cardiac index greater than $1.8 \text{ L min}^{-1}\text{m}^{-2}$. Cardiogenic shock develops in 5–10% of STEMI; its prevalence has slightly declined in the past 10 years and mortality remains high, usually more than 50% [28, 29].

Mechanical complications

Mitral regurgitation may be caused by papillary muscle dysfunction of ischaemic origin, by papillary muscle rupture, or by severe left ventricular dysfunction with left ventricular dilatation [30]. It is more commonly a complication of an inferoposterior infarction than of an anterior one. Papillary muscle rupture usually presents as acute mitral regurgitation with a typical systolic murmur and pulmonary oedema.

Ventricular free wall rupture is a particularly severe complication. In most instances, it manifests as electromechanical dissociation and is rapidly fatal. It may also present as subacute rupture, characterized by extreme hypotension, often coexisting with recurrent chest pain; signs of cardiac tamponade may appear. Echocardiography shows pericardial fluid and may detect the site of myocardial rupture. Rarely, the haemopericardium collects in a closed space that will later turn into a false aneurysm.

Ventricular septal rupture presents as abrupt haemodynamic deterioration, with signs of both right and left heart failure; recurrent chest pain is not unusual. A new, loud systolic murmur is heard. Echocardiography can identify the site of the ventricular septal defect, and evidence and quantify the left-to-right shunt. Right-sided chambers are enlarged. Although small ventricular septal ruptures may heal spontaneously and leave only a mild to moderate shunt, most cases deteriorate rapidly and the patients go into shock.

Conduction disturbances

The prognostic significance of atrioventricular block differs according to infarct location. High degree atrioventricular block during inferior MI usually resolves spontaneously and does not need specific therapeutic measures when the escape rhythm is more than 40–45 beats/min. In contrast, atrioventricular block developing in patients with anterior MI usually persists and usually requires artificial pacing [31]. Left bundle branch block is not rare, and is associated with poorer outcomes, mainly related to older age and comorbidities [32].

Arrhythmias

Atrial fibrillation occurs frequently at the acute stage of MI; it is more frequent in older individuals and may reflect left ventricular dysfunction, atrial infarction, or pericarditis. In most instances, atrial fibrillation is well tolerated and does not require specific therapy. Ventricular fibrillation develops in less than 5% of patients, once hospitalized. It requires emergency cardioversion. Ventricular premature beats are common. Accelerated idioventricular rhythm is frequent at the time of myocardial reperfusion and is benign.

Right ventricular infarction

Right ventricular infarction is the consequence of acute occlusion of the proximal right coronary artery. The clinical signs include low blood pressure, increased jugular venous pressure, and normal pulmonary auscultation. It is contemporary with an inferior infarction, and ECG tracings show ST-segment-elevation in V_3R and V_4R; ST-segment elevation may also be present in V_1–V_2. Echocardiography usually shows a dilated right ventricle, with localized or diffuse hypo- or akinesis. Conduction disturbances are not rare, as is atrial fibrillation. Even now, right ventricular infarction remains a marker of poorer prognosis [33].

Iatrogenic complications

Iatrogenic complications are not uncommon; most are related to the use of invasive procedures. The most common are bleeding complications. Bleeding may start at the puncture site in patients who have undergone coronary angiography/PCI; it may present as large haematomas, arterial pseudo-aneurysms, arteriovenous fistulas, or retroperitoneal bleeding. Intracerebral haemorrhage may also occur, in up to 1% of patients on fibrinolysis. Bleeding complications are highly correlated with the use of antithrombotic medications, including fibrinolysis; they are more frequent in older individuals and in those with poor renal function or other comorbidities [34]. Beyond their immediate hazard, bleeding complications are markers of poor long-term outcome [35].

Biomarkers and imaging

Neither biomarkers nor cardiac imaging are required to make the diagnosis of STEMI. In particular, the results of neither should not be awaited before taking the appropriate therapeutic measures, and deciding on the use of reperfusion therapy. They can, however, be used to quantify necrosis and to assess prognosis [36]. Several markers can be used, the kinetics of which differ. Myoglobin rises and decreases rapidly; the MB (myocardium–brain) fraction of creatine kinase (CK-MB) is more specific, but increased levels are only detectable a few hours after the onset of necrosis. Troponin is currently the most widely used marker of myocardial necrosis, because of its excellent sensitivity; both troponin T and troponin I can be used. Their release is slower than that of myoglobin or CK-MB, but increased levels persist for several days. Recently, ultrasensitive troponin measurement has become available for routine clinical use; increased levels are detected earlier, but the specificity in a broad spectrum of clinical circumstances has not yet been extensively studied [37, 38]. The utility of cardiac markers is more fully discussed in ❍ Chapter 33.

The most useful imaging technique at the acute stage of STEMI is echocardiography [39]. The infarcted area is seen as a severely hypokinetic or akinetic zone. Echocardiography provides an estimate of the area at risk and of left ventricular ejection fraction. Global haemodynamics can be assessed, with estimates of cardiac output and pulmonary artery pressures. It also constitutes the easiest way to confirm the presence of mechanical complications or of right ventricular infarction. Finally, it may be used to eliminate differential diagnoses, such as aortic dissection. Other imaging techniques include chest radiography, which can assess the presence of pulmonary congestion, MRI, or CT, which may be used for differential diagnosis assessment, and particularly aortic dissection or myocarditis [40].

Management

Reperfusion therapy

Reperfusion therapy modalities

The main goal of treatment in STEMI is to re-establish the patency of the infarct-related coronary artery (i.e. reperfusion therapy). From a historical perspective, fibrinolytic treatment was initially proposed by Chazov, and Rentrop was the first to use the intracoronary administration of a fibrinolytic agent; indeed, the first demonstration of the efficacy of coronary artery reperfusion in reducing clinical complications was brought about by intracoronary thrombolysis (❍ Table 41.1) in the early 1980s [41].

Because the intracoronary administration of lytic therapy was difficult to implement in routine clinical practice, the intravenous administration of lytics was tested in large randomized controlled trials. Both the GISSI [53] and the ISIS-2 [54] trials showed a marked reduction in clinical endpoints with the use of streptokinase, compared with placebo. Later on, several trials studied the efficacy and safety of fibrin-specific fibrinolytic agents, compared with streptokinase. The GUSTO trial [55] compared four regimens of fibrinolytic treatment combined with anticoagulants: 30-day mortality (the trial's primary endpoint) was 14% lower with tissue plasminogen activator (tPA) compared with the streptokinase-only arms of the trial, establishing accelerated

Table 41.1 Randomized trials of intracoronary fibrinolysis

Trial	Reference	N	Infarct size reduction (method used)	Improved LV function	Decreased early mortality	Decreased 1-year mortality
Khaja	[42]	40	–	No	No	–
Anderson	[43, 44]	50	Yes (radionuclide)	Yes	No	No
Kennedy	[45, 46]	250	–	No	Yes	Trend (p = 0.10)
Leiboff	[47]	43	–	No	No	No
Rentrop	[48, 49]	124	–	No	No	No (6-month)
Raizner	[50]	63	–	No	No	–
Simoons	[51, 52]	533	Yes (enzymes)	Yes	Yes	Yes

tPA as the standard of care for STEMI. Subsequently, newer fibrin-specific agents were tested against tPA. Reteplase, administered in two bolus doses of 10 MU given 30 min apart, showed similar rates of death (odds ratio 1.03) or death or disabling stroke (odds ratio 0.97). A single bolus of tenecteplase (30–50 mg, according to body weight) yielded similar 30-day mortality and stroke-free survival to tPA, with fewer noncerebral bleeding complications [55, 56]. In the ASSENT 3 trial, tenecteplase and reduced dose heparin was compared with tenecteplase combined with either abciximab or enoxaparin; death or ischaemic endpoints were significantly more frequent with the conventional unfractionated heparin regime; bleeding complications, however, were more frequent with abciximab or enoxaparin, compared with unfractionated heparin [57].

Finally, the concept of prehospital administration of fibrinolytic treatment, which was developed in the mid-1980s [58], was compared to in-hospital administration in several trials, the largest of which was the EMIP trial [59]. A 13% reduction in 30-day mortality was observed with prehospital treatment ($p = 0.08$), and cardiac death, a secondary endpoint of the trial, was significantly reduced by 16%. A subsequent meta-analysis of 6 randomized trials comparing prehospital and in-hospital fibrinolysis, including 6434 patients (of whom 5469 belonged to the EMIP trial), yielded a significant 17% reduction in mortality with prehospital fibrinolysis; the prehospital strategy was associated with a 1-h time gain for the administration of fibrinolytic treatment [60]. Contraindications for the use of fibrinolytic therapy are listed in ➲ Box 41.2.

The efficacy of fibrinolytic therapy, however, is not optimal, and adequate reperfusion of the infarct-related arteries is achieved only in approximately 60% of the patients, with relatively high rates of reinfarction. This led to the development of primary PCI (i.e. PCI performed without up-front fibrinolytic treatment). Finally, in the recent past, several trials investigated a strategy of 'facilitated' PCI (i.e. patients en route for primary PCI, in whom intravenous fibrinolysis and/or glycoprotein (GP)IIb/IIIa medications are administered in an attempt to achieve quicker reopening of the infarct-related artery) or a combined 'pharmaco-invasive strategy' (i.e. patients treated with fibrinolysis, in whom coronary angiography ± PCI is subsequently performed, in order to achieve higher rates of reperfusion and to limit the risk of reinfarction).

Fibrinolytic therapy vs primary percutaneous coronary intervention

The results from randomized clinical trials have formed the basis of the current reperfusion practices and of

---

Box 41.2 Contraindications for the use of fibrinolytic therapy

Absolute contraindications

- Any history of intracranial bleeding
- Known cerebral vascular lesions
- Known malignant brain tumour
- Ischaemic stroke within 6 months (except ischaemic stroke in the first 3 h)
- Suspected aortic dissection
- Active bleeding or bleeding diathesis
- Significant head trauma in past 3 months

Relative contraindications

- History of severe hypertension or severe hypertension on admission
- Any history of stroke, dementia, or intracranial abnormality
- Prolonged or traumatic resuscitation
- Major surgery in past 3 weeks
- Recent internal bleeding (in last 4 weeks)
- Noncompressible vascular punctures
- Pregnancy
- Active peptic ulcer
- Use of vitamin K antagonists (particularly with high INR)

---

international and national guidelines. Keeley and colleagues [61] performed a quantitative analysis of 23 trials and demonstrated that primary PCI compared with fibrinolytic therapy resulted in reduced mortality (7% vs 9%, $p = 0.0002$), reinfarction (3% vs 7%, $p <0.0001$), stroke (1% vs 2%, $p = 0.0004$), and their combination (8% vs 14%, $p <0.0001$). Among these trials, the CAPTIM trial [62] was the only one to compare primary PCI and prehospital thrombolytic therapy and it was also the only one to find a trend toward reduced mortality at 30 days and 1 year with prehospital fibrinolysis compared to primary PCI. Conversely, comparing primary PCI with thrombolytic treatment in patients admitted to hospitals without PCI capability showed a clear advantage to the interventional technique. In particular, the DANAMI-2 trial [63, 64] indicated that transferring a patient for primary PCI (provided that the transfer took less than 2 h) was beneficial, particularly in terms of reinfarction, compared with treating with intravenous thrombolytic therapy in the primary hospital. Of note, however, in all these trials, the use of coronary angiography and angioplasty in fibrinolytic-treated patients was limited to a minority of the patients, although there were large differences between trials: in CAPTIM, rescue PCI was performed in 26% of the patients receiving prehospital fibrinolysis, whereas in DANAMI-2, only 1.9% of patients had a rescue procedure; for any subsequent PCI during the hospital stay, the respective figures in the two trials were 34.5% and 16.4%. Most of the trials thus compared a strategy of stand-alone fibrinolysis with primary PCI. Real-world observations confirm the excellent results achieved with prehospital fibrinolysis, and with a combined strategy of fibrinolysis followed by later angioplasty [65–68] (➲ Fig. 41.1).

Newer techniques, such as thrombectomy, may improve the clinical outcomes after primary PCI [69, 70]. Likewise, interventions used in the case of no-reflow phenomenon (injection of adenosine, verapamil, nicorandil, nitroprusside, or papaverine) have been shown to improve coronary flow, but their impact on clinical outcomes has not been studied in large clinical trials [71]. Finally, the concept of myocardial postconditioning, using either balloon reinflation after reopening of the coronary artery, or medications such as ciclosporin, might constitute novel ways to further improve the results of primary PCI [72–74].

Percutaneous coronary intervention after fibrinolytic treatment

In spite of the disappointing results achieved with angioplasty following intravenous fibrinolysis in trials carried out in the late 1980s, new attempts were made in the 2000s, because considerable progress had been made with adjunctive antithrombotic therapy and in particular the combined use of aspirin, thienopyridine therapy, and intravenous GPIIb/IIIa inhibitors. Those attempts were made in two directions: improving the efficacy of primary PCI by administering fibrinolytic treatment or GPIIb/IIIa inhibitors en route for the interventional procedure (so-called 'facilitated' PCI); or improving the result of fibrinolysis by performing subsequent PCI in all or selected patients [67, 75].

Facilitated percutaneous coronary intervention

A number of randomized trials have compared primary PCI with PCI 'facilitated' by either fibrinolytic treatment, GP IIb/IIIa inhibitors, or both. A meta-analysis published in 2006 showed that, although more patients assigned to facilitated PCI had initial TIMI 3 flow, there was no clinical benefit, compared with primary PCI [76]. Recently, facilitated PCI was evaluated in two large randomized trials. The ASSENT-4 PCI trial compared primary PCI with PCI immediately preceded by tenecteplase and was interrupted prematurely because an excess of events was observed in the facilitated arm, despite the fact that more patients had an open infarct-related artery before the angioplasty procedure [77]. Two factors may have explained these findings: first, concomitant antithrombotic therapy may have been insufficient in the tenecteplase arm of the trial; second, PCI was performed very soon after administration of fibrinolytic treatment, at a time when platelet reactivity was still increased. Both factors may have played a role in the increased reinfarction rate observed in the facilitated arm. In the FINESSE trial [78], patients were randomized in a 1:1:1 fashion to primary PCI with in-laboratory abciximab, up-front abciximab-facilitated primary PCI, or half-dose reteplase/abciximab-facilitated PCI. Although ST-segment resolution was more frequently observed in the combination-facilitated PCI arm, no difference was found in the primary outcome of the trial (death, late ventricular

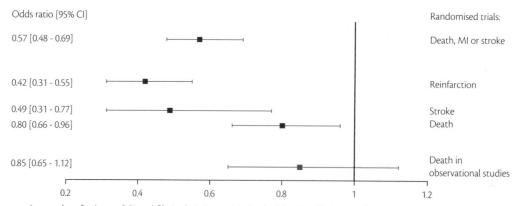

Figure 41.1 Comparative results of primary PCI and fibrinolysis in randomized trials using fibrin-specific agents (red) and in observational studies (purple). Data from Keeley EC, Boura JA, Grines CL. Primary angioplasty versus intravenous thrombolytic therapy for acute myocardial infarction: a quantitative review of 23 randomised trials. *Lancet.* 2003;**361**(9351):13–20 and Huynh T, Perron S, O'Loughlin J, *et al.* Comparison of primary percutaneous coronary intervention and fibrinolytic therapy in ST-segment-elevation myocardial infarction: bayesian hierarchical meta-analyses of randomized controlled trials and observational studies. *Circulation.* 2009;**119**(24):3101–3109.

fibrillation, cardiogenic shock or congestive heart failure at 90 days). In patients admitted to non-PCI hospitals and with a high risk score, however, 1-year survival was better with the facilitated strategy [79].

Rescue percutaneous coronary intervention

Several trials addressed the question of the benefit of coronary angiography and PCI after fibrinolytic treatment. The REACT trial showed that, in patients who had failed fibrinolytic therapy, documented by the absence of ST-segment resolution after fibrinolysis, rescue PCI was better than a conservative approach or repeated fibrinolysis [80].

Routine percutaneous coronary intervention after fibrinolysis

Beyond rescue PCI, the role of systematic PCI within 24 h of fibrinolysis was investigated in the GRACIA-1 trial [81], the CAPITAL-AMI trial [82], the SIAM-III tial [83], and the larger CARESS-in-AMI trial [84]. In all instances, a strategy of systematic PCI after intravenous fibrinolytic treatment yielded better results than conservative management. The CARESS-in-AMI trial demonstrated that a strategy of immediate PCI was better than the standard of rescue-only angioplasty after fibrinolysis, with a significant and marked reduction in the primary endpoint of death, reinfarction, or refractory ischaemia at 30 days (10.7% vs 4.4%, $p = 0.005$). More recently, the TRANSFER-AMI trial enrolled 1030 patients less than 12 h after acute MI who received fibrinolytic treatment and were randomly assigned to transfer for angioplasty within 6 h or to a strategy limiting emergency angiography to rescue angioplasty, associated with elective late angiography in those not needing rescue angioplasty [85]. There was no difference in mortality between the standard and pharmaco-invasive treatment (3.4% vs 4.5%, $p = 0.39$), but the composite endpoint of death, MI, or recurrent ischaemia strongly favoured the pharmaco-invasive strategy (17.2% vs 11.0%, $p = 0.004$). The WEST study further strengthens this concept by suggesting that rapidly applied pharmacological reperfusion with follow-up (rescue and routine) PCI within 24 h produces results equivalent to those of PPCI [86].

All these data have led to the current STEMI guidelines of the European Society of Cardiology (ESC) recommending coronary angiography in all patients treated with intravenous fibrinolysis (grade IIa recommendation) [87].

The importance of time delays

The success of reperfusion in STEMI is dependent on the time of administration. For all recent guidelines, including the ESC and the American College of Cardiology/American Heart Association (ACC/AHA) guidelines [87, 88], time delays are central in the decision-making process. There is no evidence that fibrinolysis is beneficial beyond 12 h of symptom onset [89]; likewise, the benefits of primary PCI are seen essentially in patients undergoing coronary angiography within 12 h of chest pain onset [90]. The OAT trial failed to show a clinical advantage to PCI performed on totally occluded arteries 3–28 days after STEMI [91]. In fibrinolytic-treated patients, mortality reduction is the greatest in patients seen within 3 h of chest pain onset [89]. The impact of time delays on the efficacy of reperfusion therapy is also observed in patients treated with primary PCI, although the influence of time delays on outcomes is rather less apparent than with fibrinolysis [90].

Time delays are therefore crucial in determining the best reperfusion strategy: the superiority of primary PCI over fibrinolysis exists only as far as the time to reperfusion is not too greatly increased by opting for PCI rather than the simpler approach of intravenous fibrinolysis. From their review of the National Registry of Myocardial Infarction database, Pinto *et al.* found that the balance between the two reperfusion techniques varied according to time from symptom onset, location of MI, and age of the patient [92]. Primary PCI yielded better results than fibrinolysis when the excess time delay for delivering reperfusion therapy (PCI-related delay) did not exceed 114 min on average; however, the benefit of PCI was lost when the PCI-related delay was longer than 40 min for patients younger than 65 years of age with an anterior MI presenting within 2 h of symptom onset, while a PCI-related delay of 179 min still yielded equivalent results for both reperfusion techniques in patients over 65 years of age, with a nonanterior MI seen more than 2 h from symptom onset.

Anticoagulant and antiplatelet therapy

Anticoagulants and antiplatelet agents are used in most patients with STEMI. They are part of the mandatory therapeutic regimen in patients undergoing PCI. The evidence for using anticoagulants in patients treated with fibrinolysis, however, is more debatable.

Antithrombotic agents in fibrinolytic-treated patients

The ISIS-2 trial demonstrated the benefit of aspirin in patients receiving fibrinolytic treatment for suspected MI [54]. The trial had a 2×2 factorial design, assessing the impact of streptokinase and aspirin. The 35-day vascular mortality was similarly decreased by streptokinase only (odds reduction 25%) or aspirin only (odds reduction

23%), compared to the group on placebo; patients on combined fibrinolytic and aspirin therapy had the lowest rates of vascular death (odds reduction 42%). Much more recently, the CLARITY [93] and COMMITT [94] trials assessed the efficacy and safety of clopidogrel on top of aspirin in STEMI patients receiving fibrinolysis or without reperfusion therapy. In CLARITY, treatment with clopidogrel (300 mg loading dose, followed by 75 mg/day) improved infarct-related artery patency and was associated with a trend to reduced rates of reinfarction, with no effect on mortality. In the large COMMITT trial (45 852 patients), clopidogrel (75 mg/day) reduced mortality by 7% (95% CI 1–13%) and the combination of death, reinfarction, or stroke by 9% (95% CI 3–14%), without increased risk of bleeding. The favourable effect of clopidogrel was of the same magnitude in patients receiving fibrinolysis or those without reperfusion therapy.

GPIIb/IIIa inhibitors, particularly abciximab, have been studied in patients receiving fibrinolytic treatment for STEMI. Because the initial trials combining full-dose lytics and GPIIb/IIIa inhibitors led to unacceptable bleeding rates, the most recent (and largest) trials have used half-dose lytics. In the GUSTO 5 trial, a half-dose of reteplase combined with abciximab was compared with standard dose reteplase [95]; combination therapy was not inferior to full-dose reteplase in terms of hard clinical events (OR 0.95 for 30-day mortality), with a significant reduction in reinfarction and reischaemia, but caused more nonintracranial bleeding. In addition, a significant interaction with age was found for the risk of intracranial bleeding; in patients over 75 years of age, the risk of intracranial bleeding was twice as high with the combination regimen. For the whole population, 1-year mortality was similar in both groups. In the ASSENT 3 trial, tenecteplase with unfractionated heparin was compared with half-dose tenecteplase, reduced dose heparin, and a 12-h infusion of abciximab [57]. There was a reduced incidence of the efficacy endpoint with combination therapy, but the major bleeding rate was twice as high. There was no difference in 1-year mortality. A meta-analysis of trials assessing the impact of abciximab on top of fibrinolytic treatment showed no benefit in both short-term and long-term mortality with the adjunction of the antiplatelet agent [96].

Two randomized trials, GISSI 2 and ISIS 3, individually found no significant difference in mortality or acute MI rates between unfractionated heparin plus fibrinolytics and fibrinolytics alone [97, 98]. The combined analysis of these trials, however, showed a small but significant reduction in mortality during the on-treatment period, but no difference in mortality at 1 month, thus suggesting a possible rebound effect after the end of heparin administration [98]. In patients receiving alteplase, heparin was shown to improve infarct-related artery patency [99]. Because high doses of heparin were associated with an increased risk of bleeding, the dosing regimen used in the ASSENT 3 trial, which led to 'reasonable' increases in bleeding, is now considered standard, in association with fibrinolytic treatment: 60 U/kg intravenous bolus (maximum 4000 U), followed by a maintenance infusion of 12 U/kg per hour (maximum 4000 U/h) [57]. The optimal duration of heparin treatment is not known. Only one small randomized trial compared the administration of heparin for 1 day to its prolonged administration: no difference was observed in any of the clinical endpoints, nor in the infarct-related artery patency on coronary angiography performed at 7–10 days [100]. Low-molecular-weight heparin (and particularly enoxaparin) has been compared with unfractionated heparin in patients receiving fibrinolysis. In the ASSENT 3 and ASSENT 3 plus trials, ischaemic events at 1 month were reduced by enoxaparin, but more patients on low-molecular-weight heparin had intracranial bleeding [57, 101, 102]. This increased risk of intracranial bleeding led to an adjustment in the dose of enoxaparin in the large EXTRACT TIMI 25 trial (30 mg IV bolus, followed by 1 mg/kg SC in 12 h in patients <75 years of age; no bolus and a dose of 0.75 mg/kg in 12 h in patients ≥75 years of age) [103]. The risk of death or nonfatal recurrent MI was lower in enoxaparin-treated patients, but major bleeding was increased; the overall net clinical benefit was in favour of enoxaparin. Enoxaparin is usually administered for a period of 4–8 days. These results reinforce the findings of the Eikelboom meta-analysis, which showed a significant reduction in AMI or death with enoxaparin, compared with either placebo or unfractionated heparin in patients receiving fibrinolytic treatment [104]. Overall, the evidence supports the preferential use of enoxaparin for a period of 4–8 days, rather than unfractionated heparin for 24–48 h, as adjunctive anticoagulant treatment in patients receiving fibrinolysis. The newer anticoagulant fondaparinux, a synthetic factor Xa inhibitor, was evaluated in a STEMI population in the OASIS 6 trial [105]. In the subgroup of 5436 patients receiving fibrinolytic therapy, fondaparinux was compared to placebo in 4415 patients (receiving streptokinase or urokinase) and against unfractionated heparin in 1021 patients (84% receiving a fibrin-specific agent) [106]. Overall, fondaparinux reduced the primary endpoint (death or reinfarction at 30 days); the benefit was found only in patients receiving non-fibrin-specific lytic agents (HR 0.75; 95% CI 0.62–0.90), while there was no risk reduction in patients treated with fibrin-specific agents. Severe bleeding was significantly less frequent in patients receiving fondaparinux. Of note, in this trial, very few patients underwent rescue PCI after lysis (<3%), a rate considerably lower than contemporary practice in most European countries.

Antithrombotic regimen in patients undergoing primary percutaneous coronary intervention

Aspirin and clopidogrel are standard procedure for patients undergoing PCI. In the setting of primary PCI, current discussions focus on the impact of the loading dose of clopidogrel and of newer antiplatelet agents. Most trials have used a 300-mg loading dose at the time of or immediately after PCI. The recent CURRENT-OASIS 7 trial compared a loading dose of 300 mg followed by 75 mg once a day versus 600 mg followed by 150 mg once a day for 5–7 days, in a 2 × 2 factorial design also comparing a high (300–325-mg) and a low (75–100-mg) dose of aspirin [107]. The higher dose clopidogrel regimen is associated with a nonsignificant reduction in the combined endpoint of cardiovascular death, recurrent MI, or stroke, in the 6346 patients who underwent PCI for STEMI (4.2% vs 5.0%); the combined endpoint of MI or stent thrombosis is significantly reduced (2.8% vs 4.0%). In the whole CURRENT-OASIS 7 population (i.e. including patients with non-STEMI and patients not treated with PCI), high-dose clopidogrel is associated with an increased risk of bleeding. There is no indication, however, of a reduction in cardiovascular death at 1 month with the higher loading dose, whether the patients have had PCI or not. Doubling the dose of aspirin has no impact.

Recently, new antiplatelet agents acting on the ADP pathway have been studied in large clinical trials. The thienopyridine prasugrel was used in the TRITON trial, which included patients undergoing PCI for STEMI and non-STEMI [108]. In the subgroup of 3534 patients with STEMI, of whom 69% underwent primary PCI, patients on prasugrel (60 mg loading dose, then 10 mg once a day) had a reduced risk of cardiovascular death, MI, or stroke at 30 days (OR 0.68; 95% CI 0.54–0.87), compared with patients on clopidogrel (300 mg loading dose, then 75 mg once a day) [109]. At 15 months, the odds ratio for the combined primary endpoint was 0.79 (95% CI 0.65–0.97). All-cause mortality was not significantly reduced (OR 0.76; 95% CI 0.54–1.07). There was no increase in bleeding events, except in the few patients who underwent urgent coronary artery bypass grafting (CABG). In the subset undergoing primary PCI, however, the reduction in the primary endpoint of the trial at 15 months was smaller (13%) and not statistically significant. The nonthienopyridine antiplatelet agent ticagrelor (180 mg loading dose, then 90 mg twice a day) was compared to clopidogrel (300–600 mg loading dose, then 75 mg once a day) in the large PLATO trial, including patients with STEMI and non-STEMI, irrespective of the use of PCI [110]. In the whole cohort, a significant reduction in the primary endpoint of the trial at 12 months (cardiovascular death, MI, or stroke) was observed with ticagrelor: HR 0.84; 95% CI 0.77–0.92. All-cause death was significantly reduced (HR 0.78; 95% CI 0.69–0.89). In the STEMI subgroup, the hazard ratio for the primary endpoint was 0.85, and all-cause mortality was also significantly reduced (HR 0.82; 95%CI 0.68–0.99) [111]. In both the TRITON and PLATO trials, there was no interaction with the use of GPIIb/IIIa inhibitors.

GPIIb/IIIa inhibitors have been studied in a number of trials in patients undergoing primary PCI. In a meta-analysis of 8 trials in 3949 patients undergoing PCI for STEMI, both 30-day (OR 0.68) and 6-month to 1-year (OR 0.69; 95%CI 0.52–0.92) mortality were significantly lower in patients treated with abciximab (0.25 mg/kg IV bolus, then 0.125 µg/kg per minute, maximum 10 µg/min, for 12 h) [96]. The largest benefit of abciximab was observed in patients with the highest risk profile [112]. Small molecules have been studied less extensively in the setting of primary PCI. In a meta-analysis including six trials comparing high-dose tirofiban or eptifibatide with abciximab, no difference in mortality, reinfarction, or bleeding complications was observed, suggesting a similar efficacy and safety profile for all types of intravenous GPIIb/IIIa inhibitors [113].

Unfractionated heparin has been the most widely used anticoagulant in patients undergoing primary PCI for STEMI. Pending the results of ongoing trials, there is only limited experience with the use of enoxaparin in this setting. In the EXTRACT TIMI 25 trial, patients who underwent PCI after fibrinolysis and were on enoxaparin had a lower risk of ischaemic events and a similar risk of bleeding, compared with those on unfractionated heparin [114]. In the subgroup of 3788 patients who underwent primary PCI in the OASIS 6 trial, there was no benefit of fondaparinux over unfractionated heparin: the composite of death or reinfarction at 30 days and at study end (90–180 days) showed a nonsignificant excess of events in fondaparinux-treated patients [105]. There also was a trend to increased risk of severe bleeding in the fondaparinux group. Higher rates of catheter thrombosis and coronary complications were observed in patients on fondaparinux. The direct thrombin inhibitor bivalirudin was compared to a combination of unfractionated heparin and abciximab in 3602 patients treated with primary PCI for STEMI in the HORIZONS trial [115, 116]. Bivalirudin significantly reduced the risk of severe bleeding and of net clinical adverse events (bleeding and cardiovascular ischaemic events). Consequently, a significant reduction in cardiac death (1.8% vs 2.9%) and all-cause death (2.1% vs 3.1%) was observed with bivalirudin therapy. In addition, 1-year rates of cardiac death (HR 0.57; 95% CI 0.38–0.84) and all-cause mortality (HR 0.71; 95% CI 0.51–0.98) were significantly lower with bivalirudin. Stent thrombosis within 24 h of the primary PCI procedure, however, was more frequent on bivalirudin than on heparin and abciximab. Overall the benefit/risk balance was strongly in favour of bivalirudin.

Antithrombotic medications in patients without reperfusion therapy

The ISIS 2 trial [54] demonstrated a reduction in 1-month mortality in patients with suspected MI receiving aspirin, even in the absence of concomitant fibrinolytic treatment. In the COMMIT trial, clopidogrel (75 mg once a day) was associated with a nonsignificant reduction in the primary endpoint (death, reinfarction, or stroke at one month: 9.7% vs 10.3%), compared with placebo, in patients who had no reperfusion therapy; there was no interaction between clopidogrel treatment and fibrinolysis [94].

A meta-analysis of 21 small randomized trials comparing heparin and placebo in patients with STEMI showed both a 25% reduction in the risk of death, and a reduction in stroke and pulmonary emboli in patients receiving heparin; reinfarction also trended lower [117]. Most of the patients in these trials, however, did not receive concomitant aspirin therapy. In the OASIS 6 trial, the primary endpoint of death or reinfarction at 30 days was significantly reduced with fondaparinux, compared with control in 2867 patients who had no reperfusion therapy (HR 0.80; 95% CI 0.65–0.98). The results were no different when fondaparinux was compared to placebo or unfractionated heparin. Severe bleeding was nonsignificantly reduced (HR 0.82) [105].

Other medications at the acute stage

At the acute stage, relief of pain and anxiety is particularly important as they cause sympathetic activation, which increases cardiac workload. Opioids are widely used (morphine 4–8 mg IV, with additional doses of 2 mg at 15-min intervals, as dictated by symptoms). Antiemetics may be used as necessary. Atropine (0.5–1 mg IV, up to 2 mg) is used when bradycardia and hypotension are present. Oxygen therapy (mask or nasal prongs) is traditionally used in patients who are breathless or have signs of heart failure or shock, although there is little evidence of its true

usefulness. Noninvasive monitoring of arterial saturation may help to decide on using respiratory support in severely ill patients.

Early use of β-blockers has been studied in relatively old trials [118]. Recently, however, the COMMIT trial addressed the issue of the efficacy of intravenous metoprolol in a large population of patients with STEMI receiving fibrinolysis or no reperfusion therapy [119]. Although administration of the β-blocker resulted in fewer reinfarctions or ventricular fibrillations, there was an excess of left ventricular failure and cardiogenic shock, so that overall survival was not improved by β-blocker therapy. Current recommendations suggest starting β-blockers only when the patient is haemodynamically stable.

Three important trials (GISSI 3, ISIS 4, and the Chinese study) have shown that the administration of ACE inhibitors at the acute stage of MI reduces mortality at 1 month [120–122]. They should not, however, be administered when signs of shock are present.

The routine use of nitrates has shown no benefit in both the GISSI 3 and ISIS 4 trials [121, 122]. Likewise, calcium channel blockers have no beneficial effect, and a meta-analysis even shows a trend to more adverse events with their use at the acute stage [123].

Finally, although hyperglycaemia at the acute stage is a potent risk marker for adverse events [124], there is no evidence that the routine use of insulin therapy improves outcomes in patients with acute MI: the results of the DIGAMI 2 trial [125] did not confirm the initial findings of DIGAMI [126]. Likewise, the combined results of the CREATE-ECLA [127] and OASIS 6 GIK trials, which included 22943 patients with STEMI, showed that glucose–insulin–potassium (GIK) infusion was associated with an increased risk of death at day 3 (HR 1.13), which was no longer significant by day 30 (HR 1.04) [128].

Medications that are not useful or may be harmful in STEMI are listed in ➲ Box 41.3.

Management of early complications
Right ventricular infarction

Because right ventricular infarction causes hypotension, vasodilator medications (opioids, nitrates, ACE inhibitors, or angiotensin receptor blockers)) and diuretics should be avoided. Fluid infusion is often necessary to maintain the haemodynamic balance. However, care should be used not to overexpand the already dilated right ventricle, which might be detrimental. When the amount of fluids to be administered is uncertain, invasive haemodynmamic monitoring might be useful. Occasionally inotropic support, preferably with dobutamine, might be necessary, Cardioversion of atrial fibrillation or dual chamber pacing may be required, when rhythm or conduction disturbances are present. In the first hours, primary PCI is usually extremely efficacious to treat right heart infarction, often resulting in prompt restoration of adequate haemodynamics [129].

Conduction disturbances

First degree atrioventricular block requires no specific treatment. High degree atrioventricular block during inferior MI usually resolves spontaneously and does not need specific therapeutic measures when the escape rhythm is above 40–45 beats/min. In contrast, atrioventricular block developing in patients with anterior MI usually persists and may require temporary pacemaking, eventually leading to permanent pacemaker implantation.

Arrhythmias

In most instances, atrial fibrillation is well tolerated and does not require specific therapy. β-Blockers are helpful to lower heart rate. Class Ic antiarrhythmic agents should be avoided.

Ventricular fibrillation requires emergency cardioversion. The use of beta-blockers decreases the risk of ventricular fibrillation. Prophylactic lidocaine may reduce the risk of ventricular fibrillation, but it may increase mortality, by causing excessive bradycardia and asystole [130]. Ventricular tachycardia associated with haemodynamic compromise requires treatment: amiodarone, sotalol, lidocaine, or electrical stimulation may be useful; cardioversion may be necessary. Ventricular premature beats do not require specific treatment. Accelerated idioventricular rhythm is frequent when myocardial reperfusion occurs; it requires no specific treatment.

Mechanical complications

Surgical treatment (usually mitral valve replacement) is required for papillary muscle rupture; the timing of surgery depends on the severity of haemodynamic compromise. An IABP might be very helpful to stabilize the patient until surgery can be undertaken. Functional mitral regurgitation, if not severe, usually does not require surgical treatment. Vasodilator therapy, in particular with ACE inhibitors, should be used if arterial blood pressure is adequate.

Ventricular free wall rupture is usually lethal. Subacute rupture requires immediate surgery. False aneurysms have become rare; they usually require surgical treatment.

Although small ventricular septal ruptures may heal spontaneously and leave only a mild to moderate shunt, most cases deteriorate rapidly and the patients go into shock. When shock is absent, vasodilators can be used; an IABP is helpful to stabilize the haemodynamic condition. Surgical repair is usually indicated, but its timing is debated: very early intervention is usually preferred; however, the earlier the intervention, the more fragile the surrounding tissues are, and repair may be particularly difficult. Inferobasal ruptures are difficult to treat, because of the immediate vicinity of the mitral valve apparatus. Cases of percutaneous closure have been reported, but the technique is not currently validated.

Left ventricular failure and cardiogenic shock

Lesser degrees of left ventricular failure (Killip class 2 or 3) require the use of loop diuretics, nitrates, and/or ACE inhibitors (or ARBs if ACE inhibitors are not tolerated); inotrope support may be used when arterial blood pressure is low.

The management of cardiogenic shock is detailed in ➲ Chapter 47. Briefly, intravenous inotropes (dopamine or dobutamine) and IABP form the basis of treatment. Rarely, ventricular assist devices may be used. The role of emergency revascularization (mostly PCI) has been studied in small randomized trials comparing early angiography and conservative management [131, 132]. The largest of these trials (SHOCK) included 302 patients, in the mid-1990s; 30-day mortality was nonsignificantly lower with the early revascularization strategy (47% vs 56%); mortality at 6 months, however, was significantly lower in the revascularization group (50.3% vs 63.1%) and the benefit persisted over the following 6 years [133]. Of note, a significant interaction with age was observed: in patients 75 years of age or older, a trend to higher mortality with the revascularization strategy was observed. The interaction was no longer significant over the long-term, however.

Secondary prevention

It is not the object of this chapter to discuss in depth secondary prevention after MI. Several objectives, however, must be fulfilled.

Lifestyle

Appropriate lifestyle is highly advisable after STEMI, as in all coronary artery disease patients. Smoking cessation is essential. Regular physical activity should be encouraged, as well as weight control/loss. A Mediterranean-type diet seems advisable. There is no indication that dietary supplements, including additional fish oil, are beneficial: although the open-label GISSI-prevenzione trial showed a reduction in clinical events of borderline significance [134], a meta-analysis of trials studying ω-3 supplementation failed to document a significant benefit on arrhythmias and all-cause mortality [135]. The results of the SU.FOL. OM3 trial which will be released in 2010 should clarify the situation [136]. All of the above lifestyle measures also contribute to the control of risk factors, such as hypertension, hyperlipidaemia, or diabetes.

Medications

Antithrombotic medications are necessary. Usually, these include lifelong low-dose aspirin, combined with clopidogrel or newer antiplatelet agents, for 1 year. Vitamin K antagonists can be used, preferably on top of aspirin, in patients at specific thrombotic risk (atrial fibrillation, mechanical heart valves, left ventricular thrombus). In the future, newer anticoagulants could find a place in post-MI therapy.

β-Blockers have been tested in rather old trials (usually in patients without reperfusion therapy) and have documented a consistent reduction in late mortality. They are recommended for all patients, in the absence of specific contraindication.

ACE inhibitors have a documented beneficial effect in patients with poor left ventricular function, as well as in patients with chronic coronary artery disease. Valsartan showed results similar to those of captopril after MI in the VALIANT trial. It therefore constitutes an alternative in patients with contraindications or intolerance to ACE inhibitors. Aldosterone blockers should be considered in patients with left ventricular ejection fraction less than 40%, in the absence of severe renal failure and with routine monitoring of serum potassium.

Statin therapy is recommended, irrespective of the baseline lipid levels, as for all patients with coronary artery disease.

Cardiac resynchronization therapy can be considered in patients with poor left ventricular function and increased QRS duration. Prophylactic implantable cardioverter–defibrillator reduces the risk of sudden death in patients with left ventricular ejection fraction 30% or less, symptoms of heart failure beyond 40 days after the acute episode of MI, and in patients with left ventricular ejection fraction 40% or less and spontaneous nonsustained ventricular tachycardia or sustained monomorphic ventricular tachycardia during electrophysiological testing.

Finally, additional medications are often necessary to adequately control blood pressure and diabetes mellitus.

Organization of care and networks

The organization of care and networks is discussed in ➲ Chapter 40. The current challenge for STEMI is to organize care in order to optimize the implementation of early reperfusion therapy, with a tailored approach for each patient [137]. Two main routes can be envisaged, depending on the local environment: either bringing the patient to treatment (i.e. bringing the patient in a timely manner to a catheterization laboratory, where primary angiography will be performed), or bringing treatment to the patient (i.e. administering intravenous fibrinolytic treatment in the prehospital setting) [138]. These methods can be used jointly, as concomitant antithrombotic medications can be administered in the prehospital setting, en route for the catheterization laboratory. In the past few years, the results achieved with several types of networks have been reported, with satisfactory clinical results, and emphasize that there is no unique way to deliver reperfusion therapy for STEMI patients (see ➲ Chapter 40).

Finally, many networks monitor their day-to-day practice, and the benchmarking process appears extremely useful to improve the overall quality of care, beginning with the optimization of time delays [139].

STEMI treatment in the real world: data from registries and evolution of outcomes over the past two decades

Registries document actual practice and its changes over time. The international GRACE registry has thus shown a marked increase in the proportion of patients treated with primary PCI from 1999 (15%) to 2006 (44%), with a decrease in the use of fibrinolysis (from 41% to 16%) [140];

there was no improvement, however, in the time from onset of symptoms to PCI during this time period (in 2006, the median time from symptom onset to PCI was 228 minutes). During the same time period, hospital mortality decreased from 6.9% to 5.4% [141]. Mortality has decreased over the last 10–20 years in most countries, including the United States, United Kingdom, Israel, and France [3, 142–145]. Interestingly, mortality seems to have declined in a similar fashion in patients treated with primary PCI or intravenous fibrinolysis, or receiving no reperfusion treatment. This is likely explained by the changes in medications used at the acute stage. For instance, the early use of statin therapy in STEMI patients in France increased from 10% in 1995 to 78% in 2005 [3, 145]. One of the main challenges for the coming years will be to find ways to shorten time delays between symptom onset and administration of reperfusion; this will require both improvement in the organization of care, and increasing public awareness of the initial symptoms of MI [146, 147].

Personal perspective

There are four main challenges for the future, in order to improve the outcome of STEMI patients. The first challenge is to decrease time delays and improve the delivery of reperfusion therapy; this will involve both improved organization of medical care and public awareness campaigns. The second challenge is to improve the results of primary PCI, and in particular to avoid or limit the consequences of the no-reflow phenomenon; in this regard, mechanical procedures, such as thrombectomy, are likely to play a positive role, but much is awaited from pharmacological approaches and in particular from the concept of myocardial postconditioning, which is particularly attractive in an acute setting such as that of primary PCI. The third challenge will be to improve the outcome of patients developing cardiogenic shock; at the acute stage, this may require both new pharmacologic approaches and the use of new haemodynamic support devices; in the long term, 'myocardial repair', possibly using cell therapy, might change the prognosis of patients with profound post-MI left ventricular dysfunction. Last but not least, it is estimated that up to one-third of patients with STEMI die of ventricular fibrillation before reaching the hospital. Efforts should therefore be made to better treat out-of-hospital cardiac arrest, combining the broad diffusion of resuscitation techniques into the public, and implementing new ways to treat resuscitated cardiac arrest. But most importantly, prevention of sudden cardiac death is needed, and that will involve the early detection and treatment of coronary artery plaques prone to rupture, many of which are not tight enough to provoke symptoms before the acute event.

Disclosures

Dr Danchin has received research grants from Pfizer, Servier, and The Medicines Company. He has also received fees for speaking in industry-sponsored symposia and/or consulting for Astra-Zeneca, BMS, Boehringer-Ingelheim, GSK, Lilly, Menarini, MSD-Schering, Novartis, Novo, Pfizer, sanofi-aventis, Servier, and The Medicines Company.

Further reading

Alexander KP, Newby LK, Armstrong PW, et al. Acute coronary care in the elderly, part II: ST-segment-elevation myocardial infarction: a scientific statement for healthcare professionals from the American Heart Association Council on Clinical Cardiology: in collaboration with the Society of Geriatric Cardiology. Circulation 2007;115(19):2570–2589.

Antman EM, Anbe DT, Armstrong PW, et al. ACC/AHA guidelines for the management of patients with ST-elevation myocardial infarction—executive summary: a report of the American College of Cardiology/American Heart Association Task Force on Practice Guidelines (Writing Committee to Revise the 1999 Guidelines for the Management of Patients With Acute Myocardial Infarction). Can J Cardiol 2004;20(10):977–1025.

Goodman SG, Menon V, Cannon CP, S et al. Acute ST-segment elevation myocardial infarction: American College of Chest Physicians Evidence-Based Clinical Practice Guidelines (8th edition). Chest 2008;133(6 Suppl):708S–775S.

Libby P. Current concepts of the pathogenesis of the acute coronary syndromes. Circulation 2001;104(3):365–372.

Van de Werf F, Bax J, Betriu A, et al. Management of acute myocardial infarction in patients presenting with persistent ST-segment elevation: the Task Force on the Management of ST-Segment Elevation Acute Myocardial Infarction of the European Society of Cardiology. Eur Heart J 2008;29(23):2909–2945.

⊃ For additional multimedia materials please visit the online version of the book (http://www.esciacc.oxfordmedicine.com).

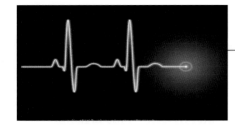

CHAPTER 42

Fibrinolytic, antithrombotic, and antiplatelet drugs in acute coronary syndrome

Peter R. Sinnaeve and Frans J. Van de Werf

Contents

Summary

Antithrombotic therapy is a major cornerstone of treatment for acute coronary syndromes (ACS), as thrombus formation upon plaque rupture or erosion plays a pivotal role in non-ST-segment elevation (NSTE) as well as ST-segment elevation ACS. Both acute and long-term oral antiplatelet therapies targeting specific platelet activation pathways have demonstrated significant short- and long-term benefits. The use of antithrombin agents is currently largely confined to the acute setting, except in patients with a clear indication for long-term treatment, including atrial fibrillation or the presence of intraventricular thrombi. Despite the benefit of primary percutaneous coronary intervention (PCI) in ST-segment elevation myocardial infarction (STEMI), fibrinolysis continues to play a major role throughout the world as well. In this chapter, fibrinolytic, antiplatelet, and anticoagulant agents used in the management of ACS patients are discussed.

Introduction

In atherosclerosis, platelets and prothrombotic pathways are activated, which contributes to disease progression and increases the risk of acute coronary syndromes (ACS) [1]. As a result, antithrombotic treatment was shown to decrease the risk of ischaemic complications in stable as well as unstable atherosclerotic patients. ACS are in essence caused by thrombus formation, following spontaneous atherosclerotic plaque rupture or erosion. Despite the proven efficacy of long-term dual antiplatelet therapy with aspirin and clopidogrel or prasugrel, residual morbidity and mortality is considerable. This may be partly due to incomplete inhibition of platelet activation with current agents, interference of other therapies, and/or lack of long-term anticoagulant therapy. Improvements in patient outcomes could be achieved by developing agents that inhibit other platelet activation pathways or by adding new anticoagulants for a prolonged period of time after the acute event. In this chapter, fibrinolytic, antithrombotic, and antiplatelet agents used today are discussed, as well as several new agents currently in development. The agents are listed in ◈ Table 42.1 and their mechanism of action is illustrated in ◈ Figs 42.1 and 42.2.

Fibrinolytic agents

Fibrinolytic agents are categorized as fibrin-specific agents and non-fibrin-specific agents (◈ Table 42.2). Fibrin-specific drugs are more efficient in dissolving thrombi and do not deplete systemic coagulation factors, in contrast to non-fibrin-specific agents. First-generation fibrinolytic regimens, including streptokinase and tissue-type plasminogen activator (alteplase), require continuous intravenous infusion. Contemporary lytic strategies, however, consist of an intravenous bolus administration of second and third generation fibrinolytics. Time delays to treatment initiation remain a crucial factor in the treatment of STEMI. Since mortality rates in randomized fibrinolytic trials are consistently lower when patients are treated within 2 h of symptom onset, early prehospital detection and treatment is an attractive approach to improve outcome in STEMI. A meta-analysis of six trials including 6434 patients shows that the time gained with prehospital treatment resulted in a significant 17% mortality reduction compared to in-hospital fibrinolysis [2]. Bolus fibrinolytic agents undoubtedly facilitate prehospital reperfusion protocols. Less complicated fibrinolytic regimens might also facilitate initiation of prehospital fibrinolytic treatment by trained paramedical staff [3].

Contraindications for fibrinolytic therapy are listed in ◈ Table 42.3, and antithrombotic cotherapies are listed in ◈ Table 42.4. Unfortunately, fibrinolytic regimens also suffer from several limitations. Fibrinolytics need 30–45 min on average to recanalize the infarct-related artery, and complete patency is only achieved in 60–80% of patients. Also, reocclusion due to prothrombotic side effects is common, occurring in 5–15% of previously recanalized arteries [4]. Furthermore, even when blood flow to the infarct-related artery is restored, microcirculatory reperfusion can still be absent ('no-reflow' phenomenon) [5]. Finally, bleeding complications, especially intracranial haemorrhages, remain a concern (📹 42.1).

Streptokinase

Streptokinase is a non-fibrin-specific fibrinolytic agent that indirectly activates plasminogen. Because of its lack of fibrin specificity, streptokinase induces a systemic lytic state.

Table 42.1 Antithrombotic and fibrinolytic agents in ACS

Fibrinolytic agents		
Fibrin specific	Alteplase	
	Reteplase	
	Tenecteplase	
Non-fibrin specific	Streptokinase	
Antiplatelet agents (◈ Fig. 42.2)		
Oral	Aspirin	
	P2Y12 inhibitor	
		Clopidogrel
		Ticlopidine
		Prasugrel
		Ticagrelor
	Thrombin receptor inhibitor	
		Thrombin receptor antagonist
Intravenous	Glycoprotein IIb/IIIa inhibitor	
		Abciximab
		Eptifibatide
		Tirofiban
	P2Y12 inhibitor	
		Cangrelor
Anticoagulant agents (◈ Fig. 42.2)		
Oral	Anticoagulant	
		Warfarin
		Coumadin
	Direct thrombin inhibitor	
		Ximegalatran
		Dabigatran
	Factor Xa inhibitor	
		Rivaroxaban
		Apixaban
Subcutaneous—intravenous	Unfractionated heparin	
	Low-molecular-weight heparin	
		Enoxaparin
		Dalteparin
		Nadroparin
	Direct thrombin inhibitor	
		Lepirudin
		Bivalirudin
		Argatroban
		Efegatran
		Inogatran
	Factor Xa inhibitors	
Indirect	Fondaparinux	
Direct	Otamixaban	

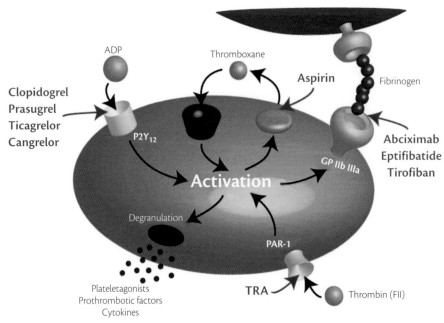

Figure 42.1 Antiplatelet agents

Although newer fibrin-specific fibrinolytics have advantages, streptokinase remains widely used, in part because of its low cost. Pre-existing antistreptokinase antibodies, induced by streptococcal infection or previous streptokinase administration, may impede reperfusion after treatment with streptokinase [6].

The first large trial to show a significant reduction in mortality with a fibrinolytic agent was the landmark GISSI-1 trial [7]. In this study, 11 806 patients with an acute myocardial infarction (MI) were randomized to either reperfusion therapy with streptokinase or standard nonfibrinolytic therapy. In-hospital mortality was 10.7% in patients treated with intravenous streptokinase versus 13.1% in control subjects, resulting in 23 lives saved per 1000 patients treated. This benefit in mortality was preserved long term [8]. Another landmark trial, ISIS-2, corroborated these results [9]: 17 187 patients received streptokinase, aspirin daily for 1 month, both treatments, or neither. Treatment with aspirin or streptokinase alone resulted in a significant reduction in mortality (23% and 24%, respectively), an effect that was additive, as demonstrated by a 43% reduction in the combination group.

Alteplase

Recombinant tissue-type plasminogen activator (rt-PA or alteplase) is a single-chain tissue-type plasminogen activator molecule. It has considerably greater fibrin specificity than streptokinase but induces mild systemic fibrinogen depletion. Because of its short half-life, alteplase requires a continuous infusion.

In two mortality trials, ISIS-3 and GISSI-2, alteplase, given as a 3-h continuous infusion, was not superior to streptokinase [10, 11]. However, in the first GUSTO trial [12] a 'front-loaded' 90-min dosing regimen of alteplase was used, which had earlier been shown to achieve higher patency rates than the 3-h scheme. The 30-day mortality was 6.3% in patients receiving alteplase compared to 7.4% in patients treated with streptokinase ($p = 0.001$). The 1% lower mortality rate at 30 days with front-loaded alteplase corresponded to a significantly higher TIMI flow grade 3 rate at 90 min [13].

Reteplase

Reteplase, a second-generation fibrinolytic agent and a mutant of alteplase which is a given as a bolus, was a first

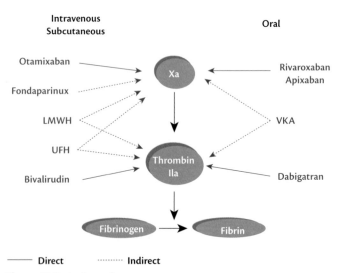

Figure 42.2 Anticoagulant agents

Table 42.2 Fibrinolytic agents

	Streptokinase	Alteplase	Reteplase	Tenecteplase
Fibrin specificity	–	++	+	+++
Half-life (min)	18–23	3–4	18	20
Administration	1-h infusion	90-min infusion	Double bolus	Single bolus
Antigenicity	+++	–	–	–

attempt to improve on the shortcomings of alteplase. It has diminishes fibrin specificity, while inactivation by plasminogen activator inhibitor (PAI-1, ⊃ Fig. 42.1) remains similar to that with alteplase.

In the GUSTO-III trial, 15 059 patients were randomized to double-bolus reteplase, or front-loaded alteplase [14]. Mortality at 30 days was similar in both treatment arms (7.47% vs 7.24%, respectively), as was the incidence of major bleeding [15]. Thus, higher TIMI 3 rates at 90 min with reteplase, as seen in the pilot studies, did not translate into lower short-term or long-term mortality rates. The reason for this incongruity remains unclear, but might be explained in part by increased platelet activation and surface receptor expression with reteplase compared to alteplase.

Tenecteplase

Tenecteplase (TNK-t-PA) is derived from alteplase after mutations in three places, increasing fibrin binding and specificity, plasma half-life, and resistance to PAI-1. Its slower clearance allows single-bolus administration. Tenecteplase leads to faster recanalization compared to alteplase, and

also has higher fibrinolytic potency on platelet-rich clots than its parent molecule.

In the ASSENT-2 trial, 16 949 patients were randomized to weight-adjusted single-bolus tenecteplase or standard front-loaded alteplase [16]. Specifically designed as an equivalency trial, this study showed that tenecteplase and alteplase had equivalent 30-day as well as 1-year mortality rates [17]. Although the rates of intracranial haemorrhage were similar, female patients, older people, and patients weighing less than 67 kg tended to have lower rates of intracranial haemorrhage with tenecteplase [18].

Anticoagulant agents

Vitamin K antagonists

Oral anticoagulants or vitamin K antagonists (VKA: warfarin, coumadin) depress the synthesis of the four vitamin K-dependent procoagulant factors II, VII, IX and X. The effect

Table 42.3 Contraindications for fibrinolysis

Absolute	Relative
Previous haemorrhagic stroke at any time	Transient ischaemic attack <6 months
Non-haemorrhagic (ischaemic) stroke <6 months	Uncontrolled or refractory hypertension on presentation (blood pressure >180/100 mmHg)
Intracranial neoplasm or damage	Traumatic cardiopulmonary resuscitation
Recent surgery or trauma (including head trauma) within 2–4 weeks	Current use of anticoagulant
Active internal bleeding	Recent internal bleeding (2–4 weeks)
Gastrointestinal bleeding within last month	Noncompressible vascular punctures
Known bleeding diatheses	Pregnancy
Suspected aortic dissection	Active peptic ulcer
	Previous use of streptokinase

Table 42.4 Fibrinolysis: dosing and concomitant antithrombotic therapies

Antiplatelet therapy	
Aspirin	Loading dose 150–325 mg;chewable, nonenteric coated (75–100 mg daily lifelong)
Clopidogrel	Loading dose 300 mg (no loading dose if age >75 y); 75 mg daily for1 year
Fibrinolysis	
Tenecteplase	Single bolus: <60 kg, 30 mg; 60–69.9 kg, 35 mg; 70–79.9 kg, 40 mg; 80–89.9 kg, 45 mg; >90 kg, 50 mg
Reteplase	Double bolus: 10 + 10 MU, 30 min apart
Streptokinase	1.5 MU in 1-h infusion
Anticoagulation	
Enoxaparin	Bolus: 30 mg IV 1mg/kg SC (>75 y no bolus) 1 mg/kg per 12 h (max 100 mg for first 2 doses) (0.75 mg/kg if >75 y)
or UFH	60 U/kg (max 4000 U) 12 U/kg per h (max 1000 U/h) 50–70 s first measurement at 3 h
Fondaparinux	Bolus 2.5 mg IV 2.5 mg SC per 24 h

of warfarin can differ considerably among patients and over time in the same individual. Also, various intercurrent illnesses, drugs, and food can influence the extent of anticoagulation. Therefore, monitoring of the anticoagulant effect using the prothrombin time (expressed as INR) is necessary. Oral VKA have been tested in several non-ST-elevation and ST-elevation ACS trials in the pre-clopidogrel era. On aggregate, these studies suggest that although aspirin alone is superior to VKA alone in preventing ischaemic events, moderate to high-dose VKA on top of aspirin further reduces the risk of ischaemic complications [19–24]. Unfortunately, there is a price to pay: VKA are associated with an up to threefold increase in bleeding complications. As a consequence, VKA are rarely used in standard care for ACS patients who do not have another specific indication for their use.

Unfractionated heparin

Traditionally, unfractionated heparin (UFH) has been the standard antithrombin (➲ Table 42.5). UFH is a preparation of heparin molecules that are heterogeneous with respect to molecular weight. The anticoagulant effect of UFH is mediated by binding to circulating antithrombin III, which augments its inhibitory activity towards several coagulation factors, primarily activated thrombin (factor IIa), and activated factor X (factor Xa). Multiple studies consistently demonstrated the benefit of UFH (➲ Table 42.5) as an adjunct to aspirin in patients with ACS. In a meta-analysis including 17 157 patients with non-ST-segment elevation (NSTE) ACS from 12 trials, heparin use was associated with a 47% reduction in death or MI, representing 29 events prevented per 1000 patients treated [25]. Although there are no randomized clinical trials, UFH is also considered standard therapy during primary PCI [26]. Intravenous UFH has also been the standard adjunctive antithrombotic therapy with fibrin-specific fibrinolytics since GUSTO-I, although no effect on mortality was observed [12].

UFH has several drawbacks. The effectiveness of UFH is highly variable in patients, because of low bioavailability due to nonspecific binding to plasma proteins and variable clearance. Therefore aPTT monitoring is required. UFH is also relatively ineffective in inhibiting clot-associated thrombin and factor X and does not reduce the generation of thrombin associated with fibrinolysis. This can result in rebound activation of the coagulation cascade after cessation of an infusion, increasing the risk of reocclusion. In addition, short-term UFH use is associated with a higher risk of bleeding complications which is directly proportional to the aPTT [27]. Finally, the binding of UFH to platelet factor 4 on platelets can result in heparin-induced thrombocytopenia (HIT) [28].

Low-molecular-weight heparin

As the name ssuggests, low-molecular-weight heparins (LMWH) are preparations comprising only heparin molecules of lower molecular weight. Like UFH, LMWHs bind and activate antithrombin III, although the relative inhibitory activity of LMWHs towards factor Xa is greater than that of thrombin. LMWH has several advantages over standard UFH, including greater bioavailability, better resistance to inhibition by activated platelets, lower incidence of HIT, and increased antifactor Xa activity. LMWH also are easier to administer, and do not need monitoring. Better anti-Xa:IIa ratio than that of UFH more efficiently promotes the inhibition of thrombin generation. Furthermore, subcutaneous administration and a longer half-life greatly facilitate administration. Because LMWH can be conveniently administered in an outpatient setting, several trials have examined the effect of prolonged LMWH use after ACS but failed to show a benefit [25, 29, 30].

Several trials evaluated the efficacy and safety of enoxaparin versus UFH in non-ST-elevation ACS patients, with inconsistent results. In contrast to older trials [31, 32], two more recent large trials, SYNERGY and A-to-Z, failed to show superiority of enoxaparin over heparin [33, 34]. Moreover, enoxaparin was associated with a higher risk of major bleeding complications in SYNERGY, which has been in part attributed to postrandomization crossover of

Table 42.5 Dosing scheme for unfractionated heparin

Indication	Bolus	Infusion	Target aPTT/ACT
NSTE ACS	60 U/kg (max 5000)	12–15 U/kg per hour (1000 U/h max)	aPTT 50–70 s
STEMI (with fibrinolysis)	60 U/kg (max 4000)	12 U/kg per hour for 24–48 h (1000 U/h max)	aPTT 50–70 s
STEMI (with primary PCI)	100 U/kg 60 U/kg if GPIIb/IIIa	–	ACT 250–300 or 200–250 if GPIIb/IIIa

antithrombin therapy [34]. A meta-analysis of 6 trials and 21 945 patients with non-ST-elevation ACS confirmed that there was no significant difference in the clinical endpoint of death, MI, or major bleeding at 30 days [35]. In the setting of an early invasive strategy, the 2007 non-ST-elevation ACS guidelines recommend enoxaparin (➲ Table 42.6) as an alternative to UFH; when an invasive evaluation is pending, enoxaparin should only be considered in patients with a low bleeding risk [36].

In the setting of STEMI, LMWH was associated with higher early patency rates and lower rates of reocclusion [37–40]. In ASSENT-3, a significant improvement in the primary combined efficacy and safety endpoint was seen with tenecteplase and enoxaparin when compared to tenecteplase and UFH [41, 42]. Unfortunately, a significant increase in intracranial haemorrhage was seen in the ASSENT-3 PLUS trial, using the same combination [43]. The excess of intracranial bleeding was predominantly observed in elderly patients. Using an age-adjusted dose (➲ Table 42.6) enoxaparin did not increase the risk of intracranial haemorrhage after fibrinolytic therapy while still reducing the risk of ischaemic complications in the ExTRACT-TIMI 25 study [44]. Meta-analyses of STEMI trials comparing LMWH to UFH confirm that LMWH reduces the risk of death and reinfarction, but is associated with a higher risk of bleeding [35, 45]. The 2008 European Society of Cardiology (ESC) STEMI guidelines recommend enoxaparin in lytic-treated patients, but not in primary PCI [26].

Factor Xa inhibitors

Fondaparinux, a synthetic pentasaccharide, is a selective indirect antithrombin-dependent factor Xa inhibitor. The pentasaccharide–antithrombin complex is active against factor Xa but not against thrombin, resulting in the inhibition of thrombin generation without the direct inhibition of thrombin activity [46]. Compared to UFH and LMWH, fondaparinux is associated with less biological variability, immunogenic reactivity, and risk of contamination. As with LMWH, fondaparinux does not need monitoring of its

anticoagulant effect. Fondaparinux does not bind to platelet factor 4 and eliminates the risk of platelet activation.

The efficacy and safety of fondaparinux was evaluated in the OASIS-5 trial, in which 20 078 patients with non-ST-elevation ACS were randomized to receive either fondaparinux [2.5 mg/day sc] or enoxaparin [47]. The rate of primary-outcome events (death, MI, or refractory ischaemia) at 9 days was comparable in the fondaparinux and enoxaparin groups (5.8 vs 5.7%, respectively), satisfying the noninferiority criteria. The rate of major bleeding at 9 days was significantly lower with fondaparinux than for enoxaparin. At 30 days, the rate of the primary endpoint was comparable between groups (8.0 vs 8.6%), while the rate of death was significantly lower with fondaparinux (2.9 vs 3.5%). Remarkably, the majority of excess deaths in the enoxaparin group occurred in patients who bled [48]. In patients undergoing PCI, additional UFH was administrated to prevent catheter-related thrombus formation, but this did not negate the benefit of fondaparinux over enoxaparin [49].

Fondaparinux was also evaluated in STEMI patients. In the OASIS-6 trial, fondaparinux was compared to UFH or placebo in 12 092 STEMI patients [50]. Lytic therapy was given to 45% of patients (n = 5436), most of them receiving a non-fibrin-specific agent, while 37% underwent primary PCI. In lytic-treated patients, fondaparinux was associated with a significant 21% lower risk of death or MI when compared to standard heparin or placebo [51]. Nevertheless, the risk of bleeding, including intracranial haemorrhage, was considerably lower with fondaparinux, irrespective of the type of fibrinolytic agent. In PCI patients, fondaparinux was associated with a nonsignificant 1% higher incidence of death or MI. In contrast, fondaparinux was found to be superior to UFH in patients not receiving reperfusion therapy. The 2008 ESC guidelines recommend fondaparinux as adjunctive therapy to streptokinase (class IIa B) but not to fibrin-specific agents, and for conservatively treated but not primary PCI patients [26].

Several direct factor Xa inhibitors are currently being developed. Two oral agents, rivaroxaban and apixaban, were evaluated in a phase II trial (ATLAS and APPRAISE, respectively) [52, 53]. Both showed a dose-dependent increase in bleeding complications, and a trend towards fewer ischaemic events. Similarly, the intravenous direct factor Xa inhibitor otamixaban was associated with a dose-dependent increased risk of bleeding complications and a trend towards a lower rate of ischaemic endpoints, compared to UFH and eptifibatide [54]. These agents are currently being evaluated in large phase III trials.

Table 42.6 Dosing scheme for enoxaparin

Indication	Dose	Duration
NSTE ACS	1 mg/kg SC twice a day	2–8 days
STEMI (fibrinolysis)	30 mg IV bolus (no bolus if >75 y of age) 1 mg/kg SC twice a day (max 100 mg for first 2 doses) 0.75 mg/kg SC twice a day if >75 y of age (max 75 mg)	Up to 7 days

Direct thrombin inhibitors

Unlike UFH, LMWH, and fondaparinux, direct thrombin inhibitors (DTI), including lepirudin, bivalirudin, argatroban, ximelagatran, and dabigatran, exert their anticoagulant effect by binding directly to thrombin. DTI do not require monitoring and have not been associated with thrombocytopenia. Clot-bound thrombin is protected from inactivation by heparin–antithrombin III, but can be inactivated by DTI. Likewise, thrombin bound to soluble fibrin degradation products is not inhibited by heparin, but remains susceptible to inactivation by DTI [55]. DTI inhibit thrombin activity better than heparin and improve protection against reactivation of thrombin after cessation of therapy [56]. Several DTI are available for intravenous administration, including lepirudin, bivalirudin, inogatran, argatroban and efegatran.

Several studies examined the benefit of DTI in ACS patients. In a meta-analysis, including 35 970 patients from 11 non-STEMI and STEMI trials, bivalirudin or lepirudin, but not other agents, were associated with a 16% lower risk of death or MI compared to UFH [57]. This benefit was most pronounced in patients undergoing early PCI, versus delayed or no PCI [58]. Interestingly, a reduction of bleeding was observed with the reversible DTI bivalirudin, but not with lepirudin. Of the intravenous DTI, only bivalirudin has been further studied in ACS patients.

The efficacy and safety of bivalirudin were evaluated in the ACUITY trial, an open-label study that randomized 13 819 patients with non-ST-elevation ACS to UFH or enoxaparin plus a GPIIb/IIIa inhibitor, bivalirudin plus a GPIIb/IIIa inhibitor, or bivalirudin alone with provisional GPIIb/IIIa inhibitor [59]. Bivalirudin alone, when compared with heparin plus a GPIIb/IIIa inhibitor, was associated with a noninferior comparable 30-day rate of the composite ischaemia endpoint of death, MI, or unplanned revascularization for ischaemia and significantly less major bleeding (3.0 vs 5.7%, *p* <0.001). The net clinical outcome endpoint (defined as the occurrence of the composite ischaemia endpoint or major bleeding) was significantly lower with bivalirudin alone. The reduction in in-hospital bleeding associated with bivalirudin appears to improve long-term outcome [60]. In patients not pre-treated with clopidogrel, however, bivalirudin alone appeared to be inferior to the combination of UFH/LMWH plus a GPIIb/IIIa inhibitor.

Bivalirudin was also studied as an adjunct to fibrinolytic therapy. In the HERO-2 trial, 17 073 patients received streptokinase and were randomized to UFH or bivalirudin [61]. Mortality at 30 days was not different, but the reinfarction rate was significantly lower in the bivalirudin group (1.6% vs 2.3% for UFH), suggesting that early and more efficient inhibition of thrombin can inhibit reocclusion. Mild to moderate bleeding complications were higher in the bivalirudin group. Bivalirudin has not been studied as an adjunct to fibrin-specific agents.

Although ximelagatran improved outcome in the ESTEEM trial, this agent was withdrawn from the market because of liver toxicity [62]. A similar agent, dabigatran was recently studied in a phase II ACS trial (REDEEM). It was associated with a favourable safety profile (unpublished), and needs to be evaluated in a large outcome trial.

Antiplatelet agents

Aspirin

Aspirin irreversibly inhibits cyclooxygenase (COX), blocking the formation of thromboxane A_2, a promoter of platelet aggregation [63]. Several studies clearly demonstrated the benefit of aspirin versus placebo in patients with NSTE ACS [64–66], while the landmark ISIS-2 trial clearly showed a benefit of adding aspirin to streptokinase [9]. A meta-analysis of 287 trials including 135 000 patients in comparisons of antiplatelet therapy versus control and 77 000 in comparisons of different antiplatelet regimens by the Antithrombotic Trialists' Collaboration (ATC), showed a 22% reduction in vascular events with aspirin [67]. This benefit was mainly driven by a 34% reduction in MI and a 25% reduction in stroke.

The optimal maintenance dose of aspirin after an ACS has long been a matter of debate. The ATC's meta-analysis suggests that doses between 75 and 150 mg offer the greatest reduction in ischaemic events [67]. Retrospective analyses from the CURE and CHARISMA trials suggest that long-term aspirin doses between 75 and 100 mg are associated with optimal efficacy [68, 69]. Higher doses do not further decrease the risk of ischaemic complications, but appear to increase the risk of bleeding, especially in conjunction with clopidogrel. This issue was recently prospectively assessed in the CURRENT (OASIS-7) trial [70]. Patients with a NSTE ACS or STEMI were randomized to low-dose (75–100 mg) versus high-dose (300–325 mg) aspirin during the first month after the event. The primary endpoint of cardiovascular death, MI, or stroke at 30 days was similar in both groups. During this short period, bleeding complications were not more frequent with higher doses of aspirin. On aggregate, aspirin doses of more than 100 mg do not appear to be warranted.

P2Y$_{12}$ inhibitors

P2Y$_{12}$ ADP receptor antagonists inhibit ADP-induced platelet activation [71]. Available agents include ticlopidine; clopidogrel and prasugrel, which are thienopyridine prodrugs (📹42.2); and ticagrelor and cangrelor, which are reversible and do not require metabolism (➲ Table 42.7). Ticlopidine and clopidogrel have been on the market for many years, whereas prasugrel has been recently approved by the regulatory authorities in Europe. Ticlopidine is rarely used in ACS patients because of its less attractive safety profile.

Clopidogrel

To test the hypothesis that combining two distinct antiplatelet drugs improves outcome, clopidogrel was evaluated as adjunct therapy to aspirin after an ACS in the CURE and PCI-CURE trials [72, 73]. In this trial, 12 562 patients with a NSTE ACS received aspirin and were randomized to placebo or clopidogrel (300 mg loading dose followed by 75 mg daily) for a mean duration of 9 months. Clopidogrel resulted in a 20% reduction in the primary composite endpoint of cardiovascular death, MI, and stroke (9.3% vs 11.5%, p <0.001). The benefit of clopidogrel occurred very early (<24 h) after randomization and was consistent among low, intermediate, and high-risk patients [74]. Patients in the clopidogrel arm had a 1% absolute increase (3.7% vs 2.7%) in major bleeding compared to aspirin alone with no significant difference in fatal bleeding. In PCI-CURE, patients undergoing PCI who were pretreated with clopidogrel for a median of 10 days also had a significantly lower rate of the primary endpoint of cardiovascular death, MI, or urgent target vessel revascularization within 30 days of PCI (4.5 vs 6.4%) [72]. These results demonstrate that the addition of clopidogrel to aspirin reduces risk of adverse ischaemic outcomes in patients with NSTE ACS. However, the residual morbidity and mortality in patients treated with aspirin plus clopidogrel remains high, and the risk of

bleeding is increased. The recommendation to administer clopidogrel for 1 year following non-STEMI or unstable angina has been incorporated in the 2007 ESC NSTE ACS guidelines [36]. Clopidogrel is also recommended for patients who are allergic to aspirin.

Despite clopidogrel's ability to reduce ischaemic events in clinical studies, a significant proportion of patients demonstrate little or no platelet inhibition with this drug [75–77]. Moreover, clopidogrel's onset of action is delayed because of the intricate hepatic metabolization from prodrug to the active compound. Studies have suggested that doubling the bolus and/or maintenance dose of clopidogrel can accelerate the onset of its action and increase the proportion of patients with sufficient antiplatelet response [78, 79]. This has recently been evaluated in the CURRENT (OASIS-7) study [70]. In this trial 25 087 STEMI and NSTE ACS patients planned for early invasive management were randomized to double-dose (600 mg bolus, 150 mg for 1 week followed by 75 mg) versus standard-dose clopidogrel (300 mg bolus, 75 mg daily). The primary endpoint of cardiovascular death, MI, or stroke at 30 days was not significantly different between the two regimens. An interaction with PCI was observed, however: PCI patients receiving the double dose appeared to have a significant 15% risk reduction for the primary endpoint. Likewise, a subanalysis from the HORIZONS-AMI study suggests that a 600-mg clopidogrel loading dose is associated with a lower risk of ischaemic complications when compared to a 300-mg dose [80].

The CLARITY trial examined whether the addition of clopidogrel was associated with higher rates of infarct-related artery patency in patients treated with a fibrinolytic agent [81]. At angiographic follow-up at least 2 days after fibrinolytic therapy, patients treated with clopidogrel had significantly higher TIMI flow grades. Clopidogrel appeared to improve patency rates by preventing reocclusion rather than through facilitating early reperfusion [82]. No increased risk of bleeding complications with clopidogrel

Table 42.7 P2Y$_{12}$ receptor antagonists

Agent	Class	Route	Bolus	Dose	Time to peak platelet inhibition	Reversible	Half-life	Prodrug
Ticlopidine	Thienopyridine	Oral	500 mg	250 mg bid	4 d	N	–	Y
Clopidogrel	Thienopyridine	Oral	300–600 mg	75 mg	2–6 h	N	–	Y
Prasugrel	Thienopyridine	Oral	60 mg	10 mg	1 h	N	–	Y
Ticagrelor	Cyclo-pentyl-triazolo-pyrimidine	Oral	180 mg	90 mg bid	2 h	Y	3 min	N
Cangrelor	ATP analogue	IV	30 µg/kg	4 µg/kg per min for 2 h	30 min	Y	12 h	N

bid, twice a day.

was observed. Since patients over 75 years of age were excluded, it remains uncertain whether dual antiplatelet therapy following lytic therapy is safe in older patients. The 2008 STEMI guidelines recommend clopidogrel for 1 year following STE ACS, based on pathophysiological similarities with non-STEMI [26].

Prasugrel

Compared to clopidogrel, prasugrel requires one step less during metabolism to the active metabolite, and hence inhibits platelets faster and more consistently. The TRITON trial included patients with NSTE ACS and STEMI who were scheduled for PCI [83]. After diagnostic angiography patients were randomized to clopidogrel or prasugrel. The primary efficacy endpoint of cardiovascular death, MI, or stroke was in favour of prasugrel when compared with clopidogrel over the 15-month follow-up (9.9 vs 12.1%, $p < 0.001$). The reduction in the primary endpoint was more pronounced (30%) in patients with diabetes versus the overall population (19%). A total of 2.4% of patients receiving prasugrel had major bleeding, as against 1.8% of patients who received clopidogrel. Moreover, significantly more patients treated with prasugrel had a fatal bleeding (0.4 vs 0.1% for clopidogrel). On the other hand, in the 12 844 patients who received at least one coronary stent, prasugrel significantly reduced the primary endpoint with 18%. Stent thrombosis was also remarkably reduced with prasugrel: overall 1.13 versus 2.35%, (HR 0.48, $p < 0.0001$), especially in patients with drug-eluting stents (0.84 vs 2.34%, HR 0.36, $p < 0.0001$).

Ticagrelor

Ticagrelor is an oral $P2Y_{12}$ inhibitor that, in contrast with thienopyridines, is reversible and does not require hepatic metabolism [84, 85]. Compared to clopidogrel, its peak antiplatelet effect is therefore much faster ($\supset$ Table 42.7); its reversibility also allows more flexibility for surgical procedures [86]. Ticagrelor was recently tested in the large phase III PLATO trial in which 18 624 patients with NSTE ACS or STEMI were randomized to clopidogrel (300–600 mg loading dose, 75 mg daily) or ticagrelor (180 mg loading dose, 90 mg twice daily) [87]. The primary endpoint was cardiovascular death, MI, or stroke. At 12 months, the primary endpoint was significantly lower with ticagrelor (9.8%) than with clopidogrel (11.7%). All-cause mortality was also significantly lower in patients randomized to ticagrelor (4.5%, vs 5.9% for clopidogrel), as were cardiovascular death and MI. Moreover, the risk of stent thrombosis was 33% lower with ticagrelor than with clopidogrel. The overall rate of major bleeding was similar in both groups, although ticagrelor was associated with a significant higher risk of bleeding complications unrelated to coronary bypass surgery. The most common side effect of ticagrelor was dyspnoea (13.8% vs 7.8% for clopidogrel), although this rarely led to study drug discontinuation.

Cangrelor

Cangrelor is an intravenous ATP analogue that reversibly inhibits the $P2Y_{12}$ receptor [86]. It has a very short half-life and effectively inhibits platelets ($\supset$ Table 42.7). Cangrelor was recently evaluated in (predominantly) ACS patients in the CHAMPION PLATFORM and CHAMPION PCI studies [88, 89]. In the CHAMPION PLATFORM study, patients undergoing PCI were randomized to cangrelor or placebo during the procedure, with patients in the placebo group receiving 600 mg clopidogrel at the end of the procedure and cangrelor patients receiving clopidogrel at the end of the 2-h infusion [88]. In the CHAMPION PCI study, cangrelor was compared to 600 mg clopidogrel given at the start of the PCI procedure; cangrelor-treated patients were given clopidogrel at the end of the 2-hour study drug infusion [89]. The primary endpoint (death, MI, or ischaemia-driven urgent revascularization) at 48 h after PCI was not different between the two groups in both studies. Unsurprisingly, the rate of minor and major bleeding complications was higher with cangrelor.

Glycoprotein IIb/IIIa inhibitors

Binding of fibrinogen to the integrin $\alpha IIb\beta_3$ (glycoprotein (GP) IIb/IIIa) receptor on activated platelets represents the final common pathway of platelet aggregation and formation of platelet-rich thrombi [1]. By preventing the interaction of GPIIb/IIIa receptors with fibrinogen, GPIIb/IIIa inhibitors prevent platelet aggregation regardless of the agonist, and subsequent thrombus formation. GPIIb/IIIa inhibitors available include eptifibatide, tirofiban, and abciximab ($\supset$ Table 42.8). Abciximab is the large F_{ab} fragment of a chimeric mouse–human monoclonal antibody that binds and inactivates the GPIIb/IIIa receptor. Eptifibatide is a small cyclic heptapeptide that inhibits the GPIIb/IIIa receptor by mimicking certain amino acid sequences of fibrinogen. Tirofiban is a nonpeptide synthetic GPIIb/IIIa inhibitor that mimics the arginine–glycine–|aspartic acid sequence of fibrinogen. Eptifibatide and tirofiban are competitive inhibitors, whereas abciximab binds permanently to the GPIIb/IIIa receptor. These three agents have different pharmacodynamic profiles, depending on the dosing scheme [108].

GPIIb/IIIa inhibitors have been extensively tested in ACS patients. A meta-analysis of 6 trials evaluating GPIIb/IIIa

Table 42.8 Intravenous GPIIb/IIIa inhibitors: dosing in ACS

Agent	Indication	Bolus	Infusion	Duration
Abciximab	Primary PCI NSTEMI	0.25mg/kg	0.125 µg/kg per min (max 10 µg/min)	12 h
Tirofiban	NSTEMI (upstream)	0.4 µg/kg/min over 30 min	0.1 µg/kg per min	Up to 108 h
	NSTEMI (adjunct to PCI)	10 µg/kg over 3 min	0.15 µg/kg per min	18–24 h
	Primary PCI	25 µg/kg	0.15 µg/kg per min	18–24 h
Eptifibatide	NSTEMI (upstream)	180 µg/kg	2.0 µg/kg per min (1.0 µg/kg per min if GFR≤50 mL/min)	Up to 72 h
	NSTEMI (adjunct to PCI)	2 × 180 µg/kg 10 min apart		
	Primary PCI	2 × 180 µg/kg	2.0 µg/kg per min	12–24 h

GFR, glomerular filtration rate.

inhibition for NSTE ACS in 31 402 patients treated with aspirin and heparin, demonstrated a 9% reduction in the combined rate of death or MI with GPIIb/IIIa inhibitors compared with placebo or control (10.8 vs 11.8%, $p = 0.015$) [109]. The relative treatment benefit was similar in subgroups stratified by risk, resulting in a greater absolute benefit in high-risk patients. The question of whether GPIIb/IIIa inhibitors are still beneficial when patients are systematically pretreated with clopidogrel was answered by the ISAR REACT-2 study. In this trial, even after a loading dose of 600 mg clopidogrel, abciximab was associated with a significant reduction of the composite of death, MI, or urgent target vessel revascularization at 30 days [110]. Although the rate of major bleeding was higher in patients treated with GPIIb/IIIa inhibitors, intracranial bleeding rates were similar.

In the PRISM-PLUS and PURSUIT trials, upstream use of tirofiban or eptifibatide reduced the rate of ischaemic complications regardless of revascularization strategy [111, 112]. EARLY-ACS was the only large randomized study prospectively assessing the effect of early GPIIb/IIIa inhibitor versus more selective use at the time of PCI [113]. Early up-front use of eptifibatide did not result in lower rates of the primary ischaemic endpoint, compared to provisional use at the time of revascularization, but was associated with a higher risk of bleeding. There was a trend towards benefit of early up-front use of eptifibatide in troponin-positive patients, consistent with previous trials and meta-analyses. The GUSTO-IV ACS study suggested that abciximab is not beneficial in NSTE ACS patients not scheduled for PCI [114]. The lack of benefit was observed in every subgroup; moreover, patients receiving abciximab had a significant threefold increase in major bleeding.

A recent meta-analysis of 10 085 patients from 16 STEMI trials suggests that the benefit of GPIIb/IIIa inhibitors is confined to high-risk patients [115]. Overall, GPIIbIIIa

inhibitors did not significantly reduce 30-day mortality or reinfarction, while bleeding complications were more frequent. However, the authors observed a significant relation between risk profile and mortality benefits from GPIIb/IIIa inhibitors: the benefit of GPIIb/IIIa inhibitors was more pronounced in patients with a higher risk profile. Although retrospective analyses suggested that early administration of abciximab was better than administration at the time of PCI in terms of outcome, the more recent FINESSE study clearly shows that facilitation with up-front abciximab is not associated with lower rates of ischaemic complications [116, 117].

On aggregate, the 2007 ESC NSTE ACS guidelines recommend eptifibatide or tirofiban as initial, early therapy, but only in intermediate to high-risk patients [36]. Abciximab at the time of PCI is reserved for high-risk patients not pretreated with a small-molecule GPIIb/IIIa inhibitor. For STEMI patients, GPIIb/IIIa inhibitors only receive a class IIa (abciximab) or IIb (eptifibatide or tirofiban) recommendation as adjunctive therapy to primary PCI in the 2008 ESC guidelines [26].

Conclusion

In atherosclerosis, platelets and prothrombotic pathways are activated, which contributes to the progression of the disease and increases the risk of acute coronary syndromes. Thrombus formation after plaque rupture or erosion plays a pivotal role in non-ST-segment elevation as well as ST-segment elevation ACS, and in recurrent ischaemic complications during follow-up after the acute event. Antithrombotic therapy therefore remains a major cornerstone in the short- and long-term management of ACS. Both acute and chronic oral antiplatelet therapies targeting specific platelet activation pathways have demonstrated significant benefits. Despite proven efficacy of long-term dual oral antiplatelet therapy with aspirin and clopidogrel or prasugrel, residual morbidity and mortality is considerable. This may be partly due to incomplete inhibition of platelet activation with current agents, interference of other therapies and/or lack of long-term anticoagulant therapy. The use of antithrombin agents is currently confined to the acute setting, except in patients with a clear indication for long-term treatment. Also, balancing antithrombotic benefits against the increased risk of bleeding complications remains a substantial challenge. Improvements in patient outcomes could be achieved by developing safer agents that inhibit other platelet activation pathways or by adding new anticoagulants for a prolonged period of time after the acute event.

Personal perspective

Substantial residual morbidity and mortality risk remains in ACS patients despite the broad use of reperfusion strategies, mechanical interventions and pharmacologic therapy. Aspirin and clopidogrel each block only one of the many platelet activation pathways. Improvements in outcomes after ACS may be achieved with novel therapeutic approaches and greater use of guideline-recommended therapy. New therapies targeting pathways that are not affected by aspirin or $P2Y_{12}$ receptor antagonists could provide more comprehensive inhibition of platelet activation and contribute to greater inhibition of platelet-mediated thrombosis. In this respect, inhibition of the platelet PAR-1 receptor for thrombin is a new approach in the development of antiplatelet agents. PAR-1 inhibition, in combination with current dual antiplatelet therapy, could further reduce ischaemic events without significantly increasing bleeding risk. In a recent phase II trial in stable patients undergoing PCI, SCH 530348 given with aspirin and clopidogrel for 2 months was associated with a reduction in the composite endpoints of death/MACE and death/MI, as well as a reduction in the individual endpoint of MI, and no increase in major bleeding events when compared with placebo [118]. The lack of chronic anticoagulant treatment after an NSTE ACS may also be partly responsible for the high incidence of recurrent ischaemic events. Lower rates of ischaemic events have indeed been demonstrated with ximelagatran/dabigatran and the anti-Xa agents rivaroxaban and apixaban, but at the cost of more bleeding complications. Obviously, large phase III trials are needed to evaluate whether adding any of these new agents to standard dual antiplatelet therapy will result in a net clinical benefit. Other antithrombotic agents in (early) development include von Willebrand factor antagonists such as the aptamer ARC1779 and the nanobody ALX-0081 [119, 120] or RB006, an aptamer antifactor IXa inhibitor with its specific antidote (RB007) [121, 122].

Further reading

Van de Werf F. Balancing benefit and bleeding risk of antithrombotic agents in the individual patient with an acute coronary syndrome. *Circulation* 2010;**121**(1):5–7.

Bonaca MP *et al.* Antithrombotics in acute coronary syndromes. *J Am Coll Cardiol* 2009;**54**(11):969–84.

Stone GW *et al.* Bivalirudin during primary PCI in acute myocardial infarction. *N Engl J Med* 2008;**358**(21):2218–30.

Pocock SJ *et al.* Prognostic modeling of individual patient risk and mortality impact of ischemic and hemorrhagic complications: assessment from the Acute Catheterization and Urgent Intervention Triage Strategy trial. *Circulation* 2010;**121**(1):43–51.

Additional online material

42.1 Antithrombotic agents and bleeding complications

42.2 Thienopyridine $P2Y_{12}$ inhibitors

➲ For additional multimedia materials please visit the online version of the book (📖 http://www.esciacc.oxfordmedicine.com).

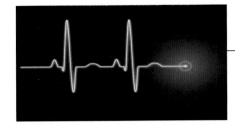

CHAPTER 43

Mechanical complications of myocardial infarction

Alexander V. Shpektor, Elena Y. Vasilieva

Contents

Summary

Mechanical complications of acute myocardial infarction (MI) include free wall rupture (FWR), ventricular septal rupture (VSR) and acute ischaemic mitral regurgitation (IMR) due to papillary muscle rupture or displacement. The frequency of ruptures has decreased to less than half of what it was in the pre-reperfusion era, but they remain the second cause of in-hospital mortality of STEMI patients, after cardiogenic shock. The risk of ruptures is increased in patients with total occlusion of the infarct-related artery and lack of collaterals. The ruptures have the a bimodal distribution, with peaks on the first day and at 5–7 days. Color Doppler echocardiography is the main diagnostic modality for all mechanical complications of MI. Surgical treatment is the main option for FWR and acute IMR with unstable haemodynamics and for all patients with VSR. The most effective prophylactic measure against all mechanical complications of MI is urgent primary PCI.

Free wall rupture

Incidence

In the last few years, the incidence of free wall ruptures (FWRs) has decreased significantly: it was about 6% in the 70s and 80s of the last century, but most recently has been only 0.5-2% (1,2). The most probable reason for this decrease is the widespread use of primary percutaneous intervention (PPCI) (3-7). Nevertheless, FWRs remain the second cause of in-hospital mortality, after cardiogenic shock, in patients with STEMI (2,8,9).

Time of occurrence

The risk of rupture exists during the first 3 weeks after the onset of MI. The distribution of ruptures is bimodal during this period: early ruptures occur during the first 24 to 48 h and late ruptures occur most often on days 5–7 (10-14). Late ruptures predominated during the prethrombolytic era (15,16). At present, early ruptures predominate (4,17) And most of them occur during the first 24 hours of disease (17).

Pathology

Ruptures of the free wall of the left ventricle (LV) are the most common ones (➲ Fig. 43.1A). Ruptures of the right ventricle are very rare. Autopsies show transmural infarctions in patients with ruptures. The area of infarction can vary considerably. FWRs occur most frequently in large infarctions occupying more than 20% of the volume of the LV (18). However, FWRs can occur in relatively small infarctions which are accompanied by considerable remodeling (15,19-22). An absence of scars is characteristic. Total occlusion of a single coronary vessel and lack of collaterals are also typical. The rupture itself can take different forms. Abrupt split-tears through the necrotic tissue are characteristic of early ruptures which occur 24–48 hours after MI (23-25). Such tears are often found near the apex at the connection with the intraventricular septum and near the base of the papillary muscles. This localisation supports the hypothesis that mechanical tension is the leading factor in this type of ruptures, since tension is greatest in the areas indicated above.

Late ruptures are associated with expansion of the infarct zone, which becomes stretched and thinned (12,15). This stretching occurs in 30% of patients with STEMI and is maximal at days 5–6, the time when most later ruptures occur. Remodelling is more common after a first AMI involving a single coronary vessel without collaterals. These usually occur in patients who did not undergo reperfusion therapy or in whom it was ineffective. When stretching is considerable, the frequency of rupture may reach 50% (15). The myocardial wall around the rupture has been found to be twice as thin as that in the unaffected zone of the myocardium. In these cases, rupture usually occurs at the boundary of the necrotic and the normal myocardium.

The reasons why MI in some patients is accompanied by myocardial expansion leading to rupture are not clear. The factors involved may include activity of metalloproteases (such as MMP-9), which are able to destroy the extracellular matrix of the myocardium. The frequency of ruptures is decreased in mice with a genetic deficiency of MMP-9 (26,27). Recently, it was demonstrated that cathenin and cadherin E, proteins responsible for cell–cell adhesion between myocytes, are significantly decreased in a ruptured myocardium (28). The authors of this work were unable to prove that this decrease has a genetic origin, so the causes of this deficiency remain obscure.

Risk factors and predictors

Risk factors and predictors of FWR are listed in Table 43.1.

Some of these factors increase the risk of early ruptures (anterior wall localisation, high arterial hypertension, preserved ejection fraction, thrombolytic therapy), while other factors increase the frequency of late ruptures (failed reperfusion, severe expansion, total occlusion of the infarct-related artery with lack of collaterals).

Despite the inconsistency of some results, there are reasons to believe that thrombolytic therapy increases the risk of rupture and shifts these ruptures to an earlier time. This effect is most pronounced when thrombolytic therapy is administered to elderly patients more than 6 hours after the onset of MI.

There is no evidence that anticoagulants and antiplatelet agents can raise the frequency of ruptures (10). PPCI decreases the risk of ruptures, with its effectiveness dependent on the promptness and efficiency of this procedure (6). When PPCI was performed during the first 12 h of MI, the frequency of FWR was only 0.7%. At the same time, when PPCI was ineffective this frequency increased to 3.8% (3).

Table 43.1 Risk factors of free wall rupture.

- Age > 65-70 years (4,6,7)
- Female gender (4,6,7)
- Low body mass index (4,29)
- History of hypertension (4)
- First myocardial infarction (2,13)
- Absence of previous angina (18,30,31)
- Single-vessel disease
- Total occlusion of the infarct-related artery (12,13,18,32,33)
- Lack of collaterals (20)
- Anterior myocardial infarction (6)
- Persistent ST-segment elevation (12,34,35)
- Preserved LV ejection fraction (36)
- Echocardiographic signs of expansion (15)
- Reperfusion failure (7,37)
- Late start of thrombolytic therapy, especially in elderly patients (7,29,38-41)
- BP > 150 mm Hg in the first 10-24 hours of hospitalization (34,35,42-44)
- Excessive physical exertion during CCU stay (straining effort, vomiting, refractory cough, excitement) (35,43)
- High levels of CRP and SAA (36,45)
- ST segment elevation in lead AVL (46)

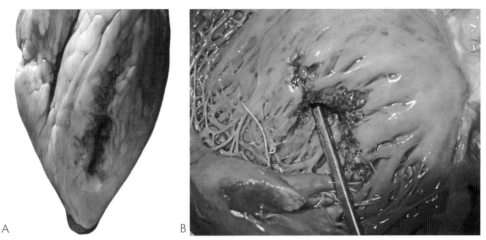

Figure 43.1 Large free wall rupture near the apex (A) and ventricular septal rupture (B) in patients with myocardial infarctions. Part A reproduced by kind permission of Dr Oleg Zayratyants.

The risk of FWR is increased in patients with high levels of C-reactive protein and of amiloid (36,45). It is not clear whether this increase reflects inflammation and remodeling or simply correlates with the extent of necrosis.

Clinical manifestation and diagnosis

Chest pain is usually the first sign of the onset of a FWR. In contrast with the initial angina, this pain is often poorly controlled by morphine. ECG can show additional and more widespread ST elevation. Echocardiography can reveal sites of severe expansion with stretching and thinning of the necrotic area. Sometimes it is possible to visualise the incomplete rupture of the ventricular wall itself (➲ Fig. 43.2 A,B). At the same time, in about half of the cases rupture manifests abruptly with signs of tamponade.

Depending on the volume of blood in the pericardium and on its haemodynamic significance, it is possible to distinguish acute and subacute ruptures (8,10,11,42,44,47-52).

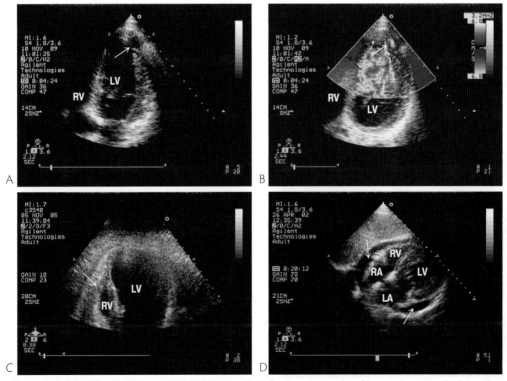

Figure 43.2 Free wall ruptures of the left ventricle in patients with myocardial infarctions: incomplete (A, two-dimensional echocardiography, B colour Doppler imaging), complete with tamponade (C), with effusion but without tamponade (D).

Acute ruptures are characterised by a rather large volume of blood in the pericardium, leading to cardiac tamponade (⊃ Fig. 43.2C). It usually manifests as cardiac arrest due to electromechanical dissociation or sustained hypotension. Diagnosis is usually made by echocardiography which demonstrates fluid in the pericardium, sometimes containing densities created by fibrin threads. Haemopericardium can be confirmed by pericardiocentesis.

A subacute course of rupture takes place when a relatively small rupture of the myocardium is temporary sealed by a fibrin clot so that a relatively small volume of blood penetrates into the pericardium without causing tamponade (⊃ Fig. 43.2D). In some cases, these ruptures can occur without obvious clinical signs. The blood in the pericardium can cause irritation of the pericardium and excite parasympathetic activation with hypotension, bradycardia and occasional syncope.

The subsequent course of subacute FWR is variable. Sometimes a final rupture with tamponade and electromechanical dissociation develops, occasionally preceded by several episodes of syncope. Nevertheless, there are numerous case descriptions in which patients remained stable over a long period without surgical treatment. This course may lead to the formation of a false aneurysm (⊃ Fig. 43.3). The wall of a false aneurysm is formed by thrombotic masses adherent to the pericardial wall, unlike the wall of a true aneurysm, formed by scars with remnants of myocardium. A false aneurysm can be differentiated from a true one by the presence of a narrow neck between the LV and the cavity. In some cases, false aneurysms can attain a considerable volume, comparable with that of the LV. Although long-term prognosis has not been well studied surgical treatment is usually recommended (53).

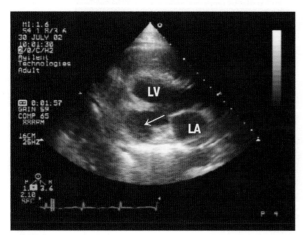

Figure 43.3 False aneurysm of left ventricle (arrow) after posterior myocardial infarction.

Treatment strategy

In the presence of tamponade it is essential to replace fluid with colloidal solutions and, if necessary, to use vasopressors. If blood pressure remains low with signs of peripheral hypoperfusion, pericardiocentesis should be performed. Removal of small amounts of pericardial fluid (40–50 ml) can be sufficient to restore haemodynamics. If pericardiocentesis is ineffective, emergent thoracotomy should be performed. Urgent surgical treatment can be life saving lives in some of these cases.

If the patient has been stabilised and it can be assumed that the rupture is covered by a thrombus, a conservative approach might be considered. This is especially true when the risk of surgery is particularly high, for instance when the patient needs to be transported to another hospital. In these cases, if the patient has been stabilised, bed rest for 1–2 weeks can be recommended; blood pressure should be carefully controlled (systolic < 120mm Hg), and beta blockers should be given unless contraindicated.

The same approach can be used when patients have a FWR without cardiac tamponade. As shown by Figueras and collaborators a conservative approach can yield better results in such cases than immediate surgery (52). According to these authors' data, only 2 of 15 patients survived emergency surgery while 13 of 19 patients survived with conservative treatment.

Surgical treatment traditionally included infarctectomy and suturing of a prosthetic patch for repair of the ventricular wall, under cardiopulmonary bypass. Mortality in these cases was as high as 33%–61% (54-60).

Gluing of an autologous patch to the defect has recently gained popularity. This is simpler and faster than suturing and can be performed off pump. An additional advantage of this technique is the restoration of the geometrical shape of the heart. Data from different reports indicate that in-hospital mortality was 15.6% and 30-day mortality was 23.5% (61-63). There were no ruptures during follow-up.

Percutaneous intrapericardial fibrin-glue injection (PIFGI) is a promising approach and may replace surgical treatment in some cases. This technique involves introduction of a pigtail catheter into the pericardial space, removal of bloody fluid and injection of fibrin glue into the pericardium. Terachima and co-authors (64) reported the application of this technique in 9 patients with FWR. In seven cases, the procedure was initially successful. During a median follow up of 4 years five patients were free of cardiovascular events.Additional data concerning the effectiveness and safety of this procedure are needed.

As FWRs lead to very high mortality, prevention is most important. Timely PPCI is the best method of prevention. Traditional methods of rupture prevention include avoidance of sternous efforts in CCU and control of blood pressure. The drugs that decrease the risk of rupture include beta-blockers and ACE-inhibitors (65). Thrombolytic therapy later than 6 hours after the onset of AMI in elderly patients should be avoided. There are no data indicating that other antithrombotic therapies, increase the risk of FWR.

It has been suggested that corticosteroids and NSAIDS increase the risk of FWR (66). However a subsequent meta-analysis did not confirm this effect of corticosteroids (67). Nevertheless, it is better to avoid the use of corticosteroids and NSAIDS (apart from aspirin) in patients with acute MI.

Ventricular septal rupture

Incidence

The incidence of ventricular septal rupture (VSR) before the reperfusion era was 1%–3% (68-72). With thrombolysis this incidence decreased to 0.2%–0.6% (73,74). The frequency of VSR after PPCI was reported to be as low as 0.2%, (75).

Time of occurrence

Like FRWs, VSRs have a bimodal distribution, with one peak on the first day and the other between days 3 and 5. Ruptures after 14 days are very rare. After thrombolysis or PPCI, most ruptures are early. Among patients included in the GUSTO-1 trial and treated with thrombolytic therapy, 94% of all ruptures took place during the first day of MI (73).

Pathology

The size of ruptures varies from several millimetres to a few centimeters (◑ Fig. 43.1B). In patients with anterior MI these ruptures usually are localised near the apex, while in patients with inferior MI they are usually in the basal part of the septum (70,76,77). Morphologically, simple and complex ruptures can be distinguished. Simple ventricular ruptures are direct defects across the septum, while complex ruptures exhibit extensive haemorrhage with serpentine tracts within the necrotic tissue (76,77).

Haemodynamics

VSR leads to a left-to-right shunting of blood. The degree of shunting depends on the size of the defect, the contractility of the ventricles, the level of pulmonary vascular resistance, and systemic vascular resistance. Considerable shunting leads to a significant decrease of forward cardiac output and shock. Simultaneously, overstretching of the right ventricle takes place and right ventricular failure develops. Pulmonary oedema is not typical, because blood shunting occurs from the left to the right.

Risk factors and predictors

Risk factors of VSR are similar to those of FWR. They include advanced age, female sex, anterior MI, low body mass index and absence of a history of angina and MI (68,69,73-83). Additional predictors include total occlusion of the infarct related artery and absence of collaterals (70,73,81,82). Persistent ST elevation is common (84,85).

Clinical presentation

With haemodynamically significant shunting, the main clinical signs of rupture are associated with right ventricular failure and low cardiac output. Cardiogenic shock is the extreme manifestation of right and LV failure. Auscultation reveals a typically harsh loud holosystolic murmur along the left parasternal area radiating towards the base, apex, and right parasternal area. About half of patients develop a parasternal thrill (86,87). If blood pressure and cardiac output decrease substantially, the murmur becomes weaker and the thrill disappears; right and LV S3 gallops are common. The pulmonic component of the second heart sound is accentuated.

Color Doppler echocardiography is the main diagnostic modality (◑ Fig. 43.4). The sensitivity and specificity of this method were reported to be as high as 100% (88,89). This method also allows assessment of the size of the rupture and of the shunting. Transoesophageal echocardiography may give additional information, which can be important for management. Real-time 3D-echocardiography can be useful for this purpose.

Modern echocardiography decreased the diagnostic importance of ventriculography and of right heart catheterisation for the diagnosis and quantification of VSR. These tools may still be employed if echjocardiographic imaging is inadequate.

Treatment strategy

Medical therapy of patients with VSR without signs of shock consists of afterload reduction and administration of diuretics. Hypotension calls for use of an intraaortic balloon pump (IABP) and vasopressors if necessary.

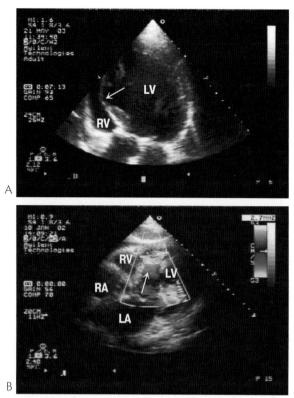

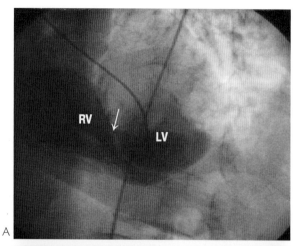

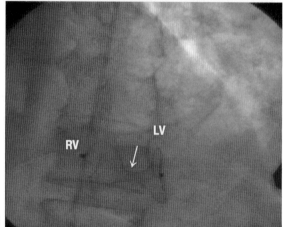

Figure 43.4 Ventricular septal ruptures in patients with myocardial infarctions: incomplete with formation of aneurysm (A) and complete with left-to-right shunting of blood visualized by colour Doppler imaging (B).

Attempts to stabilise patients medically usually have only a temporary effect And mortality with conservative treatment is as high as 90% (70,73,90-92). Surgical treatment may significantly decrease mortality. Infarctectomy with subsequent reconstruction with fabric graft are the traditional operative techniques. However, hospital and 30-day mortality are as high as 35%–59% (93-,97). The newer endocardial patch technique reduced mortality to 13.5%–24% (94,98,99). CABG can be performed in multivessel disease and it is not mandatory to bypass the artery which supplied the infarcted septum (100). Patients who survive the operation have a good long-term prognosis. The timing of the surgery is of critically important. There are reasons to believe that immediately after rupture the myocardium is too fragile for surgery. However, in the presence of cardiogenic shock immediate operation is the only option. Even in patients whose condition is relatively stable, haemodynamics may deteriorate abruptly because of an increase of the size of the rupture (70). Improved survival with rapid intervention has been described in several publications (101-103).

Percutaneous closure of septal ruptures with catheter-based devices may be an alternative to surgery or a bridge to it in selected patients (➲Fig. 43.5). This approach is most applicable to patients with relatively small, simple defects

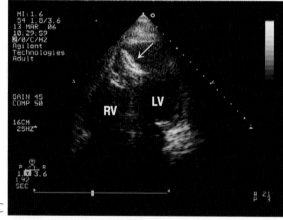

Figure 43.5 Percutaneous closure of the ventricular septal rupture (A) with Amplatz device: radiography (B) and echocardiography (C) visualization.

who do not require revascularisation. The rupture should not be too close to the apex and cardiac valves. transoesophageal and real-time three-dimentional echocardiography are useful for patient selection and for precise positioning of the occluder (104). It is prematureto recommend routine percutaneous closure of septal ruptures, because 30-day mortality, is still rather high at 28–65%, (103,105).

Acute mitral regurgitation

Epidemiology

Acute mitral regurgitation (MR) occurs in about 40%–50% of patients after MI (106-109) and in one series 12% of patients had severe MR (109). PostMIMR is an adverse prognostic marker. Outcome is worse with increasing severity of MR, but even mild post MI MR is an independent predictor of long-term mortality (110). The SAVE study reported that in post-MI patients with mild MR, mortality was 29% after 3.5 years, compared with 12% in those without MR (107). The dynamic nature of IMR may explain why small amounts of regurgitation at rest are associated with adverse outcomes.

Risk factors

The occurrence of MR is associated with advanced age, female gender, LV dysfunction and triple-vessel disease (111). Reports on the association between MR and the location of MI are conflicting (112,113).

Mechanisms

Acute MR after MI can be due to the papillary muscle rupture (PMR) or to functional disorder of the mitral valve (MV).

PMR is a rare but catastrophic complication of AMI leading to acute severe MR, pulmonary oedema, and cardiogenic shock (114,115). It typically involves the posterior PM, as this usually has a single blood supply from the posterior descending branch of the RCA and is most susceptible to infarction. The anterior PM usually has a dual blood supply from the diagonal branches of the LAD and the marginal branches of the circumflex artery, and infarction and rupture are uncommon.

Ischaemia or infarction of the PM without rupture does not appear to cause significant MR (116,117). Functional acute MR in MI patients usually occurs as a result of local LV wall motion abnormality in the region where the PM are attached (➲ Fig. 43.6A,B). Local distortion leads to displacement of the PM. Displacement of the anterior PM is rare, because of the anatomical pattern. Typically, posterior-lateral displacement of the posterior PM occurs as a result of RCA or circumflex occlusion (112,116,118,119). As the PM contributes chordae to both leaflets, the displacement of the posterior PM causes tethering of both, but more significantly of the posterior one (asymmetric tethering). The result is systolic separation of the leaflets leading to MR (116,119). Reduced or absent contraction of the

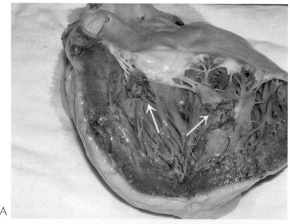

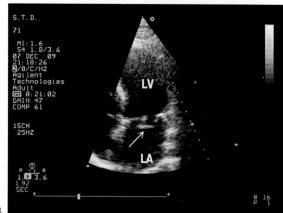

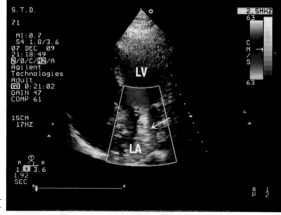

Figure 43.6 Papillary muscles ruptures in patient with acute posterior myocardial infarction. A, anterior and posterior papillary muscle ruptures (arrows); B, two-dimensional echocardiography; C, colour Doppler imaging. The arrow shows the severe mitral regurgitation.

PM may paradoxically alleviate the tethering effects on the MV (120,121). Conversely, global LV dysfunction increases the severity of MR. This is the result of incomplete valve closure caused by decrease of systolic pressure in the LV. When the mitral leaflets are tented away from the annulus, more force is needed to close them; therefore a reduced systolic function superimposed on tethering of leaflets further reduces systolic closure (117,122).

A synchronised contraction of the anterior and posterior PM also contributes to IMR (123,124). Later in the post-AMI period, MR may be increased because of scarring and shortening of the PM and because of global LV remodeling (➲Fig.6C). LV dilation leads to apical displacement of the PM, resulting in apical tethering of both leaflets and central MR (110,119,125). Dilatation of the mitral ring may additionally facilitate MR. This typically occurs after anterior MI with LV dysfunction (110,119).

Haemodynamics

In acute post MI MR, compensatory mechanisms are less effective than in chronic MR. In chronic cases, the left atrium gradually dilates. Itscompliance therefore increases, allowing greater volumes of regurgitation without severe rises in left atrial and pulmonary venous pressure. In contrast, with acute MR, the left atrium is not initially dilated and hence there is an abrupt increase of left atrial and pulmonary venous pressures. Furthermore, in chronic MR LV volume overload leads to a a compensatory increase of forward stroke volume which partly compensates for the decrease of stroke volume due to MR. In acute MR, absence of LV dilation permits a critical decrease of forward stroke volume and cardiogenic shock.

Clinical presentation

The main physical sign of MR is the systolic murmur. In contrast to chronic MR the murmur in acute IMR is less pronounced and its intensity correlates poorly with the degree of regurgitation, because of decreased ventricular systolic function and atrial compliance (126). In the non-compliant left atrium, the regurgitant volume tends to be smaller and is associated with a higher pressure but a less intense murmur. As a result, acute IMR is often unrecognisable on physical examination.

As MR is often clinically silent, it should be systematically evaluated by echocardiography. Color Doppler imaging is a sensitive method for the detection of even mild degrees of MR. To estimate the severity of MR, regurgitant volume and effective regurgitant orifice area (EROA) have been widely used. Current guidelines recommended as thresholds to define severe MR a regurgitant volume of 60 ml and an EROA of 40 mm^2. For IMR, however, adverse outcomes are associated with lower volumes and areas a, suggesting that 30 ml for regurgitant volume and 20 mm^2 for EROA should be the preferred thresholds of severity (110). To assess the degree of MV apparatus deformation, calculation of the distance between leaflet coaptation and mitral annular plane (coaptation depth) and the area enclosed during systole between the annular plane and mitral leaflets (tenting area) are useful. These parameters correlate with the severity of MR and LV dysfunction (127).

Although transthoracic echocardiography (TTE) may be used initially to assess the MR, transoesophagical echocardiography is much more sensitive in the assessment of acute MR and should certainly be used if questions regarding lesion severity remain following TTE (➲Fig. 43.7). To specify the pattern of MV leaflet tethering, three-dimensional echocardiography can be useful. This method also makes it possible to calculate not only tenting area but tenting volume: the volume between the mitral leaflets and the annular plane during systole. It has been demonstrated that tenting volume is a better index of MV remodeling than

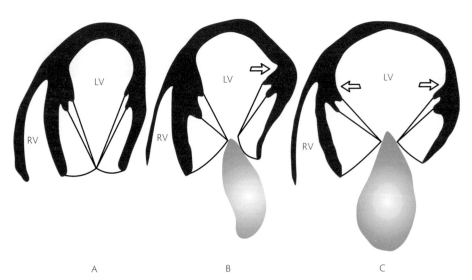

Figure 43.7 Mechanisms of ischaemic mitral regurgitation. A, normal mitral valve closure; B, asymmetric tethering due to local displacement of the lateral wall; C, symmetric tethering due to left ventricle dilation.

tenting area because it takes into account all the geometric components of tethering and tenting (128,129)

Treatment strategy

Acute MR following PM rupture warrants urgent surgical intervention following initial medical stabilisation. Medical treatment alone is associated with mortality as high as 80% (130-134).Nitrates and diuretics can help to reduce filling pressure. Nitroprusside may be useful in normotensive and especially hypertensive patients, helping to increase forward cardiac output and reducing the degree of MR. In hypotension patients, inotropic agents should be given if required. The IABP can increase forward output and reduce the amount of regurgitation, helping to achieve haemodynamic stabilisation before surgery. In most cases, MV replacement or repair, in addition to CABG, will be needed (129). Unfortunately, surgical treatment, although recommended by guidelines, is often considered too risky (especially for elderly patients with severe clinical presentations). However, operative mortality decreased from 67% before 1990 without CABG to 8.7% after 1990 with CABG. Overall, 5-year survival was 65% and 30-day operative survival was 79% (135). MVRep consists of reattachment of the ruptured PM with or without ring annuloplasty.

The approach to severe functional MR is not definitively determined. Several authors have suggested that the severity of MR in acute MI may decrease after successful reperfusion ((136-142). PCI is effective in patients in whom MR is caused by ischaemia in the base of the papillary muscle (139,140). Even after successful PPCI, however, mortality in patients with MR remains high. According to the CADILLAC study, 30-day mortality after PPCI was 1.4% in patients with no MR vs. 3.7% in those with mild MR vs. 8.6% in those with moderate-to-severe MR (*p*<0.0001), and 1-year mortality was 2.9% vs. 8.5% vs. 20.8%, respectively (*p*<0.0001). These disappointing results may be due to multivessel disease, which is present in most patients with IMR (107,143); Ellis (143) reported that only 28% of patients with IMR were fully revascularised by PCI. by. Urgent surgery cannot be recommended in patients with

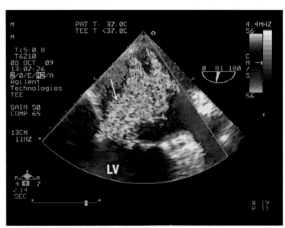

Figure 43.8 Transoesophageal echocardiography in patient with posterior myocardial infarction. The arrow shows the severe mitral regurgitation.

mild IMR, especially when asymptomatic. In more severe degrees of MR a decision regarding surgery should be based on symptoms, the degree of LV dysfunction and viability, the ability to achieve complete revascularization and the ability to repair rather than to replace the valve.

In the post-MI period, revascularisation does not itself improve the MR grade. Only 9%–11% of post-AMI patients achieved a significant reduction of MR after revascularisation (144,145). In these patients, reduction in MR probably occurs as a result of restoration of blood flow to an area of hibernating myocardium. Revascularisation is not effective in this regard when alteration of LV geometry lead to MR. Most studies did not find any prognostic advantages of MV surgery (MVS) in post-AMI patients who had undergone CABG (146-149). Operative mortality is higher than in organic MR, and long-term prognosis is less satisfactory, with a higher recurrence of MR after surgery (150-152). Benedetto et al., in a meta-analysis of 2,479 patients who had undergone CABG with or without MVS, found that MVS did not improve late mortality or NYHA class (146). According to these data, MVS for functional MR, even when severe, cannot be routinely recommended.

In selected patients with chronic IMR, CRT reduces the amount of MR and improves cardiac output and symptomatic status (153). The role of CRT in cases of acute MR is unknown.

Personal perspectives

Treatment of mechanical complications of MI is a challenging problem. Urgent surgery is still associated with considerable mortality. In some subacute cases of FWR a conservative technique is preferable. New methods of FWR treatment such as pericardial gluing show promise. The optimal timing for surgery of VSR has yet to be determined. Results of percutaneous treatment of VSR are currently not satisfactory. The criteria for surgery in patients with severe acute IMR who are hemodynamically stable need to be defined. The results of percutaneous repair of chronic MR are promising, and the extension of this approach for acute MR in MI patients may prove useful.

Considering the high mortality in patients with mechanical complications of MI, the main challenge is prevention. Primary PCI significantly decreases the rate of mechanical complications of MI. Conceivably, future specific anti-inflammatory interventions may alleviate the cellular processes which are the basis of mechanical complications of MI.

Acknowledgement

We would like to thank Dr. Dmitriy Skripnik for his contribution for this chapter.

Further reading

Birnbaum Y, Fishbein MC, Blanche C, Siegel RJ. Ventricular Septal Rupture After Acute Myocardial Infarction. *N Engl J Med.* 2001; **347**:1426–1432.

Bursi F, Enriques-Sarano M, Jacobsen SJ, Roger VL. Mitral Regurgitation after Myocardial Infarction: a Review. *Am J Cardiol.* 2006; **119**:103–112.

Chan J, Amirak E, Zakkar M *et al.* Ischemic Mitral Regurgitation: In Search of the Best Treatment for a Common Condition. *Progress in Cardiovasc Dis.* 2009; **51**:460–471.

Figueras J, Alcalde O, Barrabés JA *et al.*, Changes in hospital mortality rates in 425 patients with acute ST-elevation myocardial infarction and cardiac rupture over a 30-year period. *Circulation.* 2008; **118**: 2783–9.

Marwick TH, Lancelloti P, Pierard L. Ischemic Mitral Regurgitation: Mechanisms and diagnosis. *Heart.* 2009; **95**:1711–1718.

Vahanian A, Baumgartner H, Bax J *et al.* Guidelines on the management of valvular heart disease: The Task Force on the Management of Valvular Heart Disease of the European Society of Cardiology. *Eur Heart J.* 2007; **28**: 230–268.

Van de Werf F, Bax J, Betriu A *et al.* Management of Acute Myocardial Infarction in Patients Presenting with Persistent ST-segment Elevation. The Task Force on the Management of ST-segment Elevation Acute Myocardial Infarction of the European Society of Cardiology. *Eur Heart J.* 2008; **29**: 2909–2945.

➲ For additional multimedia materials please visit the online version of the book (✎ http://www.esciacc.oxfordmedicine.com).

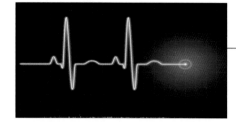

CHAPTER 44

Non-ST-elevation acute coronary syndromes

Diego Ardissino, Daniela Lina,
and Francesca Notarangelo

Contents

Summary

Acute coronary syndromes (ACS) represent a broad spectrum of ischaemic myocardial events associated with high morbidity and mortality rates, thus making them a major public health problem worldwide. Almost all ACS are due to coronary atherosclerosis, generally with superimposed coronary thrombosis. An accurate diagnosis has life-saving implications and requires the detailed assessment of a patient's history, physical examination, 12-lead ECG findings, and cardiac biomarker assays. A careful early risk stratification is mandatory and permits the identification of the moderate- and high-risk patients who gain the greatest benefit from potent antithrombotic therapies and early revascularization. To optimize the treatment of ACS, adherence to the current guidelines significantly improves clinical outcomes by reducing mortality and morbidity.

Introduction

Acute coronary syndromes (ACS) are the most common cause of cardiac-related hospital admissions worldwide, leading to more than 2.5 million hospitalizations a year and accounting for 50% of coronary care unit admission diagnoses [1]. Although significant improvements have been made to the management of ACS over the last 20 years, they remain a major public health problem especially in Western countries [2].

The term ACS covers a wide spectrum of clinical conditions ranging from unstable angina, to non-ST-elevation and ST-elevation myocardial infarction (STEMI), all of which share a common pathophysiological substrate: the development of complications at the site of unstable atherosclerotic plaque followed by various degrees of superimposed thrombosis.

In practice, patients with acute chest pain are classified into one of two categories on the basis of ECG changes:

- Patients with persistent (>20 min) ST-segment elevation (STE-ACS), who will develop STEMI and in whom the therapeutic objective is to achieve rapid coronary reperfusion by means of primary angioplasty or fibrinolytic therapy [3].

- Patients without persistent (<20 min) ST-segment elevation (NSTE-ACS), who will develop non-ST-elevation myocardial infarction (non-STEMI) when the ischaemia is sufficiently severe to cause myocardial necrosis and the subsequent release of cardiac biomarkers (if no such markers are detected in circulating blood, the patients are considered to have unstable angina); in these patients, the therapeutic objective is to relieve ischaemia by means of medical therapy and stratify short-term risk in such a way as to select the optimal subsequent invasive strategy [4].

Epidemiology

Registry data suggest that the annual incidence of NSTE-ACS in Europe is about 3/1000 inhabitants, although it varies from country to country: the highest incidence and mortality rates are observed in central–eastern Europe [5–7]. The ratio between NSTE-ACS and STEMI has changed over time, and NSTE-ACS is now more frequent than STEMI [8], possibly because of the changes in disease management and greater efforts to prevent coronary artery disease (CAD) over the last 20 years (⊃ Fig. 44.1). Registry data also show that the in-hospital mortality rate is higher in patients with STEMI than in those with NSTE-ACS (7% vs 5%), but 6-month mortality rates are similar (12% vs 13%), and 4-year mortality is twice as high among patients

with NSTE-ACS, possibly because they tend to be older and affected by more comorbidities, especially diabetes and renal failure [9–12].

Pathophysiology

Almost all ACS are due to coronary atherosclerosis, generally with superimposed coronary thrombosis (⊃ Fig. 44.2). Plaque rupture is considered to be the common pathophysiological substrate and, if this leads to the exposure of a sufficient amount of thrombogenic substances, the coronary artery lumen may become obstructed by a combination of platelet aggregates, fibrin and red blood cells, thus reducing coronary blood flow and giving rise to myocardial ischaemia.

The central role of thrombosis in the development of ACS has been demonstrated by means of autopsy data [13, 14], angiographic findings [15], the detection of markers of thrombin generation and platelet activation [16–17], and the evidence of improved outcomes after antithrombotic treatments[18]. Coronary thromboses usually develop at the sites of vulnerable plaques characterized by a thin fibrous cap, a large lipid core, a high density of macrophages and T lymphocytes, a relative paucity of smooth muscle cells, the locally increased expression of matrix metalloproteinases, eccentric outward remodelling, and neovascularization; such plaques are usually nonobstructive and clinically silent until rupture [19–21]. Endothelial erosion is another but less frequent triggering mechanism [22].

After plaque rupture or endothelial erosion, the thrombogenic components of the lipid core (particularly tissue factor)[23, 24] are exposed to circulating blood, which leads to platelet adhesion, activation, and aggregation, and

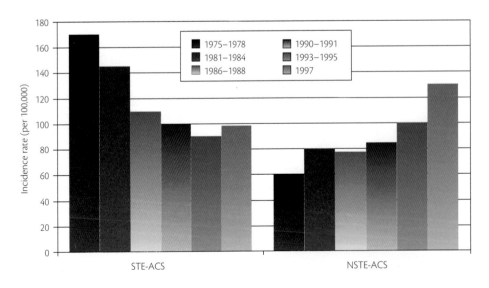

Figure 44.1 Incidence of acute coronary syndromes in Europe over time.

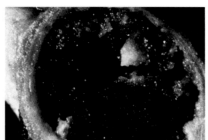
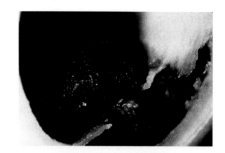
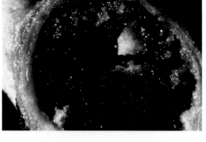
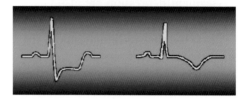

STE ACS

NSTE ACS

Figure 44.2 Coronary artery thrombosis in the pathogenesis of acute coronary syndromes (ACS). In ST-segment elevation ACS the coronary artery lumen is completely obstructed, whereas in non-ST-segment elevation ACS thrombus is usually nonocclusive.

the activation of the clotting cascade with fibrin generation and thrombus formation [25, 26].

In addition to local plaque-induced injury, the development of thrombosis critically depends on the presence of a systemic prothrombotic and pro-inflammatory state as there is clinical evidence that, although they are frequent, only a few episodes of plaque rupture actually cause ACS [27–29]. Furthermore, the fact that complicated plaques are found at multiple sites other than that of the culprit coronary lesion suggests a systemic prothrombotic state [30, 31]. In this context, vulnerable plaque should be considered as part of a vulnerable artery, a vulnerable arterial bed, and a vulnerable patient.

Finally, rare cases of ACS may have a nonatherosclerotic aetiology such as arteritis, trauma, dissection, thromboembolism, congenital anomalies, cocaine abuse, or a complication of cardiac catheterization.

Diagnosis and risk assessment

History and physical examination

Careful history taking is essential to diagnose NSTE-ACS and evaluate the risk of an adverse outcome. Patients usually describe chest discomfort as intermittent or persistent pressure or heaviness often occurring at rest, located in the retrosternal region and radiating to the left arm, neck, or jaw; they may also report other symptoms (alone or in association with chest pain) such as diaphoresis, nausea, abdominal pain, dyspnoea, and syncope [32]. Some patients, particularly elderly people, women, and patients with diabetes, chronic renal failure or dementia, may present without chest

pain or have atypical symptoms such as epigastric pain, a stabbing chest pain, or chest pain with pleuritic features and increasing dyspnoea [33, 34]. In any case, the exacerbation of symptoms upon physical exertion, or their relief at rest or after the administration of nitrates, supports a diagnosis of myocardial ischaemia, and the presence of tachycardia, hypotension, or heart failure needs rapid diagnosis and management as it indicates a poor prognosis. It is also important to identify clinical conditions that may precipitate NSTE-ACS such as anaemia, infection, inflammation, fever, and metabolic or endocrine disorders [35].

Physical examination findings are frequently normal in patients with NSTE-ACS; it is always important to search for signs of haemodynamic instability and left ventricular dysfunction such as diaphoresis, a cool skin, sinus tachycardia, a new or increasing mitral regurgitation murmur, or a third heart sound because these indicate a high risk of an adverse clinical outcome. Physical examination may also provide clues that help in establishing a differential diagnosis such as pericarditis, pneumothorax, aortic dissection, or pulmonary embolism [36]; e.g. the presence of unequal pulses, a murmur suggesting aortic regurgitation, a friction rub, or an abdominal mass may suggest a diagnosis other than NSTE-ACS.

ECG

A 12-lead ECG should be obtained within 10 min of a patient's arrival in the emergency department, and immediately interpreted by a qualified physician [37]. ECG recordings should be repeated at least after 6 h and 24 h, in the case of the reoccurrence of chest pain, and before discharge [4]. The ECG findings associated with NSTE-ACS include

ST-segment depression, transient ST-segment elevation (<20 min), T-wave inversion, or some combination of these. However, a normal ECG does not exclude the diagnosis of ACS as up to 5% of such patients have high biomarker levels indicating a myocardial infarction (MI) [38, 39]. The number of leads showing ST-segment depression and the magnitude of the depression are indicative of the severity of myocardial ischaemia and correlate with prognosis. Patients with ST-segment depression are at higher risk of cardiac events than those with isolated T-wave inversion [40–45].

ECG has a number of limitations in the evaluation of patients with NSTE-ACS, because it does not adequately represent the inferobasal (posterior), lateral, and apical walls of the left ventricle. This means that traditional 12-lead ECG frequently misses ischaemia in the territory of the circumflex artery, although it may be detected by nonstandard V4R, V3R, and V7–V9 leads. Furthermore, as myocardial ischaemia is a dynamic process of which a single ECG can only provide a snapshot: almost two-thirds of all ischaemic episodes are clinically silent and undetected by conventional ECG; hospitalized patients should therefore undergo serial ECG recordings or continuous ST-segment monitoring, which adds independent prognostic information to the findings of resting ECG [46, 47].

Markers of myocardial injury

Blood levels of the troponins and the MB isoenzyme of creatinine kinase (CK-MB) must be measured in all patients who report chest pain suggesting ACS because these cardiac biomarkers are essential for diagnosis and risk stratification. Troponin T and I are more sensitive than CK-MB in revealing myocardial injury, which may remain undetected on the basis of CK-MB alone in about one-third of patients with NSTE-ACS [48, 49]; they are also more specific. In this setting, measuring myoglobin is not recommended because of its poor specificity and sensitivity [50]. Troponin T or I can be used indifferently as their release kinetics are similar: both typically increase at least 6 h after symptom onset, and peak values are observed after 12–48 h. Serial sampling is therefore recommended: at baseline and 6–12 h after symptom onset [4]. As troponin levels remain high for 14 days after myocardial necrosis, they are not ideal for detecting a reinfarction after the index event, but they can be helpful in detecting myocardial damage in a patient who presents for assessment several days after the onset of symptoms [2]. CK-MB levels increase 3–4 h after symptom onset, peak after 10–20 h, and return to normal after 48–72 h: the shorter half-life of CK-MB makes its measurement useful for diagnosing periprocedural MI or reinfarction (➲ Fig. 44.3).

It is important to stress that ACS should never be diagnosed on the basis of cardiac biomarker levels alone. Any increase needs to be interpreted in the clinical context, as other conditions presenting with chest pain (such as dissecting aortic aneurysm or pulmonary embolism) may lead to high troponin levels [35], which may also be due to non-coronary-related myocardial injuries, including severe acute heart failure, cardiac contusion, ablation, cardioversion, inflammatory diseases, a hypertensive crisis, stroke, or a subarachnoid haemorrhage. High troponin levels are also frequently found when serum creatinine levels are higher than 2.5 mg/dL in the absence of proven ACS [51].

Troponin measurements are a powerful means of risk stratification across the spectrum of patients presenting with the symptoms of acute cardiac ischaemia. Troponins are the best biomarkers for predicting the short-term (30-day) outcomes of MI and death, and their long-term prognostic value (1 year and beyond) has also been confirmed [52].

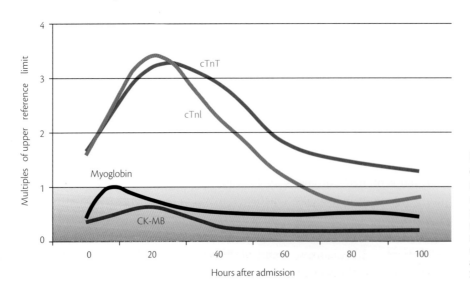

Figure 44.3 Kinetics of release of creatine kinase MB (CK-MB), myoglobin, and cardiac troponin in myocardial necrosis (shaded area indicates normal range).
From Bassand JP, Hamm CW, Ardissino D, *et al*. Guidelines for the diagnosis and treatment of non-ST-segment elevation acute coronary syndromes. *Eur Heart J* 2007;**28**:1598–1660.

The increased risk associated with high troponin levels is independent of and in addition to that associated with other risk factors such as ECG changes at rest or during continuous monitoring, which is why troponin release guides medical and interventional management choices in the setting of ACS [53, 54].

Biochemical markers of long-term prognosis

A number of biochemical markers have been evaluated in an attempt to identify ACS patients at high risk of cardiovascular events after the index event; however, they are not routinely used in clinical practice.

Among the markers of inflammation, high C-reactive protein (hsCRP) levels measured by means of highly sensitive assays predict an increased risk of mortality during long-term follow-up, and its predictive value is independent and additive to that of troponin. Even among patients with troponin-negative ACS, high hsCRP levels predict 6-month mortality [55, 56].

The B-type natriuretic peptide and its N-terminal prohormone fragment, which are sensitive and specific markers of left ventricular dysfunction, are associated with short- and long-term mortality in ACS patients [57, 58].

Risk scores

Patients with ACS are an extremely heterogeneous population at varying risk of early and late adverse events. Early risk stratification at admission is essential in order to select the site of care, define tailored management, and decide on the type of invasive strategy and its optimal timing. The risk scores used in everyday clinical practice are the GRACE, TIMI, and PURSUIT scores [59]. The GRACE score, which is currently the preferred classification upon admission and discharge, is based on a large and unselected population of the full spectrum of ACS patients in an international registry, and predicts the risk of death during hospitalization and after 6 months on the basis of easily assessed variables such as age, heart rate, systolic blood pressure, creatinine level, Killip class, ST-depression, and cardiac biomarkers [60–62]. However, as the GRACE score requires special tools for estimating risk at the bedside, the TIMI risk score is also widely accepted because of its simplicity, even though it is less accurate in predicting events [63].

Management strategies

NSTE-ACS encompasses a heterogeneous spectrum of patients at different levels of risk in terms of death or recurrent of MI. The treatment of individual patients is tailored on the basis of the risk of subsequent events, which should be assessed at the time of initial presentation and repeatedly thereafter. Risk assessment is an important component of the decision-making process and should be constantly reviewed; furthermore, the timing of catheterization should also be continuously re-evaluated and modified on the basis of clinical evolution and new clinical findings.

A clear management strategy based on the initial risk stratification distinguishes three levels of risk: life-threatening, moderate–high risk, and low risk (◆ Fig. 44.4).

Life-threatening conditions are rare at presentation, and account for only 4–5% of the total NSTE-ACS population. However, these patients are at very high risk of death or further MI, and often present with recurrent or refractory angina despite intense antianginal treatment, major ST-segment modifications and/or clinical symptoms of heart failure or haemodynamic instability, and/or life-threatening arrhythmias. They need to be managed very rapidly (within 2 h of referral) using an urgent invasive strategy [1, 4].

Moderate–high-risk patients have high troponin levels, dynamic ST-segment changes, diabetes mellitus, reduced renal function (GFR <60 mL/min), depressed left ventricular function (LVEF <40%) and/or early post-MI angina, have undergone percutaneous coronary intervention (PCI) in the previous 6 months or previous coronary artery bypass grafting (CABG), and are at intermediate/high risk on the basis of a risk score such as GRACE. They should be managed using an early invasive strategy, and be taken to the catheterization laboratory within 72 h for angiography and revascularization whenever possible [2, 4].

Low-risk patients are those without any recurrence of chest pain or signs of heart failure, who show no ECG changes in two recordings separated by an interval of 6–12 h, and in whom high troponin levels are not found in two samples separated by an interval of 6–12 h. They should be managed conservatively and undergo noninvasive evaluation in order to demonstrate the presence of ischaemia. They may be treated invasively if necessary, but this is not a first line option [4, 35].

Treatment

Anti-ischaemic drugs

These drugs decrease myocardial oxygen consumption and/or induce vasodilatation, thus relieving ischaemic chest pain.

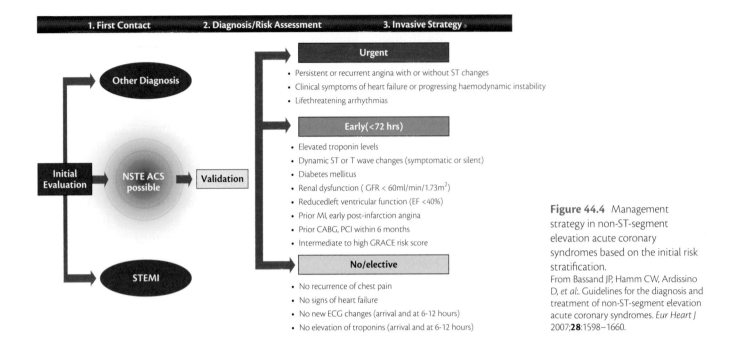

Figure 44.4 Management strategy in non-ST-segment elevation acute coronary syndromes based on the initial risk stratification.
From Bassand JP, Hamm CW, Ardissino D, et al. Guidelines for the diagnosis and treatment of non-ST-segment elevation acute coronary syndromes. *Eur Heart J* 2007;**28**:1598–1660.

β-Blockers

These inhibit the effect of circulating catecholamines by affecting β_1 receptors and decreasing myocardial oxygen consumption. Two randomized placebo-controlled trials have shown that they reduce the incidence of reinfarction, recurrent ischaemia, or both [64, 65]. They are recommended for all NSTE-ACS patients, except those with impaired atrioventricular conduction, or a history of asthma or acute left ventricular dysfunction [4].

Nitrates

Nitrates dilate veins, arteries, and arterioles. Their main therapeutic effect is related to venodilation, which decreases myocardial preload and oxygen consumption, but they also dilate coronary arteries and increase collateral flow [66, 67]. There are no randomized placebo-controlled trials confirming their benefits. Intravenous nitrates are recommended for symptom relief in the acute management of angina, but one limitation of continuous nitrate therapy is the development of tolerance [4].

Calcium channel blockers

Calcium channel blockers are vasodilators but there are conflicting data concerning their use in ACS patients [68, 69]. However, nondihydropyridine calcium channel blockers are useful treatment options in patients already receiving nitrates and β-blockers but still symptomatic, in those with contraindications to β-blockers, and in the subgroup of patients with vasospastic angina [4]. They should not be administered to patients with severe left ventricular dysfunction or pulmonary oedema.

Antithrombotic therapy

Antithrombotic therapy is the cornerstone of treatment for patients with NSTE-ACS.

Platelet inhibition and anticoagulation are effective in reducing the incidence of short- and long-term events related to atherothrombosis, and the combination of the two is more effective than either treatment alone. Antiplatelet therapy reduces platelet activation and aggregation, which are integral steps in the development of thrombosis after plaque disruption, whereas anticoagulation prevents the deposition of fibrin strands in the clot. It should always be considered that antiplatelet and anticoagulant agents are associated with an increased risk of bleeding which raises exponentially with the combination of drugs. Therefore, to optimize antithrombotic therapy, the ischaemic risk is always to be carefully balanced with the bleeding risk, particularly in some special populations such as elderly people and patients with chronic kidney disease (Fig. 44.5).

Antiplatelet agents

Platelets play a key role in the short- and long-term events related to atherothrombosis, and so antiplatelet therapy is necessary for the acute event and subsequent maintenance therapy. Three classes of antiplatelet agents play important roles in the management of NSTE-ACS patients: aspirin, thienopyridines, and platelet GPIIb/IIIa inhibitors.

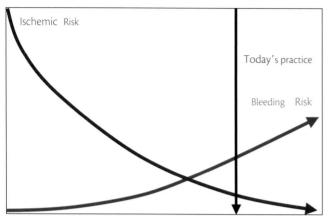

Aggressiveness of Antithrombotic therapy →

Figure 44.5 The optimal antithrombotic therapy derives from a careful balance between the ischaemic risk and the bleeding risk.

Aspirin

Aspirin irreversibly inhibits the platelet COX-1 enzyme, thus preventing the formation of thromboxane A_2 and inhibiting platelet aggregation.

Aspirin is recommended for all patients presenting with NSTE-ACS and without any contraindications to the initial loading dose of 160–325 mg (nonenteric) and the long-term maintenance dose of 75–100 mg [4, 70, 71]. Intravenous aspirin is an alternative, but it has never been validated in clinical trials. In a meta-analysis including four studies, the reduction in the rate of vascular events was 53% (➲ Fig. 44.6) [72].

The benefit of aspirin is established over a wide range of doses, whereas the risk of bleeding appears to be dose-dependent. In the CURE trial, aspirin was given in combination with clopidogrel at doses ranging from 75 to 325 mg and there was no evidence of any greater efficacy at the higher doses; however, the incidence of major bleeding increased with the dose, and was lowest at doses of up to 100 mg [73].

P2Y12 ADP receptor antagonists

P2Y12 ADP receptor antagonists inhibit ADP-dependent platelet activation. Ticlopidine and clopidogrel have both been marketed for many years but the former has been largely replaced by clopidogrel because of its more favourable safety profile. The combination of clopidogrel and aspirin became the standard dual antiplatelet therapy in patients with NSTE-ACS.

The first clinical evidence of the benefit of clopidogrel in NSTE-ACS patients came from the CURE trial in which patients received placebo or clopidogrel at an initial loading dose of 300 mg and a maintenance dose of 75 mg, plus aspirin for up to 12 months. Clopidogrel significantly reduced the primary combined endpoint of death, MI, or stroke by 20% (9.3% vs 11.4%; *p* <0.001); this benefit was obtained as early as 24 h after drug administration and throughout the 12 months of the study period [74, 75] (➲ Fig. 44.7). A 300 mg loading dose followed by 75 mg daily for 12 months is therefore recommended

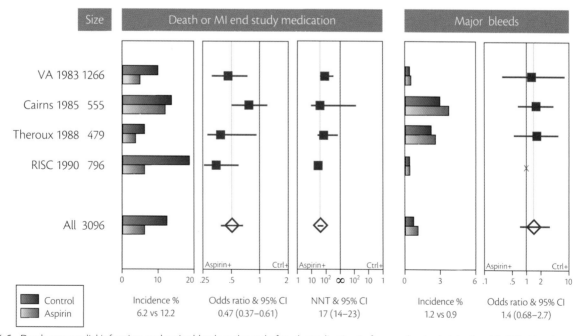

Figure 44.6 Death, myocardial infarction, and major bleeds at the end of study medication in four randomized trials of aspirin (filled bars) versus control (open bars). NNT, number of patients who needed to be treated to avoid one event.

From Bassand JP, Hamm CW, Ardissino D, *et al*. Guidelines for the diagnosis and treatment of non-ST-segment elevation acute coronary syndromes. *Eur Heart J* 2007;**28**:1598–1660.

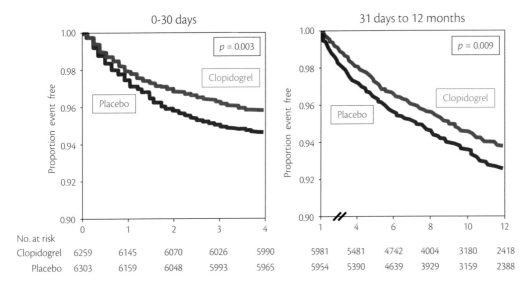

Figure 44.7 Impact of clopidogrel compared with placebo in cardiovascular death, myocardial infarction, or stroke within first 30 days (left) (RR 0.79, 95% CI 0.67–0.92, p = 0.003) and from 31 days to 12 months (right) (RR 0.82, 95% CI 0.70–0.95, p = 0.009). CI, confidence interval; RR, relative risk. Reproduced with permission from Yusuf S, Mehta SR, Zhao F, et al. Early and late effects of clopidogrel in patients with acute coronary syndromes. *Circulation* 2003;**107**:966.

for all patients with NSTE-ACS [4]. A loading dose of 600 mg leads to even more rapid and potent platelet inhibition, and may be considered in patients undergoing early invasive treatment [76].

On the basis of the CHARISMA trial results, there is no evidence that dual antiplatelet therapy should be continued for more than 12 months [77]. The benefit of dual antiplatelet therapy is associated with a significant increase in bleeding events. In the CURE trial, major bleeding occurred more frequently with clopidogrel and aspirin than with aspirin alone (3.7% vs 2.7%; p <0.001), particularly in patients undergoing CABG, although the two groups had similar rates of fatal or life-threatening bleeding [78]. Nevertheless, it is worth underlining that the therapeutic benefit of dual antiplatelet therapy outweighs the increased risk of bleeding because treating 1000 patients leads to 21 cases of cardiovascular death, MI, or stroke at the cost of an excess of 7 patients requiring transfusion and a trend towards 4 patients experiencing life-threating bleeds [78]. To minimize the risk of bleeding and its consequences, clopidogrel should be discontinued 5 days before CABG [4].

New antiplatelet drugs

Dual antiplatelet therapy with clopidogrel and aspirin is the standard of care in NSTE-ACS patients. However, the efficacy of clopidogrel is hampered by a number of potential limitations: its delayed onset of action, the modest level of platelet inhibition and its irreversibility, the increased risk of bleeding, and the wide variability in pharmacodynamic responses [79–82]. Accumulating data have shown that about 30% of patients continue to show increased platelet reactivity despite clopidogrel therapy, and that they are at increased risk of ischaemic events and stent thrombosis in the short and long term [83–85].

It has been hypothesized that clopidogrel's antiplatelet effect may be influenced by genetic variations in one or more of the hepatic cytochromes that generate its active metabolite, particularly CYP2C19*2 [86, 87]. A recent genome-wide association analysis found compelling evidence that genetic variations (*2 allele) causing CYP2C19 loss of function are associated with decreased clopidogrel activation and a subsequent decrease in its antiplatelet effect [88–93]. It has also been clearly demonstrated that the CYP2C19*2 genotype is associated with poorer clinical outcomes in clopidogrel-treated patients, particularly an increased risk of ischaemic events and a threefold risk of stent thrombosis [94–98].

Over the last few years, many attempts have been made to improve the safety and efficacy of dual antiplatelet therapy, and new drugs have been developed to overcome some of the potential limitations of clopidogrel [99].

Prasugrel, a novel thienopyridine, inhibits platelet aggregation more rapidly, more consistently, and to a greater extent than standard doses of clopidogrel [100]. On the basis of the results of the TRITON-TIMI 38 trial [101] in July 2009, the United State Food and Drug Administration [102] approved its use in patients with unstable angina or MI who undergo PCI. However, although it was associated with significantly reduced rates of ischaemic events (9.9% vs 12.1%; p <0.001), including stent thrombosis, it was also associated with a greater risk of major bleeding (2.4% vs 1.8%; p = 0.03), particularly in patients who were elderly, underweight, or had suffered a previous stroke or transient ischaemic attack. The balance between efficacy and risk therefore needs to be carefully assessed when choosing treatment for individual patients [103].

Ticagrelor, a reversible and direct-acting oral P2Y12 ADP receptor antagonist, also provides faster, greater and more consistent P2Y12 inhibition than clopidogrel. The PLATO trial has clearly demonstrated that, in comparison with clopidogrel, ticagrelor significantly reduces the rate of death, MI, or stroke (9.8% vs 11.7%; $p <0.001$); this is accompanied by an increase in the rate of non-procedure-related bleeding, but there is no increase in the rate of major bleeding (11.6% vs 11.2%; $p = 0.43$) [104, 105].

Glycoprotein IIb/IIIa receptor inhibitors

Glycoprotein (GP) IIb/IIIa receptor inhibitors are potent antiplatelet agents that inhibit fibrinogen-mediated platelet–platelet binding, the final common pathway of platelet aggregation. The three currently available agents for intravenous administration, which are eptifibatide, tirofiban, and abciximab, have been tested in the context of both conservative and invasive strategies.

In the case of a conservative approach, a meta-analysis by Boersma et al. [106] demonstrated a significant benefit over placebo in terms of death or MI after 30 days, particularly in high-risk subgroups such as patients with high troponin levels, ST-depression, or diabetes. The use of GPIIb/IIIa receptor inhibitors was associated with an increase in major bleeding complications, but there was no significant increase in intracranial bleeding. Another meta-analysis by Roffi et al. [107] confirmed this benefit only in patients referred for invasive procedures. The GUSTO-IV study found that abciximab did not offer any benefit and led to an increased risk of bleeding, and so it cannot be recommended for NSTE-ACS patients unless they undergo PCI [108]. However, on the basis of the results of the PRISM [109] and PURSUIT [110] studies, either eptifibatide or tirofiban can be recommended for the initial treatment of high-risk patients.

In the setting of an invasive strategy, two meta-analyses found a significant reduction in the risk of death and MI after 30 days in patients undergoing PCI when GPIIb/IIIa receptor inhibitors were administered before coronary angiography and continued during and after the procedure [111, 112]. The benefit of this therapy has also been confirmed in the case of patients pretreated with clopidogrel. In the ISAR-REACT 2 trial [113], abciximab was evaluated on a background of 600 mg of clopidogrel and reduced the relative risk of the primary composite endpoint of 30-day death, MI, or urgent revascularization by 25% without increasing the rate of major bleeding. In the case of high-risk patients undergoing PCI who have not been pretreated with GPIIb/IIIa receptor inhibitors, abciximab is recommended immediately following angiography [4]. The optimal timing for starting GPIIb/IIIa receptor inhibitors in the context of an invasive strategy has long been debated.

It was hypothesized that their upstream use before revascularization might reduce the risk of death and MI at 30 days in comparison with their provisional downstream use. However, the results of the EARLY-ACS trial showed that early eptifibatide offered no statistically significant benefit in reducing the composite endpoint of adverse cardiovascular events but was associated with a significant increase in bleeding [114]. These data do not support the routine upstream use of GPIIb/IIIa inhibitors in NSTE-ACS.

Anticoagulant agents

In addition to antiplatelet therapy, anticoagulant therapy is recommended in all patients with NSTE-ACS, and the type and dose should be selected bearing in mind the risk of ischaemic and bleeding events. Standard treatments are indirect thrombin inhibitors such as unfractionated heparin (UFH) or low-molecular-weight heparin (LMWH), but alternatives are the direct thrombin inhibitor bivalirudin, or the factor Xa inhibitor fondaparinux.

Unfractionated heparin

Intravenous UFH, a glycosaminoglycan made of polysaccharide chains whose molecular weight ranges from 2000 to 3000 Da, exerts its anticoagulant effect by binding antithrombin and inactivating factor Xa and thrombin [115]. Its unpredictable pharmacokinetics requires the frequent monitoring of APTT with an optimal target level of 50–70 s. An initial bolus of 60–70 IU/kg is recommended for NSTE-ACS patients, followed by an infusion of 12–15 IU/kg per hour [4]. The anticoagulant effect is rapidly lost within a few hours of discontinuation and there is a risk for reactivation of coagulation during the subsequent 24 h. The anticoagulant effect can be rapidly reversed by protamine. UFH can be safely administered in cases of renal failure with creatinine clearance levels of <30 mL/min provided that aPTT is carefully monitored.

A meta-analysis of six randomized and placebo-controlled trials of short-term UFH in NSTE-ACS patients showed a significant (33%) reduction in the risk of death and MI ($p = 0.045$) (➲ Fig. 44.8) [116], and trials comparing UFH plus aspirin with aspirin alone have found that the former is superior, albeit at the cost of increased bleeding [117].

Low-molecular-weight heparin

LMWH is derived from heparin and consists of short-chain fragments whose molecular weight ranges from 2000 to 10 000 Da. It is active against factors Xa and IIa, but its low molecular weight means that its anti-IIa activity is less than that of UFH [118].

The advantages of LMWH over UFH include greater bio-avaiability, less plasma protein binding, a higher anti-factor

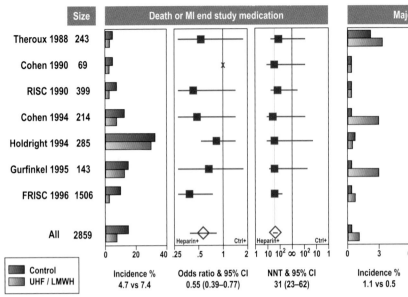
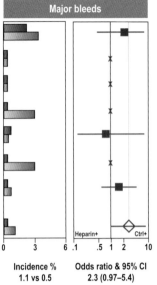

Figure 44.8 Death, myocardial infarction, and major bleeds at the completion of study medication in randomized trials of unfractionated heparin/low-molecular-weight heparin (filled bars) versus control (open bars). NNT, number of patients who needed to be treated to avoid one event.
From Bassand JP, Hamm CW, Ardissino D, et al. Guidelines for the diagnosis and treatment of non-ST-segment elevation acute coronary syndromes. *Eur Heart J* 2007;**28**:1598–1660.

Xa:IIa activity ratio, less platelet activation, a lower rate of thrombocytopenia, and a more predictable dose–effect ratio that allows the subcutaneous administration of fixed doses without the need to monitor its anticoagulant effect. The dose of LMWH is adjusted to body weight and has to be administered every 12 h. LMWH is contraindicated in the case of renal failure with creatinine clearance levels of less than 30 mL/min.

Various forms of LMWH (dalteparin, enoxaparin, and nadroparin) have been compared with UFH in the treatment of NSTE-ACS, but only enoxaparin has shown a clear benefit (◑ Fig. 44.9) [119–121]. In the setting of a conservative strategy, a pooled analysis of the ESSENCE and TIMI11b trials showed a significant reduction in the incidence of death and MI after 8, 14 and 43 days (4.1% vs 5.3%, *p* = 0.02; 5.2% vs 6.5%, *p* = 0.02; 7.1% vs 8.6%, *p* = 0.02) at the cost of

a significant increase in minor but not major bleeding complications [122, 123].

The SYNERGY trial compared enoxaparin with UFH in a contemporary invasive setting involving PCI, stent implantation, and active antiplatelet therapy with aspirin, clopidogrel and glycoprotein IIb/IIIa receptor inhibitors, and found no significant difference in terms of death and MI after 30 days (14% vs 14.5%; p=NS) but an increase in the rate of TIMI major bleeding (9.1% vs 7.6%; *p* = 0.08) [124]. A meta-analysis of six major trials comparing enoxaparin with UFH found no significant difference in terms of 30-day mortality (3.0% vs 3.0%; *p* = NS), but a significant reduction in the combined endpoint of death and MI after 30 days in favour of enoxaparin in patients who had not received UFH before randomization; there was no significant difference in major bleeding (4.7% vs 4.5%; *p* = NS) [125].

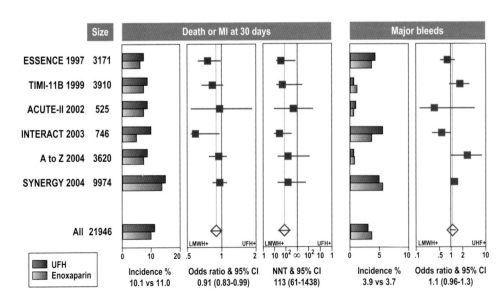

Figure 44.9 Death, myocardial infarction, and major bleeds at 30 days in randomized trials of enoxaparin (filled bars) versus unfractionated heparin (open bars). NNT, number of patients who needed to be treated to avoid one event.
From Bassand JP, Hamm CW, Ardissino D, et al. Guidelines for the diagnosis and treatment of non-ST-segment elevation acute coronary syndromes. *Eur Heart J* 2007;**28**:1598–1660.

Factor Xa inhibitors

Fondaparinux is a synthetic pentasaccharide that leads to the selective antithrombin-mediated inhibition of factor Xa. It is administered subcutaneously once daily at a fixed dose of 2.5 mg, and no monitoring of anti-Xa activity is required. However, it is contraindicated if creatinine clearance levels are less than 30 mL/min.

Fondaparinux is recommended for patients at high risk of bleeding and those awaiting a decision about early invasive or conservative strategy [4]. These recommendations are based on the results of the OASIS-5 trial, which found that fondaparinux was not inferior to enoxaparin in reducing the 9-day incidence of the primary outcome of death, MI, or refractory ischaemia and that it led to a lower rate of major bleedings (2.2% vs 4.1%; p <0.001); furthermore, an analysis of the composite variable of primary outcome and major bleeding after 9 days demonstrated an advantage in favour of fondaparinux (7.3% vs 9.0%; p <0.001). Fondaparinux was also associated with a significant reduction in 30-day (2.9% vs 3.5%; p = 0.02) and 6-month mortality rates (5.8% vs 6.5%; p = 0.005) [126, 127]. However, in the subset of patients undergoing PCI, the risk of catheter-related thrombi was more than three times higher in the fondaparinux arm, and so supplementary UFH at the time of catheterization is recommended to minimize this risk.

Direct thrombin inhibitors

Direct thrombin inhibitors (DTIs) bind directly to both soluble and fibrin-bound thrombin, and inhibit the conversion of fibrinogen to fibrin. They also act on platelets by reducing thrombin-induced platelet activation. The anticoagulant effect of DTIs is predictable because of the lack of plasma protein binding, and can be monitored by measuring aPTT and ACT.

Bivalirudin is the only DTI that can be used as an alternative anticoagulant in NSTE-ACS. It is administered intravenously and the dose needs to be adjusted in the case of renal failure with creatinine clearance levels of less than 30 mL/min. Its administration to patients with NSTE-ACS was studied in the ACUITY trial, which randomly assigned patients to UFH or enoxaparin plus GPIIb/IIIa inhibitors, bivalirudin plus GPIIb/IIIa inhibitors, or bivalirudin alone. Bivalirudin alone was found not to be inferior to standard treatment with UFH/LMWH plus GPIIb/IIIa inhibitors in terms of the composite ischaemia endpoint (7.8% vs 7.3%; p = 0.32), and led to a significantly lower rate of major bleeding (3.0% vs 5.7%; p < 0.001); subsequently the rate of 30-day net clinical outcome was significantly lower (10.1 vs 11.7%; p = 0.015). However, in the patients who did not receive clopidogrel before coronary revascularization, there was a significant excess of the composite ischaemia endpoint [128, 129].

Coronary revascularization

A number of trials have compared the benefits of an early invasive strategy with a conservative strategy [130–132]. An early invasive strategy involves routine cardiac catheterization (generally within 72 h of admission) followed by revascularization with PCI or CABG depending on coronary anatomy, whereas a conservative strategy involves initial medical management followed by catheterization and revascularization only if ischaemia recurs. A meta-analysis of randomized clinical trials comparing routine angiography followed by revascularization with a conservative strategy in NSTE-ACS patients found that the former reduced the rate of death and MI at the end of long-term follow-up (12.2% vs 14.4%; p = 0.001); however, this overall benefit came at the cost of an increased risk of death and MI during the initial hospitalization (5.2% vs 3.8%; p = 0.002) and only emerged between discharge and the end of follow-up (7.4% vs 11.0%; p < 0.001) [133]. The reduction in long-term mortality obtained using an early invasive strategy was confirmed in the 5-year follow-up of the RITA-3 and FRISC-II trials [134, 135].

The greatest benefit (a >50% reduction in relative risk) of an early invasive strategy is observed in NSTE-ACS patients at moderate or high risk, which is why current practice guidelines recommend it in such patients. Patients with severe ongoing angina, dynamic ECG changes, major arrhythmias or haemodynamic instability should undergo coronary angiography as soon as possible [4].

Bleeding complications

Bleeding complications are the most common noncardiac complications of therapy in patients with NSTE-ACS. The bleeding complication rates reported in trials and registries vary widely because different definitions are used to grade the severity of bleeding. Given these limitations, the estimated incidence of major or severe bleeding in clinical trials ranges from 0.8% to 11.5% [136, 137]. Furthermore, the bleeding rates recorded in registries are generally higher than those observed in clinical trials; in the GRACE registry, the overall incidence of major bleeding was 4.7% [138].

Many factors are independent predictors of bleeding, including an older age, female gender, a lower body weight, chronic kidney disease, the use of GPIIb/IIIa receptor inhibitors, invasive procedures, and a previous history of bleeding. In addition, inadequate drug doses may also lead to excess bleeding [138]. The predictors of ischaemia and bleeding largely overlap, and so the frailest patients are exposed to the highest risk of both.

It has been consistently shown that bleeding in the setting of NSTE-ACS is associated with an adverse prognosis. One meta-analysis has found that major bleeding is associated with an increased risk of both short- and long-term adverse events, including MI, stroke and death [139–142].

The mechanisms by which bleeding influences outcomes are still poorly understood, although factors such as hypovolaemia, renal failure, a hyperadrenergic and pro-inflammatory state, and the potentially deleterious effect of transfusion contribute to the worse outcomes. Furthermore, the discontinuation of antithrombotic therapy can also have catastrophic consequences, with a risk of the recurrent thrombotic events and subacute stent thrombosis.

Blood transfusions are also associated with an increased risk of death, MI, and refractory ischaemia in NSTE-ACS patients [143–146]. This deleterious effect may be due to erythrocyte alterations or high haemoglobin/oxygen affinity due to a low rate of 2,3-diphosphoglyceric acid, which leads to decreased oxygen delivery to tissues. It is now increasingly recommended to consider transfusions in haemodynamically stable patients undergoing acute cardiac care only if baseline haemoglobin values are less than 8 g/dL [4].

In conclusion, stratification of the risk of bleeding should form part of the evaluation of NSTE-ACS patients, and risk assessments need to consider both thrombotic and bleeding complications. Bleeding preventing involves choosing the safest drug and the appropriate dose, reducing the duration of antithrombotic treatment, using combined antiplatelet and anticoagulant agents on the basis of proven indications, and choosing the radial rather than femoral approach if angiography is planned.

Long-term management

Patients with NSTE-ACS are at high risk of recurrence of ischaemic events. Active secondary prevention, including both lifestyle modification and medical therapy, are therefore essential in the long-term management. Five classes of drugs have been shown in large randomized trials to improve outcomes following NSTE-ACS and are recommended for long-term treatment. Statins and angiotensin converting enzyme (ACE) inhibitors are indicated for plaque stabilization. Statin therapy is associated with a significant reduction in long-term ischaemic events [147–155]. ACE inhibitors have greater efficacy in patients at high risk, such as patients with diabetes, hypertension, chronic renal failure, and depressed ventricular function (LVEF<40%) [156–159]. β-Blockers are indicated for anti-ischaemic therapy. For antiplatelet therapy, the combination of aspirin with either clopidogrel, prasugrel or ticagrelor for at least a year has been shown to be beneficial in reducing the risk of ischaemic events.

Personal perspective

Acute coronary syndromes represent a broad spectrum of ischemic myocardial events associated with high morbidity and mortality rates; despite improvements in their management, the re-occurrence of cardiovascular events is still a public health problem.

Antithrombotic therapy is the cornerstone of treatment for patients with NSTE-ACS. In this setting, it is known that the benefit due to reduction of major adverse cardiovascular events may be partially offset by the increased incidence of bleeding. Therefore, it is critically necessary to optimise the selection of antithrombotic therapy, carefully balancing the ischemic and the bleeding risk.

Recent data suggest that individual response to antithrombotic drugs is influenced by a genetic basis, particularly the response to clopidogrel.

As a number of new antiplatelet drugs are now entering the market, it is essential to choose the best drug for each individual patient by carefully assessing its potential effectiveness and safety on the basis of the patient's specific genotype.

Genotype-guided antiplatelet therapy may be considered the first step towards the establishment of individualized medicine in the field of cardiovascular therapy.

Further reading

Antithrombotic Trialists' Collaboration. Collaborative meta-analysis of randomised trials of antiplatelet therapy for prevention of death, myocardial infarction, and stroke in high risk patients. *BMJ* 2002;**321**:71–86.

Bassand JP. Bleeding and transfusion in acute coronary syndromes: a shift in the paradigm. *Heart* 2008;**94**:661–666.

Bassand JP, Hamm CW, Ardissino D, *et al*. Guidelines for the diagnosis and treatment of non-ST-segment elevation acute coronary syndromes. *Eur Heart J* 2007;**28**:1598–1660.

Bhatt DL. Tailoring antiplatelet therapy based on pharmacogenomics: how well do the data fit? *JAMA* 2009;**302**:896–897.

Boden EW, Shah PK, Gupta V, *et al*. Contemporary approach to the diagnosis and management of non-ST-segment elevation acute coronary syndromes. *Progr Cardiovasc Dis* 2008;**50**:311–351.

Bonaca MP, Steg GP, Feldman LJ, *et al*. Antithrombotics in acute coronary syndromes. *J Am Coll Cardiol* 2009;**54**:969–984.

Kumar A, Cannon CP. Acute coronary syndromes: diagnosis and management, Part 1. *Mayo Clin Proc* 2009;**84**:917–938.

Marin F, Gonzalez-Conejero R, Capranzano P, *et al*. Pharmacogenetics and antithrombotic therapy. *J Am Coll Cardiol* 2009;**54**:1041–1057.

Nguyen TA, Diodati JG, Pharand C. Resistance to clopidogrel: a review of the evidence. *J Am Coll Cardiol* 2005;**45**:1157–1164.

Van de Werf F. New antithrombotic agents: are they needed and what can they offer to patients with a non-ST-elevation acute coronary syndrome? *Eur Heart J* 2009;**30**:1695–1702.

Wenaweser P, Windecker S. Acute coronary syndromes. Management and secondary prevention. *Herz* 2008;**33**:25–37.

⮕ For additional multimedia materials please visit the online version of the book (🔗 http://www.esciacc.oxfordmedicine.com).

CHAPTER 45

Percutaneous coronary interventions in patients with acute coronary syndromes

Viktor Kočka, Petr Toušek, and Petr Widimský

Contents

Summary

Three different guidelines of the European Society of Cardiology (ESC) cover the field of percutaneous coronary interventions (PCI). Their main recommendations are the following:

◆ All patients with ST-segment elevation myocardial infarction (STEMI) should undergo immediate coronary angiography and PCI as soon as possible after first medical contact. Thrombolysis can be used as alternative reperfusion therapy only for patients presenting early (<3 h from symptom onset) with expected time to PCI longer than 60–90 min.

◆ Patients with high risk non-ST-segment elevation (NSTE) acute coronary syndromes (ACS) (recurrent or ongoing chest pain, profound or dynamic ECG changes, major arrhythmias, or haemodynamic instability) should undergo coronary angiography within <2 h after the initial hospital admission.

◆ Moderate risk NSTE ACS patients should undergo coronary angiography within <3 days after the initial hospital admission.

◆ Low risk NSTE ACS patients may be treated conservatively and the decision on invasive evaluation can be based on evidence of ischaemia during exercise stress testing.

◆ Stents should be used during all PCI procedures whenever technically feasible.

◆ Drug-eluting stents decrease the risk of restenosis, but do not influence mortality when compared with bare metal stents.

◆ Triple pharmacotherapy (most frequently aspirin, clopidogrel, and heparin or their therapeutic equivalents) should be used in all PCI procedures, with GPIIb/IIIa inhibitors added in patients with high thrombotic and low bleeding risk.

Introduction

Percutaneous transluminal balloon coronary angioplasty (PTCA) was first performed by Andreas Grüntzig in 1977. During the next 15 years it developed into an effective treatment method for chronic stable coronary artery disease. In 1993 Felix Zijlstra and the Zwolle group (in the Netherlands) demonstrated the superiority of PTCA over thrombolysis in the treatment of acute myocardial infarction. Almost simultaneously, ticlopidin (and later clopidogrel) was introduced as an effective and safe antithrombotic therapy (on top of aspirin), which enabled the rapid development of coronary stents (previously, without thienopyridines, limited by 5–8% stent thrombosis rates). As a result of all these achievements, percutaneous coronary intervention (PCI)—the new name for the procedure emerged after stents became a routine part of it—was more and more used for the treatment of acute coronary syndromes (ACS), including ST-elevation myocardial infarction (STEMI). The PRAGUE-2 and DANAMI-2 trials in 2002 proved that PCI (after immediate transport to a PCI-capable hospital) should be used as the primary reperfusion therapy of STEMI also for patients presenting initially to non-PCI hospitals. Many large trials proved that very early coronary angiography followed by immediate PCI whenever suitable is also the best therapy for moderate to high risk patients with non-ST-elevation (NSTE) ACS. Thus, modern therapy for all forms of ACS involves PCI as the most effective treatment method, saving many lives and also improving symptoms for most survivors. The more severe clinical presentation of a patient with ACS, the higher benefit from emergent coronary angiography/PCI.

Primary percutaneous coronary intervention for STEMI

Primary percutaneous coronary intervention

Primary PCI is defined as intervention in the culprit vessel within 12 h after the onset of chest pain or other symptoms, without prior (full or concomitant) thrombolytic or other clot-dissolving therapy. In the 1980s, few case reports of successful primary PCI were published [1, 2]. In the 1990s, several randomized studies were performed comparing fibrinolytic therapy with direct balloon angioplasty [3–8], and a meta-analysis by Weaver *et al.* [9] clearly demonstrated reduction in mortality, reinfarction, and stroke with mechanical intervention. This benefit is mainly derived from over 90% success rate in opening the infarct-related artery by angioplasty, as compared to 50–60% success rate with thrombolysis which also comes at cost of 1–2% rate of intracranial bleeding. One study had long-term 5 year follow-up and demonstrated a highly significant 46% reduction in mortality [10]. The introduction of stenting did not have any significant influence on 6–12-month mortality compared to balloon angioplasty only, but showed a trend for a reduction in the number of reinfarctions and significantly reduced the incidence of target vessel revascularization by decreasing restenosis, and stenting became routine [11]. Most patients with STEMI present to hospitals not equipped for primary PCI, but urgent transfer to a tertiary centre for primary PCI was proved to be effective and safe, which extended the availability of the primary PCI strategy [12–14].

These data lead to the question of timing: how much time can be lost in transport before the benefit of primary PCI is lost? Several time points need to be defined first. The time of symptom onset is reported by the patient; first medical contact is typically the emergency medical service or primary care doctor. Other important moments are time of hospital admission, time of arrival at the cardiac catheterization laboratory, and time of first balloon inflation, which typically results in restoration of blood flow in the infarct-related artery. Thrombolytic therapy is more effective when the clot is fresh, i.e. time from onset of symptoms to first medical contact is less than 3 h. It must be emphasized that although thrombolytic therapy can be administered faster, its onset of action is not immediate—reperfusion occurs after 30–60 min [15]. Thus the only situation where thrombolytic therapy might be better is if the patient presents early (ischaemia <3 h) to a non-PCI hospital with estimated transport time longer than 60 minutes (⊃Fig. 45.1). The main reason favouring primary PCI even in this setting would be stroke prevention—stroke is reduced from 2% to 1% by primary PCI [16].

Except for patients in cardiogenic shock, only the culprit lesion should be dilated in the acute setting; any further intervention is not risk free. Complete revascularization of the nonculprit lesions may be performed later, depending on the remaining ischaemia.

Other benefits of primary PCI over thrombolytic therapy include the fact that early (3 days) discharge of low risk patients (defined as age <70 years, left ventricular ejection fraction >45%, one- or two-vessel disease, successful PCI, no persistent arrhythmias) is safe and cost effective [17]. These data are summarized in the form of a flow diagram in ⊃Fig. 45.2.

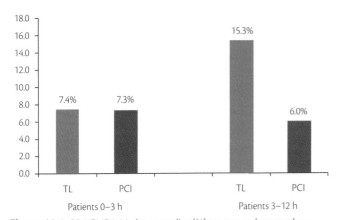

Figure 45.1 PRAGUE 2 30-day mortality (%) among early versus late presenters. PCI, primary PCI; TL, thrombolysis.
Adapted with permission from Widimsky P, *et al*. Long distance transport for primary angioplasty vs immediate thrombolysis in acute myocardial infarction. Final results of the randomized national multicentre trial—PRAGUE-2. *Eur Heart J* 2003;**24**(1):94–104.

Rescue percutaneous coronary intervention

Rescue PCI is defined as urgent PCI performed on a coronary artery which remains occluded despite thrombolytic therapy. The identification of these patients remains a challenging issue, but <50% ST-segment resolution in the lead(s) with the highest ST-segment elevations 60–90 min after start of thrombolysis and persistent symptoms is a useful marker. A clinical suspicion is confirmed at angiography by demonstrating a culprit lesion in an epicardial artery with impaired flow (<TIMI 3). A recent meta-analysis showed that rescue PCI is associated with a significant reduction in heart failure and reinfarction and a trend towards lower all-cause mortality when compared with a conservative strategy, at the cost, however, of an increased risk of stroke and bleeding complications [18, 19]. Rescue PCI

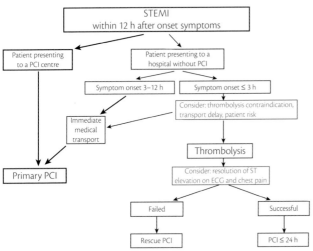

Figure 45.2 Flow diagram of patient care in STEMI.
Adapted with permission from Silber S, Albertsson P, Avilés FF, *et al*. Guidelines for percutaneous coronary interventions. The Task Force for Percutaneous Coronary Interventions of the European Society of Cardiology. *Eur Heart J* 2005;**26**(8):804–847.

should certainly be considered when clinical or ECG evidence of a large infarct is present.

Facilitated percutaneous coronary intervention

Facilitated PCI is defined as a pharmacological reperfusion treatment delivered prior to a planned PCI, in order to bridge the PCI-related time delay. This concept is intuitive and logical. Full-dose thrombolytic therapy, half-dose thrombolytic therapy with a glycoprotein (GP)IIb/IIIa inhibitor and GPIIb/IIIa inhibitor alone have all been tested for this indication. There is no evidence of a significant clinical benefit with any of these agents [16, 20–22]. In spite of the fact that pre-PCI patency rates were higher with thrombolytic-based treatments, no mortality benefit but more bleeding complications were observed. The pre-PCI patency rates with upfront abciximab or bolus dose tirofiban alone were not higher than with placebo. Facilitated PCI, as tested so far, cannot be recommended.

Late percutaneous coronary intervention

There are patients who present late, more than 12 h after onset of symptoms. Should there be clinical or ECG evidence of ongoing ischaemia, then primary PCI can still be performed till 24 h from symptom onset. However, a number of patients (estimated to be as many as 30%) present late with signs of fully developed infarction. The open artery hypothesis suggests that late patency of an infarct artery is associated with improved left ventricular (LV) function, increased electrical stability, and provision of collateral vessels to other coronary beds for protection against future events. The OAT (Occluded Artery Trial) tested the hypothesis that routine PCI performed at least 24 h from symptom onset on a totally occluded infarct-related artery with poor or absent antegrade flow would improve clinical outcome [23]. The 3-year cumulative incidence of death, reinfarction, or class IV heart failure was 17.2% in the PCI group and 15.6% in the medical therapy group (HR 1.16; 95% CI 0.92–1.45; $p = 0.2$). The OAT exclusion criteria included NYHA class III or IV heart failure, rest angina, left main or three-vessel disease, clinical instability, or severe inducible ischaemia on stress testing if the infarct zone was not akinetic or dyskinetic. In these patients we have no scientific data regarding late PCI. In summary, late PCI in stable patients cannot be routinely recommended.

Adjunctive antithrombotic medication

This topic is discussed in detail in ➲ Chapter 42 and we therefore briefly describe here a practical approach with

Table 45.1 Doses of adjunctive medication with primary PCI

Antiplatelet agents	
Aspirin	Oral dose of 150–325 mg or IV dose of 250–500 mg if oral ingestion is not possible
Clopidogrel	Oral loading dose of at least 300 mg, preferably 600 mg
GPIIb/IIIa inhibitors	Abciximab: IV bolus of 0.25 mg/kg followed by 0.125 mg/kg per min infusion (maximum 10 mg/min for 12 h), or
	Eptifibatide: IV bolus 180 μg/kg followed by 2 μg/kg per min infusion, orTirofiban: IV bolus 25 μg/kg followed by 0.15 μg/kg per min infusion
Antithrombin agents	
Heparin	IV bolus 100 IU/kg (60 IU/kg if GPIIb/IIIa antagonists are used). If the procedure is being performed under activated clotting time (ACT) guidance, heparin is given at a dose able to maintain an ACT of 250–350 s (200–250 s if GPIIb/IIIa antagonists are used)
Bivalirudin	IV bolus of 0.75 mg/kg followed by an infusion of 1.75 mg/kg per hour not titrated to ACT

Modified from Van de Werf F, Bax J, Betriu A, *et al.* Management of acute myocardial infarction in patients presenting with persistent ST-segment elevation: the Task Force on the Management of ST-Segment Elevation Acute Myocardial Infarction of the European Society of Cardiology. *Eur Heart J* 2008;**29**(23):2909–2945.

more detailed coverage of newer agents only. Indication and dosing is summarized in ⊃Table 45.1 (modified from the ESC guidelines).

Aspirin is usually administered in the prehospital phase. Unfractionated heparin (UFH) is ideally administered in 60 IU/kg dose to allow safe use of GPIIb/IIIa inhibitors if needed in the catheterization laboratory. Clopidogrel 300–600 mg oral dose has evolved into the standard regimen. As very few patients with STEMI require coronary artery surgery, clopidogrel can also be administered in the prehospital phase. Coronary angiography is performed and the decision regarding use of GPIIb/IIIa inhibitors is made based on thrombus load, expected extent of infarction, and risk of bleeding. Then either a bolus of GPIIb/IIIa inhibitor or an added bolus of heparin (to total dose 100 IU/kg) is given.

Abciximab has been studied in the setting of STEMI, and a recent meta-analysis demonstrated reduction in mortality and major adverse cardiovascular events (MACE) after 6 months [24]. The long-term benefits of abciximab in the setting of STEMI are not clear [25]. The role of abciximab administered after pretreatment with clopidogrel 600 mg has not been studied in the setting of primary PCI. Based on two recent meta-analyses, it seems that various GPIIb/IIIa antagonists demonstrate similar effectiveness in the setting of primary PCI [26, 27]. Intracoronary abciximab bolus application results in high local drug concentrations and may be more effective than a standard intravenous bolus.

Several single-centre studies have demonstrated its safety. The superiority of intracoronary to intravenous abciximab application with respect to infarct size and extent of microvascular obstruction is demonstrated in a few studies but not all [28–31]. None of these studies was sufficiently powerful to detect clinical endpoints; larger randomized trials have recently started. In summary, GPIIb/IIIa inhibitors might provide some benefit for patients with a large thrombus burden and low risk of bleeding, or for patients not pretreated with dual antiplatelet medication.

There is no evidence to support the preference for low-molecular-weight heparin (LMWH) over unfractionated heparin (UFH) for primary PCI. The direct thrombin inhibitor bivalirudin is unanimously recommended as a replacement for UFH in patients with heparin-induced thrombocytopenia [32]. Recently the HORIZONS-AMI trial compared bivalirudin alone to UFH in combination with GPIIb/IIIa inhibitors and demonstrated significant reduction in all-cause mortality. This was predominantly driven by a lower bleeding rate in the bivalirudin group (5.8% vs 9.2%; 0.61; 0.48–0.78; $p < 0.0001$). A limitation of this trial is the exclusion of patients with large thrombus where the benefit from GPIIb/IIIa inhibitors might be apparent. In summary, bivalirudin-based therapy provides a major reduction in bleeding events without any increase in thrombotic events and could be considered in patients undergoing primary PCI for STEMI who are at higher risk of bleeding [33].

Prasugrel is a specific, oral irreversible antagonist of the platelet ADP $P2Y_{12}$ receptor. Laboratory studies have shown prasugrel to be associated with more prompt, potent, and predictable degrees of platelet inhibition compared with clopidogrel. The recently published TRITON-TIMI 38 trial demonstrated that prasugrel is superior to clopidogrel in preventing ischaemic events in ACS patients who are undergoing PCI, but it is associated with an increased risk of major bleeding, especially in patients with history of stroke or transient ischaemic attack (TIA), age over 75 years, or weight less than 60 kg [34, 35].

Ticagrelor is an oral, reversible, direct-acting inhibitor of the ADP receptor $P2Y_{12}$ that has a more rapid onset and more pronounced platelet inhibition than clopidogrel. The recent PLATO study compared ticagrelor with clopidogrel and showed a significantly reduced rate of death from vascular causes, MI, or stroke without an increase in the rate of overall major bleeding but with an increase in the rate of non-procedure-related bleeding [36, 37].

Measurement of platelet activity has become quick and routinely available and will probably play significant role in the future.

Microvascular obstruction: definition, prevention, and therapy

The 'no-reflow' phenomenon in STEMI patients is characterized by inadequate myocardial reperfusion at microcirculatory level after successful reopening of the epicardial infarct-related artery without evidence of persistent mechanical obstruction. The mechanisms of no-reflow are not fully understood: distal thrombotic microembolization, vascular reperfusion injury, adrenergic microvascular constriction, and myocardial oedema may possibly contribute [38]. Some 10–40% of patients undergoing reperfusion therapy for STEMI may show evidence of no-reflow [39, 40]. A grading system was developed by the TIMI study group for epicardial flow in the infarct-related coronary artery [41] (see ⊃Box 45.1). However, a substantial number of patients with TIMI 3 flow have persistent ST-segment elevation on the post-angioplasty ECG and the primary objective of reperfusion therapies is not only restoration of blood flow in the epicardial coronary artery but also reperfusion of the infarcted myocardium. This can be judged angiographically by 'myocardial blush grade' (MBG) which uses myocardial contrast density as a measure of functional integrity of microvascular bed. The microcirculation was classified as either closed (MBG 0 or 1) or open (MBG 2 or 3). The diagnosis of no-reflow is usually made when post-procedural TIMI flow is less than grade 3, or in the case of a TIMI flow 3 when MBG is 0 or 1, or when ST-segment resolution on ECG within 4 h of the procedure is less than 70%. [42] No-reflow can cause prolonged myocardial ischaemia, may result in severe arrhythmia and critical haemodynamic deterioration, and is associated with a significantly increased risk of clinical complications [42–44]. Intracoronary administration of vasodilators such as adenosine, verapamil, nicorandil, papaverine, and nitroprusside during and after primary PCI has been shown to improve flow in the infarct-related coronary artery and myocardial perfusion, and/or to reduce infarct size, but large prospective randomized trials with hard clinical outcomes are lacking [38] (⊃Table 45.2).

Adjunctive devices

The presence of coronary thrombus creates special challenges in the performance of primary PCI. Large thrombus burden is associated with an increased incidence of distal embolization and no-reflow, and may limit reperfusion at the microvascular level. A number of adjunctive strategies have been tried. Unfortunately, the use of mechanical thrombectomy systems such as AngioJet was associated with larger infarct size and an unexpected increase in mortality. Consequently, mechanical thrombectomy is now used infrequently with primary PCI [45].

Distal protection devices are represented by filters or proximal balloon occlusion systems. There are nine randomized trials comparing primary PCI with distal protection using filters or balloon occlusion compared with primary PCI alone; they found that distal protection did not improve myocardial reperfusion or clinical outcomes. Distal protection is not thought to be beneficial with primary PCI for STEMI except in saphenous vein graft lesions [45].

All manual aspiration catheters are similar and have two lumens—one for passage of the catheter over a coronary wire, and the other for manual aspiration of thrombus and atheromatous debris. They are available in 6 French or 7 French sizes. The large TAPAS trial and smaller EXPIRA trials randomized over 1200 STEMI patients to aspiration

---

Box 45.1 TIMI flow grades

- TIMI 0: no antegrade flow beyond the point of obstruction

- TIMI 1: slow flow with contrast material not reaching the distal coronary bed in one cine run

- TIMI 2: antegrade flow opacifies all the coronary bed but more slowly than in other coronary artery

- TIMI 3: normal flow

From Sheehan FH, et al. The effect of intravenous thrombolytic therapy on left ventricular function: a report on tissue-type plasminogen activator and streptokinase from the Thrombolysis in Myocardial Infarction (TIMI Phase I) trial. *Circulation* 1987;**75**(4):817–829.

Table 45.2 Doses of medication used to prevent or treat the no-reflow phenomenon

Prevention	
Abciximab IV	0.25 mg/kg bolus and 0.125 mg/kg per min infusion for 12–24 h
Treatment	
Adenosine IV infusion	70mg/kg per min for 3 h
Adenosine intracoronary bolus	30–60 mg
Verapamil intracoronary bolus	0.5–1 mg
Papaverine intracoronary bolus	10–20 mg
Nicorandil intracoronary bolus	2 mg
Nitroprusside intracoronary bolus	50–200 µg

Modified from Van de Werf F, Bax J, Betriu A, et al. Management of acute myocardial infarction in patients presenting with persistent ST-segment elevation: the Task Force on the Management of ST-Segment Elevation Acute Myocardial Infarction of the European Society of Cardiology. *Eur Heart J* 2008;**29**(23):2909–2945.

thrombectomy followed by stenting versus stenting alone [46, 47]. Aspiration was successfully performed in 90% of patients, thrombus or atheroma was retrieved in 72% of patients, and direct stenting (without predilatation) was performed in 59% of patients. The frequency of MBG 3 (the primary endpoint) and complete ST-segment resolution on ECG (the secondary endpoint) was significantly higher with aspiration thrombectomy. These improved results in myocardial reperfusion were associated with clinical benefit at 1 year, with a lower incidence of cardiac death (3.6% vs 6.7%, $p = 0.02$) and cardiac death or MI (5.6% vs 9.9%, $p = 0.008$) [46]. Recent meta-analysis of 9 randomized trials with 2417 patients comparing PCI with aspiration thrombectomy versus PCI alone found that patients treated with thrombectomy had fewer distal emboli, a higher frequency of TIMI 3 flow and MBG 3 post-PCI, and lower 30-day mortality (1.7% vs 3.1%, $p = 0.04$) [48]. These results are certainly promising, but meta-analyses have limitations, one of which is that negative trials are often not reported or not published. Therefore large randomized trials with aspiration thrombectomy or newer generation thrombectomy devices, which are powered for clinical endpoints and possibly focused on patients with moderate or large thrombus burden, are needed to determine the optimum adjunctive device for primary PCI. In the meantime aspiration thrombectomy with primary PCI appears to improve myocardial reperfusion, may improve clinical outcomes, is relatively easy to perform, and seems to be safe. It appears reasonable to perform manual thrombectomy with primary PCI in patients with moderate to large thrombus burden. Figures 45.3 and 45.4 demonstrate thrombus aspiration by angiography, macroscopy and histology.

Logistics of care

Currently primary PCI is the preferred therapeutic option when it can be performed expeditiously by an experienced team, including not only interventional cardiologists but also skilled supporting staff. This means that only hospitals with an established interventional cardiology programme (open 24 h/7 days) should use primary PCI as a routine treatment option. High-volume operators have better results than low-volume ones, even in the era of routine

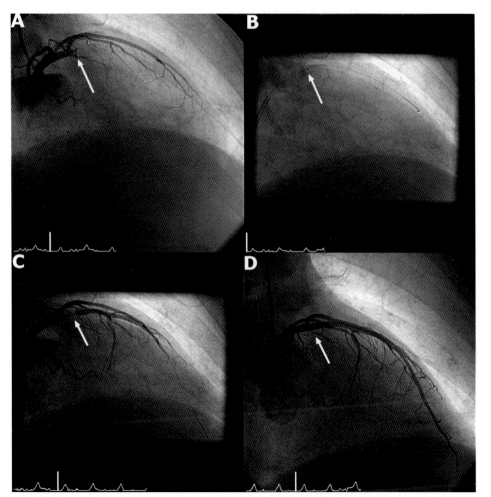

Figure 45.3 Primary PCI for anterior STEMI 3 h after symptom onset. (A) Occluded LAD just after diagonal branch. (B) Aspiration thrombectomy catheter *in situ*. (C) Critical LAD stenosis unmasked after aspiration. (D) Final result after stent implantation. For further video documentation of this case, see 🎥 45.1.

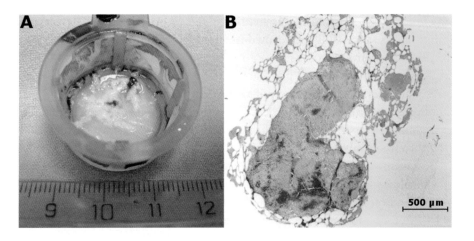

Figure 45.4 Aspiration thrombectomy from the same patient as in ➲ Fig. 45.3. (A) Macroscopic view of white thrombus with few small red thrombi. (B) Histological examination (HE stain) confirms presence of white, platelet-rich thrombus.
Histology courtesy of Tomáš Jirásek MD, Prague.

coronary stenting [49]. Many PCI centres do not have on-site cardiac surgery backup, and time to treatment with primary PCI can be significantly shortened when treating STEMI patients there compared with transport for PCI to a referral centre with on-site surgery. PCI at hospitals with off-site cardiac surgery backup can improve access to primary PCI for a larger sector of the population and can be delivered with a very favourable safety profile [50–54].

The use of primary PCI worldwide has significant limitations, both financial and geographical. Currently it is widely available in rich, densely populated countries with well-organized health care system. Within Europe, the recently launched Stent 4 Life campaign set an ambitious goal that 100% of patients in each country should be admitted to a PCI centre within the first 24 h, the large majority of them for primary PCI and a minority after thrombolysis [55]. Excellent cooperation between emergency medical services, local hospitals, and PCI centres is vital in avoiding delays.

Drug-eluting or bare metal stents?

When drug-eluting stents (DES) are implanted in ruptured plaques with a large necrotic core, typical for STEMI, they may impair vascular healing responses. A large thrombus burden may result in late stent malapposition. Both these mechanisms might potentially result in increased rates of stent thrombosis associated with DES in the STEMI setting. STEMI patients were excluded from most original trials with DES. Two large nonrandomized observational registries suggested a significant reduction in mortality and repeat revascularization with DES use [56, 57]. However, these registries have significant limitations, including inappropriate timing of benefit (much of the relative survival benefit with DES occurred within 30 days after stent implantation, before the known benefits of DES in reducing restenosis are apparent). One large randomized study

(Horizons-AMI) [57] with 1-year follow-up demonstrated no difference between bare metal stents (BMS) and DES in mortality or MI rates and no difference in stent thrombosis risk. A reduction in repeat revascularization rates favouring DES was smaller in the setting of primary PCI than in randomized trials in elective procedures. A smaller observational study with 3-year follow-up failed to demonstrate any benefit with DES use; on the contrary, a higher frequency of stent thrombosis was observed in both DES groups [58]. The greatest challenge in selecting patients for DES implantation, however, is determining in an emergency situation whether the patient is a candidate for prolonged thienopyridine therapy. As with elective procedures, DES should be avoided in the presence of doubt regarding patient compliance with dual antiplatelet medication, or medical issues that involve bleeding risks or the need for invasive or surgical procedures in the following year that would interrupt antiplatelet therapy. In summary, data regarding DES use in STEMI are conflicting, and its use should be very selective.

Specific situations and conditions

Cardiogenic shock

Emergency PCI in cardiogenic shock may be life-saving and should be considered at an early stage and performed as soon as possible. There are two important differences from routine primary PCI: the usually recommended time window of 12 h after onset of chest pain is wider, and multivessel PCI on all critical lesions should be strongly considered. The SHOCK trial randomized 300 patients to medical therapy or revascularization (PCI or surgery). 86% of patients received intra-aortic balloon counterpulsation (IABP). The 6-month mortality was lower in the revascularization group than in the medical therapy group (50.3% vs 63.1%, $p = 0.027$). This trial finished enrolment in November 1998, when routine stenting for primary PCI was just beginning, and therefore revascularization with current technology might provide even better results [59]. Real life utilization of IABP during primary PCI for cardiogenic shock is low (20–39%) [60]. Recently published meta-analysis of IABP in cardiogenic shock did not show any efficacy benefit. Rather, IABP use resulted in significant increase in bleeding complications and increase in stroke [61]. All current data regarding IABP in the setting of cardiogenic shock are importantly hampered by bias and confounding, and randomized trials are needed to clarify the situation. Recently available percutaneous LV assist devices like TandemHeart or Impella are technically feasible and provide superior hemodynamic support, but so far have not been proved to improve clinical outcomes [62]. Mechanical ventilation with high positive end-expiratory pressure should be considered early for patients with hypoxia; it is helpful to stabilize patients prior to PCI [63, 64]. In summary, despite significant efforts, cardiogenic shock remains the leading cause of in-hospital mortality for STEMI patients.

Post coronary artery bypass grafting

Patients presenting with STEMI after coronary artery bypass grafting (CABG) are challenging, and have a poorer outcome [65]. Information on the number and type of grafts is not always available, and this could result in high contrast and radiation dose. Saphenous vein graft disease behaves quite differently from native coronary atheroma. Thrombolytic therapy has poor efficacy in thrombotic vein graft occlusions. In recent primary PCI trials, the number of patients enrolled with prior CABG has been low[20]. There is a high risk of no-reflow and a higher probability of vessel rupture. Embolic protection devices—both proximal balloon occlusion systems and distal filter based systems— have demonstrated a reduced rate of periprocedural complications. GPIIb/IIIa inhibitors have not shown any benefit in vein graft PCI.

No clear culprit lesion

As a result of our collaborative effort to minimize ischaemic time and delays, occasionally a patient undergoes urgent coronary angiography with no clear culprit lesion identified. We present here a brief differential diagnostic approach to such patients. Coronary artery spasm may result in temporary coronary artery occlusion with ST elevation on ECG, and serial ECGs are usually helpful. Stress-induced cardiomyopathy of the takotsubo type is easily diagnosed with left ventriculography demonstrating a dyskinetic segment which does not correspond to a single coronary artery territory. Pulmonary embolism can result in ST elevation in anterior leads [66, 67]. Haemodynamically unstable patients with clinical suspicion of pulmonary embolism might benefit from right heart catheterization, pulmonary angiography, and possibly local thrombolytic therapy. Aortic dissection may present with ST elevation, and aortography might be diagnostic.

Percutaneous coronary intervention for non STE acute coronary syndrome

Invasive or conservative strategy

Approximately 30–38% of patients with unstable coronary syndromes have single-vessel disease and 44–59% have multivessel disease (>50% diameter stenosis) [68, 69]. The role of coronary angiography and revascularization for patients admitted with NSTEMI was first studied in randomized fashion in 1994, comparing an 'early invasive' to an 'early conservative' strategy. The Thrombolysis in Myocardial Ischaemia (TIMI) IIIB trial hypothesized that early angiography and revascularization would be beneficial in preventing subsequent cardiac events [69]. Since then, numerous trials have addressed this question with—at first sight—conflicting results. Cardiac catheterization is a significant part of an 'early conservative' strategy, and is used in approximately 20–40% of patients in large randomized trials [70]. After adjusting for real difference in coronary revascularization there appears to be a direct relationship between higher use of revascularization and lower mortality [70]. A randomized trial with strictly no revascularization in the 'early conservative' arm would not be ethical. The Global Use of Strategies to Open Occluded Arteries (GUSTO) IV-ACS investigators performed a complex analysis in a population with NSTE ACS. They observed that the mortality rate was approximately 50% lower among those who had undergone revascularization within the first 30 days. These data are again consistent with previous randomized trials (⊃Fig. 45.5). As such, the added use of revascularization appears to provide benefit in improving mortality. Thus, the old belief that revascularization does not improve mortality in coronary disease but just improves symptoms, is no longer true for patients with NSTE ACS.

Timing of angiography

Coronary angiography should be performed as soon as possible (urgent invasive strategy, <2 h) in patients with severe ongoing angina, profound or dynamic ECG changes, major arrhythmias, or haemodynamic instability. These

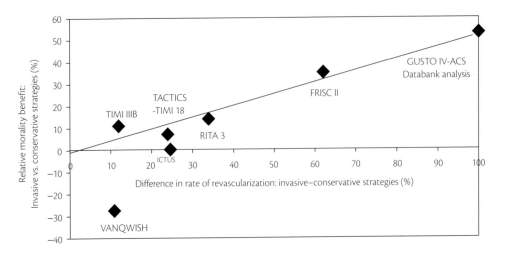

Figure 45.5 Trials comparing invasive and conservative strategies in NSTE ACS: difference in rate of revascularization versus relative benefit on mortality. The greater the difference in the rate of revascularization between the invasive and conservative strategies in the trial, the greater the benefit on mortality.
From Cannon CP. Revascularisation for everyone? *Eur Heart J* 2004;**25**(17):1471–1472. With permission.

patients represent 2–15% of the patients admitted with NSTE ACS [71–73]. In patients without these life-threatening features, the ideal timing of coronary angiography is not clear. Early intervention might prevent ischaemic events that could occur while the patient awaits a delayed procedure. Alternatively, with intensive antithrombotic therapy for few days, procedure-related complications might be avoided by intervening on a more stable plaque. The results of the ISAR-COOL [74], TIMACS [75], and ABOARD [95] studies can be summarized as follows: (1) high risk patients, defined as having GRACE risk score [76] over 140, derive benefit from early angiography within 12–24 h; (2) very early (primary PCI-like, <2 h) angiography does not add any incremental benefit; (3) timing of angiography is not important in low to intermediate risk patients and the strategy may be chosen individually according to patient, physician, or institution preference (e.g. efficiency, cost savings, etc.).

Special situations and conditions

Elderly patients

A large observational study of ACS patients (with both STEMI and NSTE ACS) determined that 30-day mortality rates were higher in older age groups (65–69, 10.9%; 70–74, 14.1%; 75–79, 18.5%; 80–84, 23.2%, 85 or older 31.2%; $p = 0.001$ for trend) [77]. Patients over 75 years of age are frequently excluded from randomized clinical trials and therefore evidence-based medicine is lacking. Primary PCI seems to be safe but less successful in elderly patients [78]. GPIIb/IIIa are associated with increased risk of bleeding and if needed, their dose should be adjusted according to renal function.

Bleeding after percutaneous coronary intervention: importance, definition, and prevention

In the past, bleeding was considered an inevitable consequence of effective antithrombotic therapy and the avoidance of bleeding therefore received little attention. However, recently it has become clear that approximately 5% of patients presenting with ACS experience major bleeding during the next 30 days and this is associated with a 3.5-fold increased mortality risk which is prolonged and steady throughout 1 year [79–82]. Different classifications of bleeding severity have been developed, some of them based on laboratory values (e.g. TIMI bleeding score), some clinical such as the GUSTO definition of bleeding: life-threatening (fatal, intracranial, or resulting in hemodynamic compromise), moderate (requiring transfusion), and mild [83, 84]. The possible mechanisms responsible for the association between bleeding and mortality include bleeding itself, discontinuation of antiplatelet or antithrombotic medication, and anaemia with reduced oxygen delivery. There are also previously unforeseen possible consequences of blood transfusion, such as nitric oxide depletion resulting in vasoconstriction or decreased oxygen tissue delivery [85]. All data regarding consequences of bleeding in the setting of ACS are obviously not randomized, but are observational with many potential confounders and therefore require cautious interpretation. Older age, female sex, renal insufficiency, baseline anaemia, LMWH administration and use of GPIIb/IIIa and IABP are among known factors predicting bleeding [86]. Early sheath removal, very careful arterial puncture site management, and properly adjusted dosing of antithrombotic medication are critical issues. Persistent hypotension with no obvious explanation after femoral artery puncture is suggestive of retroperitoneal haemorrhage, and urgent CT is indicated. Blood transfusions should be used cautiously based on clinical rather than laboratory parameters. Antiplatelet medications should be restarted as soon as the risk of bleeding allows.

Radial versus femoral approach

Cardiac catheterization using the radial artery access has become routine in many centres. The radial approach results in quick mobilization of the patient and minimizes the risk of local bleeding complications, which make it especially attractive in the setting of ACS with aggressive antithrombotic and antiplatelet medication [87]. A recent meta-analysis demonstrated significant reduction in bleeding, trend for better outcome but also trend for lower procedural success with radial compared to femoral access [88]. There is a 5–10% conversion rate due to failed radial access, and in this situation significant time delay may occur [89]. There is also concern regarding increased operator and patient radiation with the radial approach [90]. In summary we recommend that in the absence of conclusive data, operators should select the access route individually for every patient based on their experience and the predicted risk of bleeding.

Contrast nephropathy

Contrast medium induced nephropathy (CIN) is a recognized complication of PCI, defined as an increase in the serum creatinine concentration of 25% or more from the baseline up to 3 days. It can lead to acute renal failure and is associated with a significantly increased mortality rate. Patients with STEMI treated with primary PCI are at higher risk of CIN (possibly up to 20% of patients) than are those undergoing elective interventions, possibly due to impaired systemic perfusion, a large volume of contrast medium, and the impossibility of starting renal prophylactic therapies before exposure to contrast medium [91]. So far, the only strategies that are proven to be effective in preventing CIN are meticulous patient hydration, minimizing the volume of contrast agent, stopping the intake of nephrotoxic drugs, and avoiding short intervals between procedures. The role of other drugs such as N-acetylcysteine in CIN prevention is still controversial. High-osmolar contrast agents have higher risk of CIN development; regarding other contrast agents, a recently published study did not show any benefit of nonionic iso-osmolar iodixanol when compared with the ionic low-osmolar ioxaglate [92].

Personal perspective

The Czech Republic was one of a handful of countries pioneering the large-scale use of PCI for all patients with STEMI. Several Czech hospitals completely abandoned thrombolysis for their STEMI patients as early as 1995. The whole country abandoned thrombolysis in 2002, shortly after the presentation of the PRAGUE-2 study results [13] and after the STEMI guidelines of the Czech Society of Cardiology [94] declared primary PCI as the treatment of choice for all STEMI patients in the country. Between 1998 and 2005 the use of primary PCI increased from 7% of all STEMI patients to 92%. Many other countries in Europe followed a similar development. The 'Stent For Life' initiative launched by the European Association for Percutaneous Cardiovascular Interventions (EAPCI) in 2009 published data from 30 European countries and showed that primary PCI is the dominant strategy in more than 50% of these countries [93]. Surprisingly, countries with widespread use of primary PCI are able to offer reperfusion (as such) to a much larger proportion of STEMI patients than countries where thrombolysis still is the dominant reperfusion treatment.

Developments in the near future will certainly continue in this direction. Patients with ACS will make up the vast majority (>60–70%) of all PCI procedures due to the following reasons:

- ACS (and especially AMI) patients benefit most from PCI: they are actually the only group where survival benefit from PCI has been very clearly demonstrated. No other treatment can offer similar efficacy in these acutely ill patients.
- On the other hand, due to the success of pharmacotherapy and the high effectiveness and safety of cardiac surgery in chronic stable coronary artery disease, PCI will be used only for patients with limiting symptoms or for patients with very large demonstrable ischaemia (prognostically severe coronary angiography findings).

Future technological developments may introduce new stent materials (e.g. biodegradable/bioactive stents). Several very promising new antithrombotic drugs are in the late phases of development.

Further reading

Bassand JP, Hamm CW, Ardissino D, *et al*. Guidelines for the diagnosis and treatment of non-ST-segment elevation acute coronary syndromes. *Eur Heart J* 2007;**28**(13):1598–1660.

Hochman JS, Sleeper LA, Webb JG, *et al*. Early revascularization in acute myocardial infarction complicated by cardiogenic shock. SHOCK Investigators. Should we emergently revascularize occluded coronaries for cardiogenic shock. *N Engl J Med* 1999;**341**(9):625–634.

Keeley EC, Boura JA, Grines CL. Primary angioplasty versus intravenous thrombolytic therapy for acute myocardial infarction: a quantitative review of 23 randomised trials. *Lancet* 2003;**361**(9351):13–20.

Knot J, Widimsky P, Wijns W, *et al*. How to set up an effective national primary angioplasty network: lessons learned from five European countries. *EuroIntervention* 2009;**5**(3):299, 301–309.

Silber S, Albertsson P, Avilés FF, *et al*. Guidelines for percutaneous coronary interventions. The Task Force for Percutaneous Coronary Interventions of the European Society of Cardiology. *Eur Heart J* 2005;**26**(8):804–847.

Van de Werf F, Bax J, Betriu A, *et al*. Management of acute myocardial infarction in patients presenting with persistent ST-segment elevation: the Task Force on the Management of ST-Segment Elevation Acute Myocardial Infarction of the European Society of Cardiology. *Eur Heart J* 2008;**29**(23):2909–2945.

➔ For additional multimedia materials please visit the online version of the book (✎ http://www.esciacc.oxfordmedicine. com).

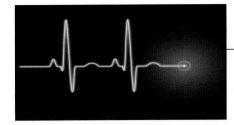

CHAPTER 46

Coronary artery bypass graft surgery

Ardawan J. Rastan, Ömür Akhavuz,
and Friedrich W. Mohr

Contents

Summary

According to current guidelines, percutaneous coronary intervention (PCI) represents the first-line approach for emergency coronary revascularization in acute coronary syndromes (ACS). However, in the setting of complex coronary pathology, unsuccessful PCI, complicated PCI, or cardiogenic shock, emergency surgical coronary revascularization may be preferable. Beyond emergency revascularization, there is no indication that the choice of revascularization technique should deviate from that applicable to stable angina pectoris patients. The timing of surgical intervention is based on clinical symptoms, coronary artery pathology, and the type of underlying ACS. Coronary artery bypass grafting (CABG) strategies may involve beating-heart revascularization, with or without cardiopulmonary bypass support. In addition, modern perioperative management enables improved outcomes for elderly patients with significant comorbidities, as well as for patients presenting with haemodynamic instability. In cardiogenic shock, a variety of different cardiopulmonary assist devices are available today, including intra-aortic balloon pump (IABP), various ventricular assist device (VAD) options and extracorporeal membrane oxygenation (ECMO).

Results of CABG in ACS patients vary significantly in the literature because of heterogeneous patient populations, as well as variable operative timing, and haemodynamic status. Thus, comparison of surgical outcomes is almost impossible. Randomized surgical trials for ACS patients are pending. However, a hospital survival of more than 95% is reported even in emergency CABG patients during the last 5 years, but increases significantly in cardiogenic shock. For surgical candidates, a close and immediate communication between interventionalist and cardiac surgeon is mandatory to quickly identify the best treatment strategy and achieve optimal revascularization results.

Introduction

Acute coronary syndrome (ACS) represents a continuum of myocardial ischemia ranging from unstable angina pectoris (UA) and non-ST-segment elevation myocardial infarction (NSTEMI) to ST-segment elevation myocardial infarction (STEMI) [1]. Common to these forms is acute myocardial ischaemia leading to symptoms and to (impending) myocardial cell necrosis, which thereby necessitates acute intervention. The treatment of ACS requires an interdisciplinary integrated approach among emergency physicians, family physicians, and internists, as well as cardiologists and cardiac surgeons.

An expeditious cardiac diagnosis and the earliest possible implementation of treatment are key determinants of successful short- and long-term outcomes. Not least because of the differing urgency of the necessary invasive diagnostics and therapy, it is important to distinguish between UA and NSTEMI on the one hand, and STEMI on the other; both the European [2–4] and American [5–7] guidelines are structured in this way.

The treatment of ACS encompasses a multitude of medical treatment options. Among these are new and refined treatment strategies with glycoprotein (GP)IIb/IIIa receptor antagonists, thienopyridines, and antithrombin agents [7]. Depending on the type of ACS and the patient's symptoms, timely coronary angiography and a prompt invasive revascularization strategy play a significant role in patient outcomes. Because of its immediate availability, lesser invasiveness, and great advances in stent technologies the revascularization strategy today primarily follows catheter-based percutaneous coronary intervention (PCI) [3, 7]. However, depending on the patient's status, and complexity of coronary artery disease (i.e. left main stem stenosis, in-stent restenosis, or bifurcational stenosis of the left anterior descending (LAD) coronary artery) as well as for chronic total coronary artery occlusion (CTO) or in unsuccessful or complicated PCI, an urgent or emergency operative coronary bypass procedure may be indicated. Operative options in addition to a conventional coronary artery bypass grafting (CABG) operation include procedures that maintain native coronary perfusion such as beating-heart and off-pump surgery, as well as the implementation of mechanical assist systems by impending or manifest cardiogenic shock, with the possibility of short- and mid-term circulatory support. The aim here is to describe the indications of coronary bypass surgery in the management of different forms of ACS, and thereby to emphasize certain operative points.

Indication and timing of the operation

Unstable angina pectoris and non-ST-segment elevation myocardial infarction

Based on the results of the TACTICS, FRICS II, and RITA-3-trials, and independent of the success of the primary pharmacological treatment, the goal of current treatment strategies is a timely diagnosis and revascularization [8–10]. This is even more important for high-risk patients presenting elevated troponin values, in diabetic patients, or in the presence of ST-segment alterations. The optimal time point of cardiac catheterization remains the object of intense research [11, 12], but as a rule, it should be done within 72 h from the onset of symptoms [2]. With UA and NSTEMI, there is no indication that the choice of revascularization technique should deviate from that applicable to stable angina [3, 13–15]. In summary, a CABG procedure rather than PCI is primarily recommended when there are prognostically relevant coronary lesions, which include multivessel coronary artery disease, left main stenosis, and involvement of the proximal LAD. Certainly, the results from the Syntax study [16] have provoked an intense and controversial discussion about the optimal treatment modality of left main stenosis, but a final conclusion can only be drawn when results are available from adequately powered studies with a focus on isolated left main diseases versus left main disease in combination with single or multivessel coronary artery disease. Indeed, it is apparent that interventionally accessible left main coronary lesions, in particular within the mid-body, in the face of otherwise minimal coronary pathology, are being increasingly approached interventionally, even if current guidelines indicate that such treatment has not been found to be equivalent to operation. However, one must consider that the risks of PCI for left main stem coronary lesions are much higher for complex coronary artery disease, and the results are highly dependent on the experience of the operator [16].

Nevertheless, once a consensus has been reached on the operative indication, the timing of the operation must be determined based on the patient's symptom complex, individual coronary pathology, and haemodynamic stability, as well as the need for routine and additional diagnostics (echo, duplex carotid ultrasound, CT, etc.; see ⊃Table 46.1). An emergency indication (i.e. operation before the beginning of the next working day) includes persisting or recurrent pain/complaints refractory to medical management, subtotal noncollateralized

Table 46.1 Mandatory and optional preoperative diagnostics before CABG surgery

Examination	Mandatory	Indicated in	Impact for treatment
Cardiac catheterization	Y		
Coronary angiography	Y		
Laevocardiography		Heart valve disease	Additional heart valve surgery
		Cardiomyopathy	Assessment for ECMO/cardiac assist device
Right heart catheterization		Pulmonary hypertension	
		Cardiomyopathy	
Echocardiography	Y		
Transthoracic	Y		Exclusion of heart valve disease, assessment of LV function
Transoesophageal		Heart valve disease	Additional heart valve surgery
		Cardiogenic shock	Preop assessment of VSD, papillary muscle rupture, cardiac function
		Suspected cardiac thrombus	Surgical thrombus removal
		Atrial fibrillation	Surgery for atrial fibrillation
12 channel ECG, 1 s/50 mm	Y		
Chest X-ray	Y		
Doppler measurement	Y		
Carotid arteries	Y		In case of carotid stenosis further diagnostics
			Consideration of periop stenting or surgical endarteriectomy
Subclavian arteries		Clinical signs of stenosis	Kind of IMA use, consideration of preop stenting
Radial arteries		Pathological Allen test, diabetes	Vessel quality and collateralization
Computed tomography		Cardiac Redo surgery	Imaging of adhesions
		Unclear findings in chest X-ray	Identification of thoracic tumours
		Pulmonary hypertension	Exclusion of pulmonary embolism
		Aortic aneurysms	Quantification of extention and diameter of aortic aneurysms
Pulmonary function test	Y		Not essential in emergeny indication
Cardiac scintigraphy		Myocardial hybernation, scarring	Identification of vital myocardium in borderline CABG patients
Nuclear magnetic resonance		Myocardial hybernation, scarring	Identification of vital myocardium
		Cardiomyopathy	Assessment of ventricular and valve function
Abdominal sonography		History of abdominal surgery or abdominal organ disease	Critical indication in severe liver cirrhosis
			Exclusion of gallbladder disease
Gastroscopy		History of peptic ulcer	Exclusion of active ulcer, malignacies, bleedings
		History of gastric surgery	
		Liver cirrhosis	Grading of oesophageal varices
Laboratory tests	Y		Blood count, coagulation test, electrolytes, serum liver and kidney values
			Blood transfusion tests, HIV test, hepatitis tests

coronary stenoses, or impending or manifest cardiogenic shock (⊃Fig. 46.1). On the other hand, with medically managed symptoms, chronically well-collateralized coronary occlusions, and stable hemodynamics, the operation may be postponed. It should, nevertheless, be carried out urgently (i.e. operation within the same hospital stay) or as an early elective operation. Transfer to a cardiac surgical unit after completion of the necessary routine diagnostics is essentially the preferred strategy. As shown recently by the APPROACH study, time from admission to CABG was not associated with an increased risk of short-term mortality [17].

ST-segment elevation myocardial infarction

The treatment of acute STEMI has undergone a major change in recent years. A multitude of clinical concerns have focused on shortening the patient decision time, the prehospital phase, as well as the in-hospital time to reperfusion, referred to as the 'door-to-needle time' for in-hospital fibrinolysis, or as the 'door-to-balloon time' for PCI. In recent years, a series of studies have shown that primary PCI is routinely employed as the reperfusion strategy, instead of fibrinolysis [18]. Currently, fibrinolysis is recommended only in cases where there are long transport times to

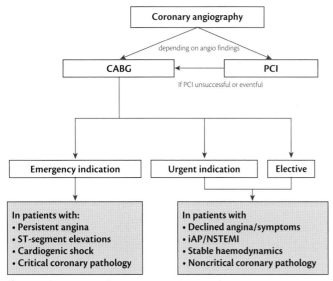

Figure 46.1 Timing of coronary artery byass graft surgery in ACS patients depending on varying clinical characteristics and ST-segment alterations.

the designated intervention centre, or a delay of more than 2 h until PCI is anticipated. Furthermore, the latest guidelines suggest that, for suitable coronary pathology, PCI of left main stem coronary lesions is equivalent to a coronary bypass operation for patients who have an elevated operative risk [7]. An indication for surgical revascularization in STEMI is therefore always considered when the infarct vessel cannot, or cannot sufficiently, become revascularized, and is therefore indicated as an immediate procedure, analogous to PCI. Not uncommonly, the infarcted vessel can be acutely reopened, but during angiography it unmasks an accompanying multivessel coronary artery disease, which *per se* represents a primary operative indication. In this setting an urgent operation is indicated after a cooling-off period of several days following the acute infarct, or even sooner in the case of recurrent symptoms, haemodynamic instability, or critical coronary anatomy.

Specific surgical considerations

Bypass graft material

The left internal thoracic artery (ITA) is the conduit of first choice as a bypass graft to the LAD artery. The endothelium of the ITA produces vasodilators (nitric oxide and prostacyclin), and responds well to pharmacological agents in the postoperative period [19–21]. The flow characteristics of the ITA are comparable to those of normal coronary arteries. There are two different ways to take down the ITA: either pedicled or skeletonized harvest technique. After exposure of the internal chest wall using special ITA

retractors, the thoracic artery can be identified lateral to the border of the sternum by inspection or palpation. In the pedicled technique, the artery is prepared with its accompanying veins and surrounding fatty and muscle tissue. If skeletonization of the ITA is preferred, only the artery is mobilized and the venous plexus is conserved. The sternal blood perfusion is always decreased when using ITA grafting, but it seems that sternal ischaemia is more pronounced after pedicled ITA harvest technique. There is evidence that the use of the left internal thoracic artery (LITA) as an arterial graft represents a favourable prognostic factor for short- and long-term survival for ACS patients. It is speculated that the mammary artery could be more resistant than other grafts to low-flow scenarios like the no-reflow phenomenon. Although the preparation of the LITA requires an additional 10–20 min, the anastomosis of the LITA to the LAD is favoured even under emergency conditions, and mammary take-down can also be done after the establishment of cardiopulmonary bypass.

The radial artery of the nondominant arm will be used as a conduit, after testing for adequate ulnar collateral circulation by the Allen test. It is essential that all patients with pathological or doubtful Allen test results receive noninvasive duplex ultrasonography [22]. The radial artery is dissected as a pedicle with minimal manipulation using conventional surgery, ultrasonic harmonic scalpel, or better, endoscopic techniques. Protection of the nerves is of the utmost importance, to avoid paresthesia and numbness of the thumb and the back of the fingers. The overall long-term patency of the radial artery is excellent, but more influenced by the site of the distal anastomosis and competitive flow [23]. Thus, the graft failure rate is higher in less severe native target vessel stenoses [24].

The saphenous vein is one of the most commonly used conduits in coronary bypass grafting. It is easy to harvest and resistant to vasospasms, and thus offers potential advantages in patients with vasoconstrictive medication. The saphenous vein can be identified easily and harvested by open, bridged, or endoscopic techniques [25].

Surgical access

Median sternotomy remains the standard access for operative therapy of multivessel coronary artery disease. Using this access, all options for operative procedures relevant to emergently operated patients are preserved. It is important to know that the suboptimal preparation of these patients represents a potential risk for postoperative wound complications or infections, which may occur at the sternotomy but more frequently at graft harvest sites. Thus, graft harvesting using minimally invasive techniques with preservation of multiple skin bridges or through endoscopic techniques, in particular for diabetics, leads to a lower incidence of post-operative wound infections [26, 27].

Coronary artery bypass grafting on the beating heart

Despite the recent criticism of off-pump coronary artery bypass surgery (OPCAB) compared to conventional CABG with cardioplegia-induced cardiac arrest [28], there is uniformly less myocardial trauma and release of myocardial necrosis parameters with OPCAB [29, 30]. Even if these benefits of OPCAB cannot be realized in elective coronary surgery, it can be assumed that patients with acute coronary ischaemic events will profit especially from preservation of the native coronary perfusion and a correspondingly lower ischaemia–reperfusion injury. The preservation of natural coronary perfusion and avoidance of cardioplegic arrest could even prevent an aggravation of myocardial oedema, the no-reflow phenomenon, and myocardial necrosis. To date, only few post-hoc analyses have analysed the influence of beating heart techniques on morbidity and mortality in ACS patients [31–36]. In addition to the preservation of physiological coronary perfusion, one further advantage of beating heart strategy is the avoidance of transverse aortic clamping of the ascending aorta, which always carries a potential risk for aortic injury or plaque embolization. In ACS, the surgical beating-heart strategy offers the special opportunity to keep the ischaemic time of the jeopardized myocardium as short as possible [34]. This is analogous to the interventional philosophy 'time = myocardium', referring to the significance of emergent revascularization of the infarct vessel for STEMI. In this context, a bypass is first performed into the ischaemic territory, commonly the LAD, and the territory is reperfused. In this way, not only is the infarct-associated ischaemic time shortened, but also the tolerance of the heart to the ensuing manipulations is increased. Depending on the patient's haemodynamic status during the beating-heart operation, the heart–lung machine may be completely avoided, or the operation may be conducted as beating-heart surgery, with the support of a cardiopulmonary bypass (CPB). In a comparative study, CPB-supported beating-heart surgery was shown to be preferable to conventional CABG with cardioplegic arrest in ACS patients. Not only was the mortality of the beating-heart group with a heart–lung machine lower (6.5% vs 8.0%), but also there were significantly fewer perioperative complications in the form of bleeding, organic brain syndromes, or perioperative myocardial infarct [34].

Coronary artery bypass grafting in cardiogenic shock

As was demonstrated in the SHOCK trial, patients with ischaemia-related cardiogenic shock benefit both short- and long-term from acute coronary revascularization [37, 38]. Thus, in the PCI guidelines of the European Society of Cardiology (ESC), relatively early revascularization is recommended in cardiogenic shock [3]. PCI recommendations in cardiogenic shock include a liberalization of the usually recommended PCI window of 12 h and, if appropriate, multivessel PCI should be entertained [3, 39]. An emergency CABG operation should be subsequently considered if the multivessel disease is not amenable to relatively complete PCI, or in unsuccessful or complicated PCI. Additionally, implantation of an intra-aortic balloon pump (IABP) is recommended [3]. If operative therapy is chosen to treat a patient in cardiogenic shock, then CPB with the heart–lung machine is inevitably required to ensure adequate organ perfusion. Nevertheless, as mentioned above, there is the possibility of carrying out coronary revascularization on the beating heart. Until recently, there has been limited reported experience regarding the strategy of on-pump beating-heart surgery in cardiogenic shock patients [32, 40]. At the Heart Centre in Leipzig we have been routinely applying this strategy for patients in cardiogenic shock for the last 6 years. For a total of 107 patients between 2002 and 2005, we showed that the on-pump beating-heart strategy, when compared to a conventional CABG, resulted in a lower perioperative mortality, and a significant decrease in perioperative morbidity. The long-term survival and the rate of major adverse cardiac events of these patients were comparable in terms of completeness of revascularization, but there was a trend towards improved long-term survival for the patients treated with the on-pump beating-heart strategy [34]. In contrast to PCI, coronary bypass surgery with the heart–lung machine offers the possibility of acute volume unloading of the left ventricle (LV) until revascularization is achieved, as well as the option of implanting an assist device in case of insufficient ventricular recovery (◗Fig. 46.2).

Intra-aortic balloon pump

As mentioned above, one further option in infarct-related cardiogenic shock is temporary circulatory support by intra-aortic counterpulsation (◗Fig. 46.3). Through IABP use an improvement in diastolic coronary perfusion is achieved and the reduced afterload leads to reduction of myocardial oxygen consumption. These pathophysiological mechanisms indicate an early use in acute myocardial

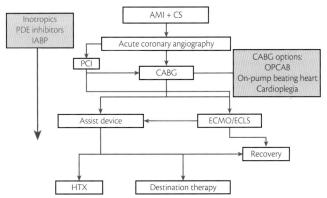

Figure 46.2 Further surgical options for patients presenting with AMI complicated by cardiogenic shock (for abbreviations, see text).

infarction complicated by manifest or impending cardiogenic shock. However, there is only limited scientific evidence of the benefit of IABP, and its role in STEMI and in cardiogenic shock is currently controversial [41–43]. At present a large multicentre trial including 600 patients is re-evaluating the impact of IABP support in acute ischaemic cardiogenic shock (clinicaltrials.gov IACP-SHOCK II Trial). However, IABP implantation at least in the context of surgical coronary revascularization remains a class I indication [13]. At the first sign of cardiac failure, the IABP should be employed. The IABP is normally placed by percutaneous femoral artery approach using a Seldinger technique, and advanced into the descending thoracic aorta, with its final position controlled with transoesophageal echocardiography or, when placed during cardiac catheterization, by C-arm fluoroscopy. If possible, the IABP

should be implanted before surgery or, if logistic reasons make a preoperative IABP insertion inopportune, during the CABG operation.

Extracorporeal membrane oxygenation/assist device implantation

If cardiogenic shock is present preoperatively, then use of the CPB, in addition to IABP, is necessary. Furthermore, the use of an additional suction catheter achieves volume unloading of the LV and pulmonary circulation. Under the protection of the CPB and LV unloading, coronary revascularization is performed as a requisite for myocardial recovery, followed by prolonged reperfusion with CPB support. If an early resumption of cardiopulmonary function is not safely possible, however, a temporary circulatory support may be considered during or after the index bypass procedure. This decision for prolonged support always required a careful balance of all individual risks and benefits. One option is the implantation of a veno-arterial extracorporeal membrane oxygenation (avECMO) or an isolated blood pump to support left and/or right heart function. Both assist modalities offer the advantage of mostly using the intraoperatively placed cannulae from the CPB and bridging the patient for further decision-making. The latter is especially helpful in patients in whom the entire medical history and comorbidities are unknown, as well as in patients with unclear neurological status in the event of preoperative resuscitation. ECMO moreover offers the advantage of supporting cardiac and also pulmonary function, but is associated with a comparably high complication rate [44].

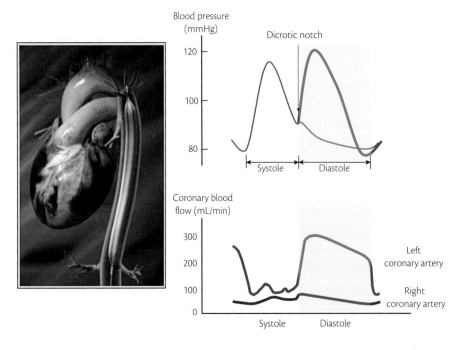

Figure 46.3 Effects of intra-aortic balloon pump (IABP) on arterial blood pressure and coronary blood supply. In the upper part unaugmented pressure is depicted by thin lines, arterial pressure and coronary blood supply under IABP augmentation are depicted by bold lines.

In the following postoperative days, the ECMO or left/right heart bypass allows the support of cardiac function until cardiac recovery occurs [44]. If cardiac recovery is not primarily anticipated, or if it does not occur within a few days, then the patient's general condition, age, and co-morbidities can be considered to decide whether implantation of a permanent assist device is appropriate, or circulatory support is stopped knowing that survival is unlikely. Depending on the patient's age, an assist device may serve as a bridge to heart transplantation or as final destination therapy (see ⬦Fig. 46.2). In particular, nonpulsatile assist devices (⬦Fig. 46.4) are associated with acceptable long-term survival rates [45].

Treatment of mechanical infarct complications

Mechanical infarct complications include free wall rupture, post-infarct ventricular septal defect (VSD), and acute mitral valve regurgitation (MR). Free wall rupture leads to acute pump failure within minutes, and a life-saving operation is only possible in selected cases.

Post-infarct VSD is seen in roughly 1% of acute MI patients, occurs mostly within the first week, and has a 1-year mortality of >90% if left unoperated. In addition to

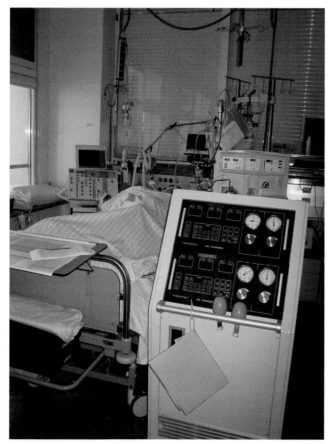

Figure 46.4 48-year-old patient with biventricular assist device support due to ischaemic acute cardiogenic shock and biventricular heart failure.

IABP implantation for reduction of the left-to-right shunt volume, treatment consists of an emergency surgical patch closure, which is still associated with a hospital mortality of about 50% [46, 47]. Alternatively, there are reports of transcatheter VSD closure using interventional occluder devices with comparably bad outcome [48].

Acute MR can be aetiologically subdivided into papillary muscle rupture, papillary muscle dysfunction, and dilation of the mitral valve annulus due to infarct-related LV dysfunction. Treatment of acute MR with pulmonary oedema or cardiogenic shock consists of an immediate mitral valve operation and IABP support until the operation. Surgical treatment most commonly consists of mitral valve replacement to keep additional global myocardial ischaemia time short. Alternatively, mitral valve repair can be performed in suitable valve pathologies using chordae transfer or chordae replacement techniques in combination with ring annuloplasty. However, it should be kept in mind that valve repair in these patients always bear a higher than average risk of repair failure. Overall 30-day mortality in emergency ischaemic mitral valve surgery is about 26% [49].

Coagulation management

CABG procedures in ACS require a more demanding coagulation management, because the overwhelming majority of patients have been acutely treated with platelet aggregation inhibitors. Although routine aspirin is not associated with an increased bleeding risk [50], a heightened postoperative bleeding risk is present in patients who have received additional thienopyridine or GPIIb/IIIa receptor antagonists within the preceding 5 days [51]. Nevertheless, all ACS patients should receive dual antiplatelet therapy according to the guidelines, and timing and indication of the CABG should be decided regardless of elevated bleeding risks. With continuation of dual therapy, an operation with low rate of bleeding complications can be achieved nowadays, thanks to a variety of options available to optimize coagulation [51]. For urgent operative indications, cessation of clopidogrel for 3–5 days prior to operation should be carefully considered. In a subanalysis of the ACUITY-study focusing on 1539 NSTEMI patients requiring urgent CABG procedure after a 5-day washout period of clopidogrel versus no clopidogrel administration, a comparably low bleeding rate but a reduced 30-day incidence of composite ischaemic events was found for clopidogrel patients. Thus, upstream clopidogrel administration even in those NSTEMI patients who subsequently undergo CABG was recommended [52].

In emergency CABG patients, preoperatively administered GPIIb/IIIa receptor antagonists has also to be considered. The half-life of abciximab is about 10–30 min, but its biological effects continue up to 48 h because of the irreversible receptor binding. Thus abciximab can only be antagonized by be platelet transfusion. In contrast, tirofiban and ebtifibatide are nonpeptide agents and have a shorter biological half-life of about 2 h. In these agents platelet administration is unsuited for antagonization, but perioperative hemodialysis is very effective for elimination of excess serum concentrations.

In general, in these ACS patients it is advisable to perform extended coagulation testing or thrombelastography immediately after protamine antagonization but still during the operation. This allows for specific substitution of coagulation factors, thrombocytes, protamine, or antifibrinolytic agents [53].

Results of coronary artery bypass grafting in acute coronary syndromes

Mortality

Although important, the classification of UA/NSTEMI and STEMI according to the guidelines is more relevant for interventional cardiologists than for surgeons. This is explained by the fact that cardiac surgeons usually do not see surgical candidates until after coronary angiography has been performed. In ACS patients with CABG indication the timing of the operation is then mainly driven by acute patient symptoms and coronary pathology. Thus, timing of surgery is comparable to the timing of PCI. Only in an asymptomatic patient presenting with ST-segment elevation might the indication of emergency surgery be based mainly on ECG alterations. This perhaps explains why, in the cardiac surgical literature, the patients are not categorized on the basis of ECG findings with the same stringency; most reports indicate only the total ACS population or MI patients (◆Table 46.2). Patients with ACS clearly represent a high-risk group among coronary surgical patients. The perioperative mortality is elevated when compared to patients with stable angina, in which 30-day mortality rates of about 1% are described [16]. However, despite the higher risks of ACS patients, there is an indication for surgical treatment within the acute phase, if the natural risk of the disease outweighs the risk of the operation.

The results in ACS patients in the literature are difficult to compare because patient populations vary considerably with respect to age, operative urgency, haemodynamic stability, and the type of ACS. The comparison of individual studies is complicated by the lack of a standardized definition of the emergency status. Analyses with especially good results have often excluded high-risk patient subsets. As a result of variable patient selection, the reported operative mortality of ACS varies from 1.6% to 32% [54–60]. Creswell reported a mortality rate for patients with AMI and an operation timeframe within a 6-h window of 9.1% [55]. In a multicentre analysis of 32 099 patients, who were operated on with conventional CABG within 24 h after AMI, hospital mortality was 14% [57]. Tomasco and colleagues reported a similar mortality of 13.4% [59]. In contrast to these studies, the mortality rate reported by Sergeant was remarkably low at 1.6% [58].

So far, there have been only a few nonrandomized retrospective studies that compare beating-heart procedures and cardioplegic arrest for this subpopulation [33, 34, 36, 61–64]. In most studies, there has been comparable hospital mortality for both groups, although a trend favouring OPCAB procedures is often evident. Notably, Locker and colleagues reported on 225 patients operated during acute MI (AMI) and demonstrated a significant reduction in hospital mortality with OPCAB surgery [33]. In terms of perioperative morbidity, there was a benefit for OPCAB patients with respect to perioperative MI [63], perioperative IABP implantation [61, 64], reoperation rate [34, 64], perioperative catecholamine requirement [34, 63], acute kidney injury [61, 64], stroke rate [34], and the duration of intensive care and hospital stays [34, 61–64].

For patients in cardiogenic shock, the mortality rates range between 21.3% and 46.7% [37, 58, 59]. However, the data from the SHOCK trial showed a benefit of early revascularization and the superiority of surgical intervention in comparison to PCI. Hospital mortality in this study was 39.6% [37]. In our propensity score analysis, hospital mortality for beating-heart patients was significantly lower than for patients operated with cardioplegic arrest (19.3% vs 33.3%) [34].

Long-term outcome depends on severity of coronary atherosclerosis, LV function, age, gender, overall health status, and the presence and severity of associated comorbidities [34]. The occurrence of ischaemic clinical events, stroke, or renal failure after CABG had a significant negative effect on long-term survival [65]. However, several studies have demonstrated that early mortality is the Achilles heel

Table 46.2 Results of CABG in patients presenting with ACS during the last 5 years

Author and reference	Location	Year	Period	N	Time interval to surgery	Type of ACS	Mean age (years)	Hospital survival	Follow-up survival	Remarks
Solodky A [70]	Tel Hashomer	2005	00–01	460	Primary hospitalization	All	65.2	96.5%		
Liistro F [71]	Arezzo	2005	02–04	92	Primary hospitalization	NSTEMI NSTEMI	68.2	96.7%		
Kerendi F [62]	Atlanta	2005	96–03	614	Emergency	All	62.3	93.5%	4 y: 84.1%	
Onorati F [63]	Catanzaro	2005	02–04	126	Emergency+urgent	All	61.2	88.9%		
Monteiro P [72]	Coimbra	2006	02–04	267	Primary hospitalization	All	67.0	99.0%	6 m: 97.4%	
Stamou [64]	Cleveland	2006	00–03	3487 vs 2773	Emergency+urgent	All	63.1 vs 65.1	95.8% vs. 96.5%		Cardioplegia vs OPCAB
Rastan AJ [34]	Leipzig	2006	00–05	638	Emergency <12 h	All	68.0	89.0%	1 y: 87.7%	Including cardiogenic shock
Hata M [73]	Tokyo	2006	94–04	104	Emergency	All	65.7	87.7%	1 y: 88.9%	Left main
Chen Y [74]	Melbourne	2006	01–04	441	Emergency+urgent	All	64.5	95.5%		
Kamohara K [75]	Fukuoka	2006		67	Emergency+urgent	All		90.9%	5 y: 80.3%	
Chew DP [76]	Adelaide	2008		1793	<72 h	All	67.8	96.0%	6 m: 93.7%	
Alexiou K [77]	Dresden	2008	03–05	220	Emergency <24 h	All	68.2	93.6%		
Ferrari E [78]	Lausanne	2008	05–06	290	Emergency	All	69.0	92.0%	1 y: 95.6%	Beating heart
Miyahara K [36]	Aichi	2008	99–05	61	Emergency	All	68.0	78.3 vs. 97.4%		Cardioplegia vs beating heart
Hochholzer W [79]	Krozingen	2008	96–99	74	<24 h	UAP/ NSTEMI	65.6	91.3%	3 y: 94.7%	
Darwazah AK [80]	Jerusalem	2009	99–05	31	<12 h	All		87.1%		After unsuccessful PCI

of ACS in CABG patients, and long-term outcome is comparably good to elective patients (see ➲Table 46.2).

Operative risk assessment

To better estimate the individual operative risk for hospital mortality and morbidity, two major risk stratification systems are currently available [66–68]. Both the Society of Thoracic Surgery (STS) score and the EuroSCORE allow online and offline risk calculation of an individual patient (see ➲Online resources). Whereas the STS score allows for estimation of the procedural risk for mortality and morbidity in a reliable way, it is widely accepted that the EuroSCORE overestimates the procedural risk by a factor of approximately 2.5 [69]. Several individual patient variables are entered into the calculators to obtain a predicted risk percentage before the operation. The variables include timing and extend of the operation, age, prior heart surgery, gender, race (STS only), left ventricular ejection fraction (LVEF), haemodynamic status, percentage of stenosis of the left main coronary artery, and number of major coronary arteries with more than 70% stenosis (STS only). Also chronic comorbidities like diabetes (STS only), vascular diseases, chronic renal insufficiency, and chronic obstructive pulmonary disease are included in the calculation.

However, neither the STS score nor the EuroScore has been sufficiently validated on emergency ACS patients, and their validity is thus limited.

Conclusion

Based on current guidelines, CABG in ACS is indicated whenever PCI is not suitable to relieve the patient's angina symptoms or to prevent further progression of coronary symptoms or vessel disease. Thus, CABG is most commonly indicated when a relatively complete PCI is not suitable in multivessel disease, or the risk of PCI is prohibitively high in patients with total chronic occlusion or complex bifurcational or trifurcational lesions.

The timing of surgery has to be based on ECG features ongoing angina symptoms, complexity of coronary artery disease, haemodynamic status, and availability of a cardiac surgery unit. If an operative indication arises in ACS, it is generally indicated emergently or urgently. With the onset or presence of cardiogenic shock, an immediate operation without delay is indicated and offers advantages over PCI [37, 39].

Surgery is guided by general strategies of CABG surgery, using at least one mammary artery to the LAD artery and further arterial grafts in younger patients. Surgical approaches not only involve a coronary revascularization, but also enable haemodynamic stabilization through various options for mechanical circulatory support. The use of an IABP should be freely considered whenever signs of haemodynamic compromise, ongoing angina, or high myocardial enzyme release are evident. There is some evidence that beating-heart surgery with or without the use of CPB is advantageous over conventional CABG using CPB and cardioplegic arrest in these critical patients. Early hospital results depend strongly on preoperative patient status and risk profile. Although asymptomatic patients with stable haemodynamics have an operative mortality risk of less than 2% comparable to elective CABG surgery, early mortality increases to more than 20% in patients with large infarctions and preoperative cardiogenic shock.

Personal perspective

An expeditious diagnosis and immediate referral to a cardiac/cardiac surgical centre remains the determining prognostic factor for patients with AMI. The differential indications for coronary revascularization ultimately depend on individual patient factors such as general condition, life expectancy, age, and comorbidities.

In general, the more complex the disease, the more urgently the patient has to be treated. However, if a patient is a potential surgical candidate the cardiac surgeon should be included in the treatment decision and management as soon as possible. Even in cases of high-risk PCI, early consultation with the cardiac surgery department is helpful. Surgical backup and collaboration between cardiologist and surgeons is needed to reduce delay in management and patient transfer to obtain the best outcome.

Further reading

Antman EM, Hand M, Armstrong PW, *et al.* 2007 focused update of the ACC/AHA 2004 guidelines for the management of patients with ST-elevation myocardial infarction. *Circulation* 2008;**117**:296–329.

Bassand JP, Hamm CW, Ardissino D, *et al.* Guidelines for the diagnosis and treatment of non-ST-segment elevation acute coronary syndromes. *Eur Heart J* 2007;**28**:1598–1660.

Eagle KA, Guyton RA, Davidoff R, *et al.* ACC/AHA 2004 guideline update for coronary artery bypass graft surgery: a report of the American College of Cardiology/American Heart Association Task Force on Practice Guidelines (Committee to Update the 1999 Guidelines for Coronary Artery Bypass Graft Surgery). *Circulation* 2004;**110**:e340–437.

George I, Oz MC. Myocardial revascularization after acute myocardial infarction. In: Cohn LH, Edmunds LH, *Cardiac surgery in the adult*, 3rd edition, pp. 669–696. McGraw-Hill, New York, 2003.

Hamm CW, Möllmann H, Bassand JP, *et al. The ESC textbook of cardiovascular medicine*, 2nd edition, Oxford University Press, Oxford, 20 09.

Kouchoukos N, Blackstone E, Doty D, *et al. Kirklin/Barratt-Boyes Cardiac surgery*, 3rd edition, pp. 353–437, Churchill Livingstone, Philadelphia, 2003.

Kushner FG, Hand M, Smith SC Jr, *et al.* 2009 focused updates: ACC/AHA guidelines for the management of patients with ST-elevation myocardial infarction. *Circulation* 2009;**120**:2271–2306.

Lemmer Jr JH, Richenbacher WE, Vlahakes GJ. *Handbook of patient care in cardiac surgery*, 6th edition, Lippincott Williams and Wilkins, Philadelphia, 2003.

Libby P, Bonow RO, Zipes DP, Mann DL. *Braunwald's heart disease*, 8th Edition, pp. 1344–1351, Saunders Elsevier, Philadelphia, 2008.

Patel MR, Dehmer GJ, Hirshfeld JW, *et al.* ACCF/SCAI/STS/AATS/AHA/ASNC 2009 appropriateness criteria for coronary revascularization. *J Am Coll Cardiol* 2009;**53**:530–533.

Silber S, Albertsson P, Avilés FF, *et al.* Guidelines for percutaneous coronary interventions. The Task Force for Percutaneous Coronary Interventions of the European Society of Cardiology. *Eur Heart J* 2005;**26**:804–847.

Van de Werf F, Bax J, Betriu A, *et al.* Management of acute myocardial infarction in patients presenting with persistent ST-segment elevation: the Task Force on the Management of ST-Segment Elevation Acute Myocardial Infarction of the European Society of Cardiology. *Eur Heart J* 2008;**29**:2909–2945.

Online resources

- ClinicalTrials.gov. http://www.clinicaltrials.gov/
- EuroSCORE. http://www.euroscore.org/
- Online STS Risk Calculator. http://209.220.160.181/STSWebRiskCalc261

⊃ For additional multimedia materials please visit the online version of the book (⟆ http://www.esciacc.oxfordmedicine.com).

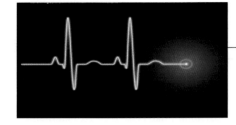

CHAPTER 47

Cardiogenic shock in patients with acute coronary syndromes

Zaza Iakobishvilli and David Hasdai

Contents

Summary

Cardiogenic shock is a clinically defined condition, often with dire consequences. Acute coronary syndromes (ACS) are the most common precipitating factors for shock, and effective revascularization is the only effective means that has been clinically proven to ameliorate outcomes in these circumstances.

Definition and diagnosis

Cardiogenic shock (CS) is defined in the presence of decreased cardiac output and, systemic perfusion in the presence of sufficient intravascular volume, and tissue hypoxia [1]. There is no single laboratory or clinical marker that can fully define this condition, making it primarily a clinically defined entity. As early as 1912, Herrick described the classic presentation of a CS patient with severe coronary artery disease—a weak, rapid pulse, feeble cardiac tones, pulmonary rales, dyspnoea, and cyanosis [2]. CS may develop as a consequence of different cardiovascular disorders other than ACS and occurs even in the presence of well-preserved left ventricular function [2].

Systemic hypotension is considered essential for the diagnosis of CS with common cut-off values for systolic blood pressure of less than 90 mmHg [3], or less than 80 mmHg [4] in different series and guidelines. If haemodynamic status is maintained solely by pharmacological or mechanical means, the diagnosis of CS may also be considered. A patient, usually with pre-existing hyperstension, may initially have clinical signs of CS in the presence of systolic blood pressure measurements greater than 90 mmHg, but a drop of more than 30 mmHg in the systolic blood pressure accompanied by clinical signs of CS may also define shock. It is important that the measurement be accurate and authentic; brachial cuff pressure measurements are often inaccurate in states of shock, and intra-arterial cannulas are used for more accurate monitoring.

Typical signs of systemic hypoperfusion in patients with shock include altered mental state, cool skin, and/or oliguria. Rales, indicating pulmonary congestion, may or may not be present. Neither auscultation nor chest radiograph detects pulmonary congestion in 30% of patients with CS [5].

Menon *et al.* [6] described severe left ventricular failure patients who have 'nonhypotensive CS'—a unique subgroup with preserved systolic blood pressure measurements (>90 mmHg without vasopressor support) but with the clinical signs of peripheral hypoperfusion, often among patients with large anterior wall myocardial infarctions. Mortality in this scenario of CS is substantial, albeit lower than that of patients with classic CS.

Measurement of cardiac output can be helpful for shock definition, but there is no universally accepted cut-off value. Some have considered cardiac index measurements of less than 2.2 L min^{-1} m^{-2} as confirmatory of the diagnosis [3], while others use a cut-off of 1.8 L min^{-1} m^{-2} [4]. The most accepted method of cardiac output determination is using pulmonary artery catheters, but because of the rare, but measurable, inherent risks of the procedure, it is not universally used in patients with CS [7]. Non-invasively derived haemodynamic parameters, such as left atrial pressure approximated by transmitral flow patterns and cardiac output computed by echocardiography (derived stroke volume multiplied by heart rate), are gaining acceptance, obviating the need for right heart catheterization [8].

There are possible pitfalls in interpreting haemodynamic data. For example, cardiac output measurements may be supernormal in patients for whom the underlying cause of CS is ventricular septal defect, or pulmonary capillary wedge pressure may be unexpectedly high in patients with right ventricular infarction caused by the leftward shift of the intraventricular septum (reversed Bernheim effect) or by concomitant left ventricular systolic dysfunction. Additionally, by the time right heart catheterization is performed, the patient with shock is typically already receiving supportive pharmacological treatment that can alter haemodynamic measurements. For example, treatment with a positive inotropic agent may improve a patient's subsequent cardiac output measurements, and treatment with diuretics may decrease subsequent pulmonary capillary wedge pressure measurements.

Tissue hypoxia is considered as another hallmark of CS, but it is difficult to assess by bedside assays and surrogate clinical and laboratory indices are sought. As the shock state persists, hypoperfusion of both the myocardium and peripheral tissues will induce anaerobic metabolism in these tissues and may result in lactic acidosis. Hyperlactataemia

as a result of hypoperfusion is independently associated with increased in-hospital mortality [9]. Another emerging technology for the assessment of tissue perfusion is side-stream dark-field imaging [10].

Aetiology of cardiogenic shock

A wide variety of cardiac disorders (ACS, valvular disease, myocardial and/or pericardial disease, congenital lesions (in both children and adults), or mechanical injuries to the heart can be complicated by CS. Because of the wide prevalence of coronary artery disease, CS as a complication of ACS is the predominant aetiology. In the international 'SHould we emergently revascularize Occluded Coronaries for cardiogenic shocK?' (SHOCK) trial registry of 1190 patients with CS, the predominant cause of shock was left ventricular failure (78.5%), while isolated right ventricular shock occurred in only 2.8% of patients. Mechanical complications of acute myocardial infarction (AMI) were observed among the remaining patients: severe mitral regurgitation (6.9%), ventricular septal rupture (3.9%), and tamponade (1.4%) [11] (➲Fig. 47.1).

Any noncoronary cause of left or right ventricular dysfunction may lead to CS. Inflammatory disorders (myopericarditis), stress-induced cardiomyopathy, hypertrophic cardiomyopathy, acute valvular regurgitation (due to endocarditis/trauma/degenerative causes), severe valvular stenosis exacerbated by acute stress, dysfunction of prosthetic valves ('stuck' valve), and massive pulmonary embolism are the examples of noncoronary causes that should be recognized in a timely manner. Adequate history, focused physical examination, prompt performance and adequate interpretation of the ECG and the echocardiogram in these very sick patients may alter treatment plans and decisions, and as a result improve survival.

Incidence of cardiogenic shock in acute coronary syndromes

Although CS occurs more frequently in the setting of ST-segment elevation ACS [12–14], it also occurs, albeit less commonly, in patients with non-ST-segment elevation ACS, even without positive cardiac biomarkers [15, 16].

Data on the incidence of shock are derived from large population-based analyses as well as from subset analyses of randomized clinical trials examining effects of different treatment modalities in the various forms of ACS. Due to differences in the definition of CS and criteria for including patients, the reported incidence of CS complicating ACS varies from 2.6% in the prethrombolytic era [17] to 6.7% in

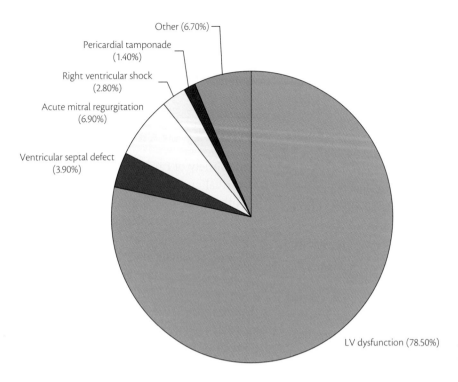

Figure 47.1 Predominant cause of cardiogenic shock in the SHOCK trial.

a contemporary cohort of consecutive AMI patients managed noninvasively [18].

ST-segment-elevation acute coronary syndrome and cardiogenic shock

In three large international thrombolytic therapy trials for ST-elevation AMI (STEMI), the incidence of shock ranged from 4.2% to 7.2% [12–14]. However, the reported incidence of CS among STEMI patients receiving thrombolytic therapy may be biased, since patients with shock are often not enrolled in multicenter randomized trials. Indeed, Zeymer and colleagues reported a 14.2% incidence of CS in 9422 patients in an 80-hospital primary percutaneous coronary intervention (PCI) German registry [19].

Until recently, the incidence of CS among STEMI patients appeared to be quite stable, despite increasing use of early reperfusion therapy, including primary PCI. Goldberg and colleagues [4] evaluated trends in the incidence of CS complicating STEMI in a single community from 1975 to 1997. The overall annual incidence for this period was 7.1% and ranged from 4.5% to 8.6%. In their more recent report, they demonstrate a decline in the incidence rates of CS from 1990, reaching a nadir of 4.1% in 2003 [20]. In a large observational study [21] from the National Registry of Myocardial Infarction (NRMI-2, 3, 4) that analysed data from 1.97 million acute STEMI patients hospitalized in the United States between 1994 and 2004, the incidence of CS was 8.6% overall, and was quite stable over the study period. In the Euro Heart Survey of Acute Coronary Syndromes,

the incidence of shock was 8.5% in the STEMI group [22]. In Global Registry of Acute Coronary Events (GRACE) registry, a reduction in the incidence of CS associated with STEMI was observed: 7.1% in 1999, subsequently decreasing significantly to 4.7% in 2005 [23].

Non-ST-elevation and cardiogenic shock

Limited data are available about the incidence of CS in the setting of non-ST-elevation ACS (NSTE ACS). In the Global Use of Strategies to Open Occluded Coronary Arteries (GUSTO IIb) trial [14], of the 7986 patients with NSTE ACS, CS occurred in 2.6% of cases. This was about half the incidence observed in the subgroup with ST-elevation ACS in the same trial. Of 9449 patients in the 'Platelet glycoprotein IIb/IIIa in Unstable angina: Receptor Suppression Using Integrilin Therapy' (PURSUIT) trial of patients with NSTE ACS [15], 237 (2.5%) developed shock after enrolment. In the large Euro Heart Survey of Acute Coronary Syndromes, the incidence of CS among patients admitted with NSTE ACS was 2.4% (of whom 1.7% developed it during hospitalization) [22]. In the GRACE registry, the incidence of shock among patients with NSTE ACS decreased significantly over a 6-year period, from 2.1% to 1.8% [23]. However, the 'Can Rapid Risk Stratification of Unstable Angina Patients Suppress Adverse Outcomes With Early Implementation of the ACC/AHA Guidelines' CRUSADE quality improvement initiative evaluated care patterns and outcomes for 17 926 high-risk NSTE ACS patients (as determined by positive cardiac markers and/or ischaemic ECG changes per ACC/AHA guidelines recommendations) at 248 United States hospitals with catheterization and revascularization facilities between March 2000 and September 2002, and found an incidence of CS that was remarkably consistent with all prior reports (2.6%) [16].

Right ventricular infarction and cardiogenic shock

Data about the frequency of right ventricular infarction as a cause of CS is very limited, because most patients with right ventricular infarction were excluded from randomized trials. In the SHOCK registry, the proportion of patients with shock complicating AMI who had shock due to 'isolated' right ventricular failure was 2.8% [11], even though in different ACS registries, right ventricular CS was rather frequent, ranging from 16.0% [24] to 19.6% [25].

Time to development of cardiogenic shock in acute coronary syndromes

In the prethrombolysis era, Leor and colleagues [17] reported that shock developed at a median of 2 days after admission (range 3 h to 16 days) in patients admitted without heart failure. Hands *et al.* [26] reported that CS developed after hospitalization in 60 (7.1%) of 845 patients presenting with AMI. Half of the patients who did not have shock upon admission developed shock within the first 24 h.

In large thrombolytic trials, the median time to the occurrence of shock among patients with persistent ST-segment elevation who developed in-hospital shock was 10 or 11 h [13,14], with most experiencing shock within the first 48 h after enrolment. Shock occurred later after symptom onset in patients without ST-segment elevation compared with those with ST-segment elevation and is often associated with reinfarction (◗Fig. 47.2). In GUSTO IIb, NSTE ACS patients developed shock a median of 76.2 h after enrolment, in contrast to ST-elevation ACS patients for whom the median time to onset was 9.6 h [14]. In the SHOCK Trial Registry [27], time from AMI onset to shock onset was also different: 8.9 h for NSTE ACS patients versus 5.9 h for ST-elevation ACS patients. In the PURSUIT database of NSTE ACS, shock most commonly developed >48 h after enrolment (median 94.0 h) [15]. The difference in time to development of shock between patients with versus those without ST elevation suggests variation in the underlying

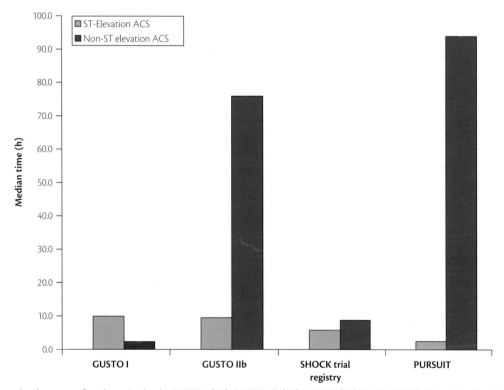

Figure 47.2 Time to development of cardiogenic shock: GUSTO-I [13], GUSTO IIb [14], SHOCK [27], PURSUIT [15]. (Clearly, by the inclusion criteria non-ST-elevation myocardial infarction patients were not included in GUSTO I trial nor were STEMI patients included in PURSUIT trial; their appearance in the figure is only for comparison purposes among two subgroups of ACS).

mechanisms of the condition. Moreover, it may reflect differences in the baseline clinical and demographic characteristics, differences in antecedent cardiac function, and differences in the extent and nature of the coronary artery disease.

Risk factors for development of cardiogenic shock

Timely recognition of high-risk ACS patients prone to develop CS is the one way to improve survival. Older age, anterior location of AMI, and previous hypertension, diabetes mellitus, AMI/angina, and heart failure, and ST-elevation ACS and left bundle branch block indicate increased risk for shock [18]. Low admission systolic blood pressure, high heart rate, and advanced Killip class combined with the patient's age provided 85% of the information needed to predict shock in the model derived from the GUSTO-I dataset [28]. Women may have a higher incidence of CS than men [29].

Pathophysiology

Left ventricular dysfunction as a cause of cardiogenic shock

There are several determinants of left ventricular dysfunction in CS: new irreversible injury, reversible ischaemia, and scar from previous AMI. Thus the index event is often, but not always, severe. Decrease in coronary flow with resulting compromise of cardiac output causes a vicious cycle, which further decreases systemic blood flow. Disease in nonculprit arteries may exacerbate myocardial ischaemia ('remote ischaemia') and haemodynamics.

A concept that CS develops in the case of severe left ventricular dysfunction with resultant low left ventricular ejection fraction was challenged in the analysis of the SHOCK trial and registry [30]. The mean left ventricular ejection fraction in the SHOCK trial was approximately 30% [31]. Similar values of left ventricular ejection fraction in shock and in the subacute/chronic phases of AMI indicate that the magnitude of myocardial insult that causes CS need not be profound. However, among patients with CS, the left ventricular ejection fraction remains a prognostic factor [32]. Altered diastolic function (ventricular relaxation and compliance) probably plays an important contributory role in the pathophysiology of CS.

Right ventricular dysfunction as a cause of cardiogenic shock

Adequate right ventricular filling pressure maintains cardiac output and left ventricle preload. In cases of CS due to predominant right ventricle infarction, very high end-diastolic pressure is observed in the affected ventricle [33]. Aggressive volume replacement therapy for right ventricular CS can cause the leftward shift of the intraventricular septum (reversed Bernheim effect), with resultant impaired left ventricle filling and systolic function [34].

Inflammation and cardiogenic shock

Decreased cardiac output in CS and ongoing ischaemia cause increased release of catecholamines and other vasopressors (vasopressin and angiotensin II) with transient afterload augmentation and improvement in coronary and peripheral perfusion. Reflex mechanisms of increased systemic vascular resistance are not fully effective in CS, as demonstrated by variable values of systemic vascular resistance, with a median value in the normal range, despite use of vasopressors in the SHOCK trial [35]. Indeed, in some shock patients, the systemic vascular resistance may be low, similar to values found in the systemic inflammatory response syndrome. Along with increased secretion of cytokines, complement, procalcitonin, neopterin, and C-reactive protein, the increased expression of inducible NO synthase is thought to be involved in CS pathogenesis [36].

Iatrogenic cardiogenic shock

In some cases of ACS, the use of vasoactive medications may contribute to the development of CS. In the 'Clopidogrel and Metoprolol in Myocardial Infarction' trial (COMMIT), increased risk of CS was observed during the first day after the early use of intravenous followed by oral β-blocker [37]. The large meta-analysis of early use of angiotensin-converting enzyme (ACE) inhibition found an excess of CS of 4.6 patients per 1000 treated [38]. Uncontrolled use of diuretics and nitrates, especially in inferior wall myocardial infarction with right ventricular infarction, can also result in haemodynamic instability.

Treatment

General measures

Patients in CS due to ACS deserve the accepted and well-proved antithrombotic treatment (heparins, aspirin, clopidogrel). Some authorities recommend postponing clopidogrel pretreatment before coronary angiography is performed [43]. Adequate oxygenation by face mask or endotracheal tube should be instituted.

Intra-aortic balloon counterpulsation

The intra-aortic balloon pump (IABP) increases diastolic coronary artery perfusion and decreases systemic afterload without increasing myocardial oxygen demand. Little data are available to support its use in improving outcomes of patients with shock. In the SHOCK registry, patients treated with IABP in conjunction with thrombolytic therapy had the lowest in-hospital mortality rate (47%). Patients with STEAMI who did not receive IABP and/or thrombolytic therapy had the worst baseline risk status [44]. The SHOCK registry data suggests that initial stabilization of CS patients using an IABP may be associated with a 20% absolute risk reduction in mortality.

In the Thrombolysis and Counterpulsation to Improve Cardiogenic Shock Survival (TACTICS) trial, the only randomized trial examining the role of IABP deployment (within 3 h of thrombolysis), mortality at 6 months was 39% in the patients randomly assigned to receive IABP, whereas it was 80% in those randomly assigned to thrombolysis alone [45].

IABP was recommended in the SHOCK trial protocol and used in 87% of patients for a median duration of approximately 3 days. Overall, IABP usage was not an independent predictor of mortality at 12 months. However, in patients with systemic hypoperfusion whose haemodynamics and end-organ perfusion were improved by IABP, the mortality rates were lower at 12 months in both the initial medical stabilization and the early revascularization treatment groups.

IABP use is firmly advocated in current guidelines for the treatment of CS patients [41]. Despite this, a perplexingly low rate of utilization of IABP in CS patients was observed in the EuroHeart Survey of ACS [22].

In summary, all patients having CS without contraindications should receive IABP for at least 3 days or longer if clinically indicated, for recovery from myocardial stunning.

Right heart catheterization

The role of right heart catheterization in the management of CS patients remains controversial. On the one hand, there are retrospective data on mortality hazard associated with this procedure [39]. On the other hand, there is positive experience from GUSTO-I and the SHOCK registry [40].

Due to the paucity of evidence-based evidence proving its efficacy, current European guidelines recommend right heart catheterization as a class IIb indication for patients with ST-elevation ACS who have CS [41].

Echocardiography

Echocardiography with Doppler imaging has become a readily available modality for bedside haemodynamic assessment and for the evaluation of cardiac function, valvular status, and mechanical complications of ACS [42]. Its use has steadily increased over the years, and currently it is performed routinely among ACS patients in many institutions. This noninvasive, readily available method has replaced right heart catheterization use in most situations.

Inotropes

In patients with CS, a mean arterial pressure of 60 mmHg is generally necessary for tissue perfusion. Experience in patients with septic shock has shown that further elevation of the mean blood pressure by noradrenaline (norepinephrine) did not improve further systemic perfusion but did increase myocardial oxygen demands [46]. The use of inotropes is recommended immediately after recognition of shock despite euvolaemic status having been achieved, before instituting IABP and revascularization and until CS resolution. Data on comparison of vasopressor are scant. The European Society of Cardiology (ESC) guidelines recommend the use of high-dose dopamine or dobutamine for improving or stabilization of the haemodynamic state [41]. Newer drugs (levosimendan, vasopressin) warrant further investigation in clinical trials.

Diuretics and fluids

The estimated left ventricular filling pressure directs use of diuretics and fluids in the setting of CS. For an estimation of filling pressure readily available different clinical parameters can be used: hourly monitored urinary output in conjunction with clear lung fields and absence of pulmonary congestion on chest radiograph may indicate a need for volume replacement therapy, especially in the setting of right ventricular infarction, whereas progressive desaturation and pulmonary congestion obviate the need for diuretic therapy. It should be mentioned that patients in CS might need optimization of left ventricular filling pressures even in the presence of a priori elevated pulmonary capillary wedge pressure to ensure maximal performance on the Starling curve. In these difficult cases right heart catheterization may be of value (see ➜ Right heart catheterization).

Glycoprotein IIb/IIIa receptor antagonists and bivalirudin

There is some evidence that CS outcomes are improved by the use of GPIIb/IIIa receptor antagonists. In the PURSUIT trial, shock patients who received eptifibatide had a 50% reduction of 30-day mortality (58.5% vs 73.5% for placebo, OR 0.51, 95% CI 0.28, 0.94, $p = 0.03$) [15]. The available data favor administration of GPIIb/IIIa antagonists, particularly abciximab, in patients with CS who are undergoing percutaneous intervention, unless the risk of bleeding is considered to be too great. In the REO-SHOCK trial, 40 patients with STEMI and CS were treated with primary revascularization, abciximab, heparin, and aspirin. The mortality rate observed at 30 days was 42.5%. Abciximab seemed to improve outcomes of younger (<75 years) versus elderly patients (>75 years), with mortality rates of 24% and 91%, respectively [47]. To test this hypothesis, the Czech PRAGUE-7 trial (80 patients) was conducted which compared routine up-front abciximab versus standard periprocedural therapy in patients undergoing primary PCI for CS [48]. The primary endpoint was reached in 17 patients in the up-front treatment group (42.5%) and 11 in the standard therapy arm (27.5%; $p = 0.24$). Thus routine use of abciximab in CS patients is not supported by this (as yet unpublished) trial.

Another antithrombotic drug, bivalirudin, was shown to be safe and effective with provisional use of abciximab in patients undergoing primary PCI for AMI complicated by CS [49].

Other pharmacological therapy

N-Monomethyl-L-arginine (L-NMMA) was tested in a large trial of CS that was stopped for futility by the steering committee and showed no benefit in addition to revascularization [36]. Adenosine, sodium/hydrogen exchange inhibitors, antioxidants, and glucose–insulin–potassium (GIK) infusion were not found to be useful in the treatment of patients with CS.

Reperfusion therapy

Thrombolytic therapy is less effective but is indicated when PCI is impossible or if a delay has occurred in patient transfer for PCI and when AMI and CS onset is within 3 h. The use of IABP may increase the efficacy of thrombolytic therapy in patients with hypotension by increasing perfusion pressure.

Bypass surgery

Early studies of coronary revascularization for cardiogenic chock focused on surgical revascularization. Several small surgical series reported relatively good outcomes in patients with CS [49, 50]. According to SHOCK trial data, surgically revascularized patients benefited most: the 30-day mortality was 45.3% among the 75 patients who underwent angioplasty alone and 42.1% among 57 patients who underwent bypass surgery. The trial was not designed to compare percutaneous and surgical revascularization strategies [31]. In the large nation-wide Society of Thoracic Surgeons National Cardiac Database, 708 593 patients were referred for coronary artery bypass grafting (CABG) with and without concomitant valvular surgery; 2.1% of them had preoperative CS [51]. Operative mortality for CS was high and depended on the surgery type, ranging from 20% for isolated CABG to 33% for CABG combined with valvular surgery and 58% for CABG plus ventricular septal repair. It is worth noting that although age was strongly associated with operative mortality, fully 70% of patients even in the oldest age group (≥75 years) survived CABG for CS with 22% overall in-hospital mortality. The National Registry of Myocardial Infarction (2002–2004) reported in-hospital mortality of 16.7–28.6% in a small number of patients with CS undergoing CABG [21]. Similarly, the SHOCK trial registry (884 patients) reported 24% in-hospital mortality for CABG [52]. These data are often criticized for referral bias (healthier patients were sent for CABG than for coronary angioplasty) and the characteristic drawback of registries—unmeasured risk factors influencing operative risk. In conclusion, although only a minority of CS patients are referred for CABG and mortality is high, operative treatment should be considered in carefully selected individuals with multivessel disease and/or severe valvular problems.

Coronary angioplasty

Two prospective randomized trials evaluated the role of revascularization among patients with CS. The 'Swiss Multicenter trial of Angioplasty for Shock' (SMASH) trial involved 55 patients with AMI complicated by CS. They were randomized to undergo revascularization (surgical or percutaneous) versus medical therapy alone [53]. SMASH was stopped prematurely because of low enrolment; partly because of the perception of physicians that revascularization was beneficial based on retrospective analyses of registries. In this small, undersized cohort, a 9% absolute reduction in 30-day mortality was seen among patients treated with revascularization (69% vs 78%), a difference that did not achieve statistical significance.

In the second randomized study, the 'Should We Emergently Revascularize Occluded Coronaries for Cardiogenic Shock' (SHOCK) trial, patients who developed CS within the first 36 h of AMI (either ST-segment elevation, or new left bundle branch block) were eligible for enrolment; patients with mechanical causes for shock or predominantly right ventricular infarction were excluded [31]. In SHOCK, an aggressive, invasive approach (angioplasty or coronary artery bypass surgery, generally with IABP) was compared with medical treatment—initial medical stabilization, including thrombolytic therapy and IABP. Randomization was required within 12 h of shock onset. Most patients randomized to the invasive arm (n = 152) underwent coronary angiography (97%), and 87% underwent revascularization (surgical or percutaneous). The primary endpoint of the study was 30-day mortality. In the invasive arm, the mortality was 46.7%, as compared to 56.0% in the conservative arm ($p = 0.11$). The mortality difference at 6 months achieved statistical significance and was lower in the invasive arm (50.3% vs 63.1%, $p = 0.027$). The survival curves continued to diverge at 12 months of follow-up [54]. In a prespecified subgroup analysis, the benefit of the invasive strategy were seen only in patients younger than 75 years of age, in whom the 30-day mortality was 56.8% for the conservative arm versus 41.4% for the invasive arm. However, 30-day survival among medically treated patients older than 75 years tended to be better than that of older patients in the invasive arm.

The 13% absolute reduction in mortality at 6 months associated with the aggressive revascularization strategy (50.3% vs 63.1%, $p = 0.027$) was both statistically and clinically significant. On the basis of the SHOCK trial, the ESC and American College of Cardiology/American Heart Association (ACC/AHA) guidelines for the treatment of patients with AMI have included early revascularization for shock as a class I indication, particularly for those less than 75 years of age [41, 55].

Of note, while analysing the subgroup of elderly patients in the SHOCK registry, Dzavik et al. [56] found that those who underwent early revascularization had lower in-hospital mortality rates (48% vs 81%, $p = 0.0003$) and after exclusion of 65 early deaths and covariate adjustment, the relative risk was 0.76 (0.59, 0.99; $p = 0.045$) in patients

aged less than 75 years and 0.46 (0.28, 0.75; $p = 0.002$) in patients aged 75 years or more. In a prospective registry of consecutive PCI in northern New England [57] the mortality rate for elderly shock patients undergoing PCI was 46%, which is significantly less than previously reported in randomized clinical trials. The management of elderly people with AMI complicated by CS requires good clinical judgement.

Several clinical, angiographic, and procedural characteristics determining survival were derived by the analysis of percutaneous revascularization data from the SHOCK trial [58]. Restoration of coronary blood flow appeared to be a major predictor of survival in CS. Coronary revascularization benefits shock patients beyond the accepted 12-h postinfarction window. Severe mitral regurgitation in shock patients after PCI was associated with 67% 1-year mortality, so surgery should be considered in shock patients with severe mitral insufficiency or multivessel disease not amenable to relatively complete PCI. In another analysis [59] of the same dataset, left ventricular function and culprit vessel patency were independent correlates of 1-year survival in revascularized patients.

In GRACE, PCI with coronary stenting was the most powerful predictor of hospital survival among shock patients [60].

There are very limited data on revascularization for NSTE ACS shock. In the SHOCK registry, the authors found a nonsignificant survival benefit for patients with NSTE ACS who underwent revascularization after adjustment for patient age and several treatment characteristics [61].

Thus, rapid revascularization, whether percutaneous or surgical, seems to reduce mortality in patients with AMI complicated by CS. It is perplexing that in the Euro Heart Survey of ACS less than one half of CS patients received any revascularization [22]. It is proposed that that the previous functional status, especially for elderly patients, should determine a revascularization approach [43].

Left ventricular assist devices

There are several surgically and percutaneously implanted devices beyond standard treatment for haemodynamic support of CS patients, but experience is limited [62 –64]. Use of left ventricular assist devices in CS is recommended by the ESC guidelines as a class IIa indication with level of evidence C [41].

Conclusion

Cardiogenic shock is the most dire complication of ACS with very high mortality rate even in the modern era. Mechanical revascularization has been proved as the only effective treatment for this condition. Thus, prevention of the shock by providing timely reperfusion and aggressive intervention (pharmacologic support and percutaneous/surgical revascularization) at the early stages of its development are the keys for improving outcomes.

Personal perspective

Although CS is the leading cause of mortality among patients with ACS, its prognosis remains ominous. It seems that any significant improvement in the outcomes of ACS is going to entail improved outcomes of shock. Pharmacotherapy has so far been disappointing in this condition. It seems that the mechanical relief of ischaemia currently plays a major role in the treatment of shock. Given the complexity of the pathogenesis of shock, it seems that there are still several areas for possible pharmacological intervention that warrant investigation. It is high time that new drugs, other than conventional inotropes, were developed to assist in the management of these difficult patients. Concomitantly, the development of more efficient assist devices may improve outcomes, as compared with the conventional IABP.

Further reading

Hasdai D. *Cardiogenic shock: diagnosis and treatment*, Humana Press, Totowa, NJ, 2002.

Hasdai D, Califf RM, Thompson TD, *et al.* Predictors of cardiogenic shock after thrombolytic therapy for acute myocardial infarction. *J Am Coll Cardiol* 2000;**35**(1):136–143.

Hochman JS, Buller CE, Sleeper LA, *et al.* Cardiogenic shock complicating acute myocardial infarction—etiologies, management and outcome: a report from the SHOCK Trial Registry. SHould we emergently revascularize Occluded Coronaries for cardiogenic shocK? *J Am Coll Cardiol* 2000;**36**(3 Suppl A):1063–1070.

Hochman JS, Sleeper LA, Webb JG, *et al.* Early revascularization in acute myocardial infarction complicated by cardiogenic shock: SHOCK investigators: Should We Emergently Revascularize Occluded Coronaries for Cardiogenic Shock. *N Engl J Med.* 1999;**341**:625–634.

Thiele H, Smalling RW, Schuler GC. Percutaneous left ventricular assist devices in acute myocardial infarction complicated by cardiogenic shock. *Eur Heart J* 2007;**28**:2057–2063.

Van de Werf F, Bax J, Betriu A, *et al.* Management of acute myocardial infarction with persistent ST-segment elevation. Task force on the management of ST-segment elevation acute myocardial infarction of the European Society of Cardiology. *Eur Heart J* 2008;**29**:2909–2945.

⊃ For additional multimedia materials please visit the online version of the book (⌘ http://www.esciacc.oxfordmedicine.com).

CHAPTER 48

Gender considerations in acute coronary syndromes

Eva Swahn, Joakim Alfredsson, and Sofia Sederholm Lawesson

Contents

Summary

Gender differences in ACS have been increasingly recognized. Although women are 5–10 years older than men in an ACS population, mortality rates from cardiovascular causes are similar. Risk factors for coronary heart disease appear to be virtually the same in men and women. Gender differences in symptoms associated with an acute MI have been intensively debated. There seem to be some differences but later studies have shown that chest pain is the most frequent symptom in both women and men.

Gender differences in treatment intensity, including differences in level of care, have been reported. Also differences in benefit from certain treatments, especially invasive treatment, and side effects have been discussed but in the ACS area treatment guidelines make no difference between the genders.

Finally, difference in outcome between men and women, have been proposed. Results have been inconsistent, partly depending on if and how adjustment for differences in background characteristics has been made. Fewer women than men have been included in cardiovascular trials and consequently the evidence base regarding several treatments is less firm for women. Prospective studies to elucidate whether there are true differences in the effects of different treatment strategies according to gender, and the importance of differences in underlying pathophysiology and comorbidity are strongly needed to identify the most appropriate treatment for men and women respectively.

Introduction

In both women and men, cardiovascular disease (CVD) remains the leading cause of death in Europe. This is true in spite of a continuous decrease in morbidity as well as mortality during recent decades. The most common manifestation of ischaemic heart disease is acute coronary syndrome (ACS) which includes sudden cardiac death, ST-elevation myocardial infarction (STEMI), non-ST-elevation MI (NSTEMI), and unstable angina pectoris (UA). Because of similarities in their pathophysiology and treatment, NSTEMI and UA are often referred to as non-ST-elevation ACS (NSTE ACS). Although in-hospital mortality is higher in STEMI than NSTE ACS, long-term mortality is comparable [1].

The ACS population is very heterogeneous, with wide variations in risk of death and new ischaemic events as well as in ACS type. Early risk stratification is therefore a key part of the management of these patients.

It has been shown in numerous trials that women with STEMI, even after adjustment for their greater age and more frequent comorbidities, are less intensively investigated and have a worse outcome than men. These gender differences might be explained by the lower use of evidence-based treatment. On the other hand, we do not know if today's evidence-based medicine is applicable to both genders, as fewer women than men have been included in most clinical studies of CVD. Whether this reflects a lower incidence in women or actual exclusion of women from the trials is debatable, but the consequence is that the evidence regarding several of the established treatments is less clear for women than it is for men.

The clinical challenge today is to identify individual patients with the highest risk for ischaemic events, without unreasonably elevated early risk for complications with treatment. For example, actions to minimize bleeding complications including dose adjustments according to renal function, weight, and age are of the utmost importance for both genders, but particularly for women. However, an individually tailored treatment strategy to balance early procedural risk with long-term reduction of cardiac events will benefit both men and women with ACS.

Our aim in this chapter is to focus on gender-specific similarities and differences that are important to identify and learn in order not to harm our patients.

Epidemiology

During the last two decades MI mortality has decreased by about 50% in most industrialized countries. The decrease is evident for both men and women, although somewhat more pronounced in men. Explanations for the marked decrease in mortality are a combination of improved risk factor status, acute treatment, and prevention. Even so, incidence of MI has remained high and CVD, with coronary heart disease (CHD) being the most prevalent, are the most common causes of death in both men and women [2, 3].

Pathophysiology and risk factors

The pathogenesis of ACS involves two different processes: a slow atherosclerotic process, with low degree of reversibility, that lasts for decades, and a fast, dynamic, and potentially reversible process characterized by plaque rupture or erosion, with subsequent thrombus formation. Studies have shown that endothelial erosion is more common in women [4, 5]. In patients with NSTE ACS several studies have shown less obstructive coronary artery disease in women, [6–8] even in patients with elevated markers [9]. Both these findings indicate different pathophysiological backgrounds to ACS, with different impact in men and women.

Early longitudinal studies revealed that there are gender differences in risk factor prevalence, especially in young and middle-aged individuals. Although there are differences between men and women in the impact of certain risk factors (diabetes and smoking being the most obvious), there is a striking similarity between the genders in relative risk associated with most of the classical risk factors [10].

The INTERHEART study, a case–control study from 52 populations all over the world, investigated the association of nine potentially modifiable risk factors for a first MI [11, 12]. The six factors positively associated with increased risk for a first MI were hyperlipidaemia, smoking, hypertension, diabetes, abdominal obesity, and psychosocial stress. The three factors negatively associated with MI (i.e. protective) were physical activity, low-risk diet (daily vegetables and fruits), and moderate alcohol consumption. The study confirmed that CHD determinants were the same in women and men, and these nine factors accounted for 90% of the population attributable risk in men and 94% in women. However, there were small differences between the genders in the strength of a certain risk factor. Hypertension, diabetes, physical inactivity, and lack of alcohol intake were more strongly associated with MI in women than men. Several longitudinal studies have also indicated that smoking is a more powerful risk factor in women than in men [10, 13].

Risk stratification

The ACS population is very heterogeneous, with a large variation in risk for future ischaemic events or death. Therefore, stratification of patients according to risk for future cardiac events, but also in order to identify patients with the highest benefit from intensive treatment, have become an integrated part of the management of NSTE ACS patients [14].

The two best-established objective findings used in risk stratification are ECG changes (in NSTE ACS, mainly ST depression) and elevation of myocardial damage markers (today, preferably troponins). Several studies have confirmed ST depression as a marker of risk of death and MI [15, 16] and as a marker to properly identify patients who will benefit most from a more intensive treatment [17]. In the same way, troponins are established markers for prediction of MI and death and benefit from an invasive strategy [18]. In a meta-analysis of 7 clinical trials and 19 cohort studies on patients with NSTE ACS, patients with elevated troponin had higher mortality [19]. Little is known about the differences between men and women in the prognostic value of ECG changes and biomarkers.

Since ACS is a complex event, different markers may reflect different pathophysiological aspects of the disease. Combining markers for myocardial necrosis, inflammation, neurohormonal activation, and renal dysfunction in a multimarker approach has been proposed and studies have demonstrated that such an approach improves risk stratification [20]. Wiviott *et al.* reported in a substudy from the TACTICS-TIMI 18 trial that a multimarker approach identified a higher proportion of high-risk women, but lack of any marker elevation also identified very low-risk women. Men were more likely to have elevated CK-MB or troponin, while women were more likely to have elevated C-reactive protein or B-type natriuretic peptide [21].

A number of risk factor scores have been constructed, among them the GRACE score, the TIMI score, and the FRISC score. In one rather small study the TIMI score was shown to correctly predict 30-day death, MI, or revascularization in both men and women [22]. Whether the GRACE and FRISC-scores perform equally in men and women is not well known.

Clinical presentation and symptoms

In a chest pain population, a substantially higher proportion of men compared to women have ACS [23]. A possible sex difference in symptoms in the ACS population has been debated for a long time and is still somewhat controversial but new knowledge tends in the opposite direction, i.e. more similarities than differences. A recent Swedish study with MI patients aged 25–74 years could not find any statistically significant sex difference in the proportion of patients with chest pain, which was 90–95%. Nausea, back pain, dizziness, and palpitations were significantly more common in women, and women as a group reported a greater number of symptoms than men did [24]. A recent study from the GRACE registry showed similar results: over 90% of both men and women with ACS had chest pain [24, 25].

Two earlier large meta-analyses reviewing ACS studies, reporting symptom data from 1989–2002 and 1970–2005, showed a somewhat higher prevalence of chest pain in men than in women [26, 27]. In the cumulative summary of the large cohort studies in the meta-analysis of Canto *et al.*, 37% of the women compared to 27% of the men had no chest pain [27]. There are several confounders that or less could explain these differences. As women present 5–10 years later than men, age is an important factor: older patients present less often with chest pain and more often with atypical symptoms such as dyspnoea, confusion, or fatigue [28–31]. This could be due to a higher pain threshold [32] or changes in autonomic function among older patients [33, 34]. Another important confounding factor is diabetes. It is well known that women with ACS have a higher prevalence of diabetes than men. Patients with diabetic neuropathy have been found to have impaired perception of cardiac ischaemia [35], and diabetic patients thus have higher frequencies of silent MI [36].

As in the two recent studies cited above, some studies have found a higher prevalence of atypical symptoms in women [25, 37–39], and this was also found in two meta-analyses [26, 27]. Women have more symptoms than men, and more often had back, neck, or jaw pain; nausea and vomiting; shortness of breath; palpitations; dizziness; and fatigue. During an acute coronary occlusion, women has been shown to react with more vagal activation than men [40]. This could be one possible reason why nausea and dizziness are more common symptoms in women than in men with MI.

Several studies have found longer patient delay in women compared to men [41, 42], but there are also earlier studies supporting a longer doctor's delay for female MI patients, such as longer time from admission to the first ECG [43], to thrombolytic therapy [44, 45], or to percutaneous coronary intervention (PCI) [46]. It has been proposed that difficulties in proper identification and interpretation of symptoms by both patients and health care professionals could cause this delay [47]. Thus it is important to acknowledge that chest pain is the most important and common symptom in both sexes, but atypical symptoms could also be present slightly more often in women.

Medical treatment

β-Blockers

Evidence for β-blockers in the context of ACS is based on a very limited amount of randomized trial data, and most of the studies were performed more than two decades ago. Although there is a lack of gender-specific data, no obvious differences in effect between the genders have been shown [48].

β-Blockers are recommended for secondary prevention in the absence of contraindications, without difference between the genders. The indication is stronger in patients with left ventricular systolic dysfunction.

Lipid-lowering treatment

Statin therapy improves long-term outcome [49] and is recommended to be initiated early in all patients with ACS [50]. Men were in the majority in most statin trials, and gender-specific data are still scarce, with somewhat contradictory results. There are studies reflecting secondary prevention [51], primary prevention in high-risk individuals [52], and primary prevention in individuals with low cholesterol but elevated CRP [53], with no apparent difference in effect between the genders. However, with a lower event rate in women, benefit was more uncertain.

Angiotensin converting enzyme inhibitors/ angiotensin receptor blockers

Several studies have shown that angiotensin converting enzyme (ACE) inhibitors are beneficial in reducing remodelling and improving survival in patients with reduced left ventricular systolic function after MI [54–56]. In patients who are intolerant to ACE inhibitors, angiotensin-2 receptor blockers (ARBs) are indicated [57]. Treatment is indicated in all ACS patients with left ventricular dysfunction, diabetes, or hypertension [54–56]. A meta-analysis (based on 10 267 men and 2396 women) indicated similar effect in men and women [58].

Antithrombotic treatment

Antithrombotic therapy is fundamental in the acute treatment of ACS to prevent progression of the thrombotic process in the afflicted coronary artery, and it is also essential in long-term treatment to prevent new ischaemic events. Antithrombotic treatment is especially important in clinical settings involving PCI and should be implemented as early as possible.

Aspirin

Randomized trials of aspirin compared with placebo, dating from the 1980s, showed consistent benefit for patients with UA/NSTEMI by reducing the risk of nonfatal MI by approximately 50% [59, 60].

Indirect comparison of maintenance doses has shown similar effects in a broad range (75–1500 mg) but a dose-dependent increase in bleeding [61]. Hence a maintenance dose of 75–162 mg/day is recommended. A recent meta-analysis revealed similar effect in men and women in secondary prevention, driven by a reduction in ischaemic stroke in women and MI in men and similar degrees of bleeding [62].

ADP receptor antagonists

Clopidogrel proved effective in combination with aspirin after NSTE ACS in the CURE study, with a 20% reduction of the composite endpoint cardiovascular death, MI, or stroke. Risk reduction was directionally the same in men and women, but lower and not statistically significant in women [63]. In the TRITON trial, prasugrel was compared to clopidogrel in ACS patients (74% NSTE ACS), on top of aspirin and it was shown that prasugrel was more effective in reducing death and ischaemic endpoints but with significant more major bleedings [64]. Gender differences parallelled those in the CURE trial, with less pronounced and statistically not significant, although directionally the same, risk reduction in women. In a recent meta-analysis of all blinded randomized clinical trials comparing clopidogrel and placebo, the relative efficacy and safety of clopidogrel in reducing CVD events in women and men was analysed. This analysis showed that there were no significant gender differences in either treatment effect, reducing CVD by 14% or in increasing bleeding risk by 42% [65]. In the recently published PLATO trial the reversible ADP receptor antagonist ticagrelor proved superior to clopidogrel in ACS patients (38% STEMI), with a lower rate of the primary endpoint (cardiovascular death/MI or stroke). Subgroup analysis revealed similar, and statistically significant, benefits in both men and women [66].

Nonresponders to antiplatelet treatment

Substantial interindividual variation in effect of both aspirin and clopidogrel has been observed [67, 68], and these so called 'nonresponders' or 'low responders' appear to be at increased risk of new ischaemic events [69, 70]. Optimal individual management of antiplatelet therapy may therefore in the near future involve monitoring of platelet activity and individual tailoring of treatment (i.e. choice of drug or dose adjustment) based on individual responsiveness.

There are reports on differences in the proportion of men and women who could be defined as nonresponders, which is why monitoring of responsiveness might be even more important in women [71].

Glycoprotein IIb/IIIa antagonists

A meta-analysis of the six large randomized glycoprotein (GP)IIb/IIIa antagonist trials in patients with UAP/NSTEMI, not routinely scheduled to undergo coronary angiography, showed a modest benefit by reducing the combined endpoint (death/MI) by 30 days (11.8% vs 10.8%, OR 0.91, 95% CI 0.84–0.98). The effect was mainly restricted to patients with high-risk features such as elevated troponin or ST depression. Patients undergoing PCI or coronary artery bypass grafting (CABG) had greater risk reduction compared to those not revascularized [72]. In the same meta-analysis, a subgroup analysis revealed significant interaction with gender. Although men had a significant benefit in reduction of death/MI by 30 days, harm was indicated in women (OR = 0.81 vs 1.15, p for interaction <0.0001) [72].

Low-molecular-weight heparin

Trials of low-molecular-weight heparin (LMWH) added to treatment with aspirin have generally shown favourable results for the combination in the acute phase, but extended treatment after hospital discharge has been less convincing [73].

The FRISC trial indicated an independent relation between anti-Xa activity and gender, resulting in a more pronounced effect of dalteparin treatment in women [74].

Direct thrombin inhibitors

The synthetic hirudin analogue bivalirudin was compared to UFH/enoxaparin in ACS patients (65% NSTE ACS) in the ACUITY trial. Bivalirudin alone was not inferior to bivalirudin+GPIIB/IIIa or UFH/LMWH+GPIIb/IIIa in the composite ischaemic endpoint, but with lower rate of bleeding [75]. A subgroup analysis according to gender showed no difference in effect but higher net clinical adverse events in women due to more bleeding complications than in men [76].

In another large scale prospective study (HORIZONS-AMI), patients with high-risk STEMI undergoing primary PCI were randomly assigned to receive bivalirudin alone or heparin plus a GPIIB/IIIa inhibitor where bivalirudin reduced the rates of net adverse clinical events and major bleeding at 1 year; no gender analyses were performed [77].

Factor Xa inhibitors

In the OASIS 5 and 6 trials, it was shown that compared with a heparin-based strategy, fondaparinux reduced mortality, ischaemic events, and major bleeding across the full spectrum of ACS and was associated with a more favourable net clinical outcome in patients undergoing either an invasive or a conservative management strategy [78, 79].

Subgroup analyses regarding net clinical benefit revealed no gender interaction.

Reperfusion therapy and coronary angiography in STEMI

Several studies have shown that women with STEMI present at the hospital after a significantly longer delay after symptom onset than their male counterparts [80, 81]. This could be one reason why women with STEMI were treated with thrombolytic therapy less often than men during the thrombolytic era, as time from symptom to treatment is crucial when using this type of reperfusion therapy. Thrombolytic therapy for STEMI has been associated with a higher risk of stroke and bleeding in women compared to men, but also with a greater relative reduction in mortality [82, 83].

Primary PCI has been shown to significantly improve the survival of patients with STEMI and to be superior to thrombolytic therapy in both men and women [84]. Primary PCI more often restores normal coronary flow in the infarct-related artery as well as reducing the incidence of recurrent ischaemia or reinfarction compared to thrombolysis. PCI studies have also showed a longer symptom-to-door time in women than in men [85–87], in spite of public education programmes. Although time to treatment is more crucial for thrombolytic therapy, there is evidence that if this time to treatment delay could be minimized to less than 2 h, this would be expected to have a beneficial impact on left ventricular function after primary PCI [88].

The success rate of PCI in STEMI is not different between the sexes [87], but major adverse cardiac events such as bleeding occur more often in women than in men [86]. The use of intracoronary stents has been significantly lower in women than in men [85], but primary stenting has been shown to be associated with a reduction in major adverse cardiac events (MACE) in women [86].

The lower incidence of stenting in women is at least in part due to the sex difference in underlying coronary artery disease (CAD) severity. In STEMI as well as in NSTE ACE, men have more often two- or three-vessel or left main disease whereas women more often have one-vessel disease [89]. Although more notable in NSTE ACE, coronary angiograms with no significant stenosis are reported more frequently in women than in men in STEMI [89]. In a recent large series from 600 United States hospitals in more than 450 000 patients with ACS, the adjusted odds for obstructive CAD were 50% lower for women than for men [90]. For patients presenting with STEMI, 10% of women compared to 7% of men had no obstructive CAD [91] as compared 25% of women and 16% of men in NSTE ACS [92].

Several possible mechanisms have been proposed for the higher incidence of MI with normal angiograms in women, such as higher prevalence of vasospastic syndromes and/or pure thrombotic disease due to coagulation disorders or oral contraceptive use [93]. It has also been shown that young women have plaque erosions instead of plaque rupture more often than older women and men [94]. Recent studies with intravascular ultrasonography and coronary vascular reactivity assessment have demonstrated more microcirculation disturbances in women with CAD than in men [95].

The addition of abciximab to primary stenting reduced the need for repeat revascularization in one STEMI study comparing the genders. In the CADILLAC study, the addition of abciximab significantly reduced ischaemic target vessel revascularization at 30 days in women after primary PCI, without an increased risk of major bleeding or stroke [86].

Gender differences in benefit from invasive treatment in non-STEMI acute coronary syndromes

An early invasive treatment strategy, with coronary angiography and revascularization if feasible, has become the treatment strategy of choice in patients with NSTE ACS, and is a class 1-recommendation in European Society of Cardiology (ESC) guidelines on NSTE ACS, at least for patients with medium- or high-risk features [14].

Gender differences in benefit from an invasive strategy have been intensively debated, and data are conflicting. Three earlier randomized trials comparing a routine invasive strategy with a selective invasive strategy in NSTE ACS have reported outcomes separately for women and men. In the FRISC II and RITA 3 trials, although there was a clear favourable outcome with a routine invasive strategy in men, there was no benefit in women [6, 96]. In contrast, the TACTICS-TIMI 18 trial indicated similar benefit in men and women with a routine invasive strategy, but mainly restricted to those with elevated markers [8]. Finally, the OASIS 5 Women Substudy included women only. There was no difference between the routine invasive strategy and the selective invasive strategy in the primary outcome measure (death/MI/stroke) or the secondary outcome (death/MI within 1 year). However, a higher rate of death was found with a routine invasive strategy [97].

A meta-analysis presented together with data from the OASIS 5 WSS suggested a clear benefit with a routine invasive strategy compared to a selective invasive strategy in men for death/MI that could not be seen in women [97]. Another meta-analysis included 8 trials (3075 women and 7075 men) and showed no significant difference in outcome with a routine invasive strategy versus a more selective invasive strategy in the endpoint of death/MI, for either men or women [98].

There are several possible reasons for less benefit from an invasive strategy in women with NSTE ACS, and for difference in outcome between earlier studies. A common finding in the three randomized trials was that women have less obstructive CHD. In the FRISC II trial patients without significant stenosis had an excellent prognosis, with no deaths during 1-year follow-up. The relative paucity of obstructive CHD may obviously dilute the treatment benefit with an invasive strategy.

Both in the FRISC II trial and the TACTICS-TIMI 18 trial, men were significantly more likely to have elevated troponin than women. Troponin is a marker of myocardial necrosis and is predictive of degree of CHD and even probability of visible thrombus on the angiogram, indicative of plaque rupture [99]. In a subgroup analysis of high-risk patients in the TACTICS-TIMI-18, there was a similar benefit for the primary endpoint (death/MI/revascularization) in troponin-positive female and male patients. These data were further supported in the meta-analysis by O'Donoghue et al., where benefit with an invasive strategy in women appeared to be restricted to patients with elevated markers [98].

Several earlier trials have indicated higher risk associated with an invasive strategy for women, especially regarding CABG, and the higher event rate in women than in men treated with a routine invasive strategy in the FRISC II trial seemed to be largely due to an increased rate of death and recurrent MI in women who had CABG surgery.

Complications

Overall, women are more likely than men to have complications related to an ACS episode, such as reinfarction, recurrent ischaemia, new onset of severe congestive heart failure (CHF), and atrial fibrillation or flutter. Rates of bleeding and stroke have consequently been reported to be higher in women, as well as mechanical complications such as myocardial rupture and ventricular septal defect. One possible explanation for this increase in risk of bleeding and thrombotic complications (including reinfarction) may be related to renal dysfunction; creatinine clearance is lower in women than in men, independent of age and body weight. If ACS patients are stratified by chronic kidney disease (CKD) stage, the proportion of women gets higher as the kidney function gets worse [100–102].

Women and patients with renal insufficiency are more likely to receive an overdose of antithrombotic therapy for ACS, resulting in excess bleeding risk. Even after adjustment for overdosing, women have higher bleeding risk with GPIIb/IIIa inhibition, as shown e.g. in TACTICS-TIMI 18. The risk of bleeding events increases as creatinine clearance declines. Bleeding events commonly lead to cessation of antithrombotic therapy, which would be expected to increase risk of reinfarction. Another potential explanation for these risk differences may be sex differences in the coagulation and fibrinolytic cascades [103].

Outcome

After an acute MI, a higher short-term mortality in women is documented in several studies [44, 104–106]. Even after adjustment for age and comorbidity, some difference has usually [44], but not always [106], remained. On the other hand, most studies assessing long-term outcome have found no difference between the genders, or even better outcome in women, at least after adjustment [106, 107].

Earlier studies focusing on gender differences in outcome after an ACS have usually studied patients with MI, including both STEMI and NSTEMI. Not only does the pathophysiology and initial management differ between these two conditions [108], but also outcome according to gender [91, 109].

In contrast to STEMI, women with NSTEMI or UAP seem to have equal or better outcomes, after adjustment for age and comorbidity [110–113]. In a large cohort of patients with NSTE ACS from the Swedish RIKS-HIA register impact of age on long-term mortality was obvious,

with substantially higher mortality with increasing age (◑Fig. 48.1). Better outcome in women, after adjustment, appeared to be restricted to older patients.

Before adjustment, short-term mortality in STEMI has been shown to be higher in women in numerous previous studies before, during, and after the thrombolytic era [80, 86, 91, 114]. After adjustment, there is no sex difference in long time outcome in STEMI [87]. The unadjusted in-hospital/short-term mortality in STEMI is about twice as high in women [85, 89]. Adjustment for age eliminates most of this difference, but contrary to NSTE ACS, the short-term STEMI mortality in women has been shown to be 15–20% higher after multivariable adjustments [82, 85, 89, 114]; yet the largest mortality gap is observed in younger women, with several studies demonstrating persistent sex differences despite covariate adjustment. One reason for higher short-term mortality in women could be a higher prehospital mortality in men [115, 116]. Other possible explanations could be differences in underlying anatomy and pathophysiology, such as reduced collateral circulation due to single-vessel CAD which has been associated with worse outcome because of less collateral circulation and myocardial preconditioning.

On the other hand, several studies comparing the outcome between genders in cohorts treated mainly with primary PCI have failed to find any sex difference in short-term mortality [85, 86] especially if body surface area has been included in the multivariable adjustment. There is now conflicting evidence whether female gender is still an

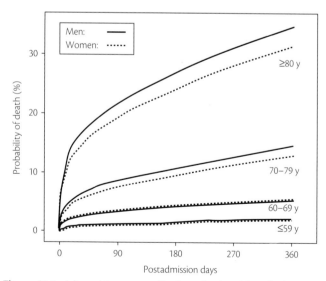

Figure 48.1 Adjusted 1-year mortality: hazard ratios with multiple adjustment using Cox regression analysis. Hazard ratios (HR) at 1 year with 95% confidence interval ≤59 years, HR 1.12 (95% CI, 0.85–1.47); 60–69 years, HR 0.99 (95% CI, 0.05–1.16); 70–79 years, HR 1.14 (95% CI 1.05–1.23); ≥80 years, HR 1.13 (95% CI 1.05–1.20).

independent predictor for poor outcome in this new primary PCI era [86, 117–119]. The relative benefit of primary PCI compared to thrombolytic therapy, at least on site, seem to be at least as good in women as in men [85].

Conclusion

It is important to shed light on gender differences and similarities in the management of patients with acute coronary syndromes (ACS). It is a fact that women have not been included in clinical trials in equal numbers to men, whatever the reason. In the future it will be necessary to individualize the management of patients as much as possible, regardless of gender. To achieve this, it is necessary to have enough patients of both genders included in trials; otherwise it is not possible to draw proper conclusions. Until now most results about women and ACS have been based on substudy analyses without enough statistical power. If gender differences have become evident in studies with gender-mixed populations, it seems obvious that the power calculated to show significant differences is not enough for men either.

There is an urgent need for more research in this area, in order not to harm patients by inappropriate theory. It is equally important not to withhold proper treatment from certain individuals when they can benefit from it.

Personal perspective

Gender is associated with differences between women and men regarding behaviour and disease, as well as with inequality of life conditions. Thus gender is, and should be, an important variable at the level of the individual physician, especially as it relates to interpersonal interactions with patients.

It is also known that men and women have well-documented differences in how they communicate, and, not surprisingly, these differences also extend to how male and female physicians interact with their patients. One of the most logical places to introduce concepts related to sex- and gender-based medicine is via the curriculum of medical, pharmaceutical, public health, and nursing schools [120].

Further reading

Regarding prognosis/outcome:

Berger JS, Elliott L, Gallup D, et al. Sex differences in mortality following acute coronary syndromes. *JAMA* 2009;**302**(8): 874–882.

Hochman JS, Tamis JE, Thompson TD, et al. Sex, clinical presentation, and outcome in patients with acute coronary syndromes. Global Use of Strategies to Open Occluded Coronary Arteries in Acute Coronary Syndromes IIb Investigators. *N Engl J Med* 1999;**341**(4):226–232.

Regarding symptoms:

Canto JG, Goldberg RJ, Hand MM, et al. Symptom presentation of women with acute coronary syndromes: myth vs reality. *Arch Intern Med* 2007;**167**(22):2405–2413.

Patel H, Rosengren A, Ekman I. Symptoms in acute coronary syndromes: does sex make a difference? *Am Heart J* 2004;**148**(1):27–33.

Early invasive treatement:

O'Donoghue M, Boden WE, Braunwald E, et al. Early invasive vs conservative treatment strategies in women and men with unstable angina and non-ST-segment elevation myocardial infarction: a meta-analysis. *JAMA* 2008;**300**(1):71–80.

Swahn E, Alfredsson J, Afzal R, et al. Regarding early invasive compared with a selective invasive strategy in women with non-ST elevation acute coronary syndromes: a sub-study of the OASIS 5 trial and a meta-analysis of previous randomized trials. *Eur Heart J* 2009.

➲ For additional multimedia materials please visit the online version of the book (♫ http://www.esciacc.oxfordmedicine.com).

SECTION VIII

Acute heart failure

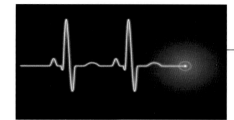

CHAPTER 49

Acute heart failure: epidemiology, classification, and pathophysiology

Marco Metra, Dirk Brutsaert, Livio Dei Cas, and Mihai Gheorghiade

Contents

Summary

Acute heart failure (AHF) is defined as a rapid onset or change in the signs and symptoms of heart failure, resulting in the need for urgent therapy. Heart failure afflicts over 15 million Europeans, and AHF is the most important cause of hospitalization for individuals over 65 years of age. It is characterized by severe symptoms, often related to fluid overload, requiring immediate hospitalization and treatment. The prognosis of the patients with AHF is poor, with a 4–7% in-hospital mortality and 3–6 months postdischarge mortality and rehospitalization rates reaching 15% and 30%, respectively. Pulmonary congestion is an almost universal finding in patients with AHF. It may be related to fluid retention and/or to fluid redistribution to the lungs caused by increased left ventricular afterload and impairment of left ventricular diastolic function. Myocardial ischaemia and necrosis and damage of kidney function are additional mechanisms potentially related to the poor prognosis of AHF patients.

Definition

According to the recent European Society of Cardiology (ESC) guidelines for the diagnosis and treatment of heart failure (HF) [1], acute heart failure (AHF) is defined as a 'rapid onset or change in the signs and symptoms of HF, resulting in the need for urgent therapy'. Patients may present as a medical emergency such as acute pulmonary oedema. AHF may present as either new onset HF or, more often, as worsening of pre-existing chronic HF. In this case, after initial management resulting in clinical stabilization, the patients should no longer be considered acute but rather chronic HF [1]. Independently of the underlying cause and precipitant factor(s), pulmonary and/or systemic congestion due to elevated ventricular filling pressures, with or without a decrease in cardiac output, are nearly universal findings in AHF [1–5]. AHF is a heterogeneous condition and the term 'AHF syndromes' has been used to emphasize this aspect [2, 3, 6–8].

Epidemiology

HF afflicts over 15 million Europeans [1] and 5. 7 million Americans [9]. Its prevalence is strictly age-dependent, ranging between 2% and 3% in the overall adult population and rising sharply at 70–75 years of age to 10–20% in those 70–80 years old [1]. AHF is the most important cause of hospitalization for people aged over 65 years [1–3]. More than 3. 8 million hospital diagnoses of HF occurred in 2004 and more than 1 million emergency department visits for AHF occurred in the United States between 1992 and 2001 [10, 11]. Hospitalizations are the most important cause of the financial burden of HF, a disease causing up to 3–4% of the total expenditure of the health care system of most European countries and the United States [2].

Outcomes

AHF is characterized by severe symptoms, related to pulmonary and, often, systemic congestion (mainly dyspnoea but often also fatigue and peripheral oedema), and by a poor prognosis. Recent studies, based on careful patient selection (i. e. through natriuretic peptides levels) and/or more thorough assessment of dyspnoea, show that a consistent percentage of patients (40–50%) does not achieve a moderate to marked improvement in dyspnoea in the first

24 h of treatment (◑ Fig. 49.1), and/or shows relapses of symptoms, and/or maintains signs of congestion at the time of discharge. All these are ominous prognostic factors and show that current AHF treatment is still inadequate from the point of view of symptom relief also [12–16].

AHF is a lethal condition associated with high mortality and rehospitalization rates. The median length of stay in the hospital is 9 days in Europe and 4 days in the United States [2, 17–20]. This has an influence on in-hospital mortality, which is 6–7% in Europe and 3–4% in the United States [2, 19, 20]. There is wide variation, with mortality rates reaching 20% in patients with low blood pressure and renal dysfunction versus 2–3% in patients with low blood urea nitrogen (BUN) and systolic blood pressure 115 mmHg or more [21].

Poor outcomes have been universally shown after discharge, with 60–90-day mortality rates of 5–15%, and hospital readmission rates of 30% [22]. Depending on the duration of the first hospitalization and on the number of rehospitalizations that have occurred, the risk of dying after a hospitalization for HF is increased from fourfold to 16-fold, compared to before the AHF hospitalization. The risk is highest in the first months after discharge [23]. There have been no major advances in the prognosis of patients with AHF in recent years [8, 24].

Modes of death and causes of rehospitalizations differ in patients hospitalized for AHF. In the 'Efficacy of Vasopressin Antagonism in Heart Failure Outcome Study with Tolvaptan' (EVEREST) approximately 40% of post-discharge deaths were caused by worsening HF and 30%

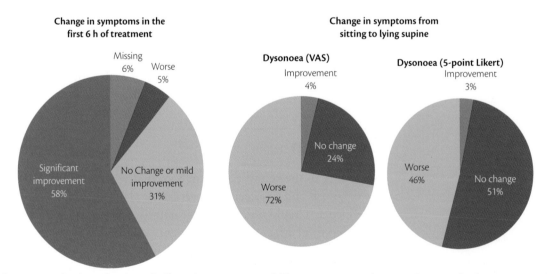

Figure 49.1 Percentages of patients showing a significant improvement, a mild improvement r no change, and a worsening in symptoms at 6 h from start of treatment for AHF (left plot) and percentages of patients with worsening symptoms changing from the sitting to the supine position in the URGENT trial.
Data from Mebazaa A, Pang PS, Tavares M, *et al*. The impact of early standard therapy on dyspnoea in patients with acute heart failure: the URGENT-dyspnoea study. *Eur Heart J* 2010;**31**(7):832–841; Figure reproduced with permission Hogg KJ, McMurray JJ. Evaluating dyspnoea in acute heart failure: progress at last! *Eur Heart J* 2010;**31**(7):771–772.

were sudden deaths. Even more important, approximately 50% of readmissions were not related to HF [2]. These data show that comorbidities may be an important cause of rehospitalizations and death in patients with AHF.

Temporal trends

Ageing of the population and advances in management of cardiovascular disease has caused a steady increase in the number of patients with HF and of HF hospitalizations. The number of hospitalizations with any mention of HF tripled in the United States from 1979 to 2004 [10], and this trend has been confirmed recently with an increase in the United States hospital discharges for HF from approximately 200 000 in 1979 to approximately 600 000 in 2006 [9].

More favourable trends have been shown in other studies [25–29]. A plateau, if not a decrease, in yearly HF hospitalizations and HF-related mortality rates has been described in the second half of the last decade and confirmed up to the year 2003 [25]. This declining trend in HF hospitalizations and mortality rates has been related to the greater use of angiotensin converting enzyme (ACE) inhibitors, β-blockers, and spironolactone in patients with HF [25]. Thus, there is an increase in the number of patients with HF although their prognosis may improve, compared with before, if they are treated with evidence-based therapies.

Causes and precipitating factors

Causes of AHF are outlined in ➲ Box 49.1 [1, 17]. The most common cause of AHF is coronary artery disease (40–65% of patients admitted for AHF) [30]. Acute coronary syndromes (ACS) cause AHF in approximately 20–30% of cases and they are the most important cause of cardiogenic shock (see ➲ Chapter 47) [2, 18–20].

Precipitating factors of AHF hospitalizations are summarized in ➲ Box 49.2 [31–34].

Classifications

The ESC guidelines divide patients into six clinical profiles, with the explicit acknowledgement that there is overlap between them (➲ Table 49.1; ➲ Fig. 49.2) [1, 35]. This classification is consistent with that previously issued in the ESC guidelines on AHF [17] and with a former classification by Cotter *et al.* [36] who distinguished four categories of AHF: exacerbated HF, pulmonary oedema, hypertensive crisis, and cardiogenic shock. The definition of hypertensive AHF is largely based on the study by Gandhi *et al.* who

---

> **Box 49.1 Causes of acute heart failure**
>
> - Acute decompensation of pre-existing chronic HF (e. g. cardiomyopathy)
> - Acute coronary syndromes
>   - With large areas of myocardial ischaemia or infarction
>   - Mechanical complications of acute myocardial infarction (papillary muscle rupture, ventricular septal defect, free wall rupture)
>   - Right ventricular infarction
> - Hypertensive crisis
> - Acute arrhythmias
>   - Atrial fibrillation or flutter, supraventricular tachycardia
>   - Ventricular fibrillation or ventricular tachycardia
> - Valvular regurgitation
>   - Endocarditis, rupture of chordate tendinae
>   - Worsening of pre-existing valve regurgitation
> - Severe aortic valve stenosis
> - Acute myocarditis
> - Post-partum cardiomyopathy
> - Takotsubo cardiomyopathy
> - Aortic dissection
> - Cardiac tamponade
> - Pulmonary embolism
> - High output syndromes
>   - Septicaemia
>   - Thyrotoxicosis
>   - Severe anaemia
>   - Shunt syndromes

---

described a group of patients with AHF and pulmonary oedema with extremely high blood pressure and preserved left ventricular (LV) ejection fraction (EF) [37].

The ESC classification has been applied to the 3580 patients with AHF enrolled in the recent EuroHeart Failure Survey (EHFS) II [20]. Decompensated chronic HF was present in 2340 (65.4%) patients whereas 407 patients (11.4%) had hypertensive HF, 581 patients (16.2%) had pulmonary oedema, 139 (3.9%) cardiogenic shock, and 113 (3.2%) isolated right HF. These different clinical presentations had a prognostic impact which was, however, mainly

Box 49.2 Precipitating factors of acute heart failure

- ◆ Lack of adherence to medical regimen
- ◆ Volume overload
- ◆ Infections, especially pneumonia
- ◆ Cerebrovascular insult
- ◆ Surgery
- ◆ Renal dysfunction
- ◆ Asthma, chronic obstructive lung disease
- ◆ Alcohol abuse
- ◆ Drugs:
  - Nonsteroidal antinflammatory drugs
  - Cyclooxygenase (COX) inhibitors
  - Thiazolidinediones
  - Antiarrhythmics (propafenone, flecainide, dronedarone, etc.)
  - Calcium antagonists (verapamile, diltiazem, nifedipine, and other dihydropyridine agents)

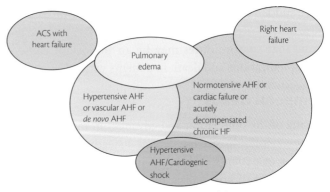

Figure 49.2 Clinical classification of acute heart failure.
Data from ESC guidelines for the diagnosis and treatment of acute and chronic heart failure 2008. *Eur J Heart Fail* 2008;**10**:933–89; and Filippatos G, Zannad F. An introduction to acute heart failure syndromes: definition and classification. *Heart Fail Rev* 2007;**12**:87–90.

that blood pressure is the most important parameter for prognostic stratification of AHF patients (see below) [22].

Two other classifications are outlined in ⊃ Table 49.2. The American College of Cardiology/American Heart Association (ACC/AHA) classification [39] is consistent with the original classification of Nohria *et al.* which assigned each patient with severe HF to one of four categories based on the presence or absence of signs of congestion and/or of signs of peripheral hypoperfusion (⊃ Fig. 49.4) [40, 41].

New onset acute heart failure versus acute decompensation of chronic heart failure

New onset AHF accounts for 20–40% of cases of AHF [2, 7, 19, 20, 38]. Patients with new onset AHF are more likely to be female, less likely to have comorbidities and a history of previous myocardial infarction, and more likely to have a history of hypertension and have higher blood pressure values at admission. Their clinical presentation is more often acute pulmonary oedema or hypertensive crisis [19, 20, 38]. Their prognosis is better than that of patients with worsening chronic HF [19, 38, 52]. This better prognosis is likely related to the greater prevalence of reversible causes of AHF (hypertension, myocardial ischaemia) and to the lower prevalence of comorbidities (diabetes, kidney dysfunction, anaemia). Many of these patients with new onset AHF have a preserved LVEF.

Acute heart failure with preserved and low left ventricular ejection fraction

Patients with AHF may have either a low LVEF or a preserved LVEF (HFpEF). In all patients hospitalized for AHF, the prevalence of HFpEF is estimated to be 50% or more [1, 39]. Compared to patients with AHF and low LVEF,

limited to the greater in-hospital mortality of cardiogenic shock and to the lower 1-year mortality of hypertensive HF. Decompensated HF, pulmonary oedema and right HF had similar outcomes (⊃ Fig. 49.3) [20, 38]. These data suggest

Table 49.1 European Society of Cardiology clinical classification of acute heart failure

Dominant clinical feature	Characteristics
Worsening or decompensated chronic HF (peripheral oedema/congestion)	History of chronic HF. Systemic and pulmonary congestion (peripheral oedema, raised jugular venous pressure, pulmonary oedema, hepatomegaly, ascites, congestion, cachexia)
Pulmonary oedema	Severe dyspnoea, tachypnoea, orthopnoea, lung rales, O_2sat <90%
Hypertensive heart failure	High BP usually LV hypertrophy, and preserved EF
Cardiogenic shock (low output syndrome)	Peripheral hypoperfusion, systolic BP <90 mmHg or drop mean BP >30 mmHg, anuria or oliguria (<0. 5 mL/kg per h)
Right heart failure	Low output no pulmonary congestion, raised JVP, hepatomegaly, low LV filling pressures
ACS and HF	c.15% of ACS have AHF.

ACS, acute coronary symdromes: BP, blood pressure; EF, ejection fraction; JVP, jugular venous pressure; LV, left ventricular

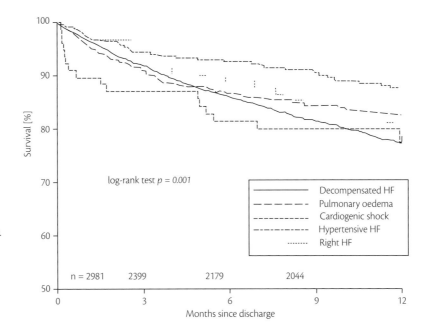

Figure 49.3 1-year mortality in patients with different clinical presentations of acute heart failure. Reproduced with permission from Harjola VP, Follath F, Nieminen MS, *et al.* Characteristics, outcomes, and predictors of mortality at 3 months and 1 year in patients hospitalized for acute heart failure. *Eur J Heart Fail* 2010;**12**:239–248.

HFpEF patients are older and more likely to be female, with a history of hypertension or arrhythmias. On admission, they often present with higher blood pressure or with atrial tachyrrhythmias [2, 42, 43]. A preserved LVEF in these AHF patients merely indicates that overall haemodynamic LV pump performance—i. e. stroke volume, stroke

work, $(+)dP/dt$, arterial blood pressure, LVEF—is still well preserved through the recruitment of numerous physiological compensatory mechanisms. However, in most of these patients, several recent studies have demonstrated the presence of substantial myocardial systolic (mainly during LV isovolumic relaxation) and diastolic (decreased late LV filling and compliance) dysfunction [44–46]. The latter diastolic and systolic abnormalities may, either alone or together, lead to pulmonary congestion or acute pulmonary oedema. It is, however, still unclear whether these

Table 49.2 Other clinical classifications of acute heart failure

ACC/AHA [39]	
With volume overload	Pulmonary and/or systemic congestion, frequently precipitated by an acute increase in chronic hypertension
With profound depression of cardiac output	Manifested by hypotension, renal insufficiency, and/or a shock syndrome
With signs and symptoms of both fluid overload and shock	Both
Gheorghiade *et al.* [2, 7, 8]	
Worsening chronic HF	Patients with structural heart disease with prior or current symptoms of HF (stage C of the ACC/AHA classification) [39] Includes c.75% of AHF patients
De novo HF	Patients with a structural heart disease or at high risk for HF but without prior symptoms of HF (stage B or stage A of the ACC/AHA classification) [39] Includes c.20% of AHF patients
Advanced HF	Refractory HF requiring specialized interventions (stage D of the ACC/AHA classification) [39] Includes c.5% of AHF patients

ACC, American College of Cardiology; AHA, American Heart Association; HF, heart failure.

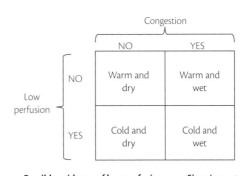

Figure 49.4 Clinical presentations of acute heart failure.
Data from Nieminen MS, Böhm M, Cowie MR, *et al.* Executive summary of the guidelines on the diagnosis and treatment of acute heart failure: the Task Force on Acute Heart Failure of the European Society of Cardiology. *Eur Heart J* 2005;**26**:384–416; Nohria A, Tsang SW, Fang JC, *et al.* Clinical assessment identifies hemodynamic profiles that predict outcomes in patients admitted with heart failure. *J Am Coll Cardiol* 2003;**41**:1797–1804; Nohria A, Lewis E, Stevenson LW. Medical management of advanced heart failure. *JAMA* 2002;**287**:628–640.

Possible evidence of low perfusion
- Narrow pulse pressure
- Sleepy/obtunded
- Low serum sodium
- Cool extremities
- Hypotension with ACE inhibitor
- Renal/hepatic dysfunction

Signs/symptoms of congestion
- Orthopnea/PND
- JV distension
- Hepatomegaly
- Oedema
- Rales
- Abdominal–jugular reflex

abnormalities can be the sole primary cause of AHF [47, 48]. A sudden increase in LV afterload and peripheral vascular resistance, as in a hypertensive crisis, or the occurrence of transient atrial tachyrrhythmias, are indeed more likely to provoke AHF with preserved LVEF in these patients [47]. Whether the prognosis of patients with AHF and preserved LVEF is different from that of patients with a low LVEF is still a matter of debate [42, 43, 49–51].

Prognostic factors

A thorough discussion of prognostic factors goes beyond the aims of this chapter. The main prognostic factors which have been related to in-hospital mortality, postdischarge mortality, or hospital readmission rates are summarized in ➲ Box 49.3 [2, 4, 17–21, 52–58]. The administration of life-saving therapies, such as β-blockers and renin–angiotensin–aldosterone system antagonists [59, 60], as well as the performance of invasive procedures, i.e. coronary angiography and revascularization [61], when indicated, have an important prognostic value. Postdischarge reassessment in the first weeks after hospitalization may allow the best prediction of future events [62–64].

Pathophysiology

The pathophysiology of AHF is complex and, from many points of view, still poorly understood. We do not know the exact mechanism(s) causing decompensation of chronic HF or the new onset of AHF in patients at risk.

Pulmonary congestion

Pulmonary congestion causing dyspnoea with or without fluid overload and peripheral oedema is an almost universal finding in patients with AHF [1–6, 8, 12, 19–22, 52, 58, 65]. Studies with continuous monitoring of right ventricular or pulmonary artery pressure have shown that an increase in intracardiac pressures precedes an episode of acute decompensation, independently of whether the patient has a low or a normal LVEF [66, 67]. LV pressure, when estimated either directly or through surrogates (natriuretic peptides, restrictive pattern of LV filling at Doppler echocardiography) is also a major prognostic factor when measured at the time of discharge and/or in the following weeks [62, 63, 68–71].

Changes in body weight are often used to detect fluid overload, and an increase of body weight has generally been

Box 49.3 Prognostic variables in patients with acute heart failure

- Demographic:
  - Advanced age
  - Male gender
- Clinical:
  - Frequent rehospitalizations
  - NYHA class IV
  - Intolerance to neurohormonal antagonists (hypotension, worsening renal function)
  - Persistent/relapsing signs of pulmonary or peripheral congestion during the initial hospital stay (worsening heart failure)
  - Hypotension
  - Low oxygen saturation
  - Comorbidities (diabetes, renal failure, hepatic failure, anaemia, COPD, cardiac cachexia, etc.)
- ECG:
  - Resting tachycardia
  - Wide QRS complex
- Laboratory:
  - Hyponatraemia
  - Renal insufficiency (BUN/serum creatinine)
  - Anaemia
  - Hepatic insufficiency
- Doppler echocardiography and right heart catheterization:
  - Low LVEF/increased LVESVI
  - Mitral regurgitation/Increased left atrial volume
  - Signs of increased LV filling pressure
  - RV dysfunction
- Functional capacity:
  - Inability to perform an exercise test before discharge
  - Low 6-min walk test distance
  - Others[a]
- Coronary angiography:
  - Extension and severity of coronary artery disease

COPD, chronic obstructive pulmonary disease; ESVI, end-systolic volume index; RV, right ventricular.
[a] Cardiopulmonary exercise testing has never been formally used for prognostic assessment in patients hospitalized for AHF.

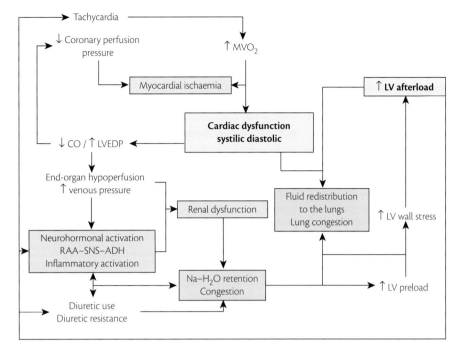

Figure 49.5 Mechanisms of acute heart failure. Initial mechanisms are shown with a light blue background, further major mechanisms with a light green background, and final outcomes (i.e. clinical presentations of AHF) with a light purple background. RAA, renin-angiotensin-aldosterone; SNS, sympathetic nervous system; ADH, antidiuretic hormone.

shown to precede HF hospitalizations [63, 72]. However, because of the possibility of fluid redistribution to the lungs causing AHF in the absence of fluid accumulation, body weight is less sensitive than monitoring of intracardiac pressures. Accordingly, changes in body weight were not predictive of mortality and the decrease in body weight with non-potassium-sparing diuretics or vasopressin antagonists was not associated with better outcomes [63, 73, 74].

Mechanisms of congestion: fluid overload and fluid redistribution to the lungs

The mechanisms of fluid overload are multiple and poorly understood. Congestion may be ascribed to two main initial mechanisms: an abnormal LV function with increased ventricular filling pressures, peripheral hypoperfusion, and renal sodium and water retention, and/or an excessive increase in LV afterload with concomitant LV diastolic dysfunction and increased intraventricular filling pressures (●Fig. 49.5). These two mechanisms may coexist, making different contributions in each patient. The two extremes of this spectrum are represented by patients with severe LV systolic dysfunction and low cardiac output and blood pressure [22] and by patients with hypertensive crisis [37], in whom heightened peripheral resistance and LV afterload predominate whereas LVEF is often normal (●Table 49.3) [2, 4, 17, 22, 35, 36, 58, 75, 76].

Patients with acutely decompensated chronic HF and LV systolic dysfunction generally present a progressive gain in body weight, consistent with fluid retention, in the

days, or weeks, preceding the hospitalization or emergency visit. Renal sodium and water retention is probably the main mechanism leading to fluid overload, pulmonary and peripheral oedema, dyspnoea and hospitalization. Renal sodium and water retention generally develops gradually, over days or weeks. It is a characteristic abnormality of patients with chronic HF. It is caused by haemodynamic mechanisms, both reduced cardiac output with renal hypoperfusion, and increased central venous and renal venous pressure [77–79], as well as by neurohormonal activation (●Fig. 49.5). Activation of the renin–angiotensin system leads, both directly and indirectly, through increased aldosterone secretion, to increased sodium and water retention in the kidney [4, 5, 76, 80]. Increased vasopressin secretion causes increased water reabsorption in the nephron collecting duct and hyponatraemia [80].

In some cases AHF may occur without salt and water retention and weight gain and the underlying mechanism is rather a redistribution of fluids to the lungs with pulmonary, but not systemic, congestion [4, 5, 58, 76]. This is likely to occur mostly in patients with HF and preserved LVEF and with clinical presentations of pulmonary oedema or hypertensive AHF. Venous and arterial constriction, rather than fluid retention, may play a pivotal role in these cases. Venoconstriction causes an increase in venous return to the right heart which, by interacting with poorly compliant ventricles, may lead to a rise in their end-diastolic pressures. Arterial vasoconstriction increases LV afterload with a reduction of stroke volume and a further increase in intraventricular pressures. Thus, excessive peripheral

Table 49.3 Spectrum of pathophysiological mechanisms causing acute heart failure

	Vascular (peripheral)[a]	Cardiac (central)
Main mechanism of onset	↑ afterload and/or predominant LV diastolic dysfunction	↓ contractility Sodium and water renal retention
Clinical characteristics		
LVEF	Normal	Low
Main cause of symptoms	Fluid redistribution to the lungs	Fluid accumulation
Gain in body weight	No	Yes
Onset	Rapid (hours)	Gradual (days)
Main symptom	Dyspnoea	Fatigue
Main sign(s)	Pulmonary congestion (rales, oedema)	Peripheral oedema, jugular venous stasis, hepatomegaly
Systolic BP	Normal or high	Normal or low
LV filling pressure	High	May be reduced by low CO
Cardiac output	Normal or high	Low
Mortality/morbidity		
In-hospital mortality	Low (<5%)	High (≥5%)
3-month mortality	Relatively low (5–7%)	High (10–15%)
3-month rehospitalizations	High (30%)	High (30%)
Relative frequency of clinical presentations		
ESC classification [1]	Pulmonary oedema: often Hypertensive HF: always acute coronary syndromes and AHF: sometimes	Decompensated chronic HF: often Cardiogenic shock: always Right HF: always
ACC/AHA classification [39]	With volume overload: often	With profound depression of cardiac output: always
Gheorghiade et al. [2, 7, 8]	De novo HF: often	Worsening chronic HF: often Advanced HF: always

[a] Abnormalities of LV diastolic function may be a major cause of symptoms in these patients.

vasoconstriction, particularly in the presence of diastolic dysfunction, may cause an increase in pulmonary capillary pressure, pulmonary congestion, and pulmonary oedema. This may occur even in the absence of volume retention through a redistribution of fluid from the peripheral to the pulmonary circulation. The mechanisms underlying excessive vasoconstriction are not yet fully elucidated, but neurohormonal activation and inflammation may have a pivotal role [81, 82].

Blood pressure

Measurement of blood pressure plays a central role in the assessment and treatment of the patients with AHF [1, 17]. Most patients admitted for acute HF present with normal or high blood pressure. Elevated systolic blood pressure during AHF episodes may have at least two different implications: (1) a precipitating factor of AHF through excessive vasoconstriction and increased afterload; or (2) a consequence of neurohormonal activation and cardiac stimulation due to AHF itself (➲ Table 49.6).

The presence of a normal to high systolic blood pressure in patients with AHF shows maintenance of an adequate cardiac contractile reserve and cardiac output. Systolic blood pressure has been consistently shown to be one of the most important, if not the most important, independent predictor of both in-hospital and postdischarge outcomes in patients with AHF (➲ Fig. 49.6) [22, 52, 56–58, 83, 84].

Acute heart failure and outcomes: additional mechanisms

Despite their importance as a cause of patients' symptoms and of hospitalization, pulmonary congestion and fluid overload remain poorly related to long-term (i. e. >3 months) outcomes [2, 7, 63, 74]. This may be related to limitations of current treatment [8, 83, 85, 86], but may also be ascribed to a weak relation of congestion to long-term outcomes. Additional mechanisms activated in AHF should therefore be taken into account. To date, the two most studied are myocardial damage and renal dysfunction. It must be pointed out, however, that, until

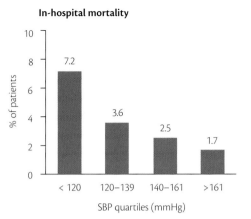

In-hospital mortality

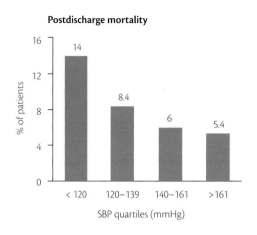

Postdischarge mortality

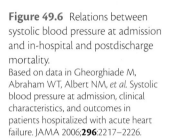

Figure 49.6 Relations between systolic blood pressure at admission and in-hospital and postdischarge mortality.
Based on data in Gheorghiade M, Abraham WT, Albert NM, *et al.* Systolic blood pressure at admission, clinical characteristics, and outcomes in patients hospitalized with acute heart failure. JAMA 2006;**296**:2217–2226.

targeted therapies can favourably affect these mechanisms and hence the patients' prognosis, their role remains hypothetical: we cannot exclude the possibility that they are only epiphenomena of the most severe forms of the syndrome.

Myocardial ischaemia and cell death

Coronary artery disease is the most common cause of AHF in Europe and the United States. There are many potential connections between coronary artery disease and AHF [2, 30]. Myocardial ischaemia and myocyte necrosis may constitute either a trigger for AHF (i.e. acute coronary syndrome leading to AHF), or alternatively the HF event itself may lead to myocardial ischaemia or necrosis even in the absence of frank ACS. This may occur during an episode of AHF as a consequence of an increase in myocardial oxygen consumption and a reduction in oxygen supply and coronary perfusion due to increased LV filling pressure, reduced systemic arterial blood pressure, tachycardia,

endothelial dysfunction mediated by neurohormonal activation (angiotensin, noradrenaline, endothelin), inflammatory mechanisms, and platelet activation (➲ Fig. 49.7). Subjects with pre-existing coronary artery disease are particularly vulnerable, especially because of the possible presence of areas of hibernating myocardium. However, ischaemia may also occur in patients with nonischaemic cardiomyopathy (➲ Fig. 49.8) [69, 87].

The clinical relevance of myocardial necrosis in AHF has been demonstrated by studies based on plasma troponin measurements. An increase of plasma troponin levels has been reported in 40–70% of patients admitted for AHF [69, 87–89] and is associated with a poor prognosis [69, 87, 88].

Comorbidities

The prevalence of comorbidities is high in patients with acute HF and the most common ones are summarized in ➲ Box 49.4. Chronic kidney disease has been reported in 30–35%, chronic obstructive pulmonary disease in 10–30%, diabetes mellitus in 35–40%, and anaemia in 15–20% of patients with AHF. Of the various comorbidities, renal dysfunction seems the most likely to play a major role in AHF. A mild to moderate impairment of renal function is present in most patients with acute HF. Renal function is highly dependent on the patient's haemodynamic conditions (both low cardiac output and increased central venous pressure) as well as on neurohormonal activation and concomitant therapy (namely, diuretics) (➲ Fig. 49.9) [77–79, 90].

Kidney dysfunction may contribute to the poor prognosis of patients with AHF through multiple mechanisms: neurohormonal activation and inflammation, intolerance to renin–angiotensin–aldosterone antagonists, increased fluid and sodium retention, and resistance to loop diuretics. Multiple studies have shown that renal dysfunction is

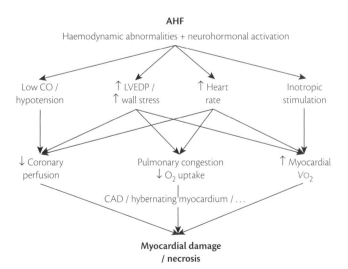

Figure 49.7 Mechanisms of ischaemia and necrosis in patients with acute heart failure.

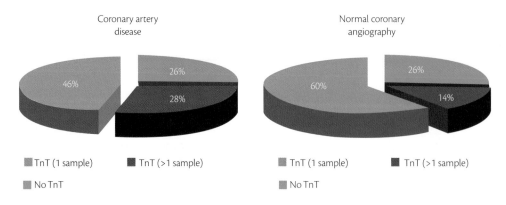

Figure 49.8 Prevalence of detectable serum troponin T levels (TnT) in one or more than one blood samples in patients hospitalized for AHF who underwent daily measurements until discharge.
Data from Metra M, Nodari S, Parrinello G, *et al.* The role of plasma biomarkers in acute heart failure. Serial changes and independent prognostic value of NT-proBNP and cardiac troponin-T. *Eur J Heart Fail* 2007;**9**:776–786.

an independent prognostic factor in AHF [19–21, 90, 91]. Worsening renal function may also occur in 20–30% of patients hospitalized for AHF and be related to a poor prognosis [90, 92]. Serum BUN, rather than serum creatinine, has been selected as the most important prognostic variable in most of the studies in which it was measured [19, 21, 53, 93]. This likely reflects the fact that BUN, but not serum creatinine, is related to the patient's overall condition and metabolic status.

All the comorbidities listed in ➲ Table 49.7 have been reported to be associated, generally independently, with a

worse prognosis in patients with acute HF and have been included in multivariable models of risk prediction [1, 19, 24, 30, 38, 53]. However, only intervention studies with drugs selectively targeting them may finally demonstrate whether such conditions directly contribute to the progression of HF or are just epiphenomena of a more severe disease state.

Conclusion

AHF is a devastating clinical condition. It is the most important cause of hospitalization for people over 65 years of age. It is a medical emergency, with a 4–6% mortality rate during the hospitalization and a 10–20% mortality rate and 30–40% readmission rate in the first months after discharge. Despite its importance, no major advances in medical treatment have occurred in recent decades. Pulmonary congestion, excessive LV afterload, and cardiac dysfunction are the hallmarks of AHF. Myocardial damage and kidney dysfunction also frequently occur and may contribute to the poor prognosis of these patients.

Box 49.4 Comorbidities in patients with acute heart failure

Cardiac

- Coronary artery disease
  - Acute coronary syndrome
  - Chronic ischaemic cardiac disease
- Arrhythmias (atrial fibrillation, etc.)
- Valvular disease (mitral regurgitation, etc.)

Noncardiac

- Chronic kidney disease
- Chronic obstructive pulmonary disease
- Diabetes mellitus
- Peripheral vascular disease
- Liver disease, cirrhosis
- Cancer
- Anaemia
- Cachexia
- Cerebrovascular disease
- Dementia, cognitive dysfunction

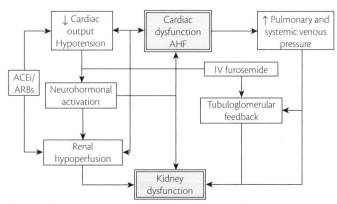

Figure 49.9 Relations between cardiac and renal dysfunction in heart failure.

Personal perspective

Due to ageing of the population and better treatment of cardiovascular disease, the number of subjects hospitalized with a diagnosis of AHF is likely to further increase in the coming years. Their prognosis may slightly improve through the earlier and more widespread administration of evidence-based therapies. However, no further major improvement is likely to be possible until we can identify the main pathophysiological mechanisms causing HF decompensation and the poor prognosis of patients with AHF. Pulmonary congestion, myocardial damage, and kidney dysfunction remain major causes of the symptoms and poor prognosis of AHF patients. Our knowledge of these mechanisms is due to the availability of specific biomarkers: natriuretic peptides, troponins, and creatinine, respectively. Almost a hundred new biomarkers are currently about to be tested in patients with AHF. The discovery of new biomarkers will probably allow better insight into old and new pathophysiological mechanisms. It is therefore likely that better assessment of fluid status, myocardial and renal damage, and/or the identification of new mechanisms (inflammation, metabolic–nutritional requirements) will allow the development of new therapies, the major unmet need for patients with AHF.

Further reading

Banerjee P, Clark AL, Nikitin N, Cleland JG. Diastolic heart failure. Paroxysmal or chronic? *Eur J Heart Fail* 2004;**6**:427–431.

Brutsaert DL, De Keulenaer GW. Diastolic heart failure: a myth. *Curr Opin Cardiol* 2006;**21**:240–248.

Colombo PC, Onat D, Sabbah HN. Acute heart failure as 'acute endothelitis'—Interaction of fluid overload and endothelial dysfunction. *Eur J Heart Fail* 2008;**10**:170–175.

Cotter G, Metra M, Milo-Cotter O, *et al*. Fluid overload in acute heart failure—redistribution and other mechanisms beyond fluid accumulation. *Eur J Heart Fail* 2008;**10**:165–169.

Cotter G, Moshkovitz Y, Milovanov O, *et al*. Acute heart failure: a novel approach to its pathogenesis and treatment. *Eur J Heart Fail* 2002;**4**:227–234.

Damman K, Navis G, Smilde TD, *et al*. Decreased cardiac output, venous congestion and the association with renal impairment in patients with cardiac dysfunction. *Eur J Heart Fail* 2007;**9**:872–878.

Damman K, Navis G, Voors AA, *et al*. Worsening renal function and prognosis in heart failure: systematic review and meta-analysis. *J Cardiac Fail* 2007;**13**:599–608.

De Keulenaer GW, Brutsaert DL. Diastolic heart failure: a separate disease or selection bias? *Progr Cardiovasc Dis* 2007;**49**:275–283.

De Keulenaer GW, Brutsaert DL. The heart failure spectrum: time for a phenotype-oriented approach. *Circulation* 2009;**119**:3044–3046.

European Society of Cardiology; Heart Failure Association of the ESC (HFA); European Society of Intensive Care Medicine (ESICM), *et al*. ESC guidelines for the diagnosis and treatment of acute and chronic heart failure 2008: the Task Force for the diagnosis and treatment of acute and chronic heart failure 2008 of the European Society of Cardiology. Developed in collaboration with the Heart Failure Association of the ESC (HFA) and endorsed by the European Society of Intensive Care Medicine (ESICM). *Eur J Heart Fail* 2008;**10**:933–989.

Filippatos G, Zannad F. An introduction to acute heart failure syndromes: definition and classification. *Heart Fail Rev* 2007;**12**:87–90.

Flaherty JD, Bax JJ, De Luca L, *et al*. Acute Heart Failure Syndromes International Working Group. Acute heart failure syndromes in patients with coronary artery disease early assessment and treatment. *J Am Coll Cardiol* 2009;**53**:254–263.

Gheorghiade M, Pang PS. Acute heart failure syndromes. *J Am Coll Cardiol* 2009;**53**:557–573.

Gheorghiade M, De Luca L, Fonarow GC, *et al*. Pathophysiologic targets in the early phase of acute heart failure syndromes. *Am J Cardiol* 2005;**96**:11G–17G.

Gheorghiade M, Zannad F, Sopko G, *et al*. Acute heart failure syndromes: current state and framework for future research. *Circulation* 2005;**112**:3958–3968.

Harjola VP, Follath F, Nieminen MS, *et al*. Characteristics, outcomes, and predictors of mortality at 3 months and 1 year in patients hospitalized for acute heart failure. *Eur J Heart Fail* 2010;**12**:239–248.

Hogg KJ, McMurray JJ. Evaluating dyspnoea in acute heart failure: progress at last! *Eur Heart J* 2010;**31**:771–772.

Jessup M, Abraham WT, Casey DE, *et al*. 2009 focused update: ACCF/AHA Guidelines for the Diagnosis and Management of Heart Failure in Adults: a report of the American College of Cardiology Foundation/American Heart Association Task Force on Practice Guidelines: developed in collaboration with the International Society for Heart and Lung Transplantation. *Circulation* 2009;**119**:1977–2016.

McMurray JJ. Clinical practice. Systolic heart failure. *N Engl J Med* 2010;**362**:228–238.

Mebazaa A, Pang PS, Tavares M, *et al*. The impact of early standard therapy on dyspnoea in patients with acute heart failure: the URGENT-dyspnoea study. *Eur Heart J* 2009;**31**:832–841.

Metra M, Dei Cas L, Bristow MR. The pathophysiology of acute heart failure—it is a lot about fluid accumulation. *Am Heart J* 2008;**155**:1–5.

Metra M, Teerlink JR, Voors AA, *et al*. Vasodilators in the treatment of acute heart failure: what we know, what we don't. *Heart Fail Rev* 2009;**14**:299–307.

Nohria A, Hasselblad V, Stebbins A, *et al.* Cardiorenal interactions: insights from the ESCAPE trial. *J Am Coll Cardiol* 2008;**51**:1268–1274.

Nohria A, Lewis E, Stevenson LW. Medical management of advanced heart failure. *JAMA* 2002;**287**:628–640.

Pang PS, Cleland JG, Teerlink JR, *et al.* A proposal to standardize dyspnoea measurement in clinical trials of acute heart failure syndromes: the need for a uniform approach. *Eur Heart J* 2008;**29**:816–824.

Pang PS, Komajda M, Gheorghiade M. The current and future management of acute heart failure syndromes. *Eur Heart J* 2010;**31**:794–805.

Paulus WJ, Tschöpe C, Sanderson JE, *et al.* How to diagnose diastolic heart failure: a consensus statement on the diagnosis of heart failure with normal left ventricular ejection fraction by the Heart Failure and Echocardiography Associations of the European Society of Cardiology. *Eur Heart J* 2007;**28**:2539–2550.

Teerlink JR, Metra M, Zacà V, *et al.* Agents with inotropic properties for the management of acute heart failure syndromes. Traditional agents and beyond. *Heart Fail Rev* 2009;**14**:243–253.

⊃ For additional multimedia materials please visit the online version of the book (http://www.esciacc.oxfordmedicine. com).

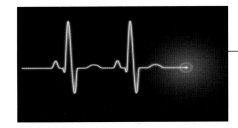

CHAPTER 50

Acute heart failure: early pharmacological treatment

John T. Parissis and Dionysia Birmpa

Contents

Summary

Acute heart failure (AHF) concerns a highly heterogeneous patient population that needs urgent treatment. Many agents are used in the management of this condition, but their use is largely empiric and based on expert consensus. Their effectiveness is based on matching the most appropriate therapy to specific clinical profiles. Diuretics seem to be beneficial in patients with volume overload and systemic congestion. These patients usually have normal systolic blood pressure (SBP) at presentation. Vasodilators are frequently used in patients with congestion and elevated SBP. Patients with severe systolic dysfunction and hypotension (SBP ≤90 mmHg) and symptoms and signs of peripheral hypoperfusion are treated with inotropic agents. Despite the symptomatic and haemodynamic improvement, none of the recommended therapies are effective in improving the short- or long-term prognosis of AHF patients.

Introduction

Acute heart failure (AHF) is defined as a rapid onset of signs and symptoms of pulmonary congestion and/or peripheral hypoperfusion, resulting in the need for urgent therapy [1]. This condition is a common discharge diagnosis in patients over 65 years of age, with extremely high readmission and mortality rates [1–4]. It appears to be a challenge for clinicians but, paradoxically, AHF treatment remains empirical because of the paucity of data from randomized clinical trials [5].

Several pharmacological agents have been used to manage AHF, but treatment success is limited [6–9]. Despite the improvement of symptoms and haemodynamic status, none of these agents has been shown to improve postdischarge outcomes [10]. This fact may be attributed to our incomplete understanding of the pathophysiology of AHF, which has been viewed as a disease of low cardiac output due to systolic dysfunction and fluid overload [6, 7, 11].

Data from recent registries and surveys have revealed that there are multiple types of AHF patients with different clinical presentations and prognosis, and various management strategies [11, 12]. Diuretics and vasodilators have been adopted in the management of acute pulmonary oedema, whereas inotropes have become the standard care in cardiogenic shock. Moreover, some of the currently used drugs can cause harmful cardiac and peripheral effects, and increase mortality [6, 13–15]. Thus, emphasis should be on minimizing the deleterious effects of these agents.

This chapter is an overview of the recommended therapies for the acute and poststabilization care of patients with an AHF episode. It should be mentioned that these recommendations are mainly based on observational data. Dosing, indications and contraindications of the most commonly used drugs are provided in ➲ Tables 50.1–50.3 [1].

Classification

AHF is not represented by a homogeneous group of patients, but rather various types of heart failure patients, classified into six clinical conditions [1]:

◆ Worsening or decompensated chronic heart failure: there is a history of heart failure on treatment, and evidence of gradually increased systemic and pulmonary congestion.

◆ Acute pulmonary oedema: patients present with severe respiratory distress and oxygen saturation less than 90% on room air, as a result of rapid pulmonary congestion. This is a clinical condition that requires urgent pharmacological treatment and oxygen therapy, and in severe cases, ventilatory support.

◆ Hypertensive heart failure: patients, usually with preserved systolic function, present with signs of pulmonary congestion accompanied by high blood pressure.

◆ Cardiogenic shock: this is defined as inadequate tissue perfusion and characterized by low SBP (<90 mmHg or drop of mean arterial pressure >30%) and absence of diuresis or oliguria (<0.5 mL/kg per hour). Organ hypoperfusion and pulmonary congestion develop rapidly.

◆ Right heart failure: this is characterized as a low output condition due to right ventricular dysfunction, presented with elevated systemic venous pressures in the absence of pulmonary congestion.

◆ Acute heart failure due to acute coronary syndromes (ACS): many patients with signs of pulmonary congestion and/or low cardiac output present with a clinical picture of an ACS, documented by ECG and other laboratory findings (biochemistry, echocardiography evaluation, coronary angiography) [1, 16].

A simpler classification is based on systolic blood pressure (SBP) at presentation [15, 17–19]:

◆ Hypertensive acute heart failure (SBP >140 mmHg): this condition represents 43–50% of all AHF cases. Most patients are elderly women with preserved left ventricular ejection fraction (LVEF). The main target is blood pressure control and response to therapy is rapid. In-hospital mortality is low, approximately <2% [15, 20].

◆ Normotensive acute heart failure (SBP 90–140 mmHg): this condition represents 48–52% of all AHF cases. These patients have gradual worsening of symptoms and signs of heart failure, with reduced LVEF. In-hospital mortality is estimated to be 8–10% [15, 21].

◆ Hypotensive acute heart failure (SBP<90mmHg): approximately 2–8% of AHF patients have severe left ventricular systolic dysfunction with symptoms and signs of peripheral hypoperfusion and impaired renal function. In-hospital mortality is more than 15% (>30% in ACS) [15, 22].

Table 50.1 Intravenous vasodilators used in management of acute heart failure: dosing, indications, and adverse effects

Drug	Indications	Regimen	Adverse effects	Limitations
Nitroglycerine	Acute pulmonary oedema Pulmonary congestion in normotensive and hypertensive AHF	Initial regimen 10–20 µg/min, Increasing dose up to 200 µg/min	Hypotension Headache	Tolerance is common after 24–48 h, requiring adjustment of dosing
Isosorbite dinitrate	Pulmonary oedema Pulmonary congestion	Initial regimen 1 mg/h Increase up to 10 mg/h	Hypotension Headache	Tolerance as for nitroglycerine
Nitroprusside	Acute hypertensive congestion Congestion due to acute mitral regurgitation	Starting $0.3 \text{ mg kg}^{-1} \text{ min}^{-1}$, Increase up to5 mg kg^{-1} min^{-1}	Hypotension Isocyanate toxicity	Light sensitive Arterial line is required for SBP monitoring
Neseritide	Pulmonary oedema Pulmonary congestion	Bolus 2 µg/kg plus continuous infusion 0.015–0.030 µg kg^{-1} min^{-1}	Hypotension Worsening of renal function	Not currently available in many European countries

Reproduced with permission from Dickstein K, Cohen-Solal A, Filippatos G, *et al.* ESC guidelines for the diagnosis and treatment of acute and chronic heart failure 2008. *Eur Heart J* 2008;**29**:2388–2442.

Table 50.2 Main diuretics used in management of acute heart failure: indications, dosing, and adverse effects

Drug	Indication	Dosing	Adverse effects	Recommendations
Furosemide	Severe fluid retention Moderate fluid retention	40–100 mg IV bolus 5–40 mg/h (continuous infusion) 20–40 mg IV bolus	Hypovolaemia, Electrolyte disturbances Worsening of renal function	Up-titrate dosing of diuretics according to clinical response Check serum sodium, potassium, magnesium, urea, creatinine frequently
Torasemide	Fluid retention	10–100 mg oral	Electrolyte disturbances	
Buetanide	Fluid retention	0.5–4 mg oral or IV	Electrolyte disturbances	
Thiazides	Fluid retention refractory to loop diuretics	50–100 mg oral (combined with high doses of loop diuretics)	Severe hypokalemia	If there is resistance to this combination consider IV vasodilators or inotropes (according to SBP) and/or peripheral haemofiltration
Metolazone	Fluid retention refractory to loop diuretics	25–100 mg oral	Severe hypokalemia	Consider if creatinine clearance is <30 mL/min

Reproduced with permission from Dickstein K, Cohen-Solal A, Filippatos G, *et al.* ESC guidelines for the diagnosis and treatment of acute and chronic heart failure 2008. *Eur Heart J* 2008;**29**:2388–2442.

Table 50.3 Main inotropic agents used for the treatment of low output state in patients with acute heart failure: mechanisms, dosing, and adverse effects

Drug	Indication	Dosing	Adverse effects	Recommendations
Dobutamine (β-agonist) Dopamine (β-agonist)	Low output syndromes with peripheral hypoperfusion	2–20 mg kg^{-1} min^{-1} <3 mg kg^{-1} min^{-1}: renal effect 3–5 mg kg^{-1} min^{-1}: inotropic action >5 mg kg^{-1} min^{-1}: vasopressor	Increased myocardial oxygen consumption Myocardial injury Arrhythmiogenesis Increased heart rate Tachyphylaxis Increased mortality Increased heart rate Arrhythmias	Should be considered as a short-term treatment (48–72 h) in AHF patients for alleviation of symptoms
Milrinone (phosphodiesterase inhibitor)	Low output syndromes with peripheral hypoperfusion	25–75 mg/kg over 10–20 min plus 0.375–0.75 mg kg^{-1} min^{-1}	Hypotension Arrhythmiogenesis	Should be avoided in ischaemic heart failure
Enoximone (phosphodiesterase inhibitor)	Low output syndromes with peripheral hypoperfusion	0.25–0.75 mg/kg bolus plus 1.25–7.5 mg kg^{-1} min^{-1}	Hypotension Arrhythmiogenesis Increased mortality in ischaemic heart failure	Should be avoided in ischaemic heart failure
Levosimendan (calcium sensitizer)	Low output syndromes with peripheral hypoperfusion	6–12 mg/kg over 10 min (optional) plus 0.1mg/kg/min which can be decreased to 0.05 or increased to 0.2 mg kg^{-1} min^{-1}	Hypotension Ventricular arrhythmias Headache	Bolus dosing should be avoided if SBP is <100 mmHg. Not currently available in USA and some European countries
Adrenaline Noradrenaline	Cardiac arrest Restoration of peripheral hypoperfusion through vasoconstriction	Bolus: 1 mg can be given IV during resuscitation, repeated every 3–5 min 0.2–1.0 mg kg^{-1} min^{-1} (without bolus)		Consider adrenaline as a rescue therapy in cardiac arrest Consider noradrenaline in cardiogenic shock when the combination of an inotropic agent and fluid challenge fails to restore SBP >90 mmHg, with inadequate organ perfusion, despite improved cardiac output

Reproduced with permission from Dickstein K, Cohen-Solal A, Filippatos G, *et al.* ESC guidelines for the diagnosis and treatment of acute and chronic heart failure 2008. *Eur Heart J* 2008;**29**:2388–2442.

Precipitating factors

Box 50.1 summarizes the most common precipitating factors of AHF. Many conditions may precipitate an AHF episode, such as increased afterload due to systolic or pulmonary hypertension, increased preload due to volume overload, circulatory failure attributed to high output conditions, noncompliance with medical treatment, and drugs. Noncardiovascular conditions are also included, such as chronic obstructive pulmonary disease (COPD) and asthma. It is essential to identify and manage these factors in order to stabilize the patient and prevent new heart failure exacerbations (e.g. revascularization for coronary artery disease, correction of valvulopathies, management of arrhythmias or infections, blood pressure control) [15].

Goals of treatment

Treatment concerns both short-term and long-term management (◆Box 50.2). Traditionally, the primary therapeutic goals are to alleviate the patient's symptoms and stabilize their haemodynamic status. Many patients will require long-term therapeutic strategies, which are

recommended to be combined with management programmes that are designed to coordinate patients' postdischarge care, through structured follow-up plans [15].

Early pharmacological treatment of hypertensive acute heart failure

It is generally recommended to restore low oxygen saturation (>95%, >90% in patients with COPD) through oxygen administration or early use of noninvasive ventilation (NIV) [15] (see ◆Chapter 23). NIV should be considered in patients with acute pulmonary oedema and hypertensive AHF, as it improves left ventricular function by reducing afterload. It is reported that this modality reduces

---

Box 50.1 Precipitating factors for episodes of acute heart failure

- Acute coronary syndromes
- Valvular disease
- Acute myocarditis
- Uncontrolled hypertension
- Arrhythmias
- Infections (e.g. pneumonia)
- High output conditions (anaemia, sepsis, thyrotoxicosis)
- Acute pulmonary embolism
- Renal dysfunction
- COPD, asthma
- Postsurgical
- Noncompliance with medical treatment
- Drugs (NSAIDs, corticoids)
- No diet restrictions
- Unknown cause

Box 50.2 Goals of treatment in acute heart failure

Immediate (ER, ICU, CCU)

- Alleviate symptoms
- Improve low oxygenation
- Restore peripheral organ perfusion
- Improve central haemodynamics
- Avoid vital organ damage
- Limit ICU/CCU length of stay

Intermediate (cardiology ward)

- Achieve clinical stabilization and optimization of IV therapies
- Start oral life saving chronic medications (e.g. ACE inhibitors, β-blockers, aldosterone antagonists)
- Detect the subpopulations that need CRTs and/or ICDs
- Minimize in-hospital stay

Predischarge and long-term management

- Optimize predischarge fluid status
- Refer to outpatient heart failure clinic and cardiac rehabilitation centre
- Educate and give instructions for lifestyle modification
- Support psychosocial status
- Improve quality of life and prognosis

Modified from Dickstein K, Cohen-Solal A, Filippatos G, *et al.* ESC guidelines for the diagnosis and treatment of acute and chronic heart failure 2008. *Eur Heart J* 2008;**29**:2388–2442.

the need for intubation, but its effects on short-term mortality remain controversial [23–25].

Patients who have AHF with elevated blood pressure and symptoms and signs of congestion are mainly treated with vasodilators (nitrates, neseritide, nitroprusside) and secondarily with low doses of diuretics.

Nitroglycerine is widely used in AHF, exerting a predominantly venodilator effect at low doses and a mild arteriolar dilation at higher doses [26, 27]. It reduces left ventricular filling pressures, wall stress, pulmonary congestion, without compromising stroke volume or increasing myocardial oxygen consumption [28]. It is available for intravenous use, and as sublingual and topical preparations. Adverse events include headache and hypotension. Careful titration and monitoring of nitroglycerine administration is needed, as patients often develop tolerance (➲ Table 50.1).

There are no large-scale randomized clinical trials focusing on the use of nitrates in AHF. Some small studies have proved a dose-dependent improvement in haemodynamic function, whereas others have demonstrated that high doses of intravenous nitroglycerine or isosorbide dinitrate are more effective than furosemide in the management of acute pulmonary oedema due to hypertensive crisis [28, 29–36].

Nesiritide, a recombinant form of human brain natriuretic peptide(BNP), is also used in AHF. This agent exerts vasodilatory effects on arterial, venous, and coronary vessels. It also has a modest natriuretic effect, enhancing diuresis. These actions lead to increased cardiac output through the reduction of both preload and afterload [37–39]. Hypotension is the main adverse event. In the 'Vasodilation in the Acute Management of Congestive Heart Failure' (VMAC) trial, nesiritide produced a greater reduction in pulmonary capillary wedge pressure (PCWP) than nitroglycerine, while most improvements in symptoms, hospitalization, and mortality rate did not differ significantly between these two agents [40].

Sodium nitroprusside is a potent arterial vasodilator which is used in AHF patients with increased afterload due to severe hypertension as well as in those with pulmonary congestion due to acute mitral regurgitation. It reduces systemic vascular resistance and improves symptoms [41, 42]. In patients with renal dysfunction this drug may cause an increase in thiocyanate levels, and should be avoided. There is some evidence derived by myocardial infarction trials that sodium nitroprusside can cause reflex tachycardia or lead to coronary steal. It is therefore contraindicated in patients with AHF secondary to ACS, as it may exacerbate myocardial ischaemia [1, 43].

Clinical use of vasodilators

About 50% of patients with AHF typically present in the emergency department with an elevated SBP (>140 mmHg). They are usually elderly women with preserved LVEF. Symptoms present abruptly, and dyspnoea is the main manifestation [1, 6, 11, 12]. The main target is to control blood pressure rapidly. Pulmonary congestion is attributed to maldistribution of fluids rather than fluid overload and is rapidly managed with aggressive vasodilation [1, 3, 6].

It is generally recommended to administer nitroglycerine sublingually or as a spray during first patient contact; this leads to a dramatic improvement of symptoms, and can be followed by intravenous vasodilatory therapy (nitroglycerine or nesiritide) [44]. The initial recommended dose of intravenous nitroglycerine is 10–20 µg/min, increased in increments of 5–10 µg/min every 3–5 min as needed. Nesiritide may be started with a bolus infusion of 2 µg/kg, followed by a continuous infusion of 0.015–0.03 $\mu g\ kg^{-1}\ min^{-1}$ [1]. Nesiritide, which is not currently available in many European countries, should not be combined with other intravenous vasodilators. Frequent blood pressure measurement is needed in order to avoid hypotension episodes.

In patients with persistent pulmonary congestion or systemic volume overload in spite of blood pressure control, an intravenous loop diuretic should be added at the lowest possible dose.

The response to therapy should be continuously assessed. If the patient responds to initial treatment, admission to an observation unit is appropriate. If clinical improvement continues, discharge from hospital should be considered. If patients fail to respond adequately, particularly those with renal insufficiency or poor urine output, admission to the intensive care unit (ICU) may be appropriate [45].

Patients with near normal levels of SBP at presentation and no satisfactory response to diuretic therapy should also be treated with intravenous vasodilators. The emphasis should be upon maintenance of adequate perfusion. If a hypotensive episode occurs, the dose of vasodilator should be reduced or discontinued. Initiation of an intravenous inotropic agent may be necessary if there is evidence of hypoperfusion at any time.

Other vasoactive agents

Morphine

Morphine is a long-standing therapy in AHF, despite a lack of supporting data. More specifically, it is used for the treatment of patients who present with severe pulmonary congestion, dyspnoea, and anxiety or chest pain, as it reduces preload through the production of mild venodilation. Furthermore, morphine relieves breathlessness and exerts a calming effect [46–48]. An intravenous dose of 2.5–5 mg may be infused, and can be repeated as necessary. Blood pressure and respiratory function should be monitored carefully, and as nausea or vomiting is frequent, an antiemetic agent should be added. Caution is required in patients with hypotension, bradycardia, advanced atrioventricular block, or CO_2 retention [1].

There are retrospective data which suggest that morphine is associated with increased adverse events, such as prolonged hospitalization, increased need for ICU admission and/or endotracheal intubation, and, finally, higher in-hospital mortality [49]. Because of these emerging safety concerns, additional studies are required to clarify whether the use of morphine is beneficial.

Angiotensin converting enzyme inhibitors

Angiotensin converting enzyme (ACE) inhibitors are used as first line treatment in chronic heart failure patients, especially in those with impaired left ventricular systolic function. ACE inhibitors have been proved to significantly prolong survival and attenuate the symptoms, and they are associated with reduced hospitalization rates and decreased mortality [50–52]. Despite their beneficial effects in chronic heart failure, limited data exist for the acute setting, and they are not generally indicated in the early phase of stabilization of patients with AHF [1] although a few studies have demonstrated symptomatic and haemodynamic improvement in AHF after administration of ACE inhibitors [53,54]. However, as these agents attenuate remodelling and reduce morbidity and mortality, they should be initiated before discharge from hospital in acute *de novo* heart failure patients. In addition, patients receiving ACE inhibitors for chronic heart failure should be continued on this treatment during the AHF episode, unless they exhibit symptomatic hypotension, renal dysfunction (serum creatinine >2.5 mg/dL), or elevated potassium levels (>5 mmol/L), or there is evidence of cardiogenic shock.

Early pharmacological treatment of normotensive acute heart failure

Loop diuretics play a pivotal role in the management of AHF, as they can rapidly control symptoms secondary to fluid retention. Although clinicians are quite familiar with diuretics, their use in AHF remains empirical because of the paucity of large-scale randomized controlled clinical trials. Emerging data underline the potential adverse events of diuretics, including maladaptive activation of the renin–angiotensin–aldosterone system, impairment of renal function, hypovolaemia and electrolyte abnormalities, when used at high doses [55–58]. Moreover, these agents are associated with increased morbidity and mortality when used on a chronic basis [55–57].

Clinical use of diuretics

Loop diuretic therapy is recommended in patients who have volume overload and systemic congestion. These patients usually present with gradual worsening of symptoms and signs of chronic heart failure, and have normal SBP (90–140 mmHg) and reduced LVEF [1, 6, 12].

Table 50.2 describes the dosing, main indications, and most frequent adverse effects of diuretics used for the treatment of AHF. The lowest effective dose should be used, with a starting dose equivalent to the daily outpatient oral dose. A starting dose of 20 mg of intravenous furosemide may be used in patients who have never been treated with loop diuretics before. The total furosemide dose should be less than 100 mg in the first 6 h and less than 240 mg during the first 24 h. High initial doses of diuretics should be avoided, as these drugs can induce renal dysfunction, lead to hypovolaemia and hyponatraemia, and increase the likelihood of hypotension on initiation of ACE inhibitors or angiotensin II receptor I blockers (ARBs) [1]. It has been reported that patients receiving lower doses of furosemide exhibit a lower risk of in-hospital mortality, ICU stay, prolonged hospitalization, or adverse renal effects [59, 60]. Evidence is emerging to suggest that the combination of low-dose intravenous dopamine and oral furosemide, despite similar improvement in symptoms and urine output, is associated with fewer deleterious effects [59]. Another randomized trial demonstrated that high-dose furosemide plus low-dose nitrates in the treatment of severe pulmonary oedema was associated with higher in-hospital mortality and increased need for mechanical ventilation [61].

In cases of diuretic resistance, loop diuretics can be combined with thiazides, as well as with aldosterone antagonists (spironolactone, eprelenone) [1]. These combinations are associated with a lower incidence of side effects than that caused by higher doses of each agent alone. Close monitoring of blood pressure and urine output as well as frequent evaluation of renal function are necessary. Patients who respond adequately to treatment may be transmitted to an observation unit. Patients who are not improved, or develop hypotension and/or renal impairment, should be admitted to the ICU.

Early pharmacological treatment of hypotensive acute heart failure

Several registries have shown that 2–8% of patients with AHF have severe left ventricular systolic dysfunction with SPB less than 90 mmHg and symptoms and signs of peripheral hypoperfusion and impaired renal function [12, 62]. These patients exhibit a fourfold greater risk for adverse outcomes in the next 6 months than those with high blood pressure [63]. Immediate enhancement of cardiac contractility is crucial for this group of patients in order to achieve clinical stabilization. The cardinal targets of treatment in patients who are in a low-output state are the restoration of SBP to normal levels, the improvement of peripheral tissue perfusion, the protection of renal function, and the prevention of new heart failure exacerbations. Inotropic agents are suitable to be administered in these type of AHF patients. Traditional inotropes, such as β-agonists and phosphodiesterase (PDE) inhibitors, improve clinical and haemodynamic status of AHF patients with low output state, but may accelerate injurious biochemical pathways (increased apoptotic cell death, myocardial ischaemia, malignant arrhythmias) leading to increased mortality [64, 65]. The novel inodilatory agent levosimendan appears to be superior to traditional inotropes in improving the haemodynamic and clinical status of AHF patients, and also exerts cardioprotective actions [66, 67]. However, in recent randomized trials, levosimendan failed to improve prognosis, in spite of the aforementioned advantages [66, 67].

Traditional inotropes

Classical inotropes such as dopamine, dobutamine, and milrinone are used in the management of AHF patients with low cardiac index and marked peripheral hypoperfusion. These agents may also serve as a life-sustaining bridge to more definitive therapies such as cardiac transplantation or left ventricular mechanical support, or can be used in a pulsed fashion for the palliative care of patients with endstage heart failure [68, 69].

Mechanisms of action

Traditional inotropes exert their actions through different pathways that lead to an increase in intracellular levels of cyclic adenylate monophosphate (cAMP) [70]. The cAMP increase is caused by the β-adrenergic mediated stimulation of adenylate cyclase by β-agonists, or by the selective inhibition of PDE III (the enzyme that catalyses the breakdown of cAMP) in the case of PDE inhibitors [70]. Elevated levels of cAMP lead to an increase in calcium release from the sarcoplasmic reticulum, resulting in an enhancement of cardiac contractility. PDE inhibitors also have vasodilatory effects due to inhibition of PDE into vascular smooth muscle cells. As their cellular site of action is distal to the β-adrenergic receptors, their effects are maintained even during concomitant β-blocker therapy.

More specifically, dobutamine is a stimulator of β_1 receptors, producing inotropic and chronotropic effects. It is usually started with a 2–3 $\mu g\ kg^{-1}\ min^{-1}$ intravenous infusion rate without a loading dose, and can be gradually up-titrated to 20 $\mu g\ kg^{-1}\ min^{-1}$ according to the patient's clinical response [1, 71].

Dopamine has a dose-dependent mechanism of action. At doses below 3 mg $kg^{-1}\ min^{-1}$ it acts on peripheral dopaminergic receptors, causing peripheral vasodilation especially in the renal, splachnic, coronary, and cerebral vessels. At doses of 3–5 mg $kg^{-1}\ min^{-1}$ it acts as a β-adrenergic agonist, enhancing cardiac contractility, and at doses higher than 5 mg $kg^{-1}\ min^{-1}$ it acts as an α-adrenergic agonist, causing peripheral vasoconstriction [72]. Dopamine and dobutamine should be used carefully in patients with a heart rate greater than 100 beats/min [73].

Milrinone and enoximone are the two currently used PDE inhibitors. These agents have both inotropic and vasodilating effects, thus increasing cardiac output and decreasing pulmonary artery pressure, pulmonary wedge pressure, and systemic and pulmonary vascular resistance. Milrinone and enoximone are administered by a continuous infusion preceded by a bolus dose in patients with well-preserved SBP, and their action is maintained even during concomitant β-blocker therapy [74].

Clinical efficacy and safety

Mortality data from retrospective analyses of large-scale clinical trials showed that dobutamine, compared to placebo or other agents, led to higher occurrence of ventricular arrhythmias and was associated with higher 6-month mortality rate [75, 76]. Moreover, the 'Outcomes of Prospective Trial of Intravenous Milrinone for Exacerbations of Chronic Heart Failure' (OPTIME-CHF) showed that patients who received milrinone had significantly higher rates of hypotensive episodes requiring intervention, new atrial arrhythmias, and higher rates of adverse clinical outcomes in the cases of heart failure secondary to ischaemic aetiology than those who received placebo treatment [77].

All the accumulated data suggest that despite the symptomatic and haemodynamic improvement, traditional inotropes may increase long-term mortality in AHF. β-Adrenergic stimulation appears to have deleterious effects, as elevated levels of catecholamines are associated with adverse prognosis. β-Adrenergic agonists, such as dobutamine, enhance cardiac contractility, consequently increasing myocardial oxygen consumption. This fact may lead to exacerbation of underlying myocardial ischaemia. In the case of hibernating myocardium, an increase in cardiac contractility without a restoration in blood flow may induce apoptotic cell death and promote further myocardial injury [78]. Furthermore, cardiomyocyte calcium overload predisposes to an increased occurrence of ventricular arrhythmias [79]. Finally, PDE inhibitors can also induce arrhythmias and hypotensive episodes [80, 81].

Levosimendan

Levosimendan is a pyridazinone dinitrile derivative molecule that has positive inotropic properties by increasing the sensitivity of the cardiomyocyte contractile apparatus to intracellular calcium [82, 83]. Additionally, it is a powerful opener of ATP-sensitive potassium channels, causing peripheral arterial and venous dilatation. This biological action is responsible for the drug-induced reduction of peripheral vascular resistance and cardiac afterload. Thus, levosimendan provokes a significant increase of cardiac output through its combined positive inotropic and peripheral vasodilatory actions [84–86].

Levosimendan may be administered as a intravenous bolus dose (3–12 μg/kg), followed by a continuous infusion (0.05–0.2 μg kg^{-1} min^{-1} for 24 h). It is recommended that in patients with SBP less than 100 mmHg, levosimendan infusion should be started without a bolus dose to avoid hypotension [85, 87]. The effects of levosimendan are maintained for 1–2 weeks, following the single intravenous administration [88]. The main side effects include hypotension, headache, and hypokalaemia.

Clinical efficacy and safety

Data from recent randomized clinical trials demonstrated that administration of levosimendan in patients with low output AHF results in significant improvements of haemodynamic parameters, neurohormonal activation, and symptoms when compared with placebo or dobutamine [76]. However, these trials showed no superiority of levosimendan versus dobutamine or placebo in terms of improving 6-month event-free survival [87, 89]. On the other hand, in selected AHF patients such as those with previous history of heart failure and receiving chronic treatment with β-blockers, levosimendan seems to be superior to dobutamine in improving central haemodynamics and short-term mortality [87, 90, 91]. As there is no evidence for class I effective inotropic therapies in AHF, research for novel inotropic agents is essential.

Clinical use of inotropes

Patients with systolic dysfunction, hypotension (SBP ≤90 mmHg), and peripheral hypoperfusion may require invasive haemodynamic monitoring and management in the ICU [1]. The use of a pulmonary artery catheter use does not improve prognosis and can be employed only in order to evaluate fluid status, distinguish between cardiogenic and noncardiogenic shock, and guide vasoactive treatment in unstable patients who do not respond to traditional therapies [1]. Inotropic agents have become standard care for this clinical condition. In patients with persistent pulmonary congestion and poor urine output, addition of diuretics and application of peripheral haemofiltration may be appropriate. If inotropic therapy fails to improve hypoperfusion despite an increase in cardiac output, a vasopressor agent such as noradrenaline (norepinephrine)should be added. Noradrenaline is not recommended as first line treatment, and is only indicated in cardiogenic shock, when inotropes and fluid administration fail to restore organ perfusion. Intra-aortic balloon counterpulsation (IABP) and intubation should be considered in resistant cases. Finally, left ventricular assist devices may be considered as a bridge to more definite strategies such as heart transplantation, or as a bridge to recovery.

Therapeutic approaches in acute heart failure: a summary

In this section therapeutic approaches are summarized according to the initial SBP [1, 17].

Hypertensive acute heart failure (SBP≥140 mmHg)

- Restoration of low oxygen saturation (>95% in patients without COPD or >90% in patients with COPD) using oxygen supply or continuous/bilevel positive airway pressure (CPAP/BiPAP) or mechanical ventilation.

- Alleviation of patient anxiety and pain using intravenous opioids (e.g. morphine).

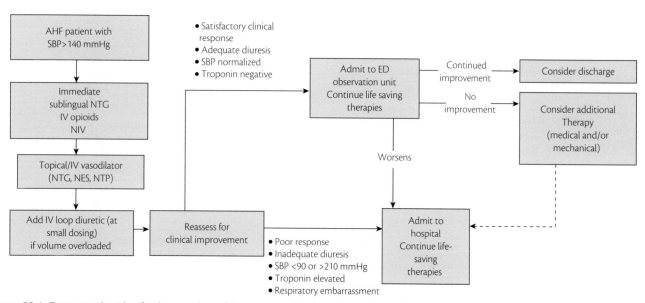

Figure 50.1 Treatment algorithm for the acute heart failure patient with elevated systolic blood pressure (>140 mmHg). AHF, acute heart failure; ED: emergency department; IV, intravenous; NES, nesiritide; NIV, noninvasive ventilation; NTG, nitroglycerine; NTP, nitroprusside; SBP, systolic blood pressure. Adapted with permission from Kirk JD, Parissis JT, Filippatos G. Pharmacologic stabilization and management of acute heart failure syndromes in the emergency department. *Heart Fail Clin* 2009;**5**:43–54.

◆ Improvement of pulmonary congestion using high doses of intravenous vasodilators and low doses of intravenous diuretics.

◆ Restoration of sinus rhythm or achievement of satisfactory heart rate control in the presence of atrial fibrillation (or other supraventricular tachycardias) using electroversion or intravenous antiarrhythmics (e.g. digoxin, amiodarone, diltiazem).

See treatment algorithm in ➲ Fig. 50.1.

Normotensive acute heart failure (SBP 90–140 mmHg)

◆ Improvement of fluid overload using high doses of intravenous diuretics (consider combination of different classes of diuretics in resistant cases).

◆ Reduction of elevated cardiac filling pressures and afterload (if SBP>100 mmHg) using low doses of intravenous vasodilators (e.g. nitrates) with parallel close monitoring of SBP.

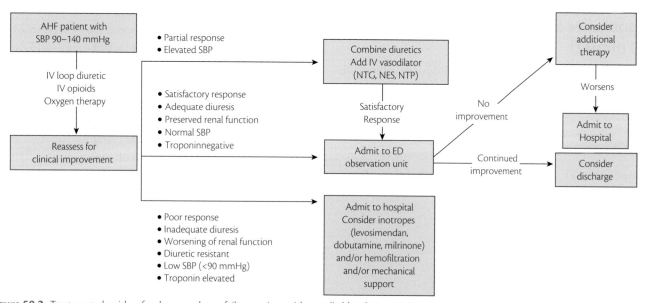

Figure 50.2 Treatment algorithm for the acute heart failure patient with systolic blood pressure 90–140 mmHg. AHF, acute heart failure; ED: emergency department; IV, intravenous; NES, nesiritide; NTG, nitroglycerine; NTP, nitroprusside; SBP, systolic blood pressure. Adapted with permission from Kirk JD, Parissis JT, Filippatos G. Pharmacologic stabilization and management of acute heart failure syndromes in the emergency department. *Heart Fail Clin* 2009;**5**:43–54.

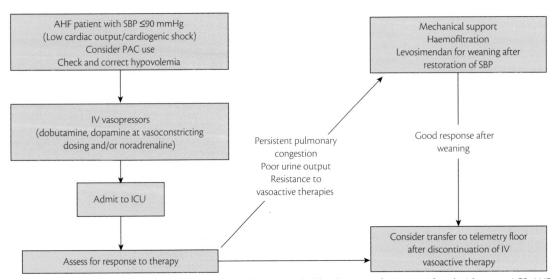

Figure 50.3 Treatment algorithm for the acute heart failure patient with low systolic blood pressure (<90 mmHg) and without an ACS. AHF, acute heart failure; ICU, intensive care unit; IV: intravenous; PAC, pulmonary artery catheter; SBP, systolic blood pressure.
Adapted with permission from Kirk JD, Parissis JT, Filippatos G. Pharmacologic stabilization and management of acute heart failure syndromes in the emergency department. *Heart Fail Clin* 2009;**5**:43–54.

- Improvement of peripheral organ hypoperfusion using intravenous inotropes (e.g. levosimendan, dobutamine) in cases resistant to the above therapies or as initial approach in the cases with low output symptoms and 120 >SBP >90 mmHg.

- Mechanical regulation of fluid status using peripheral haemofiltration devices in patients with renal function worsening under the recommended intravenous medications.

See treatment algorithm in ➲ Fig. 50.2.

Hypotensive acute heart failure (SBP ≤90 mmHg)

- Evaluation of fluid status using a pulmonary artery catheter (exclusion of hypovolaemia).

- Restoration of SBP and peripheral hypoperfusion using intravenous vassopressors (e.g high doses of dopamine and/or dobutamine, noradrenaline).

- Improvement of coronary and peripheral perfusion using mechanical support (implantation of IABP or other portable devices).

- Improvement of oliguria/anuria using portable peripheral haemofiltration devices in cases resistant to the above strategies.

- When the cause of hypotensive AHF is an ACS, immediate reperfusion treatment and implantation of an IABP are the first line therapeutic strategies.

See treatment algorithm in ➲ Fig. 50.3.

Conclusion

AHF is a complex clinical condition that has only recently received attention, and which has extremely high mortality and readmission rates. Due to the lack of many randomized controlled trials and highly heterogeneous patient population, recommendations for the management of AHF are mainly based on observational data and expert opinions. All the currently used agents have failed to improve short- and long-term prognosis in AHF, despite the alleviation of symptoms and improvement of central haemodynamics. Thus, further investigation is needed for the development of novel, more targeted treatment strategies, with an emphasis on the safety of patients.

Personal perspective

Several new pharmacological agents are under evaluation and may be helpful in the future management of AHF. Data from phase II or III clinical trials indicate that therapies with novel mechanisms of actions may effectively reduce pulmonary congestion or improve cardiac function in AHF patients [90]. Despite these promising findings, there is still no evidence that any new agent has beneficial effects on short- and long-term prognosis of AHF patients. While we await the results of ongoing research, the early pharmacological treatment of AHF should be individualized in accordance with the patient's clinical phenotype (levels of SBP, existence of congestion, peripheral perfusion status, management of comorbidities or precipitating factors).

Further reading

Cotter G, Moshkovitz Y, Milovanov O, *et al.* Acute heart failure: a novel approach to its pathogenesis and treatment. *Eur J Heart Fail.* 2002;**4**:227–234.

De Luca L, Fonarow GC, Mebazaa A, *et al.* Early pharmacological treatment of acute heart failure syndromes: a systematic review of clinical trials. *Acute Card Care 2007;***9**:10–21.

De Luca L, Mebazaa A, Filippatos G, *et al.* Overview of emerging pharmacologic agents for acute heart failure syndromes. *Eur J Heart Fail* 2008;**10**(2):201–213.

Dickstein K, Cohen-Solal A, Filippatos G, *et al.* ESC guidelines for the diagnosis and treatment of acute and chronic heart failure 2008: the Task Force for the diagnosis and treatment of acute and chronic heart failure 2008 of the European Society of Cardiology. Developed in collaboration with the Heart Failure Association of the ESC (HFA) and endorsed by the European Society of Intensive Care Medicine (ESICM) *Eur Heart J* 2008;**29**:2388–2442.

Felker GM, O'Connor CM. Inotropic therapy for heart failure: an evidence-based approach. *Am Heart J* 2001;**142**:393–401.

Gheorghiade M, De Luca L, Fonarow GC, *et al.* Pathophysiologic targets in the early phase of acute heart failure syndromes. *Am J Cardiol* 2005;**96**(suppl 6A):11G–17G.

Kirk JD, Parissis JT, Filippatos G. Pharmacologic stabilization and management of acute heart failure syndromes in the emergency department. *Heart Fail Clin* 2009;**5**(1):43–54.

Parissis J, Farmakis D, Nieminen M. Classical inotropes and new cardiac enhancers. *Heart Fail Rev* 2007;**12**(2):149–156.

Parissis J, Filippatos G, Farmakis D, *et al.* Levosimendan for the treatment of acute heart failure syndromes. *Exp Opin Pharmacother* 2005;**6**(15):2741–2751.

Shin DD, Brandimarte F, De Luca L, *et al.* Review of current and investigational pharmacologic agents for acute heart failure syndromes. *Am J Cardiol* 2007;**99**(2A):4A–23A.

⮑ For additional multimedia materials please visit the online version of the book (🕮 http://www.esciacc.oxfordmedicine.com).

CHAPTER 51

Non-pharmacologic therapy of acute heart failure: when drugs alone are not enough

Pascal Vranckx, Wilfried Mullens, and Johan Vijgen

Contents

Summary

Pharmacologic agents remain the mainstay of therapy for acute heart failure syndromes (AHFS). However, at all time during the early diagnostic, aetiologic, and therapeutic work-up non-pharmacologic therapy may be indicated. In patients not responding to the standard pharmacologic regimen, with or without non-invasive ventilation, myocardial ischaemia should be excluded.

Management of the complex cardiac patient with advanced heart failure (HF) and/or (potential) haemodynamic compromise has become a special dimension for specialized myocardial intervention centres (MICs) providing 24/7 state-of-the-art facilities for (primary) percutaneous coronary intervention (PCI) *and* advanced (intensive) cardiac care including mechanical ventilation, ultrafiltration with or without dialysis, and extracorporeal circulatory assist.

Through the understanding of the underlying pathophysiology and approaches to the problems of acute HF, one should be better prepared to understand and treat its many facets.

Introduction

The intent of this chapter is to give a readable, concise clinical overview of the non-pharmacologic treatment of different AHFS, providing a basis for clinical algorithms and the clinical use of evidence-based treatment guidelines.

The framework for the utilization of different treatment modalities will be discussed. There will be a focus on physiologic approaches addressing the balance between oxygen demand and delivery, and the manipulation of cardiopulmonary interactions to optimize ventricular function, including the use of mechanical circulatory support which might serve as a method of achieving a state of myocardial rest.

Cross references, mainly to *The ESC Textbook of Cardiovascular Medicine* (second edition) to related chapters in this textbook, and to the ESC Practice Guidelines, will be provided. The 'Background' section summarizes the basic knowledge which the interested reader should have before starting this journey, which will integrate related concepts of pathophysiology, (haemodynamic) monitoring, and technology.

Background

The heart can be conceptually approached as a hydrodynamic input–output system, a haemodynamic compression pump, a muscular pump, or a pluricellular tissue pump [1]. The heart acts, in close relationship to the lungs and circulation, with the ultimate goal to preserve adequate tissue oxygenation and function (see ➲ Chapter 35 Heart failure, ESC Textbook of Cardiovascular Medicine, 2nd edition, 2009.) The primary physiological task of the cardiorespiratory system is to deliver adequate oxygen (O_2) to meet the metabolic demands of the body (VO_2) (➲ Fig 51.1).

Oxygen delivery (DO_2) is the amount of oxygen delivered to the peripheral tissue, and is obtained by multiplying the arterial oxygen content (CaO_2) by the cardiac output (CO):

$$DO_2 = CaO_2 \times CO \qquad \text{Eqn. 1}$$

The oxygen content of blood is the volume of oxygen carried in 100mL of blood. It is calculated by:

$$(O_2 \text{ carried by Hb}) + (O_2 \text{ in solution}) = (1.34 \times Hb \times SaO_2 \times 0.01) + (0.023 \times PaO_2) \qquad \text{Eqn. 2}$$

where:

- SaO_2 = percentage saturation of Hb with oxygen
- Hb = haemoglobin concentration in grams per 100mL blood
- PaO_2 = partial pressure of oxygen (0.0225 = mL of O_2 dissolved per 100mL plasma per kPa, or 0.003mlL per mmHg).

AHFS may occur de novo or as a complication of worsening chronic HF at different pathophysiological stages of the disease (➲ Fig. 51.2). In its severest form, AHFS consist

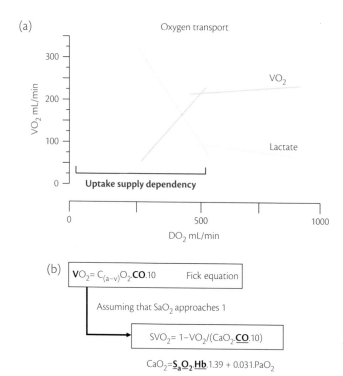

Figure 51.1 (a) Oxygen uptake-supply dependency (b) Physiology of mixed venous and central venous oxygen saturation: SvO_2 is directly proportional to the ratio of VO_2 to CO. SvO_2 is well correlated with the ratio of O_2 supply to demand. $C(a-v)O_2$ is arterio venous oxygen difference, CaO_2 is arterial oxygen content: oxygen bound to hemoglobin [product of hemoglobin concentration (Hb) and arterial O_2 saturation (SaO_2)] + physically dissolved oxygen [arterial PO_2 (PaO_2)]. SvO_2 reflects CO when Hb and SaO_2 are constant(bold)

of a life-threatening medical emergency that presents with severe circulatory failure and symptoms of impaired organ perfusion and resulting damage The syndrome is complex and often is the result of multiple contributing diseases. The symptoms of HF may be aggravated by non-cardiovascular comorbidities such as obstructive lung disease or coexisting end-organ disease, especially renal dysfunction. HF might be caused by ischaemia, hypertension, atrial fibrillation (AF), or other non-cardiac conditions (e.g. renal insufficiency, diabetes, sepsis), or untoward drug effects (see ➲ Chapter 49–50, Acute heart failure classification and pathophysiology; Chapter 35, Heart failure, ESC Textbook of Cardiovascular Medicine, 2nd edition, 2009) leading to a failure of the heart to meet metabolic demands [2].

The management of AHFS is challenging given the heterogeneity of the patient population in terms of clinical presentation, pathophysiology, prognosis, and therapeutic options. The main goals of the acute management of the patient with AHFS are to:

◆ Resuscitate the patient. Stabilize and treat life-threatening conditions and prevent further deterioration (pre-hospital, initial in-hospital phase up to 24h)

◆ Improve haemodynamics, often leading to an amelioration of symptoms (in-hospital phase)

◆ Determine the possible aetiology and provide further risk assessment. Enable early intervention when an acute reversible problem exists (in-hospital phase)

◆ Ensure implementation of evidence-based guidelines (pharmacological, surgical, interventional, and implantable cardiac-defibrillator/cardiac resynchronization therapy [CRT]) to reduce future readmissions. (pre-discharge, early post-discharge phase)

◆ Monitor your patient on an ongoing basis, triage early among alternative levels of hospital care, and allocate right hospital resources whenever needed.

Pharmacologic agents traditionally have been the mainstay of therapy for AHFS; however, at each phase of hospital evaluation and management concomitant non-pharmacologic therapy should be considered (⮑ Fig. 51.2). The initial AHFS evaluation should begin with a careful history and physical examination. Early triage and management may be guided by vital signs, physical findings, and urinary output (⮑ Table 51.1). A standard 12-lead electrocardiogram might indicate potential myocardial ischaemia, rhythm, or conduction abnormalities warranting an early invasive approach [2]. Conventional echocardiography, supplemented by tissue Doppler imaging (TDI), is a highly valuable non-invasive tool for the assessment of cardiac anatomy and function [3]. In addition to established critical roles in the early diagnostic, aetiologic, and therapeutic work-up in AHFS [2,4,5], echocardiography plays an important clinical role in early 'prognostication' and triage to more oriented therapy [3,4,6]. (For details see ⮑ Chapter 20 Echocardiography; chapter 35 heart failure, ESC Textbook of Cardiovascular Medicine, 2nd edition 2009)

A more definitive resuscitation strategy in advanced AHFS not responding to standard pharmacologic therapy, and/or patients (at high risk of) developing circulatory failure, may require invasive monitoring and a *goal-oriented* manipulation of cardiac preload, afterload, and contractility to achieve a balance between systemic oxygen delivery and oxygen demand (⮑ Fig. 51.1a). Endpoints used to confirm the achievement of such a balance include normalization of values for mixed venous oxygen saturation, arterial lactate concentration, base deficit, and pH [9]. Mixed venous oxygen saturation (⮑ Fig. 51.1b):

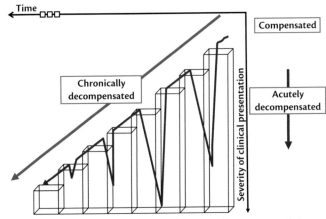

Figure 51.2 Worsening chronic heart failure at different stages of disease.

$$SvO_2 = SaO_2 - [VO_2/(CO \times [Hb \times 13.9])] \qquad Eqn. 3$$

has been shown to be a surrogate for the cardiac index as a target for haemodynamic therapy. In cases in which the insertion of a pulmonary-artery catheter is impractical, venous oxygen saturation (central venous oxygen saturation, SvO_2) can be measured in the central circulation [10]. Importantly, trends of haemodynamic measures in the right direction are as important as targeting preset specific numbers. In addition, while inotropic therapy is often used in such situations to improve haemodynamic measures, its use is eclipsed by a higher number of adverse events (Optimize-HF: the Organized Program to Initiate Lifesaving Treatment in Hospitalized Patients with Heart Failure program [59]).

In the critically ill (cardiac) patient the cardiocirculatory system is mainly challenged by two different conditions. Firstly, a drop in DO_2 which can be induced by anaemia, hypoxia, hypovolaemia, HF, or any combination of these. Secondly, fever, pain, stress, and/or respiratory failure, etc. may further decrease SvO_2 or $ScvO_2$ by increasing whole-body VO_2. It is of pivotal importance that the physician

Table 51.1 Vital signs and clinical symptoms to guide early management in AHFS (7,8)

Heart rate >100bpm
Systolic blood pressure <100(–120)mmHg
Proportional pulse pressure ≤25 (CI <2.2L/min/m²)
(If) orthopnoea (PCWP >22mmHg)
Killip class II–IV
Age

Proportional pulse pressure: systolic blood pressure (BP) – diastolic BP/ systolic BP.
CI cardiac index in L/min per square metre (normal: 2.6–4.2).
PCWP: pulmonary capillary wedge pressure.
Orthopnoea: cough, especially during semi-recumbency may be the equivalent of orthopnoea.

dealing with this type of patient understands these basic principles. Three items should be evaluated in the early stabilization period:

1 The need for sedation and ventilatory support. (*Ventilation*)

2 The need for inotropic/vasopressor support. Does the patient need a central venous access? (*Infuse*)

3 The need for mechanical circulatory support. (*Pump*)

In the context of non-pharmacologic therapy of AHFS, the 'I' may become 'Intervention' including cardioversion, revascularization, etc.

Non-pharmacologic therapy of acute heart failure

The pathway from stabilization to intervention

Patient care in AHFS is a dynamic process, requiring ongoing simultaneous diagnosis and treatment. Four phases for patient evaluation and management are proposed: 1) the initial or early phase (i.e. emergency department); 2) the in-hospital phase; 3) the pre-discharge phase; and 4) the early post-discharge phase (◆ Fig. 51.3) [11].

The goal of treatment in the pre-hospital setting or in the emergency room is to improve tissue oxygenation and optimize haemodynamics in order to improve symptoms, permit transport to a higher-level hospital, and ensure

survival. After the initial assessment which should be performed quickly, all patients should be considered for oxygen therapy and non-invasive ventilation (NIV: e.g. continuous positive airway pressure [CPAP] or bilevel positive airway pressure [BiPAP]). Escalation to ETI and an invasive approach may be required in cases of severe sensorial impairment (including coma), (high risk of) circulatory failure, life-threatening arrhythmia, progressive hypoxia, or life-threatening complications like pneumothorax etc. However, the majority of patients respond well to an initial goal-directed pharmacologic therapy with or without NIV and one should not intubate and ventilate only for the comfort of the doctor to work with a sedated patient.

Portable circulatory mechanical assist (intra-aortic balloon pump [IABP]) may be indicated early during the initial resuscitation and stabilization phase, in refractory (within 6–12h) or advanced AHFS, especially when drug-resistant hypotension and pulmonary congestion sustains. However, at all stages myocardial ischaemia should be excluded and treated whenever possible [2,12,13].

Patients with AHFS complicating acute coronary syndromes (ACS) requiring emergent PCI are at considerable risk for haemodynamic compromise or collapse at the time of intervention. Management of the complex cardiac patient with (potential) haemodynamic compromise has become a special dimension for specialized MICs providing state-of-the-art facilities for (primary) PCI, including experienced senior operators available on a 24h/7 days a week basis and critical care physicians experienced in all aspects of

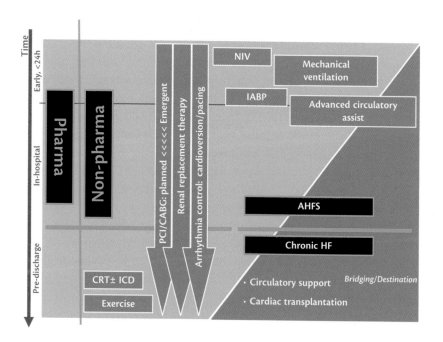

Figure 51.3 Phases for patient evaluation and management in AHFS

diagnosing and treating complex cardiac patients. If these facilities are not available on site, upgrading and transfer to a specialized MIC should be initiated early (within the first 12h) [14]. These patients may require invasive monitoring and ETI for comfort (both patient and investigator) and clinical reasons. Portable mechanical circulatory assist may provide a valuable safeguard to increase (transport and) procedural safety. Early intervention in response to physiological instability might prevent further deterioration in many patients.

Other comorbidities including (supra-)ventricular arrhythmias, bradycardia, infections, pulmonary diseases, severe anaemia, and renal or hepatic dysfunction must be addressed, and corrected when appropriate, on a ongoing base during the hospital stay (see ➲ Fig. 51.3).

Mechanical ventilation and oxygen transport

In AHFS, pulmonary and systemic congestion due to elevated ventricular filling pressures with or without a decrease in cardiac output and tissue hypoperfusion is frequent [11]. Lung dysfunction can be evaluated in terms of lung mechanics and gas diffusion (see ➲ Chapter 20, respiratory monitoring). It is recommended to administer oxygen as early as possible in hypoxaemic patients to achieve an arterial oxygen saturation ≥95% (>90% in patients with chronic obstructive pulmonary disease [COPD]) [69].

Following the formula to calculate DO_2 (see ➲ Eqns. 1 and 2), tissue oxygen delivery could be increased just by administering supplemental oxygen to increase the arterial oxygen tension (PaO_2) provided there is an adequate Hb concentration. However, spontaneous ventilatory efforts require muscular activity, thereby consuming O_2 and producing carbon dioxide (CO_2), which represents a extra metabolic load on the cardiovascular system. The inspiratory effort used by patients with acute respiratory failure is about four to six times the normal value [15–17]. Increased work of breathing will stress the cardiovascular response to maintain adequate tissue perfusion and will result in increased cardiac output to meet the increased oxygen demand (VO_2).

Mechanical ventilatory support can directly alter oxygen homeostasis in the human body by its effect on the arterial oxygen content, cardiac output, and VO_2 of the respiratory system. Ventilation affects the circulation primarily by altering the preload and afterload conditions of the heart through changes in intrathoracic pressure (ITP) and lung volume [18].

In other words, ventilation is exercise, since it consumes O_2 and produces CO_2.

Mechanical ventilation (see also Chapter 24 Procedures in ICCU)

In patients with severe cardiopulmonary distress for whom the effort of breathing is intolerable or inefficient, mechanical ventilation will artificially replace the action of the respiratory muscles. The objectives of mechanical ventilation are primarily to decrease the work of breathing (VO_2 of the respiratory system) and reverse life-threatening hypoxaemia or acute progressive respiratory acidosis. The need for mechanical ventilation and artificial airways can be reduced by substituting non-invasive ventilatory support when appropriate. However, one has to bear in mind that the mechanically-assisted inspiration will result in increased ITPs and mechanically-assisted expiration in decreased ITPs which is the opposite of normal ventilation.

NIV, delivered through tight-fitting face masks, has been shown to maintain adequate gas exchange, reduce the work of breathing, and to limit the need for ETI in patients with acute respiratory failure due to acute pulmonary oedema, status asthmaticus, or COPD [19–23]. Although its use has been associated with decreased resource utilization, mortality benefit over oxygen for either continuous or bilevel NIV remains questionable [24,25]. NIV can be safely used, even outside the intensive care unit, by experienced nurses, respiratory therapists, and physicians. However, relative haemodynamic stability, full patient cooperation and the ability of the patient to protect their own airway are important prerequisites when choosing a NIV mode. NIV should never be used when there is a need for emergent intubation. Appropriate initial settings for NIV in AHFS are listed in ➲ Fig. 51.4. The response to NIV should be assessed after 60min and thereafter on a continuous basis by trained personnel. Parameters of interest are respiratory rate (>35 beats/min and above the value at admission), blood pressure, pulse rate, pH (pH ≤7.20 and above the value at admission on two consecutive arterial blood gas samples), PCO_2 ($\pm PO_2$) and level of consciousness.

Fortunately, endotracheal intubation (ETI) and mechanical ventilation are only required in a minority of AHFS patients. Patients at risk are: non-responders to NIV; those with (profound) circulatory failure; or those at high risk of haemodynamic deterioration during intervention or inter-hospital transport.

Ventilatory mode and settings directly relate to outcome in patients suffering from acute respiratory failure [26,27]. Although there is still a debate as to whether a tidal volume of 6–8mL/kg should be applied to all patients ventilated for

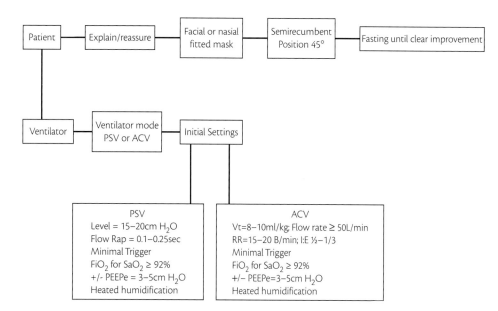

Figure 51.4 NIV implementation and settings.

acute lung injury, there is a general agreement that end-plateau pressures should be kept below 30cmH$_2$O whenever possible. Cyclic closing and re-opening of alveolar units during mechanical ventilation should be avoided.

BiPAP/airway pressure release ventilation (APRV) (see ➲Chapter 24) with superimposed spontaneous breathing improves gas exchange, often with lower maximal airway pressures, compared with controlled mechanical ventilation. Therefore, it is an attractive mode of ventilation in 'hypervolaemic' HF patients. Positive-pressure ventilation (PPV), by abolishing the negative swings in ITP, will selectively decrease left ventricular (LV) afterload, as long as the increases in lung volume and ITP are small (28). Spontaneous inspiration and spontaneous inspiratory efforts will decrease ITP. An increase in ITP compresses the vena cava and thus decreases venous return. Lung hyperinflation may further negatively affect cardiac output by altering right ventricular (RV) preload and afterload.

Applying this knowledge, ventilator settings may even prove to be more important than ventilator mode.

Static end-inspiratory pressures of ≤25cmH$_2$O are safe, >30cmH$_2$O dangerous. Considering the potential worsening effect of positive end-expiratory pressure (PEEP) on venous return and cardiac output, in AHFS only moderate levels (3–5cmH$_2$O) should be applied initially and adjusted upon haemodynamic tolerance. Respiratory rate will be set between 25–20/min and adjusted according to the patient's rate demand and PCO$_2$. Patients with acute hypoxaemic respiratory failure usually have small lung volumes. Decreases in lung volume induce alveolar collapse and hypoxia, stimulating an increased pulmonary vasomotor tone by the process of hypoxic pulmonary vasoconstriction [29].

Recruitment manoeuvres, PEEP, and CPAP may reverse hypoxic pulmonary vasoconstriction and reduce pulmonary artery pressure [29].

Transfusion of red blood cells

Anaemia is common among patients with HF, probably occurring in approximately 20% of patients, depending on the definition of terms and severity of patient illness [30]. The human tolerance of anaemia is dependent on the recruitment of physiologic reserve, a major component of which is the ability to increase cardiac output. Patients with chronic HF lack normal physiological reserve to compensate for decreased haemoglobin and may manifest decreased aerobic capacity in response to mild degrees of anaemia [31]. The clinical utility of blood transfusion in anaemic cardiovascular disease populations remains controversial [32–34]. Balancing risks and benefits, transfusion should only be considered as an acute treatment for severe anaemia on an individualized basis.

Revascularization and surgical therapy

Coronary artery disease (CAD), or its atherothrombotic complications, has emerged as the dominant underlying aetiologic factor in patients with HF and the presence of ischaemic and/or stunned/hibernating myocardium may have a profound impact on the initial, in-hospital, and post-discharge management and prognosis [35–37]. In patients with AHFS and evidence of myocardial ischaemia, the diagnosis or suspicion of obstructive CAD should lead to the consideration of early myocardial revascularization [38]. The treatment approaches for AHFS with CAD are discussed elsewhere (see ➲Chapter 45–46).

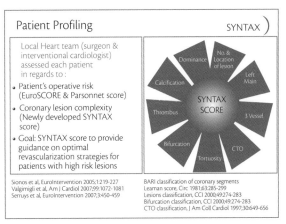

Figure 51.5 Syntax score components

With increasing operator experience, refinement of angioplasty hardware and technique, and adjunctive pharmacological treatment, the morphologic and the clinical profile of patients acceptable for coronary angioplasty has widened considerably. However, even in the acute setting, the benefits of a specific percutaneous procedure should be weighed against the risks involved, taking into account alternative treatment strategies, including the individual operator's and overall institution's (interventional and intensive care team) experience [39]. As indicated in the background section of this chapter, in such circumstances, transfer to a 'centre of excellence' that routinely performs complex PCI may be the most effective and efficient course of action. Clinical and angiographic characteristics are proven to be equally important in determining procedural risk with PCI (➲Fig. 51.5) [40–42].

Management of the complex cardiac patient with (potential) haemodynamic compromise has become a special dimension for specialized MICs.

Very high-risk procedures are, of course, often inevitable because of the inherent risk and presentation of the underlying disease. Knowledge of very high-risk procedural complications should alert the operator and should trigger measures to reduce the extent of the risk whenever possible. A strategy of early angiography and revascularization, where appropriate, in AHFS must also take into account the potential costs.

Revascularization with either PCI or coronary artery bypass grafting (CABG) can improve the perfusion of viable myocardium but does not restore function in areas of infarction. Surgical procedures to eliminate or exclude areas of infarction (surgical ventricular restoration), repair mitral regurgitation, or support the failing myocardium are discussed in ➲Chapter 52.

Portable cardiac assist

Percutaneous mechanical circulatory support (MCS) can be provided by a variety of devices and modalities designed to increase forward blood flow and reduce filling pressures (see ➲Chapter 30). Since IABP is incapable of supporting a patient with complete haemodynamic collapse, immediate triage to more advanced percutaneous (or implantable) circulatory support modalities is warranted when needed. Therefore, treatment options for MCS must be tailored to each patient in order to optimize the benefits and minimize the risk of detrimental effects. Experience with these systems continuous to grow, with leading centres and investigators contributing meaningful information towards the application and development of the latest technologies.

A minimal flow rate of 70mL/kg body weight/min is required to provide adequate organ perfusion. To make percutaneous insertion realistic, the maximum diameter of cannulae should be downsized to a maximum of around 10F. Pre-insertion abdominal and iliofemoral angiography is useful to assess feasibility of insertion and to select the appropriate insertion site, thereby minimizing complications. In case of emergency in patients with severe atherosclerotic disease, percutaneous transluminal angioplasty of the femoral artery or surgical placement may be considered. In order to prevent limb ischaemia caused by femoral cannulation, distal leg perfusion with a small catheter placed in the distal artery is often used.

MCS can be used to resuscitate patients, as a stabilizing measure for angiography and prompt revascularization, or to buy time until more definite measures can be taken [40]. In this setting, the revival of extracorporeal circuitry and hardware that can provide both respiratory and circulatory support to patients for periods up to several weeks is of particular interest (➲Fig. 51.6).

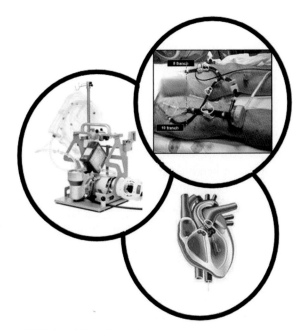

Figure 51.6 Portable cardiac assist

In addition there is experimental evidence that ventricular unloading of the left ventricle can significantly reduce infarct size. Mechanical support combines the beneficial effects of the myocardial unloading and an increase in tissue perfusion pressure [43–45].

Fluid management beyond diuretics: haemofiltration with or without dialysis

The pathophysiology of the cardiorenal interaction in the setting of advanced decompensated heart failure (ADHF) is poorly understood. Renal impairment is often present at time of admission [46]. Structural renal dysfunction due to diabetes, hypertension, and arteriosclerosis are common. Worsening renal function occurs in 20–30% of patients during hospitalization [47–50]. This worsening during or after discharge may result from further neurohormonal and haemodynamic abnormalities (low cardiac output and/or high venous pressure), which may be aggravated by high-dose loop diuretics [51–54].

Isolated ultrafiltration has recently gained great interest in the non-pharmacological management of congestion in HF [55–57]. The rationale for use of extracorporeal methodologies centres on three aspects: fast removal of fluid; avoidance of maladaptive renal tubular autoregulatory responses induced by diuretics; and higher magnitude of sodium clearance. In the acute setting it may even improve lung mechanics through body fluid content reduction (⮕ Fig. 51.7). However, excessively high ultrafiltration rates may lead to decreased effective blood volume, hypotension, renal hypoperfusion, pre-renal azotemia, and possibly acute renal failure necessitating dialysis.

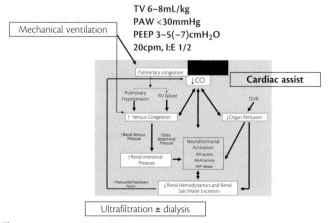

Figure 51.7 Cardiorenal interactions in advanced decompensated heart failure TV denotes Tidal Volume (ml), PAW: Airway Pressure (mmHg), PEEP: Positive End Expiratory Pressure (cmH2O), I:E inspiratory:expiratory time ratio, RV: Right Ventricle, SVR: Systemic Vascular Resistance, CO: cardiac output, AHFS: Acute Heart Failure Syndromes.

Sinus rhythm and arrhythmia devices in heart failure

Arrhythmia may frequently precipitate or aggravate AHFS and should be treated aggressively.

AHFS are often associated with electrical and conduction abnormalities [58]. AF and HF often coexist [59,60]. The prevalence of AF increases with the severity of HF and worsens its course by loss of atrial contraction, poor rate control, and irregular rhythm [61].

Some component of (reversible) tachycardia-induced myopathy is seen in up to 50% of patients with LV dysfunction and AF [62–64]. Furthermore, the detrimental effects of AF on HF also may derive from the negative inotropic effects of antiarrhythmic drugs. Over the last decade the non-pharmacologic armamentarium for HF patients has expanded.

Direct current cardioversion

When a rapid ventricular response AF does not respond promptly to pharmacological therapy, or in case of severe haemodynamic compromise, intractable myocardial ischaemia, immediate direct-current cardioversion (biphasic, synchronous, high energy: 200–360J) is recommended. In patients who relapse after successful cardioversion, it can be useful to repeat the procedure following administration of appropriate antiarrhythmic medication.

Ablation therapy

When in selected patients the rapid ventricular response is refractory to pharmacological therapy and/or cardioversion, ablation of the atrioventricular (AV) junction by catheter radiofrequency energy with subsequent pacemaker implantation can improve cardiac performance. The choice between single- or dual-chamber pacemaker depends on the probability of restoring sinus rhythm. When in the chronic, pre-discharge phase, curative AF ablation seems to be a better therapeutic option [65,66].

Creating heart block and implanting a permanent pacemaker provides regularization of the ventricular rate, and the use of biventricular pacemakers may prevent an adverse effect of RV pacing on LV function.

Pacing and cardiac resynchronization therapy

In case of atropine (Isuprel®)-resistant bradycardia, transvenous pacing may be used as an interim measure. If pacemaker implantation is indicated, CRT should be considered as well. A large body of evidence has emerged recently that underscores the harmful effects of long-term RV pacing. LV dyssynchrony imposed by RV pacing can lead to LV remodelling with further dilatation and decrease in LV ejection fraction.

CRT is an innovative, pacemaker-based approach to the treatment of patients with HF who have a QRS interval of at least 120ms on 12-lead electrocardiography [67,68]. The purpose of resynchronization is to provide electromechanical coordination and improved ventricular synchrony in symptomatic patients who have severe systolic dysfunction and clinically significant intraventricular conduction defects, particularly left bundle branch block. With CRT, pacemaker leads are placed to stimulate both ventricles, thus bypassing the conduction block in the left bundle branch (see ➲ Chapter 35 Heart failure, ESC Textbook of Cardiovascular Medicine, 2nd edition 2009). Beneficial effects include reverse remodelling, resulting in decreased heart size and ventricular volumes, improved ejection fraction, and decreased mitral regurgitation.

Most biventricular devices are programmed to sense spontaneous activity (i.e. sinus rhythm) in the atrium and provide pacing in the ventricles. Native (non-paced) atrial contraction is preferred, since atrial pacing induces intra-atrial conduction delay, which can lead to alterations in the optimal AV delay and reduced overall effectiveness of biventricular pacing. Pacing in the atrium will be provided only if the patient has an indication for this, such as sinus-node dysfunction. A short AV pacing delay most often is programmed to ensure consistent pacing of the ventricles. However, it is recommended to assess the optimal AV delay with echocardiography on easy to obtain transmitral Doppler flow.

Loss of biventricular pacing can also occur with lead disruption or malfunction of the LV lead. This may be evidenced by widening of the QRS complex with or without a significant shift in the QRS axis. However, it is not always possible to recognize loss of LV pacing from the surface electrocardiogram alone. If, after a period of clinical improvement, the patient has a sudden deterioration of symptoms, the function of the device should be reassessed. Arrhythmias or inappropriate device settings should be ruled out. Measuring of the stimulation threshold using the pacemaker programmer is recommended. Fine tuning of the pacing output, AV delay, and interventricular timing (preferably with the help of ultrasound) should be performed.

Personal perspective

A variety of non-pharmacologic approaches complement drug therapy of AHFS. In the early phase, patient management should be directed to the primary pathophysiologic problem. The development of targeted ('goal-directed') therapy will require a combination of imaging and therapy, which will permit individualized management decisions and hopefully facilitate better clinical outcomes in AHFS.

A combined cardiorenal approach may yield the greatest advances in the contemporary management of acutely decompensated HF. There is a high volume of ongoing research efforts focused on the early treatment of AHFS, including its non-pharmacologic aspects and mechanical circulatory support.

Further reading

Cleland JG, Daubert JC, Erdmann E, et al. The effect of cardiac resynchronization on morbidity and mortality in heart failure. N Engl J Med 2005;352:1539–49.

Flaherty JD, Bax JJ, DeLuca L, et al. Acute heart failure syndromes in patients with coronary artery disease: early assessment and treatment. J Am Coll Cardiol 2009;53:254–63.

Fonarow GC, Adams Jr. KF, Abraham WT, Yancy CW, Boscardin WJ. Risk stratification for in-hospital mortality in acutely decompensated heart failure: classification and regression tree analysis. JAMA 2005;293:572–80.

Gheorghiade M, Zannad F, Sopko G, et al. Acute heart failure syndromes: current state and framework for future research. Circulation 2005;112:3958–68.

Gheorghiade M, Pang PS. Acute heart failure syndromes. J Am Coll Cardiol 2009;53:557–73.

Kirkpatrick JN, Vannan MA, Narula J, Lang RM. Echocardiography in heart failure: applications, utility, and new horizons. J Am Coll Cardiol 2007;50:381–96.

Luce, JM. The cardiovascular effects of mechanical ventilation and positive end-expiratory pressure. JAMA 1984;252:807–11.

Mullens W, Abrahams Z, Skouri HN, et al. Elevated intra-abdominal pressure in acute decompensated heart failure: a potential contributor to worsening renal function? J Am Coll Cardiol 2008;51:300–6.

Wilson Tang WH, Mullens W. Cardio-renal syndrome in decompensated heart failure. Heart 2009 Apr 27. [Epub ahead of print]

➲ For additional multimedia materials please visit the online version of the book (🖑 http://www.esciacc.oxfordmedicine.com).

CHAPTER 52

Cardiac surgery and transplantation in acute heart failure

Antonis A. Pitsis and Aikaterini N. Visouli

Contents

Summary

Cardiac surgery should be considered in all cases of acute heart failure that is attributed to surgically correctable causes. Surgical revascularization, repair of mechanical complications of myocardial infarction, valve repair or replacement, left ventricular aneurysmectomy (in case of a discrete left ventricular aneurysm), mechanical circulatory support, and heart transplantation represent the main surgical interventions that may be offered in the setting of acute (*de novo* or decompensated chronic) heart failure.

Introduction

Cardiac surgery mechanically intervenes to restore the functional abnormality caused by coronary anatomical lesions, to repair or replace abnormal anatomical structures that cause significant functional cardiac compromise, the most severe form of which is heart failure (HF). In the presence of HF all potentially surgical correctable conditions should be identified and, if indicated, surgically corrected. With the advent of mechanical circulatory support (MCS) and heart transplantation, cardiac surgery offers temporary or long-term, partial or total, ventricular support of one or both failing ventricle(s), but also biological or mechanical replacement of the heart itself, when all other means have failed. Cardiac surgery in acute heart failure (AHF) is usually required in life-threatening situations that cannot be addressed otherwise, therefore it is associated with increased mortality; nevertheless it can be life saving.

The role of surgery in acute heart failure due to acute coronary syndromes

Percutaneous coronary intervention (PCI) and coronary artery by pass grafting (CABG) are alternative methods of mechanical revascularization. In acute coronary syndromes (ACS) the role of CABG is interwoven with the role of PCI; both methods aim to prevent or minimize myocardial tissue necrosis, while in severe or life-threatening circumstances they also aim to achieve haemodynamic and/or electrical stability, to aetiologically treat HF, and to preserve life [1]. When there is indication for revascularization in ACS patients, early PCI is the preferred treatment if it can be applied to coronary lesions amenable to it. The role of PCI in ACS has been gradually increased, while the role of CABG is becoming complementary, being applied when PCI is contraindicated, is not considered optimal or possible, or has failed [1–8]. The choice of the revascularization method (PCI or CABG) in patients with HF should be based on the coronary anatomy, the presence of haemodynamically significant valvular disease, the left ventricular (LV) function, the extent of the viable myocardium, potential comorbidities, and procedural risk [9]. In the acute phase of myocardial infarction (MI), CABG may be indicated in cardiogenic shock (CS), in the presence of symptoms uncontrollable by other means, in coronary occlusion not amenable to PCI, after failed PCI, and at the time of surgical correction of mechanical complications of MI [7]. In significant left main [2–4, 8] or severe three-vessel disease [3, 8] CABG may be indicated particularly in the presence of poor LV function [7], unless there is very high surgical risk [2, 4, 8].

There is consensus that surgical repair is indicated in mechanical complications of acute MI that cause HF, including severe acute mitral regurgitation, ventricular septal rupture, and free wall rupture [3, 5, 7, 9].

Revascularization strategy in cardiogenic shock complicating acute myocardial infarction

In the ACC/AHA/SCAI 2005 guideline update for PCI [2], it was stated that CABG could be considered as the revascularization strategy in CS after MI for patients with significant left main or severe three-vessel disease, without right ventricular infarction or major comorbidities (such as severe pulmonary disease or renal insufficiency). If CABG is considered a poor option because of high surgical risk, PCI was considered a reasonable strategy [2]. A recommended algorithm [2] (modified from Hochman [10]) for treatment of CS after MI suggested intra-aortic balloon pumping (IABP) (or consideration of MCS) to stabilize haemodynamics and allow performance of angiography and revascularization procedures. In single- and two-vessel disease as well as in moderate three-vessel disease PCI (of the infarct-related artery, followed by staged multivessel

PCI or CABG) was suggested, while in severe three-vessel and left main disease immediate CABG was suggested (PCI being the second choice if CABG could not be performed) [2]. Hochman considered as moderate three-vessel disease the presence of 100% occlusion of the infarct-related artery (IRA) and less than 90% stenoses in two other major coronary arteries, or more severe stenoses in second-order arteries [10]. A similar algorithm was suggested in the ACC/AHA/(SCAI) 2009 Joint STEMI/PCI Focused Update. The decision about PCI or CABG is taken after coronary angiography based on coronary anatomy [8].

In the ESC 2008 guidelines for STEMI a staged procedure with PCI of the IRA and later CABG under more stable conditions is recommended for patients with an indication for CABG (e.g. multivessel disease). The use of bare metal stents is recommended at emergency PCI of the IRA if CABG is predicted in the near future [7].

Revascularization of the LAD with use of the left internal mammary artery (IMA) should be given primary consideration in every patient undergoing CABG [3], and should be performed whenever possible in CABG after STEMI [5] (➲Fig. 52.1).

Emergent revascularization in patients with cardiogenic shock after myocardial infarction

CS is the first cause of death for patients hospitalized with acute MI [11, 12]. The multicentre, randomized 'Should We Emergently Revascularize Occluded Coronaries for

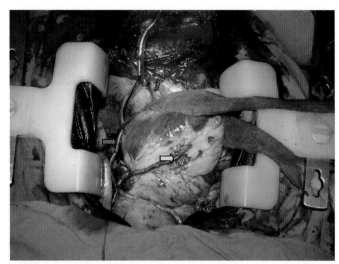

Figure 52.1 Revascularization with bilateral internal thoracic arteries (yellow arrow, left internal thoracic artery anastomosed to the left anterior descending artery; blue arrow, right internal thoracic artery anastomosed to the obtuse marginal branch of the circumflex artery) can offer exemplary long-term results with very low reintervention rates.

Cardiogenic Shock' (SHOCK) trial showed reduced mortality of CS patients with early revascularization by either CABG or PCI [12].

The SHOCK trial randomized 302 patients with predominant LV failure following an acute MI to emergency revascularization or initial medical stabilization. Of these, 128 patients underwent emergency revascularization performed by either CABG or PCI, the choice being dependent on the coronary anatomy [11]. Patients who underwent emergent revascularization (by PCI or CABG) had significant survival benefit at 6 and 12 months (50% vs 37%, $p = 0.027$ and 47% vs 34%, $p = 0.025$, respectively). [12] Thus an early invasive strategy was recommended for CS patients [12].

Any comparison between the PCI and the CABG groups of the SHOCK trial and/or registry is of an observational nature. Although the SHOCK trial patients treated with CABG had a greater prevalence of multivessel disease and diabetes mellitus than those treated with PCI, they had similar survival rate [13]. Among PCI treated patients of the SHOCK trial, multivessel PCI was significantly and independently correlated with mortality ($p = 0.040$) [14].

Patients with severe mitral regurgitation (MR) who underwent PCI experienced high mortality (67%). Thus, consideration of surgical treatment was suggested in CS patients with severe MR [14]. Multivessel disease was associated with more severe MR ($p = 0.005$) [15].

Revascularization was more complete in patients who underwent CABG than in those who underwent PCI (87.2% vs 23.1%). Among CABG patients of the SHOCK trial, those who had complete revascularization had higher survival rates than those who had incomplete revascularization (63.4% vs 16.7% at 30 days, $p = 0.07$) [13].

Results from the SHOCK registry were even more favourable for surgical revascularization in CS patients with multivessel disease. Among patients with two- and three-vessel disease, those treated with PCI had significantly higher in-hospital mortality than those treated with CABG (two-vessel disease, 42.2% PCI vs. 17.7% CABG, $p = 0.025$; three-vessel disease: 59.35% PCI vs 29.6% CABG, $p < 0.0001$). Patients with single-vessel disease had similar mortality regardless of the selected method [16].

Results from the SHOCK trial and registry showed that among CS patients with left main disease those treated with CABG had higher survival than those treated with PCI. There was a higher prevalence of three-vessel disease in the CABG group compared to the PCI group. The overall 30-day survival was significantly higher in the CABG group (54% CABG vs 14% PCI, $p \leq 0.001$). CABG was independently associated with 30-day survival (hazard ratio 0.41, 95% confidence interval 0.22–0.77, $p = 0.006$). The SHOCK investigators concluded that CABG appeared to provide a 30-day survival advantage over PCI in patients with left main disease [17].

Surgery in cardiogenic shock patients after myocardial infarction

Among a total of 708 593 patients who underwent CABG and were enrolled in the Society of Thoracic Surgeons National Cardiac Database (STS NCD, 2002–2005) [18], patients with preoperative CS constituted 2.1% yet accounted for 14% of all deaths. The overall operative mortality (in-hospital and 30-day out-of-hospital mortality) of CS patients (including patients with mechanical complications of MI) was 22%, more than sevenfold higher than the mortality of patients without CS ($p < 0.0001$). Left main disease was 1.5 times more common in patients with CS than in those without it. In total, 81.1% of patients underwent isolated CABG, 11.7% underwent CABG plus mitral valve surgery, 5.2% underwent CABG plus aortic valve surgery, and 2% underwent CABG and ventricular septal rupture (VSR) repair. The internal thoracic artery was used in 58.1% of patients [18].

The operative mortality was surgery specific, being 20% for isolated CABG, rising to 33% for CABG plus valve surgery, and to 58% for CABG plus repair of VSR. Although the overall CABG operative mortality declined significantly over time (3.0% in 2002, 2.8% in 2005, p for trend <0.0001), the mortality for CS patients undergoing urgent, emergent, or salvage procedures did not change significantly (22.9% in 2002, 21.2% in 2005, p for trend = 0.0675) [18].

The operative mortality was higher for patients with CS operated within 24 h of MI (26%), declining to 20% in patients operated from 1 to 21 days and to 18% in patients operated more than 21 days after MI [18].

Increasing age was associated with higher operative mortality. In patients 75 years or age or older, there was a 1.7-fold increased operative mortality compared to that of younger patients (31% vs 18%); nevertheless, almost 70% of patients older than 75 years survived this major surgery [18].

Preoperative factors independently associated with mortality were the type of surgery required (isolated CABG vs CABG plus valve surgery or VSR repair), older age, higher preoperative creatinine, lower preoperative left ventricular ejection fraction (LVEF), operative status (salvage vs emergent or urgent), female gender, IABP, prior cardiac surgery, preoperative resuscitation, MI within 1 week before surgery, and immunosuppressive therapy. IABP in CS patients may be a marker of unmeasured risk factors or worse haemodynamic status, accounting for its association with an increased risk. A simple bedside additive risk score based on the independent risk factors was developed for risk prediction [18].

The results of this observational study cannot be directly extrapolated to patients treated by PCI or receiving medical treatment. This 'has the potential of resulting in an inherent bias favouring survival after CABG over patients treated conservatively or with PCI'. Patients referred for CABG, which is a more invasive procedure, may be those with lower risk, lesser shock severity, younger age, and less comorbidity, while PCI may be preferred for sicker, older patients with more severe shock [18].

Very few patients with CS and multivessel disease are referred for surgery, the proportion ranging from 3.2% to 8.8%. Patients are mainly referred because of coronary anatomy unsuitable for PCI and for mechanical complications of MI. This may reflect the logistical challenges of timely arrangement of emergency surgery, particularly during off hours, when primary PCI can be undertaken expeditiously, and is offered in more hospitals than CABG. It may also reflect the fear of high operative mortality [18].

Surgery in mechanical complications of acute myocardial infarction

Free wall rupture after myocardial infarction

Free wall rupture (FWR) usually involves the left ventricle. In the ESC 2008 STEMI guidelines [7], ventricular FWR was classified as acute or subacute. Acute FWR causes cardiovascular collapse with electromechanical dissociation, being usually fatal within a few minutes. It does not respond to standard cardiopulmonary resuscitation and very rarely is there time to bring the patient to surgery. Subacute FWR (sealed rupture by thrombus or adhesions) can mimic reinfarction (recurrent angina and ST-segment elevation), but more frequently presents with sudden haemodynamic deterioration and signs of cardiac tamponade [7]. In the ESC 2008 [7] and the ACC/AHA 2004 STEMI guidelines [5], consideration of immediate surgical treatment was recommended in FWR.

Of 1048 patients studied from the SHOCK registry, 28 (2.7%) had FWR or tamponade. These patients presented with CS and had significantly less pulmonary oedema, prior MI, prior congestive HF, and diabetes. Most patients underwent surgery and/or pericardiocentesis (27/28), with an in-hospital survival rate after intervention similar to that of the overall group (39.3%). Women and older patients tended to survive intervention less often. Early detection of subacute rupture by echocardiography can result in increased survival by early intervention [19].

Direct closure, infarctectomy and prosthetic patch closure, and infarct-exclusion patch closure are performed on-pump in the 'blow-out' type of FWR. In patients with less catastrophic anatomy, a less invasive and simpler sutureless technique performed off-pump (with or without IABP or MCS) to avoid suturing of friable necrotic tissue yielded good results (n = 32, 1993–2006, surgery at a mean of 3.6 h from rupture, early survival 84.4%, 5-year survival 75%). Percutaneous pericardial drainage to treat tamponade may be required on preparation of surgery. There is a risk for rerupture in the acute phase. Later pseudoaneyrysm formation can be treated by surgical resection [20].

Ventricular septal rupture after myocardial infarction

In the ACC/AHA 2004 STEMI guidelines, consideration for urgent cardiac surgical repair was recommended for post-MI VSR [5]. According to the ESC 2008 STEMI guidelines [7], 'urgent surgery offers the only chance of survival' for large post-MI VSR with CS. Even in the absence of haemodynamic instability, early surgery is usually indicated, because the defect may increase; there is no consensus, though, about the exact timing of VSR repair, due to the presence of friable necrotic tissue early after MI that may hamper the results of surgery [7]. IABP was recommended during preparation of surgery [5, 7]. Short-term left ventricular assist devices (LVADs), preferably with left atrial cannulation, can be used to bridge patients to surgery, supporting end-organ function and providing some time for maturation of oedematous and haemorrhagic tissue (➲Fig. 52.2) [21]. Percutaneous closure has been reported, but more experience is required before it can be recommended [7].

Among 939 patients studied from the SHOCK registry, the incidence of VSR was 5.85%. VSR occurred at a median of 16 h after MI. VSR patients tended to be older, were more often women and less often had previous MI, diabetes, or a smoking history. Although VSR patients had less severe coronary disease (than non-VSR CS patients), they had higher in-hospital mortality (87% vs 61%, $p < 0.001$). In the surgically treated patients the survival was 19%; in the medically treated patients it was 4.2% [22].

Infarctectomy techniques (including excision of the infarct area and direct or patch closure) have been used, but an exclusion rather than excision technique better

Figure 52.2 Left ventricular assist device as a bridge to surgery in postinfarction ventricular septal defect. (A) Preoperative four-chamber midoesophageal transoesophageal echocardiography demonstrating significant left-to-right shunt. (B) Preoperative midoesophageal transoesophageal echocardiography showing the tip of the inflow cannula (arrow) of the LVAD into the left atrium. (C) One-year follow-up echocardiogram: long-axis three-dimensional echocardiogram demonstrating the left ventricular reconstruction using the bovine pericardial patch (arrow). (D) Extensive haematoma of the LV and RV during the first operation. (E) Bovine pericardial patch of the PVSD repair in he second operation, with arrow showing a dissector with the tip inserte dthrough the PVSD. IC, inflow cannula; IVS, interventricular septum; LA, left atrium; LV, left ventricle; OC, outflow cannula; RA, right atrium; RV, right ventricle; VC, venous cannula.

With kind permission from Elsevier: Pitsis AA, Kelpis TG, Visouli AN, et al. Left ventricular assist device as a bridge to surgery in postinfarction ventricular septal defect. *J Thorac Cardiovasc Surg* 2008; **135** :951–952. (Figures 1 and 2) (Copyright American Association for Thoracic Surgery)

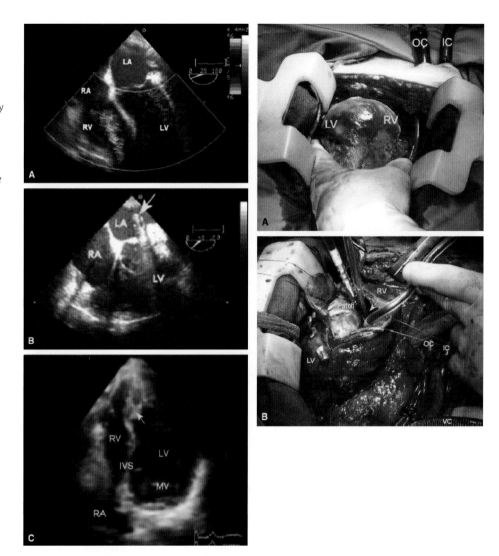

preserves the ventricular volume and geometry. Described by David, it involves endocardial patch repair and resembles the Dor technique of ventricular endoaneurysmorrhaphy. David *et al.* applied this reparative technique during the acute phase of MI with excellent results (operative mortality 14%, 6 years actuarial survival 66%±7%) [23]. Results in other centres have been mixed [24].

Mitral regurgitation after myocardial infarction

Mitral regurgitation (MR) is common after STEMI and usually occurs after 2–7 days of MI. There are three mechanisms of acute MR in this setting: (1) annular dilatation due to LV dilatation; (2) papillary muscle displacement usually due to inferior MI; and (3) (trunk or tip) papillary muscle rupture. Partial or total rupture more frequently occurs after a small infarct of the posteromedial papillary muscle in the distribution of the right coronary or the left

circumflex artery [7]. In most patients, acute MR is due to papillary muscle displacement rather than rupture.

According to the ESC 2008 STEMI guidelines, in most patients with acute MR after MI, early operation is indicated because they may deteriorate suddenly. CS and pulmonary oedema with severe MR require emergency surgery [7]. According to the ACC/AHA 2004 STEMI guidelines, in papillary muscle rupture consideration for urgent surgery is required [5]. Mitral valve replacement or repair can be done in selected cases [7]. During preparation for surgery, IABP is indicated [5, 7]. More recently, better results have been achieved with a hospital mortality of 22% or less. Improvements have been attributed to earlier operation, complete revascularization, mitral valve repair, and chordal preservation techniques when valve replacement is required [25].

In our experience there is a good chance of successful repair when the papillary muscle rupture occurs towards the muscle tip, because the presence of fibrous tissue at this area allows more secure suturing. When there is partial tip rupture (one of the usually two papillary muscle heads is ruptured) a competent valve can easily be achieved by suturing of the ruptured head to the intact one (➲ Fig. 52.3). An undersized annuloplasty by a rigid complete ring reducing the anteroposterior diameter is indicated to relieve the strain of the repaired papillary muscle. Conversely, repair of basal papillary muscle rupture is not secure, being associated with a high risk of dehiscence, thus mitral valve replacement is probably indicated (➲ Fig. 52.3) [26, 27].

CABG should be performed at the time of repair of mechanical complications of MI as needed [5, 7]. Angiography is indicated in surgical candidates with VSR and/or MR [5]. In FWR CABG should also be done if the coronary anatomy is known [5, 7], but usually there is no time to perform coronary angiography because of the unstable condition of the patient.

The role of surgery in acute heart failure due to valvular disease

In the EHFS II survey valvular heart disease was an underlying disease in 34.4% of all patients and a precipitating factor of AHF in 26.8%. Valvular disease was a precipitating factor of AHF in 30.2% of patients with acutely decompensated chronic HF, 24.1% of patients with pulmonary oedema, 17.4% in patients with CS, 12.6% in patients with hypertensive HF, and 32.7% in patients with right HF [28].

According to the ESC 2008 guidelines for acute and chronic HF [9], valvular stenosis or regurgitation (particularly aortic stenosis and mitral insufficency) can be the primary cause or a complicating factor of AHF. Gradients, regurgitant volumes, and haemodynamic consequences should be assessed and surgery may be considered. Coronary angiography and left ventriculography is indicated in patients with severe MR or aortic valve disease that may be correctable with surgery. Although poor LVEF is an important risk factor for perioperative mortality, surgery may be considered in symptomatic patients. Emergent operation should be avoided if possible; optimal medical management of heart disease and comorbities should be offered preoperatively (but without adding unnecessary delay).

In patients with HF and severe ischaemic MR, mitral surgery should be considered if revascularization is an option. Mitral valve repair appears an attractive option in selected patients [9].

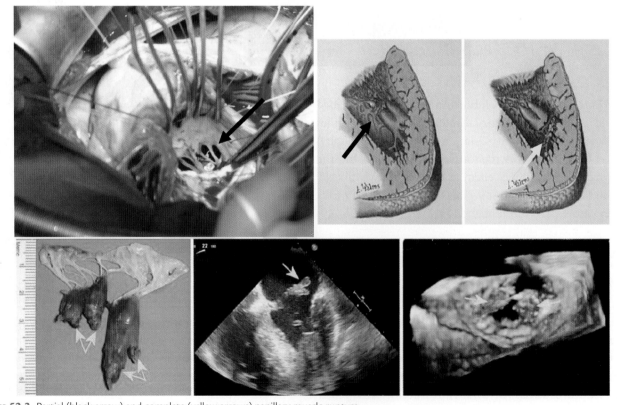

Figure 52.3 Partial (black arrow) and complete (yellow arrows) papillary muscle rupture
With kind permission from Springer Science+Business: Pitsis AA, Anagnostopoulos CE. Acute heart failure: is there a role for surgery? *Heart Fail Rev* 2007; **12** :173–178 (Top row) and Karger AG, Basel: Pitsis AA, Boudoulas H. Mitral regurgitation in acute heart failure: the role of echocardiography. *Cardiology* 2009; **113** (4):246–248 S. (Bottom row).

In organic MR (structural abnormalities or damage of the valve, usually due to rheumatic disease or endocarditis) the occurrence of HF symptoms is a strong indication for surgery. Surgery is recommended for patients with LVEF greater than 30% (I-C) and may be considered for patients with severe MR and LVEF less than 30%, although medical stabilization is preferred; in patients refractory to medical treatment and low surgical risk, surgery may be performed (IIb-C) [9].

Emergent surgery is required in refractory HF due to severe aortic regurgitation or MR (caused by endocarditis, worsening of pre-existing valvular regurgitation, aortic dissection, or rupture of mitral valve chordae tendinae) and in severe aortic valve stenosis [29] but also in severe paravalvular leak, in tissue leaflet rupture of bioprosthetic valves (due to degeneration, calcification, or endocarditis), and in mechanical valve thrombosis.

In functional MR surgery may be considered in patients with severe MR and poor LV function who remain symptomatic despite optimal medical treatment (IIb-C) [9].

Surgical ventricular remodelling on acutely decompensated chronic heart failure

The presence of a discrete ventricular aneurysm causing AHF, or an arrhythmogenic substrate in a previously infarcted akinetic or dyskinetic area, have traditionally been considered as indications for HF surgery in the acute setting, although evidence from randomized controlled trials is lacking.

Aneurysmectomy in symptomatic patients with discrete LV aneurysm has received a IIb-C recommendation. Cardiomyoplasty, partial left ventriculectomy, and external ventricular restoration are not recommended for the treatment of HF (III-C) [9].

Surgical ventricular restoration, reconstruction, or remodelling (SVR) of the anteroseptal LV wall, along with revascularization and mitral valve repair as required, have been applied in patients with ischaemic cardiomyopathy with good results according to observational data (➲ Fig. 52.4). The STICH trial [30] randomized patients with indication for revascularization, LVEF less than 35%, and no recent MI to CABG vs CABG plus surgical ventricular reconstruction (CABG+SVR). Although it showed decreased LV volume after surgical reconstruction, it also showed identical mortality and/or rehospitalization, functional class, and exercise tolerance. Surgery was offered

to patients with ischaemic heart disease and poor ventricular function not only electively but also at urgent (13%) or emergent conditions (1%), and for ongoing ischaemia (2%). Mitral valve surgery was also performed in 18% of patients. The postoperative 30-day all-cause mortality was 5% and the all-cause mortality at a median of 48 months was 28% in each group. Rehospitalization for cardiac causes was required in 42% in the CABG group and in 41% in the CABG + SVR group.

On the basis of the STICH trial, SVR can not be recommended for all patients with coronary disease and poor LV function. Further studies are required to examine whether SVR is beneficial for patients with very dilated ventricles, especially those with dyskinetic areas of myocardium.

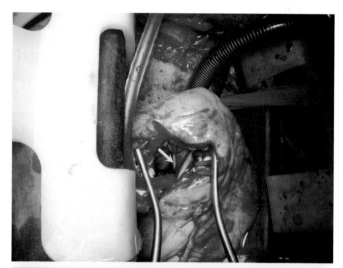

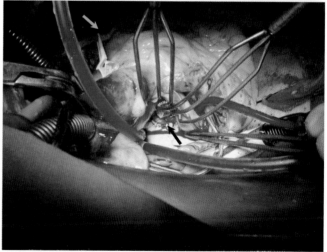

Figure 52.4 Surgical ventricular remodelling (SVR) with the use of bovine pericardial patch (yellow arrow), combined with bypass grafting (green arrow) and mitral valve repair with an undersized annuloplasty (black arrow) in a patient with decompensated heart failure due to ischaemic cardiomyopathy.

Mechanical circulatory support

MCS is applied in acute and chronic HF when all conventional measures have failed. MCS aims to preserve life, by restoring the circulation and ensuring blood flow to the vital organs, while it decompresses the heart and allows it to rest, thus assisting ventricular recovery [31–34].

According to the ESC 2008 guidelines [9], in CS, an IABP should be considered, while short-term MCS may be considered for potentially reversible causes of acute HF, as a bridge to recovery, surgery, or transplantation. MCS as a bridge to transplantation or for the management of severe acute myocarditis was given a IIa-C recommendation, and long-term treatment 'when no definitive procedure is planned' was given a IIb-C recommendation [9]. According to the ESC 2008 guidelines, there is no consensus regarding indications for MCS and patient selection. The application of MCS in terminally ill patients, who are less amenable to randomization, explains the lack of robust evidence which is reflected in the recommendations. According to the same guidelines, though, clinicians managing patients with HF 'must frequently make treatment decisions without adequate evidence or consensus expert opinion' [9]. The following description of indications and support strategies reflects the clinical practice as documented in the literature.

Short-term support is usually applied in acute *de novo* HF, while long-term support is usually applied in endstage chronic heart failure. In acute decompensation of endstage chronic HF, long-term support is best applied unless the patient is *in extremis* (profound shock and organ failure), in which case short-term support may be indicated (survivors may be then screened for long-term MCS). The indications for MCS are continuously expanding, while the boundaries between short- and long-term support and between support strategies are becoming less distinct [31–37].

Excluding uncomplicated hypertensive HF, all categories of AHF including acute decompensation of chronic heart failure can be complicated by CS, which is associated with a mortality of 40–60% [9]. MCS is indicated when all other conventional measures including IABP have failed.

Postcardiotomy HF remains the main indication for short-term MCS [31, 38, 39], other indications being AHF due to MI, acute myocarditis/cardiomyopathy, allograft failure, etc. [31, 33, 34] (➲ Box 52.1).

Bridging to recovery is the main strategy of short-term MCS. Recovery is not always achieved, though; in suitable candidates bridging to transplantation or to therapeutic operations and interventions such as revascularization may

> **Box 52.1 Indications for short-term mechanical circulatorysupport in acute heart failure**
>
> ◆ Postcardiotomy cardiac failure
> ◆ Acute MI, mechanical complications of MI
> ◆ Allograft dysfunction postcardiac transplantation
> ◆ Acute and fulminant myocarditis, postpartum cardiomyopathy
> ◆ Haemodynamic instability during cardiac catheterization procedures
> ◆ Right ventricular failure (after LVAD placement, right ventricular or biventricular MI)
> ◆ Cardiac arrest
> ◆ Massive pulmonary embolism
> ◆ Acute decompensation of chronic HF

be indicated [21, 31, 33, 34, 38] Bridging to longer-term support with or without planned transplantation are other options [38, 40, 41]. Short-term support has recently been applied to rescue patients with uncertain neurological status and/or organ function, as a rescue therapy and a bridge to decision [42]. (➲ Box 52.2). Overlap and crossover between support strategies usually occurs.

Long-term MCS is mainly applied in endstage chronic HF due to ischaemic or idiopathic dilated cardiomyopathy (➲ Box 52.3, ➲ Fig. 52.5) [32, 33, 42–46]. Long-term MCS has been rarely applied in myocarditis, postpartum cardiomyopathy, operated congenital heart disease, noncompaction cardiomyopathy, malignant refractory

> **Box 52.2 Strategies of short-term mechanical circulatory support**
>
> ◆ Bridge to recovery
> ◆ Bridge to transplantation (heart or heart/lung transplantation)
> ◆ Bridge to operations and/or interventions
> ◆ Bridge to bridge (another longer-term device, which can be used consecutively as a bridge to transplantation)
> ◆ Bridge to survival (rescue therapy)
> ◆ Bridge to decision (to all other support strategies, to operations, interventions)
> ◆ Bridge to long-term MCS

arrhythmias in transplant candidates, acute *de novo* HF (postcardiotomy or post-MI when early recovery is not anticipated and early transplantation is not an option) [33, 34, 38, 47, 48].

Bridging to transplantation remains the main strategy of long-term MCS. Bridging to possible transplantation (or to transplant eligibility or candidacy) is applied in some patients with contraindications to transplantation who may derive functional improvement during long-term MCS, such as improved organ function and amelioration of pulmonary hypertension, thus becoming transplant eligible [32–37]. Cardiac recovery in endstage chronic HF is rare, nevertheless it is desirable in all settings [33–35, 49–51] (⊃ Box 52.4). There is frequent crossover between support strategies depending on the patient's dynamic functional and clinical status, the presence of device-related adverse events, and the donor graft availability. It has been suggested that the term 'long-term circulatory support' should be used, rather than premature assignment to bridge or destination [33, 34, 36, 37].

Short- and long-term MCS can provide isolated ventricular (left or right) and biventricular (left and right) support. Short-term MCS also includes cardiopulmonary support, while long-term MCS includes total cardiac replacement [31–35] (⊃ Boxes 52.5 and 52.6).

The largest study ever to examine postcardiotomy MCS showed an overall survival of about 60% (July 2002–December 2004, n = 1585) significantly improved from about 40% (January 1995–June 1997, n = 1255). Attributable reasons may be increased experience, improved device technology, earlier application, use of longer-term support, and bridging to transplantation [38].

A review of short- and long-term MCS with various devices in patients with CS after acute/fulminant myocarditis (n = 135) showed survival rates of 30%, 47%, 53%, 70%, and 78%, with either recovery or bridging to transplantation. Patients with fulminant myocarditis have very high recovery and long-term transplant-free survival rates with aggressive treatment that may include MCS [33, 52].

A meta-analysis of three small randomized controlled trials that compared IABP versus early direct MCS with percutaneous LVADs in patients with post-MI CS showed

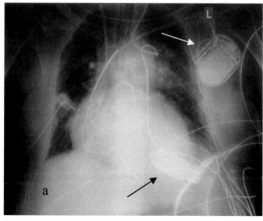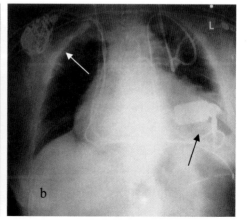

Figure 52.5 Immediate postoperative chest X rays of two patients with end stage heart failure implanted with the Jarvik 2000 LVAD as destination treatment (black arrows). a. Chest x-ray of a patient suffering from idiopathic dilated cardiomyopathy (who had been implanted with ICD in the past, white arrow). b. Chest x-ray of a patient suffering from ischemic cardiomyopathy (who had been implanted with biventricular ICD, white arrow). Device therapy is becoming increasingly common for the treatment of refractory heart failure.

Box 52.5 Categories of short-term mechanical circulatory support (types of devices)

- Left ventricular support (left ventricular assist device)
- Right ventricular support (right ventricular assist device)
- Biventricular support (biventricular assist device)
- Cardiopulmonary support (extracorporeal membrane oxygenator)

---

superior haemodynamic support with MCS but similar early survival [53].

A review of 17 major studies showed that the use of MCS in patients with CS complicating acute MI resulted in a survival rate of about 40%, similar to that of patients who received revascularization (with or without IABP) [54]. No safe conclusions can be drawn, since mechanically supported patients were probably selected on the basis of increased severity. Early revascularization combined with early MCS in carefully selected patients, for bridging to recovery, to transplantation, or to long-term support may improve the results. Short-term percutaneous devices can be used in nonsurgical patients, while newer generation short- and long-term LVADs may be preferable to older ones [35, 38, 40–42, 55]. MCS can be a significant adjunct in the surgical treatment of patients with mechanical complications of MI [21, 56].

The results of long-term support are continuously improving. The survival rate of more than 80% reported for LVAD recipients in experienced centres [34] has been achieved on a larger scale (INTERMACS registry, June 2006–March 2009, n = 1104, http://www.intermacs.org, accessed on 4 February 2010). Better patient selection, earlier application of MCS (before CS, right ventricular and/or organ failure), improved device technology, and management have contributed to improved results [32–37, 44, 45].

Box 52.6 Categories of long-term mechanical circulatory support (types of devices)

- Left ventricular support (left ventricular assist device)
- Right ventricular support (right ventricular assist device)
- Biventricular support (biventricular assist device)
- Total cardiac replacement (total artificial heart)

Heart transplantation

For decades, heart transplantation (HTx) has remained the gold standard of treatment for patients with endstage HF who remain symptomatic despite optimal medical treatment. A milestone in the history of HTx was the introduction in the 1980s of cyclosporine, which dramatically reduced acute rejection and infection [57] The surgical technique has remained virtually unchanged since the initial description by Lower and Shumway in 1960 [58]. The bicaval graft anastomosis—an alteration of the classic technique introduced in the 1990s, aiming to preserve a more normal anatomy and function of the right atrium and the tricuspid valve—has not met with universal acceptance [59].

Despite this very long history, HTx has failed to provide an epidemiologically significant impact in the treatment of endstage HF because of the critical shortage of donor hearts. The number of heart transplants reported to the International Society for Heart and Lung Transplantation (ISHLT) has followed a descending curve since the mid 1990s, although it appears to have stabilized during the last few years [60] (◊ Fig. 52.6). It is estimated that the number of heart transplants that are not entered into the ISHLT registry is more than 2000/year in recent years. Adding this to the 3300 ISHLT registered transplants indicates universal annual productivity of over 5000 [61].

In recent years, device therapy, with implantable cardioverter-defibrillator and cardiac resynchronization therapy, has been added to the treatment of HTx candidates offering improved survival. Nevertheless, many of these patients will continue to deteriorate and reach the stage of intractable HF requiring MCS as a bridge to transplantation or to transplant candidacy. The extensive use of VADs, especially the implantable ones, for the last decade, has certainly contributed to the increased survival and crash-free survival on the waiting list, especially for patients on inotropes (stable or not). This improved survival prior to HTx is without the expense of decreased survival post-HTx, as initially assumed by some. Therefore VAD-supported patients and medically treated patients appear to have similar post-HTx survival curves [62].

As far as the post-HTx survival is concerned, there is an improvement in recent years from a mean survival of 8.9 years in 1982 to 11 years in the most recent era. For recipients who live beyond the first year the mean survival is 13 years, because of the increased mortality during the first 6 months post-transplant [63].

The indications and contraindications to HTx have remained virtually unchanged in recent years. The two absolute contraindications to HTx are any systemic

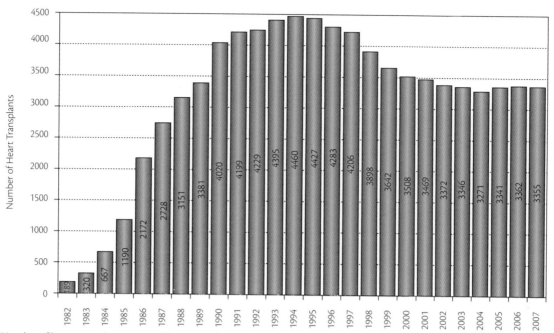

Figure 52.6 Number of heart transplants reported by year to the International Society for Heart and Lung Transplantation (ISHLT). Available at www.ishlt.org/registries/ (Slides, Overall heart and adult heart transplantation statistics - http://www.ishlt.org/downloadables/slides/2009/heart_adult. ppt#660,1,HEART TRANSPLANTATION). Reproduced with permission from *J Heart Lung Transplant* 2009; **28**: 989–1049.

illness that limits survival and fixed pulmonary hypertension (pulmonary vascular resistance greater to 4–6 Wood units and transpulmonary gradient above 15 mmHg). Of course there are several relative contraindications, such as age more than 65 years, severe peripheral vascular disease, diabetes mellitus with end-organ damage, severe lung disease, systemic infections, and psychosocial impairment to name the most important ones [60].

Patients over the age of 65 years, and other recipients who do not meet standard transplant criteria, can be accepted into alternate lists, utilizing organs from marginal donors. These marginal cardiac grafts would otherwise have been wasted. Although the survival of the transplanted patients from the alternate list appears to be worse than those from the standard list, the overall outcome of such a strategy appears to be positive [64].

Conclusion

In ACS 'time is muscle', and revascularization is required as soon as possible. In AHF due to ACS, emergency revascularization offers improved survival over the initial medical stabilization. PCI is more readily available. CABG can be applied to lesions that are not amenable to PCI (because it bypasses the lesion instead of dealing with it). In the presence of significant left main and/or severe three-vessel disease CABG may be indicated, particularly in patients with poor

LV function and acceptable surgical risk. In unstable patients with indications for CABG a staged procedure with initial PCI of the infarct-related artery and later performance of CABG has been recommended. In the presence of mechanical complications of MI, prompt surgery is clearly indicated.

Surgery may be indicated in patients with severe aortic or mitral valve disease that causes AHF or represents the major precipitating factor of AHF. Although surgery yields better results in patients with moderate LV dysfunction, it should also be considered in patients with advanced LV dysfunction refractory to optimal medical treatment, particularly in patients with a lower risk profile.

LV aneurysmectomy may be recommended in the presence of a large, discrete, and symptomatic LV aneurysm, but partial left ventriculectomy, cardiomyoplasty, and external ventricular restoration should not be done.

The established indications for MCS are rather limited, but clinicians dealing with patients facing imminent death may have to make decisions without adequate evidence or consensus of expert opinion. As the results of short- and long-term MCS are progressively improving, its indications should be accordingly revised.

Despite lack of evidence from randomized trials there is consensus that heart transplantation is the recommended surgical treatment of endstage chronic heart failure. Heart transplantation has progressively improving results, but its epidemiological impact is limited mainly by shortage of donor organs.

Personal perspective

AHF in ACS still has a grave prognosis. It should be managed by urgent revascularization. Rescue/salvage revascularization in acute terminal collapse is the most challenging goal that may be managed with rapid implementation of invasive techniques, such as primary PCI with or without (percutaneous) MCS. If the patient is saved but the results are suboptimal, a staged (hybrid) approach could be beneficial. When more time is provided by a more stable clinical status, CABG may be offered in the presence of left main and/or severe multivessel disease. Salvage primary stenting of the left main stem can be life saving and should probably be attempted in life-threatening situations, when the likelihood of death before the patient can even reach the operating theatre is high. Elective stenting of the left main, should be highly selective, however, concerning only suitable lesions in patients with high operative risk.

AHF in the presence of mechanical complications of MI is associated with a higher mortality than AHF due to ventricular failure. Surgery should be performed (with or without MCS). Acute severe mitral regurgitation is a potent predictor of death in AHF due to ACS, and surgical management (preferably by mitral valve repair) along with surgical revascularization when indicated is required.

Surgical ventricular remodelling for chronic HF due to ischaemic cardiomyopathy is still under investigation and has very limited role in the setting of AHF, unless it concerns a discrete ventricular aneurysm causing AHF (which has become rather rare in the current era of thrombolysis or revascularization).

Short-term MCS can be life saving in all AHF syndromes (ACS, acute myocarditis of any cause, postpartum cardiomyopathy, postcardiotomy, etc.). It can be used as rescue therapy, and as a bridge to decision, to interventions or operations, to recovery, to transplantation, and finally to long-term support (when recovery and transplantation are not feasible). Direct application of long-term MCS can be used in acute decompensation of chronic endstage HF and more rarely in acute *de novo* heart failure, when fast recovery or transplantation is unlikely.

Cardiac transplantation remains, for the time being, the gold standard of the surgical treatment of endstage chronic HF, but is of limited value because of the shortage of donors. Urgent transplantation in the setting of AHF (particularly in the setting of acutely decompensated chronic HF) is possible, but bridging to transplantation with inotropes or MCS is usually required.

Further reading

De Robertis F, Rogers P, Amrani M, *et al*. Bridge to decision using the Levitronix CentriMag short-term ventricular assist device. *J Heart Lung Transplant* 2008;**27**(5):474–478.

Felker GM, Rogers JG. Same bridge, new destinations. *J Am Coll Cardiol* 2006;**47**:930–932.

Hernandez AF, Grab JD, Gammie JS, *et al*. A decade of short-term outcomes in post–cardiac surgery ventricular assist device implantation. *Circulation* 2007;**116**:606–612.

Jones RH, Velazquez EJ, Michler RE, *et al*. Coronary bypass surgery with or without surgical ventricular reconstruction. *N Engl J Med* 2009;**360**:1705–1717.

Lietz K, Long JW, Kfoury AG, *et al*. Outcomes of left ventricular assist device implantation as destination therapy in the post-REMATCH era: implications for patient selection. *Circulation* 2007;**116**:497–505.

Lietz K, Miller LW. Destination therapy: current results and future promise. *Semin Thorac Cardiovasc Surg* 2008;**20**(3):225–233.

Lietz K, Slaughter M, Deng MC, *et al*. Outcomes of medical therapy and mechanical circulatory support as bridge to transplantation in UNOS status 1 heart transplant candidates—analysis of the U.S. UNOS/OPTN Data, years 1999–2007. *ISHLT Meeting* 2009.

Mehta RH, Grab JD, O'Brien SM, *et al*. Clinical characteristics and in-hospital outcomes of patients with cardiogenic shock undergoing coronary artery bypass surgery: insights from the Society of Thoracic Surgeons National Cardiac Database. *Circulation* 2008;**117**(7):876–885.

Menon V, Fincke R. Cardiogenic shock: a summary of the randomized SHOCK trial. *Congest Heart Fail* 2003;**9**(1):35–39.

Miller LW, Pagani FD, Russell DS, *et al*. Use of a continuous-flow device in patients awaiting heart transplantation. *N Engl. J Med* 2007;**357**:885–896.

Rose EA, Gelijns AC, Moskowitz AJ, *et al*. Randomized Evaluation of Mechanical Assistance for the Treatment of Congestive Heart Failure (REMATCH) Study Group. Long-term mechanical left ventricular assistance for end-stage heart failure. *N Engl J Med* 2001;**345**(20):1435–1443.

Simon MA, Kormos RL, Murali S, *et al*. Myocardial recovery using ventricular assist devices: prevalence, clinical characteristics, and outcomes. *Circulation* 2005;**112**(9 Suppl):I32–6.

Stevenson LW, Couper G. On the fledgling field of mechanical circulatory support. *J Am Coll Cardiol* 2000;**50**(8):748–751.

Taylor DO, Stehlik J, Edwards LB, *et al*. Registry of the International Society for Heart and Lung Transplantation: Twenty-Sixth Official Adult Heart Transplant Report—2009. *J Heart Lung Transplant* 2009;**28**:1007–1022.

Online resources

- ACC/AHA Joint Guidelines. http://www.americanheart.org/presenter.jhtml?identifier=3004542
- Aggarwal S, Cheema F, Oz M C, Naka Y. Long-term mechanical circulatory support. In: Cohn Lh (ed.) *Cardiac surgery in the adult*, McGraw-Hill, New York, 2008, pp. 1609–1628. http://cardiacsurgery.ctsnetbooks.org
- Agnihotri AK, Madsen JC, Daggett WM Jr. Surgical treatment of complications of acute myocardial infarction: postinfarction ventricular septal defect and free wall rupture. In: Cohn Lh (ed.) *Cardiac surgery in the adult*, McGraw-Hill, New York, 2008, pp.753–784. http://cardiacsurgery.ctsnetbooks.org
- All things INTERMACS. https://www.uab.edu/ctsresearch/mcsd
- ESC Clinical Practice Guidelines. http://www.escardio.org/guidelines-surveys/esc-guidelines/Pages/GuidelinesList.aspx
- Interagency Registry for Mechanically Assisted Circulatory Support (INTERMACS). http://www.intermacs.org.
- International Society for Heart and Lung Transplantation. http://www.ishlt.org/registries/
- McGee E, McCarthy P, Moazami N. Temporary mechanical circulatory support. In: Cohn Lh (ed.) *Cardiac surgery in the adult*, McGraw-Hill, New York, 2008, pp. 507–534. http://cardiacsurgery.ctsnetbooks.org

➲ For additional multimedia materials please visit the online version of the book (෴ http://www.esciacc.oxfordmedicine.com).

SECTION IX

Arrhythmias

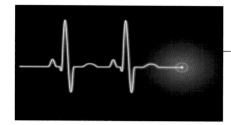

CHAPTER 53

Conduction disturbances and pacemaker

C. Lavalle, R. P. Ricci, and M. Santini

Contents

Summary

The most frequent clinical conditions complicated by bradyarrhythmias or atrioventricular (AV) blocks seen in an emergency setting are degeneration of the conduction system, acute myocardial infarction, drug toxicity, and hyperkalaemia. Pacemaker malfunction is another cause of potentially life-threatening bradyarrhythmias. The presence of signs/symptoms of hypoperfusion and the localization of the block condition the therapeutic approach. Treatment of bradyarrhythmias and AV blocks in a critical care setting may be preventive or therapeutic. A preventive approach is necessary when the risk of a sudden block with an inadequate ventricular escape rhythm is present, but the patient is asymptomatic. Symptomatic patients require immediate treatment. If the block is located at His bundle level or at bundle branch level atropine may be ineffective and may even worsen the degree of block. If drug administration is ineffective, transvenous temporary pacing is indicated. Transcutaneous cardiac pacing is another temporary method of pacing indicated in various critical clinical settings.

Introduction

Bradyarrhythmias and syncope, two conditions often correlated, represent one of the most frequent reasons for admission to emergency departments and intensive cardiac care units (ICCUs).

The first step in the management of bradyarrhythmias in an emergency setting consists in evaluating whether these such conditions represent a life-threatening event. The signs and symptoms associated with a poor prognosis are:

◆ Syncope

◆ Chest pain

◆ Alteration in the level of consciousness

◆ Hypotension (systolic blood pressure <90 mmHg)

◆ Orthostatic hypotension

- Heart rate less than 40 beats/min
- Coexisting ventricular arrhythmias which may be triggered by the bradycardia
- Acute heart failure
- Signs of cardiogenic shock related to bradycardia.

The most frequent situations complicated by bradyarrhythmias or atrioventricular blocks in an emergency setting are idiopathic degeneration of the conduction system, acute myocardial infarction (MI), drug toxicity, and hyperkalaemia.

The initial approach to patients with bradyarrhythmia requires:

- Monitoring of heart rhythm and blood pressure
- Obtaining venous access
- 12-lead ECG recording
- Monitoring of oxygen saturation, and oxygen therapy if necessary.

The treatment of bradyarrhythmias and atrioventricular blocks in a critical care setting may be preventive or therapeutic. A preventive approach is necessary when the risk of a sudden block with an inadequate ventricular escape rhythm is present but the patient is asymptomatic: this implies the use of temporary cardiac pacing, either transcutaneous or transvenous.

The therapeutic approach to patients with bradyarrhythmia or atrioventricular block in the critical care setting is conditioned by the presence of signs and symptoms of hypoperfusion (⊃Table 53.1). In this case immediate treatment with drugs (atropine, isoproterenol) or transcutaneous temporary pacing is required; if the symptoms persist, transvenous temporary pacing is indicated in order to establish a valid heart rhythm.

Table 53.1 Signs and symptoms of hypoperfusion correlated with bradyarrhythmia or AV block and particular situations associated with conduction disturbances which require a specific therapeutic approach

Symptoms	Signs	Particular situations
Vertigo	Hypotension	Ventricular arrhythmias triggered by the bradycardia
Syncope or presyncope	Heart failure	Hypovolaemic shock
Intense fatigue	Shock	MI
Dysponea/shortness of breath		
Chest pain	Pulmonary oedema	Cardiac tamponade

MI, myocardial infarction.

Clinical conditions

Sinus node dysfunction

The sinus node is a structure located in the right atrium characterized by the ability to generate electrical impulses that trigger cardiac contraction (automaticity); it is the heart's pacemaker. Since it is richly innervated from both the parasympathetic and sympathetic nervous system, it is able to regulate heart rate depending on the autonomic tone.

Causes of sinus node dysfunction

The causes of sinus dysfunction and atrioventricular node dysfunction (AV blocks) can be classified as intrinsic (i.e. primarily concerning the heart) or extrinsic (i.e. due to extracardiac disease) (⊃Table 53.2).

Clinical presentation

This may present as sinus bradycardia or sinoatrial block.

Sinus bradycardia

This is defined as a sinus rhythm at a rate <60 beats/min. A relative bradycardia is defined as a heart rate which is low considering the haemodynamic state of the patient. In the clinical evaluation of a sinus bradycardia, some physiological causes of bradycardia must be taken into consideration since they do not require specific treatment:

- Well-trained athletes can attain heart rates at rest of less than 40 beats/min in absence of symptoms
- During sleep
- Vagal stimulation (e.g. vomiting, pain).

ECG criteria

- Presence of normal P waves (morphology and axis)
- The number of P waves is equivalent to the number of QRS complexes

Table 53.2 Cardiac (intrinsic) and extracardiac (extrinsic) cause of bradyarrhythmias and conduction disturbances

Intrinsic	Extrinsic
Idiopathic degeneration	Iatrogenic (due to drugs such as digoxin, amiodarone, β-blockers, diltiazem, propaphenone, clonidine)
Ischaemic cardiomyopathy	
Degenerative disease	
Myocarditis	Electrolyte abnormalities
Myopathies	Hypothyroidism
Vasculitis due to collagenopathies	Neuromediated
Post-surgery	Endocranial hypertension

- The P wave precedes the QRS complex, with a constant PR interval
- Regular PP and RR cycles.

Therapeutic approach

Sinus bradycardia generally does not require treatment unless associated with the symptoms described in ➲ Table 53.1. It generally responds to drug administration and does not require temporary pacing. When treatment is required, the following approach is recommended:

1 Atropine 0.5 mg intravenously every 5 min up to the maximum permitted total dose of 3 mg or 0.04 mg/kg.

2 Adrenergic drugs (isoproterenol $0.050–0.1\ \mu g\ kg^{-1}\ min^{-1}$ up to $2\ \mu g\ kg^{-1}\ min^{-1}$; dopamine $5\mu g\ kg^{-1}\ min^{-1}$ up to the maximum dose of $20\ \mu g\ kg^{-1}\ min^{-1}$; adrenaline $2–10\ \mu g/min$).

3 Temporary pacing.

Sinoatrial block

This is characterized by the inability of the impulse generated in the sinus node to propagate to the adjacent myocardium; the obstacle is located inside the sinus node or at the sinoatrial junction.

Aetiology

Some particular conditions must be kept in mind as possible cause of sinoatrial blocks: inferior myocardial infarction as an intrinsic cause, and hyperkalaemia and drug toxicity as extrinsic cause.

ECG criteria

As for AV blocks, depending on how the impulse propagation is blocked from the sinus node to the atria, sinoatrial blocks are classified as follows:

- First degree sinoatrial block: the conduction time inside the sinus node is prolonged; an ECG diagnosis is not possible.
- Second degree sinoatrial block: periodic absence of the impulse conduction from the sinus node to the atria. It can be further divided into:
  - Type 1: with Luciani–Wenckebach periodism; a progressive lengthening of the PP interval until a P is missing. The asystolic pause is less than twice the baseline PP interval.
  - Type 2: sudden absence of P wave with regular PP intervals before the pause. The pause is a multiple of the baseline PP interval.
  - Type 2:1: one impulse out of two is not conducted to the atria; if the 2:1 sinoatrial block is constant, a

differential diagnosis with sinus bradycardia is not possible; in the paroxysmal form the frequency of the P wave doubles and then reduces to half its value.

- Third degree sinoatrial block: no impulse is conducted from the sinus node to the atria. P is missing for variable periods so that it is not possible to distinguish this from sinus arrest (the impulse is not generated).

From the clinical point of view, in a young person with no structural cardiomyopathy these are benign conditions that do not require specific treatment. In older patients or in patients with structural cardiomyopathy they can be associated with:

- symptoms due to cerebral hypoperfusion: syncope, fatigue, impairment of cognitive function
- heart failure
- coronary artery disease
- hyperkinetic ventricular arrhythmia triggered by the bradycardia and by the relative long QT.

Rarely, these conditions require acute treatment. The underlying cause should be treated. Specific treatment is indicated only if signs and symptoms are present. In this case the treatment is similar to that of sinus bradycardia, described earlier.

Atrioventricular node dysfunction (atrioventricular block)

The atrioventricular node is a structure formed from slow conduction fibres which determines an activation delay between the atria and the ventricles. An AV block is defined as the interruption or slowing down of impulse propagation between the atria and the ventricles. The conduction defect can be localized either in the atrioventricular node or in the bundle of His. Blocks localized at the AV node may be 'functional', due to an imbalance between the sympathetic and the vagal nerve system. These are generally transitory and benign and respond to atropine treatment. Blocks localized in the bundle of His or further down are generally due to structural damage, are not transitory, and have a worse prognosis. In this latter case atropine treatment determines an increase of P rate and therefore worsens the degree of block.

First degree atrioventricular block

This is defined as a delay of impulse conduction, generally at the AV node (80% of cases), rarely at the bundle of His.

- ECG criteria: prolongation of the PR interval >0.20 s.

- Aetiology:
  - Increase of vagal tone
  - Drugs: β-blockers, digoxin, calcium antagonists, class I antiarrhythmic drugs
  - Acute MI
  - Senile degeneration of the conduction pathway
- Therapeutic approach: a specific treatment is not required. If a first degree AV block appears in the acute setting the patient should be monitored for possible progression to a more advanced AV block.

Second degree atrioventricular block

This is defined as an intermittent interruption of the conduction of one or more impulse from the atria to the ventricles. Three subtypes are identified, distinguished by their ECG presentation: type 1 (Mobitz 1), type 2 (Mobitz 2), and advanced.

Second degree atrioventricular block type 1 (Mobitz 1)
ECG criteria

Progressive prolongation of the PR interval until a P is not conducted (Luciani–Wenckebach periodism).

Localization

Anatomically the block is localized either within the atrioventricular node (in most cases), in the bundle of His or in the distal fascicles of the bundle of His (infranodal block). A narrow QRS complex suggests that the block is localized in the AV node; with a wide QRS complex, a bundle branch block usually coexists with an AV node block. The block can be localized by the use of procedures that act on the autonomic nervous system (⊃ Table 53.3):

- Atropine improves conduction if the block is localized in the AV node, and worsens it if the block is infranodal.
- Carotid sinus massage (CSM) worsens the conduction if the block is located in the AV node, whereas it may improve or produce no change if the block is infranodal.

Unlike infranodal blocks, an AV nodal block rarely evolves toward a more advanced block.

Aetiology
- MI (especially inferior)
- Digoxin

Table 53.3 Localization of a type 1 second degree AV block

	Nodal block	Infranodal block
CSM	↓	↑
Atropine	↑	↓

CSM, cardiac sinus massage.

- Enhanced vagal tone
- Chronic coronary disease
- Myocarditis.

Therapeutic approach

Generally no specific treatment is required and only cardiac monitoring is recommended. If hypoperfusion signs and symptoms are due to the reduced heart rate induced by the AV block, treatment includes:

- atropine (0.5 mg repeated if necessary every 5 min till the maximum dose of 3 mg)
- transcutaneous and/or transvenous temporary pacing if there is no response to atropine.

Second degree atrioventricular block type 2 (Mobitz 2)
ECG criteria

Sudden blocked sinus P wave (i.e. not followed by a QRS complex); the preceding conducted beats have all the same PR interval. The pause determined by the blocked P wave is equal to twice the sinus cycle length. The PR interval of the first beat after the block is the same as the PR interval of the previous beat. The conduction ratio is generally 1:1 with an occasional and/or intermittent blocked P wave. Sometimes a regular conduction pattern of 2:1 (2P and 1 QRS complex), 3:1 and so on can be observed.

Localization

The second degree AV block type 2 is generally infranodal and indicates structural damage of the conduction system. This implies a worse prognosis than type 1, since it more frequently evolves towards a total AV block. A particular type of AV block is the 2:1 AV block, which can be either Mobitz 1 or Mobitz 2 type. Since it is characterized by the alternation of a conducted P wave and a blocked P wave the Luciani–Wenckebach periodism can not be observed and an ECG diagnosis is not possible. Nonetheless, in 2:1 AV block it is better to assume the worst and consider the block a type 2 unless proved otherwise, bearing in mind the relatively unfavourable course of a type 2 AV block.

Advanced second degree atrioventricular block
ECG criteria

More than two consecutive blocked P waves in the context of normal AV conduction. It is frequently paroxysmal and may cause prolonged asystole. This pattern implies advanced conduction disease and high risk for sudden development of complete heart block. These patients most often have wide QRS complexes and a ventricular escape rhythm (20–40 beats/min).

Aetiology
- MI (especially anterior)

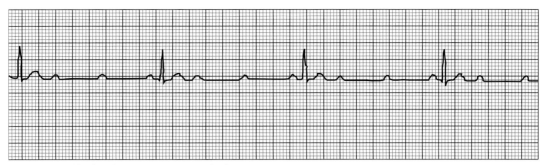

Figure 53.1 Third degree AV block with narrow QRS escape rhythm.

- Drugs: digoxin, calcium antagonists, β-blockers

- Degenerative disease of the conduction system.

Therapeutic approach

Patients with second degree type 2 AV block or advanced second degree AV block can be unstable at the time of assessment or suddenly develop a third degree block. In this case transvenous pacing is indicated. In patients with anterior MI and type 2 block the risk of progression to complete block is high, so prophylactic transvenous pacing is indicated. In patients with inferior MI the risk is lower and the patients are generally haemodynamically stable: transcutaneous pacing in standby mode is recommended. Transvenous pacing is indicated only if the block progresses or the patient becomes unstable. Atropine should not be used in type 2 or advanced second degree block since it increases the sinus rate while not affecting AV conduction, therefore increasing the degree of AV block.

Third degree atrioventricular block

This is characterized by nonconduction of the atrial impulse to the ventricles. The ventricular activity is therefore guaranteed by a substitute pacemaker. The atrial rate is always greater than the ventricular rate and no apparent relationship is present between the P waves and the QRS complex. The location of the block may be nodal or infranodal. In nodal blocks, the escape rhythm originating from the junctional or high septal region is characterized by narrow QRS

complexes at a rate of 40–60 beats/min (⮕ Fig. 53.1); often functional, it may be transitory and is associated with better prognosis. In infranodal blocks, the escape rhythm originates from the Purkinje net and is characterized by wide QRS complexes at a rate of less than 40 beats/min (⮕ Fig. 53.2). This reflects structural damage of the conduction system. The block is not transitory and is characterized by an electrical instability, so may evolve toward asystole; it is associated with a worse prognosis, requiring a pacemaker implant.

ECG criteria

Regular P-P interval. Some P may be hidden in the ventricular depolarization or in the repolarization phase and therefore may be identified as distortions of the QRS complex or T wave. No relationship is observed between the P and the QRS complex (AV dissociation). The number of Ps is generally greater than the number of QRS complexes. The width of the QRS complex and the ventricular rate reflect the localization of the escape pacemaker.

- Narrow QRS: the escape pacemaker is localized before the split of the bundle of His.

- Wide QRS: the escape pacemaker is localized after the split of the bundle of His.

Therapeutic approach

See ⮕ Table 53.4

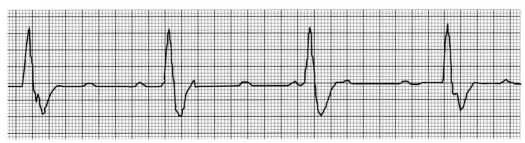

Figure 53.2 Third degree AV block with wide QRS escape rhythm.

Table 53.4 Third degree AV blocks: therapeutic approach

	Nodal block	Infranodal block
Transcutaneous pacing	For monitoring and in standby mode	For monitoring and in standby mode, or for pacing if symptomatic or asystole as bridge to transvenous pacing
Drug treatment	If signs /symptoms of hypoperfusion: atropine (0.5 mg, repeated if necessary every 5 min till the maximum dose of 3 mg)	If signs/symptoms of hypoperfusion as bridge to transvenous pacing: adrenergic drugs (isoproterenol 0.05–0.1 µg kg^{-1} min^{-1} up to 2 µg kg^{-1} min^{-1}, dopamine 5 µg kg^{-1} min^{-1} up to the maximum dose of 20 µg kg^{-1} min^{-1}, adrenaline 2–10 µg/min)
Temporary transvenous cardiac pacing	If signs/symptoms of hypoperfusion and no response to atropine	As a bridge to permanent pacing

Acute conduction disturbances in particular settings

Acute coronary syndrome

Myocardial ischaemia represents one of the major causes of conduction disturbances. Conduction abnormalities may, in fact, result from the ischaemia and/or necrosis of the conduction structure or from an autonomic imbalance.

Data from clinical trials suggest that AV block occurs in about 7% of patients with acute myocardial infarction (AMI); patients who manifest such conduction disturbances during the immediate period following AMI have a higher in-hospital and late mortality. In these cases, the long-term prognosis is related primarily to the extent of myocardial injury and the higher incidence of haemodynamic complications. The location of the infarct influences the type of conduction disturbances in the setting of AMI. The AV block associated with an inferior wall infarction is generally localized near or in the AV node. The escape rhythm is junctional (narrow QRS) with a rate ranging between 40 and 60 beats/min and a rare tendency toward an asystole. It is generally transitory and resolves spontaneously (within 7 days). In the anterior wall AMI the AV block is generally infranodal; in this case the conduction pathway which runs along the interventricular septum is involved. The escape pacemaker is at ventricular level with a wide QRS; the heart rate is about 30 beats/min, with electrical instability and a tendency towards a cardiac arrest.

Therapeutic approach

For an inferior wall infarction with narrow QRS and a rate greater than 40 beats/min:

◆ Observation and cardiac monitoring are recommended.

◆ If symptoms of hypoperfusion are present, atropine administration is recommended at a dose of 0.5 mg repeated every 5 min if needed till a maximum dose of 3 mg (0.04 mg/kg).

◆ If no response to drug treatment and symptomatic, transcutaneous pacing is indicated.

◆ If symptoms persist, transvenous temporary pacing is indicated.

In case of an anterior wall MI with a wide QRS escape rhythm at a rate of less than 40 beats/min, atropine is contraindicated and temporary transvenous pacing is mandatory.

Prophylactic pacing is indicated in case of:

◆ newly developed right bundle branch block associated with left anterior or left posterior hemiblock

◆ newly developed left bundle branch block with first degree AV block

◆ alternating left and right bundle branch block.

All these cases may evolve into a total AV block; transcutaneous pacing is indicated, maintaining the pacemaker in standby mode until pacing is required. A second degree type 2 AV block or total AV block requires immediate transvenous temporary pacing. Transcutaneous pacing is indicated as a bridge to transvenous pacing. Indications for permanent pacing after AMI are related to coexistence of AV block and intraventricular conduction defects and persistence (>14 days) of the conduction disturbances.

Drugs and electrolyte imbalance

Conduction disturbances can be caused by cardiovascular drug toxicity, including β-blockers, calcium channel blockers (CCB), and digoxin. CCB toxicity, in particular due to verapamil and diltiazem, is characterized by hypotension and conduction disturbances, including sinus bradycardia and varying degree of AV block. β-Blockers toxicity can cause brachycardia due to the excessive blockade of the β-receptors. For cases of β-blocker poisoning, high-dose glucagon is considered the first line antidote. For cases of CCB poisoning where cardiotoxicity is evident, a combination of calcium and adrenaline (epinephrine) should be used initially. Temporary transcutaneous pacing is indicated.

Digoxin is another cardiovascular drug commonly associated with bradycardia and AV blocks at toxic dose. Bradyarrhythmias that are haemodynamically stable may be treated just with observation and discontinuation of the drug. Haemodynamically unstable bradyarrhythmias respond best to digoxin-specific antibody fragments. Atropine may be used for temporary adjuncts because it improves AV nodal conduction. Cardiac temporary pacing has been used successfully.

Abnormal electrolytes levels also affect cardiac conduction. The electrolyte disturbance most often associated with AV node dysfunction is hyperkalaemia. The ECG abnormalities go from T wave changes to P wave flattening and PR interval prolongation; with higher levels of potassium, sinoatrial and AV blocks are observed. The fatal event is either asystole, as there is complete block in ventricular conduction, or ventricular fibrillation. In these cases the most important approach is to treat the electrolyte abnormality. A transcutaneous pacemaker in standby mode is indicated.

Postprocedural bradyarrhythmias

Alcohol septal ablation in hypertrophic obstructive cardiomyopathy

Transcoronary alcohol ablation of septal hypertrophy (TASH) is a therapeutic catheter-based option and an alternative to surgery in the treatment of patients with hypertrophic obstructive cardiomyopathy. However, delayed in-hospital sudden unexpected complete heart block after an uncomplicated intervention remains a major complication and leads to permanent pacemaker implantation in 7–38% of patients.

The onset of delayed complete heart block may occur up to several days after an uncomplicated TASH procedure. Therefore, telemetric monitoring for 8 days is recommended by some groups. The site of injury seems to be located distal to or inside the bundle of His in most cases. Temporary pacemakers are routinely placed at the time of alcohol injection, but there are no widely accepted guidelines for their management after the procedure.

Other ablation procedures

Bradyarrhythmias and in particular AV blocks represent possible complications of transcatheter ablation.

Ablation of the slow pathway is the treatment of choice in patients with episodes of AV non-re-entrant tachycardia (AVNRT). It has a high rate of success (>95%) and is safe (major complications 1.5–5%). One of the most ominous complications is a third degree AV block (0.74–4%);

it presents with a narrow QRS and is, therefore, a nodal block due to damage of the AV node determined by radiofrequency. The block may be transitory, but if it lasts more than 24–48 h a permanent pacemaker is necessary. It is generally not associated with severe symptoms or signs. Cardiac monitoring is therefore necessary in the 24–48 h after the procedure.

Ablation of the accessory pathway is also the treatment of choice in patients with Wolff–Parkinson–White syndrome or AV re-entrant tachycardia (AVRT) and the procedure is very effective (rate of success 90% with about a total of 5% of complications). The septal accessory pathways (midseptal, anteroseptal, and parahissian) are the ones most often complicated by blocks (*c.*28%). These are generally infranodal blocks, less often transitory, and with a wide QRS escape rhythm. Cardiac monitoring is indicated for 24–48 h after the procedure and if the block does not resolve, a pacemaker implant is recommended. One of the catheters used for the ablation procedure can be left and used for transvenous pacing.

Percutaneous transcatheter valve implantation

Transcatheter aortic valve implantation is becoming established as an alternative treatment for some patients with symptomatic severe aortic stenosis who are not considered suitable for surgical aortic valve replacement because of prohibitive surgical risks. One of the potential complications is complete AV block, requiring definitive pacemaker implantation.

Acute pacemaker malfunction: detection and management

Pacemaker (PMK) malfunction, especially in patients who are PMK dependent, is an important cause of bradyarrhythmias and potentially life threatening. The symptoms and signs are those of the bradyarrhythmias, but more often PMK malfunction manifests with a syncope. The symptoms and signs are due to defects of electric stimulation of the heart when this is expected and asystole and/or severe bradycardia develops. The principal stimulation defects can be classified as capture defects or sensing defects.

ECG criteria

Two different ECG patterns characterize pacemaker malfunction:

- An atrial and/or ventricular spike is present (PMK stimulation artefact) not followed by depolarization

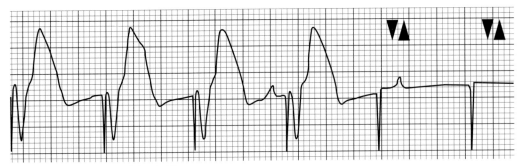

Figure 53.3 Loss of capture due to increase of threshold.

(⬭ Fig. 53.3). In this case the energy delivered by the device is not sufficient to determine a depolarization; there is an increase of the stimulation threshold (minimum quantity of energy necessary to determine depolarization of the heart). A loss of capture is present.

◆ The PMK spike is not present where it is expected (⬭ Fig. 53.4). In this case there are two possibilities:

• The impulse is correctly developed by the PMK but is not able to reach the endocardium: this is mainly due to damage of an element of the system.

• The impulse is not delivered by the generator; the most frequent cause is oversensing.

The principle causes of stimulation defects are:

◆ Increase of the stimulation threshold due to medications, metabolic abnormalities, inflammation, MI involving the portion of the myocardium where the lead is placed, or lead perforation. In these cases a threshold test must be carried out and the PMK's output reprogrammed to the maximum output (7.5 V, 1.5 s). Since the threshold may not be stable, the patient must be monitored. A transcutaneous pacemaker in standby mode must also be placed. If the loss of capture persists, a temporary transvenous pacemaker is indicated.

◆ Interruption of electrical continuity; the impulse cannot be transmitted to the heart and therefore the spike is missing on the ECG. This can be due to lead fracture, loose set-screw, or disconnection of the lead from the pacemaker. In this case the problem cannot be resolved by reprogramming the pacemaker and a temporary transvenous pacemaker is indicated.

◆ The generator does not create the impulse. On the ECG, the spike is missing where it is expected. It can be due to:

• end of life of the pacemaker

• oversensing with improper pacing inhibition: the pacemaker incorrectly senses noncardiac potentials (myopotentials, noise from PMK lead fracture) as cardiac activity (depolarizations) and is inhibited from pacing.

◆ On the ECG the spike is missing either constantly or intermittently. Interrogation of the device can identify the 'noises' that determine improper pacing inhibition. The malfunction can be corrected by reprogramming the pacemaker so as to exclude sensing in the chamber where the defect is present (i.e. V00, D00). If reprogramming is not possible and the defect is intermittent, the use of a transcutaneous pacemaker in standby mode

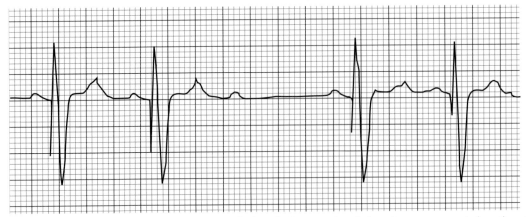

Figure 53.4 Oversensing with inhibition of ventricular pacing. Ventricular loss of capture can be ruled out because no ventricular spike artefact can be seen after the third P wave.

is sufficient; if the defect is constant and determines symptomatic bradycardia, a transvenous pacemaker is indicated.

Temporary pacing in intensive acute cardiac care

Transcutaneous temporary pacing

This represents a noninvasive technique of temporary pacing. It does not require special training and can be performed quickly in an emergency setting, which gives it an advantage over invasive pacing. Most defibrillator units are equipped with transcutaneous pacing capability. The procedure is as follows:

1 Two adhesive pacing electrodes are applied to the patient's thorax: one on the anterior chest wall, on the apex, the other on the patient's back to the left of the thoracic spine, between the spine and the left scapula.

2 The electrodes are then connected to the pacing unit.

3 After the pacing unit is turned on, the pacing parameters must be determined (ventricular pacing threshold and pacing rate):

- Pacing threshold: pacing is begun at a rate slightly faster than the patient's rhythm and at a minimal output (5–10 mA) and then increased gradually. The ventricular output is increased by about 5–10 mA at a time until cardiac capture is demonstrated. The lowest output at which capture is obtained is defined as the pacing threshold. Electrical capture is identified by the presence on the ECG tracing of a wide stimulated QRS complex followed by a ST segment and a T wave. The final output setting should be about 10 mA above the pacing threshold.

- Standby mode: if the patient is asymptomatic, the pacing rate is set lower than the patient's spontaneous rhythm and the pacemaker is set in demand mode so that it generates electrical stimuli only when the patient's heart rate falls below the pacing rate.

- Therapeutic pacing: if patient is in asystole or is symptomatic, the pacing rate is set at about 70–80 beats/min.

The disadvantages of the procedure are that it may cause significant discomfort and pain to the patient; pectoral muscle twitching is often present, caused by the high voltage required for pacing; skin burns may occur and therefore periodic skin evaluation is recommended with possible repositioning of the electrodes. In conscious patients analgesia (morphine sulphate) and sedation (midazolam) should be used. This technique may not be able to guarantee stable ventricular capture and therefore this should be evaluated periodically; the pacing threshold may increase with prolonged pacing.

Transcutaneous cardiac pacing is a temporary method of pacing, indicated in various critical clinical settings. It is generally indicated in patients with symptomatic and haemodynamically unstable bradyarrhythmias, particularly in those who do not respond to drug therapy, and prophylactically in patients at high risk of evolving toward asystole. It is used in patients with reversible or transitory conditions such as digoxin toxicity, electrolyte imbalance, inferior acute MI, or when transvenous pacing is not immediately available. It is often used as a bridge to temporary transvenous pacing or a permanent PMK. It should not be relied on if temporary pacing is required for a prolonged period of time.

Transvenous temporary pacing

This is generally indicated in patients with bradycardia and AV block in asystole or with an inadequate escape rhythm and therefore symptomatic. It should be used in patients who require continuous pacing as a bridge to a permanent PMK, in reversible or transient conditions such as drug toxicity, electrolyte imbalance, or inferior acute MI. See ⤷ Chapter 25 for a detailed account.

Permanent pacing in intensive acute cardiac care

The indication for permanent pacing in the ICCU are the same as those recommended for sinus node disease and AV blocks in the current European Society of Cardiology (ESC) guidelines, which must be consulted. It is important to emphasize that the evaluation and treatment of possible transitory and reversible causes is mandatory.

Personal perspective

Conduction disturbances will increase in the future, considering that one of the most frequent cause is the degeneration of the conduction system, which is correlated with age, and the number of elderly people in the general population is increasing. Procedures such as alcohol septal ablation in hypertrophic obstructive cardiomyopathy, percutaneous transcatheter valve implantation, and ablation procedures for treatment of arrhythmias are also becoming more widely used, and this also implies an increase in conduction disturbances, which represent one of its possible complications. In our opinion, all physicians who work in an emergency setting must be familiar with this kind of arrhythmia and keep it in mind. It is important to be able to distinguish between blocks of probable nodal origin and those of infranodal origin. It must be emphasized that even though the use of atropine is often recommended in the treatment of AV blocks, it should be used only in blocks with probable nodal origin and should be avoided in the infranodal blocks. Transcutaneous pacing has become more efficient and extremely easy to use, and must therefore be considered as an important therapeutic approach in an emergency setting. It is highly relevant that the transcutaneous pacing electrodes may be used also to interrupt possible ventricular shockable arrhythmias; this renders this device of primary importance in the management of all life-threatening arrhythmias (bradycardias and ventricular tachyarrhythmias).

Further reading

Baskett P. *Pocket book of the European Resuscitation Council Guidelines for Resuscitation 2005*, Mosby Elsevier, London, 2006, pp. 66–80.

Bergfeldt L. Atrioventricular conduction disturbances. *Cardiac Electrophysiol Rev* 1997;**1**:15–21.

European Resuscitation Council Guidelines for Resuscitation 2005: Section 4: Adult advanced life support. *Resuscitation* 2005;**67**(S1):S39–S86.

Guidelines for cardiac pacing and cardiac resynchronization therapy. *Eur Heart J* 2007;**28**:2256–2295.

Peters R. Heart block. In: Rakel R (ed.) *Conn's current therapy 2005*. Elsevier Saunders, Philadelphia, 2005, pp. 349–353.

➲ For additional multimedia materials please visit the online version of the book (✆ http://www.esciacc.oxfordmedicine.com).

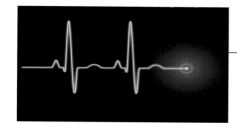

CHAPTER 54

Atrial fibrillation and supraventricular arrhythmias

Panos E. Vardas, Emmanuel P. Koutalas, and Emmanuel N. Simantirakis

Contents

Summary

Critically ill patients often exhibit cardiac arrhythmias. These arrhythmias occur with an incidence that varies according to the pathological substrate; they affect the patients' haemodynamic state, increase the rate of further complications, and are often associated with a poor prognosis.

In the main, patients who exhibit atrial arrhythmias in the intensive care unit include those with myocardial ischaemia, or more rarely acute myocarditis or pericarditis; those undergoing cardiothoracic or other surgery; and those with respiratory failure from various causes. With the gradual introduction of haemodynamic monitoring devices and myocardial pump function support devices, concerns have been raised regarding possible device dysfunction resulting from arrhythmias and, conversely, arrhythmias that may be caused by these devices.

This chapter analyses the aetiological and pathogenetic mechanisms that underlie the main supraventricular arrhythmias in different categories of patients, evaluates their prognostic significance with regard to the in-hospital outcome, and discusses strategies for the short- and mid-term management of such arrhythmias.

Mechanisms of arrhythmogenesis

The mechanisms through which arrhythmias are produced can be divided into those that involve disturbances of stimulus generation, those that involve disturbances of stimulus conduction, and combinations of the two.

Disturbances of stimulus production

Automaticity refers to the ability of certain cardiac tissue to produce automatic pacing activity. Disturbances of automaticity include both natural accelerated automaticity and pathological automaticity.

Triggered activity is a tachycardia mechanism that is associated with disturbances of the recovery or repolarization of the myocardial cell. Triggered rhythms originate via interruptions in repolarization that are called after-depolarizations. Early after-depolarizations occur before the repolarization of the myocardial tissue and are produced by the action of drugs, sympathetic discharges, or hypoxia. Delayed after-depolarizations have been observed in atrial tissue and in mammalian cells exposed to mechanical or neurohormonal stress, or digitalis [1].

Disturbances of stimulus conduction

Re-entry is the most common mechanism of arrhythmogenesis. The generated pulse propagates to a piece of tissue that has already been repolarized, after its depolarization (circuit creation).

Types of supraventricular arrhythmias

Atrial fibrillation is the most common supraventricular arrhythmia and manifests itself as uncoordinated atrial electrical activity leading to a deterioration of atrial mechanical function [2]. It is thought to be triggered by depolarizations that usually originate from the pulmonary veins, and sustained by re-entry wavelets in the atria.

Other supraventricular arrhythmias include rhythms originating from the sinus node, from atrial tissue (atrial flutter, atrial tachycardia), and from junctional tissue, as well as reciprocating or accessory-pathway tachycardias. The latter term includes re-entrant tachycardias that involve the atrioventricular junction (atrioventricular nodal reciprocating tachycardia, the atrium (atrial tachycardia), as well as atrioventricular reciprocating rhythms (atrioventricular reciprocating tachycardia) [3].

The mechanisms of production of the main supraventricular arrhythmias are shown in ⮡ Table 54.1.

Table 54.1 Supraventricular arrhythmias and the mechanisms that produce them

Arrhythmia	Mechanism
AVNRT	Re-entry
AVRT	Re-entry
Atrial tachycardia	Automatic activity or re-entry
Atrial flutter	Re-entry
Atrial fibrillation	Started by triggered activity and sustained by multiple wavelet re-entry

AVNRT, atrioventricular nodal reciprocating tachycardia; AVRT, atrioventricular reciprocating tachycardia.

Supraventricular arrhythmias in acute heart diseases

Acute myocardial infarction

Acute myocardial ischaemia is accompanied by significant ionic and metabolic changes, both inside and outside the myocardial cell, interfering with the inward and outward flow of ion currents, causing depolarization of the resting membrane potential, reduced upstroke velocity, slowing of conduction, decreased excitability, shortening of the action potential duration, altered refractoriness, dispersion of repolarization, and abnormal automaticity [4].

Atrial fibrillation is the most frequently occurring supraventricular arrhythmia [4]. In the era of thrombolysis, the incidence of atrial fibrillation in patients with acute myocardial infarction (AMI) ranged from 6.6% to 21% [5, 6]. Similar figures are noted in studies with primary percutaneous coronary intervention (PCI). Published data from the OACIS study show an incidence of atrial fibrillation of 12% [7]. The Cooperative Cardiovascular Project (CCP), a study of patients aged over 64 years, reported that 22.1% of cases suffered from atrial fibrillation, with half of them developing the arrhythmia during their hospitalization [5].

Advanced age, the presence of symptoms of heart failure (increased Killip class), increased heart rate on admission, and systolic left ventricular dysfunction are the main prognostic indexes associated with a high rate of occurrence of atrial fibrillation [5, 7, 8].

Factors that have been implicated in the occurrence of atrial fibrillation in patients with myocardial infarction during the immediate postinfarction period (up to 48 h from the acute episode) include increased atrial tension due to dysfunction of the left or right ventricle, possible atrial infarct due to lesions in the circumflex or right coronary artery (involving the sinus node artery), increased sympathetic tone, as well as other causes such as pericarditis, hypokalaemia, hypomagnesaemia, chronic pulmonary diseases, and hypoxia [9, 10, 11]. The development of atrial fibrillation within the first 24 h after MI is usually associated with occlusion of the right coronary artery and an inferior wall infarction. In contrast, atrial fibrillation occurring after the first 24 h is associated with an anterior wall infarction and left ventricular systolic dysfunction [4]. It occurs more often in patients with large infarcted regions (anterior infarction) and in those whose hospitalization is complicated by heart failure, complex ventricular arrhythmogenesis, and high-degree atrioventricular block [12, 13].

In the CCP study, the development of atrial fibrillation during hospitalization was associated with higher in-hospital mortality (25% vs 16%) and higher 30-day mortality. On the other hand, the presence of atrial fibrillation on admission was not associated with increased mortality, suggesting that any new-onset atrial fibrillation has a deleterious effect on the patient's haemodynamic profile, in contrast to those who are already suffering from the persistent or chronic form [5]. In the OPTIMAAL trial, 30-day mortality was not significantly higher in patients who were already in atrial fibrillation on admission to hospital [14]. On a long-term basis, most studies also report higher mortality in patients with MI complicated by atrial fibrillation, compared to those who had the arrhythmia on admission [5–7].

If a patient with AMI develops atrial fibrillation, the first evaluation includes the probable cause and whether or not immediate electrical cardioversion is required, in cases with haemodynamic instability due to a drop in blood pressure, worsening ischaemia, or symptoms of pulmonary congestion (⊃ Table 54.2). Short-lasting anaesthetic agents are preferred. The initial single-phase current energy delivered should be only 50 J for the conversion of atrial flutter. Higher energy levels (100–360 J) are required for the cardioversion of atrial fibrillation with single-phase current.

If a biphasic defibrillator is available, the energy delivered may be reduced by half [12].

If drug therapy is preferred, intravenous agents such as amiodarone, β-blockers, nondihydropyridine calcium antagonists (diltiazem, verapamil), and digitalis are used (⊃ Table 54.3). Class Ic antiarrhythmic agents are not recommended [2, 12, 15]. In addition, unfractionated or low-molecular-weight heparin should be administered to prevent stroke [2, 12, 15]. The 3.1% incidence of stroke reported for patients with ST-elevation myocardial infarction (STEMI) and atrial fibrillation underlines the need for care on the part of the treating physician [6].

Finally, treatment of any electrolyte disorder is essential, since hypomagnesaemia and especially hypokalaemia predispose to unsuccessful cardioversion of supraventricular and ventricular arrhythmias.

If control of the heart rate is achieved, the treating physician should evaluate the possible benefit of the restoration of sinus rhythm. The restoration of sinus rhythm in haemodynamically stable patients with atrial fibrillation is analysed in the current guidelines for the treatment of patients with atrial fibrillation [2].

Table 54.2 ESC guidelines for the treatment (rate control) of atrial fibrillation in the setting of acute myocardial infarction

Recommendation	Class	Level
Rate control of atrial fibrillation		
Electrical cardioversion if severe haemodynamic compromise or intractable ischaemia, or when adequate rate control cannot be achieved with pharmacological agents	I	C
IV β-blockers or nondihydropyridine calcium antagonists (verapamil, diltiazem). If no clinical signs of heart failure, bronchospasm (only for β-blockers) or AV block. Verapamil and diltiazem should be used cautiously or avoided in patients with heart failure due to their negative inotropic effect	I	C
IV amiodarone to slow a rapid ventricular response and improve LV function	I	C
IV digitalis if severe LV dysfunction and/or heart failure	IIb	C
Anticoagulation for atrial fibrillation		
IV administration of a therapeutic dose of UFH or LMWH	I	C

AV, atrioventricular; LV, left ventricular; LMWH, low-molecular-weight heparin; UFH, unfractionated heparin.
From Van de Werf F, Bax J, Betriu A, et al. Management of acute myocardial infarction in patients presenting with persistent ST-segment elevation: the Task Force on the Management of ST-Segment Elevation Acute Myocardial Infarction of the European Society of Cardiology. *Eur Heart J* 2008;**29**:2909–2945.

Table 54.3 Intravenous doses of recommended antiarrhythmic medications

Drug	Bolus	Maintenance infusion
Amiodarone	150 mg over 10 min. Supplemental boluses of 150 mg may be given over 10–30 min for recurrent arrhythmias, but limited to 6–8 supplemental boluses in any 24-h period	1 mg/min for 6 h and then 0.5 mg/min may be necessary after initial bolus dose
Esmolol	500 µg/kg over 1 min, followed by 50 µg/kg per min over 4 min	60–200 µg/kg per min
Metoprolol	2.5–5.0 mg over 2 min; up to 3 doses	–
Atenolol	5–10 mg (1 mg/min)	–
Propranolol	0.15 mg/kg	–
Digitalis	0.25 mg each 2 h, up to 1.5 mg	–
Verapamil	0.075–0.15 mg/kg over 2 min	-
Diltiazem	0.25 mg/kg over 2 min	–
Adenosine	6 mg × 1 over 1–2 s; if no response, 12 mg IV after 1–2 min may be given; repeat 12-mg dose if needed	–

From Antman EM, Anbe DT, Armstrong PW, et al. ACC/AHA guidelines for the management of patients with ST-elevation myocardial infarction; A report of the American College of Cardiology/American Heart Association Task Force on Practice Guidelines (Committee to Revise the 1999 Guidelines for the Management of patients with acute myocardial infarction). *J Am Coll Cardiol* 2004;**44**:E1–E211; Van de Werf F, Bax J, Betriu A, et al. Management of acute myocardial infarction in patients presenting with persistent ST-segment elevation: the Task Force on the Management of ST-Segment Elevation Acute Myocardial Infarction of the European Society of Cardiology. *Eur Heart J* 2008;**29**:2909–2945.

The other supraventricular arrhythmias appear only rarely in the setting of AMI and are usually self-limiting [4, 10]. Atrial flutter is treated in the same way as atrial fibrillation. Paroxysmal re-entrant tachycardias, because of the rapid ventricular response, should be treated according to the following algorithm in ⮕ Box 54.1; for dosages see ⮕ Table 54.3 (class I recommendation, level of evidence C) [12]. There may be a delay of at least 1 h before any pharmacological effect is observed.

If the patient becomes haemodynamically unstable and needs immediate electrical cardioversion, this should be done in accordance with the published guidelines.

Acute pericarditis

The sinus node is tightly embedded in the locally thick parietal pericardium, just below the visceral pericardium of the right atrial wall. Because of this anatomical relationship, inflammation of the pericardium often involves at least atrial muscular tissue around the sinus node, or even the sinus node itself, and thus predisposes to rhythm disturbances [16]. However, only a minority of patients with acute pericarditis develop atrial arrhythmias[16]. In a recent study of patients with acute pericarditis, who were divided into two groups according to the presence or not of myocardial inflammation on endomyocardial biopsy, it was found that the patients who had no myocardial involvement showed fewer cases of supraventricular paroxysmal arrhythmias compared to the other group (5% vs 40%). In contrast, the patients with only pericardial inflammation had a higher incidence of atrial fibrillation (20% vs 0%) [17].

The highest risk from supraventricular arrhythmias is seen in patients with large pericardial effusions and incipient compression of the pericardial cavities, and reaches its maximum in patients with cardiac tamponade. This is because of the further reduction in diastolic ventricular filling time, which causes an even greater fall in left ventricular stroke volume and the occurrence of shock due to low cardiac output. The only therapeutic intervention in such cases, apart from treatment of the effusion (e.g. pericardiocentesis), is immediate electrical cardioversion of the arrhythmia in order to restore the patient to some degree of haemodynamic stability.

Acute myocarditis

Patients with myocarditis may exhibit the entire spectrum of atrial and ventricular arrhythmias. In one series of patients with myocarditis, reported by Morgera et al., 22% developed atrial arrhythmias. Atrial fibrillation is more frequent in patients with symptom duration of more than 1 month. Atrial fibrillation, left bundle branch block, and signs of hypertrophy are the most powerful markers of a poor prognosis in these patients [18].

Finally, the principles for treating supraventricular arrhythmias in patients who are hospitalized for myocarditis are the same as those that apply in other acute conditions, as described above, depending on the therapeutic approach and mainly on the haemodynamic profile of each individual patient.

Supraventricular arrhythmias in patients who have undergone surgery

Postoperative atrial arrhythmias, especially atrial fibrillation and flutter, occur in up to 6.1% of elderly patients who undergo noncardiothoracic surgery and in 10–65% of patients who undergo heart or thoracic surgery.

The main independent preoperative prognostic factor associated with the occurrence of atrial fibrillation postoperatively is age over 60 years [19–21]. As a result of age, inflammatory and degenerative processes are activated in the atria, which lead to changes in the atrial electrophysiological properties [22]. The paths that connect inflammation with atrial fibrillation still remain largely unknown. The inflammatory reaction to surgical intervention may be genetically determined.

It has been observed that a higher heart rate in elderly patients was an independent prognostic factor for atrial fibrillation after cardiothoracic surgery, suggesting that a reduced preoperative parasympathetic tone predisposes to atrial fibrillation [20, 21]. There are conflicting views as to whether the imbalance seen in the autonomic nervous system is due primarily to disturbances of the sympathetic or the parasympathetic system.

Box 54.1 Treatment algorithm for paroxysmal re-entrant tachycardias

1 Carotid sinus massage

2 Intravenous adenosine

3 Intravenous β-adrenergic blockade with metoprolol or atenolol

4 Intravenous diltiazem

5 Intravenous digitalis

Open heart surgery

Atrial fibrillation is the most common complication after open heart surgery. It results in a longer stay in the intensive care unit (ICU) and a longer hospitalization overall [23]. Atrial fibrillation is seen in 25–40% of cases after coronary artery bypass surgery (CABG), and this approaches 60% when the CABG is combined with valve replacement, with the peak incidence being during the second and third postoperative days [24]. In a retrospective study of patients undergoing CABG or aortic valve replacement, or a combination of the two, the total incidence of atrial fibrillation was 25.6% (from 22.7% for simple CABG to 44.0% to CABG plus valve replacement).

Postoperative atrial fibrillation does not increase in-hospital mortality. However, in patients undergoing CABG, atrial fibrillation appears to increase the 1-year mortality. This relation between atrial fibrillation and an increase in late mortality after CABG, but not after valve surgery, is a matter that needs further careful investigation [23]. Subsequent studies confirmed that post-CABG atrial fibrillation was an independent predictor of long-term mortality [25]. The influence of atrial fibrillation on long-term mortality has also been confirmed by other studies. Villareal *et al.* concluded that postoperative atrial fibrillation was an independent predictor of long-term mortality in patients undergoing isolated CABG [26].

The main risk factors for postoperative atrial fibrillation, apart from age, are the type of operation, temporary pacing, inotropic support, an advanced stage of heart failure, and complications during weaning from cardiopulmonary bypass [21, 23]. Metabolic syndrome in patients over 50 years old is also viewed as a risk factor for postoperative atrial fibrillation [27]. In one study, a left atrial volume greater than 32 mL/m ^{2} was the strongest predictor of postoperative atrial fibrillation, independently of age, and the other clinical and surgical parameters [28].

During aortic valve replacement surgery, the factors found to be significantly associated with atrial fibrillation in the early postoperative period in patients with aortic stenosis were left ventricular ejection fraction, and the end-systolic thickness of the intraventricular septum. In the case of surgery for aortic regurgitation, the corresponding factors for the whole postoperative period were age, left ventricular ejection fraction, left ventricular end-systolic diameter, end-systolic thickness of the intraventricular septum, left atrial dimension, and insignificant mitral regurgitation, while for the early postoperative period prognostic factors were left ventricular ejection fraction, and left atrial dimension [29]. Research is continuing into

a possible genetic background that might predispose to the postoperative occurrence of this arrhythmia [30].

The underlying mechanisms of postoperative atrial fibrillation have not yet been fully elucidated. As already stated, it appears that inflammation plays a primary role. Patients who took statins prior to CABG showed a lower incidence of atrial fibrillation postoperatively [31]. Also studied has been the relation between cytokines and C-reactive protein and postoperative atrial fibrillation, although no clinically significant conclusions have emerged so far [32]. Attempts have been made to reduce the inflammation burden by administering dexamethazone preoperatively, but with conflicting results [33]. Finally, another field of research concerns disturbances of the autonomic nervous system. The competition between parasympathetic tone and increasing sympathetic activity may be an important triggering mechanism of this arrhythmia [34].

Thoracic surgery

Atrial fibrillation is the most common arrhythmia after chest surgery, with an incidence ranging from 4% to 30%. Atrial fibrillation was found to be associated with a significant increase in mortality, length of hospital stay, and hospital costs [35]. In the case of thoracic aortic surgery, disruption of the aortic fat pad leads to a reduction in cardiac vagal tone, which increases the likelihood of occurrence of atrial fibrillation [36].

Postoperative arrhythmias most often occur during the first or second postoperative day [37]. Significant multivariate predictors of postoperative atrial fibrillation include male sex, increasing age, and a history of congestive heart failure, preoperative arrhythmias, or peripheral vascular disease [35]. Some specific types of operation are associated with an increased risk of the arrhythmia, including resection of a mediastinal tumour, or thymectomy, lobectomy, bilobectomy, and pneumonectomy [37] Possible triggering mechanisms of supraventricular arrhythmias are disturbances of blood gas exchange, possible autonomic enervation during the removal of pulmonary tissue, and systemic inflammation [38].

Nonthoracic surgery

In this setting the reported incidence of supraventricular arrhythmias ranges from 4% to 20% [39, 40]. In one published review, atrial fibrillation was the most common arrhythmia [41].

Surgery and anaesthesia are thought to cause a stress reaction that can lead to the development of arrhythmias [42]. In addition, inflammation is considered to play a significant role [43]. The highest incidence of supraventricular arrhythmias is seen during the first 4 days after operation, when the inflammatory reaction is at a maximum [19, 40, 44]. Sepsis may also cause arrhythmias[45]. Observed disturbances of the acid–base balance—especially metabolic acidosis—and electrolytes, tend to be contributory rather than principal causes of the arrhythmia [41, 45].

Arrhythmias prolong hospital stay and are associated with increased mortality [39, 45]. Risk factors for arrhythmia occurrence include age, male sex, congestive cardiac failure, valvular heart disease, asthma, a history of supraventricular arrhythmias, premature atrial complexes on the preoperative ECG, left anterior hemiblock, hypertension, and low preoperative serum potassium levels.

Prevention and management of postoperative supraventricular arrhythmias

Prevention of postoperative atrial fibrillation

β-Blockers, administered preoperatively, significantly reduce the incidence of atrial fibrillation [46]. In a meta-analysis by Crystal et al., it was found that controls had an atrial fibrillation incidence of 33%, compared to 19% for patients who received β-blockers, with the number needed to treat (NNT) being only 7 [46]. Sotalol, a class III antiarrhythmic agent, was more effective in reducing the postoperative incidence of atrial fibrillation than were other β-blockers or placebo [47]. Crystal et al. reported that the incidence of postoperative atrial fibrillation was 12% in patients who received sotalol, compared to 22% in patients who took another β-blocker (NNT 10) [48].

Prophylactic amiodarone (10 mg/kg per day by mouth) reduced the incidence of atrial fibrillation from 29.5% to 16.1% [49]. The meta-analysis of Crystal et al. reported an incidence of atrial fibrillation of 22.5% in groups taking amiodarone compared to 37% for controls (NNT 7) [48]. Studies that used digitalis, verapamil, or procainamide found no significant effect.

An analysis of biatrial pacing as a prophylactic measure against postoperative atrial fibrillation showed a statistically significant benefit [50]. Biatrial pacing for the prevention of atrial fibrillation in patients undergoing cardiac surgery has not been used widely [51]. As regards the prophylactic administration of magnesium, in one meta-analysis, 23% of patients who took prophylactic magnesium developed atrial fibrillation, compared with 31% of controls [52]. It also seems that patients who undergo off-pump CABG are at a lower risk of atrial fibrillation than those undergoing conventional CABG [53]. Posterior pericardiotomy is thought to reduce the incidence of atrial fibrillation after

cardiac surgery. In a meta-analysis by Biancari and Asim Mahar the incidence of atrial fibrillation was 10.8% in the posterior pericardiotomy group and 28.1% in the control group. Other supraventricular arrhythmias occurred in 13.8% of patients in the posterior pericardiotomy group and 35.4% in controls. Pericardial effusion was also significantly less common in the former group. Postoperative pericardial effusion appears to be related with the development of atrial fibrillation after cardiac surgery [54].

The guidelines for the prevention of postoperative atrial fibrillation are summarized in 📇 54.1 [3]. In procedures for the removal of a section or all of a lung, there are no clear data concerning standard prevention. Some studies have provided evidence for a possible benefit from the administration of diltiazem, magnesium, or bupivacaine epidural. The prophylactic administration of amiodarone is not recommended, because of the risk of development of adult respiratory distress syndrome [51].

Treatment of postoperative atrial fibrillation

The hypercatecholeminergic state of the postoperative patient, in combination with the coexisting comorbidities, make it difficult to control the heart rate in postoperative atrial fibrillation. Intravenous β-blockers with short-lasting action (e.g. esmolol) have been used, as have nondihydropyridine calcium antagonists (verapamil, diltiazem)—the latter with caution in view of their negative inotropic action. Intravenous amiodarone has been used in this setting, with good results. In contrast, digitalis, because of the increased adrenergic tone and its slow onset of action, is not widely used.

Cardioversion of atrial fibrillation or flutter is generally not recommended in patients who have no or only mild symptoms until possible triggering factors are corrected. In addition, since atrial fibrillation most usually resolves spontaneously, electrical cardioversion is not required unless the arrhythmia appears during the immediate hypothermal period [2]. If the patient is strongly symptomatic, cardioversion to sinus rhythm may be performed, as long as the necessary anticoagulation precautions are taken in accordance with the current guidelines. In any case, before cardioversion any electrolyte disturbances should be corrected, especially potassium or magnesium deficiency. The drugs that have usually been used for the cardioversion of postoperative atrial fibrillation are amiodarone, procainamide, ibutilide, and sotalol.

Anticoagulants increase the risk of haemorrhage after surgery. For this reason, and taking into account that the occurrence of atrial fibrillation after CABG is associated with an elevated incidence of stroke, an individualized therapeutic approach to the possibility of administering anticoagulants to these patients is required.

Drug therapy for atrial flutter is in general the same as for atrial fibrillation. If epicardial pacing electrodes remain attached to the patient cardioversion may be achieved using overdrive pacing. Other supraventricular arrhythmias are usually self-terminating, but if not may be treated as described above.

The guidelines for the treatment of postoperative atrial fibrillation are summarized in 📷54.1 [2].

Supraventricular arrhythmias in patients with respiratory failure

Patients with respiratory failure show a high incidence and a wide variety of cardiac arrhythmias. The most common arrhythmias seen in these patients are atrial and ventricular extrasystoles, multifocal atrial tachycardia, atrial flutter, and atrial fibrillation. These arrhythmias usually acquire clinical significance, may potentially become dangerous, and are associated with a poor prognosis.

Hypoxaemia, hypercapnia, a drop in pH, and electrolyte disturbances, especially potassium, are likely to promote arrhythmogenesis by disturbing cellular entropy, with changes that influence the electrophysiological properties of the cardiac stimulus conduction system and the myocardium in general. When the partial oxygen pressure in arterial blood falls sufficiently, the tissue hypoxia thus created, and the consequent anaerobic metabolism with production of lactate and lactic acid, may be avoided by an increase in haemoglobin oxygen saturation in the arterial blood and by an increase in cardiac output. If these mechanisms reach their functional limit or are inadequate, anaerobic metabolism and metabolic acidosis develop, with further deterioration due to impaired cardiac contractility. Hypercapnia, by causing acidosis and hypoxaemia, can promote the appearance of disturbances of the autonomic nervous system and potassium ion channels in myocardial cells, resulting in a prolongation of the QT interval via a slowing of the repolarization process. In addition, hypoxia and hypercapnia, via stimulation of sympathetic tone, cause vasoconstriction, and a rise in blood pressure and peripheral resistances [55–57].

Hudson et al., studying patients with respiratory failure on a substrate of chronic obstructive pulmonary disease, reported supraventricular arrhythmias in 23 of 70 patients [58]. Multifocal atrial tachycardia was a very common finding. Hypoxaemia was present in 43% of patients with multifocal atrial tachycardia in various studies [59].

In patients with respiratory failure who exhibit supraventricular arrhythmias, the first priority is to restore their blood gases to normal (oxygen, carbon dioxide) and generally to correct disturbances of the acid–base balance. It is therefore of crucial importance to identify the probable reason for the compromise of the patient's compensatory mechanisms (e.g. respiratory infection, pulmonary embolism, worsening heart failure stage, chronic obstructive pulmonary disease) and to correct it as soon as possible. The administration of any drugs, e.g. for the treatment of bronchospasm—such as theophylline or β-blockers, drugs with an arrhythmogenic effect—should be approached with caution. By reducing cAMP in myocardial cells, theophylline can cause delayed after-depolarizations [60]. β-Agonists can also cause disturbances and for that reason their administration should be reduced or stopped. Direct current cardioversion may not be effective for the conversion of atrial fibrillation to sinus rhythm when there is a severe respiratory disturbance, but it should be attempted in cases of haemodynamic instability. β-Blockers, sotalol, propafenone, and adenosine are contraindicated in the presence of bronchospasm. Control of the ventricular rate in atrial fibrillation may be achieved by the administration of verapamil or diltiazem, while digitalis is no more effective than nondihydropyridines.

The guidelines for the treatment of atrial fibrillation in patients with respiratory disorders are summarized in 📷54.1 [2].

Supraventricular arrhythmias in patients with intravascular devices or catheters

In many patients who are treated in the ICU, intravascular or endocardial devices may be inserted, either to assist the pump function of the heart (intra-aortic balloon pump counterpulsation), or to prevent bradycardic complications (temporary pacemaker), or to make measurements related to the patient's haemodynamic condition (Swan–Ganz pulmonary artery catheter). The role of these devices in causing cardiac arrhythmias and the possible effects arrhythmias may have on their function are discussed below.

Intra-aortic balloon pump counterpulsation

The intra-aortic balloon pump (IABP) is the most widely used method for mechanical support of the circulation [61]. The IABP uses a specific triggering mechanism for inflation and deflation of the balloon. The most commonly used triggers are the ECG waveform and the systemic arterial pressure waveform [61]. Poor ECG quality or electrical interference can affect the functioning of the device and reduce the support it provides to the patient. The same can happen if the patient develops an arrhythmia, such as multiple atrial or ventricular extrasystoles, or atrial fibrillation. Premature IABP inflation impairs left ventricular ejection and relaxation through an increase in afterload, and leads to mechanical dyssynchrony during the second part of the ejection phase. Thus, premature IABP inflation, as may occur during arrhythmia, can adversely affect the cardiac performance of patients who suffer from heart failure. A delay in IABP deflation increases stroke volume and stroke work by increasing afterload during early ejection and decreasing it in late ejection [62].

Temporary pacing

From one series of patients who underwent temporary pacing it was reported that complications could arise in relation to the venous access, mechanical interactions of the lead with the heart, the electrical performance of the pacemaker lead, infection, or thromboembolism caused by the presence of a foreign body. The rate of these complications is around 14–20% and in the majority of patients they will be manifested as development of a pericardial rub, ventricular arrhythmias produced during electrode positioning, or infection. No episodes of persistent atrial arrhythmias have been recorded [63].

Pulmonary artery catheter

Recently published clinical trials in patients with pulmonary catheters reported complication rates of 10% and 5%. The most common complications in the PAC-Man trial were site haematoma (4%), arterial puncture (3%), and

arrhythmias needing treatment (3%, with one cardiac arrest). In the ESCAPE trial, catheter-related infections occurred in 2.5% of cases, catheter knotting and pulmonary infarction or haemorrhage each in 1%, and ventricular arrhythmia in 0.5%. None of the complications in either study led to death [64, 65]. These studies did not report any cases of persistent atrial arrhythmias. Seguin *et al.*, in a study of 460 patients in a surgical ICU, reported that atrial fibrillation was more common in patients who had a central venous catheter or a pulmonary artery catheter. The latter catheter was an independent risk factor for atrial fibrillation. The authors hypothesized that contact between the catheter and the cardiac cavities over several days could induce atrial fibrillation through mechanical irritation of the atrium [66].

Conclusion

Atrial fibrillation and supraventricular arrhythmias present as common complications during the hospitalization of the critically ill. Their effect on morbidity and mortality depends directly on the functional and structural substrate of every individual patient. In the majority of cases they are the result of reversible causes, such as myocardial ischemia, inflammation, metabolic and electrolyte disturbances. Moreover, the prevalence and incidence of atrial fibrillation and supraventricular arrhythmias in hospitalized patients continues to rise due to population aging and an increase in the numbers of invasive procedures being performed. It is therefore vital that attending physicians pay constant attention to ensure arrhythmias are prevented or treated properly, according to existing international guidelines, so as to decrease the rate of further complications and improve short- and long-term prognosis.

Personal perspective

Critically ill patients make up a population that is at high risk for the development of arrhythmias. Supraventricular arrhythmias, and atrial fibrillation in particular, are seen at an ever-increasing rate in these patients, mainly as a result of the growing number of elderly patients and the longer survival of those with severe disease. However, research in this field still has a long way to go. The possible correlation between the occurrence of atrial fibrillation and the genetic substrate in a given patient, in

combination with further elucidation of the triggering factors for the arrhythmia under stress conditions, holds out attractive prospects for the development of strategies for both primary and secondary prevention. In addition, there must be an intensification of efforts to develop new drugs with more capabilities for the inhibition of arrhythmogenesis, without an increase in adverse effects. We believe that the future will bring us effective tools for combating supraventricular arrhythmias, and especially atrial fibrillation, on a platform of evidence-based and individualized medicine.

Further reading

Fuster V, Ryden LE, Cannom DS, *et al.* ACC/AHA/ESC 2006 guidelines for the management of patients with atrial fibrillation: full text: A report of the American College of Cardiology/American Heart Association Task Force on practice guidelines and the European Society of Cardiology Committee for Practice Guidelines (Writing Committee to Revise the 2001 Guidelines for the Management of Patients With Atrial Fibrillation) Developed in collaboration with the European Heart Rhythm Association and the Heart Rhythm Society. *Europace* 2006;**8**:651–745.

Kober L, Swedberg K, McMurray JJ, *et al.* Previously known and newly diagnosed atrial fibrillation: a major risk indicator after a myocardial infarction complicated by heart failure or left ventricular dysfunction. *Eur J Heart Fail* 2006;**8**:591–598.

Van de Werf F, Bax J, Betriu A, *et al.* Management of acute myocardial infarction in patients presenting with persistent ST-segment elevation: the Task Force on the Management of ST-Segment Elevation Acute Myocardial Infarction of the European Society of Cardiology. *Eur Heart J.* 2008;**29**:2909–2945.

Goodman S, Weiss Y, Weissman C. Update on cardiac arrhythmias in the ICU. *Curr Opin Crit Care* 2008;**14**:549–554.

Walsh SR, Tang T, Wijewardena C. Postoperative arrhythmias in general surgical patients. *Ann R Coll Surg Engl* 2007;**89**:91–95.

Crystal E, Garfinkle MS, Connolly SS, *et al.* Interventions for preventing postoperative atrial fibrillation in patients undergoing heart surgery. *Cohrane Database Syst Rev* 2004;CD003611.

Schreuder JJ, Maisano F, Donelli A. Beat-to-Beat Effects of Intraaortic Balloon Pump Timing on Left VentricularPerformance in Patients With Low Ejection Fraction. *Ann Thorac Surg* 2005;**79**:872–880.

Binanay C, Califf RM, Hasselblad V, *et al.* ESCAPE Investigators and ESCAPE Study Coordinators: Evaluation study of congestive heart failure and pulmonary artery catheterization effectiveness. *JAMA* 2005;**294**:1625–1633.

Additional online material

54.1 Atrial fibrillation: ACC/AHA/ESC guidelines

⊃ For additional multimedia materials please visit the online version of the book (✆ http://www.esciacc.oxfordmedicine.com).

CHAPTER 55

Ventricular tachyarrhythmias and implantable cardioverter/ defibrillator

Joachim R. Ehrlich and Stefan H. Hohnloser

Contents

Summary

Few scenarios in intensive coronary care are commonly associated with as much fear and apprehension as the event of a ventricular tachyarrhythmia. This chapter provides helpful information for the successful management of such situations. Residents, fellows, and physicians involved in providing acute cardiac care need broad background knowledge of diagnostic and therapeutic methods as well as prognostic implications of such events in order to provide adequate medical care to their patients.

The present chapter summarizes information on the pathophysiological basis of ventricular tachyarrhythmias and ways of detecting and correctly differentiating ventricular from supraventricular arrhythmia on the surface ECG. The chapter provides the reader with a summary of specific treatment modalities and information on indications for treatment with an implantable cardioverter/defibrillator.

Lastly, the chapter deals with the management of device interventions (appropriately delivered for ventricular tachyarrhythmias or inappropriately delivered for other reasons) within the increasing population of patients fitted with an implantable cardioverter/defibrillator.

Introduction

Ventricular tachyarrhythmias are common and important complications among patients hospitalized in intensive coronary care units (ICCU). There is significant variability in aetiology and clinical presentations and correct diagnosis is therefore always pivotal to guide optimal therapy. Classification of the type of arrhythmia represents the *sine qua non* for adequate acute treatment and for long-term management of affected patients. As a general rule, ventricular tachyarrhythmias need to be viewed separately from their haemodynamic consequences (i.e. haemodynamic instability is not a criterion for the presence of ventricular tachycardia). Perhaps the most important prerequisite for further correct management of patients with ventricular tachyarrhythmias is the documentation of the presenting arrhythmia in a 12-lead surface ECG whenever possible. Whenever this is not feasible because of the need for immediate emergency treatment, documentation of the arrhythmia (a printout from the monitor) is mandatory. Failure to document the arrhythmia holds up other physicians in verifying the diagnosis and may prolong the time to adequate treatment.

Pathophysiology of ventricular tachyarrhythmias

Ventricular tachyarrhythmias can occur in a continuous spectrum from unsustained to sustained arrhythmias. Sustained ventricular tachyarrhythmia (VT) is defined as VT lasting longer than 30 s or needing immediate termination (i.e. electrical cardioversion) because of haemodynamic compromise. VT can occur as a haemodynamically stable episode or as an unstable emergency leading to cardiac arrest and death. The most important determinant of clinical consequences of VT is the type and the degree of underlying structural heart disease.

Structurally normal hearts

Several types of VTs originate from otherwise healthy myocardium—so-called idiopathic VTs—and there is considerable heterogeneity among this group. Careful analysis of the ECG allows classification of most types of idiopathic VT. Invasive electrophysiological studies including pharmacological testing (i.e. assessment of sensitivity of the VT to adenosine or verapamil administration [1, 2]) may further elucidate the underlying mechanisms of the rhythm disturbance and allow differentiation between the different types of idiopathic VTs.

The most common forms of idiopathic VTs originate from the ventricular outflow tracts with the most common origin being from the right-sided outflow tract (RVOT) (➔ Fig. 55.1A, B). RVOT VT typically shows left bundle branch block configuration in the precordial leads and an inferior axis in the limb leads. In some cases the origin of VT may be located in the left ventricular outflow tract (LVOT), so-called idiopathic left ventricular tachycardia (ILVT) [3]. ILVT typically shows right bundle branch block with left axis deviation, often with relatively narrow QRS complexes. R-wave pattern in lead V_1 is important for differentiating various origins of outflow tract VT. V_1 is a right-sided and anterior lead and accordingly RVOT originating close to this electrode will have a negative deflection as the propagation waves travels away from the electrode. If an R-wave is present in V_1, together with rapid R/S transition, this may rather suggest LVOT. Patients with such arrhythmias typically present repetitive monomorphic premature beats in the surface ECG and arrhythmias are often induced by physical exercise (➔ Fig. 55.1C) [4]. The prognosis of RVOT tachycardia (in the absence of structural heart disease) is usually excellent and catheter ablation is the treatment of choice. However, early forms of arrhythmogenic right ventricular dysplasia may present with RVOT type tachycardia and accordingly carry a less benign prognosis [5]. In such cases, arrhythmias may trigger polymorphic VT or ventricular fibrillation (VF), subsequently leading to sudden cardiac death. Malignant forms of RVOT VT are more frequently polymorphic, have shorter cycle length, and patients have more often reported malignant syncope. Radiofrequency ablation may be effective in patients with both types of arrhythmias, but an implantable cardioverter/defibrillator (ICD) is always indicated in patients with documented VF or aborted sudden death. The underlying cellular substrate of idiopathic VTs is generally based on triggered activity mediated through (catecholamine-sensitive) delayed afterdepolarizations [4]. Accordingly, idiopathic VTs are often sensitive to β-blockade or calcium channel blocker therapy. This effect is mediated through a reduction of intracellular calcium. Adenosine works in a mechanistically similar fashion, terminating arrhythmias that are cAMP-dependent through modulation of adenosine receptors that in turn reduce intracellular levels of cAMP [6].

Genetically determined arrhythmias such as the long or the short QT syndrome, Brugada syndrome, or catecholaminergic polymorphic ventricular tachycardia each have a specific pathophysiological basis often represented by abnormalities in ion channel function/expression or changes in intracellular proteins involved in trafficking or calcium handling. All of these syndromes are associated with an increased risk of malignant VTs and cardiac arrest. The QT and Brugada syndromes are characterized by specific changes in the resting ECG. Long QT syndrome may be suspected if QTc intervals exceed 450 ms in men or 470 ms in women [7]. Short QT syndrome may be suspected if QTc is shorter than 330 ms [8]. Characteristic ECG findings similarly lead to the diagnosis in Brugada syndrome and may be present either spontaneously or during febrile illness or after exposure to specific drugs. This syndrome was originally described as a syndrome of right bundle branch block and ST-segment elevation in the

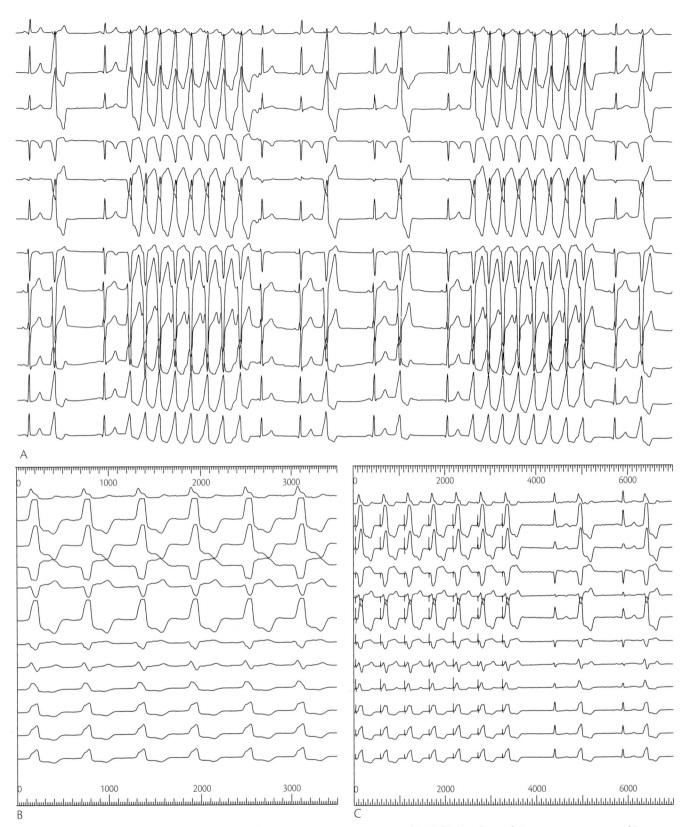

Figure 55.1 Panel A shows the typical repetitive type of spontaneous, incessant monomorphic VT (Galaverdin type). Spontaneous monomorphic ventricular tachycardia (shown at high resolution in B) has the same morphology as paced beats (in C) confirming the focal site of origin of the tachycardia. C illustrates catheter-based pace-mapping with the ablation catheter localized in the right ventricular outflow tract. Paper speed for ECGs is 25 mm/s in panels A and C, 100 mm/s in B; voltage scale is 1 mV/cm.

right precordial leads [9]. Two types of spontaneous ECGs ('coved type' and 'saddleback type') can be differentiated in Brugada syndrome representing so-called type 1 and type 2 ECG patterns, respectively [10] (➲Fig. 55.2A–C). While saddleback type ECG (type 2) may be transformed to the diagnostic coved type ECG (type 1) with application of class I antiarrhythmic agents (ajmaline, flecainide, procainamide), the development of a type 1 ECG always carries prognostic implications for patients [11]. Re-entry due to shortened repolarization or dispersion of action potential duration plays a role for arrhythmogenesis in short QT and Brugada syndrome, and conduction slowing within the ventricular wall has been observed in Brugada syndrome [8, 12]. In contrast, triggered activity contributes to arrhythmias in long QT syndrome (early after-depolarizations) and catecholaminergic polymorphic VT

(delayed after-depolarizations) [13, 14]. In long QT syndrome the prolonged cardiac repolarization period allows reopening of inactivated calcium channels that carry positive charge into the cells triggering repetitive depolarizations. Catecholaminergic polymorphic VT is often caused by mutations in ryanodine receptors which physiologically mediate calcium release from the sarcoplasmic reticulum and thus lead to delayed after-depolarizations. We refer the interested reader to respective detailed review articles as an in-depth discussion of these syndromes is beyond the scope of this chapter.

Cardiomyopathies

Dilated cardiomyopathy (DCM) can give rise to all types of VTs. Clinically, DCM is characterized by biventricular

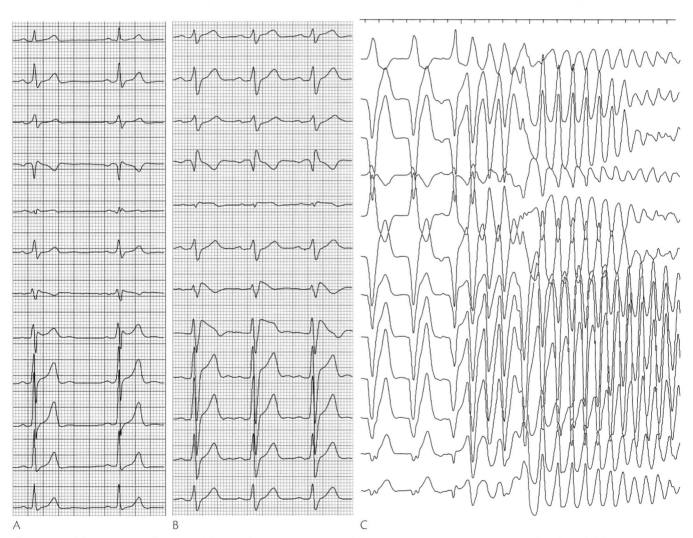

Figure 55.2 (A) Resting ECG of a 36-year-old man with status post syncope demonstrating type 2 Brugada ECG pattern (saddleback). (B) The ECG after intravenous administration of ajmaline (1 mg/kg) in the same patient; the drug reveals a type 1 Brugada ECG pattern (coved type). (C) ECG recordings during an electrophysiological study illustrating the inducibility of a polymorphic VT degenerating into VF in this patient, who received an ICD. Paper speed is 25 mm/s, voltage scale 1 mV/cm for all ECG tracings.

enlargement and impaired systolic function with diverse underlying aetiologies such as myocarditis, valvular heart disease, hypertension, or metabolic/toxic aetiologies (such as chronic alcohol consumption). In few cases, DCM may present as a heritable disorder [15]. Multiple factors (such as chamber enlargement with elevated wall-stretch or intraventricular fibrosis) contribute to the arrhythmia substrate in this setting. Importantly, there is diffuse intramyocardial scarring owing to replacement fibrosis in DCM and such areas may act as sources for re-entry [16]. Besides nonspecific arrhythmias, bundle branch re-entry tachycardia is a characteristic arrhythmia in DCM that deserves special mention. (◗ Fig. 55.3A, B). The VT usually is very rapid and shows relatively narrow QRS complexes and patients typically present with syncope. Bundle branch re-entry VT is based on a macro-reentrant circuit within the Purkinje system, often with antegrade conduction through the right fascicle and retrograde conduction through the left. It is important to recognize this type of arrhythmia, as ablation of the right bundle branch is curative in this setting.

Heritable diseases such as hypertrophic or arrhythmogenic right ventricular cardiomyopathy are other important substrates of VTs in particular among younger patients [17–19]. There are regional variations in the prevalence of these diseases. Studies in the United States identified a high percentage of hypertrophic cardiomyopathy among young patients and athletes with aborted sudden cardiac death [20]. VT may be the initial presentation of these patients. In contrast, arrhythmogenic right ventricular cardiomyopathy is common in previously unaffected young individuals in Italy [17]. This disease entity is characterized by progressive structural alterations involving cell coupling proteins of the right ventricle leading to right-sided heart failure and arrhythmogenesis. It is important to recognize heritable disease entities, as affected patients are typically young and otherwise healthy.

Coronary artery disease

VT or VF most often occurs in patients with coronary artery disease (CAD) or an old myocardial infarct (MI). CAD has the most likely pathological substrate, consisting of scar tissue, and represents the most frequent cause of VTs. Up to three-quarters of patients who died from sudden cardiac death have underlying CAD [21]. Sustained monomorphic VT typically arises from electrical activity of surviving cells within the border zone of extensive healed infarcts. Slow impulse propagation and unidirectional conduction block within these areas are prerequisites for the occurrence of reentrant arrhythmias in this clinical setting. The extent of myocardial scarring, involvement of septal sites, and presence of left ventricular dysfunction are major determinants of VT occurrence [22]. With the advent of improved cardiac care through optimized rapid coronary revascularization, the incidence of VT after MI has declined from approximately 3% to 1% of affected patients [22].

Types of ventricular tachyarrhythmias

Accelerated idioventricular rhythm

Accelerated idioventricular rhythm (AIVR) is defined as a ventricular rhythm with a rate between 50 and 120 beats/min (◗ Fig. 55.4A,B). It is caused by enhanced automaticity and has a benign short-term prognosis. AIVR is usually not associated with haemodynamic compromise because of its relatively slow rate. The occurrence of AIVR after initiation of reperfusion therapy has been considered a marker of successful reperfusion in patients with ST-segment elevation myocardial infarction (STEMI) treated with fibrinolysis. This notion apparently does not hold true for patients undergoing primary percutaneous interventions (PCI). In this setting, AIVR was associated with longer time to normalization of ST segments and larger overall infarct size; however, as an arrhythmia *per se* it does not warrant specific treatment [23].

Ventricular tachycardia

VT is defined as a wide complex (QRS >120 ms) tachycardia (heart rate >100 beats/min) originating from the ventricles. Symptoms occurring during VT depend on ventricular rate and duration of the arrhythmia as well as the extent of underlying cardiovascular disease. Rapid VT may lead to loss of consciousness, as short diastolic filling time is insufficient to sustain adequate cardiac output, and eventually it may degenerate into VF. If the ventricular rate of VT is very fast (>250 beats/min) this has been previously termed 'ventricular flutter'. However, this classification should be avoided as it does not provide any additional information [24]. QRS morphology during the VT may be constant (i.e. monomorphic—cf. ◗ Figs 55.1, 55.3, 55.6]) or may morphologically vary in a repetitive manner (polymorphic, e.g. torsade de pointes, ◗ Fig. 55.5). Torsade de pointes tachycardia is defined as a specific form of polymorphic VT undulating QRS axis ('twisting of the pointes') in the presence of baseline QT prolongation. It is important to note this specific entity, as therapy diverges from the general management of VT (see below).

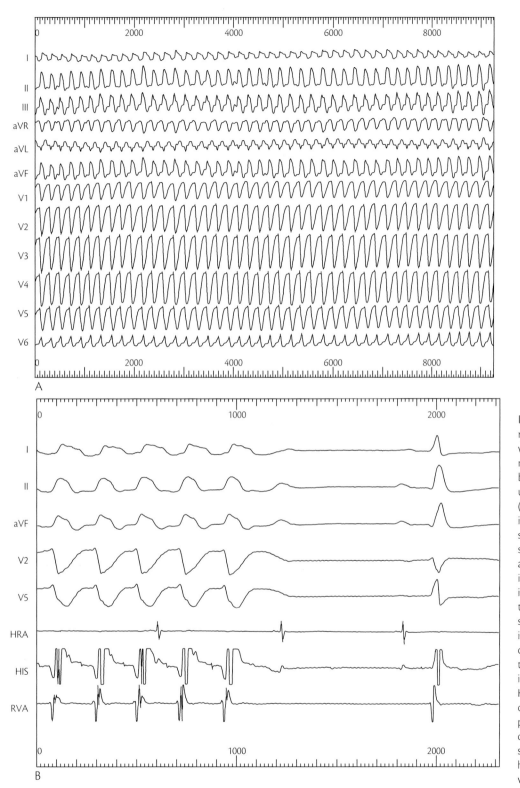

Figure 55.3 (A) Bundle branch re-entry ventricular tachycardia with a rapid rate (*c.*280 beats/min) and a left bundle branch block configuration with a sharp upstroke of the QRS complex (paper speed 25 mm/s). The intracardiac electrograms (paper speed 100 mm/s) illustrate several important features of this arrhythmia: clear A-V dissociation is visible comparing activation in high right atrium to that in the right ventricular apex or the surface ECG; prolongation of H-H interval proceeds prolongation of the R-R interval prior to VT termination. In sinus rhythm, there is borderline prolongation of the H-V interval (*c.*60 ms). This type of arrhythmia typically occurs in patients with some form and signs of intraventricular conduction slowing. HIS, bundle of His; HRA, high right atrium; RVA, right ventricular apex.

Ventricular fibrillation

During VF, the surface ECG shows no discernible QRS complexes but undulating fibrillation waves of varying form and amplitude. VF is the final common pathway of cardiac substrate depletion during sustained VTs and represents the most important cause of sudden cardiac death. VF results in loss of consciousness within a few seconds, due to cerebral hypoperfusion.

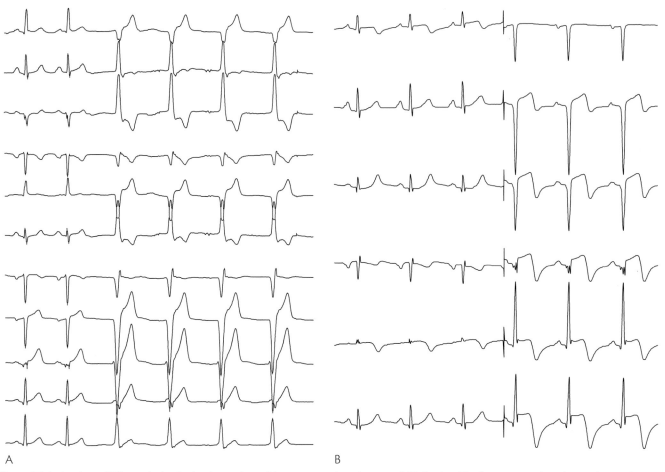

A   B

Figure 55.4 Accelerated idioventricular rhythm in a patient with acute anterolateral myocardial infarction. The first two complexes in panel A are sinus beats then overtaken by an accelerated idioventricular rhythm. Panel B illustrates the ECG changes following percutaneous coronary intervention in the same patient. Paper speed is 25 mm/s, voltage scale 1 mV/cm.

The mechanisms of arrhythmia and their therapeutic implications are summarized in ➲ Table 55.1.

ECG diagnosis of ventricular tachycardia

Various criteria and algorithms have been proposed to diagnose VT from the surface ECG. Many are not helpful to the physician in day-to-day practice, and substantial uncertainty remains. Beyond ECG findings, haemodynamic stability is often considered an argument against the presence of VT and in favour of the presence of supraventricular tachycardia with aberration or pre-existing bundle branch block [25]. However, this assumption is erroneous and may lead to contraindicated use of verapamil to slow ventricular response rate (in a presumed supraventricular tachycardia), with deleterious haemodynamic consequences [26].

When describing VTs it is important to use consistent terminology: 'wide complex tachycardia' describes any rhythm with QRS duration of 120 ms or more and a rate of 100 beats/min or more. Wide QRS complex tachycardia may be regular or irregular. VT is a wide complex tachycardia that originates from below the level of the bundle of His and does not include supraventricular structures. For assessment of wide complex tachycardia, all 12 leads of the surface ECG must be analysed. A firm diagnosis of VT can be made if atrioventricular (AV) dissociation is visible (➲ Fig. 55.6A) or fusion and capture beats can be identified (➲ Fig. 55.6B). Fusion beats indicate that the ventricles are activated from two different sites: one ventricular and one supraventricular. Atrial activity can be 1:1 with ventricular activation in the case of retrograde VA conduction (present in *c*.25% of all VTs). Several other rules may help to diagnose VT in the ECG. However, none of these are specific for the presence of VT. If QRS duration is greater than 140 ms the diagnosis of VT is very likely, as supraventricular tachycardia rarely has such prolonged QRS complexes [27]. Furthermore, the QRS axis may provide a hint. If the QRS axis points to the right upper quadrant of the Cabrera

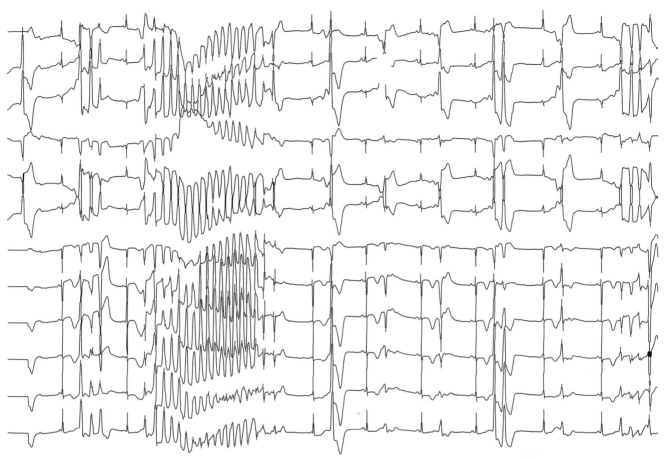

Figure 55.5 Repetitive polymorphic ventricular ectopic beats and onset of polymorphic VT (torsade de pointes) in a patient treated with sotalol for atrial fibrillation. There is prominent baseline QT prolongation (QTc >500 ms). Of note, ectopic beats occur during the QT interval, probably related to early after-depolarizations. This tracing represents a typical example of drug-induced acquired long QT syndrome. Paper speed 12.5 mm/s, voltage scale 1 mV/cm.

circle ('the North-West territory', 'no man's land'), the diagnosis again is most likely VT. If the arrhythmia can be modulated by vagal manoeuvres it may be more likely to be supraventricular in nature. If the wide complex tachycardia is due to supraventricular tachycardia with aberration or pre-existing bundle branch block, typically some form of fascicular block is present, and if no such morphology is observed the diagnosis is rather VT. However, none of these criteria are proof of VT.

Specific ECG algorithms have been proposed for the diagnosis of VT, and two warrant special mention [28, 29] (➲ Fig. 55.7A, B). The classical algorithm proposed

Table 55.1 Arrhythmia mechanisms and therapeutic implications

Arrhythmia	Mechanism	Heart disease	ECG findings	Acute therapy	Long-term management
AIVR	Automaticity	Acute MI	HR <100 beats/min, broad complexes	None	None
VT	Re-entry	Mostly CAD, DCM	Monomorphic	IV ajmaline, DC cardioversion	ICD, ablation, AAD
RVOT	Automaticity	None	Inferior axis LBBB	Adenosine, verapamil, ajmaline	Ablation
ILVT	Automaticity	None	Superior axis RBBB	Verapamil	Ablation
Torsade de pointes	Automaticity and re-entry	Congenital or drug-induced LQTS	Polymorphic	Discontinue precipitating drugs, Mg^{2+}, K^+	ICD, β-blocker
VF	Multiple re-entry	Mostly CAD, DCM	Polymorphic	Defibrillation	ICD, ablation

AAD, antiarrhythmic drug treatment; AIVR, accelerated idioventricular rhythm; CAD, coronary artery disease; DC, direct current; DCM, dilated cardiomyopathy; HR, heart rate; ILVT, idiopathic left ventricular tachycardia; ICD, implantable cardioverter/defibrillator; LBBB, left bundle branch block; RBBB, right bundle branch block; RVOT, right ventricular outflow tract; LQTS, long QT syndrome.

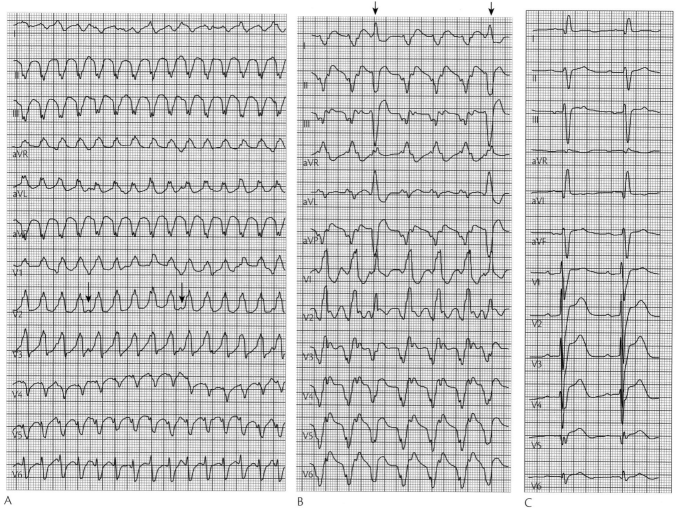

A   B   C

Figure 55.6 ECG features of VT diagnosis. Panel A illustrates the presence of AV dissociation. P-waves can be seen in leads V_2/V_3 (arrows) This VT has broad right bundle branch block morphology and a superior QRS axis ('no man's land') further suggestive of VT. Panel B illustrates fusion beats (arrows) during sustained monomorphic VT. C shows a recording from the same patient and illustrates QRS morphology during sinus rhythm for comparison of QRS axis and morphology during VT. Paper speed is 25 mm/s, voltage scale 1 mV/cm for all ECGs.

by Brugada *et al.* applied the following four criteria: (1) absence of an RS complex in all precordial leads; (2) when an RS complex is present, an RS interval of more than 100 ms is highly specific for VT (3), presence of AV dissociation, and (4) morphology criteria in leads V_1, V_2, and V_6 are examined (➲ Table 55.2). If any of these is present, the diagnosis of VT is made. However, these criteria have been established only for VT in the context of CAD [28]. A rapid downslope to the nadir of the S wave in V_1 and V_2 or a triphasic QRS morphology in V_6 hint at supraventricular tachycardia with aberration (➲ Fig. 55.7C). In contrast, a slow, possibly notched downslope in V_1 and V_2 and any Q-wave in V_6 is suggestive of VT.

In the Vereckei *et al.* algorithm the following criteria were included: (1) the presence of AV dissociation—a definite criterion for the presence of VT; (2) the presence of an initial R wave in lead aVR suggests VT; (3) whether the morphology of the wide complex tachycardia corresponds to a typical bundle branch or fascicular block pattern, which would suggest supraventricular tachycardia; and (4) estimation of initial (v_i) and terminal (v_t) ventricular activation velocity ratio (v_i/v_t) by measuring the voltage change on the ECG tracing during the initial 40 ms (v_i) and the terminal 40 ms (v_t) of the one QRS complex. A v_i/v_t ratio greater than 1 was associated with the presence of supraventricular tachycardia and a ratio of 1 or less was suggestive of VT [29].

An important ECG differential diagnosis of regular wide complex tachycardia is atrial flutter with 1:1 conduction in the presence of bundle branch block (➲ Fig. 55.8). Since in untreated patients, atrial flutter is usually conducted in a 2:1 fashion to the ventricles, the ventricular rate is most often between 150 and 180 beats/min. Careful inspection of the ECG is of utmost importance to detect the arrhythmia. Simple vagal manoeuvres or the administration

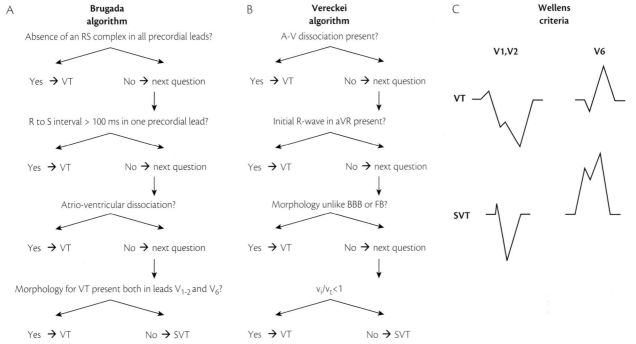

Figure 55.7 Algorithms for systematic approach to ECG diagnosis of VT: (A) Decision tree of the Brugada algorithm (morphology criteria in ➡ Table 55.2). (B) The Vereckei algorithm, for comparison. (C) Schematic of Wellens morphology criteria for supraventricular tachycardia (SVT) relative to VT. A slow, possibly notched downslope to the nadir of S (V1, V2) as well as any Q in V$_6$ are suggestive of VT. SVT is often characterized by a narrow R wave and a rapid downslope in V1, V2 or triphasic QRS in V6..

of adenosine (12–18 mg IV) may help to unmask these flutter waves. The second important differential diagnosis of irregular wide QRS complex tachycardia concerns the presence of an arrhythmia which is antegradely conducted via an accessory pathway. Specifically if the tachycardia is irregular in rate (so-called 'FBI' tachycardia: 'fast, broad, irregular') and presents in a young otherwise healthy individual, presence of atrial fibrillation in the setting of a Wolff–Parkinson–White (WPW) syndrome should be considered (➡ Fig. 55.9).

Ventricular tachycardia/ ventricular fibrillation: therapy

Acute therapy of monomorphic/ polymorphic ventricular tachycardia

➡ Figure 55.10 illustrates a schematic approach to patients with wide complex tachycardia. If the patient is clinically stable, a 12-lead ECG of the arrhythmia should always be obtained first and analysed as with the default mechanism, the assumption being that there is VT. After acute management, patient characteristics, ECG findings, and initial therapy should be discussed with an electrophysiologist to choose optimal long-term therapy [24].

If the diagnosis of VT has been established in a haemodynamically stable patient, pharmacological conversion of the arrhythmia may be attempted by intravenous administration of a single antiarrhythmic drug. For instance, ajmaline (a class IA drug) may be given at a dose of 1 mg/kg. However, this agent should not be used in patients who have been on chronic therapy with amiodarone; in such cases, massive QRS widening with the occurrence of incessant VT has been described. If VT recurs soon after cardioversion, continuous intravenous antiarrhythmic drug therapy should be initiated at least until sinus rhythm can be stabilized. In most instances, intravenous amiodarone administration is started via a central venous access. A single bolus of 200 mg amiodarone is infused over 30 min, followed by 1200 mg over 24 h. This dose can be maintained for several days, or until the patient has received a cumulative dose of approximately 10–12 g. At this point, therapy can usually be switched to oral drug administration.

Table 55.2 QRS morphology suggestive of VT

Tachycardia with RBBB-like QRS	Tachycardia with LBBB-like QRS
Lead V$_1$: monophasic R, QR or RS	Lead V$_1$ or V$_2$: R >30 ms, >60 ms to nadir S, notched S
Lead V$_6$: R/S <1, QR or QS, monophasic R	Lead V$_6$: QR or QS

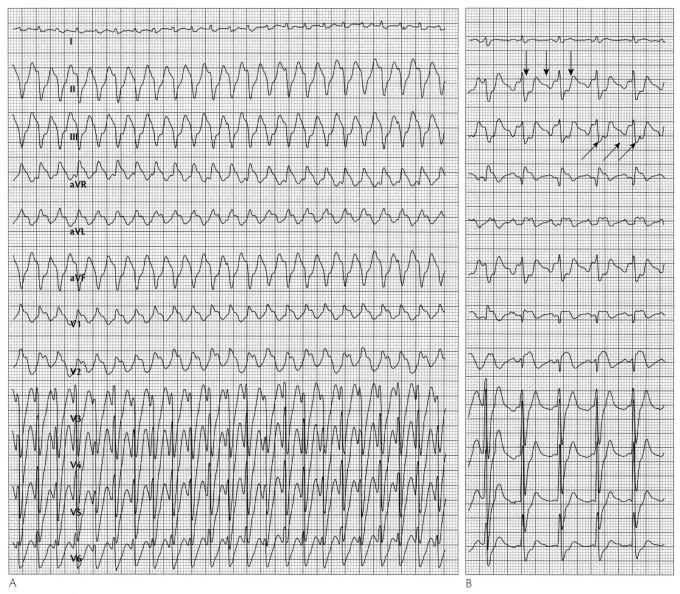

Figure 55.8 (A) Wide complex tachycardia caused by atrial flutter with 1:1 AV conduction in a patient treated with class IC antiarrhythmic drugs for paroxysmal atrial fibrillation. With carotid sinus massage, slowing of the AV conduction occurs unmasking the atrial flutter (B, arrows indicating flutter waves).

If monomorphic VT results in hypotension, loss of consciousness, angina, or heart failure, immediate R-wave triggered electrical cardioversion (≥100 J) is performed with mild sedation. Continuous documentation (by ECG, or at least rhythm strip) of the cardioversion is mandatory. Unstable polymorphic VT is treated as VF using defibrillation. Synchronized cardioversion is generally not recommended to treat unstable polymorphic VT because of unreliable synchronization to QRS complexes. If there is any doubt whether monomorphic or polymorphic VT is present in unstable patients, defibrillation should be applied

and should not be delayed for rhythm analysis. The initial recommended shock energy with a biphasic defibrillator is 150–200 J and an equal or higher dose is recommended for second and subsequent shocks [30]. If a monophasic defibrillator is used, 360 J is recommended for all shocks. After shock delivery, physicians should be prepared to provide measures according to advanced cardiac life support algorithms if necessary [31].

In polymorphic VT, underlying baseline prolongation of the QT interval may be present, which of course is a contraindication to repolarization-prolonging drugs such

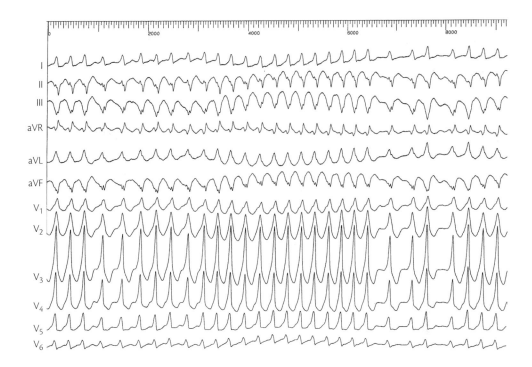

Figure 55.9 Irregular wide complex tachycardia due to antegrade conduction via a left-sided postero-lateral accessory pathway in a young patient: 'fast, broad, irregular' (FBI) ECG. Paper speed is 25 mm/s, voltage scale is 1 mV/cm.

as amiodarone or sotalol. In this case normalization of electrolytes (supplemental IV potassium to a high normal level) and application of intravenous magnesium should be considered until the QT interval is below 500 ms (2 g magnesium sulphate within 15 min, followed by continuous infusion of 2 g within 1 h and use of 2 g magnesium sulphate within 24 h) [32]. Besides defibrillation, pharmacological measures (isoproterenol infusion, initially at a rate of 2 µg/kg/min with subsequent titration to patient response (2–10 µg/kg/min)) or temporary transvenous pacing should be initiated in order to raise the heart rate if the patient has bradycardia, which is often a precipitating factor for polymorphic VT. Administration of isoproterenol should be avoided if there is a suspicion of CAD.

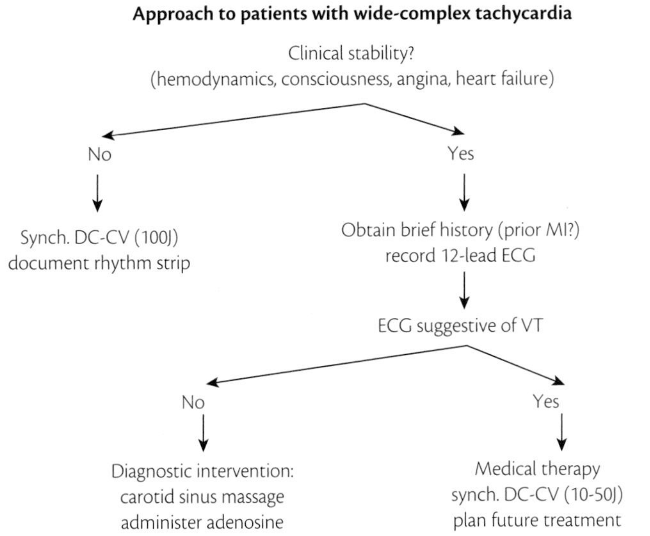

Acute therapy of ventricular fibrillation

VF-induced cardiac arrest mandates immediate cardiopulmonary resuscitation aiming at restoration of spontaneous circulation [31]. If cardiac arrest is witnessed, it is adequate to treat directly with electrical defibrillation. A precordial thumb may be attempted if the onset of VF has been witnessed [33]. If VF has been present for an unknown period of time (in case of resuscitation of a person with an unwitnessed cardiac arrest) the delivery of chest compressions and mask ventilation for a period of approximately 5 minutes before defibrillation are encouraged. This relates to significant substrate deprivation within the heart during VF, and chances of returning spontaneous circulation are much greater with a previous set of basic life support [34]. In case of refractory VF amiodarone is typically applied during resuscitation. It is the safest and most effective agent in the setting of structural heart disease and has replaced most other compounds for medical management of unstable VT/VF [35–37]. Long-term therapy with an ICD is usually indicated in survivors of VF cardiac arrest (see next section).

Approach to patients with wide-complex tachycardia

Clinical stability?
(hemodynamics, consciousness, angina, heart failure)

No → Synch. DC-CV (100J) document rhythm strip

Yes → Obtain brief history (prior MI?) record 12-lead ECG

ECG suggestive of VT

No → Diagnostic intervention: carotid sinus massage administer adenosine

Yes → Medical therapy synch. DC-CV (10-50J) plan future treatment

Figure 55.10 Practical approach to patients with sustained wide complex tachycardia. DC-CV, direct current electrical cardioversion; MI, myocardial infarction; VT, ventricular tachycardia.

Long-term treatment of patients with ventricular tachycardia/ventricular fibrillation

Subacute management of the patient presenting with VT or VF involves treatment of the underlying disease as well as specific antiarrhythmic treatment. In all patients with known CAD or signs of acute coronary syndromes, coronary angiography is mandatory to optimize revascularization where needed. Left ventricular function needs to be optimized as well, particularly when signs of congestive heart failure are present. Other arrhythmia-precipitating factors such as electrolyte imbalances or therapy with potentially proarrhythmic medications need to be carefully corrected. Once these general treatment rules are considered and therapy with respect to this is optimized, specific considerations concerning further arrhythmia therapy must be made.

Implantable cardioverter/defibrillator treatment

The development of the ICD has revolutionized the treatment of patients with life-threatening VTs. Indications for ICD treatment are divided in primary and secondary prevention of sudden cardiac death, the latter being defined as prevention of VT/VF in patients with previous episodes of VT or VF or survived cardiac arrest (⮞ Table 55.3) [38]. Three randomized controlled trials have shown clear benefit from ICD implantation for secondary sudden death prevention, regardless of the type of underlying structural heart disease. Primary prevention of sudden cardiac death refers to the use of ICDs in patients who are deemed to be at risk for VT/VF but have not yet experienced an event. ICD implantation leads to improved survival in some [39–43], albeit not all [44, 45] selected patient populations studied. ICD treatment should be in accordance with current guidelines and initiated in cooperation with an electrophysiologist [38].

Catheter ablation

Catheter ablation can be applied in the treatment of VT in patients with coronary disease, cardiomyopathy, bundle branch re-entry, and various forms of idiopathic VT [24]. In patients with extensive structural abnormalities, especially those with prior infarction, multiple VT morphologies may be present [46]. Accordingly, ablation of a single VT morphology can reduce the arrhythmia burden but may not eliminate the need for an ICD or pharmacological antiarrhythmic therapy. This approach is of particular value among ICD patients with repetitive VT to reduce the number of device interventions [24].

In patients with so-called idiopathic VF (without evidence of structural or electrical heart disease) arrhythmogenic foci within the Purkinje system have been described and successfully ablated [47]. However, not all catheter-based approaches have been systematically compared to ICD therapy as primary therapy for prevention of recurrence of VTs and risk of sudden death, and may accordingly only be applied as adjunct therapy [30]. For further information we refer the reader to specific review articles.

Pharmacological therapy

β-Blockers reduce the incidence of sudden cardiac death in a spectrum of cardiac disorders. These compounds are safe and effective and should be considered the mainstay of antiarrhythmic drug therapy [48]. Sotalol is effective in suppressing atrial and ventricular arrhythmias. It has been of value to reduce arrhythmia episodes in patients with an ICD to avoid repetitive device therapy ('electrical storm', see next section) [49]. The combination of β-blockers and amiodarone is an alternative approach [50]. Because many affected patients have impaired systolic LV function and poor renal function, amiodarone and β-blockers rather than sotalol should be considered. Sotalol should be avoided in patients with reduced renal function or significant heart failure.

Management of implantable cardioverter/defibrillator patients with device interventions

Appropriate device therapy, electrical storm

There is a high prevalence of patients previously fitted with an ICD being admitted to an ICCU. Whereas single ICD-treated VT/VF episodes in the absence of acute coronary syndromes or exacerbated heart failure do not warrant admission to ICCU, arrhythmia episodes causing complications, predominantly acute heart failure, often lead to admission. In such patients, immediate interrogation of the ICD is mandatory to obtain detailed information on the type of arrhythmia, its morphology and rate, and its rate of recurrence.

Table 55.3 Clinical trials of implantable cardioverter/defibrillator therapy for primary and secondary prevention of sudden cardiac death

Trial	Publication year	Patients (n)	Inclusion criterion LVEF (%)	Other inclusion criteria	HR	95%CI	*p* value
Primary prevention trials							
MADIT I [39]	1996	196	35	NSVT and positive EP	0.46	0.26–0.82	0.009
MADIT II [40]	2002	1232	30	Prior MI	0.69	0.51–0.93	0.016
CABG-Patch [41]	1997	900	36	Positive SAECG and CABG	1.07	0.81–1.42	0.63
DEFINITE [42]	2004	485	35	NICM, PVCs, or NSVT	0.65	0.40–1.06	0.08
DINAMIT [44]	2004	674	35	6–40 d post MI and HRV	1.08	0.76–1.55	0.66
IRIS [45]	2009	898	40	HR >90 beats/min or NSVT	1.04	0.81–1.35	0.78
SCD-HeFT [43]	2005	1676	35	Prior MI or NICM	0.77	0.62–0.96	0.007
Secondary prevention trials							
AVID [57]	1997	1016	n.a.	Prior cardiac arrest, sustained VT, LVEF <40%	0.62	0.43–0.82	<0.02
CASH [58]	2000	288	n.a.	Prior cardiac arrest	0.77	?–1.11[a]	NS
CIDS [59]	2000	659	n.a.	Prior cardiac arrest, sustained VT and syncope, sustained VT and LVEF<35%, unclear syncope and inducible VT at EPS	0.82	0.60–1.10	NS

[a] Only 95% CI upper bound reported (ICD vs antiarrhythmic therapy).

CABG, coronary artery bypass grafting; EP, electrophysiological study; HR, heart rate; HRV, heart rate variability; LVEF, left ventricular ejection fraction; MI, myocardial infarction; n.a., not applicable; NICM, nonischaemic cardiomyopathy; NS, not significant; NSVT, nonsustained ventricular tachycardia; SAECG, signal averaged ECG; VT, ventricular tachycardia.

A particular clinical syndrome in ICD recipients called an 'electrical storm' (ES) represents a medical emergency and must lead to ICCU hospitalization. An ES is usually defined as three or more appropriate VT/VF episodes in 24 h, treated by the device by antitachycardia pacing or shock delivery [51]. Contrary to common belief, ES is a relatively frequent complication affecting up to 25% of ICD patients within the first year after implantation [50]. Patients with LVEF less than 25% and QRS greater than 120 ms are at greater risk for ES [52]. Potential triggers can be identified only in a minority of patients and include worsening of heart failure, changes in antiarrhythmic medication, acute myocardial ischemia, contact with other illnesses, psychological stress, and electrolyte imbalance. In most patients, ES is caused by VT while recurrent VF is less often encountered. Although the acute management of this serious complication is usually successful, the occurrence of ES was found to be an independent predictor of poor outcome in ICD patients in some studies [53].

The key therapeutic intervention in ES is a reduction of elevated sympathetic tone which can be achieved by mild sedation and application of β-blockers. Occasionally, application of an external magnet over the implanted device is necessary to withhold ICD therapy in case of repetitive appropriate (in a stable patient) or inappropriate device action. This intervention stops antitachycardia therapy, leaving the antibradycardia pacing modalities of the device unaffected. Application of intravenous amiodarone has also been successful and azimilide seems promising, while class I antiarrhythmic drugs are not recommended [54]. Substrate mapping and VT ablation may be mandatory during the acute situation if recurrence of VT/VF cannot be suppressed by pharmacological therapy alone. If no experienced electrophysiology laboratory is at hand, patients with otherwise unresponsive ES should be transferred to an institution at which catheter ablation of such patients can be performed.

To reduce the incidence of ES in ICD recipients before such devastating events occur, specific antiarrhythmic drug therapy can be considered. In particular, amiodarone, sotalol and azimilide have been shown in randomized controlled clinical trials to significantly reduce the incidence of ES when given prophylactically [49, 50, 55].

Inappropriate implantable cardioverter/ defibrillator interventions

Inappropriate ICD therapy (i.e. antitachycardia pacing or shock delivery by the device for non-VT/VF reasons) may result from several causes. Most importantly, ICD therapy may be delivered for supraventricular arrhythmias falsely detected as VT by the device. On the other hand, technical problems such as defective lead insulation, fracture, or oversensing of cardiac (T-waves) and extracardiac signals (myopotentials) can lead to erroneous arrhythmia detection by the device and trigger the respective therapy. With optimized programming the rate of inappropriate interventions can be reduced and prevention of inappropriate shocks has important implications for the quality of life of affected patients [56]. Technical problems are systematically looked for at each device interrogation follow-up visit.

Conclusion

Among ICCU patients there is a high prevalence of potentially life-threatening VTs. Adequate detection and correct diagnosis are essential for initiation of proper treatment. Acute termination of any haemodynamically compromising arrhythmia is performed according to current resuscitation guidelines. Unless clinically unstable, all arrhythmias must be documented on 12-lead ECG—a point that cannot be stressed enough—for later consultation of electrophysiology specialists. ECG appearance may be mono- or polymorphic, and ECG signs of VT include presence of AV dissociation and/or fusion/capture beats. VT may occur in a broad spectrum of disease entities from structurally normal hearts to genetically determined arrhythmia syndromes (such as long QT or Brugada syndrome) to VT in ischaemic heart disease, which is the most common underlying cause. Medical management consists of the use of amiodarone or ajmaline in haemodynamically stable patients with sustained VT. In patients presenting with torsade de pointes tachycardia (particularly in case of baseline QT prolongation) repolarization-prolonging antiarrhythmic drugs such as amiodarone are contraindicated and intravenous magnesium should be given. Ultimately, cardioversion under mild sedation is successful in terminating episodes. Subsequently, most patients qualify for implantation of an ICD as a secondary preventive measure unless a clear cut reversible cause (such as acute myocardial infarction) is identified. Specific consideration needs to be given to patients with a preimplanted ICD in the case of appropriate device intervention. ES is present if three or more episodes in 24 h are terminated by the device (antitachycardia pacing or shock delivery). This entity may be managed acutely by sedation and application of β-blockers and/or amiodarone. Inappropriate device interventions are stressful for affected patients and need to be rapidly detected and treated. Application of an external magnet to the ICD pocket interrupts antitachycardia treatments without an effect on antibradycardia pacing, and may be helpful in such situations.

Personal perspective

VTs will continue to represent an important clinical entity complicating almost all forms of cardiac diseases. Treatment options will be further refined, particularly in the area of ablative therapy. Furthermore, ICD technology will also continuously be improved and its clinical use is likely to increase. Thus, ICU physicians will have to deal with such patients perhaps even more often than in the past. Continuous medical education regarding various acute and chronic treatment options for VTs is mandatory. Treatment guidelines will be updated as new results from controlled clinical trials, but also from basic electrophysiology studies, become available.

Further reading

Aliot EM, Stevenson WG, Almendral-Garrote JM, *et al.* EHRA/HRS Expert Consensus on Catheter Ablation of Ventricular Arrhythmias: developed in a partnership with the European Heart Rhythm Association (EHRA), a Registered Branch of the European Society of Cardiology (ESC), and the Heart Rhythm Society (HRS); in collaboration with the American College of Cardiology (ACC) and the American Heart Association (AHA). *Heart Rhythm* 2009;**6**:886–933.

Amin AS, Tan HL, Wilde AA, Cardiac ion channels in health and disease Heart Rhythm 2010;**7**:117–126

Epstein AE, DiMarco JP, Ellenbogen KA, *et al.* ACC/AHA/HRS 2008 Guidelines for Device-Based Therapy of Cardiac Rhythm Abnormalities: a report of the American College of Cardiology/American Heart Association Task Force on Practice Guidelines. *J Am Coll Cardiol* 2008;**51**:e1–62.

Lehnart SE, Ackerman ME, Benson Jr. DW *et al.* Inherited Arrhythmias: a National Heart, Lung, and Blood Institute and Office of Rare Diseases Workshop Consensus Report about the Diagnosis, Phenotyping, Molecular Mechanisms, and Therapeutic Approaches for Primary Cardiomyopathies of Gene Mutations Affecting Ion Channel Function Circulation 2007;**116**:2325–2345.

Nolan JP, Deakin CD, Soar J, *et al*. European Resuscitation Council guidelines for resuscitation 2005. Section 4. Adult advanced life support. *Resuscitation* 2005;**67**, Suppl 1:S39–86.

Zipes DP, Camm A, Borggrefe M, *et al*. ACC/AHA/ESC 2006 Guidelines for Management of Patients With Ventricular Arrhythmias, the Prevention of Sudden Cardiac Death. *Circulation* 2006;**114**:e385–e484.

⮕ For additional multimedia materials please visit the online version of the book (〰 http://www.esciacc.oxfordmedicine.com).

SECTION X

Other acute cardiovascular conditions

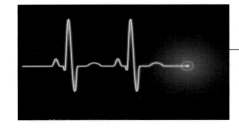

CHAPTER 56

Myocarditis, cardiac tamponade, and pericarditis

Michel Noutsias, Sabine Pankuweit, and Bernhard Maisch

Contents

Summary

Acute myocarditis (AMC) and its sequelae, dilated cardiomyopathy (DCM) and inflammatory cardiomyopathy (DCMi) are most often caused by cardiotropic viral infections in the Western world. Immunohistological detection of inflammation and anticardiac autoantibodies have proven adverse prognostic impact in AMC. Endomyocardial biopsies (EMBs) are now indispensable diagnostic procedures for the selection of DCMi patients who are likely to benefit from immunosuppression or antiviral (interferon) treatment. Intravenous immunoglobulin (IVIG) and immunoadsorption (IA) are further promising therapeutic options for DCM patients.

Acute pericarditis is labelled idiopathic or suspected viral without adequate proof of the respective aetiology. Many cases respond to nonsteroidal anti-inflammatory drugs (NSAIDs) and/or colchicine. Pericardioscopy and epicardial biopsies can contribute to aetiological differentiation of pericardial effusions. Pericardiocentesis is a life-saving treatment of cardiac tamponade.

Cardiac magnetic resonance (CMR) has emerged as a valuable diagnostic approach for AMC and pericarditis, but is not suitable for the detection of viral infections.

Myocarditis

Definition and pathogenesis

Formerly, a diagnosis of classical myocarditis was restricted to the acute myocarditis (AMC) stage. With increasing knowledge of the intimate pathogenic link between AMC and dilated cardiomyopathy (DCM), the 1995 WHO/ISFC Task Force Report introduced among other specific cardiomyopathies the new entity 'inflammatory cardiomyopathy' (DCMi), which is characterized by myocarditis in association with cardiac dysfunction [1].

Infectious agents, toxicity, and other conditions have been associated with AMC and DCM ($\Rightarrow$ Table 56.1).

Detailed knowledge of virus-induced myocardial damage has been unravelled with respect to Coxsackie B virus (CBV) in experimental and human myocarditis (❯ Fig. 56.1) [2, 3]. Intense but time- limited myocardial inflammation during the AMC presumably aims at viral elimination and spontaneous recovery, and is not primarily detrimental to the heart. A complex network of adaptive and innate immune responses is involved, encompassing direct cytopathic effects of the virus, virus-induced anticardiac immune responses, and genetic susceptibility of the host. These mechanisms are not mutually exclusive, and can contribute to the transition from AMC to DCMi [2–4].

After viral invasion facilitated by receptors [5–7], the ensuing antiviral immune response is mainly maintained by T lymphocytes, macrophages, and NK cells [8–11]. This early stage of viral infection may be accompanied by viraemia and the appearance of IgM antiviral antibodies, which can subsequently switch to persisting antiviral IgG antibodies

in the subacute and chronic phases of the disease, paralleled by a substantial decrease of viral loads. Neutralizing antiviral antibodies are involved in viral elimination, and immunosuppressive treatment is rather detrimental at this stage [12]. Cytokines exert cardiodepressive effects, and promote remodelling by inducing an imbalance of metalloproteinases (MMPs) and their tissue inhibitors (TIMPs) [13–16]. This AMC-associated type of fibrosis is rather localized and to some extent is potentially reversible as shown by cardiac magnetic resonance (CMR) in human AMC [17, 18]. Moreover, cytokines induce cell adhesion molecules (CAMs), which mediate the migration of infiltrates [19]. Myocytolysis exerted by cytotoxic T lymphocytes (CTLs) is also mediated by CAM–ligand interactions [20]. AMC can be paralleled by pericarditis in terms of 'myopericarditis'. Acute mortality, mostly due to sudden cardiac death (SCD)/ malignant arrhythmias and severe cardiac failure, can be witnessed in both experimental and human AMC [21, 22].

Table 56.1 Infectious agents, toxic agents, and conditions associated with AMC, DCMi, and DCM

Infectious agents	
Viruses	Adenovirus (ADV), arbovirus, arenavirus, coxsackievirus (especially coxsackie B virus, CBV), cytomegalovirus (CMV), dengue virus, echovirus, encephalomyocarditis, enteroviruses (EV), Epstein–Barr virus (EBV), flavovirus, hepatitis A virus, hepatitis B virus, hepatitis C virus (HCV), herpes simplex virus, herpes zoster virus, HIV, human herpes virus type 6 (HHV-6), influenza virus, Junin virus, lymphocytic choriomeningitis virus, lyssavirus, measles virus, mumps virus, parvovirus B19 (B19V), poliomyelitis virus, rabies virus, respiratory syncytial virus, rubella virus, rubeola virus, vaccinia virus, varicella–zoster virus, variola virus, yellow fever virus
Bacteria	Actinomyces, *Borrelia* species, *Brucella* species, *Chlamydia pneumoniae, Chlamydophila psittaci, Clostridium tetani, Corynebacterium diphtheriae, Coxiella burnetii, Francisella tularensis, Haemophilus influenzae, Legionella pneumophila*, leptospira, *Neisseria gonorrhoea*, meningococcus, *Mycobacterium tuberculosis, Mycoplasma pneumoniae*, pneumococcus, Rickettsiae, *Salmonella typhi, Serratia marcescens*, staphylococcus, *Streptococcus pneumoniae, Streptococcus pyogenes, Treponema pallidum, Tropheryma whippelii, Vibrio cholerae*
Fungi	Actinomyces species, aspergillus, blastomyces, candida, coccidioides, cryptococcus, histoplasma, mucormycosis, nocardia, *Sporothrix schenkii*
Protozoa	Ascaris, *Entamoeba histolytica*, echinococcosis, leishmania, helminthic diseases, malaria, *Paragonimus westermani, Schistosoma* species, *Strongyloides stercoralis, Taenia solium, Trichinella spiralis, Toxoplasma gondii*, trichinosis, *Trypanosoma cruzi*, sleeping sickness/African trypanosomiasis, visceral larva migrans, *Wuchereria bancrofti*
Toxic conditions	
Animal toxic agents	Bee stings, wasp stings, scorpion bites, snake bites, spider bites
Medications	Acetazolamide, amitriptyline, aminophylline, amphotericin B, amphetamines, ampicillin, benzodiazepines, bumatenide, carbamazepine, catecholamines, cefaclor, cephalosporins, chemotherapeutics (especially anthracyclines), chloramphenicol, chlorthalidone, clozapine, colchicine, cocaine, cyclophosphamide, ciclosporin, dobutamine, ethanol, fluorouracil, furosemide, hemetine, hydralazine, hydrochlorothiazide, interleukin-2, isoniazid, lidocaine, lithium, metalazone, methyldopa, methysergide, nitroprusside, oxyphenbutazone, para-aminosalicylic acid, penicillin, phenindione, phenylbutazone, phenytoin, reserpine, spironolactone, sulfadiazine, sulfamethoxypyridine, sulfisoxazole, sulfonyureas, streptomycin, tetracycline, thiazides, triazolam, trastuzumab, tricyclic antidepressants
Natural mediators and conditions	Catecholamines, various cytokines (i.e. tumour necrosis factor, interleukin-2), electric shock, hyperpyrexia, radiation, sepsis
Toxic agents	Alcohol, arsenic, carbon monoxide, copper, diverse inhalants, iron, lead, lithium, phosphorus, tetanus toxoid
Cardiac involvement in systemic disorders	Coeliac disease, Churg–Strauss syndrome, collagen vascular diseases, inflammatory bowel disease, diabetes mellitus, hypereosinophilia, Kawasaki's disease, myasthenia gravis, polymyositis, sarcoidosis, scleroderma, systemic lupus erythematosus, thyrotoxicosis, Wegener's granulomatosis

The table is not claimed to present all known or suspected associations with AMC, DCMi, and DCM completely. In parts, the associations are based on case reports only, and a robust 'proof of principle' causative relationship or pathogenic pathway is not established.

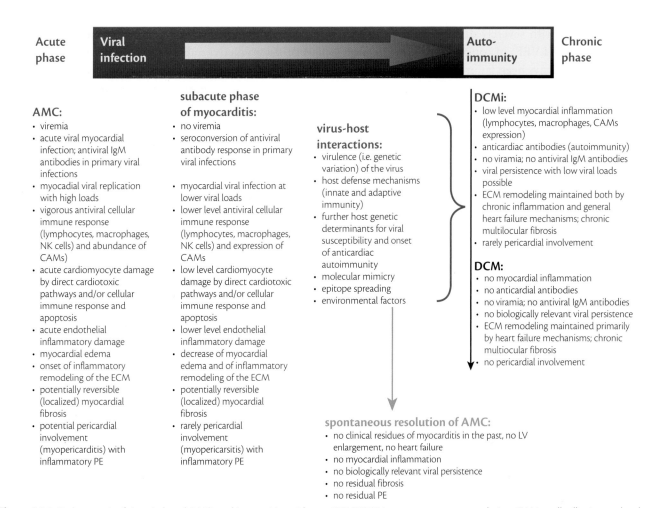

Figure 56.1 Pathogenesis of virus-induced AMC, and its transition either to DCMi/DCM or to spontaneous resolution. CAMs, cell adhesion molecules; ECM, extracellular matrix; LV, left ventricular; NK cells, natural killer cells.

These intricate virus–host interactions guide AMC over its subacute phase either to spontaneous recovery without any substantial long-term clinical residues, or to transition to DCMi. The latter is characterized by low-level intramyocardial inflammation, accompanied by low-level persistence of viral loads in the absence of viraemia. Anticardiac autoantibodies, induced among others by molecular mimicry, can frequently be detected in this later stage of DCMi in both experimental myocarditis and human DCM [23–27]. At this stage, sustained effects of general heart failure pathways become prominent, leading among other things to irreversible extracellular matrix (ECM) remodelling with the chronic multilocular fibrosis pattern typical for DCM, even after cessation of inflammatory and/or biologically relevant viral persistence.

Epidemiology

No detailed epidemiological survey is available for human AMC because of its frequently insidious clinical presentation. However, systematic surveys available from symptomatic patients and post-mortem analyses of young SCD patients have reported myocarditis accounting for approximately 20%, with an incidence of 0.17 per 1000 person-years [28–31]. The prevalence of DCM is 29 per 10^6 persons/year, and the incidence is 131 cases per 10^6 persons/year [32]. Along with ischaemic cardiomyopathy, DCM is the leading indication for heart transplantation [33].

Clinical presentation and prognosis

AMC can further present with an acute myocardial infarction (AMI)-like situation, with chest discomfort, arrhythmias, acute heart failure, palpitations, syncope, and SCD. AMC patients may report a close temporal association (days to a few weeks) with an antecedent flu-like illness (respiratory or gastrointestinal tract infection) before the onset of symptoms. However, AMC may frequently be missed because its symptoms are subtle or virtually absent [34–38]. In AMC with preserved systolic function, regional wall motion abnormalities, diastolic dysfunction, wall oedema, and pericardial effusions can be detected by echocardiography.

Patients presenting with severely depressed left ventricular ejection fraction (LVEF) in concert with LV dilatation report rapidly progressive heart failure symptoms. The most severe presentation is acute fulminant myocarditis, which by definition requires inotropic or mechanical support, i.e. a left ventricular assist device (LVAD). LV function in patients with acute fulminant myocarditis usually improves dramatically and may even normalize under heart failure regimens, with an excellent long-term outcome [39].

The clinical presentation of DCM patients is dominated by chronic and often progressive heart failure (CHF) symptoms (i.e. dyspnoea on exertion or at rest, peripheral oedema). Cardiomegaly, pulmonary congestion/oedema, and pleural effusions are frequently observed in the chest radiograph. Systolic and diastolic dysfunction and LV or biventricular dilatation can be confirmed by echocardiography. LV thrombi can cause thromboembolic complications.

Both AMC and DCM/DCMi can present with various types of ECG abnormalities (right or left bundle branch block, ST-segment depression, Q-waves and T-wave inversions, AV block) and rhythm disturbances on Holter monitoring (sinus tachycardia/bradycardia, supra-/ventricular extrasystoles, atrial fibrillation/flutter, and ventricular tachycardia/flutter/fibrillation). AMC is a frequent cause of SCD (up to 40%) especially in the young, and is often associated with strenuous physical exertion [22, 29].

Clinical findings in AMC and DCM patients are summarized in ⬚ 56.1.

After AMC, highly heterogeneous clinical courses have been observed. Transition of AMC to DCM/DCMi has been reported in approximately 20% of patients [34, 40]. After AMC, transplantation-free survival has been determined as 78% within a mean follow-up of 59±42 months [41], and is no different from the survival of DCM patients [42]. Clinical characteristics are not valuable for the aetiological differentiation of the disease, and have limited value for the prognostic assessment of AMC patients. NYHA class III/IV and elevated LV filling pressures may predict a worse prognosis [40, 41, 43–45].

Evidence emerging from recent observations confirms the decrease of mortality and hospitalization of DCM patients under heart failure treatment [40, 46]. The reported 5-year survivals of DCM patients vary between 36% and 70% [47, 48].

Pathogenic substrates of DCMi, namely the immuno-histological proof of intramyocardial inflammation, cardiotropic viral persistence/viral replication, the presence of autoantibodies and late gadolinium enhancement (LGE) in CMR are associated with adverse outcome [41, 49–55].

In contrast, histological morphometric analyses have limited or no predictive value [42, 44, 56]. Investigations on soluble Fas and soluble TNF-receptor suggest that the extent of cellular apoptosis may provide important prognostic information [57, 58], as well as marker cytokines of immune dysregulation such as IL-10 [59]. Furthermore, there is an emerging role for genetic mutations with prognostic impact in DCM patients [60].

Diagnosis

Endomyocardial biopsies

Refined endomyocardial biopsy (EMB) investigations have contributed substantially to progress in understanding the pathogenesis of AMC and DCMi. Complications of the obtaining of EMBs are rare in experienced centres, and serious periprocedural complications have been reported as less than 0.5% in large series studies [41, 61, 62].

Histology

The histological Dallas criteria differentiate 'active' (interstitial infiltrates with myocytolysis with/without fibrosis; ➲ Fig. 56.2) from borderline myocarditis (increased infiltrates with/without fibrosis) [63]. By histological assessment, myocarditis can be revealed only in a minority of the patients (c.5–20%). Histological assessment of myocarditis is hampered by the substantial sampling error and interobserver variability [64–66]. These diagnostic obstacles, as well as the neglect of viral persistence, have likely contributed to the failure of immunosuppression in the Myocarditis Treatment Trial [67, 68]. The Dallas criteria

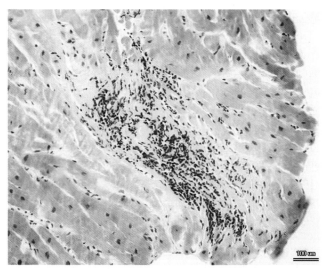

Figure 56.2 Histological aspect of myocarditis. Focal lymphomononuclear infiltrate with adjacent myocytolysis (active myocarditis; original magnification ×200).
Reproduced with permission from Hess OM, McKenna W, and Schultheiss H, Myocardial Disease. In: Camm AJ, Lüscher TF, Serruys PW (eds) The ESC textbook of cardiovascular medicine 2nd Edition , pp. 665–716 Oxford University Press, 2009.

are not relevant for prognostic assessment or the selection of patients who will likely profit from immunosuppression [41, 42]. Notwithstanding these pitfalls, histological assessment of EMBs is still mandatory for the diagnosis of 'active myocarditis', and also for the detection of further pathologies (e.g. giant-cell myocarditis, storage diseases) [69–71].

Immunohistology

Immunohistological evaluation, as opposed to simple histological haematoxylin and eosin staining, enables the specific detection and exact quantification of infiltrates, a detailed phenotypic characterization of infiltrates, and the assessment of endothelial CAM abundance. One immunohistological approach determined a level of more than 7.0 $CD3^+/CD2^+$ lymphocytes/mm^2 myocardial tissue area as the diagnostic threshold for DCMi, with concurrent abundance of several CAMs [19, 72]. The World Heart Federation (WHF) consensus elaborated a combined approach with lymphocytes and macrophages (>14.0 leucocytes/mm^2) and facultative CAM abundance, which has been used by several independent groups [73–79].

A homogeneous infiltration pattern is present in most DCMi cases (➲ Fig. 56.3a), but focal infiltrates, consistent with histologically detected 'active myocarditis', with predominance of CTLs, can also be observed in approximately 10–20% of the EMBs of DCM patients (➲ Fig. 56.3b) [19, 20]. Abundance of several CAMs, with typically homogeneous expression pattern (➲ Fig. 56.3c), which likely reduces the sampling error, can be observed in approximately 60% of DCM patients [19, 80, 81]. Additionally, sarcolemmal induction of several CAMs has been observed in DCMi [19, 80]. HLA sarcolemmal expression was used as a selection criterion for DCMi patients who responded favourably to immunosuppressive treatment [80, 82]. In contrast to the histological Dallas criteria, the immunohistological EMB evaluation has shown prognostic impact in AMC patients (➲ Fig. 56.4), and has been confirmed as a suitable diagnostic approach for the selection of DCMi patients who will likely benefit from immunosuppression treatment [76, 80]. Digital image analysis (DIA) systems have been employed to standardize quantification of immunohistological EMB staining [83]. A synopsis comparing the histological Dallas criteria of myocarditis with the immunohistological diagnosis of DCMi is summarized in ➲ Table 56.2.

Virological analyses

Amplification of viral genomes by polymerase chain reaction (PCR) has confirmed viral aetiology in a major proportion of AMC and DCM patients (➲ Fig. 56.5) [36, 38, 41, 49, 50, 77, 84–89]. DCM patients with viral persistence have a progressively deteriorating LVEF under conventional

under heart failure medication. In contrast, DCM patients with viral elimination show an improvement of LVEF (🎥 56.2) [85]. Viruses may either reside by latent infection, or actively replicate within the host tissue [50, 90].

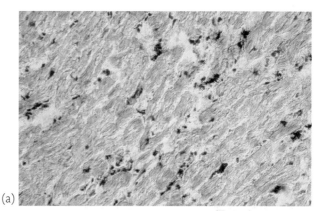

(a)

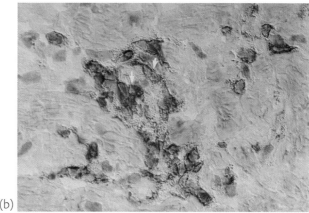

(b)

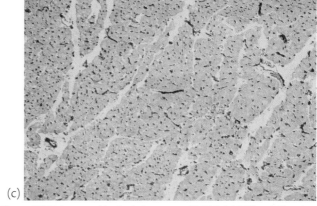

(c)

Figure 56.3 Immunohistological aspects of DCMi: (a) Diffuse infiltration pattern of LFA-1$^+$ lymphocytes in DCMi (original magnification ×400). (b) Focal infiltration pattern of perforin$^+$ CTLs in DCMi, encircling and entering (white arrows) a cross-sectioned cardiomyocyte, suggesting myocytolysis (original magnification ×630). (c) Homogeneous ICAM-1 abundance in DCMi (original magnification ×200).
(a) Reproduced from Noutsias M, Seeberg B, Schultheiss HP, Kühl U. Expression of cell adhesion molecules in dilated cardiomyopathy: evidence for endothelial activation in inflammatory cardiomyopathy. *Circulation* 1999;**99**(16):2124–2131, with permission from Wolter Kluwer Health; (b), (c) Reproduced from Noutsias M, Pauschinger M, Schultheiss HP, Kühl U. Cytotoxic perforin$^+$ and TIA-1$^+$ infiltrates are associated with cell adhesion molecule expression in dilated cardiomyopathy. *Eur J Heart Fail* 2003;**5**(4):469–479, with permission from Oxford University Press.

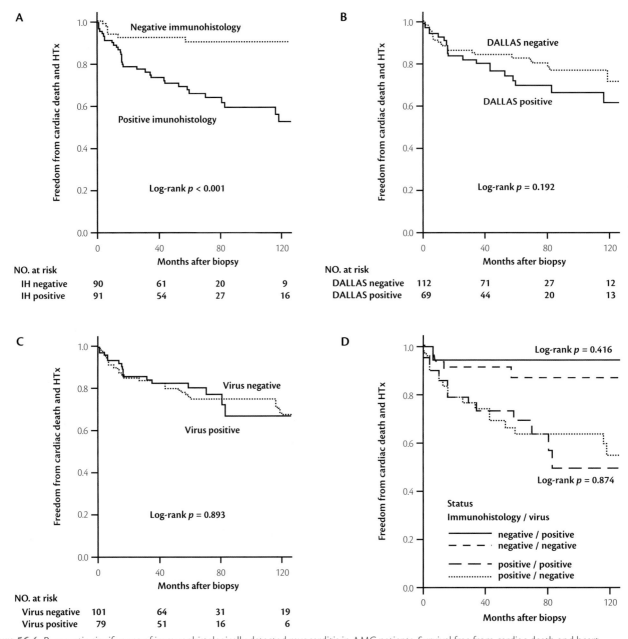

Figure 56.4 Prognostic significance of immunohistologically detected myocarditis in AMC patients. Survival free from cardiac death and heart transplantation according to the findings of EMBs: (A) Immunohistological results. (B) Histopathological results according to the Dallas criteria. (C) Viral genome detection. (D) Combination of immunohistological and PCR findings. HTx, heart transplantation.
Reproduced from Kindermann I, Kindermann M, Kandolf R, *et al.* Predictors of outcome in patients with suspected myocarditis. *Circulation* 2008;**118**(6):639–648, with permission from Wolter Kluwer Health.

In particular, DCMi patients with active enterovirus (EV) replication have a substantially worse prognosis than DCMi patients with EV latency [50].

Viral loads can be determined by quantitative real-time PCR (qPCR). The parvovirus B19 (B19V) loads in EMBs range widely, between 10 and 10^8 viral copies/μg nucleic acids, with higher B19V loads in acute infections and substantially decreasing B19V loads after B19V viraemia in AMC [84, 91–94]. Direct sequencing of positive PCR results allows the identification of the genotype and

mutations of the viral genomes. Genotype analysis showed that B19V genotype 1 was associated with significantly reduced LVEF compared to patients with B19V genotype 2 (24.4±10.4% vs 31.0±9.5%, $p = 0.0001$) [95]. The additional determination of the antiviral T-cell specificity and of the epitope-specific anti-B19V humoral response [96, 97] and the immunohistological characterization of B19V protein-expressing cells [98–100] may be helpful to detect biologically relevant from latent B19V infections. This differentiation gains importance in light of the high

Table 56.2 Comparison of the histological of myocarditis and of the immunohistological evaluation of DCMi

	Histological evaluation of myocarditis (Dallas criteria)	Immunohistological evaluation of inflammatory cardiomyopathy (DCMi)
Interobserver variability	High [65, 67]	Not precisely known, but expected to be substantially lower, especially using DIA [19, 80, 83]
Sampling error	High [66]	Not precisely known, but expected to be substantially lower [19, 80, 174]
Variability of detection of inflammation	High [67, 175]	Lower [19, 80, 176]
Specific identification and quantification of infiltrates	Impossible	Feasible [19, 72, 128, 177, 178]
Phenotypic characterization of infiltrates	Impossible	Broad phenotypic characterization feasible (i.e. T-lymphocytes, CTLs, macrophages, specific activation markers) [19, 20, 51, 72, 128, 177–179].
Evaluation of CAMs expression	Impossible	Feasible [19, 20, 80, 83, 128, 174, 176, 177, 180]
Prognostic relevance	No prognostic relevance [41, 42]	Patients with immunohistologically proven DCMi have a worse prognosis [41, 51]
Clinical relevance	No discrimination of DCM patients who benefit from immunosuppression [67]	Patients with immunohistologically proven DCMi benefit from immunosuppressive treatment [80, 116, 181]

Adapted and updated from Noutsias M, Pauschinger M, Poller WC, *et al.* Immunomodulatory treatment strategies in inflammatory cardiomyopathy: current status and future perspectives. *Expert Rev Cardiovasc Ther* 2004;**2**(1):37–51.

detectability of B19V genomes in cardiac tissues from non-AMC/non-DCM patients [96, 101].

Diagnosis by cardiovascular magnetic resonance

Since its first publication in 1998 by Friedrich *et al.* [102], followed by several landmark publications, consensus diagnostic CMR approaches have been elaborated for myocarditis [103]. The LGE pattern in myocarditis differs from ischaemic, hypertrophic heart disease and amyloidosis, being located typically subepicardially in the posterolateral wall in acute myocarditis, and midventricularly within the septum in DCM [104, 105]. In addition, T_1- and

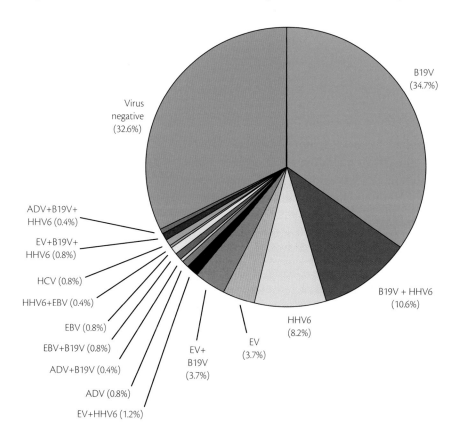

Figure 56.5 Spectrum of cardiotropic viruses in patients presenting with DCM. Reproduced from Kühl U, Pauschinger M, Noutsias M, *et al.* High prevalence of viral genomes and multiple viral infections in the myocardium of adults with 'idiopathic' left ventricular dysfunction. *Circulation* 2005;**111**(7):887–893, with permission from Wolter Kluwer Health.

T_2-weighted CMR detects oedema and hyperaemia. CMR can noninvasively monitor the dynamics of the natural course of myocarditis [17, 106]. CMR-LGE has demonstrated an adverse prognostic impact in DCM patients [54, 105]. In AMC patients with AMI-like presentation, the combination of EMB diagnostics and CMR-LGE can contribute to synergistic diagnostic effects, overcoming some of the limitations of both approaches used separately. The particular strength of immunohistological EMB investigations is the detection of more subtle AMC presentations with lesser release of cardiac injury markers, compatible with 'borderline myocarditis', which may be missed by CMR-LGE [78]. However, viral infections cannot be detected specifically by CMR [107].

Relevance of autoantibodies

A series of autoantibodies targeting different myocardial structures has been described for DCM patients (🎥 56.3). Anticardiac autoantibodies are also involved in familial DCM [24]. Experimental 'proof of principle' on the functional relevance and discrimination from noncardiac diseases and healthy controls has not been established for all these autoantibodies. Binding to the Fc receptor of the cardiomyocytes may be a common pathway of virtually all anticardiac autoantibodies contributing to DCM [108]. The presence of anticardiac autoantibodies has been associated with more aggressive prognosis in AMC patients [53]. In particular the IgG3 fraction of antibodies seems to be relevant for pathogenesis and immunoadsorption of DCM patients [109, 110].

Treatment

Conventional heart failure treatment

The general guidelines for heart failure treatment apply equally to AMC and DCM, including assist devices and cardiac transplantation as a last resort [111]. Cardiotoxic agents (e.g. alcohol, anthracyclines) should be discontinued [112]. In AMC, exercise should be avoided during the first weeks after the initial diagnosis, since both experimental data and observations in human indicate that SCD is associated with strenuous physical activity [28–31] and early decompensation. In contrast, moderate exercise training can contribute to alleviation of heart failure symptoms and improve prognosis in noninflammatory DCM patients [113]. Genetic counselling and noninvasive cardiological screening (ECG, echocardiography) is advisable in patients with familial DCM and their first-degree relatives [60].

AMC/DCM patients should be followed regularly by clinical assessment and noninvasive examinations. Especially in cases with progressively deteriorating or failure of improving LV function despite symptomatic heart failure medication (i.e. within 2 weeks), EMBs should be obtained in these patients and subjected to contemporary diagnostic techniques, preferably in experienced centres and/or in the framework of multicentre studies [70].

Immunomodulatory treatment

Immunosuppression

The indication for immunosuppression (corticosteroids and ciclosporin) in histologically diagnosed giant-cell myocarditis for prolonging transplantation-free survival is well defined [70, 114, 115]. Although immunosuppression did not show beneficial effects in histologically confirmed active or borderline myocarditis without exclusion of viral persistence [67], sustained beneficial effects of immunosuppression on CHF symptoms, LV dimensions, and LVEF have been confirmed in immunohistologically proven DCMi in two randomized trials [76, 80]. Further data on immunosuppression in DCMi should be expected from the ongoing 'European Study of Epidemiology and Treatment of Cardiac Inflammatory Diseases' (ESETCID) trial [75]. In DCMi patients with viral persistence, however, immunosuppression has been associated with treatment failure and even deleterious outcome [2, 116].

Intravenous immunoglobulin treatment

The immunomodulatory effects of intravenous immunoglobulins (IVIG) are multifaceted [117–119]. The randomized 'Intervention in Myocarditis and Acute Cardiomyopathy' (IMAC) trial failed to confirm beneficial effects of IVIG in acute DCM [120]. However, a 26-week course of IVIG treatment led to a significant improvement of LVEF from $26\pm2\%$ to $31\pm3\%$ ($p <0.01$), accompanied by a marked rise of anti-inflammatory mediators (IL-10, IL-1 receptor antagonist) in CHF patients (both ischaemic cardiomyopathy and DCM) [121]. These data imply that the anti-inflammatory effects of IVIG may not be restricted to intramyocardial inflammation, but also affect the systemic inflammatory response in CHF [122]. A trial with 20 g of intravenous Pentaglobin (IgG and IgM) is ongoing for DCMi patients with B19V persistence [123].

Antiviral immunomodulation with interferon

Type I interferons such as IFN-β are pivotal for the antiviral immune response in experimental CBV-induced myocarditis [124]. In a phase II study, 22 DCMi patients with EMB-proven enteroviral (n = 15) or adenoviral (n = 7) persistence were treated with IFN-β for 24 weeks [125]. IFN-β was initiated with 2×10^6 U IFN-β three times a week on alternate days, and increased to 12×10^6 U during the second week and 18×10^6 U during the third week. Elimination of viral genomes was proven in follow-up EMBs in all enrolled patients. This was paralleled by a significant raise of LVEF (from 44.7±15.5% to 53.1±16.8%) and amelioration of CHF symptoms. IFN-β treatment was safe and well tolerated, and influenza-like side effects could be efficiently suppressed by nonsteroidal anti-inflammatory drugs (NSAIDs) [125]. The randomized multicentre 'Bioferon in Chronic Viral Cardiomyopathy' (BICC) trial has been concluded in 143 patients with PCR proof of enterovirus, adenovirus, or B19V in EMBs. Results presented at the American Heart Association meeting in 2008 showed a significant improvement of NYHA functional class and of the subjective assessment according to the Minnesota Heart Failure Questionnaire [126].

Immunoadsorption

Immunoadsorption (IA) extracts immunoglobulins from the patients' plasma. The immediate beneficial haemodynamic effects of IA in DCM patients are attributed partly to the removal of cardiodepressive anticardiac autoantibodies [127]. However, further mechanisms such as decrease of lymphocytic infiltration and CAM expression [128] and inhibition of oxidative stress [129] may be relevant. In several IA studies, the plasma IgG levels were restored by 0.5 g/kg polyclonal IgG in several studies, which might also have contributed to the results in terms of an IVIG effect in DCM patients [130]. The beneficial effects of immunoadsorption on LVEF and CHF symptoms last for 2.5 years or more after treatment, and contribute to a significant reduction of hospitalization days and morbidity [131, 132]. Notwithstanding these promising data, IA investigations have clearly shown heterogeneous effects in DCM patients, with 'responders' versus 'nonresponders' [130]. The deciphering of the prognostically relevant patient profiles is ongoing [133, 134]. A randomized multicentre trial has been initiated for DCM patients.

Cardiac tamponade

Definition, pathogenesis, clinical presentation, and diagnosis

Cardiac tamponade is the decompensated phase of cardiac compression caused by accumulation of pericardial effusion and the increased intrapericardial pressure [135].

Up to 30% of patients with asymptomatic large chronic pericardial effusions develop unexpected cardiac tamponade [136]. Detailed cross-sectional epidemiological data on the prevalence of cardiac tamponade are not available.

The prevalence of different aetiologies of pericardial effusion accessed by pericardiocentesis results are listed in Chapter 26, ⊃ Table 26.1.

Patients can present with orthopnoea, cough, and dysphagia, and occasionally with episodes of unconsciousness. Insidiously developing tamponade may present with complicating sequelae (renal failure, abdominal plethora, shock liver, and mesenteric ischaemia). Pulsus paradoxus may be found (⊃ 56.4). The clinical presentation of cardiac tamponade and diagnostic pathways are summarized in Chapter 26, ⊃ Table 26.4. Pericardial effusions detected by transthoracic echocardiography (TTE) are classified by the Horowitz criteria (⊃ Fig. 56.6) [137]. The size of effusions can be graded as: (1) small (echo-free space in diastole <10 mm), (2) moderate (10–20 mm), (3) large (≥20mm), or (4) very large (≥20mm and compression of the heart). In large pericardial effusions, the heart may move freely within the pericardial cavity ('swinging heart') [138, 139]. In 'iatrogenic' tamponade, intrapericardial pressure is rising rapidly (i.e. haemorrhage, in minutes to a few hours) and this is usually highly symptomatic. In contrast, an inflammatory process developing days to weeks before cardiac compression occurs ('medical' tamponade) can be remarkably asymptomatic. Triggers for tamponade include hypovolaemia, paroxysmal tachyarrhythmia, and intercurrent acute pericarditis. Tamponade without two or more inflammatory signs (typical pain, pericardial friction rub, fever, diffuse ST-segment elevations) is usually associated with a malignant effusion. CT and especially CMR have taken over the leading diagnostic role for the determination of size and extent of both simple and complex pericardial effusions, encompassing the sensitive detection of pericardial inflammation by LGE-CMR [140–142].

Treatment and prognosis

Cardiac tamponade is an absolute indication for pericardiocentesis under fluoroscopic or echocardiographic guidance (level of evidence B, class I indication) [135, 139]. For procedural details on pericardiocentesis and the corresponding indications, see Chapter 26, ⊃ Box 26.1. Intermittent pericardial aspiration with prolonged pericardial drainage is performed until the effusion volume obtained every 4–6 h falls to less than 25 mL/day. In 'idiopathic' pericardial effusions, extended pericardial catheter drainage (mean 3±2 days, range 1–13 days) is associated with a lower recurrence rates (6% vs 23% during follow-up of 3.8±4.3 years) [143]. A surgical approach is recommended only in patients with very large chronic pericardial effusions with impending or ensuing tamponades, in whom repeated pericardiocentesis

Table 56.3 Differential diagnosis of specific entities of pericarditis

	Viral	Bacterial	Tuberculous	Autoreactive	Malignant
Microbial agents	EV, ADV, B19V, EBV, CMV, HIV, echovirus, herpes simplex virus, hepatitis virus A, B, C	Staphylococci, pneumococci, streptococci, neisseria, proteus, Gram-negative rods, legionella	Mycobacterium tuberculosis	autoimmune process in the absence of viral and bacterial agents	none
Aetiological evidence by	PCR or in situ hybridization (evidence level B, indication IIa)	Gram-stain, bacterial culture, PCR for borrelia and Chlamydia pneumoniae (evidence level B, indication I)	Ziehl–Neelsen, auramin 0 stain, culture, PCR (evidence level B, indication I)	Ig-binding to peri- and epicardium, negative PCR for cardiotropic agents, epicarditis (evidence level B, indication IIa)	malignant cells in PE and primary tumour
Incidence (%) in Western countries	30	5–105 per 100 000	<4 (much more in Africa and South America)	20–30	30–40
Male: female ratio	3:1	1:1	1:1	1:1	1:1
Predisposition	Unknown	Chronic alcohol abuse, immunosuppression	Alcohol abuse, HIV, immunosuppression	Association to autoimmune disorders	primary tumour
Clinical features	Identical to acute pericarditis, often subfebrile	Spiking fever, fulminant, tachycardia, pericardial rubs	Subfebrile, chronic	subfebrile, chronic	chronic, ranging from insidious to tamponade
Effusion size	Variable, mostly small	Variable	Variable, mostly large	variable	variable, mostly large
Tamponade	Infrequent	80%	Frequent	infrequent	frequent
Spontaneous remission	Frequent	None	None	rare	none
Recurrence rate	30–50%	Rare	Frequent	frequent (>25%)	frequent
Aspect of PE	Serous/serosanginous	Purulent	Serosanginous	serous	often sanginous
Protein content	>3 g/dL	High	High/intermediate	intermediate	>3g/dL or high
Leucocyte count (PE)	>5000/mL	>>10 000/mL	Intermediate (>8000/mL)	intermediate (<5.000/ml)	low to intermediate
Pericardial fluid analyses	Activated lymphocytes and (sparse) macrophages, ADA-negative	Granulocytes and (massive) macrophages, ADA-negative	Granulocytes and (intermediate) macrophages ADA positive (>40 U/mL)	activated lymphocytes and (sparse) macrophages, ADA-negative	malign cells, tumour markers (i.e. CEA, NSE) can be increased [204, 205]
Peri- and epicardial biopsy	Lymphocytic peri-/ epicarditis, PCR positive for cardiotropic virus	Leucocytic epicarditis	Caseous granuloma, PCR	lymphocytic peri-/ epicarditis, PCR for cardiotropic virus negative	malign cells
Mortality if untreated	Depending on agent and tamponade	100%	85%	in untreated tamponade	100%
Intrapericardial treatment	Drainage, if needed, no IP corticoids	Drainage and rinsing (saline), gentamycin 80 mg IP	Drainage, if needed	drainage, i.p. triamcinolone (evidence B, indication IIa)	drainage, i.p. cisplatin or thiotepa
Pericardiotomy/ pericardiectomy	Rarely needed	Promptly needed (evidence level B, indication I)	Rarely needed	rarely needed	rarely needed
Systemic treatment	IVIG, in enteroviral pericarditis IFN SC	Antibiotics	Tuberculostatic treatment, combination with prednisone to be considered	NSAIDs, colchicine, rather obsolete: prednisolone, and its optional combination with azathioprine	treatment of primary tumour
Constriction	Rare	Frequent	Frequent (30–50%)	rare	rare

ADA, adenosine deaminase; ADV, adenovirus; B19V, parvovirus B19; CBV, coxsackie B virus; EBV, Epstein–Barr virus; EV, enteroviruses; IFN, interferon; IP, intrapericardial; IV, intravenous; NSAIDs, nonsteroidal anti-inflammatory drugs; PCR, polymerase chain reaction; SC, subcutaneous.

Adapted with permission from Maisch B, Seferovic PM, Ristic AD, et al. Guidelines on the diagnosis and management of pericardial diseases executive summary; The Task force on the diagnosis and management of pericardial diseases of the European Society of Cardiology. *Eur Heart J* 2004; **25** (7):587–610.

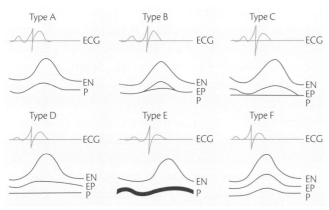

Figure 56.6 Horowitz classification of PEs. Type A, no effusion; type B, separation of epicardium and pericardium (3–16 mL); type C1, systolic and diastolic separation of epicardium and pericardium (small effusion >16 mL); type C2, systolic and diastolic separation of epicardium and pericardium with attenuated pericardial motion; type D, pronounced separation of epicardium and pericardium with large echo-free space; type E, pericardial thickening (>4 mm). EN, endocardium; EP, epicardium; P, pericardium. Reproduced from Maisch B, Karatolios K. [New possibilities of diagnostics and therapy of pericarditis.]. *Internist* (Berlin) 2008;**49**(1):17–26. With permission from Springer, Belin/Heidelberg.

and/or intrapericardial therapy has had no sustained success. Surgical drainage is preferred in traumatic haemopericardium and purulent pericarditis. Resistant neoplastic processes require intrapericardial treatment (Chapter 26, ➲ Table 26.4), percutaneous balloon pericardiotomy, or rarely pericardiectomy [144–147]. However, prognosis in malignant pericardial effusions is limited by the primary disease [148]. Malignancy is the primary cause of medical tamponade (65%), with the poorest 1-year mortality (76.5%) compared to patients with nonmalignant tamponade (13.3%) [149].

Pericarditis

Definition, pathogenesis, clinical presentation, and diagnosis

Independently of its aetiology, pericarditis can be subdivided in terms of clinical stage and course into acute, chronic (>3 months), and recurrent pericarditis. Acute pericarditis may be dry, fibrinous, or effusive. Chronic pericarditis includes effusive (inflammatory or hydropericardium in heart failure), adhesive, and constrictive forms. The term 'recurrent pericarditis' encompasses (1) the intermittent type (symptom-free intervals without therapy) and (2) the incessant type (discontinuation of anti-inflammatory therapy ensures a relapse).

Detailed cross-sectional epidemiological data on the prevalence of pericarditis are not available. As in myocarditis,

the majority of cases are presumably not diagnosed because their course is asymptomatic or subclinical. The prevalence of the different pericardial effusion aetiologies based on pericardiocentesis results are listed in Chapter 26, ➲ Table 26.1. In up to 60% of the patients, the cause of pericardial effusions is a known medical condition [150]. In developing countries, tuberculous pericarditis is quite common, and is often associated with HIV infections.

The diagnostic algorithm for pericarditis is summarized in Chapter 26, ➲ Table 26.2. A prodrome of fever, malaise, and myalgia may precede acute pericarditis. Major symptoms are retrosternal or left precordial chest pain and shortness of breath. The pericardial friction rub can be transient, mono-, bi-, or triphasic in cardiac auscultation. Symptoms are usually milder in chronic pericarditis (chest pain, palpitations, fatigue). ECG changes are usually reversible after pericardial effusion drainage and/or successful anti-inflammatory treatment [151]. Echocardiography is essential to detect pericardial effusion according to the Horowitz classification (➲ Fig. 56.6) [137, 141]. Myopericarditis can be furthermore evidenced by global or regional myocardial dysfunction. Laboratory findings include elevations of myocardial injury markers (troponins I and T, creatine kinase MB, myoglobin). In viral or idiopathic acute pericarditis, troponin I elevation is frequently observed but has no prognostic impact [152–154]. Furthermore, inflammatory markers (i.e. CRP, ESR, LDH, leucocytes) can be increased [148]. When detailed clinical diagnostic workup (📷 56.5) is undertaken, the rate of 'idiopathic' pericardial effusions remains less than 5% [148]. The spectrum of cardiotropic viruses in pericardial biopsies and in pericardial effusion resembles findings in EMBs of AMC and DCMi/DCM patients, which argue for similar causal infections in the endo- and the pericardium as well as the pericardial effusion in the context of 'myopericarditis' [155]. Neoplastic aetiology was found in 7% of 450 patients with acute pericardial disease. Acute pericardial disease was the first manifestation of previously unknown malignancies in 4% of the patients, with lung cancer being the most common malignancy (72%) [156]. Typical aspects of pericardial effusion investigations for cytomegalovirus (CMV) and tuberculous pericarditis, as well as pericardial involvement in Hodgkin's disease, are presented in ➲ 56.6. An approach for the differential diagnosis of viral, bacterial, tuberculous, and autoreactive pericarditis is summarized in ➲ Table 56.3.

For recurrent myocarditis, massive pericardial effusion, overt tamponade, or constriction are rare. Evidence for an immunopathological process includes (1) the latent period lasting for months; (2) the presence of antiheart antibodies; (3) the similarity and coexistence of recurrent pericarditis with other autoimmune conditions [148].

For details on further rare pericardial diseases, see the corresponding European Society of Cardiology guidelines [148] and ➲ Chapter 26.

Treatment and prognosis

Prognostic indicators for poor clinical outcome in acute pericarditis are fever (>38°C), subacute course, large effusion or tamponade, and failure of NSAIDs [157]. After exclusion of these relevant prognostic conditions, acute pericarditis has generally a brief and benign course under NSAIDs and/or colchicine [158]. Myopericarditis is a relatively common disease in patients presenting with acute pericarditis (14.6% = 40/274 consecutive patients) and shows a relative benign evolution [159]. Hospitalization is warranted to determine the aetiology and observe for tamponade as well as the initial effect of treatment [148, 160].

The primary medical treatment of acute pericarditis is NSAIDs (level of evidence B, class I). Because of its rare side effects, its beneficial effects on coronary flow, and the large dose range, ibuprofen is preferred (300–800 mg every 6–8 h, best until disappearance of pericardial effusion). Gastrointestinal protection must be provided [148]. Several randomized trials have shown that colchicine as monotherapy or added to NSAIDs is effective both for the treatment of acute pericarditis and for the prevention of recurrent pericarditis (level of evidence A, class I indication; 2 mg/day for 1–2 days, followed by 0.5–1 mg/day for 3–6 months) [160–163]. Intrapericardial application of triamcinolone avoids systemic side effects and is highly effective (level of evidence B, class IIa indication) [148, 164]. The formerly usual treatment of 'idiopathic' pericarditis with systemic corticosteroids has to be regarded as obsolete, since it has been identified as an independent predictor for recurrent pericarditis [165–167]. Systemic corticosteroid therapy should be restricted to autoreactive or uraemic pericarditis, and pericardial involvement in connective tissue diseases [148]. In patients in whom treatment with prednisone has already been initiated, ibuprofen and/or colchicine should be introduced early to taper off prednisone [168]. Whenever possible, treatment should target the underlying aetiology. This is valid for acute, chronic, and recurrent pericardial effusion. Indications and regimens of systemic and intrapericardial treatment of pericardial effusion are summarized in Chapter 26, ➲ Table 26.4. Pericardiocentesis is not necessary if a definitive diagnosis can be made otherwise or the pericardial effusions are small or resolving under anti-inflammatory treatment (➲ Chapter 26). A scheme showing the diagnostic and therapeutic pathways for pericardial effusions is illustrated in Chapter 26, ➲ Fig. 26.1.

Symptomatic treatment of chronic and recurrent pericarditis is as in acute pericarditis. Recurrent chest pain without clinical evidence of acute pericarditis after a documented event of acute pericarditis is a risk condition for recurrent pericarditis and the development of constrictive pericarditis. This constellation was recorded in 3.5–10% of patients with previous viral or 'idiopathic' acute pericarditis [169, 170]. Female gender (OR 4.3; 95% CI 1.8–10.6), previous use of corticosteroids (OR 5.2; 95% CI 2.2–12.3), and previous recurrent pericarditis (OR 3.7; 95% CI 1.3–10.2) were identified as risk factors [169]. The medical treatment of recurrent pericarditis is the same as for acute pericarditis (see above) [161, 163, 168]. Corticosteroids should be restricted to selected patients with poor general condition or in frequent crises at low doses (0.2–0.5 mg/kg per day; level of evidence C, indication IIb) [148, 166, 167]. Corticosteroids are associated with an increased risk of recurrent pericarditis (OR 10.35; 95% CI 4.46–23.99; p <0.001) [165]. Azathioprine (75–100 mg/day) or cyclophosphamide can be added if patients do not respond adequately [171]. In cases with frequent and symptomatic recurrences despite medical treatment, balloon pericardiotomy or pericardiectomy can be considered as options of last resport (level of evidence B, indication IIb) [146, 148, 172, 173].

Personal perspective

Myocarditis and pericarditis remain challenging diseases for cardiologists. Progress in the last two decades has substantially improved our understanding of these diseases. In addition, innovative diagnostic procedures and novel therapeutic approaches have lead to new evidence in this area of cardiovascular medicine.

After decisive drawbacks resulting from the negative results of the Myocarditis Treatment Trial, there is an increasing interest and progress in immunomodulatory treatment of DCMi. EMB-based diagnosis of DCMi is undertaken by an increasing number of investigators. However, consensus guidelines for standardized protocols and diagnostic tools for EMBs and for anticardiac autoantibodies are awaited, and essential. Results of ongoing multicentre trials will likely affect evidence-based guidelines. There is a need for frequent noninvasive monitoring of intramyocardial inflammation and viral activity. CMR is an acknowledged powerful diagnostic tool for the noninvasive detection of inflammation, and guidelines have been established for CMR in AMC. However, CMR cannot detect viral infection specifically. The value of CMR for monitoring DCMi in its natural course and possibly also during immunomodulatory treatment strategies remains an intriguing future task, as well as molecular imaging.

Diagnostic and treatment guidelines, as well as prognostic criteria, have been elaborated for pericarditis, which help to standardize its management. Insights from pericarditis research have contributed to decrement of recurrent pericarditis. Colchicine has proven as first-choice therapy for recurrent pericarditis in addition to NSAIDs, while systemically administered corticosteroids have proven an independent risk factor for further recurrences and should be reserved for autoimmune cases. There is an increasing value of CMR for diagnosis and possibly also for noninvasive monitoring of pericarditis.

Further reading

Cooper LT, Baughman KL, Feldman AM, *et al*. The role of endomyocardial biopsy in the management of cardiovascular disease: a scientific statement from the American Heart Association, the American College of Cardiology, and the European Society of Cardiology. *Circulation* 2007;**116**(19):2216–2233.

D'Ambrosio A, Patti G, Manzoli A, *et al*. The fate of acute myocarditis between spontaneous improvement and evolution to dilated cardiomyopathy: a review. *Heart* 2001;**85**(5):499–504.

Dorffel WV, Wallukat G, Dorffel Y, *et al*. Immunoadsorption in idiopathic dilated cardiomyopathy, a 3-year follow-up. *Int J Cardiol* 2004;**97**(3):529–534.

Esfandiarei M, McManus BM. Molecular biology and pathogenesis of viral myocarditis. *Annu Rev Pathol* 2008;**3**:127–155.

Friedrich MG, Strohm O, Schulz-Menger J, *et al*. Contrast media-enhanced magnetic resonance imaging visualizes myocardial changes in the course of viral myocarditis. *Circulation* 1998;**97**(18):1802–1809.

Frustaci A, Russo MA, Chimenti C. Randomized study on the efficacy of immunosuppressive therapy in patients with virus-negative inflammatory cardiomyopathy: the TIMIC study. *Eur Heart J* 2009;**30**(16):1995–2002.

Imazio M, Bobbio M, Cecchi E, *et al*. Colchicine in addition to conventional therapy for acute pericarditis: results of the COlchicine for acute PEricarditis (COPE) trial. *Circulation* 2005;**112**(13):2012–2016.

Kindermann I, Kindermann M, Kandolf R, *et al*. Predictors of outcome in patients with suspected myocarditis. *Circulation*. 2008;**118**(6):639–648.

Maisch B, Seferovic PM, Ristic AD, *et al*. Guidelines on the diagnosis and management of pericardial diseases executive summary; The Task force on the diagnosis and management of pericardial diseases of the European society of cardiology. *Eur Heart J* 2004;**25**(7):587–610.

Wojnicz R, Nowalany-Kozielska E, Wojciechowska C, *et al*. Randomized, placebo-controlled study for immunosuppressive treatment of inflammatory dilated cardiomyopathy: two-year follow-up results. *Circulation* 2001;**104**(1):39–45.

Additional online material

⦾ For additional multimedia materials please visit the online version of the book (👁 http://www.esciacc.oxfordmedicine.com).

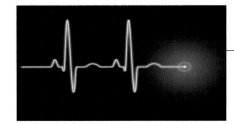

CHAPTER 57

Acute valve disease and endocarditis

Gregory Ducrocq, Franck Thuny, Bernard Iung, and Alec Vahanian

Contents

Summary

The management of patients with acute valve disease is now a rare situation but remains a very challenging one, as valvular patients are often elderly with severe comorbidities. Furthermore, there is a proportion of previously operated patients who present with valve dysfunction. The aim in this situation is to establish rapid diagnosis based on clinical examination and echocardiography followed by early intervention. The main treatment is valve replacement, but a more conservative surgical approach is being developed and more recently percutaneous interventional techniques have been introduced. In the future every effort should be made to avoid interventions in an acute situation as they are always risky.

Introduction

Valvular heart disease (VHD), although not as common as coronary disease or hypertension, is an important and challenging clinical entity. There have been important changes in the distribution of the aetiologies of VHD in Western countries over the last 50 years, and the degenerative aetiology is now the most frequent [1]. In addition, increased age is associated with a higher frequency of comorbidity, rendering decision-making for intervention more complex [2–6].

The main surgical treatment is valve replacement, but the conservative surgical approach is being developed, and, more recently, percutaneous interventional techniques have been introduced.

In current practice the incidence of emergency cases with VHD is rare overall. For example, valve surgery performed in an emergency setting represents only 2% of the total number of cases of surgical intervention in the EuroHeart Survey [1], but it is a major clinical challenge owing to its consequences in terms of mortality and morbidity [6].

This review will concentrate on acute presentation in adult patients with acquired VHD or valve prosthesis, and finally acute endocarditis.

General considerations

Decompensation in patients with VHD may occur at the endstage of a chronic disease due to continued deterioration of the condition or may be precipitated by cardiac complications such as atrial fibrillation, acute myocardial ischaemia, endocarditis, or noncardiac complications such as respiratory infection. Alternatively, an acute situation may occur in patients without previous significant VHD, mainly due to endocarditis, or more rarely myocardial infarction (MI) or trauma. In such cases acute regurgitations are poorly tolerated because of the absence of previous adaptative mechanisms.

Taking into account the population of patients with severe VHD, especially with aortic stenosis (AS), who are now elderly with comorbidities, and the high risk of surgery, the selection of candidates should involve multidisciplinary consultation between cardiologists, surgeons, and anaesthesiologists [3, 4].

When patients present in an emergency setting their valvular disease status may or may not be known; thus, rapid diagnosis, relying mainly on clinical examination as well as echocardiography, is key.

The aim of echocardiography is to confirm the diagnosis of VHD, to assess its severity, mechanisms, and consequences, and to search for associated lesions. Echocardiography also enables the measurement of pulmonary pressures and the degree of the combined lesions and measurements of left ventricular (LV) function.

Cardiac catheterization has virtually no indication in these patients except for coronary angiography, which should be done preoperatively according to guidelines, [3, 4] except in rare circumstances such as when the haemodynamic condition does not allow for it or when there is a large vegetation in front of the left main coronary.

Across the spectrum of VHD, patients with severe heart failure, especially when presenting in an acute setting, have a dismal spontaneous prognosis and a worse postoperative outcome than those who are at an earlier stage of the disease [6]. This argues in favour of considering intervention at first glance, except in patients with limited life expectancy due to severe comorbidity, but this may be difficult to estimate in the acute setting if the patient's history is not already known.

Aortic stenosis

AS is the most common valvular disease in Europe and North America and is increasing in prevalence because of the ageing of the population [1].

Diagnosis

In practice, AS may be discovered during attempted diagnosis of unexplained congestive heart failure or even at the onset of shock or after cardiac arrest. Clinical examination is particularly difficult in patients with low output since there is no slowly rising pulse; the murmur may become softer or even disappear and auscultation could be limited to a soft murmur of functional mitral regurgitation (MR) and S3 sound at the apex and signs of heart failure.

Doppler echocardiography confirms the presence of AS, and is the preferred technique for assessing its severity. For clinical decision-making, valve area should be considered in combination with flow velocity, pressure gradient, and ventricular function, as well as functional status. The thresholds generally recommended for the definition of severe AS are aortic jet velocity greater than 4 m/s; mean gradient greater than 40–50 mmHg; aortic valve area less than 1 cm². Indexing to body surface area (BSA), with a cut-off value of 0.6 cm²/m² BSA, is helpful [3, 4]. Low flow is frequent in patients with heart failure, usually due to depressed LV function, and may be associated with low pressure gradients even with severe AS. As soon as the mean gradient is less than 40 mmHg, even a small valve area does not definitely confirm severe AS, since mild to moderately diseased valves may not open fully resulting in a 'functionally small valve area' ('pseudosevere AS') [2–4].

Stress echocardiography, using low dose dobutamine, cannot be done in emergency situations. In such cases severe valve calcification implies the presence of severe AS, while the opposite is most often true in elderly patients. Transoesophageal echocardiography carries a high risk in this setting and is not recommended if transthoracic echocardiography is adequate.

Treatment strategy

Inotropic agents and diuretics may transiently improve heart failure; however, intervention should always be considered and not be deferred. In selected patients with pulmonary oedema, nitroprusside can be used under haemodynamic monitoring.

Early valve replacement should be strongly recommended in patients who are otherwise candidates for surgery. Unfortunately, repeated observations worldwide show that a large proportion of potentially suitable candidates are not referred for surgery at present [7]. As long as the mean gradient is still over 40 mmHg, there is virtually no lower ejection fraction (EF) limit for surgery.

In patients in shock or in severe heart failure, data are limited but consistently show that aortic valve replacement

(AVR) carries a very high risk, with a perioperative mortality ranging from 25% to 50%; however, recent improvements in surgical and postoperative care are now able to provide better results [8–10].

More recently, transcatheter aortic valve implantation (TAVI) has emerged as a potential alternative in patients with a contraindication or high risk for surgery [11–13]. Current knowledge shows that TAVI is feasible and provides significant clinical and haemodynamic improvement up to 3 years, but this technique is still under evaluation with questions remaining on safety and long-term results. TAVI can be considered only if the patient's life expectancy is at least 1 year, and if there are no contraindications to the technique. TAVI has been used in patients with severe heart failure, but very seldom in emergency settings because only a limited number of centres have experience and are also able to prepare the devices independently, which requires the participation of technical specialists in most centres.

Percutaneous balloon aortic valvuloplasty (PAV) has a limited role as its efficacy is low, its complication rate is quite high, and restenosis with clinical deterioration occurs within a couple of months [14–17]. PAV can be considered as a bridge to surgery or TAVI in haemodynamically unstable patients who are at high risk for surgery. This type of bridging PAV could be proposed if the institution has experience in PAV, patients have acceptable, or at least uncertain, life expectancy, and the contraindication for surgery is temporary. If PAV is successful, aortic valve surgery or TAVI should be done early [2, 3].

On the other hand, medical treatment is probably the best option in definitely inoperable patients such as frail octogenarians or those with severe comorbidities compromising life expectancy in the short term [11].

Aortic regurgitation

Aortic regurgitation (AR) is observed in 13% of patients with native valve disease in the EuroHeart Survey [1].

Acute AR may be due to active endocarditis or more rarely dissection, trauma (either blunt chest or more rarely after percutaneous intervention), dissection of the ascending aorta, or prosthetic dysfunction [18].

Diagnosis

Acute AR rapidly leads to disabling dyspnoea or pulmonary oedema due to the rapid elevation of end diastolic pressures in the nondilated, noncompliant LV. In acute AR, patients are tachycardic and an S3 sound may be heard at the apex with clinical signs of pulmonary oedema. The diastolic

murmur and peripheral signs are attenuated because the pulse pressure is narrow.

Transthoracic and/or transoesophageal echocardiography enables the anatomy of aortic leaflets and the aortic root to be accurately assessed, thereby contributing to the identification of the aetiology and mechanisms of AR. Quantitative measurements are favoured but are less validated than for MR. The criteria for defining severe AR are an effective regurgitant orifice area (ERO) of more than 0.30 cm^2, regurgitant volume greater than 60 mL, or a regurgitant fraction of more than 50% [2–4] (➲ Fig. 57. 1).

The most frequent signs in severe acute AR are vena contracta greater than 6 mm, pressure half-time <200 ms, holodiastolic flow reversal in abdominal aorta, and premature mitral valve closure (➲ Fig. 57.2). In acute AR the variability of the loading conditions decreases the value of the quantitative criteria.

Treatment strategy

Chronic aortic regurgitation

In patients with severe LV dysfunction, as long as AR is severe, the current trend is to favour AVR over heart transplantation because recent series have shown satisfactory postoperative outcomes which are likely to be superior to the dismal spontaneous prognosis [19]. In patients with major LV dysfunction, the final choice between valve replacement, heart transplantation, or medical therapy is made on an individual basis [3, 4].

Acute aortic regurgitation

The presence of acute heart failure (HF) is an indication for urgent surgery because of poor haemodynamic tolerance and the dismal spontaneous prognosis. Surgery should not be delayed in favour of efforts at medical management.

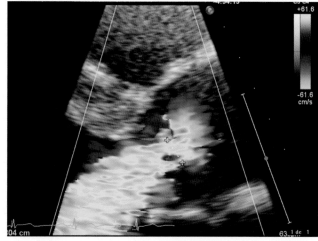

Figure 57.1 Severe aortic regurgitation. Colour Doppler flow imaging.

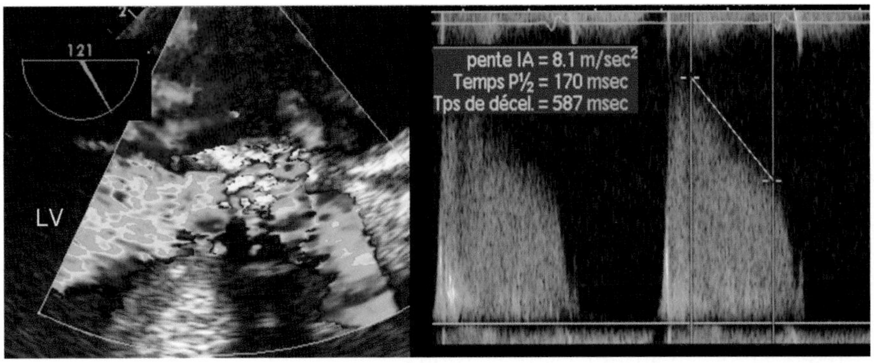

Figure 57.2 Acute aortic regurgitation. On the left, severe regurgitation shown by transoesophageal echocardiography. On the right, transthoracic echocardiography showing short pressure half-time (<200 ms).

Nitroprusside and inotropic agents are useful in poorly tolerated acute AR to stabilize the clinical condition en route to surgery [20].

If acute AR is seen in the context of dissection of the ascending aorta, a replacement of the ascending aorta should be associated with valve replacement (➲ Fig. 57.3).

Severe acute AR could be due to blunt trauma, usually a motor vehicle accident. After trauma, even if reconstructive repair has been described, valve replacement is usually necessary [21, 22].

Massive AR seldom occurs after PAV but requires emergency AVR, or in the future, TAVI, if the clinical condition of the patient permits [14].

Mitral stenosis

Although the prevalence of rheumatic fever has greatly decreased in Western countries, mitral stenosis (MS) still results in significant morbidity and mortality worldwide [1].

Emergency presentation of these patients is very rare, which explains the lack of data. MS may deteriorate, causing patients to present in shock.

◆ In developing countries where rheumatic disease is still frequent, young patients may be seen initially at an advanced stage of the disease with pulmonary oedema, low cardiac output, and shock.

◆ In the Western world, patients with refractory HF are usually at the endstages of the disease with advanced age, poor general condition, and frequent comorbidities.

In both situations there is often a precipitating factor such as respiratory infection, anaemia, atrial fibrillation, or more specifically pregnancy in developing countries. Finally, in some cases MS may not yet be diagnosed [2].

Diagnosis

In patients with HF the diastolic murmur may be of low intensity or even inaudible in patients with low output. Pulmonary hypertension causes both a louder second heart sound at the base and a murmur of tricuspid regurgitation located at the xyphoid. Pulmonary oedema or—at a more advanced stage—respiratory failure, severe pulmonary hypertension, or cachexia may dominate the examination.

Echocardiography is the main method of assessing the severity and consequences of MS, as well as the extent of anatomic lesions. The severity of MS should be quantified using two-dimensional planimetry and the pressure half-time method, which are complementary. MS is considered significant when valve area is less than 1.5 cm^2 or less than 1 cm^2/m^{2}BSA. A transthoracic approach provides sufficient information for decision-making; however, transoesophageal examination should also be done when transthoracic visualization is suboptimal or to exclude left atrial thrombosis, in particular in the appendage, before

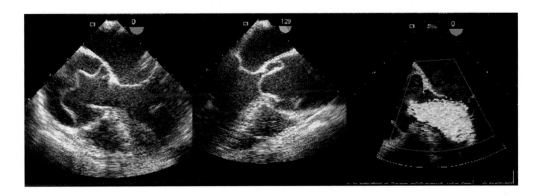

Figure 57.3 Aortic dissection. On the left and middle panels, transoesophageal echocardiography showing in horizontal (left) and longitudinal planes (middle) an intimal flap prolapsing into the left ventricle which causes severe aortic regurgitation (right panel).

percutaneous mitral commissurotomy or in case of suspicion such as after an embolic complication [3, 4].

Treatment strategy

Diuretics or nitrates ameliorate dyspnoea transiently. β-Blockers or calcium channel blockers are useful to slow the heart rate. Anticoagulant therapy is indicated in patients with atrial fibrillation and is recommended in patients with sinus rhythm, when there has been prior embolism or a thrombus is present in the left atrium. Cardioversion is not indicated before intervention in patients with severe MS, as it does not robustly restore sinus rhythm.

Intervention is indicated in highly symptomatic patients with severe MS [14, 23–28]. When patients are in a critical clinical condition the threshold for percutaneous mitral commissurotomy (PMC) over surgery is lower since the mortality of surgery is very high (20–50%) and PMC can be used as a life-saving procedure serving as a bridge to lower the risk of secondary surgery [23–25]. PMC can be performed as a life-saving procedure in critically ill patients, as the sole treatment when there is an absolute contraindication to surgery, or as a bridge to surgery in other cases. In this context dramatic improvement has been observed in young patients, but the outcome is very bad in elderly patients presenting with endstage disease who would probably be better treated conservatively. In pregnant patients, PMC can be proposed after 20 weeks by experienced teams.

Surgery is the only alternative when PMC is contraindicated, the most important contraindication being left atrial thrombosis. Other contraindications for PMC include more than mild MR, severe bicommissural calcification, absence of commissural fusion, combined severe aortic or tricuspid valve disease, or coronary disease requiring bypass surgery. In such patients, valve replacement is performed. On the other hand, coexisting moderate aortic valve disease and functional tricuspid regurgitation are not considered as contraindications for the technique.

Mitral regurgitation

MR is the second most frequent valve disease after AS in hospitalized patients. It is essential to distinguish between primary organic MR, in which abnormalities of the mitral valve apparatus are the cause of the disease, and secondary MR, which results from LV disease and remodelling.

Severe acute MR is mainly due to rupture of the chordae in degenerative disease, endocarditis, or rupture of a papillary muscle (which occurs less frequently since the use of immediate reperfusion strategies in acute MI), traumatic lesions, prosthetic dysfunction, or, rarely in Western countries, acute rheumatic fever [18]. Acute MR induces an immediate decrease in afterload, LV emptying increases, and left atrial pressure rises acutely, which is transmitted back to the pulmonary circulation. Forward stroke volume is reduced in clinical presentation, shock, or severe dyspnoea with acute pulmonary oedema.

Diagnosis

Acute severe MR usually results in acute pulmonary oedema [29]. In patients with papillary muscle rupture during acute MI, the presence of shock contrasts with a hyperdynamic heart on echocardiography (📷 57.1). Dynamic chronic ischaemic MR can lead to acute pulmonary oedema in the absence of acute myocardial ischaemia [30]. In acute MR, the murmur is shortened by a rapid reduction in the pressure gradient between LV and the left atrium; it may even be inaudible in papillary muscle rupture with low output. Finally, pulmonary oedema may be localized to one segment and confused with pneumonia [29].

Echocardiography makes it possible to establish aetiology and mechanisms, quantify severity, and assess the reparability of the valve (➲ Figs 57.4–57.6). In experienced hands, transthoracic echocardiography is highly accurate for a precise localization of the involved scallops in the case of degenerative MR. In ischaemic MR, the apical displacement of the leaflets can be quantitated by measuring the tenting area and the distance between the annulus and the coaptation point.

Finally in functional MR, the evaluation of the degree of LV dysfunction is key. The assessment of severity requires an approach integrating blood flow data from Doppler with morphologic information, and careful cross-checking of the validity of such data against the consequences on LV and pulmonary pressures. Organic MR is considered severe when the regurgitant orifice area is 40 mm² or more and regurgitation volume is 60 mL or more. In secondary MR, the corresponding thresholds of severity are 20 mm² and 30 mL respectively [3, 4].

In acute MR the most frequent signs are vena contracta less than 7 mm, reversed pulmonary vein flow, and decreased aortic valve opening.

Treatment strategy

Chronic primary mitral regurgitation

Intervention is only indicated in patients with severe MR. In patients who have severely decompensated severe chronic MR when LVEF is less than 30%, the decision whether to

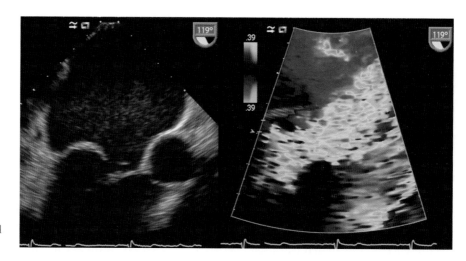

Figure 57.4 Severe mitral regurgitation. Transoesophageal echocardiography shows a flail leaflet (segment P2), due to chordal rupture.

operate will take into account the response to medical therapy, comorbidity, and the likelihood of valve repair [3, 4].

Functional mitral regurgitation

There is a continuing debate on the indications for surgery in functional MR because it has yet to be demonstrated in a randomized clinical trial that suppression of MR minimizes mortality and HF [29, 31–34].

In patients with severe MR, surgery is indicated if coronary bypass is performed [3, 4]. The preferred surgical procedure remains controversial, although there is a trend in favour of repair even if results are less satisfactory than in other aetiologies [31]. The limited data available suggest that isolated mitral valve surgery, in combination with LV reconstruction techniques, may be considered in selected patients with severe functional MR and severely depressed LV function [35]. Such patients include those with coronary disease where bypass surgery is not indicated, who remain symptomatic despite optimal medical therapy, and where comorbidity is low—the aim being to avoid or

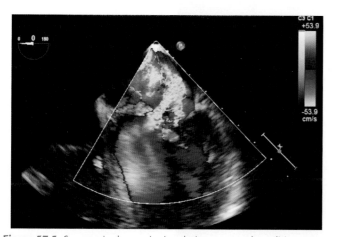

Figure 57.5 Severe mitral regurgitation during acute endocarditis. Transoesophageal echocardiography shows perforation of the anterior leaflet of the mitral valve.

postpone transplantation. Ongoing trials are expected to better define appropriate strategies. In other patients medical therapy, followed by transplantation when this fails, is probably the best option.

Surgery on the regurgitant mitral valve should not be considered in patients who are *in extremis* with low output, severe right ventricular failure, and high comorbidity.

The techniques of percutaneous mitral valve repair are at an early stage and it is not currently possible to make any recommendations for their use.

Acute mitral regurgitation

Urgent surgery is indicated in patients with acute MR. Acute MR is poorly tolerated and carries a poor prognosis in the absence of intervention, which is indicated urgently.

Reduction of filling pressures can be obtained using vasodilators such as nitroprusside. In the presence of systemic hypotension, an intra-aortic balloon pump (IABP) helps to stabilize the patient before surgery. Inotropic agents should be added in cases of hypotension.

The rupture of the papillary muscle necessitates urgent surgical treatment, which is most often valve replacement, even if valve repair can be successfully performed in selected circumstances, such as younger patients, if the rupture is partial and the surrounding tissue is of good quality. Myocardial revascularization is associated in most cases [36].

Traumatic mitral valve injury occurs less frequently than tricuspid trauma [21, 22]. It is more commonly associated with dramatic haemodynamic compromise, and most cases are operated on within hours of the injury. Mitral valve replacement is often used, but repair can be performed more successfully than in MI because the rupture of papillary muscle is often associated with less myocardial necrosis and diffuse injuries in an ischaemic setting.

Severe MR after balloon commissurotomy seldom necessitates urgent surgery, except in cases with poor

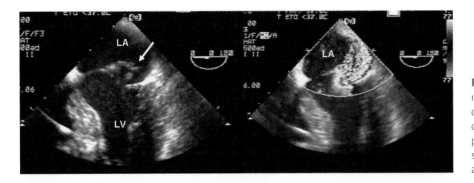

Figure 57.6 Rupture of papillary muscle. On the left, severe prolapse of the mitral valve due to rupture of papillary muscle. On the right panel, Doppler colour flow shows severe mitral regurgitation. LA, left atrium; LV, left ventricle.

haemodynamic tolerance. Surgery will mostly necessitate valve replacement due to the severity of underlying disease rather than the presence of the valvular tear itself [14].

Patients after prosthetic valve surgery

Patients who have undergone previous valve replacement represent an important proportion of patients with VHD [1]. Functional deterioration during follow-up requires prompt echocardiographic examination.

Treatment of specific prosthetic complications

Prosthetic thrombosis

Occlusive prosthetic thrombosis is characterized by impaired motion of the mobile part of the prosthesis. It is more frequent in patients with a mechanical prosthesis and should be suspected promptly in any patients with any type of prosthetic valve who present with a recent increase in shortness of breath or embolic event. Inadequate anticoagulation is the most important risk factor [2]. The diagnosis should be immediately confirmed by echocardiography (either transthoracic or transoesophageal) (➲ Fig. 57.7), and also fluoroscopy showing an increase in gradient and decreased mobility of the leaflets. Clinical examination is often difficult in this setting because of frequent pulmonary oedema.

The management of prosthetic thrombosis is high risk, whatever the option taken [37–40]. Surgery is high risk as it is most often done in emergency conditions and represents reintervention. On the other hand, fibrinolysis carries a risk of bleeding, systemic embolism, and recurrent thrombosis. The risk/benefit analysis of each approach should be adapted to patient characteristics and local resources. (➲ Fig. 57.8). Emergency valve replacement is the treatment of choice in obstructive thrombosis in critically ill patients without serious comorbidity [38–40]. If the thrombogenicity of the

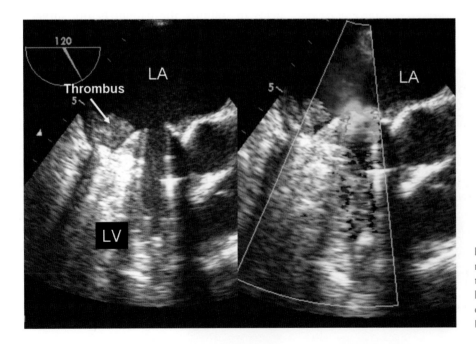

Figure 57.7 Thrombosis of a mitral prosthesis. In the left panel, thrombus is seen blocking one leaflet. In the right panel, there is only one colour jet. LA, left atrium; LV, left ventricle.

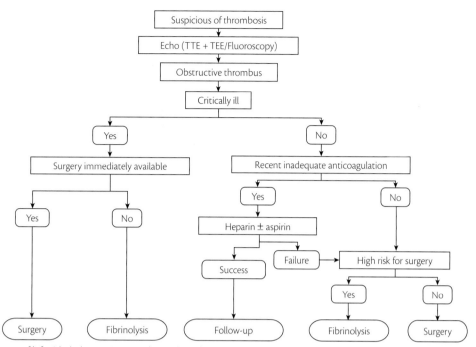

Figure 57.8 Management of left-sided obstructive prosthetic thrombosis. Risks and benefits of fibrinolysis versus surgery should be individualized. The presence of a first-generation prosthesis is an incentive to surgery.
Adapted with permission from Vahanian A, Baumgartner H, Bax J, et al . Guidelines on the management of valvular heart disease: The Task Force on the Management of Valvular Heart Disease of the European Society of Cardiology. *Eur Heart J* 2007; **28** :230–268

prosthesis is an important factor, it should be replaced by a less thrombogenetic prosthesis. Fibrinolysis should be considered in critically ill patients unlikely to survive surgery [37, 40] because of comorbidities or severely impaired cardiac function; situations in which surgery is not immediately available and patients cannot be transferred; and thrombosis of tricuspid valve because of the higher success rate and lower incidence of embolism. Fibrinolysis is less likely to be successful with mitral prosthesis, chronic thrombosis, and in the presence of pannus, which can be difficult to distinguish from thrombus [41].

If the patient presents with thromboembolism thorough investigation is essential, including cardiac and noncardiac imaging, to allow for appropriate management [4].

Structural dysfunction

Emergency intervention for bio-prosthesis failure is rare and carries very high risk due to the cardiac condition and also the noncardiac condition, because these patients are often elderly. It is again mandatory to avoid such situations and to envisage reintervention when there are clear signs of valve failure and if the condition of the patient allows for it [42, 43]. In the future, TAVI is a promising way forward for research, but so far only a few procedures have been performed [44]. Structural dysfunction of mechanical valves such as disc escape, which occurred with the Björk–Shiley convex or concave prosthesis, is now extremely rare.

Decompensation from other causes

If decompensation occurs in a patient with a valve prosthesis and is not related to prosthetic dysfunction, another cause such as systemic hypertension, coronary disease, sustained arrhythmias, anaemia, or thyrotoxicosis must be considered. If these causes have been eliminated, decompensation is most often due to LV systolic dysfunction resulting from an operation being carried out too late (in particular after correction of a regurgitation) with or without additional perioperative myocardial damage. In such cases medical treatment, cardiac resynchronization, and cardiac transplantation should follow the guidelines on the management of HF [5].

Acute endocarditis

The management of acute infectious endocarditis (IE) has changed as a result of the recent changes in the epidemiological profile of the disease, with an increase in complicated situations owing to a greater incidence of more virulent organisms and intracardiac material infections [45, 46]. In parallel, the development of surgical techniques has encouraged physicians to offer surgical treatment to an increasing number of patients.

As a general principle, close collaboration between all the specialists implicated in the management of IE is key [47].

Risk stratification

On admission, the prognosis should be assessed immediately to identify patients at high risk of developing severe complications and to determine their operative risk [47–49].

In-hospital mortality ranges from 9% to 26%. Several markers have previously been identified as predictors of worse outcome, including age, diabetes mellitus, occurrence of complications, staphylococcal infection, vegetation length, neurological symptoms, and prosthetic valve IE. On the other hand, operative mortality in active IE is 6–25%. Preoperative shock, HF, renal insufficiency, impaired LV function, prosthetic valve IE, perivalvular abscess, and high logistic Euroscore have been identified as the strongest predictors of operative mortality [50–52].

Treatment strategy

General principles

If a medical strategy is chosen, the situation should be reassessed regularly using close clinical, biological, and echocardiographic monitoring because IE can rapidly progress even under antibiotics.

Although no randomized trials have evaluated the benefit of surgery, the recently published 2009 European guidelines provide clear recommendations on the surgical indications during the active phase of the disease [4, 7]. HF or high risk of HF, uncontrolled infection, and high embolic risk are the three main situations in which cardiac surgery is required [47, 53, 54] (◒ Table 57.1). These guidelines have also have established an optimal timing for each indication: emergency surgery (within 24 h) or urgent surgery (within a few days) basis, irrespective of the duration of antibiotic treatment. In other cases, surgery can be postponed to allow 1 or 2 weeks of antibiotic treatment under careful clinical and echocardiographic observation before an elective surgical procedure is performed.

Indications for surgery

Heart failure

Moderate to severe HF is the strongest predictor of mortality and is present at admission in most cases. In mild HF with a good response to diuretic therapy, surgery is also indicated because of the high risk of relapse of HF. Echocardiography is useful for identifying criteria suggestive of a high risk of severe HF in patients with severe valvular regurgitation: acute valvular regurgitation associated with signs of elevated left filling pressures (early mitral valve closure) (◒ Figs 57.2, 57.5) valvular obstruction by vegetations, large prosthetic dehiscence, pulmonary

Table 57.1 Indications and timing of surgery in native and prosthetic valve infective endocarditis

Indications	Timing	Class[a]
Heart failure		
Aortic or mitral IE or PVE with severe acute regurgitation or valve obstruction or fistula causing refractory pulmonary oedema or cardiogenic shock	Emergency	I
Aortic or mitral IE with severe acute regurgitation or valve obstruction and persisting HF or echocardiographic signs of poor haemodynamic tolerance (early mitral closure or pulmonary hypertension)	Urgent	I
Aortic or mitral IE or severe prosthetic dehiscence with severe regurgitation and no HF	Elective	IIa
Right HF secondary to severe tricuspid regurgitation with poor response to diuretic therapy	Urgent/elective	IIa
Uncontrolled infection		
Locally uncontrolled infection (abscess, false aneurysm, fistula, enlarging vegetation)	Urgent	I
Persisting fever and positive blood cultures >7–10 days not related to an extracardiac cause	Urgent	I
Infection caused by fungi or multiresistant organisms	Urgent/elective	I
PVE caused by staphylococci or Gram-negative bacteria (most cases of early PVE)	Urgent/elective	IIa
Prevention of embolism		
Aortic or mitral IE or PVE with large vegetations (>10 mm) following one or more embolic episodes despite appropriate antibiotic therapy	Urgent	I
Aortic or mitral IE or PVE with large vegetations (>10 mm) and other predictors of complicated course (HF, persistent infection, abscess)	Urgent	I
Aortic or mitral or PVE with isolated very large vegetations (>15 mm)	Urgent[b]	IIb
Persistent tricuspid valve vegetations >20 mm after recurrent pulmonary emboli	Urgent/elective	IIa

HF, heart failure; IE, infective endocarditis; PVE, prosthetic valve endocarditis.

[a] Class I, evidence and/or general agreement that a given treatment or procedure is beneficial, useful, effective; class IIa, weight of evidence/opinion is in favour of usefulness/efficacy; class IIb, usefulness/efficacy is less well established by evidence/opinion.

[b] Even more so if valve repair is feasible.

Data from Habib G, Hoen B, Tornos P, et al. Guidelines on the prevention, diagnosis, and treatment of infective endocarditis (new version 2009): the Task Force on the Prevention, Diagnosis, and Treatment of Infective Endocarditis of the European Society of Cardiology (ESC). *Eur Heart J* 2009; **30**:2369–2413.

hypertension, LV dysfunction, and perivalvular abscess exposing to a risk of intracardiac fistula. Elevated NT-proBNP has a potential value in predicting HF. Since poor surgical outcome is predicted by HF, the early identification of these criteria would allow surgery to be performed urgently with a lower operative risk.

Uncontrolled infection

In some situations, especially in case of prosthetic valve IE, antibiotic therapy is not sufficient to control the infection leading to a high risk of death by HF, embolism, severe sepsis, or complete atrioventricular block.

There are several reasons for fever that persists for more than 7–10 days after the initiation of appropriate antimicrobial therapy, including inadequate antimicrobial therapy, resistant organisms, locally uncontrolled infection, embolic complications or extracardiac site of infection, infected lines, and adverse reaction to antibiotics. When fever persists, the intravenous lines should be replaced; extracardiac complications such as visceral infarction, abscess, or infectious aneurysms should be looked for; blood cultures should be repeated; and echocardiography must be done to detect a perivalvular or myocardial abscess [55, 56].

Locally uncontrolled infection includes increasing vegetation length and perivalvular complications that can be diagnosed by transthoracic and transoesophageal echocardiography. Obviously, the increasing size of vegetations is associated with a high risk of embolism. Perivalvular complications include abscess, pseudo-aneurysm, and fistula; they are more frequently observed in cases of staphylococcal IE, aortic IE and prosthetic valve IE. They could be suspected in the presence of a persistent fever, a new heart murmur, or a new atrioventricular block.

Embolic events

Embolic events develop in 20–50% of patients. Although embolism can arise at any time of the disease, the majority occur before the initiation of the antimicrobial treatment and during the first 2 weeks of therapy [48, 57]. Echocardiography plays a major role in the prediction of embolic risk, because vegetation size and mobility have been proved to be the strongest predictors of embolic events (➲Figs 57.9–57.11). The type of micro-organism involved can also influence the risk of embolism. *Staphylococcus aureus* infection has been associated with a higher incidence of embolic events. Thus, the decision to perform surgery in order to avoid embolism in high risk patients should take all these factors into account.

In case of right-sided native valve IE, the prognosis is better and surgery should generally be avoided [47].

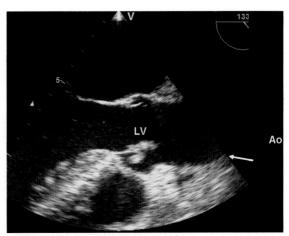

Figure 57.9 Acute aortic endocarditis. Presence of an aortic vegetation. LV, left ventricle.

Management of neurological complications

Neurological complications occur in 20–50% of all patients with IE and are usually related to vegetation embolism [50]. *Staphylococcus aureus* is the causative microorganism most frequently involved. The management of patients developing these complications is difficult and should be multidisciplinary including cardiologists, neurologists, microbiologists, cardiac surgeons, and neurosurgeons. After the first neurological event, the majority of patients still have at least one indication for cardiac surgery, and keep a poor prognosis if this intervention is not performed or cannot be performed.

The impact of valvular surgery on outcome in patients with cerebrovascular complications in IE has been widely debated. In the most recent series, the risk of postoperative neurological deterioration was low (0–6%) even when surgery was done very early after the first neurological symptoms appeared. In fact, the risk of postoperative neurological

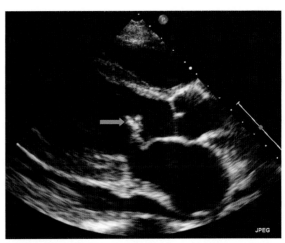

Figure 57.10 Endocarditis of the mitral valve. Echocardiography shows vegetation on the anterior mitral leaflet (arrow).

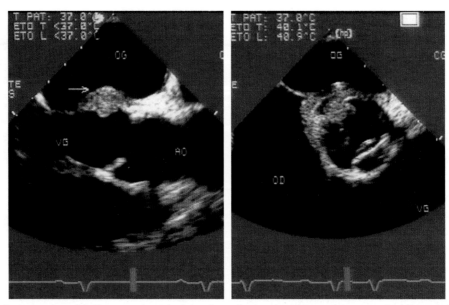

Figure 57.11 Aortic and mitral endocarditis. Transoesophageal echocardiography shows an abscess of the aortomitral fibrosa in longitudinal (left panel) and short-axis (right panel) views.

deterioration seems to depend more on the severity of cerebrovascular complications than on the timing of surgery.

Surgery can be done early after neurological complications if cerebral haemorrhage has been excluded by cranial CT scan and neurological damage is not severe [58]. Conversely, in cases with large intracranial haemorrhage, neurological prognosis is worse and surgery must be postponed for at least 1 month. However, if urgent cardiac surgery is needed, close cooperation with the neurosurgical team is mandatory [47].

The management of intracranial infectious aneurysms in case of indication of cardiac surgery is difficult. They should be looked for in any patients with neurological symptoms using CT, MRI, or conventional angiography. Since ruptured aneurysms with severe haemorrhage carry a very poor prognosis, they should be treated by neurosurgery or endovascular therapy before cardiac surgery. In case of unruptured aneurysm, cardiac surgery can be performed first, especially if there is haemodynamic impairment.

Conclusion

The management of patients with acute valve disease is now rare but remains a very challenging problem which requires a multidisciplinary collaboration between cardiologists, surgeons, and other specialists when needed. The key to success is establishing a rapid diagnosis, based mainly on echocardiography, followed by early intervention. Such intervention performed in an emergency setting will always carry a high risk and every effort should be made to avoid such circumstances by using better prevention.

Personal perspective

First of all, the most important progress to be expected in the management of patients with acute valve disease is its prevention. This will be based first on the better education of patients and physicians in order to decrease the incidence of endocarditis and prosthetic-related complications such as thromboembolism, and secondly on earlier intervention when symptoms or objective signs of LV dysfunction are observed in patients with known valve disease.

In the unfortunate case of presentation only in the acute stage, the key to success is establishing a rapid diagnosis and evaluation of the risk. Echocardiography will remain the preferred tool besides clinical assessment. It is expected that improvements in imaging, using three-dimensional techniques, will improve its performance. Risk stratification can also be improved by elaborating risk scores specific to valve surgery which have to be tested prospectively in a large contemporary patient population. It is likely that surgical valve replacement will remain the preferred treatment in such situations; however, further improvement in conservative surgical techniques is to be expected, as well as developments in percutaneous interventional techniques. PMC will remain the established treatment for MS in most cases. TAVI is likely to become widely used in the emergency treatment of AS, and this is also likely to be the case for acute dysfunction of bioprostheses excluding acute endocarditis and thrombosis.

The future of percutaneous mitral valve repair globally and especially in this setting is not clear at presents; however, it may well be that percutaneous mitral valve replacement will have a role in the future.

Finally, continuous improvements are to be expected in the pre-, peri-, and postoperative/interventional care of these very high risk patients.

Further reading

American College of Cardiology/American Heart Association Task Force on Practice Guidelines, *et al.* ACC/AHA 2006 guidelines for the management of patients with valvular heart disease. *Circulation* 2006;**114**:e84–231.

Botelho-Nevers E, Thuny F, Casalta JP, *et al.* Dramatic reduction in infective endocarditis-related mortality with a management-based approach. *Arch Intern Med* 2009;**169**:1290–1298.

Habib G, Hoen B, Tornos P, *et al.* Guidelines on the prevention, diagnosis, and treatment of infective endocarditis (new version 2009): the Task Force on the Prevention, Diagnosis, and Treatment of Infective Endocarditis of the European Society of Cardiology (ESC). *Eur Heart J* 2009;**30**:2369–2413.

Iung B, Baron G, Butchart EG, *et al.* A prospective survey of patients with valvular heart disease in Europe: The EuroHeart Survey on Valvular Heart Disease. *Eur Heart J* 2003;**24**:1231–1243.

Laplace G, Lafitte S, Labeque JN, *et al.* Clinical significance of early thrombosis after prosthetic mitral valve replacement: a postoperative monocentric study of 680 patients. *J Am Coll Cardiol* 2004;**43**:1283–1290.

Russo A, Suri RM, Grigioni F, *et al.* Clinical outcome after surgical correction of mitral regurgitation due to papillary muscle rupture. *Circulation* 2008;**118**:1528–1534.

Stout KK, Verrier ED. Acute valvular regurgitation. *Circulation* 2009;**119**:3232–3241.

Thuny F, Beurtheret S, Mancini J, *et al.* The timing of surgery influences mortality, morbidity in adults with severe complicated infective endocarditis: a propensity analysis. *Eur Heart J* 2009 Mar 26. [Epub ahead of print].

Vahanian A, Alfieri O, Al-Attar N, *et al.* Transcatheter valve implantation for patients with aortic stenosis: a position statement from the European Association of Cardio-Thoracic Surgery (EACTS) and the European Society of Cardiology (ESC), in collaboration with the European Association of Percutaneous Cardiovascular Interventions (EAPCI). *Eur Heart J* 2008;**29**:1463–1470.

Vahanian A, Baumgartner H, Bax J, *et al.* Guidelines on the management of valvular heart disease: The Task Force on the Management of Valvular Heart Disease of the European Society of Cardiology. *Eur Heart J* 2007;**28**:230–268.

Additional online material

57.1 Severe mitral regurgitation due to papillary muscle rupture during acute MI

➲ For additional multimedia materials please visit the online version of the book (✍ http://www.esciacc.oxfordmedicine.com).

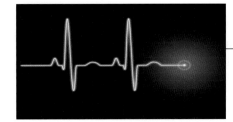

CHAPTER 58

Congenital heart disease in adults

Susanna Price, Brian F. Keogh, and Lorna Swan

Contents

Summary

The number of patients with congenital heart disease surviving to adulthood is increasing, with many requiring ongoing medical attention. Although recommendations are that these patients should be cared for in specialist centres, the clinical state of the acutely unwell patient may preclude transfer prior to instigation of life-saving treatment. Although the principles of resuscitation in this patient population differ little from those with acquired heart disease, the acutely unwell adult congenital heart disease (ACHD) patient presents a challenge, with potential pitfalls in examination, assessment/monitoring, and intervention. Key to avoiding error are to know the primary pathophysiology, any interventions that have been undertaken, residual lesions present (static or dynamic), and the normal physiological status for that patient; to determine the precise cause for acute deterioration; and to appreciate the effects (detrimental or otherwise) that any supportive and/or therapeutic interventions might have. Expert advice should be sought at the earliest opportunity.

Introduction

The number of adult patients with congenital heart disease (CHD) is estimated at 20 000 in the United Kingdom today, and is expected to increase at a rate of around 2500 per year [1, 2]. Many at the more complex end of the spectrum will inevitably require ongoing medical attention, presenting not only to specialist centres for repeat surgery or catheter interventions, but also to their local hospitals, particularly when more acutely unwell. Urgent/emergency medical admissions in the adult congenital heart disease (ACHD) population are usually for common cardiological indications (e.g. arrhythmia and heart failure).

It is generally recommended that ACHD patients be managed in specialist cardiac centres, but on occasions the acute nature of the admission and the clinical status of the patient may preclude transfer [3]. Thus, knowledge of the principles and potential pitfalls of immediate assessment and intervention in the acutely unwell ACHD patient is important for all cardiologists involved in acute cardiac care, as failure to recognize and appropriately manage seemingly benign conditions may have catastrophic consequences. This chapter will outline these principles, and the common causes for presentation to the acute cardiac care unit/ intensive cardiac care unit (ICCU), in particular where they differ from standard care. The general, critical care and postoperative management of the ACHD patient are considered the remit of experts in CHD, and are therefore beyond the scope of this chapter.

Classification and principles

CHD is generally divided into simple, moderately complex, and complex [4] (⊃Table 58.1; see also ⊃ *The ESC Textbook of Cardiovascular Medicine*, Chapter 10). In the critically ill ACHD patient, mortality and morbidity have been shown to increase with increasing complexity [5], and expert advice should always be sought, particularly at the more complex end of the spectrum. The first principles of assessment and treatment of the acutely unwell ACHD patient include:

◆ Understanding the cardiopulmonary anatomy, including the primary lesion(s), effects of any previous intervention(s), and presence of any residual lesion(s).

◆ Appreciating the normal physiology of each individual patient, including heart rate, systemic blood pressure, oxygen saturations, haemoglobin concentration, and pulmonary artery pressures.

◆ Diagnosing the underlying cause for the acute deterioration.

◆ Anticipating the effects (beneficial or otherwise) that supportive and/or therapeutic interventions may have on the circulation. This is of particular importance in the univentricular circulation, and/or in the presence of significant pulmonary hypertension.

The more common interventions in patients with complex ACHD are shown in ⊃ Table 58.2. All patients on admission to the ICCU should have an electrocardiogram, chest radiograph, standard labs, and, where indicated, haematinics (if cyanotic, with automated electronic particle counts), coagulation screen (citrate adjusted if erythrocytotic), pregnancy test (women of child-bearing age), blood cultures, serum/faecal α_1-antitrypsin (Fontan circulation with ascites), transthoracic echocardiogram (new/acute deterioration). In general, the principles of monitoring do not differ from patients with acquired cardiac disease, but potential pitfalls are outlined in ⊃ Table 58.3.

Clinical presentations

The most common acute presentations in different groups of ACHD patients relate to arrhythmia, ventricular failure, and endocarditis. Although less common, other potentially catastrophic complications of CHD (i.e. haemoptysis, syncope, cerebrovascular accident) may present acutely to the non-ACHD cardiologist. The common indications for acute admission related to the relevant ACHD diagnosis are shown in ⊃Table 58.4. Many admissions can be managed initially in the ICCU; however, in all cases the patient should be discussed early with an expert in ACHD, and where there is not immediate improvement in clinical status in response to therapeutic interventions, consideration should be made for transfer to a higher intensity of care. As with non-ACHD patients, when considering transfer to tertiary level care, the appropriateness of transfer should be considered, taking into account the potential reversibility of any deterioration and the patient's wishes, where known.

Arrhythmia

Arrhythmias are an inevitable part of the long-term sequelae of many ACHD patients, occurring in 5–50% at long-term follow-up [6–11]. The diagnosis may prove difficult because of the underlying anatomical and electrophysiological abnormalities, and may be associated with significant haemodynamic compromise at only modest elevations of heart rate. In all cases a 12-lead ECG should be obtained and compared with previous recordings. In the more complex patients the unpredictable response to anaesthetic and sedative agents and to direct current (DC) cardioversion, and the difficulty of obtaining access to the heart for transvenous pacing, means that cardioversion is not without significant risk. However, thromboembolic complications are common, particularly in the Fontan circulation where these contribute to late mortality [12, 13], and progressive haemodynamic deterioration may be catastrophic, meaning that any delay in anticoagulation and cardioversion may also put the patient at risk. Where haemodynamic compromise is significant, urgent cardioversion should be undertaken; however, sedation and anaesthesia will reduce sympathetic and vasomotor tone. These effects can be profound in a sympathetically driven circulation, and may result in major circulatory collapse, necessitating cardioversion without delay, as inotropic agents may simply potentiate the arrhythmia and pressor agents worsen atrioventricular valve regurgitation/ pulmonary hypertension where present. External pacing facilities must always be available, as access for transvenous pacing may be obstructed (multiple previous surgeries)

Table 58.1 Classification of congenital heart disease

Complexity of disease	Native disease	Repaired conditions
Simple	Isolated congenital AV disease	Previously ligated/occluded PDA
	Isolated congenital MV disease	Fully repaired secundum/SV ASD
	Isolated PFO/ASD	Repaired VSD with residua
	Isolated small VSD	
	Mild pulmonary stenosis	
Moderately severe	Aorto-left ventricular fistulae	
	Anomalous pulmonary venous drainage, partial or total atrioventricular canal defects (partial or complete)	
	Ostium primum ASD	
	Ebsteins's anomaly	
	Coarctation of the aorta	
	Tetralogy of Fallot	
	Pulmonary valve regurgitation (moderate to severe)	
	RVOTO	
	Aortic regurgitation	
	PDA (not closed)	
	Mitral disease	
	Subvalvar or supravalvar aortic stenosis (except HOCM)	
	Subaortic stenosis	
	VSD with absent valve or valves straddling TV/MV	
	Sinus of Valsalva fistula/aneurysm	
	Sinus venosus ASD	
	Infundibular RVOTO of significance	
Complex	Conduits, valved or nonvalved	
	Cyanotic congenital heart (all forms)	
	Double-outlet ventricle	
	Eisenmenger's syndrome	
	Fontan procedure	
	Mitral atresia	
	Single ventricle (double inlet or outlet, common or primitive)	
	Pulmonary atresia (all forms)	
	Pulmonary vascular obstructive disease	
	Transposition of the great arteries	
	Tricuspid atresia	
	Truncus arteriosus/hemitruncus	
	Other abnormalities of atrioventricular or ventriculoarterial connection not included above	

ASD, atrial septal defect; AV, aortic valve; MV, mitral valve; PDA, patent ductus arteriosus; PFO, patent foramen ovale;RVOTO, right ventricular outflow tract obstruction; TV, tricuspid valve. VSD, ventricular septal defect.

or impossible (Fontan/total cavopulmonary connection circulation), and if anticoagulation has been subtherapeutic intravenous heparin should be administered. Caution should be exercised when prescribing antiarrhythmics to patients with complex anatomy, as the degree of conduction system disease and ventricular pathology is often extensive. Polypharmacy should be avoided, and early referral for electrophysiological assessment should be considered.

Pharmacological treatment of arrhythmias is discussed in detail in ➲ Chapters 54 and 55.

Table 58.2 Common interventions in complex ACHD

Procedure	Corrective/palliative	Details	Aim
Blalock–Taussig shunt	Palliative	Anastamosis between subclavian and ipsilateral pulmonary artery	Increase/provide pulmonary blood flow
PA band	Palliative	Palliative. Surgically created main PA stenosis	Protect lungs against high pulmonary blood flow and blood pressure
Mustard/Senning (TGA)	Palliative	Atrial switch, with venous return redirected to contralateral ventricle	Relief of cyanosis (but morphological right ventricle supports systemic circulation)
Arterial switch (TGA)	Corrective	Reattachment of great arteries to contralateral ventricles with coronary artery implantation	Relief of cyanosis with restoration of normal circulation (morphological left ventricle supports systemic circulation)
Fontan	Palliative	Surgical diversion of systemic venous return to pulmonary artery	Relief of cyanosis and/or restoration of pulmonary circulation
TCPC	Palliative	Surgical diversion of IVC and SVC flow to PA	Relief of cyanosis and/or restoration of pulmonary circulation

IVC, inferior vena cava; PA, pulmonary artery; SVC, superior vena cava; TCPC, total cavo-pulmonary connection; TGA, transposition of the great arteries.

Atrial tachycardia

Atypical 'flutter' (or intra-atrial re-entry tachycardia) is a common cause of arrhythmia in those with previous atrial surgical scars or with atrial dilatation (e.g. Ebstein's anomaly) and flutter waves may be slow, inhomogeneous, and therefore difficult to diagnose [8–11]. Chemical cardioversion is often unsuccessful, and prompt electrical cardioversion is the treatment of choice; however, acute catheter ablation

Table 58.3 Pitfalls in monitoring and assessment in ACHD

Parameter	Previous intervention/pathology	Comment
Blood pressure	Previous classical/modified BT shunt	Will under-read. Place catheter/cuff on contralateral arm
	Previous bilateral shunts	Lower body pressure measurements more accurate
	Previous coarctation/residual coarctation, previous femoral bypass/multiple cardiac catheterizations	Lower limb pressures under-represent central pressure
	Radial line cannulation/surgical cutdown (esp. neonatal)	Ulnar dominant/absent radial artery. Cuff accurate, avoid ulnar cannulation
Circulating volume	Cyanotic ACHD	Tolerate hypovolaemia poorly
	Univentricular heart	Tolerate hypovolaemia poorly, but may have significantly impaired ventricular function/AV valve regurgitation
	Fontan/TCPC	'CVP' often misleading as represents pulmonary artery pressures
	Pulmonary vein stenosis	Basal crepitations not indicative of systemic ventricular failure
Pulse oximetry	Compromised arterial supply/ systemic hypotension	Digital oximeters may be unreliable, use central oximetry (ear lobe sensors/reflectance oximeters)
	Cyanotic ACHD	Oximetry may be inaccurate (calibrated to be accurate at SpO_2 >80%)
Cardiac output	Tricuspid/pulmonary atresia/Fontan/TCPC	PA catheter placement not possible
	Intra-/extracardiac shunts	PA catheter unreliable
	Chronic low CO state	Oesophageal Doppler unreliable (small aorta)
Pacing	Multiple previous access, cutdowns, etc	Expert in access required
	Fontan, TCPC, tricuspid/pulmonary atresia	Standard transvenous pacing is not possible. In an emergency transcutaneous pacing may be required
ECG	Massive atrial enlargement and univentricular circulation	Atrial tachycardia may be disguised as sinus tachycardia. High index of suspicion, comparison with previous ECGS, CSM/adenosine/pacemaker interrogation may be useful
INR	Cyanotic patients	If haematocrit >60, need citrate adjusted samples for accurate measurement

CO; cardiac output; CSM; carotid sinus massage; CVP; central venous pressure; INR; international normalized ratio; PA; pulmonary artery; SpO_2; oxygen saturations; TCPC; total cavo-pulmonary connection.

Table 58.4 Common acute presentations in patients with ACHD

Diagnosis	Acute presentation	Comments
ASD	Atrial arrhythmia	May occur whether repaired/unrepaired Standard antiarrhythmic treatment recommended acutely Should be referred for further investigation/intervention
	LVF	Older patients may have significant LV disease
	Pulmonary hypertension	May be disproportionate to the size of the shunt May persist after closure
VSD	Endocarditis	On VSD, VSD patch, and/or related anomaly (e.g. bicuspid aortic valve) Early liaison with multidisciplinary ACHD team recommended
	Unrepaired: LVF	If unrepaired, treat in standard way and refer for further investigation/intervention
AVSD	Unrepaired: LVF	If VSD small, may present with ventricular failure and/or left AV valve regurgitation Degree of pulmonary hypertension key Urgent treatment is standard, with early discussion with ACHD specialist
	Unrepaired: Eisenmenger's	Surgical repair contraindicated Standard Eisenmenger's management Seek expert ACHD advice
	Endocarditis	Diagnosis may be challenging due to calcification related to previous repair: expert echocardiography indicated Early liaison with multidisciplinary ACHD team recommended
AS	Angina/dyspnoea/ syncope	Heralds rapidly worsening prognosis, refer for work-up for urgent surgery Symptomatic 'low gradient' AS should be urgently referred for expert investigation
Sub-AS	Angina/dyspnoea/syncope	May re-present after previous successful intervention Early liaison with multidisciplinary ACHD team recommended
Coarctation	Uncontrolled upper body hypertension	
	CVA	Association with berry aneurysm: urgent neurological investigation required
Marfan's	Aortic dissection	Standard immediate management required Redissection can occur
RVOTO	Dyspnoea/syncope	Higher degrees of obstruction usually better tolerated than left-sided lesions Symptoms may be precipitated by development of arrhythmia
	Endocarditis	Echocardiographic diagnosis may be challenging Early liaison with multidisciplinary ACHD team recommended
Tetralogy of Fallot	VF/VT and aborted sudden cardiac death	Atrial and ventricular arrhythmias are common SCD reported in 1–6% (VF/VT) Standard emergency treatment and early liaison with ACHD specialist recommended
PA+VSD	Haemoptysis	Usually due to rupture of small collaterals or thrombus in a small pulmonary artery
	Heart failure	Response to standard dilators and inotropic agents unpredictable May be precipitated by new arrhythmia: underlying cause should be sought & discussion with ACHD specialist recommended
TGA + Mustard/ Senning	Atrial tachyarrhythmias	Generally tolerated poorly (systemic right ventricle) so early cardioversion recommended (see text) May precipitate rapid decline in systemic ventricular function
	Sinus node dysfunction	Pacing specialist intervention in these patients
	Systemic AV valve regurgitation	Associated with systemic ventricular failure Support with standard agents recommended IABP may not be helpful in younger patients (NB may also have small aortic diameter)
TGA + Rastelli	Syncope/dyspnoea	Atrial and ventricular arrhythmias common Conduit stenosis may occur and be severe
TGA + arterial switch	Ventricular failure and arrhythmias	Generally relate to inadequate coronary perfusion (usually longstanding), but coronary investigation is indicated and stenting/surgery recommended for ongoing ischaemia Standard support recommended initially Early referral to ACHD specialist recommended

(Continued)

Table 58.4 Common acute presentations in patients with ACHD

Diagnosis	Acute presentation	Comments
ccTGA	Syncope	AV block not uncommon
	Heart failure	May be presentation in young adults with undiagnosed ccTGA Immediate standard therapy, and referral to ACHD specialist recommended
Cyanotic patients	Hyperviscosity symptoms	Unusual if iron replete and with HCT <65%
	Dyspnoea/fatigue	Commonly related to iron deficiency
	Haemoptysis	Usually represents pulmonary haemorrhage (see text)
	CVA	Degree of erythrocytosis not risk factor per se Risk increased in iron deficiency with inappropriate venesection
	Arrhythmia	Maintain sinus rhythm where possible Avoid transvenous pacing leads Anticoagulation individualised to patient
Univentricular circulation	Arrhythmia	May be challenging to diagnose (see text) Restore sinus rhythm as soon as possible Early referral for expert ACHD opinion recommended
	Heart failure	Cause for underlying deterioration should be aggressively sought Response to standard inotropic and dilator agents unpredictable (see text) Early referral for expert ACHD opinion recommended

ACHD, adult congenital heart disease; AS, aortic stenosis; ASD, atrial septal defect; AV valve, atrioventricular valve; AVSD, atrioventricular septal defect; ccTGA, congenitally corrected transposition of the great arteries (or double discordance); CVA, cerebrovascular accident (including transient ischaemic attack and prolonged residual ischaemic neurological deficit); HCT, haematocrit; LV left ventricle; LVF, left ventricular failure; PA+VSD, pulmonary atresia + ventricular septal defect; RVOTO, right ventricular outflow tract obstruction; SCD, sudden cardiac death; TGA, transposition of the great arteries; VF, ventricular fibrillation; VSD, ventricular septal defect; VT, ventricular tachycardia.

may be an alternative. Postcardioversion referral for elective ablation should be considered routinely [14, 15].

Ventricular tachycardia

Ventricular tachycardia (VT) is more common with previous surgical ventriculotomies and/or impaired ventricular function, and patients with a broad QRS complex [8–11, 16, 17] appear to be at increased risk. The treatment of acute VT is similar to that of ischaemic VT, but the indications for insertion of an implantable cardioverter/defibrillator in ACHD patients remain contentious. The treatment of a VT storm is as in acquired heart disease (➲ Chapter 55).

Arrhythmia in complex congenital heart disease

Sustained arrhythmia in complex CHD should be treated urgently, even where the patient appears well, as rapidly progressive and profound haemodynamic deterioration can and does occur, particularly in those with a univentricular (including Fontan) or Eisenmenger circulation (see ➲ Table 58.4). Here cardioversion should not be delayed where anticoagulation has been subtherapeutic. As the diagnosis can be challenging, rate control is rarely appropriate, standard guidelines do not apply, and expert advice should be sought urgently. The priorities are to assess the degree of haemodynamic compromise, ascertain the urgency for cardioversion, determine the need for anticoagulation/stroke risk, and ensure that back-up pacing and treatment by the most

experienced clinicians are available. Cardioversion should in general be performed on the day of presentation.

Pacing

The most common pacing emergencies presenting to the ICCU are new high-level atrioventricular (AV) block, and lead failure/battery depletion in patients with existing pacemakers (see also ➲ Chapter 25). Infusions of isoprenaline/external pacing may stabilize the situation temporarily but are not reliable. The patient's anatomy may not allow transvenous pacing, access may be challenging, right-sided valves may have been repaired/replaced and, residual shunts may complicate the issue further (➲ Fig. 58.1). Oesophageal pacing, retrograde transaortic pacing, and emergency epicardial pacing are all alternatives.

Ventricular failure

The causes of acute/decompensated ventricular failure in the ACHD population also include those found in acquired heart disease. Although ischaemic heart disease has been anecdotally considered rare in these patients, with an ageing population the incidence is likely to increase. Further, as patients with previous arterial switch surgery are now reaching adulthood the incidence of ventricular failure secondary to suboptimal coronary artery perfusion is likely to increase [18]. In patients with an acute deterioration in ventricular function presenting with failure, as in all patients, the

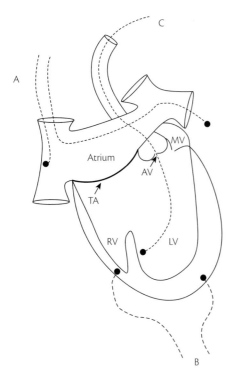

Figure 58.1 Emergency pacing in patients with a Fontan-type circulation: (A) Transvenous pacing. The atrial lead will function relatively normally. However, a ventricular lead will go through the Fontan anastomosis (RA to PA) and end up in the pulmonary circulation. (B) Epicardial pacing requires a surgical approach with either a limited thoracotomy or even a sternotomy if the anatomy is complex. (C) Retrograde pacing through the aortic valve may be associated with damage to the aortic valve and the risk of systemic embolism.

Table 58.5 Lesions that may present with left (or systemic) sided heart failure

Lesion	Examples/notes
New volume-loading shunt	e.g. acute VSD patch leak or ruptured Sinus of Valsalva aneurysm
Mitral or left AV valve disease	May be dynamic or static
Acute valvular volume loading	e.g. aortic or left AV valve regurgitation
Obstructive lesions	Decompensation to heart failure rare in young adults
Ventricular disease (systemic RV)	Mustard/Senning or congenitally corrected transposition
Late systemic LV dysfunction in elderly patient	e.g. older tetralogy patient
Pulmonary vein obstruction	May mimic pulmonary oedema
Ischaemia	e.g. coronary anomaly (i.e ALCAPA), previous aortic root surgery including arterial switch
Arrhythmia	New arrhythmia in previously stable patient, particularly in univentricular circulation, or systemic right ventricle

AV, atrioventricular; ALCAPA, anomalous left coronary artery from pulmonary artery; LV, left ventricle; VSD, ventricular septal defect.

balloon counterpulsion (IABP), particularly in younger patients, may be ineffective, and the use of mechanical and electrical interventions to support the failing ACHD heart remains unproven.

The failing morphological right ventricle

This may be subpulmonary, systemic, or the only effective ventricle. When in the subpulmonary position, the failing right heart may be supported using standard inotropic agents while avoiding pulmonary vasoconstrictors and reducing right ventricular afterload (including the use of pulmonary vasodilators, bronchodilators where relevant, and aggressive drainage of pulmonary effusions). Treatment of the failing systemic right ventricle (congenitally corrected transposition of the great arteries, and transposition following Mustard/Senning procedures) is challenging. There may be extensive subendocardial fibrosis even with angiographically normal coronary arteries, and although standard therapy (including pharmacological and mechanical support) may be used, these may be less effective than when used to treat the failing morphological left ventricle. The roles of newer inotropic agents and multisite pacing remain uncertain.

The failing univentricular heart

Assessment of univentricular function is challenging, particularly in the presence of inotropic support and

underlying cause should always be sought and treated where possible. The main causes of failure of the systemic ventricle in ACHD are listed in ● Table 58.5. Failure of the subpulmonary ventricle is common in ACHD patients, presenting subacutely with fluid overload, ascites, anorexia, weight loss, deranged liver function, and cardiac cachexia. Causes include previous cardiac surgery, pulmonary hypertension, atrial septal defects (in elderly patients), large residual intracardiac shunts, tricuspid and pulmonary valve disease. Failure of the subpulmonary ventricle is rare in the setting of isolated pulmonary stenosis unless it is very advanced. As in acquired heart failure anaemia, hyponatraemia and an elevated creatinine and B-type natriuretic peptide (BNP) are all markers of a poor prognosis [19–21]. In patients with a Fontan circulation, right-sided failure may represent obstruction in the circulation, arrhythmia, or protein-losing enteropathy and expert input should be sought [22].

When treatable causes have been excluded, management is directed towards support of the failing ventricle; however, standard interventions may acutely destabilize the ACHD patient, be less effective, and should be used with care (● Table 58.6) [23]. Specifically, the use of intra-aortic

Table 58.6 Heart failure drugs in congenital heart disease

Drug	Pros	Cons
Loop diuretics	Highly effective in symptom control	Caution if preload dependent Caution with renal function Absorption may be impaired in chronically oedematous Unlikely to impact on mortality
Spironolactone	Effective for right-sided failure symptom control	Mortality benefits in this group unknown
ACEI	Treatment of ventricular dysfunction in ACHD	Mortality benefits in ACHD? Beware if preload dependent Beware renal function Beware if obstructive lesions
ARB	Used if ACEI intolerant Rarely as add on therapy Possible role in Marfan's	As above No evidence base
Beta-blockers	Antiarrhythmic Antihypertensive Used for HR control (e.g.MS) probable benefits in heart failure in ACHD	Mortality benefits in ACHD? Caution regarding conduction defects and in slowing the HR in patients with restrictive physiology
Digoxin	Rate control of permanent AF Parallel therapy to other antiarrhythmias	Often over prescribed in ACHD Inotropic benefits unclear
Nitrates		Rarely used clinically in ACHD Patients often borderline hypotensive
IV inotropes	Perioperative role	Very limited data in setting of heart failure

ACEI, angiotensin converting enzyme inhibitor; AF, atrial fibrillation; ARB, angiotensin receptor blocker; HR, heart rate; IV, intravenous; MS, mitral stenosis.

tachycardia, and expert echocardiography is indicated, with comparison against the most recently available studies. The commonest cause of acute deterioration in this context is tachyarrhythmia. The choice and route of administration of supportive agents is challenging. Air entrainment via vascular access may result in paradoxical embolism, and all venous lines should have an air filter *in situ*. Choice of inotropic/vasoactive agents is determined by the nature of the pulmonary connections.

The unprotected pulmonary circulation with Eisenmenger physiology should be managed to minimize any increase in pulmonary artery pressure. Where the pulmonary circulation is protected (pulmonary banding/stenosis) the relative effects of pulmonary/systemic constriction/dilatation differ from cases where the pulmonary circulation is dependent upon systemic-pulmonary collaterals or shunts. Here, a small increase in pulmonary vascular resistance will result in a reduction in pulmonary blood flow and consequent desaturation. By contrast, an increase in systemic vascular resistance may result in an increase in systemic–pulmonary shunting and a fall in cardiac output. The haemodynamic effects of oxygen administration may also alter the balance between pulmonary and systemic circulation. Support of the failing univentricular heart is therefore challenging, and requires specialist expertise.

Endocarditis

Suspected endocarditis (see ➲ Chapter 57) is a relatively common reason for acute admission in ACHD patients. As with the non-ACHD population, presenting symptoms depend upon the underlying cardiac diagnosis, the degree of haemodynamic upset, the time course of the illness, and virulence of the infective organism [24,25]. Key in the complex patient is to have a low threshold of suspicion in the setting of a new haemodynamic lesion and/or functional deterioration. Significant haemodynamic deterioration is generally due to severe valvular dysfunction; however, multiorgan failure or infection-related complications (acute embolic events/heart block) may also occur. The commonest sites of infection include the stenosed pulmonary value/valved conduit, residual ventricular septal defect, or prosthetic valves [23, 24] and therefore initial evaluation requires highly specialist imaging with transthoracic and/or transoesophageal echocardiography (➲ Table 58.7, 🎥 58.1) and on occasion cardiac magnetic resonance (CMR), CT scanning, or nuclear medicine. Of note, the 'endocarditis' may be extracardiac. Patients with cyanotic heart disease are immunocompromised and unusual organisms (e.g. Q fever or fungal infections) should therefore be considered. Further, there should be a low threshold for total body imaging as cerebral and lung abscesses are not uncommon.

Table 58.7 Assessment of suspected endocarditis

Investigation	Details
Blood work	Blood cultures FBC with differential WCC Renal and liver function Immunoglobulin, antibodies (if diagnosis unclear) C-reactive protein (serial) BNP (risk stratify in the setting of haemodynamic compromise)
Specimens	Urine—urinalysis, culture and sensitivities (C&S) Other microbiology specimens as appropriate
ECG	Changes, especially new conduction defects
Imaging	CXR—Changes in cardiothoracic ration, parenchymal changes Echo—initially transthoracic but low threshold for trans-oesphageal imaging CT/MRI—for complications such as brain abscess or splenic infarcts

BNP, B-type natriuretic peptide; C&S, culture and sensitivity; CXR, chest radiograph; Echo, echocardiogram; FBC, full blood count; WCC, white cell count.

In all cases, a multidisciplinary approach is key, and advice from an ACHD surgeon should be sought early.

Haemoptysis

Haemoptysis in an ACHD patient should be considered a serious event, and early transfer to high-level care should be considered as even a minor bleed may herald a further larger bleed that may compromise the airway. In patients with Eisenmenger physiology, haemoptysis accounts for 11–15% of deaths [26]. The principles of early management include airway protection (possibly with insertion of a double-lumen endotracheal tube) and restoration of circulating volume. Early discussion with anaesthetic colleagues and transfer to tertiary care may be appropriate, as most deaths in massive haemoptysis are a result of loss of airway rather than blood. Catastrophic bleeding occurs in the context of rupture of a high-pressure vessel, e.g. a hypertensive pulmonary artery or from the aorta (Marfan's/coarctation). Specialist investigations with CT and/or angiography with a view to embolization of the bleeding vessel may be possible, but their performance remains highly specialized. Bronchoscopy carries significant risk, and seldom provides useful additional information.

Conclusion

Management of the ACHD patient on the ICCU should ideally involve a specialist team; however, patients will inevitably increasingly present to their local hospital for acute care. Where required early and appropriate assessment and management can and should be undertaken by cardiologists in the ICCU in order to avoid inappropriate and potentially detrimental delay in treatment.

Personal perspective

Future developments in the acute cardiac care of the ACHD population are likely to encompass advances in critical care, cardiology, and information technology. Acute care of the ACHD patient is a much neglected specialty within the fields of cardiology, critical care, and anaesthesia. Current recommendations are that these patients should be cared for within specialist hospitals, but with increasing numbers at the more complex end of the spectrum surviving to adulthood it is inevitable that they will present to nonspecialist centres requiring potentially life-saving treatment. Although this is addressed in curricula, the complexity of many of these patients demands immediate and expert input for optimal management. Advances in telemedicine will improve access to real-time expert advice and image interpretation, even at the more remote hospitals.

In the critically ill patient, optimization of the circulation is achieved by adjustment of global cardiac output, oxygen supply, and delivery. Development of more targeted monitoring aimed to evaluate specific organ systems that are difficult to support (i.e. liver, brain, and intestine) and that may be the drivers of multiorgan failure will revolutionize critical care management. The main indications for ICCU admission remain arrhythmia, heart failure, and suspected endocarditis. Advances in specialist electrophysiological interventions in the ACHD population will potentially reduce the frequency of admissions, even at the more complex end of the spectrum. Development of less cardiotoxic pharmacological support, together with more effective therapy for pulmonary hypertension, may reduce the incidence of heart failure, and enable the acute cardiologist to administer more effective therapy. Mechanical circulatory support continues to advance, and may further improve the mortality and morbidity in this patient population.

Further reading

ACC/AHA 2008 Guidelines for the management of adults with congenital heart disease. *Circulation* 2008;**118**:e714–e833.

Engelfriet P, Boersma E, Oechslin E, *et al.* The spectrum of adult congenital heart disease in Europe: morbidity and mortality in a 5 year follow-up period. The Euro Heart Survey on adult congenital heart disease. *Eur Heart J* 2005;**26**:2325–2333.

Gatzoulis M, Swan L, Therrien J, Pantely G. *Adult congenital heart disease: a practical guide*, Blackwell, Oxford, 2005.

Griffiths M, Cordingley J, Price S. *Cardiovascular critical care*, Wiley, Chichester, 2010.

Task Force on the Management of Grown Up Congenital Heart Disease of the European Society of Cardiology. Management of Grown Up Congenital Heart Disease. *Eur Heart J* (2003);**24**:1035–1084 [New guidelines To be published 2010?]

Online resource

🐾 European Society of Cardiology Guidelines on Management of Grown-Up Congenital Heart Disease. http://www.escardio.org/guidelines-surveys/esc-guidelines/Pages/grown-up-congenital-heart-disease.aspx

➲ For additional multimedia materials please visit the online version of the book (🐾 http://www.esciacc.oxfordmedicine.com).

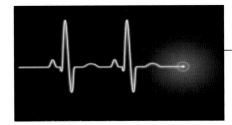

CHAPTER 59

Aortic emergencies

Laurent de Kerchove, Manuel Pirotte,
and Gébrine el Khoury

Contents

Summary

Acute aortic dissections are the leading and most feared aortic emergencies. They have a dreadful mortality rate, so accurate diagnosis and immediate treatment are mandatory. The key point of a life-saving management strategy is the distinction between acute type A dissection, uncomplicated type B dissection, and complicated type B dissection, those including contained ruptured aorta (severe pleural effusion) and/or malperfusion syndrome (by end-organ ischaemia: paraplegia, intestinal ischaemia renal insufficiency, limb ischaemia). Type A generally requires urgent surgery. Uncomplicated type B dissections are treated conservatively, while complicated type B dissections are currently managed by means of minimally invasive endovascular techniques possibly associated with a tight surgical time (e.g. in case of limb ischaemia). Surgical repair of type A dissection consists of the replacement of the ascending aorta. The repair is extended proximally towards the aortic root and valve, and distally towards the aortic arch in function of the lesions found and the clinical presentation of the patient (haemodynamic status, age, comorbidities). The emergence of endovascular techniques and the contribution of thoracic endovascular aortic repair (TEVAR), with thoracic stent-grafts deployed from the proximal descending aorta to reopen the true lumen and to seal the entry tear in type B dissections, have revolutionized the surgical treatment of this condition and thus the patient's immediate and medium-term survival.

In the same group of acute aortic syndromes, traumatic ruptures of the aortic isthmus are also a life-threatening condition and account for one of the main cause of death at the time of traumatic accidents. As in the case of complicated type B dissections, introduction of aortic stent-grafts has changed the outcome of these patients.

Introduction

One of the first description of aortic dissection was made in 1760 by Nichols on the dead body of King George II [1]. Subsequently, Morgani [2] and Laennec [3] contributed to a better understanding of the disease process, but aortic dissection remained a post-mortem diagnosis until the early 20th century. Surgical approaches to aortic dissection began in 1935 with aortic fenestration to treat malperfusion syndrome [4]. In 1955, De Bakey was the first to report aortic repair operations for aortic dissections [5]. Since that time, developments in medical management and technology have contributed to improve outcomes of patients with aortic dissection.

Definition and classification

Acute aortic dissection may be defined as a sudden-onset event in which blood flow is redirected from the true aortic lumen through an intimal tear into the media of the aortic wall. The dissection plane rapidly separates inner from outer layers of the media along a variable length of the aorta. Dissection is considered acute within the 2 weeks immediately following the process; thereafter, the terms subacute or chronic are used.

The different types of aortic dissection are distinguished on basis of the location and extent of the dissection. Two classification systems are used in clinical practice: the De Bakey and the Stanford (➲ Fig. 59.1, ➲ Box 59.1). The De Bakey classification focuses more precisely on location and extension of the dissection. The Stanford system represents a functional classification based on the principle that the clinical behaviour of patients with aortic dissection is essentially determined by involvement of the ascending aorta [6]. The Stanford systems therefore represents a basic but important algorithm for initial patient care.

Incidence

As acute aortic dissection cause sudden death in many patients, the incidence in general population is difficult to estimate. An autopsy study has shown that up to 85% of acute aortic dissections were undiagnosed before death [7]. The incidence of aortic dissection is estimated at 2.6–3.5 cases per 100 000 person-years [8, 9].

Pathophysiology

Aetiology and anatomical findings

The main mechanism causing aortic dissection is a disruption of the intima (the primary tear). The intimal tear is generally located in the ascending aorta (usually the right anterior aspect) or in the upper descending aorta just beyond the origin of the left subclavian artery [7] (🎥 59.1). Less often, the intimal tear occurs in the aortic arch, or even more rarely in the distal portion of the descending thoracic or abdominal artery [10, 11]. The dissection progress generally distally (antegrade) but may also extend proximally (retrograde).

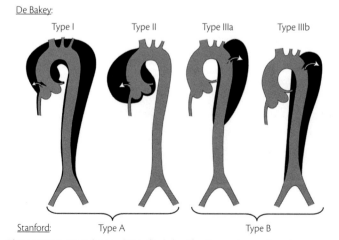

Figure 59.1 De Bakey and Stanford classification systems of aortic dissection.

> **Box 59.1** Classification of aortic dissection
>
> **De Bakey classification**
>
> - De Bakey type I dissection involves the ascending aorta, arch, and descending thoracic aorta
> - De Bakey type II dissection involves the ascending aorta only
> - De Bakey type III dissection involves the descending thoracic aorta; in type IIIa dissection is limited to thoracic aorta and in type IIIb it is extended to the abdominal aorta
>
> **Stanford classification**
>
> - Stanford type A includes any dissection involving the ascending aorta regardless of its extension to the arch or descending aorta
> - Stanford type B includes any dissection that does not involve the ascending aorta

Advanced imaging technologies have allowed to identify other mechanisms of dissection than the classical intimal tear [12, 13]. Intramural haematoma (IMH) is a CT imaging diagnosis made in 10–20% of the patients thought to have acute aortic dissection [14]. IMH may be considered as a variant as well as a precursor of aortic dissection. Originating from ruptured vasa vasorum of the media, the resulting IMH may provoke aortic wall infarct and secondary tear with evolution towards classic aortic dissection [13, 14]. IMH has grossly similar natural history to classic dissection, but spontaneous resorption has been reported in approximately 10% of cases [12, 15]. Typically associated with hypertension, IMH occurs more often in the descending aorta (50–85%) and is generally a more limited process [16].

Although atherosclerosis is not a predisposing lesion for aortic dissection, deep ulceration of atherosclerotic plaque can lead to IMH, aortic dissection, or perforation [17].

When dissection occurs, it creates a membrane floating between a true and a false aortic lumen. This membrane (the dissection 'flap') is composed of the intima and the inner thickness of the media. One wall of the false lumen consists of the dissection flap and the other of the outer thickness of the media and the adventitia. The latter may be extremely thin, and often ruptures into pericardium or pleural space (usually the left). If it does not rupture, however, blood may extravasate to form haemopericardium or haemothorax. The false lumen usually involves half to two-thirds of the circumference of the aorta. Often the distal false lumen communicates with the true lumen through one or more re-entry tear within the dissection flap. In other cases, the false lumen may end in a blind pocket which may then thrombose.

In the acute phase of dissection there is diffuse enlargement of the aorta, but the enlargement does not reach generally aneurysmal dimensions. During the following months, the dissection flap undergoes fibrous remodelling and become thicker and stronger. On the other hand, the outer wall of the false lumen remains relatively thin and weak, carrying a significant risk of progressive dilatation during the years following the acute event.

Malperfusion syndrome

The malperfusion syndrome related to acute aortic dissection corresponds to a mechanical obstruction of aortic side branches with end-organ ischaemia. Any distal organ may be affected (heart, brain, spinal cord, intestines, kidneys, limbs) (❖ Fig. 59.2). The mechanisms of obstruction are compression of the true lumen by the false lumen, or an intimal tear that creates an intraluminal flap, or intussusceptions of the intima (❖ Fig. 59.3). The resulting organ ischaemia depends on the degree and duration of the obstruction as well as the presence of a collateral circulation. In practice, the vascular harm is often subtotal and the clinical severity changes over the first few hours.

Risk factors

In many cases, the histological analysis of dissected aortic wall show only changes commensurate with the patient's age [18, 19]. This means that dissection may occur in essentially normal aortic wall, although several predisposing

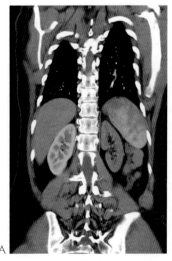
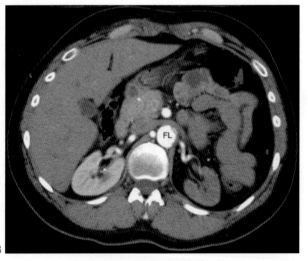

Figure 59.2 CT scan of an acute type B (De Bakey type IIIb) aortic dissection with kidney malperfusion syndrome: (a) reconstructed coronal view CT shows a 'switched-off' left kidney. (b) Malperfusion is explained by compression of the true lumen by the false lumen (FL); the left renal artery originates from the collapsed true lumen.

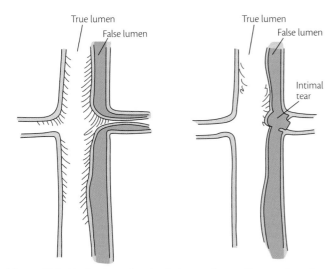

Figure 59.3 Mechanisms of malperfusion syndrome: diagram of aortic dissection. (A) An intact dissection membrane compresses the true lumen and causes malperfusion of a branch artery. (B) Rupture of the dissection membrane that may or may not restore blood flow to the branch. Reproduced with permission from Cohn LH, *Cardiac surgery in the adult*, McGraw-Hill Education, New York, 2008.

factors have been identified. Chronic arterial hypertension is the factor most often associated with dissection and is found in 70% of cases (➲ Table 59.1) [20]. Acute arterial hypertension, such as occurs in weightlifters and cocaine users, also predisposes to acute aortic dissection [21, 22]. Another important predisposing factor is connective tissues disorders such as Marfan's syndrome in which mutation of the fibrillin-1 gene results in an abnormal protein. Patients with Marfan's syndrome (1 per 5000 live births) generally develop aortic dilatation during second to the fourth decades of life and 20–40% of them experience aortic dissection [23, 24]. Ehlers–Danlos, Loeys–Dietz, Noonan's and Turner's syndromes are other connective tissue disorders which predispose to aortic dissection relatively early in life [25–28]. The frequently associated bicuspid aortic valve, ascending aorta dilatation, and coarctation are also predisposing factors [29, 30]. Familial aggregations of aortic dissection without discerned biochemical or genetic abnormalities also exist [31]. During pregnancy, the hypervolaemia and high cardiac output contribute, probably with other risk factors, to the increased incidence of dissection [32]. Catheterization procedures, aortic cannulation or cross-clamping during cardiac surgery, and placement of intra-aortic balloon pump (IABP) are all situations carrying a low risk of provoking iatrogenic aortic traumatism that may lead to dissection. Finally, closed chest trauma may rarely result in true aortic dissection.

Natural history and prognosis

Acute aortic dissection is the most lethal condition of the aorta. It is estimated that 40% of the patients suffering from acute aortic dissection die immediately. For patients who survive after the onset of dissection and reach hospital, the risk of death remains high but varies according to several risk factors. Hospital mortality is increased in older patients (≥70 years) and in patients who develop complications such as cardiac tamponade or severe hypotension with shock. Major organ malperfusion, such as cardiac ischaemia/infarction, stroke, renal failure, visceral ischaemia, or pulse deficit is another risk factor influencing survival [33, 34].

In Stanford type A aortic dissection, the mortality rate is estimated to be 1–2% per hour after onset of symptoms [7, 35]. Data from the International Registry of Acute Aortic Dissection (IRAD) show that in type A dissection, early surgical repair decreases in-hospital mortality by more than 50% in comparison to medical treatment alone (➲ Fig. 59.4). At 14 days, a repaired type A dissection has a mortality of 20% versus 49% for a nonrepaired one [20].

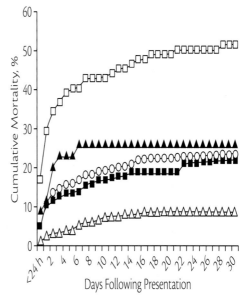

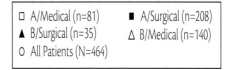

Figure 59.4 30-day mortality in 464 patients from the IRAD registry stratified by medical and surgical treatment in acute type A and type B dissection. Data issued from the International Registry of Aortic Dissection (IRAD).
Reproduced with permission from Hagan PG, Nienaber CA, Isselbacher EM, *et al*. The International Registry of Acute Aortic Dissection (IRAD): new insights into an old disease. *JAMA* 2000;**283**:897–903. Copyright 2000, American Medical Association. All rights reserved.

Table 59.1 Demographics and history of patients with acute aortic dissection

Category	No. [a] (%)	Type A, No. (%) (n = 289)	Type B, No. (%) (n = 175)	p value Type A vs B
Demographics				
Age, mean (SD). y	63.1 (14.0)	61.2(14.1)	66.3 (13.2)	<.001
Male sex	303 (65.3)	182 (63.0)	121 (69.1)	0.18
Referred from primary site to IRAD centre	280 (60.3)	177 (61.2)	103 (58.9)	0.61
Ethnicity (n = 407)				
White	337 (82.8)	205 (84.4)	132 (80.5)	
Asian	55 (13.5)	31 (12.8)	24 (14.6)	0.51
Black	7 (1.7)	2 (0.8)	5 (3.0)	
Other	8 (2.0)	5 (2.0)	3 (1.9)	
Patient history				
Marfan's syndrome	22/449 (4.9)	19(6.7)	3 (1.8)	0.02
Hypertension	326/452 (72.1)	194 (69.3)	132 (76.7)	0.08
Atherosclerosis	140/452 (31.01)	69 (24.4)	71 (42)	<0.001
Known aortic aneurysm	73/453 (16.1)	35 (12.4)	238 (2.2)	0.006
Prior aortic dissection	29/453 (6.4)	11 (3.9)	18 (10.6)	0.005
Diabetes mellitus	23/451 (5.1)	12 (4.3)	11 (6.6)	0.29
Prior cardiac surgery [b]	83 (17.9)	46 (15.9)	37 (21.1)	0.16
Aortic valve replacement	24/444 (5.4)	16 (5.8)	8 (4.8)	0.66
Aortic aneurysm and/or dissection	43/444 (9.7)	20 (7.2)	23 (14)	0.02
Coronary artery bypass graft surgery	19/442 (4.3)	14 (5)	5 |3.0i	0.32
Mitral valve surgery	3.444 1.0.7)	1 (0.3)	2 (0.1)	NA
Iatrogenic aortic dissection	20 (4.3)	14 (4.8)	6 (3.4)	0.47
Catheterization/PTCA	10/454 (2.2)	5 (1.7)	5 (2.8)	NA
Cardiac surgery	10/454 (2.2)	9 (3.1)	1 (0.6)	NA

IRAD, International Registry of Acute Aortic dissection; PTCA, percutaneous transluminal coronary angioplasty; NA. not applicable. Type A dissections involve the ascending aorta; and type B dissections occur distal to the left subclavian artery.

[a] Denominator of reported responses is given if different than stated in the column heading

[b] Prior cardiac surgery includes aortic valve surgery, coronary artery bypass graft surgery, aortic aneurysm and/or dissection, mitral valve surgery, or other aortic surgery.

Data from the International Registry of Aortic Dissection (IRAD). Reproduced with permission from Hagan PG, Nienaber CA, Isselbacher EM, et al. The International Registry of Acute Aortic Dissection (IRAD): new insights into an old disease. JAMA 2000;**283**:897–903. Copyright 2000, American Medical Association. All rights reserved.

From the same registry, data indicate that uncomplicated type A dissections have a 17% in-hospital mortality in comparison to 31% for complicated ones [36].

Acute type B dissection is less lethal than type A. Uncomplicated type B dissections, generally medically treated, have a relatively good prognosis with a 14-day mortality of less than 10%. Conversely, complicated type B dissections need surgical or endovascular repair and have much worst prognosis, with in-hospital mortality around 30% [20, 37].

Clinical presentation

Demography and syndromes

Type A dissections represent 60–65% of the acute aortic dissections and type B the remaining 35–40% (⊃Table 59.1).

Acute aortic dissection is twice as frequent in males as in females and the mean age of presentation is 63 years for men and 67 for women [38]. Patients with type A dissection tend to be younger than those with type B dissection (⊃Table 59.1). In patients with connective tissues disorders aortic dissection tend to occur at a younger age, generally during the third or fourth decade of life. In them, and in younger patients, there is likely to be no history of hypertension and type A dissection is more common.

Signs and symptoms

Patients suffering from acute aortic dissection may present with variable degrees of haemodynamic instability (⊃ Table 59.2). Hypovolaemic shock results in an important amount of blood loss into the periaortic tissues or spaces. In type A dissection with retrograde

Table 59.2 Presenting symptoms and physical examination of patients with acute aortic dissection

Category	Present, No. reported (%)	Type A, No. (%)	Type B, No. (%)	p value Type A vs B
Presenting symptoms				
Any pain reported	443/464 (95.5)	271 (93.8)	172 (98.3)	0.02
Abrupt onset	379/447 (84.8)	234 (85.4)	145 (83.8)	0.65
Chest pain	331/455 (72.7)	221 (78.9)	110 (62.9)	<0.001
Anterior chest pain	262/430 (60.9)	191 (71.0)	71 (44.1)	<0.001
Posterior chest pain	149/415 (35.9)	85 (32.8)	64 (41)	0.09
Back pain	240/451 (53.2)	129 (46.6)	111 (63.8)	<0.001
Abdominal pain	133/449 (29.6)	60 (21.6)	73 (42.7)	<0.001
Severity of pain: severe or worst ever	346/382 (90.6)	211 (90.1)	135 (90)	NA
Quality of pain: sharp	174/270 (64.4)	103 (62)	71 (168.3)	NA
Quality of pain: tearing or ripping	135/267 (50.6)	78 (49.4)	57 (52.3)	NA
Radiating	127/449 (28.3)	75 (27.2)	52 (30.1)	0.51
Migrating	74/446 (16.6)	41 (14.9)	33 (19.3)	0.2
Syncope	42/447 (9.4)	35 (12.7)	7 (4.1)	0.002
Physical examination findings				
Haemodynamics (n = 451) [a]				<0.001
Hypertensive (SBP ≥150 mmHg)	221 (49.0)	99 (35.7)	122 (70.1)	
Normotensive (SBP 100–149 mmHg)	156 (34.6)	110 (39.7)	46 (26.4)	
Hypotensive (SBP <100 mmHg)	36 (8.0)	32 (11.6)	4 (2.3)	
Shock or tamponade (SBP <80 mmHg)	38 (8.4)	36 (13.0)	2 (1.5)	
Auscultated murmur of aortic insufficiency	137/434 (31.6)	117 (44)	20 (12)	<0.001
Pulse deficit	69/457 (15.1)	53 (18.7)	16 (9.2)	0.006
Cerebrovascular accident	21/447 (4.7)	17 (6.1)	4 (2.3)	0.07
Congestive heart failure	29/440 (6.6)	24 (8.8)	5 (3.0)	0.02

SBP, systolic blood pressure; NA, not applicable. For definitions of type A and B dissections, see footnote to Table 59.1.
[a] SPB is reported for 277 patients with type A and 174 patients with type B acute aortic dissection. respectively.
Data from the International Registry of Aortic Dissection (IRAD). Reproduced with permission from Hagan PG, Nienaber CA, Isselbacher EM, *et al.* The International Registry of Acute Aortic Dissection (IRAD): new insights into an old disease. *JAMA* 2000;**283**:897–903. Copyright 2000, American Medical Association. All rights reserved.

propagation towards the aortic root, cardiogenic shock may result from myocardial ischaemia, acute aortic regurgitation, or tamponnade.

Haemodynamically compromised or not, most patients experience sudden severe pain and anxiety at the moment of dissection (◑ Table 59.2). The pain is usually described as 'ripping' or 'tearing'. Precordial pain is more often described in ascending aortic dissection, whereas interscapular or back pain is more usual in descending thoracic aortic dissection. The pain tends to migrate or radiate as the dissection extends along the aorta.

Some patients may present symptoms related to organ malperfusion such as paraparesis or paraplegia of sudden onset, abdominal pain or discomfort, or symptoms relating to an unilateral or bilateral limb ischaemia. In a few patients, the acute dissection results in no symptoms and passes unnoticed.

On physical examination, patients present tachycardia accompanied by hypotension in the case of hypovolaemia or cardiogenic shock. In the absence of such complications, tachycardia and hypertension may be found as a result of pain, anxiety, and pre-existing essential hypertension. Abnormal peripheral vascular examination is present in about 15% of cases. Pulse deficit in the upper extremities suggest involvement of the ascending aorta, whereas pulse deficit in the lower extremities (more the left than the right) suggests involvement of the aortic bifurcation and iliac arteries. Heart auscultation may reveal a diastolic murmur consistent with acute aortic regurgitation. Jugular venous distension and a pulsus paradoxus are signs of pericardial tamponade. Unilateral loss of breath sounds, usually on the left, may indicate haemothorax.

Cerebrovascular accident occurs in 5–10% of patients due to involvement of the brachiocephalic vessels [20,

39], and paraplegia occurs in 2–5% due to occlusion of the intercostal or lumbar arteries [40]. Malperfusion of peripheral nerves may yield findings similar to spinal cord malperfusion, but peripheral ischaemia has a much better prognosis after restoration of blood flow.

Acute aortic dissection may also cause superior vena cava syndrome, vocal cord paralysis, haematemesis, Horner's syndrome, haemoptysis, and airway compression as a result of local compression and mass effects.

Diagnostic studies and imaging

Routine diagnostic studies (blood tests, ECG, and chest radiograph) are necessary but are often not sufficient to establish the diagnosis of acute aortic dissection. The ECG may help to differentiate pain from acute myocardial infarction, which indicates anticoagulation, and pain from dissection, which contraindicates anticoagulation. One-third of acute dissections show no ECG anomalies (➲ Table 59.3). Nonspecific ST-segment or T-wave change and left ventricular hypertrophy are the most common anomalies observed on ECG. Ischaemia or acute myocardial infarc-

tion is observed in about 22% of acute type A and 13% of acute type B dissection. Surprisingly, one-third of patients with coronary ostia involvement may present with normal ECG [41]. Biomarkers specific for aortic dissection would be useful to differentiate the origin of the pain. Several biomarkers are under investigation (e.g. smooth muscle myosin heavy chain, D-dimer, soluble elastin fragment [42–44]), but currently they are not readily available or reliable for systematic bedside use. The chest radiograph may exhibits several features like widening of the mediastinal shadows, rightward tracheal displacement, irregular aortic contour with loss of the aortic knob, and a left pleural effusion (➲ Table 59.3, ➲ Fig. 59.5).

Diagnostic imaging is essential to determine the precise anatomy of acute aortic dissection, on which the initial management and operative planning depend. Currently, CT and transoesophageal echocardiography (TOE) are the two imaging modalities most used for this purpose (➲ Table 59.3); aortography and MRI are also used to diagnose acute aortic dissection but are second-line modalities. Aortography was the gold standard before development of

Table 59.3 Chest radiography, electrocardiography, and initial diagnostic imaging results for patients with acute aortic dissection

Category	Present, No. reported (%)	Type A, No. (%)	Type B, No. (%)	p value, Type A vs B
Radiography findings (n = 427)	427 (100)	256 (88.6)	171 (97.7)	
No abnormalities noted	53 (12.4)	26 (11.3)	27 (15.8)	0.08
Absence of widened mediastinum or abnormal aortic contour	91 (21.3)	44 (17.2)	47 (27.5)	0.01
Widened mediastinum	263 (61.6)	169 (62.6)	94 (56)	0.17
Abnormal aortic contour	212 (49.6)	124 (46.6)	88 (53)	0.20
Abnormal cardiac contour	110 (25.8)	69 (26.9)	41 (24.0)	0.49
Displacement/calcification of aorta	60 (14.1)	29 (11–3)	31 (18.1)	0.05
Pleural effusion	82 (19.2)	46 (17.3)	36 (21.8)	0.24
ElectroCardiogram findings (n = 444)				
No abnormalities noted	139 (31.3)	85 (30.8)	54 (32.1)	0.76
Nonspecific ST-segment or T-wave changes	184 (41.4)	116 (42.6)	68 (42.8)	0.98
Left ventricular hypertrophy	116 (26.1)	67 (25)	498 (32.2)	0.11
Ischaemia	67 (15.1)	47 (17.3)	20 (13.2)	0.27
Myocardial infarction, old Q waves	34 (7.7)	19 (7.1)	15 (9.9)	0.30
Myocardial infarction, new Q waves or ST segments	14 (3.2)	13 (4.8)	1 (0.7)	0.02
Initial modality (n = 453)				
Computed tomography	277 (61.1)	145 (50.2)	132 (75.4)	<0.001
Echocardiogram (TOE and/or TTE)	148 (32.7)	122 (42.2)	26 (14.9)	<0.001
Aortography	20 (4.4)	12 (4.2)	8 (4.6)	0.92
Magnetic resonance imaging	8 (1.8)	2 (0.7)	6 (3.4)	0.36
Images performed per patient, mean (SD)	1.83 (0.82)	1.64 (0.69)	2.15 (0.91)	<0.001

TOE, transoesophageal echocardiography; TTE, transthoraic echocardiography. For definitions of type A and B dissections, see footnote to Table 59.1.

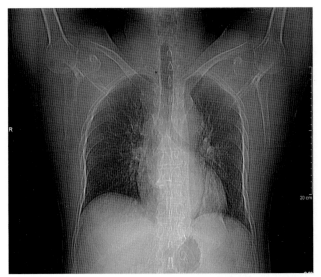

Figure 59.5 Chest radiograph of an acute type A dissection exhibiting widened upper mediastinum especially towards the left side. This feature suggests involvement of the arch or proximal descending aorta.

the other, less invasive, modalities, and remains an indispensable tool during endovascular procedures for type B aortic dissection. MRI is an excellent imaging method for any aortic disease, and avoids the use of contrast medium, but it is less widely available than CT or TOE, less accessible to monitored or ventilated patients, and takes longer to complete.

In daily practice, CT is the technique most frequently used to diagnose acute aortic dissection. Although it has slightly lower sensitivity and specificity than MRI or TOE [45, 46], CT is widely available, quickly done, and generates images familiar to most practitioners. Extension of the dissection process may be evaluated on the entire aorta and side branches (❍ Figs 59.6 and 59.7; 📹 59.2). Pleural and pericardial spaces are also imaged. One limitation of CT is the need for intravenous contrast medium, which may be contraindicated in patients with allergies to contrast agent or with renal insufficiency. Also, in the modality in which CT is used to diagnose aortic dissection, aortic regurgitation cannot be determined accurately [46].

TOE is the second most frequently used method of diagnosing acute aortic dissection. Like CT, TOE is widely available and quickly performed, but it does not requires intravenous contrast or radiation and provides precise assessment of aortic valve and left ventricular function (❍ Fig. 59.8 and 📹 59.3). TOE allows visualization of the coronary ostia and pericardial and pleural spaces but not the aortic arch, brachiocephalic vessel, and abdominal aorta. TOE requires operator expertise to acquire the images and interpret them appropriately, as well to conduct the examination safely. Patient comfort is paramount during examination, to avoid a hypertensive peak and to complete examination of the aorta, as it is necessary to exclude the diagnosis of acute

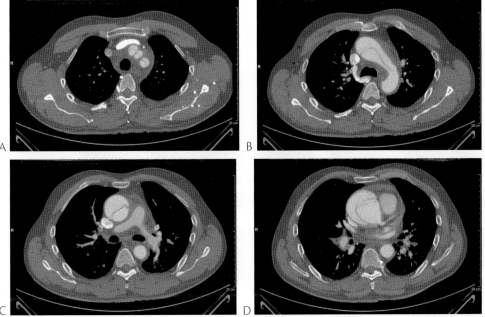

Figure 59.6 CT scan of an acute type A (De Bakey type I) aortic dissection; dissection stops in the distal aortic arch. (a) Extension of the dissection into the three brachiocephalic arteries. The dissection flap can be seen in the three vessels. (b) Dissection of the arch with re-entry tear at the level of the distal arch. (c) Dissection of the ascending aorta; the true lumen is posterior. The descending aorta is not involved in the process. (d) Dissection extend to the aortic root; the main stem ostia is not involved in the process.

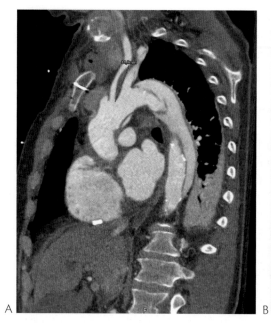
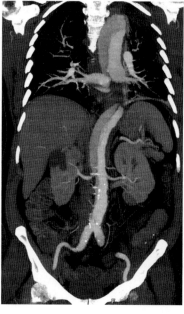

Figure 59.7 CT scan of an acute type B (De Bakey type IIIb) aortic dissection; the dissection extends as far as the renal arteries, with many fenestrations. (a) Reconstructed sagittal view. Dissection of the descending aorta with the intimal tear originating just after the emergence of the left subclavian artery. (b) Reconstructed coronal view.

dissection. Contraindications to TOE include oesophageal varices, stricture, or tumour; and a recent meal.

Transthoracic echocardiography (TTE), which provides only images of the ascending aorta and sections of the aortic arch, is generally considered insufficient to reliably establish the diagnosis of dissection. Moreover, evaluation of TTE is additionally limited by patient-related factors including body habitus, emphysema, and mechanical ventilation.

The diagnostic strategy depends essentially on the haemodynamic stability of the patient. A very unstable patient with high clinical likelihood of acute aortic dissection should be immediately transferred to the operating room. After intubation and placement of essential monitoring lines, TOE is performed and surgery may be expedited. In patients who have been stabilized in the emergency department, the choice between TOE and CT is made according to their respective availability in the hospital. In stable patients, a CT arteriogram is probably the most effective mode for therapeutic planning.

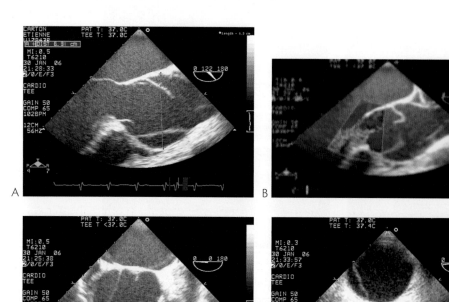

Figure 59.8 Transoesophageal echocardiography of an acute type A (De Bakey type I) aortic dissection. (a) Long axis view of the ascending aorta showing the dissection flap. The transversal diameter of the ascending aorta is 6.3 cm. (b) Long axis view of the ascending aorta with colour Doppler flow showing the aortic valve regurgitation. (c) Short axis view of the ascending aorta showing the dissection flap. (d) Short axis view of the descending aorta showing the dissection flap.

Treatment

In general, a type A acute aortic dissection must be considered as a surgical emergency. In contrast, type B dissections are generally treated medically unless the patient develops complications such as progression of dissection, intractable pain, failure of medical management to control hypertension, organ malperfusion, or contained or free aortic rupture.

Initial medical treatment

In haemodynamically unstable patients, intravenous fluid administration is usually necessary to restore the circulating blood volume and to compensate for the blood lost in the false lumen, the pericardium, or the pleural space. If the patient is not rapidly stabilized, transfer to the operating room is mandatory while the resuscitation manoeuvres are continued. In case of pericardial tamponade, pericardiocentesis as an initial therapeutic step before surgery may be harmful because it reduces intrapericardial pressure and may therefore cause recurrent pericardial bleeding and sudden death [47].

In stable patients, hypertension is the primary target of medical therapy to decrease the risk of aortic rupture or extension of the dissection. Therefore, well-targeted and aggressive antihypertensive treatment with close haemodynamic monitoring must be started quickly. The aim is to normalize blood pressure and mainly to reduce the strength of the left ventricular contraction (as reflected by the the dP/dT) thereby reducing the stress applied by the ejected blood on the aortic tear. Intravenous β-blockers (metoprolol, esmolol) are the most appropriate drugs if no contraindication exists. They should be titrated to lower systolic blood pressure to 100–110 mmHg and to slow heart rate below 60 beats/min. If blood pressure is insufficiently controlled by β-blockers, intravenous vasodilator agents such as sodium nitroprusside or urapidil can be associated. Calcium channel blockers such as nicardipine can also be used in combination. Dihydropyridine is also used in patients with contraindications to β-blockers. Angiotensin converting enzyme (ACE) inhibitors are not recommended in the initial management of an acute type B dissection, as impairment of renal perfusion due to the dissection can be difficult to exclude in the first hours.

Pain can also contribute to hypertension and tachycardia, so analgesia is necessary in such patients. However, in most cases, an effective blood pressure control will usually relieve the pain. Moreover, persistence or recurrence of pain in spite of good control of hypertension is an indicator of disease progression and of the need to take the patient to the operating room. The use of strong analgesia is in our opinion not recommended in the initial step, when beginning antihypertensive treatment. Paracetamol or tramadol can be used as first line analgesia.

Surgical management in type A aortic dissection

Operative indication

In view of the high mortality risk with medical therapy alone (50–60%) [20, 48, 49] no absolute contraindication for surgery is unanimously proposed in type A aortic dissection. However, data from the IRAD registry indicates that only 80% of the patients with type A dissection undergone surgical repair. The main reasons for abstaining from surgery were old age (mean 80 years), comorbid conditions, and patient refusal. In a multicentre study on operative outcomes in octogenarians with type A dissection, in-hospital mortality was relatively high (46%), but when compassionate surgery and total aortic arch replacement were excluded from the series the mortality dropped to 34% at 1 year [50]. Neurological status at the time of presentation is an important criterion in the surgical decision. Surgery is generally contraindicated in comatose patients, but localized neurological deficit resulting from stroke is not a contraindication, even if postoperative recovery is uncertain.

The natural history of IMH and atherosclerotic ulcer is an ongoing debate. Regression occurs in about 10% of IMH, but evolution towards classic aortic dissection occurs in 28–47% with a risk of rupture in 20–45% of cases [51]. Similarly, patients with penetrating atherosclerotic ulcer were found to have a 42% rate of acute rupture [52]. As a result of these relatively high acute rupture rates, experts recommend that IMH and penetrating ulcer should be managed similarly to acute type A or type B dissection.

Operative technique

Type A dissection repair: general considerations

As introduced by De Bakey, the general principle of aortic dissection repair is to reroute blood flow towards true lumen, to resect the primary intimal tear, and to reconstruct the aorta by interposition of a polyester aortic graft. In type A aortic dissection, because acute complications come essentially from ascending aorta involvement, the treatment consists of replacement of the ascending aorta extended more or less proximally and distally. The decision to extend the repair to the aortic root, valve, and arch are made on the basis of patient-related criteria (age, comorbidity, clinical status, Marfan's disease), intraoperative findings, and the surgeon's experience. Repair of the dissected descending aorta is not mandated during initial surgical treatment of type A dissection.

Techniques of aortic arch repair

Surgical repair of acute type A dissection is performed through a median sternotomy. After heparinization, cardiopulmonary bypass (CPB) is started using subclavian or femoral artery cannulation for arterial inflow and right atrium cannulation for venous drainage (📷59.4a).

In the rare case without involvement of the aortic arch (De Bakey type 2) repair is limited distally to the replacement of the ascending aorta (📷59.4b). When dissection involves the aortic arch, distal repair must be performed under circulatory arrest. Cerebral protection is ensured using hypothermia and continuous cerebral perfusion with oxygenated blood. Hemiarch replacement is generally adequate even if dissection extends beyond the arch (📷59.4c). In some cases, total arch replacement (📷59.4d) is indicated for anatomical reasons (intimal tears in the arch, head vessel involvement) or to avoid the risk of further dilatation as in young or Marfan's patients.

Techniques of aortic root and valve repair

If dissection does not involve the aortic root, the aortic graft is anastomosed proximally at the level of the sinotubular junction. If dissection involves the aortic root, the decision to replace the root and the aortic valve depends on several anatomical and patient-related factors. If the root is normal-sized with limited dissection and no pathological change in the aortic cusps, then the dissected aortic layers can be reunited using surgical adhesive (e.g. BioGlue) and strips of Teflon felt (📷59.5a). If the root is dissected and/or dilated and the aortic valve presents calcific degeneration, both the root and the valve are replaced using a composite graft (a valve prosthesis inserted into a polyester tube graft) (📷59.5b) If the root is dissected and/or dilated and the aortic cusps are normal, valve-sparing root replacement (📷59.5c) is an alternative to valve replacement. In patients with Marfan's syndrome or other aggressive connective tissue disorders, root replacement (with valve replacement or preservation) is recommended even in presence of a normal-sized root [7].

Aortic valve insufficiency is present in 63% of acute type A dissection [36]. The principal mechanism of aortic insufficiency in most cases is the loss of commissural support of the valve cusps, which are then generally preserved. Resuspension of the commissure within the root repair makes it possible to restore valve competence in most cases.

Outcomes after surgical repair of type A aortic dissection

In early series, long-term survival after repair of type A dissection varies from 37% to 64% at 10 years [49, 53]. Risk factors are advanced age, complicated dissection, false lumen patency, resection of aortic arch, and early year of operation. More recently, data from the IRAD registry have shown 90% survival at 3 years, with history of atherosclerosis and previous cardiac surgery as risk factors for mortality [54].

Late aortic reoperation is necessary in up to 26% at 10 years [49, 55–57]. Such morbidity is explained by the fact that the aorta remains predisposed to redissection, dilatation, rupture, or the development of false aneurysm on anastomotic dehiscence. Systemic hypertension, young age, Marfan's syndrome, initial aortic size, and false lumen patency are all risk factors for long-term complications [49, 53, 57]. Therefore, long-term management after repair of type A dissection requires optimal antihypertensive therapy to reduce aortic wall stress, serial imaging to observe pathological evolution of the aorta, and finally, reoperation when indicated. Lifelong β-blocker therapy is essential to maintain a blood pressure below 120/80 mmHg [58]. Because complications may develop on different segments of the aorta, CT and MRI are the most appropriate imaging studies for patient follow-up. Imaging should be performed before hospital discharge and every 3–6 months during the first postoperative year. Thereafter, if the aortic diameter remains unchanged at 1 year, studies are obtained yearly. Aortic enlargement of more than 1 cm within a 1-year period is considered as a high-risk change, and the interval is then decreased to 3 months if surgery is not indicated. Annual TTE is also indicated in patients with preservation of the native aortic valve, because progressive aortic insufficiency may develop in some of them.

Management in type B dissection

Endovascular procedures, described since 1999, have revolutionized the management of type B dissections [59, 60]. As a remedy for the substantial morbidity and mortality of conventional surgical aortic repair, thoracic endovascular aortic repair (TEVAR) using a stent-graft is currently and widely used in complicated type B dissections and its use in uncomplicated cases is debated. ➲Figure 59.9 summarizes the proposed treatment algorithm for acute type B dissection.

Uncomplicated type B dissection: conservative management

Medical treatment

After initial medical management in the intensive care unit (ICU), once stable blood pressure is obtained with partial or total spontaneous chest/back pain relief, the patient can be clinically followed in a cardiovascular (surgical and/or cardiological) in-hospital unit. Oral antihypertensive treatment is used: β-blockers in association with a calcium

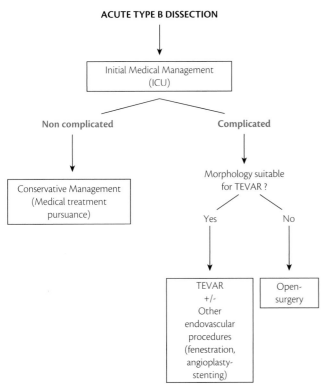

Figure 59.9 Treatment algorithm for acute type B dissection.

channel blockers, adding an ACE inhibitor or a sartan drug if there is no renal damage. Continuous clinical and haemodynamic monitoring is mandatory. The patient is usually discharged within 15 days, after a thoraco-abdominal CT scan to exclude rapid enlarging false lumen, signs of rupture, distal malperfusion, or progression of the dissection.

Prophylactic invasive treatment

In the current era, surgery for type B dissections is reserved for complications because invasive repair has not proved superior to medical treatment in stable patients [61]. Effectively, the INSTEAD trial [62, 63] compared medical therapy to stent-grafting in uncomplicated type B dissection: the 1-year mortality was 3% for medical therapy versus 10% for stent-grafting. In the medically treated group, only 11% crossed over to stent-graft or surgical treatment. Therefore, prophylactic stent-grafting does not appear to be justified in medically controlled patients with subacute or chronic type B aortic dissection. However, close follow-up is necessary and delayed endovascular treatment is indicated in patients presenting with the following signs and symptoms:

◆ Maximal thoracic aorta diameter greater than 55 mm.

◆ Documented increase of aortic diameter of more than 1 cm within a year.

◆ Resistant hypertension despite antihypertensive combination therapy associated with a small true lumen or renal malperfusion.

◆ Recurrent episodes of chest/back pain that cannot be attributed to other causes.

Complicated type B dissection: interventional considerations

About 30% of acute type B dissections are complicated at clinical presentation with a subsequent high risk of spontaneous death [64, 65]. The definition of complicated type B dissection includes one or more of the four major syndromes listed in ⊃ Box 59.2.

Open surgical repair for type B aortic dissection

Although late outcomes on young and low surgical risk patients treated with stent-graft are not yet clearly defined [66], the open surgical technique is currently no longer the treatment of choice, especially on an acute/urgent basis.

The principle of an open surgical thoracic aorta repair is to replace the proximal descending thoracic aorta by insertion of a tubular Dacron prosthesis, allowing restoration of the blood flow into the true lumen. Replacement of the distal descending aorta or the total thoracoabdominal aorta is rarely required [67].

Surgery is performed via a left thoracotomy or a left thoracophrenolaparotomy for a thoracoabdominal repair. A left heart bypass from left atrium to femoral artery is generally used for lower body perfusion during thoracic aorta clamping. To reduce spinal cord ischaemia and reduce the risk of paraplegia, intercostals or lumbar side branches are reimplanted on the aortic graft and cerebrospinal fluid drainage may be placed before the surgical procedure.

Stent-grafting technique

TEVAR requires a surgically exposed femoral (or iliac) artery, associated with a controlateral percutaneous femoral access. By means of intraoperative digital subtraction angiography and TOE the true lumen can be catheterized and the entry tear visualized, usually at the isthmic region. The optimal diameter of the stent-graft is defined using multiplanar reformation images from the CT angiography.

Box 59.2 Major complications relating to type B aortic dissection

◆ (Pre-) ruptured aorta with significant haemothorax, with or without haemodynamic instability

◆ Intractable hypertension

◆ Recurrent chest/back pain with expanding diameter of the descending aorta or extension of the dissection

◆ Distal malperfusion syndrome (end-organ ischaemia): spinal cord, bowel, kidneys, limbs

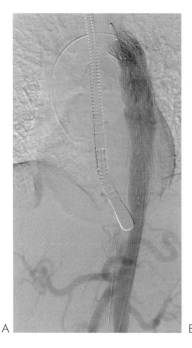
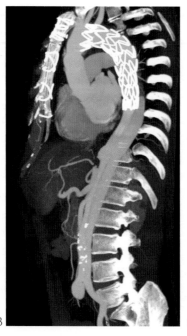
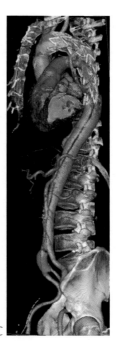

A   B   C

Figure 59.10 Imaging of an acute type B (De Bakey type IIIb) aortic dissection after a TEVAR procedure: (a) Aortography post stent-graft deployment; notice the permeability of distal aorta and abdominal side branches. (b) CT scan, reconstructed sagittal view. Distally to the stent-graft, the false lumen is still perfused via multiple natural fenestrations of the dissection flap. The proximal end (±2–3 cm) of the stent-graft, which not covered, is deployed intentionally in front of the left subclavian artery to ensure exclusion by the covered portion of the stent-graft of the intimal tear located just beyond this branch. (c) CT scan: reconstructed three-dimensional view in the same patient.

The stent-graft, a synthetic, conformable, covered stent, is advanced via the vascular access as far as the distal aortic arch, to cover the entry tear (◐ Figs 59.10, 🎥 59.6). The sealing of the entry tear reopens the true lumen (🎥 59.7). Reperfusion of the descending and abdominal aorta normalizes distal-vessel patency and makes it possible to sort out most of the prerupture and malperfusion syndromes. The depressurization and shrinkage of the false lumen leads to thrombosis and fibrous transformation, with subsequent remodelling and stabilization of the aorta.

Several technical pitfalls have to be clearly elucidated before the procedure: oversizing of the diameter and length of the device, the bending of the aortic arch, the optional covering of the ostium of the left subclavian artery to seal the proximal segment of the stent-graft, and the suitability of a balloon dilatation/impaction of the landing zones (often not recommended in dissected aortas).

The various devices available differ in technical details: some are considered as more flexible, conforming easily to a sharp aortic inner curvature (e.g. the Gore TAG Excluder); others are said to be more comfortable in the presence of short landing zones, especially with tortuous distal arches; and others target the anchoring problem (e.g. the Medtronic Valiant, with an unsheathing mechanism and a proximal bare-top barb stent; the Cook Zenith TX2 Pro-Form, with proximal and distal deployment trigger wires, also implementing the new concept of increasing conformability by enhancing the space between the 'z-stents').

Endovascular thoracic aortic repair seems to be minimally invasive, offers quicker recovery, and seems to be a relatively safe alternative to traditional open repair, although potentially lethal complications, acute or delayed, may occur: paraplegia (due to impaired perfusion of the lower spinal cord), stroke-embolization (immediate, related to the procedure, or delayed, caused by the lack of sealing of the prosthesis) retrograde extension of the dissection [68], collapse of the stent-graft [69, 70], occurrence of endoleaks, and delayed aortic ruptures.

Endovascular treatment versus open surgery

Fattori *et al.* [64] reviewed the impact on survival of different treatment strategies in 571 patients with acute complicated type B aortic dissections. Medical treatment was used in 390 patients (68.3%), open surgery in 59 (10.3%), and endovascular treatment in 66 (11.6%). In-hospital complications occurred in 20% after endovascular treatment and in 40% after open surgery; in-hospital mortality was also significantly higher after open surgery (33.9%) than after endovascular treatment (10.6%, $p = 0.002$). Open surgery was associated with an independent increased risk of in-hospital mortality (OR 3.41, 95% CI 1.00–11.67, $p = 0.05$). Thus, in complicated type B dissection, the choice of an endovascular stent-graft placement may offer a strategy to optimize management and improve in-hospital prognosis.

Early outcomes after stent-graft deployment

In the EUROSTAR/United Kingdom registry report [71], representing the first large series of patients (131) treated with thoracic aortic stent-grafts for acute aortic dissections, primary technical success was achieved in 86% of the patients, no cases of paraplegia were reported, but two patients (3.2%) sustained a periprocedural stroke. The 30-day mortality rate was only 8.4%.

In a meta-analysis [72] reviewing 609 patients subjected to endovascular stent-graft repair for aortic dissection, the procedural success rate was 98.2%. In-hospital surgical conversion rate was 2.3% and an in-hospital mortality rate was 5.2% with 21.7% of complications. Complications such as retrograde extension of the dissection into the ascending aorta were reported in 1.9% and neurological complications in 2.9% of patients. The 30-day mortality rate was 9.8%.

Late failure of thoracic endovascular aortic repair

Because TEVAR procedures have been introduced relatively recently, few data are available on the long-term outcomes after treatment of acute type B dissection. In a disease characterized by diffuse fragility of the aortic wall, the impact of a noncompliant device applying constant radial force at the treatment site, the frequency of severe complications, and the time when they occur are unknown. Alves *et al.* [66] recently published one of the longest follow-up periods for patients treated with TEVAR for type B dissection (106 patients: 45 acute, 61 chronic). They found a mean time to first event of 29±17.4 months (follow-up of 35.9±28.5 months). Late failures (including endoleaks type I and III, stent migration, proximal intimal rupture, distal aneurysmal degeneration, death after aortic rupture, or multiple organ failure) were observed in 37%. In those 27 patients, a second endovascular aortic repair was necessary in 60%, while open surgery was necessary in 11% and 18% died in relation to a TEVAR procedure. The 5-year survival was 92%.

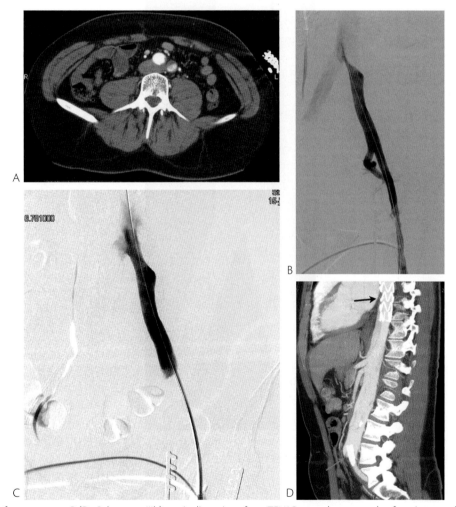

Figure 59.11 Imaging of an acute type B (De Bakey type IIIb) aortic dissection after a TEVAR procedure; example of persistent malperfusion syndrome. (a) CT scan showing subocclusion of the left common iliac artery by the dissection flap. (b) Angiographic image of the left common iliac artery subocclusion. (c) Endovascular treatment by deployment of a bare stent at the level of the subocclusion. (d) CT scanner reconstructed sagittal view showing the thoracic stent-graft (black arrow) and the bare stent (red arrow) in the left common iliac artery.

Endovascular 'rescue' for malperfusion syndrome

Deployment of a stent-graft to cover the entry tear in a type B dissected aorta is a intuitively perfect therapeutic solution and allows the management of complicated cases. But, while reopening the true lumen and collapsing the false one, stent-grafting can be responsible for hypoperfusion of the branch vessels supplied by the false lumen and thus precipitate ischaemia of the respective organs. Moreover, reperfusion of the true lumen can be distally deficient, with a lack of re-expansion at different levels (➡ Fig. 59.11a, b). These complications can be treated by different endovascular procedures, e.g.:

◆ Endovascular fenestration of the dissection membrane to increase communication between the two lumens.

Fenestration is performed by balloon angioplasty or by the 'Rousseau scissors' technique (➡ Fig. 59.12).

◆ Placement of stent to reopen a compressed side branch vessel (visceral, renal, limb) (➡ Fig. 59.11c, d).

Spinal cord malperfusion with paraplegia has a poor prognosis. We favour immediate cerebrospinal drainage to reduce spinal cord ischaemia by lowering cerebrospinal fluid over-pressure.

Primary or secondary (after TEVAR) unilateral limb ischaemia can also be treated by open surgical management such as cross-femoral bypass.

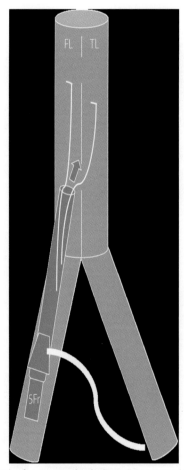

Figure 59.12 Schematic representation of an endovascular fenestration by the 'Rousseau scissors' technique: the dissection flap is cut by an introducer sheath passed over individual guide wires in each lumen. FL, false lumen; TL, true lumen.

Personal perspective

There has been considerable improvement in the treatment of patients with aortic dissection over the last 50 years. Noninvasive imaging technologies such as CT, TOE, and MRI are now indispensable tools for diagnosis, treatment and follow-up. New therapeutic technologies such as endovascular repair are nowadays, if feasible, the first line treatment for most of the descending thoracic aorta pathologies. Complex forms of dissection that include aortic root, valve, or aortic arch will, however, require surgical treatment for the foreseeable future. These patients will benefit from the diverse techniques developed for neurological protection, aortic valve preservation, and extended aortic repair as during initial surgical management. Although aortic stent-grafting has already spread worldwide, the new hybrid surgical/endovascular procedures for type A dissection need further clinical development before universal acceptance as an effective therapeutic tool. Notwithstanding these new technologies, the clinician's approach to aortic dissection must be led by the individual patient's history and clinical presentation. An old, frail, or neurologicaly compromised patient will probably not benefit from long and complex procedure as young or uncomplicated patients will do. Finally, patients surviving aortic dissection must remain under close medical follow-up for the long term as they are at high risk of develop complicationing. New treatments certainly do not relieve patients from this surveillance, as they unfortunately do not completely suppress the risk of complication and because their long-term results are still under evaluation.

Further reading

Akin I, Kische S, Ince H, Nienaber CA. Indication, timing and results of endovascular treatment of type B dissection. *Eur J Vasc Endovasc Surg* 2009;**37**:289–296.

Erbel R, Alfonso F, Boileau C, *et al*. Diagnosis and management of aortic dissection. *Eur Heart J* 2001;**22**:1642–1681.

Koutchoukos N, Blackstone E, Doty D, *et al. Cardiac surgery,* 3rd edition, Churchill Livingstone, Edinburgh.

Svensson LG, Kouchoukos NT, Miller DC, *et al*. Expert Consensus document on the treatment of descending thoracic aortic disease using endovascular stent-grafts. *Ann Thorac Surg* 2008;**85**:1–41.

Tsai TT, Nienaber CA, Eagle KA. Acute aortic syndromes. *Circulation* 2005;**112**(24):3802–3813.

Tsai TT, Trimarchi S, Nienaber CA. Acute aortic dissection: perspectives from the International Registry of Acute Aortic Dissection (IRAD). *Eur J Vasc Endovasc Surg* 2009;**37**(2):149–159.

Additional online material

59.1 Chest and abdominal angio-MRI of an acute type B (De Bakey type IIIb) aortic dissection

59.2 CT scan of an acute type A (De Bakey type I) aortic dissection

59.3 Transoesophageal echocardiography of an acute type A (De Bakey type I) aortic dissection

59.4 Illustration of surgical techniques: right subclavian canulation, ascending aorta and aortic arch repair

59.5 Illustration of surgical techniques: aortic valve and root repair

59.6 TEVAR procedure for an acute type B aortic dissection: CT scan

59.7 TEVAR procedure for an acute type B aortic dissection: transoesophageal echocardiography

Online resources

Cohn LH. *Cardiac surgery in the adult*, 3rd edition. McGraw-Hill, New York, 2008; online publication by HighWire Press: http://cardiacsurgery.ctsnetbooks.org

International Registry of Acute Aortic Dissection (IRAD): http://www.iradonline.org/index.html

➲ For additional multimedia materials please visit the online version of the book (⌘ http://www.esciacc.oxfordmedicine.com).

CHAPTER 60

Cardiac complications in trauma

Demetrios Demetriades and Leslie Kobayashi

Contents

Summary

Post-traumatic cardiac complications may occur after penetrating or blunt injuries to the heart or may follow severe extracardiac injuries. Most victims with penetrating injuries to the heart die at the scene and do not reach hospital care. For those patients who reach hospital care, an immediate operation, sometimes in the emergency room, cardiac injury repair, and cardiopulmonary resuscitation provide the only possibility of survival. Many patients develop perioperative cardiac complications such as acute cardiac failure, cardiac arrhythmias, coronary air embolism, and myocardial infarction. Some survivors develop postoperative functional abnormalities or anatomical defects, which may not manifest during the early postoperative period. It is essential that all survivors undergo detailed early and late cardiological evaluations. Blunt cardiac trauma may include a wide spectrum of injuries, ranging from asymptomatic myocardial contusion, arrhythmias, or cardiogenic shock to full-thickness cardiac rupture. Clinical examination, ECG, troponin measurements, and echocardiography are the cornerstone for the diagnosis and monitoring of these patients. Lastly, some serious extracardiac traumatic conditions, such as postpneumonectomy or after head or other severe injuries, may result in cardiac complications, which may include tachyarrhythmias, cardiogenic shock, ECG changes, and troponin elevations.

Penetrating cardiac injury

Epidemiology

About 10% of victims of gunshot wounds or stab wounds to the chest who reach hospital care have a cardiac injury. However, the real incidence is much higher because the majority of patients with cardiac injuries are declared dead at the scene, with only 10–15% of victims reaching hospital care [1, 2].

The selection of survivors is determined by numerous factors, such as the mechanism of injury (stab wound vs gunshot wound), cardiac chamber involved, size of the cardiac wound, presence of tamponade, associated injuries, and prehospital times.

Clinical presentation

Every penetrating injury to the chest, especially in the presence of hypotension, should be suspected of cardiac injury until proven otherwise (📷 60.1). Hypotension is the most common clinical presentation, although patients with small cardiac injuries and short prehospital times may be normotensive on admission. Prospective studies have shown that the Beck's triad (hypotension, distended neck veins, distant cardiac sounds) is found in about 90% of patients with tamponade [3]. In contrast, pulsus paradoxus is found in only about 10% of cases with tamponade. Tachycardia and weak pulse are usually present. Although in the presence of cardiac tamponade the neck veins are usually distended, this sign may not be present if there is associated severe blood loss. Finally, the patient is often very restless and the inexperienced physician may mistake this for intoxication with alcohol or drugs of abuse.

Investigations

Focused Assessment with Sonography for Trauma (FAST) performed by emergency physicians or trauma surgeons has become the most useful investigation in the early diagnosis of cardiac tamponade (📷 60.2). Its sensitivity and specificity are very high, although false negatives can occur, especially in the presence of significant haemothorax or pneumothorax [4–8]. A formal echocardiogram by a cardiologist should be performed in stable patients with questionable diagnosis.

Other investigations should be considered in stable patients with uncertain diagnosis. An erect chest radiograph or an ECG may be diagnostic in about 50% of cases with cardiac injury [3]. Radiological signs suggestive of cardiac trauma include an enlarged cardiac shadow, pneumopericardium and widened upper mediastinum (➲ Fig. 60.1, 📷 60.3). ECG abnormalities may include arrhythmias, elevated ST, inverted T waves, and low QRS complexes.

Invasive investigations such as pericardiocentesis and subxiphoid window have a limited role in a hospital environment. Pericardiocentesis has an unacceptably high false negative rate because of clotting in the pericardial sac [3] (➲ Fig. 60.2). In addition, there is a risk of iatrogenic injury to the myocardium, especially in the absence of tamponade. Subxiphoid window is a very invasive surgical procedure and should only be considered when FAST or echocardiography are not available. In contrast, a transdiaphragmatic window during laparotomy for associated intra-abdominal

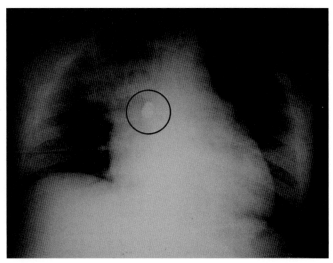

Figure 60.1 Chest radiograph shows an enlarged cardiac shadow due to cardiac tamponade after a gunshot wound (bullet in circle).

injuries is useful and expeditious in ruling out cardiac injury in the multitrauma patient [9, 10].

Management

Time is the most precious commodity in penetrating cardiac trauma. In the prehospital phase the 'scoop and run' approach should be followed in all victims with suspected cardiac trauma. In the emergency room no attempts should be made to stabilize the patient with intravenous fluids, nor should time be wasted for complex diagnostic tests, if the clinical diagnosis is obvious. A FAST examination, which takes only a few seconds to do, is the only acceptable investigation in the haemodynamically unstable patient.

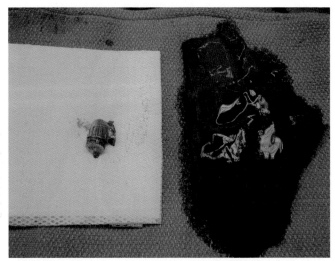

Figure 60.2 Bullet removed from the myocardium. The large clot (right) was drained from the pericardium. The formation of clot in the pericardial sac results in a high incidence of false negative pericardiocentesis.

Many patients arrive *in extremis* or full cardiac arrest and there is no time to transfer them to the operating room. Their only chance of survival is a resuscitative thoracotomy in the emergency room (➲ Fig 60.3). A left anterolateral thoracotomy is performed simultaneously with endotracheal intubation and intravenous catheter insertion. The cardiac wound is sutured, the thoracic aorta is cross-clamped to improve coronary and cerebral circulation, and cardiac resuscitation is performed with cardiac massage, intravenous fluids, adrenaline (epinephrine), and internal defibrillation as needed.

Patients with suspected cardiac injuries who are not in imminent cardiac arrest should be transferred to the operating room immediately for a median sternotomy or left thoracotomy. The techniques used to repair the cardiac wound are outside the scope of this chapter. Cardiopulmonary bypass is almost never needed during the acute stage. Any significant intracardiac defects should be repaired electively at a later stage.

A common and serious intraoperative complication is air embolism. This complication should be suspected in patients with injuries to the low-pressure cardiac chambers or in the presence of associated injuries to the lung or the major veins. In some cases air bubbles can be seen in the coronary veins. In a prospective study of 70 patients with penetrating cardiac injuries, air embolism was diagnosed in 7 (28%) of 25 patients with atrial injuries [3]. Cardiac needle aspiration should be performed for diagnostic and therapeutic purposes.

Outcomes

The prognosis after penetrating cardiac trauma is poor, and the overall mortality is in excess of 80% [1, 2]. The mortality is about 90% in gunshot wounds and 65% in stab wounds (➲ Fig 60.4, 📷 60.4). For the selected group of patients who reach hospital care the overall mortality is about 65%. The survival of patients undergoing emergency room resuscitative thoracotomy is about 14% [11, 12].

Postoperative complications

Most patients who suffered preoperative or intraoperative cardiac arrest, or those who required coronary artery ligation, experience postoperative acute heart failure. Echocardiography should be performed to assess myocardial contractility and volume status, and to monitor for pericardial effusion or recurrence of tamponade. The management is similar to that in nontraumatic cardiac failure.

All survivors should undergo routine early and late cardiological clinical, ECG, and echocardiographic evaluation, to rule out any functional myocardial abnormalities or intracardiac lesions, such as septal defects or valvular and papillary muscle damage. The troponin levels and the ECG are almost always abnormal during the early postoperative period but in most cases they return to normal within a few days. Persistent ECG abnormalities occur after ligation of a significant coronary artery branch.

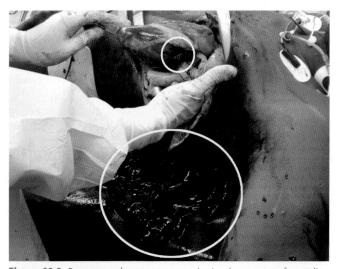

Figure 60.3 Emergency department resuscitative thoracotomy for cardiac arrest, after a gunshot injury to the heart (small circle). Note the large clot removed from the left pleural cavity and the pericardium (large circle).

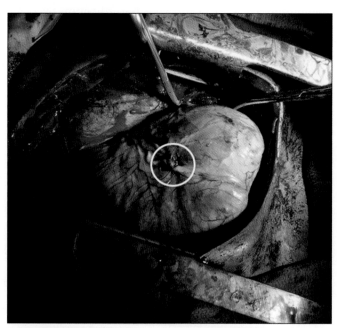

Figure 60.4 Stab wound to the heart very close to the left anterior descending artery (circle). Ligation of the coronary artery results in myocardial infarction.

The initial postoperative evaluation may miss significant abnormalities. Progression of the myocardial damage secondary to shock wave or transient cavitation injuries after gunshot wounds or progression of ischaemia after injury, thrombosis, or ligation of the coronary artery may cause focal dyskinesia or cardiac pseudoaneurysm. Early echocardiography may miss some small septal defects or other abnormalities. Localized oedema or haematoma may prevent flow through small septal defects, wall motion abnormalities may take weeks to develop, and false aneurysms may develop many weeks after the initial operation. In a study of 54 patients surviving stab wounds to the heart, late follow-up (mean 23 months) showed ECG abnormalities in 31%, echocardiographic abnormalities in 31%, and valvular or septal defects in 19% of patients, 50% of which were asymptomatic. The late echocardiographic abnormalities included valvular or septal defects in 10 cases, ventricular dilatation or dysfunction in 7, septal hypokinesia in 2, and a single case of pericardial effusion [13]. Another study of 642 survivors of penetrating cardiac trauma with early follow-up showed an incidence of 7.9% of ventricular septal defects and 7.1% of valvular lesions on routine echocardiogram in asymptomatic patients [14]. The high incidence of abnormalities in these two studies highlights the importance of early and late follow-up of all patients regardless of symptoms.

Although most patients with echocardiographic abnormalities do not require treatment [13–15], monitoring the progress of any lesions or antibiotic prophylaxis for unrelated procedures to prevent endocarditis are important issues to bear in mind. The natural history of post-traumatic small asymptomatic septal defects is unpredictable. Although many of them may heal spontaneously, others become larger and symptomatic because of the pressure gradient between the right and left heart and may need repair with open surgery or interventional techniques.

Cardiac pseudoaneurysm is a rare complication after cardiac trauma and usually occurs after ligation of a major branch of a coronary artery [16]. The presentation is generally delayed, often for many weeks or months.

Another late complication after cardiac injury is post-pericardiotomy syndrome, which is reported in up to 20% of survivors [17]. It is characterized by fever, pleuritic chest pain, friction rub, leucocytosis, high erythrocyte sedimentation rate, and ECG changes which may include diffuse ST elevation and PR depression [18]. It is thought to be an autoimmune problem and is benign in most cases. However, it can be complicated by pleural or pericardial effusion. Treatment consists of supportive measures and nonsteroidal anti-inflammatory drugs (NSAIDs). In severe cases, steroids or indomethacin may be helpful [19–21].

Retained missiles, such as bullets, pellets, or fragments from explosions are not uncommon. The missile may be embedded in the myocardium or float in the cardiac cavity (60.5, 60.6, Fig 60.5). Intracardiac missiles may embolize in the systemic or pulmonary circulation. At the acute stage the patient usually presents with signs of tamponade and haemodynamic instability, although some cases may be asymptomatic, especially if the injury is due to small pellets. If the missile is identified to be partially embedded in the myocardium during an emergency operation, it should be removed and the cardiac wound repaired. Asymptomatic patients with no obvious need for emergency operation should be evaluated by means of chest radiography, CT scan and echocardiography. Plain films may show a double shadow sign (60.5) because of the constant movement of the missile during a single exposure [22]. CT and echocardiography provide reliable information about the exact location of the missile (Fig. 60.5). At the acute stage, all retained missiles should be removed irrespective of symptoms because of the risk of erosion through the myocardium which could result in bleeding and tamponade, missile embolization, endocarditis, and pericarditis. Partially embedded missiles are removed with open surgery, while those floating free in the cardiac cavity can successfully be managed by interventional cardiology. If the diagnosis of the retained foreign body is made long after the injury and is completely embedded, asymptomatic patients

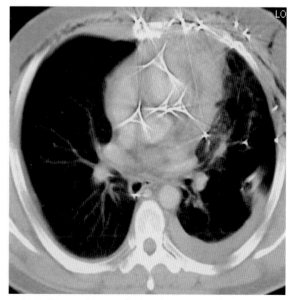

Figure 60.5 CT scan shows multiple pellets in the heart and myocardium after a shotgun injury.

may observed. However, partially embedded or symptomatic foreign bodies should be removed [20, 22, 23].

Blunt cardiac trauma

Definition and epidemiology

Blunt cardiac injury includes a wide spectrum of pathologies, ranging from asymptomatic myocardial contusion to free cardiac wall rupture. The at-risk population is broad and includes any significant blunt chest trauma. Blunt cardiac injuries can be divided into conduction abnormalities and anatomical lesions. Overall, the most commonly seen electrical abnormality is a nonspecific ST and T-wave change. The most frequent clinically significant electrical disorders are arrhythmias, usually tachyarrhythmias [24, 25]. Cardiogenic shock is a less frequent complication after blunt trauma [26, 27]. The anatomical lesions may include myocardial contusion, cardiac rupture, valvular or papillary muscle rupture, and coronary artery injury.

The incidence of symptomatic blunt cardiac trauma requiring treatment (arrhythmias or cardiogenic shock) after significant chest trauma resulting in chest wall fractures or intrathoracic injuries is about 13% [26, 27].

The reported incidence of cardiac rupture in patients reaching hospital care is about 0.05%. In a review of more than 810 000 blunt trauma patients from the National Trauma Data Bank, the incidence of cardiac rupture was 0.05% [28]. Motor vehicle collision was the most common mechanism of injury (73%), followed by pedestrians struck by a car (16%), and falls from height (8%). The right cardiac chambers are most commonly injured because of their more vulnerable location beneath the sternum and the relatively thin wall of the myocardium (→ Fig. 60.6). The low incidence of cardiac rupture in victims reaching hospital care is deceptive. The real incidence is much higher, but the vast majority of cases are declared dead at the scene and are transported to the coroner's department or morgue. In a recent autopsy study of 304 deaths after traffic injuries in the County of Los Angeles, 20% had a cardiac rupture; 85% of deaths occurred at the scene and only 15% reached medical care [29].

Valvular or papillary muscle rupture may occur as a result of direct transmission of energy by the sternum or by increased pressure within the cardiac chambers. The most frequently injured valve is the aortic, followed by the mitral [28, 30, 31]. Some studies suggest that the valvular injuries are progressive and often require valve replacement [31].

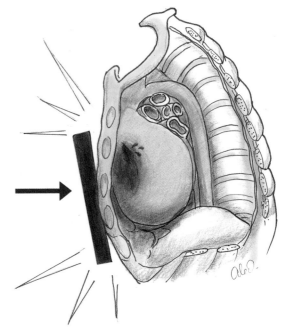

Figure 60.6 Motor vehicle injuries are the most common cause of blunt cardiac trauma. Cardiac rupture usually occurs in the right ventricle because of its close contact with overlying sternum.

Blunt coronary artery injury is found in less than 2% of cases with blunt cardiac trauma [32–35]. Direct impact may cause coronary vessel thrombosis, dissection, or rupture. The injury most often involves the left anterior descending artery, because of its location adjacent to the sternum.

Clinical presentation

The vast majority of victims with blunt cardiac rupture are dead at the scene and never reach hospital care [29]. Of those who reach the hospital alive, many are asymptomatic and the diagnosis is made by ECG or elevated troponins (🎥 60.7) Symptomatic cardiac arrhythmias or cardiogenic shock requiring treatment are diagnosed in about 13% of significant chest trauma (defined as rib, sternal, or scapular fractures; pulmonary contusion; haemo-pneumothorax; or anterior seatbelt marks) [26, 27]. Patients with cardiac rupture reaching hospital care are almost always *in extremis* or suffer a cardiac arrest in the emergency room, and they usually require a resuscitative thoracotomy. In rare occasions, with small ruptures and short prehospital times, the patient might be stable on admission and the diagnosis is made by ultrasound or CT scan (🎥 60.8).

Coronary artery rupture may present with shock, tamponade, or haemorrhage. Occlusion or dissection present similarly to acute myocardial infarction (MI) and may result in cardiac aneurysm [36].

Screening and diagnosis

All severe blunt trauma patients should be routinely evaluated for possible cardiac trauma, irrespective of clinical signs or symptoms. The routine evaluation should include trauma ultrasonography, ECG, and cardiac biomarkers. Several studies have demonstrated the superiority of troponin-I to CK-MB as a biomarker of traumatic myocardial injury [37–39], and most trauma centers use troponin-I for screening purposes. Selected patients with abnormal findings should be further evaluated by formal echocardiography.

Admission ECG and troponin-I levels may predict which patients are likely to develop a cardiac-related complications. In a large prospective study of 333 consecutive patients with severe chest trauma, the authors evaluated the diagnostic role of the initial and serial troponin and ECG evaluation. In this cohort of patients, 13% had a diagnosis of significant cardiac trauma requiring treatment or the echocardiogram showed structural abnormalities, or the cardiac index was less than 2.5 L min^{-1} m^{-2}. The sensitivity and specificity of the initial troponin-I alone were 73% and 60% respectively and those of ECG alone were 89% and 67%, respectively. However, when the two investigations were combined the sensitivity and specificity were 100% and 71% respectively. Looked from a different angle, if the troponin-I alone was abnormal the incidence of significant blunt cardiac trauma was 7%; if only the ECG was abnormal the incidence was 22%; and if both were abnormal the rate increased to 36%. Most importantly, if both investigations were normal, no clinically significant blunt trauma was observed [27]. The recommended algorithm for the cardiac evaluation in blunt multitrauma patients is shown in ➲ Fig. 60.7.

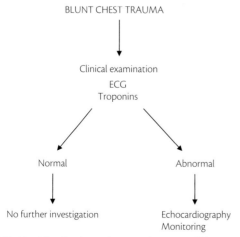

Figure 60.7 Algorithm for the evaluation of suspected blunt cardiac trauma.

Management

Asymptomatic patients with abnormal ECG or cardiac enzymes should be observed in a monitored area until return to normal. There is no need for any specific treatment in this group of patients. Echocardiography should be performed to evaluate for any underlying functional or anatomical cardiac abnormalities.

The treatment of symptomatic patients with cardiogenic shock or arrhythmias is similar to that for nontraumatic conditions and may include replacement of intravascular volume, inotropic agents, and occasionally placement of an intra-aortic balloon [24]. Serial echocardiography should be performed to rule out delayed tamponade or other complications.

Treatment of coronary artery injury includes medical management, percutaneous intervention, and operative revascularization. Fibrinolytic therapy is usually contraindicated because of associated injuries, although in isolated cardiac trauma it might be helpful [32]. Operative repair is preferably performed off bypass in order to avoid the risks of anticoagulation and because the severely contused heart is unlikely to tolerate an arrest well [3, 32].

Patients with ultrasound diagnosis of cardiac rupture and tamponade need an emergency operative repair. In the presence of severe haemodynamic instability or cardiac arrest, a left thoracotomy with cardiac repair, and resuscitation should be performed in the emergency room. Less unstable patients are transferred to the operating room for the repair of the cardiac rupture. There is no need for cardiac bypass and no effort should be made to identify any intracardiac traumatic lesion during this stage.

Prognosis

Blunt cardiac rupture is associated with very high mortality. Nearly 85% of deaths occur at the scene and the remainder en route or on arrival at the hospital [29]. Only a small number of patients with fairly small ruptures and short pre-hospital times reach the hospital alive. In a National Trauma Data Bank review of 334 cases with cardiac rupture admitted to emergency rooms, 6% were dead on arrival and 42% died in the emergency room. The overall mortality in patients arriving with signs of life was 89% [28].

The outcome in less severe blunt cardiac trauma, such as myocardial contusion, is very good. The majority of haemodynamically significant complications resolve within a few hours or days. The effects of myocardial contusion on long-term myocardial function are not known. Experimental work and case studies reported permanent damage and fibrosis of the injured part of the myocardium [40, 41]. However, another prospective study of 14 patients with diagnosed myocardial contusion reported that 3 and 12 months post-injury there were no residual abnormalities on ECG, echocardiography, and bicycle ergometry exercise test [42]. Other small series of patients utilizing the New York Heart Association classification and functional testing at 1 year demonstrated excellent recovery among survivors [43]. Long-term functional outcome studies are lacking.

In patients with myocardial contusion requiring early surgery for other associated injuries, general anesthesia and operation are safe, although consideration should be given to intraoperative haemodynamic monitoring with transoesophageal echocardiography or pulmonary artery catheters [25–27].

Cardiac complications after extracardiac injuries

Cardiac complications may occur after severe trauma to other system organs. They are particularly common after traumatic brain injury, especially in patients with severe subarachnoid haemorrhage. The cardiac complications may vary from tachycardia, arrhythmias, and nonspecific ECG changes to extreme haemodynamic lability. The serum troponin is frequently elevated and is an independent predictor of adverse outcomes. In an analysis of 420 patients with isolated severe head injuries, 30% had elevated troponin on admission. The degree of troponin elevation correlated with the severity of head injury. Multivariate analysis adjusting for injury severity, identified elevated troponin levels as an independent predictor of increased mortality [44]. Another important finding of the study was the improved survival outcome in patients who received β-blockers. The therapeutic implication of this finding needs further scientific testing in prospective randomized studies.

When traumatic brain injury progresses to brain death, a series of predictable haemodynamic changes occurs. First, mixed vagal and sympathetic stimulation cause bradycardia and hypertension, known as the Cushing response. Next, loss of parasympathetic innervation results in a 'sympathetic storm' which is characterized by tachycardia, increased myocardial oxygen demand, and coronary vasoconstrictions. Cardiac ischaemia can be diagnosed in more than 30% of brain-dead patients [45]. Finally, as herniation is completed there is loss of spinal sympathetic tone and vasodilation, which causes profound hypotension. ECG changes at this stage are common, initially bradycardia

and various stages of heart block. These are followed by tachyarrythmias and then return to sinus rhythm after completion of herniation [46]. In addition to the impaired catecholamine production, disruption of the neurohormonal axis causes deficiencies in cortisol, insulin, and thyroid hormone, resulting in severe hypotension, not responsive to vasopressors [47]. There is some clinical evidence that administration of the 'thyroxine protocol' reverses hypotension not responding to vasopressors and preserves the blood supply of crucial organs [48, 49]. This protocol consists of a bolus administration of 50 mL of 50% dextrose, 20 units of insulin, 2 g of methyprednizolone, and 20 µg of levothyroxine, followed by a continuous infusion of levothyroxine at 10 µg/L.

Other severe extracardiac injuries are also associated with troponin increases. In an analysis of 1081 critically injured intensive care unit (ICU) patients, increased troponin levels were found in 29% [51]. Independent predictors of increased troponins were the admission base deficit, injury severity score, and APACHE score. Significant increase of troponins was an independent predictor of increased mortality after controlling for age, gender, mechanism, base deficit, Glasgow Coma Scale score, and injury severity score. Use of a β-blocker was associated with a 50% reduction in mortality among patients with an increased troponin [44, 50].

Pneumonectomy following trauma is associated with a high incidence of severe acute right cardiac fracture, which is the most common cause of postoperative deaths. Pneumonectomy, especially combined with hypovolaemic shock, increases the pulmonary vascular resistance, resulting in acute right cardiac fracture [51]. Fluid restriction, inotropic agents, and in haemodynamically stable patients vasodilating agents may be helpful [52, 53]. In a National Trauma Data Bank review of 100 cases with pneumonectomy after trauma the mortality of patients with no major extrapulmonary injuries was 53% [54]. In the long term, there is some evidence that survivors of pneumonectomy after trauma are at a significant risk of cor pulmonale [55].

Conclusion

Post-traumatic cardiac complications may occur after penetrating or blunt injuries to the heart or may follow severe extracardiac injuries. Few victims of penetrating cardiac injuries survive to hospital care; for those who do, an immediate operation and resuscitation can result in a small portion surviving. Survivors may develop complications such as acute cardiac failure, arrhythmias, air embolism, and MI. All survivors should undergo detailed early and late clinical and radiographic evaluations. Blunt cardiac trauma may include a wide spectrum of injury severity, but most are asymptomatic. Clinical examination, ECG, troponin measurements, and echocardiography are essential for diagnosis. Lastly, serious extracardiac traumatic conditions, especially those involving the brain or lungs, may result in cardiac complications. The future of diagnosis and treatment of cardiac complications following trauma is vast, and includes many diverse areas of research such as post-injury pharmacotherapy, on-site surgical treatment and increasing use of cardiopulmonary bypass.

Personal perspective

There are many possible areas of research and advances in the short- to medium-term future. One exciting field in trauma is induced hypothermic cardiac arrest. Early experimental results in animal models undergoing emergency room thoracotomy for haemorrhagic cardiac arrest are encouraging [56, 57]. Patients with isolated penetrating cardiac injuries suffering cardiac arrest in the emergency room may benefit from this kind of intervention.

Another area of major interest is the use of internal cardiac pacing or cardiopulmonary bypass in the emergency room in patients with persistent cardiac arrest after resuscitative thoracotomy. Experimental work has shown the feasibility of cardiopulmonary bypass in the emergency room [58].

One of the most frustrating experiences for a trauma surgeon is the persistent cardiac arrest after repair of a small cardiac wound in a young, otherwise healthy victim. The experience gained from nontraumatic cardiac arrest may be helpful in trauma and it should be explored.

Finally, β-blockers may have a role in the management of the severe multitrauma patients. Recent retrospective studies have shown that β-blockers improve the survival outcome in severe multitrauma and head injuries. This is an area that needs to be investigated in prospective randomized studies.

Further reading

Actis Dato GM, Arslanian A, Di Marzio P, *et al*. Posttraumatic and iatrogenic foreign bodies in the heart: report of fourteen cases and review of the literature. *J Thorac Cardiovasc Surg* 2003;**126**(2):408–414.

Alam HB, Chen Z, Ahuja N, *et al*. Profound hypothermia protects neurons and astrocytes, and preserves cognitive functions in a swine model of lethal hemorrhage. *J Surg Res* 2005;**15**:172–181.

Asensio JA, Berne JD, Demetriades D, *et al*. One hundred five penetrating cardiac injuries: a 2-year prospective evaluation. *J Trauma* 1998;**44**(6):1073–1082.

Brevard S, Weintraub SL, Bronaugh H, *et al*. Effects of epoprostenol on pulmonary hypertension after pneumonectomy for trauma. *J Trauma* 2008;**64**(2):496–499.

Bruschi G, Agati S, Iorio F, Vitali E. Papillary muscle rupture and pericardial injuries after blunt chest trauma. *Eur J Cardiothorac Surg* 2001;**20**(1):200–202.

Campbell NC, Thomson SR, Muckart DJ, *et al*. Review of 1198 cases of penetrating cardiac trauma. *Br J Surg* 1997;**84**(12):1737–1740.

Cryer HG, Mavroudis C, Yu J, *et al*. Shock transfusion, and pneuonectomy. Death is due to right heart failure and increased pulmonary vascular resistance. *Ann Surg*;**212**:197–201.

Dellegrottaglie S, Pedrotti P, Pedretti S, *et al*. Persistent myocardial damage late after cardiac contusion:depiction by cardiac magnetic response. *J Cardiovasc Med* 2008;**9**:1177–1179.

Demetriades D. Cardiac wounds. Experience with 70 patients. *Ann Surg* 1986; **204**(3):315–317.

Demetriades D, Charalambides C, Sareli P, Pantanowitz D. Late sequelae of penetrating cardiac injuries. *Br J Surg* 1990;**77**(7):813–814.

Duque HA, Florez LE, Moreno A, *et al*. Penetrating cardiac trauma: follow-up study including electrocardiography, echocardiography, and functional test. *World J Surg* 1999;**23**(12):1254–1257.

Kronson JW, Demetriades D. Retained cardiac missile: an unusual case report. *J Trauma* 2000;**48**(2):312–313.

Lindstaedt M, Germing A, Lawo T, *et al*. Acute and long-term clinical significance of myocardial contusion following blunt thoracic trauma: results of a prospective study. *J Trauma* 2002;**52**(3):479–485.

Martin MJ, McDonald JM, Mullenix PS, *et al*. Operative management and outcomes of traumatic lung resection. *J Am Coll Surg* 2006;**203**(3):336–344.

Martin M, Mullenix P, Rhee P, *et al*. Troponin increases in the critically injured patient:mechanical trauma or physiologic stress? *J Trauma* 2005;**59**(5):1086–1091.

Rozycki GS, Feliciano DV, Ochsner MG, *et al*. The role of ultrasound in patients with possible penetrating cardiac wounds: a prospective multicenter study. *J Trauma* 1999;**46**(4):543–551; discussion 551–552.

Salim A, Hatzizacharia P, Braown C, *et al*. Significance of troponin elevation after severe traumatic brain injury. *J Trauma*, 2008;**64**:46–52.

Salim A, Martin M, Brown C, *et al.* Complications of brain death: frequency and impact on organ retrieval. *Am Surg.* 2006;**72**(5):377–381.

Salim A, Vassiliou P, Velmahos G, *et al.* The role of thyroxine administration in potential organ donors. *Arch Surg* 2001;**136**:1377–1380.

Salim A, Velmahos GC, Jindal A, *et al.* Clinically significant blunt cardiac trauma: role of serum troponin levels combined with electrocardiographic findings. *J Trauma* 2001;**50**(2):237–243.

Teixeira P, Georgiou C, Inaba K, *et al.* Blunt cardiac trauma: lessons learned from the medical examiner. *J Trauma* 2009;**67**(6):1259–1264.

Teixeira PG, Inaba K, Oncel D, *et al.* Blunt cardiac rupture: a 5-year NTDB analysis. *J Trauma* 2009;**67**:788–91.

Velmahos GC, Karaiskakis M, Salim A, *et al.* Normal electrocardiography and serum troponin I levels preclude the presence of clinically significant blunt cardiac injury. *J Trauma* 2003;**54**(1):45,50; discussion 50–1.

Additional online material

- 🖳 60.1 Gunshot wound to the anterior chest
- 🖳 60.2 Haemopericardium (arrows) after a knife injury to the heart
- 🖳 60.3 Pneumopericardium (arrows) after a knife injury to the heart
- 🖳 60.4 Gunshot wound to the heart
- 🖳 60.5 'Double shadow' of a bullet
- 🖳 60.6 Shotgun pellets
- 🖳 60.7 Myocardial contusion
- 🖳 60.8 Rupture of the right atrium

⮕ For additional multimedia materials please visit the online version of the book (🕮 http://www.esciacc.oxfordmedicine.com).

CHAPTER 61

Cardiac emergencies in pregnancy

Patrizia Presbitero, Dennis Zavalloni, and Benedetta Agnoli

Contents

Summary

Pregnancy leads to several changes in physiological processes. The cardiovascular system progressively adapts to modifications that may worsen pre-existing pathological conditions or unmask previously undiagnosed diseases. Furthermore, pregnancy may be complicated by specific pathological conditions that are harmful for patients with cardiac diseases.

Cardiac disease is an increasingly important cause of morbidity and mortality in pregnant women. Admission to the intensive care unit (ICU) is a rare event (0.1–0.9% of deliveries) but, in these patients, mortality rates range from 3.5% to 21%. Only 30% of patients admitted to ICU are still pregnant whereas the others present in the postpartum period (defined as 6–12 weeks after delivery) [1, 2].

When treating pregnant women we are taking care of two subjects: the mother and the fetus. The possible adverse effects on the fetus of diagnostic examination and/or therapies should be always considered and, even after delivery, the possible drug interactions on breastfeeding should be taken into account. The management of cardiac emergencies during gestation strictly depends on fetal viability. In the early stages of pregnancy, until the fetus is no longer viable, the achievement of good clinical conditions in the mother is the only way to guarantee fetal survival. When the fetus is viable, especially during the last 2 months of pregnancy, an early delivery should be always considered because survival rates are higher outside rather than inside a critically ill mother.

In this chapter, an overview on main cardiac emergencies that may affect pregnancy is provided with a particular focus on treatments allowed for both mother and fetal protection.

Cardiovascular and respiratory adaptations to pregnancy

Pregnancy induces changes in biochemistry, anatomy, and physiology to allow an adequate blood supply to the uterus and developing fetus. ➲ Table 61.1 summarizes the main cardiovascular and respiratory adaptations according to gestational periods. Circulatory adaptations lead to an increase in heart size by about 12%, and the progressive uterine enlargement causes a left-upward displacement and rotation of the heart [3, 4]. Blood flow progressively increases in maternal organs, especially in the uterus, to maintain adequate placental perfusion. This is supported by a rise of 40–50% in cardiac output, with a further 20% increase during each uterine contraction during labour. Stroke volume is sensitive to maternal position: in the supine position it progressively decreases because of compression of the inferior vena cava by the gravid uterus. After delivery, as venous return is restored, a prompt rise in cardiac preload is observed [3, 5]. The increase in plasma volume is disproportionately higher than the red cell mass, resulting in the 'physiological anaemia of pregnancy' [6, 7].

The main ventilation changes develop progressively. The hyperventilation and hyperdynamic circulation increases arterial Po_2 to sustain a 20% raise in oxygen consumption in maternal muscle tissue and in the products of the fetal genome. The increase of ventilation and the subsequent decrease in $PaCO_2$ are also in part due to progesterone effects on the central respiratory centre. Respiratory rate is only little increased and the increase in minute ventilation (50%) results mainly from the raise in tidal volume. Abdominal muscles have less tone activity, causing respiration to be progressively more diaphragm dependent. The enlargement of conceptual mass induces a raise in diaphragm level, as much as 4 cm with a concomitant muscle excursion increased by only 1.5 cm. An increase of the thorax circumference by approximately 6 cm and a progressive recruitment of costal muscles enable a compensation to the progressive reduced role of the diaphragm in respiration [4, 8].

Table 61.1 Adaptations during pregnancy
(a) Cardiovascular adaptations

	1st trimester	2nd trimester	3rd trimester
Blood volume	↑	↑↑	↑↑↑
Cardiac output	↑	↑↑	↑↑↑
Stroke volume	↑	↑↑↑	↑, ↓, or ↔
Heart rate	↑	↑↑	↑↑ or ↑↑↑
Pulse pressure	↑	↑↑	↔
Systolic systemic pressure	↔	↓	↔
Diastolic systemic pressure	↓	↓↓	↓
Systemic vascular resistance	↓	↓↓↓	↓↓

(b) Respiratory adaptations

	Changes
Volumes	
Tidal	↑ 35–50%
Inhaling reserve	↓
Expiratory reserve	↓ 20%
Residual	↓ 20%
Capacities	↓ 5%
Total lung	↔
Vital	↑ 5%
Functional	↓ 20%

Emergencies related to pregnancy

Hypertension, pre-eclampsia, and eclampsia

Hypertensive disorders are the most common causes of adverse maternal and perinatal outcomes. These disorders can be regarded as a spectrum of disease, ranging from isolated chronic hypertension to pre-eclampsia and eclampsia. All chronic hypertensive disorders predispose to development of pre-eclampsia or eclampsia [9]. Although isolated chronic hypertension appears to have little effect on pregnancy outcomes, morbidity and mortality are high among patients with severe pre-eclampsia or eclampsia. The diagnosis of hypertensive disorders complicating pregnancy [10] is shown in ➲ Table 61.2.

Pre-eclampsia is characterized by a classic diagnostic triad that includes hypertension, proteinuria, and oedema, although the latter sign may be present even during normal pregnancies. The severity of pre-eclampsia is assessed by the frequency and intensity of the abnormalities listed in ➲ Table 61.3. It should not be underestimated that apparent mild disease may progress rapidly to a severe form [9].

Eclampsia is defined as the development of convulsions and/or coma in a patient with signs and symptoms of pre-eclampsia. The estimated incidence is 1–3 in 1000 pre-eclamptic patients. It occurs more frequently in the third trimester but it may appear at any time, until up to 10 days after delivery. Maternal mortality has decreased

Table 61.2 Diagnosis of hypertensive disorders complicating pregnancy

Gestational hypertension	BP ≥140/90 mmHg first time during pregnancy
	Proteinuria absent
	BP normal in <12 weeks postpartum (final diagnosis)
	May have other signs, e.g. headaches, epigastric pain
Preclampsia	
Minimum criteria	BP ≥140/90 mmHg after 20 weeks of gestation
	Proteinuria >300m g/24 h or≥1+ dipstick
Increased certainty of pre-eclampsia	BP ≥160/110 mmHg
	Proteinuria 2 g/24 h or ≥2+ dipstick
	Serum creatinine >1.2 mg/dl unless known to be previously elevated
	Platelets <100 000/mm³
	Microangiopathic haemolysis (increased LDH)
	Elevated AST or ALT
	Persistent headache or other cerebral or visual disturbance
	Persistent epigastric pain
Eclampsia	Seizures that cannot be attributed to other cause in a woman with pre0eclampsia
Superimposed pre-eclampsia (on chronic hypertension):	New-onset proteinuria ≥300 mg/24 h but no proteinuria before 20 weeks of gestation
	A sudden increase in proteinuria or BP or platelet count ≤100 000/mm³ and proteinuria before 20 weeks of gestation
Chronic hypertension	BP≥140/90 mmHg before pregnancy or diagnosed before 20 weeks of gestation or hypertension first diagnosed after 20 weeks of gestation and persistent after 12 weeks postpartum

ALT, alanine transaminase; AST, aspartate transaminase, BP, blood pressure; LDH, lactate dehydrogenase.

Table 61.3 Severity of hypertensive disorders during pregnancy

Abnormality	Mild	Severe
Diastolic blood pressure	<100 mmHg	≥110 mmHg
Proteinuria	Trace to 1+	≥persistent 2
Headache	No	Yes
Visual disturbances	No	Yes
Upper abdominal pain	No	Yes
Oliguria	No	<500 mL/24 h
Convulsion	No	Yes
Serum creatinine	Normal	↑
Thrombocytopenia	No	Yes
Liver enzyme elevation	Minimal	Marked
Fetal growth restriction	No	Yes
Pulmonary oedema	No	Yes

from 5–10% to less than 1% in the past three decades in developed countries. All pregnant women with convulsions should be considered to have eclampsia until other causes are excluded. In most cases, seizures are self-limiting, lasting 1–2 min. The duration of coma after a convulsion is variable and in very severe cases death may result before the patient awakens [10, 11].

The aetiology of pre-eclampsia and eclampsia is not well established but it seems that an initial vasospasm may have a damaging effect on vessels, with exposure of subendothelial collagen that stimulates platelet aggregation, activation, and release of platelet-derived thromboxane A2 (TXA2). TXA2 may sustain progressive vasoconstriction and hypertension. Elevated intravascular pressure combined with damaged vascular endothelium results in movement of fluid in extravascular space and haemorrhages. These processes lead to cerebral oedema with subsequent convulsion or intracranial haemorrhage, pulmonary oedema, blindness secondary to retinal detachment or occipital ischaemia, and stretching of Glisson's capsule with abdominal pain [11, 12].

Hospitalization is mandatory for women with persistent or worsening hypertension or development of proteinuria. Initial expectant management with the aim of improving infant outcome without compromising the safety of the mother is recommended [13]. General care includes:

- scrutiny of clinical findings such headache, visual disturbances, epigastric pain, and rapid weight gain

- measurement of blood pressure every 4 h until drug control of hypertension is achieved

- measurements of creatinine, haematocrit, platelets, and serum liver enzymes with frequency to be determined by the severity of hypertension; proteinuria at least every 1–2 days.

- frequent evaluation of fetal well-being by the obstetrician.

In case of eclampsia, the first priorities are to ensure that the airway is clear and to prevent injury and aspiration of gastric contents. Invasive haemodynamic monitoring should be considered for those women with multiple clinical factors such as intrinsic heart disease and/or advanced renal disease that might cause pulmonary oedema. The following antihypertensive drugs are suggested to lower blood pressure to 130–150/80–100 mmHg:

- hydralazine, intravenous, 5–10 mg at 15–20 min intervals

- labetalol, intravenous, 10–80 mg at 10–20 min intervals

- nifedipine, orally, 10–30 mg at 15–30 min intervals.

In severe cases of pre-eclampsia/eclampsia, magnesium sulphate is the first choice anticonvulsive agent because it does not produce central nervous system depression in either the mother or the fetus. An intravenous loading dose of 4–6 g over 15–20 min is followed by continuous infusion (2 g/h). Serum magnesium levels should be monitored every 4–6 h to maintain plasmatic concentration between 4 and 7 mEq/L (4.8–8.4 mg/dL). Magnesium sulphate is generally discontinued 24 h after delivery [14–16].

The control of maldistribution of extravascular fluid, which increases the risk of pulmonary and cerebral oedema, is difficult to achieve but hyperosmotics and diuretics are usually avoided and fluid administration should be limited (lactated Ringer solution 60–125 mL/h).

When the mother has stabilized, the time of delivery should be planned with the obstetrician. Our advice is to perform a caesarian section as soon as the fetus is viable. In an attempt to enhance fetal lung maturation, glucocorticoids may be administered to severely hypertensive pregnant women who are not nearly at term.

Pulmonary embolism (see also ➲ Chapter 64)

Pregnancy is characterized by an hypercoagulable state induced by a combination of physical and hormonal physiological changes of the haemostatic system [17]. Together with the intravascular volume overload, progesterone-induced venodilatation and venous compression (pelvic veins by the gravid uterus and left leg veins by the right iliac artery) increase the rates of venous thromboembolism.

The reported risk of PE is estimated to be 0.03–0.05% in pregnant women [18], 7–10 times more frequent than in nonpregnant age-matched controls before delivery, and 15–35 times higher during the puerperium [19]. Main predictors for venous thromboembolism are thrombophilia, obesity, family or previous history of PE, need for maternal immobilization, IUGR, assisted reproduction, pre-eclampsia, haemorrhage and infections during or after delivery [20–24]. Isolated arm vein thrombosis has been reported in patients undergoing assisted reproductive techniques [19].

Clinical signs and diagnostic examinations for PE are comparable to those of nonpregnant women, although special attention is paid to reducing fetal exposure to radiation. In particular, CT pulmonary angiography seems to be the diagnostic imaging with the lowest exposure [25].

Treatment should be started as soon as diagnosis is made and carried on throughout all of pregnancy and the postpartum period. Therapy consists of low-molecular-weight or unfractioned heparin (LMWH or UFH) [17, 19]. Placental degradation increases heparin clearance [26–28], therefore drug doses should be adjusted according to the antifactor-Xa concentration, until therapeutic levels are reached (0.5–1.1 IU/mL 3–6 h after administration for LMWH and 0.35–0.67 IU/mL for UFH). Oral anticoagulants are contraindicated until postpartum to avoid fetal haemorrhages and teratogenicity [29] but are allowed during breastfeeding [30, 31].

In case of haemodynamic instability or refractory hypoxiemia, thrombolysis (rt-PA 100 mg IV in 2 h) should be administered [32, 33]. Transcatheter thrombectomy or surgical embolectomy may be attempted when thrombolysis fails or in patients with contraindication to anticoagulation [18].

UFH is preferred to LMWH [19] only in patients with impaired renal function or when a reversal of anticoagulation might be promptly required (labour, delivery, epidural anaesthesia). When PE occurs <2 weeks before delivery, the insertion of a retrievable inferior vena cava filter and induction of labour should be encouraged [34–35]. In these cases, UFH should be reversed by protamine during labour and reinitiated soon after delivery. If the risk of relapse of PE is low, it can be delayed for 12 h. Then, it should last until 6 weeks postpartum. Afterwards, prolongation of therapy should be tailored according to individual patient risk profile [19].

Bleedings may occur in 4–14% of patients treated with thrombolysis, in 2% of those treated with full dose of heparin, and in 0.4–1.5% of those treated with prophylaxis [36–38]. Other potential side effects of heparin are allergic skin reactions(2% of cases), heparin-induced thrombocytopenia (3–5%) and heparin-induced bone loss (0.04%) [39].

Hyperthyroidism and Graves' disease (see also ➲ Chapter 68)

Hyperthyroidism during pregnancy occurs in 0.1–0.4% of cases, with Graves' disease being the main cause (>95% of cases). In the other 5% of patients hyperthyroidism is secondary to gestational transient thyrotoxicosis, excessive thyroid hormone intake (iatrogenic), nodular goitre, toxic adenoma, viral thyroiditis, choriocarcinoma, tumours of the pituitary gland or ovarian neoplasia [39–41].

Diagnosing hyperthyroidism during pregnancy is cumbersome for two reasons:

- Signs and symptoms mimic normal physiological changes of pregnancy.

- Pregnancy itself modifies the normal thyroid hormone metabolism. Human chorionic gonadotropin has direct thyrotropic activity through its α-subunit which it shares with TSH [42]; oestrogens cause an increase in the synthesis and a reduction in hepatic clearance of plasmatic thyroid binding globulins. Therefore, during the first trimester, FT3 and FT4 levels are 1.5 times the normal range in nonpregnant women and their concentrations decrease to normal values at the end of pregnancy. A reciprocal fluctuation is observed in TSH serum levels. Based on the individual variability of hormone concentrations, no trimester-specific normal ranges for hormone serum concentration have been stated in available commercial assays.

Hyperthyroidism should be suspected either in patients with a previously efficiently treated hyperthyroidism, or with a relapse of the disease, or in those without an history of thyroid disease. In case of recurrence, it may develop in spite of concomitant antithyroid therapy or it may present as isolated fetal thyroid dysfunction with maternal euthyroidism. As circulating antibodies against TSH receptor may be still present and pass the placenta, fetus may develop thyroid dysfunction even if the mother has been previously treated with surgery or with radioiodine [43].

Graves' disease is associated with both maternal and fetal adverse outcomes. Main signs and symptoms are the hyperdynamic state (similar to that occurring during normal pregnancy), goitre, tremors, frequent stool and hypertension, whereas ophthalmopathy and dermopathy are less frequent. In women with pre-existing or unknown heart disease, it may exacerbate pre-eclampsia, evolve into thyroid storm and cause miscarriage, placental abruption, postpartum haemorrhage, and preterm delivery [44–47]. The main risks for the fetus are growth retardation, accelerated bone maturation, malformations, goitre, and death [48, 49].

In up to 30% of cases, clinical remission may be observed in the second and third trimesters, with a rebound of symptoms during the puerperium, because of the influence of the normal changes of the immune system that tend to minimize the maternal cell-mediated immune response to the fetus [39, 50].

Graves' disease should not be confused with gestational transient thyrotoxicosis (the second most frequent cause of hyperthyroidism), a nonautoimmune form, secondary to the physiological modifications of the thyroid induced by pregnancy, characterized by hyperemesis gravidarum and usually not requiring treatment. Antithyroid agents may be considered only for cases with worsened or prolonged symptoms. Compared to Graves' disease, it is characterized by the absence of goitre, of anti-TSH-receptor antibodies, and by normal FT3 serum levels [51].

Thyroid storm is an extremely rare (1% of pregnant patients with hyperthyroidism [52]) but life-threatening event. The syndrome, consisting of fever, confusion, seizures, vomiting, and diarrhoea, arrhythmias, shock and coma may be triggered by infections, surgery, placenta previa, pre-eclampsia, labour or delivery [53]. Diagnosis is based on symptoms and hormone sample assays. In addition to specific therapy (see below), supportive measure are required: oxygen administration, maintenance of intravascular volume, surveillance of plasma concentration of electrolytes and both maternal and fetal monitoring. An intensive care setting with invasive monitoring should be planned. Delivery has to be avoided but, when it is impending, a paediatrician should be alerted to treat the newborn.

Therapy of Graves' disease concerns either the mother and the fetus. The aim of therapy is to administer the lowest possible drug dose to keep the patient's thyroid hormone levels at the upper limit of the normal range, to avoid fetal or neonatal hypothyroidism [54]. In fact, fetal thyroid function depends on the transplacental passage of both maternal hormone and antithyroid drugs. Maternal thyroid hormone levels are therefore the most useful index even of fetal thyroid status [55]. Therapeutic options are medical treatment and surgery, because radioiodine therapy is contraindicated until postpartum period. Thionamide drugs are considered the first line therapy and are effective in about 8 weeks. Propylthiouracil (100–150 mg/8 h) is preferred to methimazole (10 mg/day) because of its higher affinity for plasma protein binding, with a consequent lower transplacental passage, and because the latter has been associated with teratogenic effects [41, 56]. After delivery both drugs may be considered without restrictions [54]. When antithyroid drugs may not be administered β-blockers may be used to relieve symptoms (propranolol 20–40 mg/8 h). ⊇ Table 61.4 shows the therapeutic options in case of thyroid storm [53]. Surgery should be considered only if necessary for the mother's health (signs of dysphagia or airways obstruction due to the goitre) or when medical therapy is not efficient. In any case, it should be carried out after the first trimester, when the rates of postintervention abortion decrease [42].

Peripartum cardiomyopathy (see also ⊇ Chapter 18 of *The ESC Textbook of Cardiovascular Medicine*)

Peripartum cardiomyopathy (PPC) has an incidence of 1 in every 3000–4000 live births [57] and usually occurs after delivery in 80% of patients, in the last month of pregnancy in 10%, and either in the last month antepartum or in the 4 months postpartum in the remaining 10%.

Its pathogenesis is unclear, but several underlying aetiological mechanisms have been proposed such as myocarditis,

Table 61.4 Thyroid storm therapy

Drug	Dose	Effect
Propylthiouracil	Bolus of 600–800 mg, orally, followed by 150–200 mg/4–6 h	Antithyroid effect
Dexamethasone	2 mg IV or IM every 6 h for the first 24 h	↓ Thyroid hormone release and peripheral conversion of FT4 to FT3
Potassium iodide	2–5 drops orally every 8 h, 1–2 h after propylthiouracil administration	Block hormone release
Sodium iodide	0.5–1 g IV every 8 h	Block hormone release
Phenobarbital	30–60 mg orally every 4–6 h	↑Hormone catabolism; sedation
Propranolol	20–80 mg orally every 4–6 hours or 6 mg IV (1–2 mg every 5 min) followed by 1–10 mg/4 h	Inhibition of adrenergic effects
Reserpin	1–5 mg IM every 4–6 h	Inhibition of adrenergic effects (when β-blocker contraindicated)
Guanethidine	1 mg/kg orally every 12 h	Inhibition of adrenergic effects (when β-blocker contraindicated)
Diltiazem	60 mg orally every 8 h	Inhibition of adrenergic effects (when β-blocker contraindicated)

abnormal immune response, or nutritional deficiency [58–59]. Actually, PPC remains a diagnosis of exclusion. The main criteria are development of heart failure signs in the last month of pregnancy or in the 5 months after delivery, absence of other causes of heart failure, lack of evidence of heart disease before the last month of pregnancy, and echocardiographic documentation of reduced left ventricular function (EF <45%, and/or fractional shortening<30%, and/or end-diastolic diameter >2.7 cm/m^2) [60]. The ECG may show supraventicular arrhythmias, atrioventricular and intraventricular conduction defects, and nonspecific ST-segment and T-wave abnormalities [61, 62].

Clinical signs and symptoms do not differ from other forms of congestive heart failure, but the NYHA classification may be not adequate to estimate severity of clinical status owing to development of symptoms even in normal pregnancies. The natural history may be characterized by a sudden deterioration of left ventricular function with signs of acute cardiac failure and shock. These patients therefore require hospitalization in a referral centre where an ICU and heart surgery unit are available.

Prognosis depends on the recovery of left ventricular function. In case of persistent low EF, prognosis is poor and mortality rates reach 25% in the first trimester after delivery. Main causes for death are shock, arrhythmias, and thromboembolism. On the contrary, when left ventricular function improves in the first 6 months postpartum, prognosis is favourable [61, 63].

ACE inhibitors should be avoided and replaced by hydralazine or nitrates (another alternative is amlodipine).

Prophylactic use of LMWH is suggested [63, 64]. In patients with evidence of myocarditis and resistant to therapy, use of immunosuppressive drugs (steroids) or immunoglobulins has been attempted with uncertain results [63, 65]. When heart failure is refractory to medical treatment, intra-aortic balloon pump and insertion of a left ventricular assist device [61] may be used as a bridge to recovery, in most cases, or to heart transplantation [66].

Acute myocardial infarction (see also ⊃Chapters 41–46)

The increasing proportion of older women having babies may explain the increasing rates of pregnancy-related acute myocardial infarction (AMI) observed in the last decade [67]. AMI occurs in 3–10 in 100 000 deliveries, with a peak of incidence during the third trimester and in the puerperium. Mortality rates range from 5% to 7% in the mother and 13% to 17% in the fetus [68, 69].

The underestimation of ischaemic chest pain in women is even more evident during pregnancy when patients' risk profile is low. Diagnostic criteria and therapeutic options are the same as for nonpregnant women except for the reduced predictive value of creatine kinase MB (CK-MB), which may also be increased by uterine contractions [70].

An underlying atherosclerotic disease is present in only one-half of cases and the main role in pathophysiology is played by hormone-related changes in composition of vessel walls, hypercoagulability, and cardiovascular overload that may lead to spontaneous coronary dissection or thrombosis and vasospasm. These pathogenetic mechanisms do not allow an adequate development of compensatory coronary collateral circulation, with subsequent large infarctions and evolution towards dilated cardiomyopathy, especially because the left anterior descending artery is the vessel most commonly involved [71].

Urgent percutaneous revascularization is considered the treatment of choice. The use of a radial approach and abdominal shielding may reduce fetal radiation exposure. Furthermore, the use of contrast should be limited to avoid fetal dysthyroidism.

Experiences with thrombolysis in this subset are scarce but data from its use in pulmonary embolism report major complications in up to 15% of cases with 6% of fetal loss [36–38, 72]. Cardiac surgery should be discouraged because of the risk of fetal loss (20–30%), mainly due to the adverse effect of hypothermia and hypotension, with subsequent fall in placental perfusion [73].

Emergencies in pregnancy due to worsening of a pre-existent cardiac disease

Valvular heart disease (see also ➲ Chapter 21 of *The ESC Textbook of Cardiovascular Medicine*)

The presence of valvular heart disease (VHD) increases the risk of pregnancy to both the mother and the fetus. Acquired VHDs are mainly represented by mitral stenosis (MS) due to rheumatic heart disease, followed by mitral regurgitation (MR) due to either rheumatic heart disease or mitral prolapse, aortic stenosis (AS), aortic regurgitation (AR), and pulmonic stenosis mainly due to congenital heart disease [74]. Physiological adaptations and the accelerated metabolism of pregnancy are scarcely tolerated by patients with valve stenoses because the pressure gradient increases proportionally with the rise in cardiac output. On the contrary, valve regurgitations are usually well tolerated because of the significant fall in systemic vascular resistance and reduced left ventricular afterload [75], and rarely lead to cardiac emergencies.

Maternal complications are related to the severity of VHD. Moderate to severe MS and severe AS may suddenly precipitate pulmonary oedema, in particular as a consequence of tachyarrhythmias. Medical therapy for MS consists of the use of a β_1-blocker (β_2-blockers should be avoided to prevent uterine relaxation) [76]. A higher drug dose than

in nonpregnant patients [79] may be necessary because of increased sympathetic activity during gestation. Diuretics may be used avoiding hypovolaemia that causes uteroplacental hypoperfusion [78]. Digoxin is considered safe for heart rate control in case of atrial fibrillation. Management of AS with medical therapy is less successful and usually requires valve repair or replacement. See the outline in ➲ Arrhythmias below for the treatment of arrhythmias.

When symptoms are resistant to medical therapy, valve repair should be attempted by either percutaneous balloon valvuloplasty or surgery. When required, the former intervention should be preferred because of the smaller risk for the mother and the fetus [74]. In the very early stages of gestation, termination of pregnancy may be necessary. Later in pregnancy, timing and mode of delivery should be discussed jointly by the obstetrician, cardiologist, and anaesthetist. During labour and delivery, haemodynamic monitoring with a pulmonary artery catheter is recommended in patients with moderate or severe VHD [74].

Percutaneous valve repair has been performed in both MS and AS, obtaining acute clinical improvement [79]. Transient maternal hypotension and fetal heart rate decrease may occur because of balloon inflation or prolonged supine position and may be treated with crystalloid infusion. Postprocedural results are maintained in MS but not sustained in AS. However, aortic balloon angioplasty enables the pregnancy to continue, and valve replacement has to be considered soon after delivery [80].

Heart surgery during gestation should be performed in patients who are refractory to optimal medical therapy but not suitable for percutaneous interventions. When fetal maturity is achieved, delivery should be carried out first and then valve repair or replacement performed. Maternal surgical mortality has been reported in 10% in the past but actually can be considered not different from that observed in nonpregnant women. Fetal loss ranges from 29% to 38% [74].

Valvular prosthesis dysfunction (VPD) represents another cause of VHD that may occur during gestation [74]. Pregnancy-related higher rates of bioprosthesis deterioration (10–30%) and mechanical prosthesis thrombosis (7–23%) have been observed [81]. The main complications are congestive heart failure, especially in patients with pre-existent ventricular dysfunction, and valve thrombosis, usually in the mitral position. Thrombolysis is the first line therapy in case of valve thrombotic obstruction. LMWH is considered as a valid alternative for small thrombi [81] (see section ➲ Pulmonary embolism for complication of thrombolysis and management of anticoagulant therapy during pregnancy).

Congenital heart disease (see also ⇥ Chapter 10 of *The ESC Textbook of Cardiovascular Medicine* and ⇥ Chapter 58)

The improvements in medical and surgical management of congenital heart disease (CHD) have enabled such patients to reach to adult life and to become pregnant. [82]. Patients with complex CHD, either repaired or not repaired, require intensive care evaluation mainly for arrhythmias, peripheral or pulmonary embolism and congestive heart failure [83–85].

Emergencies in patients with simple CHD are mainly supraventricular tachyarrhythmias and should be treated as in pregnant women without CHD [82, 86–87] (see section ⇥ Arrhythmias).

Patients with repaired CHD and extensive atrial scars (transposition of great arteries, Fontan procedure, AV canal, etc.) often present rapid atrial flutter/fibrillation alternated with bradycardias. In these conditions class IC antiarrhythmic drugs may precipitate 1:1 atrial flutter and lead to ventricular fibrillation or may cause high degree AV blocks, especially when associated with β-blockers or digoxin. In this subset of patients the best option to treat supraventricular tachyarrythmias is electric cardioversion.

LMWH and UFH should be used with caution in cyanotic patients because of their haemorrhagic tendency, mainly due to low platelet counts and probably to tissue hypervascularization secondary to chronic hypoxia.

Management of congestive heart failure in cyanotic patients should imply a careful use of diuretics, avoiding hypotension and placental hypoperfusion that increase the risk of pre-eclampsia and avoiding the relative increase in the haematocrit that may enhance thromboembolism.

In patients with pulmonary hypertension pregnancy may be complicated by progressive or sudden right ventricular failure because the fixed pulmonary circulation does not tolerate an increase in cardiac output. Sudden cardiac arrest is mostly due to acute pulmonary fibrinoid necrosis, but differential diagnosis with acute pulmonary embolism should be made. Fetal growth retardation, premature delivery, or the onset of pre-eclampsia may be observed due to placental hypoperfusion [88, 89]. Emergencies usually occurs during the second trimester and in the peripartum period (first week) and may present as cardiac shock or sudden death. Data on treatment of such patients derives from case reports and maternal mortality is reported in 30–60% of cases. Prostanoids (epoprostenol IV 5–20 ng/kg per min, nebulized iloprost 10–20 μg 7–9 times daily) and sildenafil (20–40 mg daily) have been successfully administered to reduce pulmonary vascular resistances without fetal morbidity. Bosentan should be avoided because of its teratogenicity [90]. Fetal protection mainly consists in avoiding placental hypoperfusion and potentially harmful drugs.

Aortic dissection (see also ⇥ Chapter 59)

Oestrogen-related changes in vessel wall tissue texture together with the volume overload due to physiological adaptations of cardiovascular system may enhance the risk of aortic dissection with gestational age. In fact aortic dissection usually occurs in the third trimester [91].

The main causes of aortic dissection during pregnancy are hypertension, endocrine diseases, atherosclerosis, aortic coarctation (operated or not operated) and, above all, Marfan's syndrome: this is considered the clinical condition at highest risk, especially when associated with bicuspid aortic valve and aortic root enlargement. During pregnancy type A dissection is more frequent than type B [91–93].

In healthy pregnant women, the aortic root enlarges by 2–3 mm during the course of pregnancy [87]; therefore, in patients with aortic root greater than 40 mm, especially those with Marfan's syndrome who are characterized by a 10-fold increase of risk, echocardiographic evaluation of the aorta should be done every 4–6 weeks. In patients with Marfan's syndrome and aortic root less than 40 mm, controls should be planned each trimester. MRI can be considered as a valid alternative when echocardiography does not provide reliable information [94–95].

$β_1$-Blockers should be administered to prevent complications in patients with aortic root greater than 40 mm and in those with Marfan's syndrome regardless of aortic root dimension. Medical therapy should be administered up to 3 months after delivery to prevent late dissections [91].

In case of a type A dissection, urgent surgical repair should be performed. Maternal and fetal survival after surgery have improved in the last decades, especially for the mother. The presence of Marfan's syndrome is an additive negative prognostic factor for surgery. When the fetus is viable (>30 weeks), delivery by caesarean section followed by cardiac surgery should be planned.

Type B dissection rarely requires urgent surgery and data on outcomes for both mother and fetus are scarce. Aortic dissections occurring in postpartum should be managed as in nonpregnant women [91, 96].

Arrhythmias (see also ⇥ Chapters 54 and 55)

Women have a different electrophysiological profile from men because of their different hormonal profile [97]. Oestradiol prolongs cardiac action potential duration and atrial effective refractory period [98, 99]. This reflects the prevalence of supraventricular tachycardias (SVT) during the luteal phase of the menstrual cycle and a greater predisposition to torsade de pointes when using drugs that prolong ventricular repolarization [100, 102]. Pregnancy and postpartum (in particular labour and delivery) may therefore increase the risk of developing arrhythmias owing to the hormonal changes and adaptations of cardiovascular system.

Antiarrhythmic drugs cross the placenta and should therefore not be considered completely safe [95]. ⊃ Table 61.5 shows the main permitted drugs with their potential adverse effect on the fetus. In case of untreatable tachyarrhythmias radiofrequency ablation may be attempted [103, 104] and in case of haemodynamic instability electric cardioversion may be performed [94].

Isolated premature beats do not require any treatment; a selective β_1-blocker may be considered in highly symptomatic patients [105] (β_2-blockers should be avoided because they are associated with reduced uteroplacental perfusion)[106]. As a general rule, stimulants such as coffee, smoking, and alcohol should be avoided and the main electrolyte disturbance corrected.

Supraventricular tachyarrhythmias are usually secondary to accessory pathways or AV nodal re-entry aetiology [107].

When vagal manoeuvres are ineffective, adenosine or calcium channel blockers (preferably verapamil) should be considered. Ajmaline is the first choice drug for Wolff–Parkinson–White syndrome.

Atrial fibrilliation/flutter is rare but, in case of rapid ventricular rates, diastolic filling times are shortened with potential reduction of placental perfusion. Digoxin, β_1-blockers, or nondihydropyridine calcium channel blockers may control heart rate [108]. Cardioversion may be obtained with propranolol, quinidine, or flecainide [109].

Ventricular tachycardias (VT) are less common but usually associated with an underlying cardiac disease [109]. Idiopathic VT may originate from either right or left ventricle [110] and physical and psychological stresses are considered the main triggers [111, 112]. Procainamide, ajmaline, or lidocaine are the first choice drugs, followed by sotalol, amiodarone, or magnesium sulphate. β-Blockers are indicated to prevent torsade de pointes in patients with long QT syndrome. This subset of patients may be partially protected during pregnancy from the increase of basal heart rate that reduces QT interval but, after delivery, the decrease of heart rate together with the psychological stress may potentially induce arrhythmias [113]. For this reason, medical treatment should be continued throughout pregnancy and the postpartum period [114].

Table 61.5 Antiarrhythmic therapy during pregnancy

Drug	Dose	Indication	Pregnancy-related collateral effects	Effect on fetus
Adenosine	9–18 mg IV bolus	SVT	Not significant AE	Bradycardia
Ajmaline	50–100 mg IV over 5 min	SVT-VT	Scarce data. Not significant AE	Avoid in 1st trimester for lack of specific studies
Amiodarone		VT	Pro-arrhythmic	Thyroid disease
Digoxin	0.25 mg/day monitoring plasmatic levels	AF	Not significant AE	Possible low birth weight
Disopyramide	100–150 mg every 6–8 h		Scarce data. Not significant AE	Uterine contractions
Flecainide	50–200 mg every 12 h	AF	Scarce data. Not significant AE	Scarce data. Not significant AE
Lidocaine	100–200 mg over 2 min	VT	↑ myometral tone, ↓ placental growth	Central nervous system depression, bradycardia
Magnesium sulphate	2–6 mg/kg bolus IV over 2 min followed by 0.3–1 mg/kg/h IV	VT	Not significant AE	Not significant AE
Procainamide	100 mg IV over 5 min, 300 mg orally every 4–6 h	VT	Not significant AE	Not significant AE
Quinidine	275 mg every 6–8 h	AF	Not significant AE	Thrombocytopenia, cranial nerve VIII damage
Sotalol	80–160 mg every 8 h	VT	Torsade de Pointes	Growth retardation, bradycardia, hypoglycaemia, hyperbilirubinaemia, uterine contraction
Verapamil	80–120 mg every 12 h	SVT, AF	Not significant AE	Heart block, hypotension
Electrical cardioversion	10–50 J 50–100 J 50–360 J	SVT AF VT, VF	Not significant AE	Not significant AE

AE, adverse effect; AF, atrial fibrillation; SVT, supraventricular tachycardia; VF, ventricular fibrillation; VT, ventricular tachycardia.

Cardioverter–defibrillator implantation should be considered as definitive long-term therapy [115].

Bradyarrhythmias are rare (0–0.02%) and usually well tolerated [116]. A pacemaker can be implanted at any stage of pregnancy [115, 117–118] but anticoagulation with LMWH should be considered to prevent the pregnancy-related higher risk of endocavital lead thrombosis.

All types of arrhythmias may occur in the fetus [119]. Intrauterine arrhythmias classification is different from that used during adulthood: bradycardia is defined a less than 100 beats/min and tachycardia as more than 180 beats/min. Diagnosis is obtained by measuring reciprocal atrial and ventricular motion with M-mode or Doppler echocardiography [119]. Isolated premature supraventricular or ventricular beats are the most frequent arrhythmias, followed by SVT (atrial flutter, junctional tachycardia, multifocal atrial tachycardia, atrioventricular re-entrant tachycardia), VT, and bradyarrhythmias. The main risk for the fetus is to develop hydrops fetalis and death. Therapy is usually given to the mother, with drugs crossing the placenta and acting on the fetus. Drugs may also be administered directly to the fetus by an intraperitoneal and/or umbilical intravenous route. Tachycardias are usually treated with digoxin, sotalol, flecainide, or amiodarone [127, 128]. Bradycardias, often associated with an underlying CHD or long QT syndrome, are treated with β-stimulants, such as terbutaine or salbutamol, or steroids (dexamethasone or betamethasone) in case of immune-mediated cardiac disease (myocarditis or presence of maternal SS-A antibodies) [119].

Other conditions that require cardiologic care

Some pathological conditions require a multidisciplinary approach and cardiologists may be involved in diagnosis and management of diseases that are not primarily cardiologic.

Stroke (see also ➲ Chapter 65)

Pregnancy-related stroke occurs in 4.3–210 per 100 000 deliveries [122–124]. The above-mentioned modifications of cardiovascular, haemostatic, and hormonal physiology during pregnancy increase the risk of stroke, which may be the first manifestation of an underlying cardiovascular disease such as pre-eclampsia, peripartum cardiomyopathy, spontaneous vessel dissections, or paradoxical embolism through a patent foramen ovale [124]. These pathological conditions should therefore always be suspected and

researched. The treatment of the underlying cardiac disease follows the indications as previously discussed. As far as stroke management is concerned, in the very acute phase, systemic or locoregional thrombolysis should be considered [125, 126]. Percutaneous closure of a patent foramen ovale has been safely performed during pregnancy even under echocardiographic guidance, but indication to intervene during gestation should be discussed according to the risk of relapse, to avoid fetal exposure to radiation [127]. For the management of anticoagulant therapy see Pulmonary embolism.

Amniotic fluid embolism

Amniotic fluid embolism (AFE) is a rare obstetric complication that occurs in approximately 1 in 8000–30 000 pregnancies with mortality rates ranging from 25% to 90% [128]. Amniotic fluid enters the circulation as a result of a breach in the physiological barrier between maternal and fetal compartments. There may be maternal exposures to various fetal element during pregnancy, following amniocentesis, trauma, labour, vaginal or caesarean delivery that affords various opportunities for mixture of maternal blood and fetal tissue [128]. These events may initiates a complex series of physiological reactions that are similar to those seen in human anaphylaxis and sepsis.

AFE is often difficult to diagnose [129]. Its clinical manifestation may consist of abrupt onset of maternal respiratory distress and cyanosis, hypotension, hypoxia, and consumptive coagulopathy. The main differential diagnoses include thromboembolism, congestive heart failure, hypotension, and eclampsia; therefore, cardiologists are often involved in the management of these patients [130].

Therapeutic measures [131] should be directed toward maintenance of cardiac output, minimizing hypoxaemia, and correction of coaugulopathy [132, 133]. Rapid volume infusion of isotonic crystalloid solutions may be helpful to restore preload and treat hypotension. Vasopressors and inotropes such as dopamine, dobutamine, norepinephrine, and milrinone are allowed to achieve arterial systolic values of at least 90 mmHg. In case of refractory hypoxaemia (Pao_2<60 mmHg), intubation and positive end-expiratory pressure (PEEP) may be required. The development of consumptive coagulopathy may require specific treatment (see below) [131]. Caesarean delivery is a complex decision and depends especially on the presence or absence of maternal cardiac arrest. Prognosis is ominous. Residual neurological damage is common in survivors. High perinatal morbidity and mortality rates would be expected, with a survival of approximately of 70%, but almost one-half of these infants suffer residual neurological impairments [133].

Disseminated intravascular coagulation

Disseminated intravascular coagulation (DIC) is a pathological systemic activation of coagulation that may be secondary to several diseases. In particular, during pregnancy, it may complicate the course of pre-eclampsia/eclampsia, AFE, intrauterine fetal demise, placental abruption, infections, or haemorrhages during delivery and postpartum [134]. Diagnosis requires a haematologist, because of the changes in main haemostatic parameters occurring during pregnancy. Treatment consists [134] of:

- Control of bleedings either surgically or with percutaneous intervention.
- Control of hypothermia and acidosis that may enhance coagulation.
- Restoration of fluids and blood products (O− red cells until exclusion of red cell antibodies, 1 unit of plasma and 1–2 units of platelet for each unit of red cells, 2 pools of cryoprecipitate and 4 g of fibrinogen concentrate to achieve plasma levels >1 g/L).
- Anticoagulation with UFH.
- Recombinant factor VIIa in case of massive haemorrhage (15–120 μg/kg).

Cardiopulmonary resuscitation

Cardiac arrest during pregnancy is extremely rare, with an incidence of 1 in 30 000 deliveries [135]. Modifications to basic life support (BLS) guidelines and to advanced life support have been adopted due to the physiological changes occurring during pregnancy:

- ABCDE approach as for nonpregnant women.
- Place patient in 15° of lateral decubitus and displace the uterus to the left to restore venous return (caval compression by the uterus may precipitate cardiac arrest and limit the effectiveness of chest compression during resuscitation manoeuvres) [136].
- 100% oxygen administration.
- Fluid bolus administration.
- Re-evaluate clinical status and consider any drug to be given.
- Ensure early involvement of gynaecologist and anaesthetist.

In case of cardiac arrest, chest compression has to be performed with hands slightly higher than the normal position owing to the elevation of the diaphragm. Defibrillation may be performed as usual (adhesive defibrillator pads are preferred to paddles) [137]. Early tracheal intubation is preferred because of a greater risk for gastro-oesophageal reflux and aspiration pneumonia. A tracheal tube with internal diameter 0.5–1 mm smaller than usual may be needed because of maternal oedema and swelling [138].

When maternal cardiac arrest lasts longer than 4 min, at more than 24 weeks of gestation, an early caesarean delivery may improve the outcomes of both mother and fetus, through relief of caval compression on venous return. Before 20 weeks of gestational age urgent delivery is not required and between 20 and 23 weeks hysterotomy should be performed primarily to save the mother's life [139–140].

Personal perspective

The increasing proportion of pregnancies at older ages, the recent increase of immigration from developing countries where rheumatic disease is still frequent, and the improvements in management of adult patients with CHD will progressively lead to an increase in heart-related emergencies during pregnancy. It is therefore very important that cardiologists are able to face this unusual and complex clinical condition, taking care of both the mother and the fetus. The three most frequent presentation of cardiac emergencies during pregnancy are (1) tachyarrhytmias, (2) pulmonary or systemic embolism, and (3) acute cardiac failure. A prompt diagnosis is mandatory to obtain a successful treatment. The first issue is, therefore, the awareness of the problem and of the differential diagnosis. Most diagnostic examinations can actually be performed with minimal exposure of the fetus to radiation. Drugs are safe during gestation and breastfeeding, but possible placental crossing with subsequent fetal harm should be always considered. New approaches, such as interventional procedures, may now be attempted. Even cardiac surgery, in dedicated centres, guarantees better results than in the past decades. Close cooperation between cardiologists, anaesthetists, obstetricians, and paediatricians is therefore mandatory to face this complex clinical issue.

Further reading

James AH. Pregnancy-associated thrombosis. *Hematology Am Soc Hematol Educ Program* 2009:277–285.

Lindheimer MD, Taler SJ, Cunningham FG. Hypertension in pregnancy. *J Am Soc Hypertens* 2010;**4**(2):68–78.

Moioli M, Valenzano Menada M, Bentivoglio G, Ferrero S. Peripartum cardiomyopathy. *Arch Gynecol Obstet* 2010;**281**(2):183–188.

Srinivasan S, Strasburger J. Overview of fetal arrhythmias. *Curr Opin Pediatr* 2008;**20**(5):522–531.

Tsiaras S, Poppas A. Cardiac disease in pregnancy: value of echocardiography. *Curr Cardiol Rep* 2010;**12**(3):250–256.

➲ For additional multimedia materials please visit the online version of the book (⌨ http://www.esciacc.oxfordmedicine.com).

SECTION XI

Concomitant acute conditions

CHAPTER 62

Acute respiratory failure and acute respiratory distress syndrome

Luciano Gattinoni and Eleonora Carlesso

Contents

Summary

Respiratory failure is present whenever the respiratory system fails in the gas exchange function. It is classified as 'hypoxaemic' when oxygen tension values are lower than normal, or 'ventilatory' when the elimination of CO_2 is insufficient. The acute hypoxaemic respiratory failure arising from widespread diffuse injury to the alveolar–capillary membrane is termed acute respiratory distress syndrome (ARDS).

ARDS is the clinical and radiographic manifestation of acute pulmonary inflammatory states. The cause may be of either pulmonary or extrapulmonary origin. The generalized inflammatory response process begins with the local production of cytokines by inflammatory cells, epithelial cells, and fibroblasts which increases the alveolar–capillary barrier permeability. The progression of the lung injury has been divided into three phases: exudative, proliferative, and fibrotic. To date, the definition routinely used to recruit ARDS patients includes the sudden onset of acute hypoxaemic respiratory failure (Pao_2/Fio_2 ratio <300), presence of diffuse pulmonary infiltrates that are not caused by hydrostatic pulmonary oedema, and absence of left atrial hypertension. The knowledge of ARDS pathology and mechanisms has been greatly improved by the use of CT analysis, which makes it possible to delineate the ARDS lung appearance, oedema distribution, and superimposed pressure computation, and characterize lung severity and potential for lung recruitment. The primary treatment for ARDS patients is mechanical ventilation, used to buy time while awaiting the resolution of the underlying pathology. Several randomized clinical trials have been conducted to investigate many aspects of the treatment such as the use of the prone position, the setting of ventilation parameters, and fluid resuscitation.

Introduction

Respiratory failure (RF) is defined as the acute or chronic impairment of respiratory system function to maintain normal oxygen and CO_2 values when breathing room air. 'Oxygenation failure' occurs when Pao_2 value is lower than the normal predicted values for age and altitude and may be due to ventilation/perfusion mismatch or low oxygen concentration in the inspired air. In contrast, 'ventilatory failure' primarily involves CO_2 elimination, with arterial CO_2 partial pressure ($Paco_2$) higher than 45 mmHg. The most common causes are exacerbation of chronic obstructive pulmonary disease (COPD), asthma, and neuromuscular fatigue, leading to dyspnoea, tachypnoea, tachycardia, use of accessory muscles of respiration, and altered consciousness. History and arterial blood gas analysis is the easiest way to assess the nature of acute RF and treatment should solve the baseline pathology. In severe cases mechanical ventilation is necessary as a 'buying time' therapy.

Pathophysiology of respiratory failure

Alveolar hypoxia

Alveolar hypoxia is characterized by a reduced fraction of oxygen on the alveolar side of the pulmonary units. A low alveolar oxygen concentration may be caused by breathing at a reduced barometric pressure or inhalation of gas mixture with inspired oxygen fraction (Fio_2) less than 21%. However the most clinically relevant mechanism is a ventilation/perfusion (Va/Q) mismatch. Briefly, perfusion removes a given amount of oxygen per unit of time from the alveolar units, which is granted by alveolar ventilation. This mechanism works properly when Va/Q ratio is near 1. The oxygen provided by ventilation may be calculated as:

$$Vo_2 = (Fio_2 - Feo_2) \times Va$$

Where Feo_2 is the expired oxygen concentration, Vo_2 is the amount of oxygen required, and Va is the alveolar ventilation. The equation shows that if ventilation decreases, and the subtraction of oxygen is constant, the difference between inspired and expired oxygen fractions must increase by the same percentage. If Fio_2 is not changed, Feo_2 decreases and the alveolar oxygen concentration decreases. The alveolar hypoxia, however, is simply corrected by increasing the Fio_2.

Shunt

The worst Va/Q alteration is called 'shunt', which is defined as the fraction of cardiac output perfusing unventilated regions where no gas exchange occurs ($Va/Q = 0$). Shunt may either be intracardiac or intrapulmonary. An interesting lung model developed by Riley [1] divides the lung into three ideal compartments according to Va/Q ratio: (1) ventilated and perfused; (2) perfused but not ventilated (shunt); (3) ventilated but not perfused (dead space). Hypoxaemia due to shunt can only be partially corrected by supplemental oxygen administration, as this will increase alveolar Pao_2 without affecting the unventilated regions. With shunt fractions as high as 30–35%, Pao_2 will not exceed 100 mmHg even with Fio_2 up to 100%. Correction of hypoxaemia due to shunt requires either pulmonary blood flow diversion or anatomical modification of the shunt regions. It has been shown that the same collapsed fraction of the lung corresponds to different levels of hypoxaemia in different patients, according to hypoxic vasoconstriction. This means that at the same Pao_2/Fio_2 ratio the lung parenchyma may be differently involved in the pathology.

Ventilatory failure

Hypercapnic respiratory failure or ventilatory failure is defined as the inability of the respiratory system to maintain normal levels of $Paco_2$ (i.e. $Paco_2$ <45 mmHg), due to the impaired excretion of CO_2. At steady state the rate of CO_2 production, Vco_2, equals CO_2 excretion. Moreover,

$$Faco_2 = Paco_2/(Pb - Ph_2o)$$

where $Faco_2$ is the alveolar fraction of CO_2, $Paco_2$ is the alveolar Pco_2, Pb is the barometric pressure, and Ph_2o is the saturated water vapour pressure. It follows that

$$Vco_2 = Faco_2 \times Va$$

This simple formula highlights that increased $Faco_2$, usually associated with decreased alveolar oxygen concentration, is the hallmark of ventilatory failure. In fact if Va decreases, to maintain constant CO_2 excretion $Faco_2$, i.e. $Paco_2$ and $Paco_2$, must increase in the same proportion.

Minute ventilation (Vt) is equal to the sum of Va and dead space ventilation (Vd), so rearranging the previous equation it follows that:

$$Faco_2 = Vco_2/(Vt - Vd)$$

Therefore elevated $Faco_2$ (and $Paco_2$) may result from a combination of the alteration of any of the three variables, i.e. increased CO_2 production, decreased tidal ventilation, and increased dead space.

Diagnosis

Blood gases

Pao_2 and $Paco_2$ values obtained by blood gas analysis give immediate information for the diagnosis and determination of the nature of respiratory failure (i.e. oxygenation or ventilatory). A challenge test with two different levels of Fio_2 may be useful to assess the primary mechanism of oxygenation failure. In fact if hypoxaemia is partially corrected by increasing Fio_2 the origin is alveolar hypoxia; otherwise, if hypoxaemia is only partially corrected, the most likely primary cause is shunt.

In most clinical cases pulse oximetry is an adequate surrogate for arterial Pao_2 [2, 3], while end-tidal CO_2 may reflect $Paco_2$ [4]. In steady state arterial Pco_2 is well correlated with venous Pco_2, being 4–5 cmH_2O higher [5], consequently $Pvco_2$ higher than 50 mmHg may indicate ventilatory failure [6]. Conversely, Pvo_2 is poorly correlated to Pao_2 and cannot be used a surrogate [5]. This derives from the fact that central venous oxygen saturation (Svo_2) depends not only on arterial oxygen saturation (Sao_2), but on a series of variables, such as Vo_2, cardiac output (CO), and oxygen-carrying capacity (haemoglobin concentration, Hb):

$$Svo_2 = Sao_2 - Vo_2/(CO \times [Hb])$$

Imaging

The portable chest radiograph is one of the simplest examinations used to assess the cardiopulmonary status of patients. Its great advantage is the low exposure to radiation and the possibility of performing the examination at the bedside. Chest radiographs are useful to assess device positions [7], and to detect pulmonary infiltrates, pneumothorax, and pleural effusions. Although the daily chest radiograph has been abandoned [8–11], in critically ill patients it remains a valid preliminary examination for suspected respiratory failure. On the other hand, CT allows a complete examination of lung parenchyma and quantitative analysis makes it possible to determine the degree of aeration of each lung region [12] (Fig. 62.1).

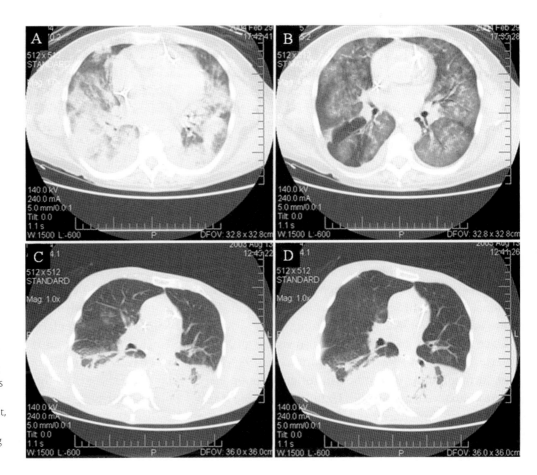

Figure 62.1 Representative CT images of ARDS lungs. Panels A and C represent CT images taken at end expiration at 5 cmH_2O PEEP. Panels B and D represent CT images taken at end inspiration at 45 cmH_2O plateau pressure. Panels A and B represent a patient with high potential for lung recruitment, while panels C and D represent a patient with low potential for lung recruitment.

Haemodynamics

The patient's haemodynamic status has to be carefully assessed in order to understand the nature of their respiratory failure. Cardiac output and pulmonary wedge pressure may provide important information for the diagnosis (e.g. pulmonary embolism, cardiac failure, etc.) Pulmonary pressure measurement is useful in patients characterized by chronic respiratory failure, to evaluate possible cardiogenic components of the pathology.

A pulmonary artery catheter (PAC) or central venous catheter (CVC) allows the precise monitoring of the patient's volaemic status, cardiac function, and haemodynamic effects of mechanical ventilation. Svo_2 is an optimal index of the adequacy of oxygen transport [13, 14]. Normal Svo_2 values are between 68% and 77% [15]; values lower than 65% indicates possible cardiovascular problems and values lower than 50% are associated with metabolic acidosis [16]. It should be remembered that PACs and CVCs give slightly different values of oxygen saturation because of their different positioning [17]. Moreover, abnormally low saturation values should be checked, as they may possibly be due to sources of error.

Acute respiratory distress syndrome

Definition

The original description of acute respiratory distress syndrome (ARDS) was published in 1967 by Ashbaugh and collegues in a cornerstone paper in the *Lancet* [18]. The authors outlined the characteristics and the clinical course of 12 patients treated for respiratory failure who did not respond to usual therapeutic modalities. 'The clinical pattern ... includes severe dyspnoea, tachypnoea, cyanosis that is refractory to oxygen therapy, loss of lung compliance, and a diffuse alveolar infiltrate seen on chest X-ray'. Seven patients died, and at autopsy the authors found that 'At necropsy in seven patients, gross inspection showed heavy and deep reddish-purple lungs ... the appearance resembled liver tissue'. In 1971, after a conference at the United States National Academy of Sciences, the same authors coined the name 'adult respiratory distress syndrome' [19].

Since then there have been several revisions of ARDS criteria to refine an working definition. In 1982 Pepe *et al.* introduced the noncardiogenic origin of pulmonary oedema into the definition [20]. Until 1988 no more major revisions were introduced and the only variations to the ARDS definition related to a combination of presence of hypoxaemia (Pao_2, Fio_2), radiographic infiltrates, low

compliance, and wedge pressure [21–23]. In 1988 Murray [24] proposed an approach based on the 'lung injury score' (LIS) to quantify the lung damage. The scoring system takes into account different components and differing degrees of their abnormality:

* Chest radiogram
* Hypoxaemia (Pao_2/Fio_2 ratio)
* Positive end-expiratory pressure (PEEP) (when ventilated)
* Respiratory system compliance.

Three levels of lung injury severity were defined: (1) absence of lung injury (LIS = 0); (2) mild to moderate lung injury (LIS = 0.1–2.5); (3) severe lung injury (ARDS) (LIS >2.5).

In 1994 the American European Consensus Conference developed a definition which is still routinely used for the recruitment of ARDS patients in clinical and epidemiological studies [25]: ARDS is characterized by the sudden onset of acute hypoxaemic respiratory failure, diffuse pulmonary infiltrates that are not caused by hydrostatic pulmonary oedema, and absence of left atrial hypertension (if measured, pulmonary artery wedge pressure must be <18 mmHg). The definition is also based on the degree of hypoxaemia defined by a Pao_2/Fio_2 ratio cut-point of 300: a ratio between 200 and 300 indicates acute lung injury (ALI), a ratio lower than 200 indicates ARDS. The Conference recommended that the syndrome be called 'acute', rather than 'adult', respiratory distress syndrome. Though this definition provided a standard way to select patients, it is not without limitations, such as the high variability of interpretation of chest radiographs [26], the problematic exclusion of the cardiogenic origin of pulmonary oedema [27], and the alteration of oxygenation by PEEP manipulation. Recent studies showed that over half of patients initially classified as having ARDS did not meet the criteria after 30 min of ventilation with a standardized PEEP [28]. Even at autopsy, the accuracy of the Conference definition was low [28]. In a recent study Gattinoni *et al.* studied 68 ALI/ARDS patients recruited according to the Conference definition and found that lung collapse, amount of lung oedema, and potential for lung recruitment (defined as the percentage of tissue regaining aeration from 5 cmH$_2$O PEEP to 45 cmH$_2$O end-inspiratory plateau pressure) have wide distributions [29]. Moreover, the authors found that the greater the alveolar collapse, the greater the potential for lung recruitment, with a distribution from nearly 0 to 65% of the lung weight. Moreover, the results showed that higher percentages of recruitment indicated higher severity, severe hypoxaemia, and more oedema.

Accordingly the ARDS definition should be updated to consider the amount of lung tissue involved in the pathology, as indicated by the amount of pulmonary oedema. ARDS should be diagnosed in those patients with extended pulmonary oedema, high potential for lung recruitment, and positive response to PEEP or pronation. At the moment no bedside method is available to obtain accurate estimation of lung recruitment; the only technique currently available is the quantitative analysis of CT images of the lung.

Risk factors

Many heterogeneous diseases, either direct or indirect lung injuries, have been reported as potential risk factors for ARDS (⊃ Table 62.1).

The major incidence of ARDS is linked to pneumonia, aspiration, sepsis and trauma. However a series of biological variables have emerged as potential risk factors for mortality, e.g. age, African-American ethnicity, and male gender. Sepsis and trauma are linked to greater mortality, and the amount of nonpulmonary organ failure, increased illness severity, shock, and hepatic failure are independent risk factors for mortality although the degree of hypoxia is not [30].

ARDS has always been considered rare. It is quite difficult to identify a specific incidence of the phenomenon, which is related to geography and to the definition used. The first epidemiological report, published in 1972 by the National Heart and Lung Institute Task Force on Respiratory Diseases [31], estimated an incidence of 150 000 cases per year (75 cases/100 000 population per year) in the United States. Other studies published in the 1980s and 1990s, however, reported an incidence between 1.5 and 8.3 cases/100 000 population [23, 32–35]. The most recent studies reported an incidence of 17.9 cases/100 000 population in Scandinavia [36], 34 in Australia [37], and 78.9 in the United States [38]. The last report from Rubenfeld et al. reported a considerably higher incidence, at least in the United States. The reliability of data is, however, guaranteed by the rigorous method of patient selection and by the particular geographical configuration of the study area (King County, Washington state, USA) which suggests that the majority of the inhabitants in need of care were treated at the study hospital.

In terms of mortality data, it is important to remember that in the initial description 7 of 12 patients died [18]. Despite nearly three decades of progress the mortality reported in the 1980s and 1990s was similar, ranging between 40% and 70% [23, 32, 33, 35]. The most recent studies, however, have reported a decline of mortality rate (29–40%) [38, 39]. An explanation of this reduction may be better general care for critically ill patients, as well as improved mechanical ventilation [39]. Most patients appear to die with ALI or from complications of their underlying risk factor as opposed to dying from unsupportable hypoxaemic respiratory failure [37]. The combination of declining short-term mortality associated with the incidence suggests that caring for survivors of ALI will be an increasingly important problem in the future. The data suggest that there is a significant increase of long-term neuromuscular, cognitive, and neurophysiological dysfunction in survivors of ALI/ARDS [40, 41] leading to possible post-traumatic stress disorders [42].

Pathophysiology

ARDS is the clinical and radiographic manifestation of acute pulmonary inflammatory states. The noxious stimulus, of either pulmonary or extrapulmonary origin, causes a generalized inflammatory response involving the whole lung. The process begins with the local production of cytokines by inflammatory cells, epithelial cells, and fibroblasts, which increases the alveolar–capillary barrier permeability. The progression of the lung injury has been divided into three phases: exudative, proliferative, and fibrotic. The exudative phase of the pathology consists in the progression of injury to the interstitium and alveolar spaces, to which inflammatory cells and proteins migrate. Protein-rich fluid enters the alveolar spaces with formation

Table 62.1 Risk factors associated with ALI/ARDS, grouped according to source of injury

Direct lung injury	Indirect lung injury
Pneumonia	Sepsis
Pulmonary aspiration	Major trauma
Near drowning	Cardiopulmonary bypass
Pulmonary contusion	Burn
Smoke inhalation	Bacteriaemia
Alveolar haemorrhage	Massive blood transfusion
Fat embolism	Bone fractures
	Disseminated intravascular coagulation
	Drug overdose
	Abdominal surgery
	Thoracic surgery
	Postanoxic coma
	Cerebral haemorrhage
	Pancreatitis
	Prolonged hypotension
	Shock
	Peritonitis
	SLE

of hyaline membranes. The generalized inflammation of lung parenchyma leads to pulmonary oedema formation of noncardiogenic origin, which causes alveolar collapse. This phase may rapidly resolve, or it may last as much as 5–7 days, up to fibrosis development. The proliferative or regenerative phase is characterized by gradual reduction of the inflammatory process and proliferation of type II pneumocytes in the reparative process. In this phase the interstitium remains oedematous and inflammatory cells are still present. The third phase (fibrotic) is characterized by dense deposition of collagen in the interstitial spaces and in the alveolar spaces of collapsed alveoli.

CT

CT analysis of the lung has proved the best way to assess the lung status during ARDS, and its degree of aeration [12]. The digital image produced by the CT scan is based on measuring the reduction of radiation intensity upon passage through matter by the attenuation coefficient (μ) [43]. By measuring the initial intensity and the emerging intensity of the X-ray, the integral function of the attenuation coefficient μ along the X-ray beam is calculated, then an attenuation number is assigned to each voxel by a mathematical algorithm. This attenuation number primarily represents the density of the voxel, i.e. the ratio of mass to volume, and is expressed as a CT number [44], which relates to the density of water (μ_{water}):

$$CT = 1000 \times [(\mu_{voxel} - \mu_{water})/\mu_{water}]$$

According to the formula, a CT number equal to zero Hounsfield units (HU) indicates that density equals that of water, −1000 HU indicates a density similar to that of gas, and +1000 HU indicates a density equal to that of bone. Note that a given CT number assigned to a voxel does not detect the composition of the voxel, but simply expresses its density as related to that of water.

Knowledge of the CT number, assuming the specific weight of the lung tissue to be equal to 1 (water), allows us to compute the volume of gas and the volume of tissue, either in the whole lung or in whatever region is of interest [45, 46]. In fact, a voxel with a CT number equal to 0 HU will consist only of tissue, a voxel with CT equal to −1000 HU will consist only of gas, and a voxel with a CT equal to −700 HU will be made up of 30% of tissue and 70% of gas. Accordingly:

$$volume\ of\ tissue = [1-(CT/1000)] \times total\ volume$$

$$volume\ of\ gas = total\ volume - volume\ of\ tissue$$

The frequency distribution of lung CT numbers, using appropriate thresholds, allows us to identify different compartments according to their degree of aeration (⮕ Table 62.2). These thresholds, however widely accepted, are arbitrary and have been introduced since 1987 by our group [47]. Slightly different thresholds have been proposed by other authors [12].

Inflammatory pulmonary oedema

The CT images of the lung during the early phase of ARDS are characterized by three vertically distributed compartments: the nondependent regions, which are usually normally aerated; the middle lung, characterized by ground glass opacification; and the almost consolidated dependent regions [12]. According to the descriptors proposed by the Fleischner Society Nomenclature Committee [48] 'ground glass opacification' means 'increase in lung attenuation, with preservation of bronchial and vascular margins', while 'consolidation' means 'homogeneous increase in lung attenuation that obscures bronchovascular margins in which an air bronchogram may be present'. The ground glass opacification reflects the active inflammatory process which involves the interstitium, filling of the alveolar space, and oedema, which corresponds to the poorly aerated tissue. Consolidation refers to the lung parenchyma being completely or almost completely airless due either to a complete filling of the alveolar spaces or to the total collapse of potentially recruitable pulmonary units (atelectasis). In quantitative analysis it corresponds to the nonaerated tissue. The late phase of ARDS is characterized by decreased densities and presence of fibrosis with distortion of bronchovascular markings, subpleural cysts, or bullae. Patients surviving ARDS present a reticular pattern at follow-up, principally in the nondependent lung regions [12].

The quantitative assessment of CT images has allowed us to understand that the amount of normally aerated tissue of the ARDS lung is of the same order of magnitude of that of a 5- or 6-year-old child. This amount has been found to be correlated with the respiratory system compliance, indicating that the ARDS lung is small and not stiff (the 'baby lung' concept) [49, 50]. The 'baby lung', however, is not an

Table 62.2 Identification of compartments by degree of aeration

Degree of aeration	CT number (HU)
Hyperinflated compartment	−1000 to −901
Normally aerated compartment	−900 to −501
Poorly aerated compartment	−500 to −101
Nonaerated compartment	−100 to +100

anatomical entity located in the nondependent regions: in fact, when patients are turned to the prone position, the densities are redistributed in the dependent lung regions [51]. On regional analysis, dividing the lung into 10 levels along the sternovertebral axis, it has been found that at each level the mass is almost doubled compared to the normal values, suggesting an even distribution of lung oedema throughout the lung parenchyma [52]. The nongravitational distribution of lung oedema apparently contrasts with the gravitational distribution of densities. However, the increased weight due to oedema accumulation raises the hydrostatic pressures transmitted throughout the lung, reducing the transpulmonary pressure (i.e. the distending force of the lung) and squeezing out the gas from the lung parenchyma. So the loss of alveolar gases is a result of compressive gravitational forces, including the weight of the heart, and not of an increase in the amount of oedema [12]. This phenomenon accounts for the mechanism of PEEP: a PEEP level higher than the superimposed pressure is necessary to keep open the most dependent lung regions. These findings led to an evolution of the ARDS model: the sponge model [53]. According to this model the ALI/ARDS lung increases its own permeability in each region with an even distribution of oedema, and the increased lung mass causes the lung to collapse under its own weight. However, there are also craniocaudal and sternovertebral gradients, which take into account the heart weight and the abdominal pressure.

The amount of nonaerated tissue measured at CT scan analysis is well correlated with hypoxaemia and shunt fraction, indicating that hypoxaemia in the case of ARDS is primarily due to shunt. Although the relationship between nonaerated tissue and hypoxaemia is straightforward, the relationship between hypoxaemia and poorly aerated tissue (ground glass opacification) is still not known. Taken together, poorly and nonaerated tissues relates to hypoxaemia, but poorly aerated tissue alone does not [12]. CT imaging does not in fact provide information on the perfusion degree or on ventilation (as it is a fixed image of a ventilatory status), so it is not known to what degree the compartment is capable of oxygenating the blood. The same holds true for normally aerated tissue. In fact, if these regions are overdistended they exchange oxygen well but do not exchange CO_2. Despite these limitations, the re-expansion of nonaerated regions is usually associated with increased oxygenation [54].

Potential for lung recruitment

The quantitative analysis of CT images provides several other kinds of information that are important in understanding ARDS pathophysiology [29]. For example, the severity of the overall lung injury may be expressed as the ratio of nonaerated lung tissue weight to total lung weight at end expiration (5 cmH_2O PEEP). This index includes both consolidation and collapsed tissue which can regain aeration. Another important index is the potential for lung recruitment, i.e. the ratio of the amount of lung tissue which regains aeration from 5 cmH_2O PEEP to 45 cmH_2O airway plateau pressure at end inspiration to the total lung weight at 5 cmH_2O PEEP. In a population of 68 ALI/ARDS patients Gattinoni et al. found that both the amount of nonaerated tissue and of potential for lung recruitment are highly variable in ALI/ARDS patients, ranging from 5% to 70% and from nearly 0 to more than 50%, respectively [29]. The PEEP response to lung recruitment depends on the amount of potential for lung recruitment: the higher the potential for lung recruitment, the higher the lung portion that remains aerated on increasing the PEEP level from 5 to 15 cmH_2O. It has also been found that increasing PEEP from 5 to 15 cmH_2O keeps open a portion of lung tissue nearly equal to 50% of the maximal potential for lung recruitment [29]. Until recent years, patients characterized by an high percentage of recruitable lung were considered less severe than those who had a lower percentage of lung recruitment with the same degree of lung damage. Actually, Gattinoni et al. found that patients with higher percentages of potential for lung recruitment had worse gas exchange and respiratory mechanics, and higher mortality rate [29]. A high potential for lung recruitment, in fact, is correlated to worse initial lung damage, defined as nonaerated tissue. This is easily understandable considering that less severe cases have a nearly completely aerated lung and a minimal percentage of potential recruitment; on the contrary, patients characterized by higher amounts of lung oedema have a higher percentage of potential recruitment. As previously mentioned, nonaerated lung tissue includes both consolidated tissue (not recruitable) and lung collapse (recruitable). The consolidated tissue represents the initial nucleus of the pathology while the lung collapse is the inflammatory response in the adjacent lung tissue and oedema. Lung collapse is due to the effect of gravity, i.e. lung weight. In the study by Gattinoni et al. lung collapse was nearly constant in all patients, amounting to 24% of the total lung weight. Patients with higher potential for lung recruitment have, however, higher amounts of collapsed tissue. These results also explain to the PEEP effect on cyclic opening and closing during tidal ventilation. Patients with less potential for lung recruitment should have less benefit from high PEEP levels, or even damage due to overdistension. Conversely, the use of high PEEP levels in patients with high potential for lung recruitment should recruit the tissue collapsed at end expiration, avoiding cycling opening and closing.

So far, CT analysis is the only reliable method of measuring potential for lung recruitment at the bedside. Different combinations of physiological variables have been tested. The best results have been obtained combining Pao_2/Fio_2 less than 150 (at 5 cmH$_2$O PEEP), increase of lung compliance, and decrease of dead space from 5 to 15 cmH$_2$O PEEP (sensitivity 79%, specificity 81%). It is worth remembering that respiratory variables measure functional recruitment of lung tissue (i.e. lung compartments participating in gas exchange), while CT imaging data represent anatomical recruitment.

Mechanical ventilation

Mechanical ventilation is an important 'buying time' manoeuvre in the treatment of ALI/ARDS patients. Through the years modalities and techniques have been considerably modified to provide ventilatory support, improving oxygenation while avoiding augmentation of the existing lung damage. In the 1970s ALI/ARDS patients were ventilated with high tidal volumes and low PEEP levels [55]. Lung damage due to mechanical ventilation was not known at that time, and the only concerns were high inspiratory oxygen concentration and haemodynamics. Clinical and experimental studies led to the development of barotrauma [56–59], i.e. lung damage due to excessive strain, and even rupture caused by high ventilating pressure. In 1875 Suter *et al.* [60] published the first study combining PEEP, respiratory mechanics, gas exchange, and haemodynamics. In the following years the concept of volutrauma, overdistension due to high tidal volumes, was developed due to the work of Dreyfuss and colleagues [61–63]. As previously described, in the 1980s the use of CT in the management of ALI/ARDS patients was fundamental to understanding a new aspect of the pathophysiology of the syndrome [64, 65], leading to the baby lung concept and its evolutions [49, 50]. The next step in the ALI/ARDS history was the use of extracorporeal CO$_2$ removal to prevent the damage caused by mechanical ventilation in lungs with extremely small aerated compartments [66, 67]. The goal of mechanical ventilation progressively shifted from the improvement of gas exchange to avoiding lung damage. Hickling *et al.* introduced the concept of permissive hypercapnia [68], which consists of ventilating the lung open to ventilation with small tidal volume even at cost of increased $Paco_2$. Several other studies have been conducted on this topic. Another mechanism that could potentially damage the lung is the cyclic opening and closing of alveoli (atelectrauma). Moreover, alveolar overdistension may give rise to a systemic inflammatory response (biotrauma) [59].

Mechanical ventilation settings

The setting of ventilator parameters involves respiratory rate, tidal volume, inspiration/expiration (I/E) ratio, and pressure.

There is no evidence that an I/E ratio other than 1 may be useful in ALI/ARDS patients. Modern ventilators provide a wide range of respiratory frequency from nearly 0 to 2000–3000 breaths/min. Animal studies on isolated lung demonstrated that low rates reduce oedema formation [69], but during spontaneous breathing, a high respiratory rate increases oedema formation [70]. High-frequency oscillation ventilation (HFOV) has been proposed as an alternative technique of providing mechanical ventilation using low tidal volume. Unfortunately none of the clinical trials demonstrated a survival benefit. The largest trial on this topic showed improved oxygenation associated with a nonsignificant reduction of mortality in the HFOV group. Experimental models, on the contrary, did not find differences in gas exchange and lung mechanics using 15, 120, and 1000 breaths/min [71]. Further investigations are needed to understand the possible effects of high frequencies on ventilator-induced lung injury.

Tidal volume (V_T) and inspiratory pressure deserves particular attention as they have been extensively studied in recent years. The scientific community agrees on the use of low V_T as it provides less injury to the lung, but the debate is still open on the PEEP setting.

Tidal volume and plateau pressure

In clinical practice V_T is normalized on patient ideal body weight (V$_T$/IBW) to avoid excessive strain on the lung parenchyma. Several clinical studies have analysed the effects of lower versus higher values of V_T/IBW. The ARDS Network tested 6 mL/kg IBW versus 12 mL/kg IBW, finding significant mortality reduction in the low tidal volume group (31% vs 40%) [72]. Other studies, on the contrary, did not find any significant mortality reduction [73–75]. These studies, however, tested intermediate V_T values in the 6–12 mL/kg range. Amato and colleagues [76] tested two different ventilator strategies, one characterized by low V_T/IBW (<6 mL/kg) and high PEEP level, the other with high V_T/IBW (12 mL/kg) and low PEEP. The authors found a significant mortality reduction in the low V_T/high PEEP group (38% vs 71%). In this study, however, it was not possible to divide the effect of V_T from the effect of PEEP and the mortality value in the high V_T/low PEEP group was unusually high. As previously mentioned, low-V_T ventilation has been widely accepted by the scientific community. However, normalizing V_T to IBW is not a precise surrogate for the strain to which the lung parenchyma is subjected. We have to remember, in fact, that according to the severity the percentage of lung open to ventilation in ALI/ARDS patients is highly variable, so the same tidal volume may be safe or dangerous in different patients. The best way to normalize tidal volume is with respect to the end-expiratory lung volume (functional residual capacity, FRC) [77].

The maximal value proposed for airway pressure (P_{AW}) is 30 cmH$_2$O [78]. This value has been successively modified in a post hoc analysis by the ARDS Network, as even lower values may cause lung damage [79]. Even airway pressure, as described for V_T/IBW, is not a good surrogate for lung stress (i.e. transpulmonary pressure, P_L, which is the real distending force of the lung). The same airway pressure, in fact, is associated to a wide range of P_L due to different ratios of chest wall elastance (E_W) to respiratory system elastance (E_{RS}):

$$P_L = P_{AW} \times E_W/E_{RS}$$

where E_W is the transpulmonary pressure variation associated with a volume variation of 1 L:

$$E_W = \Delta P_L/\Delta V$$

and E_{RS} is the airway pressure variation associated with a volume variation of 1 L:

$$E_{RS} = \Delta P_{AW}/\Delta V$$

Positive end-expiratory pressure

It is still not clear what is the best way to set an adequate PEEP level. Several methods have been proposed according to lung mechanics, pressure volume curve, or hysteresis. The ARDS Network randomized trial in an unselected ALI/ARDS population did not find significant mortality reduction and was stopped for futility [74]. Two other recent trials (the LOV [80] and ExPress [81] studies) tested low versus high PEEP levels in an unselected ALI/ARDS population and did not find mortality differences. On other hand, Villar et al. [82], in a severe ARDS population, found a significant mortality difference. The authors recruited only patients who still had severe ARDS criteria after 24 h. Even the previously described study of Amato et al. [76] found improved survival in the high PEEP group but, as for V_T/IBW, it is not possible to distinguish the effect of PEEP. The analysis conducted by Gattinoni et al. [83] in the editorial accompanying the LOV and ExPress publication evaluated

the number of patients with severe disease present in the trials. In the LOV trials, the most severe cases were characterized by P_{aO_2} less than 60 mmHg and F_{iO_2} 100%; in the ExPress trial severe cases were defined according to P_{aO_2} less than 55 mmHg, S_{aO_2} less than 88%, and F_{iO_2} greater than 80% for at least 1 h. Taken together, the severe cases recruited in the two studies were 94 (10.9%) in the high PEEP group and 184 (20.7%) in the low PEEP group. As the overall mortality was not different (60.6% vs 58.2% respectively), the different percentage of severe cases suggests that mortality in the high PEEP group is lower than the mortality rate in the low PEEP group (6.6% vs 12%). It sounds reasonable that high PEEP is effective in the most severe cases, characterized by smaller baby lung and high percentages of potential for lung recruitment. In the other patients high PEEP levels may not only be ineffective but can also overstretch the lung parenchyma. This can also explain the results of the clinical trials: the positive effects on the most severe cases may be cancelled by the nil or negative effects on the less severe ones. This suggest that a correct characterization of the patient is needed before tailoring mechanical ventilation [83].

Prone position

The prone position is suggested for ALI/ARDS patients in whom mechanical ventilation has potential injurious effects [84]. Since the first description in 1976 [85], the beneficial effect on oxygenation provided by the prone position has been proven, and other physiological mechanisms have been postulated: improvement of V/Q mismatch, recruitment of the most dependent areas, shunt reduction, less lung compression by the heart. Moreover, extensive laboratory work [86, 87] has proved that prone positioning is able to prevent or delay the development of ventilator-induced lung injury, probably because of a more homogeneous distribution of lung stress and strain. However no randomized clinical trial, to date, has demonstrated a significant improvement in mortality. Mancebo et al. [88], in a study in which prone position was prolonged for 20 h, found a significant trend towards survival mortality. The authors concluded that, 'Prone ventilation is feasible and safe, and may reduce mortality in patients with severe ARDS when it is initiated early and applied for most of the day'. A subgroup analysis of the Italian randomized trial suggested that the prone position may have beneficial effects in the most severe cases [89]. In a recent meta-analysis the subgroup analysis of the most severe ALI/ARDS patients (P_{aO_2}/F_{iO_2} <100) showed a significant reduction in mortality in the prone group, suggesting that prone position is beneficial in this kind of patients. In contrast, the lack of benefit in moderately hypoxaemic patients means that the risks of complications due to the use of long-term prone positioning are unacceptable.

Fluid management

The fluid management of ALI/ARDS patients is controversial [90–92]. These patients, in fact, usually need aggressive management to restore adequate haemodynamics [93, 94]. At present, no definite conclusions can be drawn about the use of albumin in resuscitating patients. Three meta-analyses published to date on the clinical use of albumin have demonstrated that albumin administration has adverse [95], neutral [96], or beneficial [97] effects, respectively. In order to clarify the contradictory results of these meta-analyses, a randomized double-blind trial was performed (the SAFE study) in 16 intensive care units (ICUs) in Australia and New Zealand [98]. This study clearly demonstrated that in a general ICU population 4% albumin or normal saline for intravascular fluid resuscitation (volume replacement/expansion) results in similar outcomes. The ARDS Network performed a large randomized clinical trial to evaluate liberal versus conservative fluid management in patients with ALI/ARDS [99]. Both strategies were tested on the basis of CVC versus PAC data. The use of a PAC provided similar outcomes to the use of a CVC. In contrast, conservative fluid management, although there was no significant difference in the primary outcome of 60-day mortality, resulted in significantly improved outcome. Patients treated with the conservative strategy had improvement in the oxygenation index and LIS, and improved ventilator-free days and ICU-free days, without increasing nonpulmonary organ failures. The authors concluded that these results support the use of a conservative strategy of fluid management in patients with ALI.

Basic management of acute lung injury/ acute respiratory distress syndrome

ALI/ARDS patients are subjected to a number of risk factors. Prophylaxis for pulmonary embolism and venous thrombosis should be used in all patients unless contraindicated [100]. Enteral nutrition is also important, to prevent gastrointestinal bleeding and to maintain the normal barrier function of the mucosa [100–102]. Tight glycaemic control has been proved to reduce the occurrence of multiple organ failure in a population of postoperative patients treated with intensive insulin, improving ICU and hospital outcome also [103, 104]. The same results were not translated into a general medical ICU population, but the authors found a survival improvement in patients who remained in the ICU

for more than 3 days [104]. An important goal of treatment is the prevention of nosocomial or secondary infections and ventilator associated pneumonia, which are responsible for the high mortality rate of ALI/ARDS patients [105, 106]. Several ways have been proposed to improve oxygenation while reducing inspiratory oxygen fraction [107]. Most of these techniques, including prone position, sighs, recruitment manoeuvres, and vasodilators are the subject of accurate evaluations. Lung recruitment, for example, is the gain of aeration of previously nonaerated lung tissue. However for the lung to be opened, it is necessary that part of it is collapsed, before the application of airway pressure. We may therefore expect that the recruitment manoeuvre is very effective when lung recruitability is high, and less effective, or even dangerous, when lung recruitability is low [29]. Two randomized clinical trials have failed to demonstrate a survival improvement in oxygenation associated with inhaled nitric oxide (INO) versus placebo [108, 109].

Finally the use of corticosteroids in ALI/ARDS patients has been tested by the ARDS Network [110]. The authors conducted a randomized placebo-controlled trial using corticosteroids in ALI/ARDS patients who needed mechanical ventilation for not less than 7 days and no more than 28 days. They did not find benefits in terms of survival, duration of mechanical ventilation, or ICU stay. On the contrary, in the steroid group more patients had to return to mechanical ventilation and in the subgroups of patients with ARDS for more than 14 days the rate of mortality was higher. The authors concluded that the routine use of corticosteroids is not recommended in patients with persistent ARDS.

Conclusion

Both types of respiratory failure, oxygenation failure and ventilatory failure, are common problems in the ICU. Among the diagnostic tools available, blood gas analysis is the most important as it gives immediate information for the diagnosis and the treatment of respiratory failure, while imaging techniques are used to assess the cardiopulmonary status of the patients. Haemodynamics is also fundamental to understanding the nature of the pathology.

The incidence of ARDS is most frequently linked to pneumonia, aspiration, sepsis, and trauma. However, a series of biological variables have emerged as potential risk factors. The incidence of the pathology is quite difficult to determine, as it is linked to geography and the definition used for the diagnosis. The mortality rate is still high, but the most recent studies report a decline to 29–40% from the 40–70% reported in the 1980s and 1990s.

The CT scan for quantitative analysis of the ARDS lung, introduced in the 1980s, has proven the best way to assess the status of the lung and its degree of aeration during ARDS. The quantitative assessment of CT images has allowed us to understand that the amount of normally aerated tissue of the ARDS lung has the same order of magnitude of that of a 5–6-year-old child (the 'baby lung' concept). So far, CT scan analysis is the only reliable method of measuring potential for lung recruitment at bedside.

At the moment the management of ALI/ARDS patients is mainly supportive and the specific treatment must be directed to the underlying pathology, providing adequate ventilatory, circulatory, and nutritional support. Mechanical ventilation, inevitably linked to this pathology since its first description, is an important way of 'buying time' in the treatment of these patients. Over the years modalities and techniques have been modified to provide ventilatory support that improves oxygenation without exacerbating the existing lung damage. During this time the concept of ventilator-induced lung injury has been developed and has evolved through the concepts of barotrauma, volutaruma, atelectrauma, and biotrauma. The scientific community agrees on the use of low tidal volume based on ideal body weight, as it causes less injury to the lung. The debate is still open, however, on the most effective PEEP setting. Recently the use of the prone position has proved beneficial in the most severely affected patients, but the lack of benefit in moderately hypoxaemic patients makes the risks of complications unacceptable. Correct fluid management and the use of corticosteroids are still open issues in the treatment of ARDS.

Personal perspective

The knowledge of ALI/ARDS pathophysiology is still an open issue, although several aspects have been investigated and clarified. It is clear that the accurate patient characterization is necessary to treat the pathology appropriately. The wide range of severity of lung injury (according to the tissue weight estimated at CT scan) and of the potential for lung recruitment, in fact, proof that the response to particular manoeuvres is different according to the lung status. Recruitment manoeuvres, prone position, and high PEEP levels may be effective in the most severe cases, while they can be useless or even dangerous in the less severe ones.

Further reading

Ashbaugh DG, Bigelow DB, Petty TL, Levine BE. Acute respiratory distress in adults. *Lancet* 1967;**2**:319–323.

Bernard GR, Artigas A, Brigham KL, *et al.* The American-European Consensus Conference on ARDS. Definitions, mechanisms, relevant outcomes, and clinical trial coordination. *Am J Respir Crit Care Med* 1994;**149**:818–824.

Chiumello D, Carlesso E, Cadringher P, *et al.* Lung stress and strain during mechanical ventilation for acute respiratory distress syndrome. *Am J Respir Crit Care Med* 2008;**178**:346–355.

Gattinoni L, Caironi P, Cressoni M, *et al.* Lung recruitment in patients with the acute respiratory distress syndrome. *N Engl J Med* 2006;**354**:1775–1786.

Gattinoni L, Caironi P, Pelosi P, Goodman LR. What has computed tomography taught us about the acute respiratory distress syndrome? *Am J Respir Crit Care Med* 2001;**164**:1701–1711.

Gattinoni L, Caironi P. Refining ventilatory treatment for acute lung injury and acute respiratory distress syndrome. *JAMA* 2008;**299**:691–693.

Hickling KG, Henderson SJ, Jackson R. Low mortality associated with low volume pressure limited ventilation with permissive hypercapnia in severe adult respiratory distress syndrome. *Intensive Care Med* 1990;**16**:372–377.

Kolobow T, Gattinoni L, Tomlinson T, Pierce JE. An alternative to breathing. *J Thorac Cardiovasc Surg* 1978;**75**:261–266.

Suter PM, Fairley B, Isenberg MD. Optimum end-expiratory airway pressure in patients with acute pulmonary failure. *N Engl J Med* 1975;**292**:284–289.

Ventilation with lower tidal volumes as compared with traditional tidal volumes for acute lung injury and the acute respiratory distress syndrome. The Acute Respiratory Distress Syndrome Network. *N Engl J Med* 2000;**342**:1301–1308.

➲ For additional multimedia materials please visit the online version of the book (🖰 http://www.esciacc.oxfordmedicine.com).

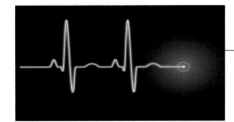

CHAPTER 63

Pulmonary hypertension

Nazzareno Galiè, Alessandra Manes,
Massimiliano Palazzini, and Enri Leci

Contents

Summary

Pulmonary hypertension (PH) is a haemodynamic and pathophysiological condition defined as an increase in mean pulmonary arterial pressure (PAP) of 25 mmHg or more at rest as assessed by right heart catheterization (RHC) [1]. In fact, although transthoracic echocardiography may provide clues to the presence of PH, the haemodynamic evaluation offers a more precise and comprehensive assessment.

PH is heterogeneous from the pathophysiological point of view and the diversity is reflected in the haemodynamic definitions. The different haemodynamic forms of PH can be found in multiple clinical conditions which have been classified into 6 main groups and at least 26 subgroups. Each main clinical group shows specific pathological changes in the lung distal arteries, capillaries, and small veins. This combination of haemodynamic and clinical heterogeneity determines the complexity of an accurate diagnosis in the individual patient, which is crucial for the prognostic assessment and the treatment strategy. In addition, the concomitant presence of different haemodynamic and clinical mechanisms cannot be excluded in individual cases (e.g. in patients with congestive heart failure and associated lung diseases).

The presence of PH as defined above is always a ominous prognostic sign, even if its severity may differ according to haemodynamic changes and the underlying clinical condition. The therapeutic approach also is markedly different according to the clinical group and the symptomatic and haemodynamic severity. For these reasons the classifications are described in the introductory section and the four most frequently encountered clinical groups are then discussed individually.

Introduction

Pulmonary hypertension (PH) is an heterogeneous haemodynamic and pathophysiological state that can be found in multiple clinical conditions which have been classified into six diagnostic groups with specific histological, clinical, and therapeutic features (see ➲ Box 63.1). Despite possible comparable elevations of pulmonary pressure in the different clinical groups, the underlying mechanisms, the diagnostic approaches, and the prognostic and therapeutic implications are completely different. There are four clinical groups that are most frequently encountered.

◆ Group 1, defined as pulmonary arterial hypertension (PAH), includes rare conditions which share comparable clinical and haemodynamic pictures and virtually identical pathological changes in the lung microcirculation. PAH comprises the idiopathic and familial forms and the forms associated with connective tissue diseases, congenital heart defects with systemic-to-pulmonary shunts, portal hypertension, and HIV infection. The treatment of the more advanced stages (deteriorating WHO functional class III or class IV) requiring intensive care includes the identification of precipitating conditions and the appropriate use of diuretics, inotropic treatment, oxygen therapy and ventilatory support, and specific PAH drug therapies (prostanoids, endothelin receptor antagonists, phosphodiesterase type 5 inhibitors). Intensive and acute care is also required in patients with lung infection and haemophthysis and in cases of elective surgery or interventional procedures such as balloon atrial septostomy and during pregnancy.

Box 63.1 Updated clinical classification of pulmonary hypertension [9]

1 Pulmonary arterial hypertension (PAH)

  1.1 Idiopathic PAH

  1.2 Heritable

    1.2.1 BMPR2

    1.2.2 ALK1, endoglin (with or without hereditary haemorrhagic telangiectasia)

    1.2.3 Unknown

  1.3 Drugs and toxins induced

  1.4 Associated with (APAH):

    1.4.1 Connective tissue diseases

    1.4.2 HIV infection

    1.4.3 Portal hypertension

    1.4.4 Congenital heart disease

    1.4.5 Schistosomiasis

    1.4.6 Chronic haemolytic anaemia

  1.5 Persistent pulmonary hypertension of the newborn

1′ Pulmonary veno-occlusive disease and/or pulmonary capillary haemangiomatosis

2 Pulmonary hypertension due to left heart disease

  2.1 Systolic dysfunction

  2.2 Diastolic dysfunction

  2.3 Valvular disease

3 Pulmonary hypertension due to lung diseases and/or hypoxia

  3.1 Chronic obstructive pulmonary disease (COPD)

  3.2 Interstitial lung disease

  3.3 Other pulmonary diseases with mixed restrictive and obstructive pattern

  3.4 Sleep-disordered breathing

  3.5 Alveolar hypoventilation disorders

  3.6 Chronic exposure to high altitude

  3.7 Developmental abnormalities

4 Chronic thromboembolic pulmonary hypertension (CTEPH)

5 PH with unclear and/or multifactorial mechanisms

  5.1 Haematological disorders: myeloproliferative disorders, splenectomy.

  5.2 Systemic disorders, sarcoidosis, pulmonary Langerhans cell histiocytosis, lymphangioleiomyomatosis, neurofibromatosis, vasculitis

  5.3 Metabolic disorders: glycogen storage disease, Gaucher's disease, thyroid disorders

  5.4 Others: tumoral obstruction, fibrosing mediastinitis, chronic renal failure on dialysis

ALK-1, activin receptor-like kinase 1 gene; APAH, associated pulmonary arterial hypertension; BMPR2, bone morphogenetic protein receptor, type 2; PAH, pulmonary arterial hypertension

- Group 2 includes patients with PH due to left heart disease. In these cases the treatment is addressed to the underlying heart condition and medications approved for PAH have not proved to be convincingly effective.

- Group 3 includes cases of PH associated with lung diseases in which the use of PAH-specific drugs is not recommended on the basis of their minimal clinical efficacy and because they may impair pulmonary gas exchange.

- Group 4 includes patients with chronic thromboembolic PH which treatment of choice is pulmonary endarterectomy, and PAH-specific drugs may be considered in nonoperable cases and/or after suboptimal surgery.

Definitions and classifications

Haemodynamic definitions

PH has been defined as an increase in mean pulmonary arterial pressure (PAP) of at least 25 mmHg at rest as assessed by right heart catheterization (RHC) [2, 3]. Recent re-evaluation of available data has shown that the normal mean PAP at rest is 14±3 mmHg with an upper limit of normal of approximately 20 mmHg [4, 5]. The significance of mean PAP between 21 and 24 mmHg is unclear. Patients presenting with PAP in this range need further evaluation in epidemiological studies. The definition of PH on exercise as a mean PAP greater than 30 mmHg as assessed by RHC is not supported by published data, and healthy individuals can reach much higher values [4, 6]. Thus no definition for PH on exercise as assessed by RHC can be provided at present.

An additional very important haemodynamic parameter which characterizes the definitions of PH is pulmonary wedge pressure (PWP). In fact, according to various combinations of values of PWP, pulmonary vascular resistance (PVR), and cardiac output (CO), different haemodynamic types of PH are shown in ➲ Table 63.1. Precapillary PH (PH with normal PWP) is found in clinical groups 1, 3, 4, and 5 while postcapillary PH (PH with elevated PWP) is found in the clinical group 2 (➲ Box 63.1) [7]. The distinction between precapillary and postcapillary PH is extremely important because the treatment strategy may differ markedly between the two haemodynamic conditions; therapies effective in the precapillary form may be detrimental in the postcapillary type, and vice versa.

Echocardiographic definitions

Doppler echocardiography is not able to measure PAP but it provides an estimate of it by the use of the Bernoulli

Table 63.1 Haemodynamic definitions of pulmonary hypertension (all values measured at rest)

Definition	Characteristics	Clinical group(s) [a]
PH	Mean PAP ≥25 mmHg	All
Precapillary PH	Mean PAP ≥25 mmHg PWP ≤ 15 mmHg CO normal or reduced [b]	1 Pulmonary arterial hypertension 3 PH due to lung diseases 4 Chronic thromboembolic PH 5 PH with unclear and/or multifactorial mechanisms
Postcapillary PH	Mean PAP ≥25 mmHg PWP >15 mmHg CO normal or reduced [b]	2 PH due to left heart disease
Passive	TPG ≤12 mmHg	
Reactive (out of proportion)	TPG >12 mmHg	

CO, cardiac output; PAP, pulmonary arterial pressure; PH, pulmonary hypertension; PWP, pulmonary wedge pressure; TPG, transpulmonary pressure gradient (mean PAP − mean PWP).
[a] According to ➲ Box 63.1.
[b] High cardiac output can be present in cases of hyperkinetic conditions such as systemic-to-pulmonary shunts (only in the pulmonary circulation), anaemia, hyperthyroidism, etc.

continuity equation and the tricuspid regurgitation velocity, which includes many theoretical assumptions (see ➲ Chapter 20). Accordingly, the evaluation of PH by Doppler echocardiography runs the risks of false-positive and false-negative diagnosis. When an exact measure of PAP is considered relevant, RHC should be performed. RHC can also provide a reliable assessment of the PWP, which allows the precise identification of the haemodynamic type of PH. The recent guidelines on PH of the European Society of Cardiology (ESC) and the European Respiratory Society (ERS) [1] have proposed arbitrary criteria for estimating the presence of PH based on tricuspid regurgitation peak velocity and Doppler-calculated PA systolic pressure at rest (➲ Table 63.2).

Other echocardiographic variables that might raise or reinforce suspicion of PH independently of tricuspid regurgitation velocity include an increased velocity of pulmonary valve regurgitation and a short acceleration time of right ventricle (RV) ejection into the pulmonary artery (PA). Increased dimensions of right heart chambers, abnormal shape and function of interventricular septum, increased RV wall thickness, and dilated main PA are also suggestive of PH, but tend to occur later in the course of the disease.

Clinical classification

A more updated clinical classification of PH is presented in ➲ Box 63.1 [8]. Clinical conditions with PH are classified according to similar pathological, pathophysiological, and

Table 63.2 Arbitrary criteria for estimating the presence of PH based on tricuspid regurgitation peak velocity and Doppler-calculated PA systolic pressure at rest (assuming a normal right atrial pressure of 5 mmHg) and on additional echocardiographic variables suggestive of PH. Exercise Doppler echocardiography is not recommended for screening of PH

Echocardiographic diagnosis	Tricuspid regurgitation velocity (m/s)	PA systolic pressure (mmHg)	Additional variables
PH unlikely	≤2.8	<36	–
PH possible	≤2.8	<36	+
	2.9–3.4	37–50	±
PH likely	>3.4	>50	±

+, presence of additional echocardiographic variables suggestive for PH; –, no additional echocardiographic variables suggestive of PH; ±, with/without additional echocardiographic variables suggestive of PH.

therapeutic characteristics. Despite possible comparable elevations of PAP and PVR in the different clinical groups, the underlying mechanisms, the diagnostic approaches, and the prognostic and therapeutic implications are completely different. The features of each main clinical group are discussed in the specific sections, with particular attention to PAH (group 1), in which PH represents the leading pathophysiological feature.

It is important to avoid the typical confusion between PH and PAH. In fact, while PH is a haemodynamic condition, PAH is a is a clinical condition characterized by the presence of precapillary PH (➲ Table 63.1) in the absence of other causes of precapillary PH such as PH due to lung diseases, chronic thrombo-embolic PH, or other rare diseases (➲ Box 63.1). PAH includes different forms that share a similar clinical picture and virtually identical pathological changes of the lung microcirculation (➲ Box 63.1). Comparative epidemiological data on the prevalence of the different groups of PH are not available. In a survey carried out in an echocardiography laboratory [10], the prevalence of PH (defined as a PA systolic pressure >40 mmHg) among 4579 patients was 10.5%. Among the 483 cases with PH, 78.7% had left heart disease (group 2), 9.7% had lung diseases and hypoxaemia (group 3), 4.2% had PAH (group 1), 0.6% had chronic thromboembolic pulmonary hypertension (CTEPH; group 4), and in 6.8% it was not possible to define a diagnosis.

Pulmonary arterial hypertension

PAH is the type of PH in which the most important advances in the understanding and treatment have been achieved in the past decade. It is also the group in which PH is the 'core' of the clinical problems and may be treated by specific drug therapy.

Pathology and pathophysiology

PAH comprises apparently heterogeneous conditions (see ➲ Box 63.2) that share comparable clinical and haemodynamic pictures and virtually identical pathological changes of the lung microcirculation. Pathological lesions affect the distal pulmonary arteries (<500 μm) in particular. They are characterized by medial hypertrophy, intimal proliferative and fibrotic changes (concentric, eccentric), adventitial thickening with moderate perivascular inflammatory infiltrates, complex lesions (plexiform, dilated lesions), and thrombotic lesions. Pulmonary veins are classically unaffected. Additional pathological changes include dilatation of the proximal elastic pulmonary arteries and of the bronchial arteries (likely due to a compensatory mechanism intended to provide supplementary blood flow to hypoperfused lung parenchyma areas). The exact processes that initiate the pathological changes seen in PAH are still unknown, although it is recognized that PAH has a multifactorial pathobiology that involves various biochemical pathways and cell types. The increase in PVR is related to different mechanisms, including vasoconstriction, proliferative and obstructive remodelling of the pulmonary vessel wall, inflammation, and thrombosis. The PVR increase leads to RV overload, hypertrophy and dilatation, and eventually to RV failure and death. The importance of the progression of RV failure on the outcome of idiopathic PAH (IPAH) patients is confirmed by the prognostic impact of right atrial pressure, cardiac index (CI), and PAP [3], the three main parameters of RV pump function. The depression of myocardial contractility seems to be one of the primary events in the progression of heart failure in a chronically overloaded RV. Changes in the adrenergic pathways of RV myocytes leading to reduced contractility have been shown in IPAH patients [11]. Afterload mismatch remains the leading determinant of heart failure in patients with PAH and CTEPH because its removal, as follows successful pulmonary endarterectomy or lung transplantation [12], almost invariably leads to sustained recovery of RV function. The haemodynamic changes and the prognosis of patients with PAH are related to the complex pathophysiological interactions between the rate of progression (or regression) of the obstructive changes in the pulmonary microcirculation and the response of the overloaded RV, which may also be influenced by genetic factors [13].

Clinical profile of advanced cases

The symptoms of PAH are nonspecific and include breathlessness, fatigue, weakness, angina, syncope, and abdominal distension [14]. The physical signs of PAH include left parasternal lift, an accentuated pulmonary component of second heart sound, a pansystolic murmur of tricuspid regurgitation, a diastolic murmur of pulmonary insufficiency, and a RV third sound. Symptoms at rest are reported only in advanced cases which show also jugular vein distension, hepatomegaly, peripheral oedema, ascites, and cool extremities. Low blood pressure and sinus tachycardia are also usually present. The clinical course may be complicated by sudden death (due to arrhythmias, rupture of the pulmonary artery, compression of the left main coronary artery by a dilated pulmonary artery) and by haemophthysis that can be life threatening (due to the rupture of dilated bronchial arteries into the bronchial tree).

Precipitating conditions

Possible causes for the deterioration of the clinical status of patients with PAH include lung infections, haemophthysis, supraventricular arrhythmias, anaemia, hypo- or hyperthyroidism, elevated fluid intake, renal failure, excessive physical exercise, reduction of diuretic dose, or withdrawal of specific PAH-approved drugs. If these events can be excluded, the clinical deterioration may be attributed to the deterioration of RV dysfunction or to the progression of the pulmonary vascular obstructive disease.

Required investigations

In addition to history and physical examination, the investigations required to detect the presence of precipitating conditions include routine haematological and biochemical investigations, ECG, and chest radiograph. The diagnostic work-up typical of patients with PH [1] is required only if it has not been done previously. To assess the severity of the clinical deterioration and the progression of the PAH, both echocardiography evaluation and RHC should be considered. The latter procedure is indicated in particular if additional invasive treatments such as parenteral prostanoids or listing for transplantation are considered.

Assessment of severity

The evaluation of severity of patients with PAH is based on a panel of parameters assessing clinical conditions, exercise capacity, and RV function.

A worse clinical status includes presence of signs of RV failure (tachycardia, gallop rhythm, cold extremities, increased jugular venous pressure, hypotension, reduced diuresis, hepatomegaly, ascites, recumbent oedema), syncope, angina, and/or a WHO functional class III or IV. The deterioration of one or more functional classes is also a bad prognostic sign. Reduced exercise capacity (e.g. 6-min walk distance <300 m or peak oxygen consumption <12 mL min^{-1} kg^{-1}) or the decline of a previous better performance as signs of a worse prognosis. RV function can be assessed by B-type natriuretic peptide (BNP or NT-proBNP) plasma levels, echocardiography, and RHC. Very elevated or rising BNP or NT-proBNP plasma levels, the presence of pericardial effusion or of a tricuspid annular plane systolic excursion less than 1.5 cm, or a CI of 2.0 L min^{-1} m^{-2} or less, or a right atrial pressure greater than 15 mmHg represent poor prognostic indicators. The concordance of multiple parameters confirms and reinforces the severity of the condition.

Treatment

The treatment of PAH in an intensive and acute care setting is required in the more severe cases (advanced WHO functional class III or class IV, multiorgan failure, severe ascites), in case of complications (e.g. lung infections with respiratory failure, haemophtysis) immediately after elective surgery or interventional procedures, and during pregnancy (when termination is not accepted).

The appropriate indications for the three classes of specific PAH drugs (prostanoids, endothelin receptors antagonists, and phosphodiesterase type-5 inhibitors) have been extensively described in the recent ESC/ERS PH guidelines [1]. Only the aspects related to the intensive care setting are discussed here.

Advanced WHO functional class III or class IV

Decompensated RV failure leads to fluid retention, raised central venous pressure, hepatic congestion, peripheral oedema, and ascites (in advanced cases) [15]. Increased intra- and extravascular volumes can markedly impair symptoms and exercise capacity. In WHO functional class III and IV patients hepatic congestion and, occasionally, ascites may reduce diaphragmatic respiratory dynamics compromising lung volumes. In this setting the initial treatment aims to restore diuresis, reduce fluid retention, and limit multiorgan failure if any.

A clear symptomatic benefit can be achieved in fluid-overloaded patients by the use of diuretic therapy. Intravenous administration of loop diuretics is temporarily preferred in the more severe cases of fluid retention, to overcome the reduced oral bioavailability. Eventually, diuretic treatment can be converted to the oral route at the dose which is able to maintain an optimal fluid balance and minimize symptoms of congestion. Furosemide oral doses may vary from 20–25 mg/day up to 500 mg/day or more. Loop diuretics with better bioavailability may present some advantages [16]. The addition of aldosterone antagonists should also be considered. The combination of loop diuretics with thiazides may be temporarily used in selected cases with refractory oedema for the synergistic effects of the two compounds. In fact, the mid- to long-term combination of these two classes of diuretics increases the incidence of severe electrolyte disturbances. Proper fluid balance can be facilitated by a controlled salt and water intake. It is important to monitor renal function and blood biochemistry in patients to avoid hypokalaemia, hyponatraemia, and the effects of decreased intravascular volume leading to prerenal failure.

Paracentesis should be considered in case of refractory ascites, if the increase in intra-abdominal pressure produces intolerable symptoms and impairs the respiratory dynamics. Similarly, thoracenthesis should be considered in the unusual cases of relevant pleural effusions due to RV failure.

In severe decompensated RV failure, the use of intravenous adrenergic support may help the recovery of blood pressure and renal function. The effects of adrenergic inotropic drugs on the failing RV have received little attention from investigators. From a theoretical point of view and from some experimental studies [17] it appears that the inotropic stimulation of these compounds is similar in the right and left ventricular myocardium. The absence of systemic hypotensive effects together with the renal blood flow increase suggests the use of dopamine, alone or in combination with dobutamine, as the inotropic strategy of choice in PAH patients. In critical cases dopamine can be used together with intravenous prostanoids for its synergistic activity on CO and its antagonistic effect on blood pressure decrease. It is not clear for how long the inotropic support remains effective (due to tolerance) and whether long-term therapy may have detrimental effects. It may be safe in the acute setting to prolong the adrenergic inotropic support only until the specific PAH drugs become effective or precipitating conditions are corrected. Although digoxin has been shown to improve CO acutely in idiopathic PAH, its efficacy is unknown when administered chronically [18]. It may be given to slow the ventricular rate in patients with PAH who develop atrial tachyarrhythmias.

Low CO may contribute to hypoxaemia due to low mixed venous oxygen saturation. Oxygen therapy is indicated in the acute setting in patients with PAH and arterial oxygen pressure measured below 55–60 mmHg (≤90% of oxygen saturation); the oxygen flow should be increased to achieve an arterial oxygen saturation greater than 90%. Noninvasive and invasive mechanical ventilation measures should be adopted if the simple administration of oxygen is not sufficient to achieve this goal.

Anticoagulant treatment in the acute setting may be limited to the prophylaxis of venous thromboembolic events. However, if the patient was already being treated with an oral anticoagulant it should be continued or converted to intravenous or subcutaneous treatment.

Continuous intravenous administration of epoprostenol (prostacyclin) by central venous catheters is the treatment of choice for WHO functional class IV PAH patients [1]. This treatment can also be adopted in addition to oral PAH-specific drugs in patients already treated with these compounds. The continuous intravenous administration of epoprostenol requires specific experience and in most cases it will be continued long-term by the use of tunnelized central venous catheters and portable pumps. Treatment with epoprostenol is initiated at a dose of 2–4 ng^{-1} kg^{-1} min, with doses increasing at a rate limited by side effects (flushing, headache, diarrhoea, leg pain). The optimal dose varies between individual patients, being between 20 and 40 ng^{-1} kg^{-1} min in most cases [19, 20].

If intravenous epoprostenol is not available, concurrent initiation of oral endothelin receptor antagonist and phosphodiesterase type 5 inhibitors may be considered [1].

Lung infection/haemophthysis

Patients with PAH are susceptible to developing pneumonia, which is the cause of death in 7% of cases [14]. Any lung infection in PAH patients can evolve in a clinical emergency which requires admission to an intensive care setting due to hypoxaemia and RV failure. Aggressive antibiotic treatment should be initiated together with the required respiratory and circulatory supports aimingto correct hypoxaemia, hypercapnia, hypotension, and reduced urine output (see above). Although there are no controlled trials, vaccination against influenza and pneumococcal pneumonia is recommended as a preventive strategy.

Haemophthysis due to the rupture of enlarged bronchial arteries may be a life-threatening complication of PAH. Mild to moderate haemophthysis may regress spontaneously and requires the withdrawal of anticoagulant therapy, if any. In cases of persistent or severe haemophthysis the urgent embolization of the culprit bronchial arteries is required. Bronchial artery embolization should be electively planned also in cases of moderate haemophthysis that has regressed spontaneously. The risk/benefit ratio of the prophylactic embolization of enlarged bronchial arteries detected in a routine thoracic CT scan is unknown.

Elective surgery or interventional procedures

Elective surgery is expected to have an increased risk in patients with PAH, and admission to an intensive care unit (ICU) in the postoperative period should be anticipated. It is not clear which form of anaesthesia is preferable, but epidural is probably better tolerated than general anaesthesia. Patients who are usually maintained on oral therapy may require temporary conversion to intravenous or nebulized treatments until they are able to both swallow and absorb drugs taken orally. Oral anticoagulant treatment, if used, should be withdrawn for the shortest possible time and deep venous thrombosis prophylaxis should be systematically adopted.

Interventional procedures in PAH patients which ideally may require intensive care include balloon atrial septostomy and angioplasty with stenting of the left main coronary artery stenosis due to the compression of the enlarged pulmonary artery.

Graded balloon atrial septostomy is intended to create a small atrial septal defect in order to allow a right-to-left shunt which ideally decompresses the right heart chambers and improves systemic output at the expense of increased hypoxaemia. This demanding procedure is indicated when all available medical treatments have been tried, and it should be done in experienced centres [12].

Left main coronary artery compression by an enlarged pulmonary artery is an increasingly often detected complication of PAH patients and may be responsible for angina symptoms and probably also sudden death. Treatment by coronary percutaneous procedures has been successful.

Pregnancy

Maternal mortality in women with PAH remains prohibitively high (c.25–38%) and contraception or early termination is recommended [21]. The patient who becomes pregnant should be informed of the high risk of pregnancy, and termination of pregnancy discussed. Those patients who choose to continue pregnancy should be treated with specific PAH therapies, bearing in mind potential teratogenic effects. Prostanoids seem to have no demonstrated teratogenic effects. Thromboprophylaxis is also required. Planning an elective delivery is recommended, and close and effective collaboration between obstetricians and the PAH team is required. Close monitoring is needed to identify maternal haemodynamic deterioration or fetal distress requiring urgent delivery. Theoretically, epidural anaesthesia and caesarean section should have less haemodynamic impact as a delivery strategy.

Pulmonary hypertension due to left heart disease

PH carries a poor prognosis for patients with chronic heart failure [22]. The mechanisms responsible for the increase in PAP are multiple and include the passive backward transmission of the pressure elevation (postcapillary passive PH, ⮕ Table 63.1). In these cases the transpulmonary pressure gradient (TPG = mean PAP minus mean PWP) and PVR are within the normal range. In other circumstances the elevation of PAP is greater than that of PWP (increased TPG) and an increase in PVR is also observed (postcapillary reactive or 'out of proportion' PH, ⮕ Table 63.1). The elevation of PVR is due to an increase in pulmonary artery vasomotor tone and/or to fixed structural obstructive remodelling of the pulmonary artery resistance vessels [23]: the former component of reactive PH is reversible under acute pharmacological testing while the latter, characterized by medial hypertrophy and intimal proliferation of the pulmonary arteriole, does not respond to the acute challenge [7]. Which factors lead to reactive (out of proportion) PH, and why some patients develop the acutely reversible vasoconstrictive or the fixed obstructive components or both, is poorly understood. Pathophysiological mechanisms may include vasoconstrictive reflexes arising from stretch receptors localized in the left atrium and pulmonary veins, and endothelial dysfunction of pulmonary arteries that may favour vasoconstriction and proliferation of vessel wall cells. The prevalence of PH in patients with chronic heart failure increases with the progression of functional class impairment. Up to 60% of patients with severe LV systolic dysfunction and up to 70% of patients with isolated LV diastolic dysfunction may present with PH [24]. In left-sided valvular diseases, the prevalence of PH increases with the severity of the defect and of the symptoms. PH can be found in virtually all patients with severe symptomatic mitral valve disease and up to 65% of those with symptomatic aortic stenosis [5, 7, 25]. Currently, there is no specific therapy for PH due to left heart diseases. A number of drugs (including diuretics, nitrates, hydralazine, angiotensin converting enzyme inhibitors, β-adrenoceptor blockers, nesiritide, and inotropic agents) or interventions (LV assist device implantation, valvular surgery, resynchronization therapy, and heart transplantation) may lower PAP more or less rapidly through a drop in left-sided filling pressures [7]. Therefore, management of PH due to left heart disease should be aimed at the optimal treatment of the underlying disease. No heart failure drugs are contraindicated because of PH [26].

Few studies have examined the role of drugs currently recommended in PAH. The use of inhaled nitric oxide has been shown to reduce PAP but also to increase PWP, increasing the likelihood of lung oedema [27]. Randomized controlled trials evaluating the effects of chronic use of epoprostenol [28] and bosentan [29, 30] in advanced heart failure have been terminated early due to an increased rate of events in the investigational drug treated group compared with conventional therapy. A small study recently suggested that sildenafil may improve exercise capacity and quality of life in patients with PH due to left heart disease [31]. The history of medical therapy for heart failure is full of examples where drugs had positive effects on surrogate endpoints but eventually turned out to be detrimental, such as the phosphodiesterase type 3 inhibitors. Thus, the use of PAH-specific drugs is not recommended until robust data from long-term studies are available, in particular in out of proportion PH associated with left heart disease.

Pulmonary hypertension due to lung disease

PH is a poor prognostic factor in either chronic obstructive pulmonary disease (COPD) or interstitial lung diseases. The pathobiological and pathophysiological mechanisms involved in this setting are multiple and include hypoxic vasoconstriction, mechanical stress of hyperinflated lungs, loss of capillaries, inflammation, and toxic effects of cigarette smoke. There are also data supporting an endothelium-derived vasoconstrictor–vasodilator imbalance. On the basis of published series, the incidence of significant PH in COPD patients with at least one previous hospitalization for exacerbation of respiratory failure is 20%. In advanced COPD, PH is highly prevalent (>50%) [32, 33], although in general it is of only mild severity. In interstitial lung disease, the prevalence of PH is 32–39% [34]. The combination of lung fibrosis with emphysema is associated with a higher prevalence of PH [35]. Currently there is no specific therapy for PH associated with COPD or interstitial lung diseases. Long-term oxygen administration has been shown to partially reduce the progression of PH in COPD. Nevertheless, with this treatment PAP rarely returns to normal values and the structural abnormalities of pulmonary vessels remain unaltered [36]. In interstitial lung diseases, the role of long-term oxygen therapy on PH progression is less clear. Treatment with conventional vasodilators is not recommended because they may impair gas exchange due to the inhibition of hypoxic pulmonary vasoconstriction

[37, 38] and their lack of efficacy after long-term use [39, 40]. The published experience with specific PAH drug therapy is scarce and consists of the assessment of acute effects [41, 42] and uncontrolled studies in small series [43–47].

The treatment of choice for patients with COPD or interstitial lung diseases and associated PH who are hypoxaemic is long-term oxygen therapy. Patients with out of proportion PH due to lung diseases (characterized by dyspnoea insufficiently explained by lung mechanical disturbances and mean PAP ≥40–45 mmHg) should be referred to expert centres and enrolled in clinical trials targeting PAH-specific drug therapy. The use of targeted PAH therapy in patients with COPD or interstitial lung diseases and mean PAP less than 40 mmHg is currently discouraged because there are no systematic data regarding its safety or efficacy.

Chronic thrombombolic pulmonary hypertension

Nonresolution of acute embolic masses which later undergo fibrosis leading to mechanical obstruction of pulmonary arteries is the most important pathobiological process in CTEPH. The obstructive lesions observed in the distal pulmonary arteries of nonobstructed areas (virtually identical to those observed in PAH) may be related to a variety of factors, such as shear stress, pressure, inflammation, and the release of cytokines and vasculotrophic mediators. Although more recent publications suggest that the prevalence of CTEPH is up to 3.8% in survivors of acute pulmonary embolism [48], most experts believe that the true incidence of CTEPH after acute pulmonary embolism is 0.5–2%. CTEPH can be found in patients without any previous clinical episode of acute pulmonary embolism or deep venous thrombosis (up to 50% in different series) [49].

Patients with CTEPH should receive life-long anticoagulation, usually with vitamin K antagonists adjusted to a target international normalized ratio of 2.0–3.0. Despite anticoagulation, CTEPH patients without additional treatments have a poor prognosis.

The decision on how to treat a patient with CTEPH should be made at an expert centre, on the basis of interdisciplinary discussion among internists, radiologists, and expert surgeons. Pulmonary endarterectomy is the treatment of choice for patients with CTEPH, as it is a potentially curative option. As a rule, a patient should not be considered inoperable until the case has not been reviewed by an experienced surgeon.

The general medical intensive treatment of advanced WHO functional class III or class IV CTEPH patients does not differ substantially from that of a patient with PAH. In this setting an urgent pulmonary endarterectomy should be planned as soon as reasonable haemodynamic conditions have been restored.

Specific PAH drug therapy may play a role in selected CTEPH patients, mainly for three different scenarios: (1) if the patient is not considered a candidate for surgery; (2) if preoperative treatment is deemed appropriate to improve haemodynamics; and (3) if the patient presents with symptomatic residual/recurrent PH after pulmonary endarterectomy surgery.

Personal perspective

PH remains a severe pathophysiological state, despite recent progress in the medical and surgical treatments of the multiple clinical conditions in which it can be found.

PAH represents the clinical group in which three classes of drugs are available but the outcome of the patients is still unsatisfactory. Current and future plans devoted to increasing our ability to treat PAH patients in both the acute and the chronic setting should include randomized controlled trials on early aggressive combination therapy and on novel compounds.

PH found in the most common clinical settings such as left heart disease and lung diseases has been recognized as a poor prognostic indicator, but no specific medical treatment strategy has been demonstrated to be consistently effective. Multicentre randomized controlled trials assessing the efficacy of new compounds, in particular in patients with out of proportion PH, are warranted in both conditions.

The treatment of choice of CTEPH is pulmonary endarterectomy: an increased rate of operable patients and reduced operative mortality is expected, with the improvement of medical and surgical management techniques.

Further reading

Badesch BD, Champion HC, Gomez-Sanchez MA, *et al*. Diagnosis and assessment of pulmonary arterial hypertension. *J Am Coll Cardiol* 2009;**54**:S55–S56.

Barbera JA, Roger N, Roca J, *et al*. Worsening of pulmonary gas exchange with nitric oxide inhalation in chronic obstructive pulmonary disease. *Lancet* 1996;**347**(8999):436–440.

Bedard E, Dimopoulos K, Gatzoulis MA. Has there been any progress made on pregnancy outcomes among women with pulmonary arterial hypertension? *Eur Heart J* 2009;**30**(3):256–265.

Galiè N, Hoeper M, Humbert M, *et al*. Guidelines on diagnosis and treatment of pulmonary hypertension: The Task Force on Diagnosis and Treatment of Pulmonary Hypertension of the European Society of Cardiology and of the European Respiratory Society. *Eur Heart J* 2009;**30**:2493–2537.

Hoeper MM, Mayer E, Simonneau G, Rubin LJ. Chronic thromboembolic pulmonary hypertension. *Circulation* 2006;**113**(16):2011–2020.

Keogh A, Benza RL, Corris P, *et al*. Interventional and surgical modalities of treatment in pulmonary arterial hypertension. *J Am Coll Cardiol* 2009;**54**:S67–S77.

Oudiz RJ. Pulmonary hypertension associated with left-sided heart disease. *Clin Chest Med* 2007;**28**(1):233–241.

Rietema H, Holverda S, Bogaard HJ, *et al*. Sildenafil treatment in COPD does not affect stroke volume or exercise capacity. *Eur Respir J* 2008;**31**(4):759–764.

Simonneau G, Robbins I, Beghetti M, *et al*. Updated clinical classification of pulmonary hypertension. *J Am Coll Cardiol* 2009;**54**:S43–54.

Vahanian A, Baumgartner H, Bax J, *et al*. Guidelines on the management of valvular heart disease: The Task Force on the Management of Valvular Heart Disease of the European Society of Cardiology. *Eur Heart J* 2007;**28**(2):230–268.

⊃ For additional multimedia materials please visit the online version of the book (⅋ http://www.esciacc.oxfordmedicine.com).

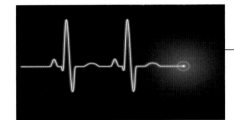

CHAPTER 64

Pulmonary embolism

Stavros Konstantinides and Adam Torbicki

Contents

Summary

Pulmonary embolism (PE) and deep vein thrombosis (DVT) are two clinical presentations of venous thromboembolism (VTE) and share the same risk factors and predisposing conditions. In most cases, PE is a consequence of DVT of the lower extremities. Nonthromboembolic causes of PE are rare. PE is a relatively common and potentially life-threatening disease if left untreated. This is due to a natural tendency towards early recurrence of pulmonary emboli which may lead to acute and often fatal right ventricular (RV) failure. Clinical presentation of PE is nonspecific and may include dyspnoea, chest pain, haemoptysis, syncope, hypotension, and shock. Patients with suggestive history, symptoms, or signs require prompt formal clinical evaluation of the probability and severity of suspected PE. This determines further management strategy. CT angiography has become the mainstay of diagnosis. However, depending on the clinical presentation, definitive treatment decisions can also be made based on other tests, which may be particularly useful under specific circumstances. Patients with PE and shock or hypotension require admission to the intensive care unit (ICU) and aggressive treatment. Such management may be also considered in normotensive patients who present with objective signs of RV dysfunction and/or myocardial injury. In case of doubt, a 'watchful waiting' strategy, based on close monitoring of clinical and biomarker trends, may help in therapeutic decisions.

Introduction

Morbidity and mortality associated with pulmonary embolism (PE) remain high despite important advances in cardiovascular diagnosis and treatment. The reported annual incidence rate of venous thromboembolism (VTE) ranges between 23 and 69 cases per 100 000 population [1, 2], with approximately one-third of patients presenting with acute PE and two-thirds with deep vein thrombosis (DVT) [3]. Case fatality rates vary widely depending on the clinical severity of the thromboembolic episode [4–7], but it is estimated that 10% of all patients with acute PE die during the first 1–3 months [8, 9], 1% of patients admitted to hospital die of acute PE, and 10% of all hospital deaths are PE-related [10–12].

The present chapter summarizes the current state of knowledge on the management of acute PE. It is compatible with the guidelines of the European Society of Cardiology [13] and considers most recent evidence, but also includes authors' opinions on some practically relevant issues, where conclusive evidence, particularly in the setting of intensive and acute care, is still missing.

Predisposing factors and pathophysiology

Major elements predisposing to thrombosis such as changes in vessel wall, blood flow, and blood composition were identified by Rudolf Virchow 150 years ago. Clinical situations which may result in those conditions are usually classified as acquired (either setting- or patient-related) or inherited [14, 15]. Recent surgery, trauma, sepsis and immobilization, particularly due to acute medical diseases, are examples of acquired setting-related predisposing factors. Advanced age, malignancy, obesity, pregnancy, and the antiphospholipid syndrome can be considered as patient-related factors. Inherited predisposing factors consist of 'thrombophilias' related to abnormal levels or quality of elements of the coagulation cascade. The concomitant presence of several predisposing factors is common, further increasing the risk of VTE (e.g. caesarean section, oncological surgery) [15, 16]. The contribution of some of the inherited thrombophilias may be difficult to assess in the acute phase of the disease, because of changes in levels of coagulation factors induced by thrombosis. In a large PE registry, 25% of patients with confirmed VTE had no identifiable predisposing factors [4].

Primary prevention applied to patients with transient predisposing factors reduces but does not eliminate the risk of VTE. The detailed recommendations regarding indications and preventive methods are periodically updated by American College of Chest Physicians [17]. Most patients requiring acute and intensive care will also need some form of prophylaxis. It should be selected depending on the level of risk of VTE and the risk of bleeding. Subcutaneous low-molecular-weight heparin or fondaparinux should be considered in acutely ill patients at high risk for VTE, and the manufacturer's suggested dosing guidelines should be followed [17]. The indications and dosing of new antithrombotic agents, particularly factor Xa and direct thrombin inhibitors, for prevention purposes, are currently being defined. Critical care patients at exceptionally high risk of bleeding should receive graduated compression stockings and/or intermittent pneumatic compression to the lower limbs. Antithrombotic agents should, however, be introduced as soon as bleeding risk falls to an acceptable level [17]. Central venous catheters increase the risk of upper body venous thrombosis, but not to the extent justifying antithrombotic prophylaxis. A subclavian or internal jugular vein catheter insertion site, and placement of its tip at the entrance to the right atrium, should decrease catheter-related thrombotic risk [17].

The most clinically relevant consequence of PE is related to acute increase of RV afterload, which depends on the extent and localization of pulmonary clots. Small, isolated thromboemboli can be haemodynamically irrelevant; multiple and large ones will disturb right ventricular (RV) performance during exercise or even at rest. Low systemic output, shock, or sudden death, usually due to electromechanical dissociation, are the most feared consequences of PE. Respiratory failure is common but usually less relevant than haemodynamic instability.

Diagnosis of pulmonary embolism

Normotensive (non-high-risk) patients

Several diagnostic tests are useful for making therapeutic decisions in patients with clinical suspicion of PE. Their interpretation usually requires previous assessment of clinical (pretest) probability of PE [18–20]. Such assessment should account for predisposing factors (particularly recent surgery, fracture, malignancy, advanced age, previous VTE) as well as symptoms and signs suggestive of PE (particularly dyspnoea of recent onset, chest pain, haemoptysis, tachycardia, unilateral leg pain, or oedema). Implicit evaluation is acceptable, but two prediction rules may help to standardize probability assessment. The Wells and Geneva scores have been prospectively validated in large populations of mostly normotensive (non-high-risk) patients with suspected PE episode [21, 22] and continue to be optimized [23–25].

Although helpful, prediction rules do not suffice to confirm or exclude PE with the reliability required for therapeutic decisions. In most cases such decisions are based on CT angiography. However, in normotensive (non-high-risk) patients with low or intermediate clinical probability (non-high probability) of PE the diagnostic assessment may be limited to D-dimer. If this is found negative with a highly sensitive test, it justifies withholding anticoagulation [26, 27] (◑ Fig. 64.1). Because D-dimer levels increase with age, comorbidities, or pregnancy [27–30], the test is more useful for evaluation of outpatients in the emergency department

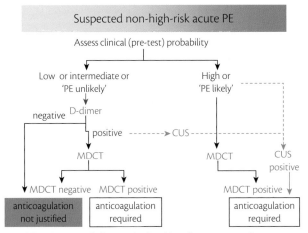

Figure 64.1 Suggested diagnostic algorithm for normotensive (non-high-risk) patients with suspected acute PE. MDCT, multidetector computed tomography (angiography).

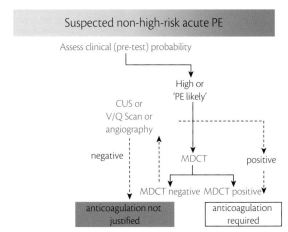

Figure 64.2 Suggested diagnostic algorithm for normotensive (non-high-risk) patients with high clinical probability of acute PE but a negative CT angiography result.

[28, 30–32], particularly if the clinical probability is low [33]. Positive compression ultrasound (CUS) of the leg veins may justify treatment, although its diagnostic yield in patients without clinical symptoms or signs of DVT is low [34]. On the other hand, in patients with high clinical probability of PE even negative CT angiography may still require additional testing to safely withhold anticoagulation [20, 35] (➲ Fig. 64.2). Strategies based on lung scintigraphy are particularly useful in pregnancy, renal dysfunction, or allergy to contrast media [36]. Recent reports on potential role of thoracic [37–39] and endobronchial ultrasound (EBUS) [40] in suspected PE are still preliminary. Also, the role of magnetic resonance imaging (MRI) as a diagnostic test in PE remains controversial [41–44].

Details on diagnostic strategies in PE can be found in the European Society of Cardiology (ESC) guidelines [13] (see 🖳 Online resource). Diagnostic strategies suggested for normotensive (non-high-risk) patients have been validated by several outcome trails [45] and verified by a large accuracy trial [20]. They should guarantee similar accuracy of management decisions to those based on pulmonary angiography: the 3-month rate of symptomatic VTE episodes should remain below 3% in patients left without anticoagulation treatment despite clinical suspicion of PE [13].

Patients with hypotension and/or shock (high risk)

The diagnostic strategy is different in the minority of patients presenting with hypotension or shock (suspected high-risk PE), who should be admitted to the intensive care unit (ICU). As evidence hardly exists, most recommendations are based on expert opinion [13]. Regardless of the cause of haemodynamic instability, such patients are at very high risk of early death and immediate differential diagnosis is an absolute priority. Emergency CT angiography provides diagnostic information on the presence of PE as well as aortic dissection, cardiac tamponade, or pneumothorax, but it may not be feasible in a highly unstable patient. Under such circumstances, bedside echocardiography is an acceptable alternative [13]. Although usually it does not provide definite diagnosis or exclusion of PE [46], echocardiography can confirm or exclude severe RV pressure overload and dysfunction. Considering its recognized value for diagnosing cardiac tamponade, aortic dissection, left ventricular and acute valvular dysfunction, and even hypovolaemia, echocardiographic examination should suffice for the initial management decision in critically ill patients (➲ Fig. 64.3). However, as RV pressure overload is not specific for acute PE, additional diagnostic testing should still be considered. If the patient can be stabilized, CT pulmonary angiography should be reconsidered. If only bedside tests are feasible, CUS [47] and/or transoesophageal echocardiography [48] may be useful to confirm proximal venous or pulmonary artery clots, thus assisting in otherwise difficult management decisions. Also, if a floating thrombus-in-transit from the venous system is detected in a right heart chamber by echocardiography, immediate treatment is needed rather than further diagnostic testing [49].

Currently recommended diagnostic algorithms for PE avoid invasive tests [13]. However, despite the lack of controlled data, invasive diagnosis (and possibly treatment) of PE may represent an option in patients directly referred for cardiac catheterization because of initial suspicion of an acute coronary syndrome (ACS). Some of these patients present with hypotension or shock but fail to show culprit lesions requiring primary coronary angioplasty. Ideally, during preparation for coronary angiography such patients

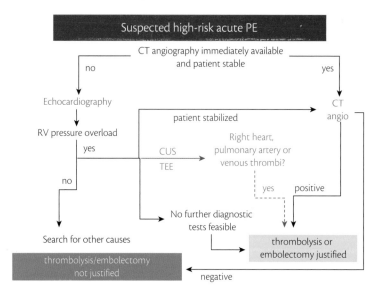

Figure 64.3 Suggested diagnostic algorithm for hypotensive (high-risk) patients with suspected acute PE.

should be evaluated by portable echocardiography to assist in differential diagnosis, including acute PE [50, 51]. A decision on whether to proceed to conventional pulmonary angiography (with the option of intrapulmonary intervention) (⊃Fig. 64.4) or rather discontinue invasive assessment and transfer the patient to the Radiology department for CT angiography should be taken on a case by case basis. Importantly, the presence of right heart thrombi should be excluded with portable echocardiography prior to inserting an angiographic catheter in order to avoid catheter-induced thrombus dislodgement to the pulmonary artery.

Specific diagnostic challenges in pulmonary embolism

Differentiation between an exacerbation of chronic obstructive pulmonary disease (COPD) and an episode of PE usually requires CT angiography, as D-dimers tend to increase in both conditions and *V/Q* scans are rarely diagnostic [27, 52, 53]. CT angiography is also most helpful in patients presenting with haemoptysis, in whom diagnosis of PE and the decision to start anticoagulation must be particularly well justified. Detection of PE in the absence of signs suggesting bronchial carcinoma could obviate the need for fibreoptic bronchoscopy (FOB), which may be difficult to perform in patients with hypoxaemia and haemoptysis.

Pregnancy poses particularly difficult problems. While being one of the predisposing factors for PE, normal pregnancy may also mimic some of its symptoms and signs: breathlessness (sometimes with hypoxaemia), unilateral (usually left sided) lower limb oedema, and even syncope [54]. Assessment of clinical probability is therefore difficult. D-dimers are rarely low [29], particularly during the second and third trimesters. Venous clots may be confined to the iliac vein and therefore may missed on standard CUS evaluation, even in a symptomatic patient [54]. Echocardiography may justify therapeutic decisions only in critically unstable patients, and diagnostic tests based on ionizing radiation therefore often have to be considered. Contrary to common belief, the radiation absorbed by the fetus remains well below the dose considered as dangerous, even if *V/Q* scan, CT, and classical contrast pulmonary angiography were to be sequentially performed [54]. Even so, reduction of radiation dose is always among priorities in pregnancy. Based on expert opinion, the currently preferred approach consists of chest radiograph followed, if normal, by perfusion lung scintigraphy [55, 56]. CT angiography delivers slightly less radiation to the fetus but is believed to increase the whole-life risk of breast cancer in the mother by approximately 15%. Also, up to one-quarter of CT examinations suffer from suboptimal opacification of pulmonary arteries due to mixing of injected contrast with an increased volume of blood returning from the inferior vena cava due to placental flow [55].

Pregnancy is also a risk factor for amniotic fluid PE. The description of clinical presentation and diagnostic strategies in this and other nonthrombotic PE (fat, air, tumour, bacterial vegetations, etc.) is beyond the scope of this chapter, but has recently been described in detail elsewhere [57].

Contemporary classification of disease severity and pulmonary embolism-related risk

Acute PE covers a wide spectrum of clinical severity, with mortality rates during the acute phase ranging between less than 1% and well over 50% in different studies [4–9, 58]. The principal factor which determines disease severity and short-term prognosis is the presence of RV dysfunction [59]. Importantly, the extent of RV dysfunction is only roughly related to thrombus burden and the severity of anatomical obstruction [60, 61]. This is due to the involvement of additional pathophysiological factors such as pulmonary vasoconstriction, platelet activation, and persistent myocardial injury despite maintained coronary flow to the right ventricle [62–65]. Because of these considerations, contemporary clinical assessment of PE severity should focus on PE-related early death risk rather than on volume, shape, or distribution of intrapulmonary emboli. The recent ESC guidelines have replaced potentially misleading terms such as 'massive', 'submassive', and 'nonmassive' PE, with 'high-risk', 'intermediate-risk', and 'low-risk' PE [13, 66].

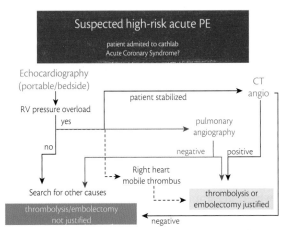

Figure 64.4 Suggested diagnostic algorithm for hypotensive (high-risk) patients admitted to the catheterization laboratory because of initial suspicion of acute coronary syndrome (ACS).

Clinical assessment of haemodynamic status

High-risk PE is defined by the presence of overt RV failure which results in haemodynamic instability, i.e. persistent arterial hypotension (systolic blood pressure <90 mm Hg, or a pressure drop by ≥40 mmHg, for at least 15 min) and shock. This condition accounts for almost 5% of all cases of acute PE and constitutes a medical emergency associated with a 15% or greater risk of in-hospital death, particularly during the first few hours after admission [5, 67–69]. On the other hand, the absence of haemodynamic collapse indicates non-high-risk PE, which is generally associated with a more favourable outcome provided that anticoagulation is instituted without delay [58, 67, 68]. It is of crucial importance to make this simple clinical distinction already when confronted with a patient suspected of having acute PE, as it will both permit a risk-adjusted diagnostic strategy and guide the initial therapeutic management.

Detection of right ventricular dysfunction

While high-risk patients with acute PE are identified by clinical assessment, normotensive non-high-risk patients may also have an elevated risk of death or major complications if they present with RV dysfunction. Echocardiography is capable of detecting the changes occurring in the morphology and function of the right ventricle. There is an association between echocardiographic parameters of RV dysfunction and a poor in-hospital outcome [58, 68, 70–72]. However, a recent meta-analysis including 475 normotensive patients with PE reported only moderate negative (60%) and positive (58%) value of echocardiography for predicting early death [73]. Overall, the therapeutic implications of cardiac ultrasound for non-high-risk patients with PE remain

questionnable, mainly due to the lack of standardization of the echocardiographic criteria [74].

Four-chamber views of the heart on the multidetector-row CT, which is currently the preferred method for diagnosing PE, may detect RV enlargement due to PE. In a retrospective series of 431 patients, 30-day mortality was 15.6% in patients with right/left ventricular dimension ratio greater than 0.9 on multidetector-row chest CT, compared to 7.7% in those without this finding [75]. A meta-analysis of two studies (with two different RV/LV diameter thresholds, 1.5 and 1.0) including 191 normotensive patients with PE reported a 58% overall negative and a 57% positive value of RV dilatation on CT for predicting early death [73].

Natriuretic peptides are sensitive indicators of neurohormonal activation due to ventricular dysfunction, and their levels have been determined in patients with acute PE [76–79]. A meta-analysis of 13 studies enrolling 1132 patients found that elevated B-type natriuretic peptide (BNP) or NT-proBNP levels were associated with an increased risk of early death (OR 7.6, 95% CI 3.4–17) [80]. However, the authors concluded that elevation of natriuretic peptides alone does not appear to justify more invasive treatment regimens. The prognostic value of natriuretic peptides may be improved if they are combined with echocardiography [81] and clinical parameters [82].

Detection of myocardial injury

Elevated levels of cardiac troponin I or T, a sensitive and specific indicator of myocardial cell damage and microscopic myocardial necrosis, are found in up to 50% of patients with acute PE [83]. A meta-analysis of 20 studies with a total of 1985 patients showed that cardiac troponin elevation was associated with an increased risk of death

(OR 5.24, 95% CI 3.28–8.38) and major adverse events (OR 7.03, 95% CI 2.42–20.43) in the acute phase [84]. However, a more recent meta-analysis focusing only on normotensive patients (1366 patients in 9 studies) was unable to confirm the prognostic value of cardiac troponins in non-high-risk PE [85]. Thus, troponin elevation alone does not suffice to identify normotensive, intermediate-risk patients who might necessitate early aggressive (e.g. thrombolytic) treatment.

Fatty acid binding proteins are small cytoplasmic proteins which are abundant in tissues with active fatty acid metabolism, including the heart [86]. Following myocardial cell damage, heart-type FABP (H-FABP) appears in the circulation 90 min after symptom onset, reaching its peak within 6 h [87]. Preliminary data suggest that H-FABP may provide prognostic information superior to that of cardiac troponins in acute PE [88, 89] also in non-high-risk patients [90].

Growth-differentiation factor 15 (GDF-15) is a member of the transforming growth factor β cytokine family. Its cardiac expression increases sharply after pressure overload or myocardial ischaemia [91, 92], and thus GDF-15 might be capable of integrating information both on RV dysfunction and myocardial injury. Elevated levels of GDF-15 were associated with an increased 30-day risk of death or major complications in PE [93].

Clinical parameters and integrated scores

Several variables collected during routine clinical and laboratory evaluation have prognostic significance in PE. Recently, the Pulmonary Embolism Severity Index (PESI;

Table 64.1 The Pulmonary Embolism Severity Index (PESI) [97]

Variable	Points
Age	1/year
Male sex	10
History of cancer	30
History of heart failure	10
History of chronic lung disease	10
Pulse rate >110 beats/min	20
Systolic blood pressure <100 mm Hg	30
Respiratory rate > ≥30 breaths/min	20
Body temperature <36 ºC	20
Altered mental status (disorientation, confusion, somnolence)	60
Arterial oxyhaemoglobin saturation <90%	20

Risk categories (30-days all-cause mortality %): Class I, <65 points (0%); class II, 66–85 points (1%); class III, 86–105 points (3.1%); class IV, 106–125 points (10.4%); class V, >125 points (24.4%). Patients in risk classes I and II are defined as low-risk.

Table 64.1) has been validated in large populations of patients with PE [94, 95]. The index appears more capable of identifying patients with very low rates of adverse events than the Geneva prediction rule [96]. It remains to be determined whether a low PESI (risk classes I or II) is by itself sufficient to permit early discharge and home treatment of low-risk patients with acute PE.

Initial treatment

In acute PE, cardiovascular mortality is highest during the first few hours [69]. In patients who survive the early phase, the risk is determined mainly by the potential for recurrent thromboembolic events. Thus management of PE must focus on two major goals: (1) the early reversal of RV dysfunction, if present; and (2) the prevention of recurrent thromboembolism.

Initial anticoagulation

Anticoagulant treatment (Table 64.2) should be administered to all patients upon clinical suspicion of acute PE, i.e. without awaiting definitive confirmation by imaging procedures. Intravenous unfractionated heparin (UFH) is the preferred mode of initial anticoagulation (1) for patients with severe renal impairment (creatinine clearance <30 mL/min); (2) for patients at high risk of bleeding; (3) for high-risk, hypotensive patients; and, as a rule, (4) for extremely overweight, underweight, or old patients. With the exception of these circumstances, UFH has largely been replaced by low-molecular-weight heparin (LMWH) or fondaparinux given subcutaneously at weight-adjusted doses. Routine anticoagulation monitoring, i.e. measurement of anti-factor Xa levels, is not necessary in patients receiving LMWH, but it should be considered during pregnancy. In this case, anti-Xa levels should be determined 4 h after the morning injection; the proposed target range is 0.6–1.0 IU/mL for twice-daily and 1.0 to 2.0 IU/mL for once-daily administration.

The risk of heparin-induced thrombocytopenia is highest (3–5%) in patients who have undergone orthopaedic surgery and those who have received UFH. In medical and surgical patients receiving LMWH, the incidence is below 1%, and for patients receiving fondaparinux the risk is negligible [66, 98]. The recommendations for platelet count monitoring under heparin treatment are summarized in Table 64.2. Upon clinical suspicion of heparin-induced thrombocytopenia, all sources of heparin should be discontinued and therapy with direct parenteral thrombin

Table 64.2 Initial anticoagulation for acute pulmonary embolism

	Dosage	Interval	Remarks
Unfractionated heparin (IV infusion)	80 IU/kg as an intravenous bolus, followed by infusion at the rate of 18 IU kg⁻¹ h⁻¹	Continuous infusion	1. Adjust infusion rate to maintain aPTT between 1.5 and 2.5 times control, corresponding to therapeutic heparin levels (0.3–0.7 IU/mL by factor Xa inhibition) 2. Monitor platelet count at baseline and every other day from day 4 to 14 or until heparin is stopped. Investigate for HIT if platelet count falls by ≥50% and/or a thrombotic event occurs
LMWH (SC)			1. LMWH not tested and thus not recommended for patients with arterial hypotension or shock 2. Monitoring of anti-factor Xa levels may be helpful in patients at increased risk of bleeding, particularly those with moderate or severe renal impairment. The need for monitoring anti-Xa levels in pregnancy remains controversial 3. Monitor platelet count at baseline and every 2–4 days from day 4 to 14 or until heparin is stopped.*
Enoxaparin	1.0 mg/kg, or	Every 12 h	If creatinine clearance <30 mL/min, reduce enoxaparin dosage to 1 mg/kg once daily; consider unfractionated heparin infusion as an alternative [10]
	1.5mg/kg	Once daily	
Tinzaparin	175 U/kg	Once daily	
Fondaparinux	5 mg (body weight <50 kg) 7.5 mg (body weight 50–100 kg) 10 mg (body weight >100 kg)	Once daily	1. Contraindicated if creatinine clearance <20mL/min 2. No routine platelet monitoring [26]

aPTT, partial thromboplastin time; HIT, heparin-induced thrombocytopenia; IV, intravenous; LMWH, low-molecular-weight heparins; SC, subcutaneous.
*This recommendation applies to postoperative patients and to medical or obstetric patients recently (within 100 days) exposed to unfractionated heparin [98, 99].
For medical or obstetric patients who have only received LMWH, some authorities recommend no routine platelet count monitoring [99].
Adapted with permission from Kostantinides S. Clinical practice. Acute pulmonary embolism. *N Engl J Med* 2008; **359** (26): 2804–2813.

inhibitors, particularly argatroban or lepirudin, initiated; bivalirudin is approved for patients undergoing percutaneous coronary interventions.

Anticoagulation with unfractionated heparin or LMWH should be continued for at least 5 days. Oral anticoagulants (vitamin K antagonists) should be initiated as soon as possible in all haemodynamically stable patients, preferably on the same day as heparin. Parenteral anticoagulation can be stopped as soon as the international normalized ratio (INR) has been in the therapeutic range (2.0–3.0) on two consecutive days.

Thrombolysis

Randomized trials performed over a 30-year period [100] have consistently shown that thrombolytic therapy of PE effectively resolves thromboembolic obstruction and promptly reduces pulmonary artery pressure and resistance with a concomitant increase in cardiac output. One of the largest trials also demonstrated a significant improvement in RV function as assessed by echocardiography, 3 h after treatment with recombinant tissue plasminogen activator [72]. In the only randomized thrombolysis trial with clinical endpoints, early thrombolytic treatment given to normotensive patients with evidence of RV dysfunction significantly reduced the need for emergency escalation of therapy during the hospital stay [101].

Overall, up to 92% of patients with PE appear to respond favourably to thrombolysis as indicated by clinical and echocardiographic improvement within the first 36 h [102]. The greatest benefit is observed when treatment is initiated within 48 h of symptom onset, but thrombolysis can still be useful in patients who have had symptoms for 6–14 days [103]. On the other hand, the haemodynamic benefits of thrombolysis over heparin alone appear to be confined to the first few days. In patients who were alive 1 week after treatment, the improvement in the severity of vascular obstruction and RV dysfunction appeared to be similar in thrombolysis-treated and heparin-treated patients [104]. Moreover, thrombolysis carries a significant bleeding risk. A cumulative rate of up to 13% for major bleeding and a 2% rate of intracranial and/or fatal haemorrhage should be anticipated [105, 106], although the risk of major or life-threatening bleeding may be lower if noninvasive imaging methods are used in the diagnostic work-up of PE [72, 101]. Taken together, these data underline that thrombolysis should be reserved for patients in whom a high risk of early PE-related death is anticipated.

Currently approved thrombolytic regimens for PE include:

- Streptokinase: 250 000 IU as a loading dose over 30 min, followed by an infusion of 100 000 IU/h over 12–24 h

- Urokinase: 4400 IU/kg as a loading dose over 10 min, followed by 4400 IU kg–1h–1 over 12–24 h

- Alteplase (recombinant tissue plasminogen activator): 100 mg infusion over 2 h, with the first 10 mg usually given as a bolus injection.

Brief (2-h) infusion regimens of streptokinase or urokinase appear preferable to the 12–24-h infusion periods mentioned above, as they achieve more rapid clot lyis while also reducing the bleeding risk. A short (over 15 min) infusion regimen of alteplase at the dosage of 0.6 mg/kg (maximum dosage 50 mg) can be used in emergency situations, e.g. during cardiopulmonary resuscitation. Satisfactory haemodynamic results also have been obtained with double-bolus reteplase, two injections (10 U) 30 min apart [107]. Furthermore, the results of a recent multicentre controlled trial appear to support the efficacy and safety of bolus tenecteplase in acute PE [108]. However, neither reteplase nor tenecteplase is officially approved for treatment of PE at present.

Surgical or catheter-based embolectomy

Pulmonary embolectomy remained a rarely performed rescue operation for several decades, and limited data existed regarding its efficacy and safety. Recent technical advances in transportable extracorporeal assist systems, and particularly the timely involvement of the cardiac surgeon as part of an interdisciplinary approach to high-risk PE, may contribute to better postoperative outcomes [109]. Currently, pulmonary embolectomy is a recommended option in patients with high-risk PE in whom there are absolute contraindications to thrombolysis, or if thrombolysis has failed. Alternatively, catheter embolectomy or thrombus fragmentation may be considered, provided that there is adequate experience with these modalities on site [110].

Inferior vena cava filters

Cava filters may be used as a means of primary or secondary PE prevention. However, the data about their relative safety and efficacy remain inconclusive. Comparison with therapeutic anticoagulation has to take into account the fact that the latter treatment is very effective in preventing recurrent thromboembolism in patients treated for symptomatic PE. For example, recurrence rates under effective anticoagulation are in the range of 3% even in the presence of free-floating thrombi in the proximal leg veins [111], and fatal PE occurs in 0.4–1.5% of patients during treatment with heparin or warfarin [112]. In one study, inferior vena cava filter placement increased the risk of recurrent leg vein thrombosis over the long term [113]. At present, temporary inferior vena cava filters have a role in the prevention of PE only if anticoagulation is absolutely contraindicated, or in cases of recurrence in spite of adequate medical treatment.

Risk-adjusted management strategy in the acute phase

High-risk pulmonary embolism

In view of the high early mortality and complication risk associated with high-risk PE, existing guidelines [13, 114] and the majority of experts agree that patients who present with persistent arterial hypotension or shock are in need of immediate pharmacological or mechanical recanalization of the occluded pulmonary arteries. Thus, haemodynamically unstable patients with suspected high-risk PE should immediately receive a weight-adjusted bolus of unfractionated heparin while awaiting the results of further diagnostic work-up; if PE is confirmed, thrombolysis should be administered without delay. If thrombolysis is absolutely contraindicated or has failed, surgical embolectomy or catheter-based thrombus fragmentation or suction is a valuable alternative (Table 64.3).

Non-high-risk pulmonary embolism

At present, LMWH or fondaparinux is considered adequate treatment for most normotensive patients with PE (Table 64.3). Thrombolysis is generally not recommended as a first-line therapeutic option. However, it may be considered in selected intermediate-risk patients, i.e. those with evidence of RV dysfunction or myocardial injury, if they are at higher risk of death (due, for example, to pre-existing cardiac or respiratory failure) and have no contraindications to thrombolytic agents. A large multinational randomized trial has set out to determine whether normotensive, intermediate-risk patients with RV dysfunction, detected by echocardiography or CT, plus evidence of myocardial injury indicated by a positive troponin test, may benefit from early thrombolytic treatment. This study, which is already under way in 10 European countries, plans to recruit a total of 1000 patients and will be completed in 2012.

It has been proposed that selected patients with 'low-risk' PE, i.e. normotensive patients with neither RV dysfunction nor myocardial injury, could be discharged early and treated

Table 64.3 Severity-adjusted management of acute pulmonary embolism

PE-related early mortality risk		Risk markers			Recommended treatment
		Clinical[a]	RV dysfunction[b]	Myocardial injury[c]	
High (> 15%)		+	(+)*	(+)†	UFH plus thrombolysis or embolectomy
Non-high	Intermediate (3–15%)[‡]	−	+	+	LMWH
			+	−	As a rule, no early thrombolysis
			−	+	Monitor clinical status and RV function
	Low (<1%)	−	−	−	LMWH
					Outpatient treatment currently not recommended

H-FABP, heart-type fatty acid binding proteins; LMWH, low-molecular-weight heparin, including fondaparinux; MDCT, multidetector CT; PE, pulmonary embolism; RV, right ventricle; UFH, unfractionated heparin.

[a] Shock or hypotension.

[b] Echo, MDCT, natriuretic peptides.

[c] Troponin, H-FABP elevation.

Adapted with permission from Torbicki A, Perrier A, Konstantinides SV, et al. Guidelines on the diagnosis and management of acute pulmonary embolism: The Task Force for the Diagnosis and Management of Acute Pulmonary Embolism of the European Society of Cardiology (ESC). *Eur Heart J* 2008; **29** :2276–3315..

as outpatients [115]. In particular, the PESI (⊃ Table 64.1) appears to identify patients with very low rates of adverse events [96]. However, a randomized study of home treatment versus hospitalization of low-risk patients with PE was recently discontinued because of high mortality in the early discharge group [116]. Indeed, current evidence suggests that only a small proportion (up to 20%) of patients with PE may be eligible for home treatment [117], and this management option cannot be recommended at present (⊃ Table 64.3).

Recurrence and long-term secondary prophylaxis

PE and particularly unprovoked PE is considered a lifelong disease, and chronic secondary prophylaxis is necessary. Without continuing anticoagulation, as many as 50% of patients with symptomatic proximal DVT or PE may suffer a recurrent episode within the first 3 months [118]. The frequency of recurrence appears to be independent of the initial clinical manifestation of VTE, but recurrent VTE is three times more likely to present as PE if the initial clinical event was PE than if it was DVT [119]. This fact emphasizes the need for effective secondary prophylaxis in patients who have suffered PE. To date, most of the studies addressing recurrence prophylaxis have included patients with DVT rather than focusing on PE alone. The available data indicate that the long-term recurrence rate may be 30% or even higher after 8–10 years [120–122], and it was found that indefinite treatment might be capable of reducing the risk for recurrent thromboembolism by up to 90% [123].

Thus, oral anticoagulants (vitamin K antagonists) are highly effective in preventing recurrent thromboembolism. However, they do not eliminate the risk of subsequent recurrence after their discontinuation, regardless of the duration of treatment [124, 125]; besides, the benefits of chronic oral anticoagulation are partly offset by the increased risk of major bleeding [123, 126].

In view of these considerations, the recommended duration of oral anticoagulation after an episode of acute PE weighs the risk versus benefits of vitamin K antagonists [13, 114]. As a rule, treatment should be continued for 3 months after a first episode of PE triggered by a transient risk factor (trauma, surgery, immobilization, pregnancy, contraceptive use, or hormonal replacement therapy), and for at least 3 months for patients with unprovoked PE. Indefinite oral anticoagulation should be considered and discussed on an individual basis for patients with a first manifestation of unprovoked PE and a low risk of bleeding, and it is clearly recommended for most patients with a second unprovoked episode of VTE. Patients with high-risk thrombophilia or active cancer are also candidates for long-term oral anticoagulation. Finally, recent data suggest that D-dimer testing 1 month after discontinuation of vitamin K antagonists could be used to resume or definitely terminate therapy in patients who have received oral anticoagulants for 3 months after the first episode of idiopathic vein thrombosis or PE [127]. Novel, vitamin K-independent oral anticoagulants are currently under investigation for both prophylaxis and treatment of VTE [128]. If eventually approved for the treatment and long-term secondary prophylaxis of VTE, the new oral anticoagulants may simplify chronic anticoagulation and increase patient compliance.

Conclusion

Contemporary management of acute PE places particular emphasis on risk-adjusted diagnostic and therapeutic strategies. For patients who present with normal arterial blood pressure (non-high-risk PE), the development and validation of structured models for assessment of clinical (pretest) probability, the use of D-dimer testing in case of intermediate or low clinical probability and the technical advances of multidetector-row CT pulmonary angiography have helped to optimize diagnostic algorithms. On the other hand, in patients presenting with haemodynamic instability, i.e. persistent arterial hypotension or cardiogenic shock (suspected high-risk PE), the detection of right ventricular dysfunction on bedside echocardiography may suffice to confirm the diagnosis and proceed to immediate treatment measures. Current treatment regimens for haemodynamically stable patients are based on LMWH followed by oral anticoagulants, while early thrombolysis and technical advances in surgical and interventional treatment permit successful removal of thrombus in high-risk PE. Finally, while current guidelines recommend considering further risk stratification of patients with non-high-risk PE based on markers of right ventricular dysfunction and/or myocardial injury (intermediate- vs low-risk PE), the therapeutic implications of further imaging or biomarker tests remain controversial at present. In this regard, prospective management trials are currently under way to investigate whether patients with intermediate-risk PE may benefit from early thrombolysis, and whether low-risk PE can safely be treated out of the hospital.

Personal perspective

In recent decades, awareness of PE has been increased, partly thanks to the promotion of primary prophylaxis supported by the pharmaceutical industry. Introduction of validated diagnostic strategies based on easily available noninvasive tests such as CT pulmonary angiography, D-dimers, and CUS, as well as identification of objective indicators of the risk of early death, greatly enhanced the chances of correct management decisions in suspected PE. The future should bring long-awaited answers regarding indications for thrombolysis beyond the group of patients with shock or hypotension, and the possible role of percutaneous interventions for the management of high-risk PE. New oral anticoagulants could facilitate treatment, particularly long-term secondary prevention. However, the universal implementation of evidence-based guidelines remains the greatest challenge and hope for patients suffering from all forms of PE around the globe.

Further reading

Anderson FA Jr, Spencer FA. Risk factors for venous thromboembolism. *Circulation* 2003;**107**(23 Suppl 1):I9–16.

Bourjeily G, Paidas M, Khalil H, *et al.* Pulmonary embolism in pregnancy. *Lancet* 2009;**375**(9713):500–512.

Geerts WH, Bergqvist D, Pineo GF, *et al.* Prevention of venous thromboembolism: American College of Chest Physicians Evidence-Based Clinical Practice Guidelines (8th edition). *Chest* 2008;**133**(6 Suppl):381S–453S.

Jorens PG, Van ME, Snoeckx A, Parizel PM. Nonthrombotic pulmonary embolism. *Eur Respir J* 2009;**34**(2):452–474.

Kearon C, Kahn SR, Agnelli G, *et al.* Antithrombotic therapy for venous thromboembolic disease: American College of Chest Physicians Evidence-Based Clinical Practice Guidelines (8th edition). *Chest* 2008;**133** (6 Suppl):454S–545S.

Konstantinides S. Clinical practice. Acute pulmonary embolism. *N Engl J Med* 2008;**359**(26):2804–2813.

Kucher N. Catheter embolectomy for acute pulmonary embolism. *Chest* 2007;**132**(2):657–663.

Torbicki A, Perrier A, Konstantinides SV, *et al.* Guidelines on the diagnosis and management of acute pulmonary embolism: The Task Force for the Diagnosis and Management of Acute Pulmonary Embolism of the European Society of Cardiology (ESC). *Eur Heart J* 2008;**29**:2276–2315.

Online resource

European Society of Cardiology (ESC) guidelines. http://www.escardio.org

For additional multimedia materials please visit the online version of the book (http://www.esciacc.oxfordmedicine. com).

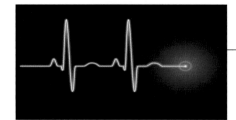

CHAPTER 65

Stroke

Didier Leys, Charlotte Cordonnier,
and Valeria Caso

Contents

Summary

Stroke is a major public health issue, and many strokes are treatable at the acute stage provided patients are admitted soon enough. The overall incidence of stroke in Western countries is approximately of 2400 per year per million inhabitants, and 80% are due to cerebral ischaemia. The prevalence is approximately 12 000 per million inhabitants. Stroke is associated with increased long-term mortality, handicap, cognitive and behavioural impairments, recurrence, and increased risk of other types of vascular events. It is of major interest to take the heterogeneity of stroke into account, because of differences in acute management, secondary prevention, and outcomes according to the subtype and aetiology of stroke. In all types of strokes, early epileptic seizures, delirium, increased intracranial pressure, and nonspecific complications are frequent. In ischaemic strokes, specific complications such as malignant infarcts, spontaneous haemorrhagic transformation, early recurrence, and a new ischaemic event in other vascular territory are frequent complications. In haemorrhagic strokes, the major complication is the subsequent increase of the bleeding.

Stroke unit care is the cornerstone of the treatment of stroke, aiming at the detection and management of life-threatening emergencies, stabilization of most physiological parameters, and prevention of early complications. In ischaemic stroke, besides this general management, specific therapies are intravenous recombinant tissue plasminogen activator given as soon as possible and before 4.5 h, otherwise aspirin 300 mg, immediately or after 24 h in case of thrombolysis. In intracerebral haemorrhages, blood pressure management and haemostatic therapy are two potential targets under investigation. Surgery does not prove effective to reduce death and disability.

Introduction

Stroke is a major public health issue, because of a high incidence rate, high case fatality rates, risks of residual physical and neuropsychological disability, and direct and indirect costs [1]. Many strokes are preventable, and many are treatable at the acute stage provided patients are admitted soon enough [2].

The term 'stroke' covers a wide range of heterogeneous disorders, depending on (1) the severity of the clinical presentation, from transient deficits to severe cases with coma and early death, (2) the underlying mechanism, i.e. cerebral ischaemia, parenchymal haemorrhage, subdural or subarachnoid haemorrhage, and (3) the cause, i.e. atherosclerosis, cardioembolism, small-vessel occlusion, rare vasculopathies, and undetermined causes in cerebral ischaemia; or vascular malformations, cerebral amyloid angiopathies, small-vessel diseases, rare vasculopathies, and undetermined causes in parenchymal haemorrhages.

This chapter focuses on acute cerebral ischaemia and parenchymal haemorrhages, which are the two types of strokes that are the most likely to be seen in cardiac intensive care units (ICUs). Several aspects of stroke medicine that are not likely to occur or to be treated in cardiac ICUs are not covered here (cerebrovascular diseases without stroke, silent strokes, subarachnoid haemorrhages, subdural and extradural haematomas). We will cover the epidemiology of stroke, a crucial issue to understand what should be expected in the future; the general assessment of stroke patients; the complications that can occur at the acute stage; the treatment of acute stroke; and finally a few situations that require specific managements and where evidence-based data are scarce.

Epidemiology of stroke

Incidence and prevalence

The overall incidence of stroke in Western countries is approximately 2400 per year per million inhabitants [3], and is now slightly higher than that of acute coronary syndromes (ACS) [4]. In Western countries approximately 80% of strokes are due to cerebral ischaemia and 20% to parenchymal haemorrhages. The incidence varies between countries, and is nowadays increasing even more in low-income countries [5]. The overall prevalence of stroke in Western countries is approximately 12 000 per million inhabitants [3].

Long-term outcome

Stroke is associated with increased long-term mortality, handicap, cognitive and behavioural impairments, recurrence, and increased risk of other types of vascular event, such as myocardial infarction (MI) [3].

Risk factors

Besides nonmodifiable risk factors such as increasing age, male gender, nonwhite ethnicity, and familial predisposition, the most important modifiable risk factors are:

- High blood pressure: there is a continuous linear relationship between systolic and diastolic blood pressure and the incidence of ischaemic and of haemorrhagic stroke; there is no threshold, and the risk of stroke is doubled for every 7.5 mmHg increase in diastolic blood pressure.
- Blood cholesterol: there is an increased risk of ischaemic stroke with increasing total and low-density lipoprotein (LDL) cholesterol levels, and decreasing high-density lipoprotein (HDL) cholesterol.
- Cigarette smoking doubles the risk of ischaemic stroke.
- Diabetes mellitus doubles the risk of ischaemic stroke, independently of other factors.
- Oral contraceptive therapies increase the risk of stroke especially in women above the age of 35 years, when they smoke and have migraine.

Stroke subtypes

It is of major interest to take the heterogeneity of stroke into account, because of differences in acute management, secondary prevention, and outcomes according to the subtype and aetiology of stroke [6]. For instance, for the same level of stenosis of the internal carotid artery, patients with cervical artery dissections have a lower risk of recurrence, sequelae, ACS, and death, than patients with atheroma. Patients with transient ischaemic attacks (TIA) have a higher risk of recurrent cerebral ischaemic event than patients with ischaemic stroke, especially if they are found to have a corresponding lesion on MRI.

The major difference between stroke and MI is the heterogeneity of stroke. Most MIs are the consequence of atheroma on the coronary arteries, but approximately 20% of strokes are the consequence of intracerebral haemorrhages (ICH) [4]. Moreover, even cerebral ischaemia is heterogeneous, because the arterial occlusion may be the consequence of various disorders such as large-vessel atheroma, various cardiac sources of embolism especially atrial fibrillation, small-vessel occlusions, or many other definite rare causes such as angeitis, dissections, or toxic angiopathies [7]. Besides, many ischaemic strokes remain of undetermined cause because of multiple causes, lack of identified cause despite an extensive diagnostic work-up, or incomplete diagnostic work-up [8]. The same heterogeneity exists for parenchymal haemorrhages.

General assessment of stroke patients

Is this patient having a stroke?

Stroke is characterized by a sudden loss of cerebral function without any other identified cause than vascular. It includes both cerebral infarcts and ICH. The classical definition requires the symptoms to last more than 24 h, except in the case of early death. More recently patients with deficits lasting less than 24 h, but associated with a corresponding infarct on imaging, have been classified as having a stroke. The following clinical characteristics are suggestive of a stroke, although one or more may sometimes be missing:

- Sudden onset of symptoms, within seconds or minutes, then stabilizing and improving over time.

- Focal symptoms and signs, i.e. neurological deficit explained by a single lesion of the brain (◑ Box 65.1). Symptoms such as faintness, dizziness, generalized weakness, light-headedness, confusion, incontinence, drop attacks, syncope, or tinnitus, are not suggestive of stroke unless they are associated with focal signs.

- Symptoms suggesting a loss of function, even if, sometimes, they may also be 'positive': i.e. jerking of a limb, seizure, paraesthesia, tingling, seeing flashing lights, visual hallucinations, or movement disorders, although these are not typical of a stroke.

- Other associated symptoms are not typical but may be useful to help in diagnosis (◑ Box 65.2).

How severe is this stroke?

The level of consciousness can be assessed by the widely used Glasgow Coma Scale (GCS) which is more appropriate than terms such as stupor, drowsiness, or coma. Its main limitation in stroke is when there is aphasia or a motor deficit (the best motor response should be evaluated in nonparetic limbs).

The severity of the neurological deficit should be assessed by the National Institutes of Health (NIH) Stroke Scale

---

Box 65.1 Focal neurological symptoms consistent with the diagnosis of stroke

Most suggestive symptoms, even when isolated

- Motor symptoms: weakness or clumsiness of one side of the body (hemiplegia or hemiparesis), or part of the body

- Sensory loss: decreased sensation on one side of the body, or part of the body

- Aphasia: impairment or loss of linguistic abilities, resulting in difficulties in speaking, understanding oral conversation, reading, and writing

- Visuospatial neglect: usually on the left side and associated with left hemiplegia and hemianopia

- Visual disturbances: monocular blindness, hemianopia or quadranopia, bilateral blindness with anosognosia

Symptoms that may be present in case of stroke, but usually with other focal symptoms

- Dysphagia

- Ataxia

- Paraparesis or paraplegia

- Dysarthria

- Diplopia

- Rotational vertigo

- Acute unilateral hearing loss

- Acute amnesia

---

[9] which quantifies different categories of neurological impairments, including consciousness. It is widely used in monitoring stroke patients, and to select candidates for thrombolytic therapy [6]. The NIH Stroke Scale is available online. Although it takes only minutes, is reliable and reproducible, and can be performed by non-neurologists, some training is still required (see ▣ Online resources).

What type or subtype of stroke is it?

Although some symptoms are more frequent in ICH (e.g. headache, impairment of consciousness at onset, epileptic seizures), none of them is specific enough for diagnosis in an individual patient. Brain imaging is therefore mandatory to differentiate ischaemic stroke from ICH in all patients. This is a crucial stage of the diagnosis because patients will require different diagnostic work-up, acute treatments, and secondary prevention measures in ICH

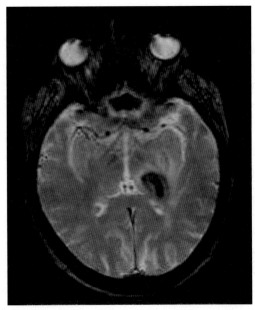

Figure 65.2 Hyposignal on $T_2{}^*$ images, in favour of a left thalamic haemorrhage.

and ischaemic strokes. The only exception, when imaging is not necessary, is for patients in palliative care for any reason.

MRI is the most appropriate technique in acute stroke, with the following sequences:

♦ T_1- and T_2-weighted images, and FLAIR sequences identify old lesions and lesions of nonvascular origin.

♦ Diffusion-weighted images (DWI) identify new ischaemic lesions (➲ Fig. 65.1). Low cerebral blood flow induces cytotoxic oedema with cellular swelling and, as a consequence, decreased movement of extracellular water which is responsible for the hyperintense signal on DWI and a decrease in the apparent diffusion coefficient of

water. These changes appear before T_1, T_2, and FLAIR changes.

♦ $T_2{}^*$ sequences to identify haemorrhages (➲ Fig. 65.2).

♦ Time-of-flight (TOF) sequences to visualize occlusions of the extra- and intracranial arteries (➲ Fig. 65.3).

♦ Perfusion-weighted images (PWI) may be useful to visualize the area at risk in cerebral ischaemia but they are not routinely used in most centres.

When an MRI scan is not available in emergency, or cannot be performed because of contraindications (pacemaker, claustrophobia, agitation, etc.), a brain CT scan without contrast should be performed without delay. It easily identifies ICH as a spontaneous hyperdensity in the brain parenchyma (➲ Fig. 65.4). In acute cerebral ischaemia, the scan may be normal, especially very early, but it may show signs of cerebral ischaemia, even within 3 h: loss

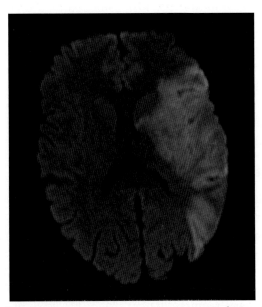

Figure 65.1 Hypersignal on diffusion-weighted images, in favour of a new ischaemic lesion in the left middle cerebral artery territory (same patient as in ➲ Figs 65.3 and 65.6).

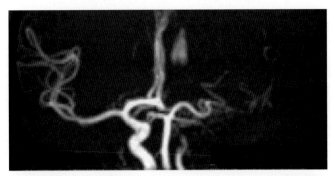

Figure 65.3 Time-of-flight (TOF) sequence revealing the occlusion of the left middle cerebral artery (same patient as in ➲ Figs 65.1 and ➲ 65.6).

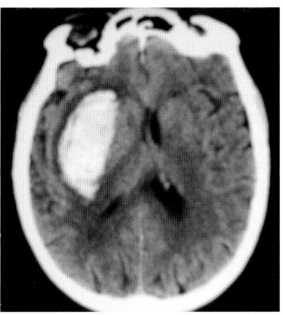

Figure 65.4 Noncontrast CT scan showing a spontaneous hyperdensity of the right lenticular nuclei, due to a deep intracerebral haemorrhage.

of the limits of the lenticular nucleus, loss of the insular ribbon, disappearance of the difference between grey and white matter (➲ Fig. 64.5). When the middle cerebral artery is occluded, the CT scan may show it as hyperdense. New generation CT scanners can now provide arterial anatomy and perfusion information, but this requires irradiation and intravenous contrast.

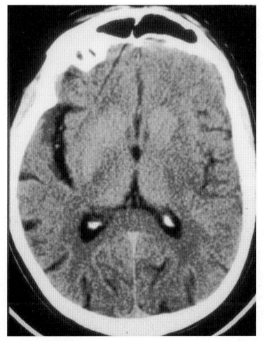

Figure 65.5 Noncontrast CT scan showing early signs of acute left middle cerebral artery ischaemia (loss of the limits of the lenticular nucleus, loss of the insular ribbon).

What is the most likely cause of this stroke?

Ischaemic strokes

In Western countries the most frequent causes are large-artery atherosclerosis, atrial fibrillation, and small-vessel occlusions of the deep perforators, and in young patients the leading cause is arterial dissection. In other parts of the world the causes have a different breakdown, with a prominent place of valvulopathies and infectious disorders.

In all patients the following investigations are necessary in the acute setting to allow an appropriate management of patients, especially for secondary prevention measures:

◆ Clinical examination, especially for cardiac abnormalities and peripheral pulses/bruits.

◆ Full blood count to detect polycythaemia and thrombocythemia.

◆ Erythrocyte sedimentation rate to detect vasculitis.

◆ Blood glucose to detect diabetes, or hypoglycaemia.

◆ ECG to detect atrial fibrillation and acute MI.

◆ Cervical and transcranial ultrasonography to detect stenosis or occlusion, or dissection.

◆ Transthoracic echocardiography to detect intracardiac thrombus or tumours, valvulopathies, valvular vegetations, decreased ventricular ejection fraction, patent foramen ovale.

Optional investigations are guided by the results of the initial investigations, age, presumed aetiology and the clinical context:

◆ Angiography (usually MR, sometimes CT and almost never via catheter).

◆ Transoesophageal echocardiography when the left atrium should be better explored.

◆ 24-h ECG if intermittent arrhythmia is suspected.

◆ Specialized biological tests when oriented towards a specific cause, such as anticardiolipin antibodies, serologies, antinuclear antibodies, etc.

Intracerebral haemorrhage

The causes of ICH are listed in ➲ Box 65.3; most cases are not due to a vascular malformation, but to small-vessel disease (usually as a consequence of chronic arterial hypertension), or cerebral amyloid angiopathy (lobar haemorrhage).

In all patients the following investigations are necessary:

◆ Careful history for hypertension, medications, alcohol consumption, family history of stroke, cancer, trauma, illicit substance use.

- MRI to identify cavernous malformations, intracranial venous thrombosis, brain microbleeds, arteriovenous malformation, tumour, indirect signs in favour of unrecognized trauma.

- Coagulation tests.

- Blood pressure recording, bearing in mind that it may also increase as a consequence of ICH.

- Search for relevant illicit drugs in blood and urine.

- MR, CT, or catheter angiography depending on age, history of arterial hypertension, and location of the ICH, with huge differences between countries and specialties.

Complications occurring at the acute stage of stroke

In any type of stroke

- Early epileptic seizures occur within 2 weeks after stroke onset in about 5% of patients, more frequently in case of cortical lesion or severe stroke [10].

- Delirium occurs in about 25% of stroke patients, especially in those with pre-existing cognitive decline and who develop metabolic or infectious complications [11].

- Increased intracranial pressure: large cerebellar strokes may lead to hydrocephalus or direct compression of the brainstem, usually within the first 4 days in infarcts and sometimes earlier in haemorrhages.

- Nonspecific complications include pressure sores, pneumonia, urinary tract infection, hyponatraemia due to inappropriate secretion of antidiuretic hormone, deep vein thrombosis, and pulmonary embolism. They are all more frequent in patients with severe neurological deficits.

In ischaemic strokes

- Malignant infarcts with swelling and raised intracranial pressure occur mainly (but not exclusively) in young patients with large hemispheric infarcts, usually within 48 h of onset, and have a high mortality (➲ Fig. 65.6).

- Spontaneous haemorrhagic transformation may occur even in the absence of antithrombotic or thrombolytic drugs, and may not increase stroke severity.

- Early recurrences become less frequent over time and depends mainly on stroke severity (the greater the severity the lower the risk) and cause (high in atrial fibrillation or severe carotid stenosis, low in dissection).

Box 65.3 Causes of nontraumatic intracerebral haemorrhage

- Morphological abnormalities of the cerebral arteries
  - Small-vessel disease of the deep perforators
  - Cerebral amyloid angiopathy
  - CADASIL
  - Intracranial dissection
  - Vasculitis
  - Mycotic aneurysm
- Vascular malformations
  - Arteriovenous malformation
  - Cavernous malformation
  - Dural arteriovenous fistula
  - Saccular aneurysm
  - Moyamoya syndrome
- Intracranial venous thrombosis
- Brain tumours
  - Metastasis
  - Primary malignant brain tumours

Haemostatic disorders (iatrogenic: thrombolytic therapy, oral anticoagulation, antiplatelet agents; congenital or acquired coagulation and haemostatic disorders) are considered not as causes but as trigger factors.

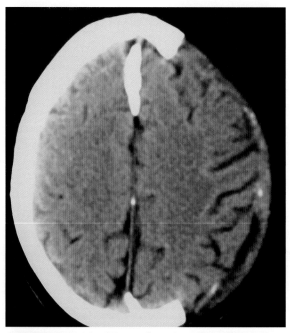

Figure 65.6 Postoperative CT scan of a patient who underwent decompressive surgery for malignant infarct in the left middle cerebral artery territory (same patient as in ➲ Figs 65.1 and 65.3).

◆ New ischaemic events in other vascular territories are also frequent (MI, aortic dissection, etc.)

In haemorrhagic strokes

◆ Subsequent increase of the bleeding is an early complication after ICH. The frequency of ICH enlargement is high: growth, defined as a 33% increase of haematoma volume on CT, occurs in 38% of 103 patients within 24 h after onset, most of the growth occurring within the first 4 h [12]. ICH growth is significantly associated with clinical deterioration [12]. Because of its prognostic value, haematoma growth is often used as a surrogate marker in clinical trials. The pathophysiology of growth is not clear: is it due to rebleeding or continuous bleeding? Predictors of haemorrhage expansion include initial early presentation, irregular shape, alcohol use, and low level of fibrinogen [13]. The presence of a spot sign on CT angiography [14] may be predictive of haematoma growth [15, 16]. In patients on oral anticoagulants, haematoma enlargement occurs more frequently [17] and the duration of the period of enlargement is increased [18]. The 30-day mortality increases with the volume of ICH (from 93% for deep ICH of 60 cm^3 or more, to 7% for lobar ICH of less than 30 cm^3), decreasing consciousness, increasing age, infratentorial location, intraventricular bleeding, and hydrocephalus.

◆ The risk of early recurrence has probably been underestimated in ICH.

Treatment of acute stroke

Nonspecific management of all types of strokes

There is a strong evidence that stroke patients should be treated in dedicated stroke units : each time 24 patients are treated in a stroke unit instead of a conventional ward, 1 death and 1 dependence is prevented [19, 20]. This effect does not depend on age, severity, or stroke subtype [19, 20]. For this reason, stroke unit care is the basis of the treatment of stroke [21, 22].

These measures should be applied to all types of strokes with persistent deficits. The term 'nonspecific management' refers to treatment strategies that aim at stabilizing the patient, to control systemic issues that may compromise recovery. This is a central part of stroke treatment [6, 23]. However, many aspects of general stroke treatment have not been adequately assessed in randomized clinical trials.

◆ Detection and management of life-threatening emergencies (risks of aspiration, occurrence of status epilepticus, respiratory failure, etc.). Airway protection should be provided in case of coma, local obstacle, or central respiratory failure.

◆ Stabilization of most physiological parameters: Sao_2 (>93%), glycaemia (<180 mg), temperature (<37.5°C), and hydration). This is necessary during the first few days to prevent a deleterious effect on the penumbra.

◆ Normal respiratory function with adequate blood oxygenation may be important in the acute stroke period to preserve ischaemic brain tissue, but there is no convincing evidence that giving oxygen to all acute stroke patients is effective [24]. In case of hypoxaemia blood oxygenation is improved by the administration of oxygen via a nasal tube, or artificial ventilation.

◆ Atrial fibrillation is frequent and heart failure, MI, and sudden death are also recognized complications [25, 26]. The frequency of these complications explains why continuous monitoring is necessary for 2–3 days.

◆ Many stroke patients are dehydrated, and this is associated with a poor outcome [27]. Although clinical trial evidence is limited, delivery of intravenous fluids (saline 0.9%) is considered part of general management of acute stroke, particularly in patients at risk of dehydration due to reduced consciousness or impaired swallowing. Experience in the management of hyperglycaemia supports the avoidance of dextrose in the early poststroke phase and strict glycaemic control [28].

◆ It has been shown in animal studies that the autoregulation of cerebral blood flow is lost in the penumbra area, and that any drop in blood pressure during the first hours, i.e. when the penumbra is still present, may decrease the cerebral blood flow and be deleterious in the ischaemic area. Therefore, although it is not possible to measure the cerebral blood flow routinely in stroke patients, and despite the lack of evidence-based data, high blood pressure should not be treated at the acute stage unless there is an associated life-threatening disorder such as aortic dissection or ICH [21, 22]. A low or low–normal blood pressure at stroke onset is unusual [29], and may be the result of a large cerebral infarct, cardiac failure, ischaemia, hypovolaemia, or sepsis. A systematic review covering a variety of blood pressure altering agents has not provided any convincing evidence that active management of blood pressure after acute stroke influences patient outcomes [30]. In the absence of reliable evidence from clinical trials, it is common practice to begin cautious blood pressure reduction when levels exceed 220 mmHg systolic and 120 mmHg diastolic.

However, in many centres blood pressure reduction is only considered in the presence of severe cardiac insufficiency, acute renal failure, aortic arch dissection, or malignant hypertension. In patients undergoing thrombolysis it is common practice to avoid systolic blood pressures above 185 mmHg. Intravenous labetalol (10 mg bolus, followed by a continuous infusion of 0.1–0.3 mg kg^{-1}h^{-1}) or urapidil (12.5 mg bolus in 20 s, repeated if necessary, followed by a continuous infusion of 6–30mg/h) are frequently used.

◆ Hyperglycaemia occurs in up to 60% of stroke patients without known diabetes [31, 32]. Hyperglycaemia after acute stroke is associated with larger infarct volumes and cortical involvement, and with poor functional outcome [33–35]. The largest randomized trial of blood glucose lowering by glucose–potassium–insulin (GKI) infusion [28], compared with standard intravenous saline infusion, found no difference in mortality or functional outcomes in patients with mild-to-moderate blood glucose elevations (median 137 mg/dL [7.6 mmol/L]). This regime was labour intensive and associated with episodes of hypoglycaemia. At present the routine use of insulin infusion regimes in patients with moderate hyperglycaemia cannot be recommended. However, based on very weak evidence, the European Stroke Organization recommend reducing blood glucose levels below 180 mg/dL (10 mmol/L) [36]. It is possible that this target level will be reduced in future if more evidence is provided, and that a recommendation to prevent large variations in glucose levels is made, as this is the case for intensive care medicine in general.

◆ Body temperature management. Hyperthermia is associated with increased infarct size and worse outcome [37]. Raised temperature is associated with poorer clinical outcomes [38–40]. A raised body temperature should prompt a search for infection and treatment where appropriate.

◆ Prevention of early complications:
  • Bed sores: appropriate caloric intake, early mobilization, and appropriate beds and nursing.
  • Aspiration pneumonia: specialized detection of swallowing impairment by physicians, nurses, or speech therapists, and nasogastric tube when necessary.
  • Deep venous thrombosis (DVT) and pulmonary embolism (PE): low-molecular-weight heparin (LMWH) at low dose reduces the risk of DVT and PE, but has no effect on mortality. As it leads to a small nonsignificant increase in risk of brain haemorrhagic changes, it should be used only in patients at risk, i.e. those with

leg immobilization, during the first hours in cerebral infarcts [21], and not before 24 h in those with ICH [41].
  • Rehabilitation can be started as soon as the patient is stable: passive measures minimize the risks of contractures, pressure sores, and pneumonia.
  • Stroke unit care provides coordinated multidisciplinary input, with continuous training of specialized staff members, and reduces mortality and dependency, in part by the prevention of nonspecific complications that occur in the first days.

Specific management of ischaemic stroke
Thrombolytic therapy

Intravenous recombinant tissue plasminogen activator (rtPA) increases the odds of a favourable outcome at 3 months about eightfold when given within 90 min, about twofold within 91–180 min, and 1.4-fold within 181–270 min [42, 43]. Mortality is not affected up to 270 min, but increases thereafter [42]. Haemorrhagic transformation is associated with increasing age, and large infarcts [42]. The main messages are the sooner rtPA is given, the greater the benefit, and even if there is still a benefit beyond 3 h, the magnitude of the benefit decreases. The dose is 0.9 mg/kg (10% as an IV bolus, 90% as a continuous IV infusion over 1 h). Thrombolytic therapy is therefore recommended as soon as possible after stroke onset, with a limit of 4.5 h, and strict limitations concerning both contraindications (increased risk of haemorrhage, delay >4.5 h, blood pressure >185 mmHg, glucose level >4 g/L) and strict conditions of use (only by a neurologist or a stroke-trained physician, and in a stroke unit) [6].

Other ways to achieve early recanalization are currently under investigation: other thrombolytic drugs, MRI criteria for selection of patients on mismatch, intra-arterial thrombolytic therapy, mechanical devices, and ultrasound-assisted intravenous thrombolytic therapy.

Antithrombotic therapies

◆ Aspirin 300 mg start and then 75–150 mg daily prevents 9 dependencies or deaths per 1000 patients treated. Because of the large number of patients who can receive aspirin, this small individual effect provides a reasonable effect in terms of public health. Aspirin should not be started until 24 h after any thrombolysis.

◆ Heparin (unfractionated or LMWH) does not provide any overall benefit because the decreased early ischaemic recurrences are counterbalanced by haemorrhagic transformations. There is no reason to recommend heparin routinely during the acute stage of ischaemic stroke, even in patients with atrial fibrillation.

Neuroprotective measures

◆ Potential neuroprotective drugs that have shown an effect in animals have so far failed in humans.

◆ Hypothermia is a potential way to achieve neuroprotection but because of adverse effects and the need for intensive care, it can only be used in severe cases, especially for patients at risk for malignant infarcts, and should now be tested in randomized trials.

Decompressive surgery

Decompressive surgery (hemicraniectomy) reduces mortality and disability in patients below the age of 60 years, who have a recent large infarct in the middle cerebral artery territory. To be effective surgery should be performed before the occurrence of malignant infarct. The best selection criterion is the volume of abnormality on DWI performed within the first 24 h, a volume of 145 cm^3 being a good predictor of further malignant infarct. Therefore good candidates for surgery are those patients with severe ischaemic strokes, less than 60 years of age, who have more than 145 cm^3 of diffusion abnormality on MRI [6, 44]. The effect of hemicraneictomy is important, the number of patients needed to be treated (NNT) to prevent 1 death being 2.

Specific management of intracerebral haemorrhages

Blood pressure management

◆ Blood pressure reduction within the first hours may prevent or retard the growth of the haematoma and may also decrease the risk of rebleeding.

◆ The possibility that early lowering of blood pressure might induce cerebral ischaemia in critically perfused or hypometabolic regions of the brain adjacent to the haematoma has been a major concern, although imaging studies have failed to identify such adverse effect or any significant rim of hypoperfusion in ICH [45, 46].

◆ The INTERACT study showed in a population of 404 ICH patients treated within the first 6 h that early intensive blood pressure lowering treatment was clinically feasible, well tolerated, and seemed to reduce haematoma growth [47]. Other studies are also encouraging from a safety point of view [48]. However, this strategy remains controversial due to the fact that there are as yet no large randomized trials to guide the management and the

European recommendations rely on low level of evidence (class IV evidence) [41]:

• No specific drug is recommended.

• Patients with known prior hypertension or signs (ECG, retina) of chronic hypertension: systolic blood pressure >180 mmHg and/or diastolic blood pressure >105 mmHg. If treated, target blood pressure should be 170/100 (or mean arterial pressure of 125 mmHg).

• Patients without known hypertension: systolic blood pressure >160 mmHg and/or diastolic blood pressure >95 mmHg. If treated, target blood pressure should be 150/90 (or mean arterial pressure of 110 mmHg).

• Reduction of mean arterial pressure by more than 20% should be avoided.

• These limits and targets should be adapted to higher values in patients with monitoring of increased intracranial pressure to guarantee a sufficient cerebral perfusion pressure >70 mmHg.

Prevention of deep venous thrombosis and pulmonary embolism

DVT and PE are feared complications in ICH patients. Only a few patients with ICH were included in trials evaluating different strategies of prevention. A small study dedicated to ICH patients suggested that intermittent pneumatic compression stockings were more efficient than stockings alone, but the study lacked power [49]. In the CLOTS trial [50], graduated compression stockings did not demonstrate any efficacy. However, only 232 ICH patients were included among 2518 stroke patients. The usefulness of heparin (fractionated or LMWH) remains to be demonstrated in a setting where the haemorrhagic risk could easily counterbalance the benefit. In clinical practice, a low dose of subcutaneous heparin or LMWH can be considered after 24 h [41].

Increased intracranial pressure

Increased intracranial pressure (ICP) has a negative impact on vital and functional outcome. Invasive ICP monitoring has not yet been proven more efficient than clinical and radiological monitoring. All randomized studies to date have failed to demonstrate any efficacy on the outcome of ICH patients [51]. Methods for medical decompression for increased ICP may be useful to bridge the time to surgery, if the latter is planned. Corticosteroids are not recommended and should be avoided in the treatment of acute phase of ICH. Recommendations rely on a low level of evidence [41]. Medical treatment of elevated ICP includes glycerol, mannitol, hyper-HAES, and short-term hyperventilation (class IV evidence). For example, mannitol (20%) in a dose of 0.75–1 g/kg may be given as intravenous bolus followed by 0.25–0.5 g/kg every 3–6 h, depending on the neurological status and fluid balance.

Haemostatic therapy

Although this is very promising, to date no haemostatic agents has proved its efficacy in the acute setting of ICH. The most recent candidate was recombinant factor VIIa (rFVIIa). After an encouraging phase IIb trial, [52] the phase III trial which recruited 841 patients failed to demonstrate an improvement of the outcome [53]. Another agent that may be a candidate is ε-aminocaproic acid. A careful analysis of current data suggests that a large randomized trial of this is justified [54]. Meanwhile, no haemostatic agent can be recommended in clinical practice.

Intracerebral haemorrhages in patients treated with oral anticoagulants

In the acute phase, every patients suffering an ICH with an INR >1.4 should be treated with intravenous vitamin K to reverse the effects of warfarin and with treatment to replace clotting factors, whatever the reason for oral anticoagulant is (i.e. including patients with mechanical heart valve) [41].

The aim of rapid reversal is to prevent secondary growth of the haematoma. The European recommendations suggest using either prothrombin complex concentrates (PCC) or fresh frozen plasma, both of them being associated with intravenous vitamin K. An example of dosage for PCC (given in unit of factor IX contained in PCC) is 10–20 U/kg when INR <3.5 or 20–30 U/kg when INR >3.5, along with vitamin K (10 mg IV).

Only a few case reports have described the use of recombinant factor VIIa in this setting. To date rFVIIa has not been used routinely outside clinical trials.

Intracerebral haemorrhages in patients treated with antiplatelet drugs

No specific strategy is recommended for patients bleeding while under antipletelet drugs. Studies evaluating the efficacy of platelet infusion failed to demonstrate a benefit [55]. Other studies are ongoing [56].

Thrombolytic therapies

In ICH patients with intraventricular extension and obstruction of the third and fourth ventricles, some data suggest that the use of rtPA injected directly in the ventricles may improve the functional outcome [57, 58]. The CLEAR III trial is currently recruiting patients.

Surgery

Infratentorial intracerebral haemorrhages

Clot evacuation should be considered if there is neurological dysfunction or radiological evidence of obliteration of cerebrospinal fluid (CSF) spaces infratentorially. Optimal timing has not been established and there are no prospective randomized controlled trials of surgery in cerebellar haemorrhage. European recommendations state that ventricular drainage and evacuation of the cerebellar haematoma should be considered if haematomas are larger than 2–3 cm in diameter or if hydrocephalus occurs, although advanced age and coma advocate against favourable outcomes [41].

Supratentorial intracerebral haemorrhages

The Surgical Trial in Spontaneous Intracerebral Haemorrhage (STICH) showed in 1033 patients that early surgery (within 24 h) did not improve outcome compared to medical management. Therefore, clinical observation and medical management is the first step in the management of ICH patients. Prespecified subgroups analyses from STICH and a recent metanalyses suggest that craniotomy could be considered in case of deterioration in consciousness (from GGS 12–9 or lower) [59], or if the ICH is superficial (≤1 cm from the surface and does not reach deep basal ganglia) [41]. Deep-seated haematomas do not benefit from craniotomy.

Specific issues

Stroke due to cerebral venous thrombosis

Diagnosis

Cerebral venous and sinus thrombosis (CVST) accounts for less than 1% of all strokes. The estimated annual incidence is 3–4 cases per 1 million persons. It results from the occlusion of a venous sinus and/or cortical vein (➲ Fig. 65.7). This may lead to cortical venous infarction with petechial or overt haemorrhagic perivascular venous infarction. The common causes of CVST are genetic and acquired prothrombotic disorders, such as pregnancy and puerperium, infections, central nervous system infections, as well as infections of the ear, sinus, mouth, face, or neck. Diagnostic and therapeutic procedures such as surgery, lumbar puncture, jugular catheter, and some drugs, especially oral contraceptives, hormonal replacement therapy, steroids, and oncology treatments, can also predispose to CVST.

Unfortunately, misdiagnoses are frequent, as well as delay in diagnosis. This is due to the wide spectrum of clinical symptoms and the usual subacute clinical

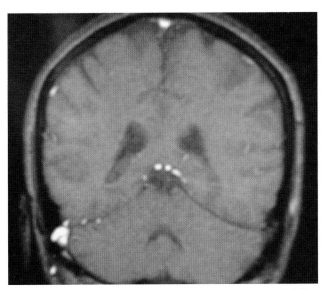

Figure 65.7 MRI of a patient with cerebral venous thrombosis: the left lateral sinus is occluded.

evolution. The clinical presentation is highly variable, but CVST should be considered in young and middle-aged patients having recent unusual headache associated with stroke-like symptoms, transient deficits, seizures, or lobar ICH. This is especially true for patients with intracranial hypertension, as well as those with evidence of haemorrhagic infarcts, especially if the infarcts are multiple and not confined to the arterial vascular territories.

The gold standard for a diagnosis of CVST is MRI which directly shows the occluded veins and sinus, and the thrombus. Sometimes, when CT is used (which cannot be recommended when MRI is feasible), a hyperdense fresh thrombus in the occluded sinus can be seen, referred to as the 'cord or dense sign'. Another sign is the 'dense delta' which is a dense triangle (from hyperdense thrombus) within the superior longitudinal sinus.

Treatment

Heparin therapy

Available treatment data from controlled trials favour the use of heparin in CVST because it can reduce the risk of fatal outcome and severe disability without promoting ICH [60, 61]. A meta-analysis of two randomized trials showed that anticoagulation led to an absolute risk reduction in death or dependency by 13% (CI −30 to +3%) with a relative risk reduction of 54% [62]. Although this difference is not statistically significant, both trials show a consistent trend in favour of heparin without causing a higher risk for ICH.

According to European guidelines [63], CVST should be treated either with bodyweight-adjusted subcutaneous LMWH or dose-adjusted intravenous heparin with an at least doubled activated partial thromboplastin time. Concomitant ICH related to CVST is not a contraindication for heparin therapy [63].

Thrombolytic therapy

There is no evidence from randomized controlled trials regarding the efficacy and safety of either systemic or local thrombolytic therapy in CVST patients. However, from uncontrolled series, positive effects have been reported when local thrombolytic therapy for CVST is used [64–67]. Additionally, a recently published systematic review on thrombolytic use in CVST suggests a benefit in comatose cases [68].

According to European guidelines [63], there is insufficient evidence to support the use of either systemic or local thrombolysis in patients with CVST. If patients deteriorate despite adequate anticoagulation and when other causes of deterioration have been ruled out, thrombolysis may be a therapeutic option in selected cases, possibly in those without ICH. The optimal substance (urokinase or rtPA), dosage, route (systemic or local), or method of administration (repeated bolus or bolus plus infusion) are not known.

Oral anticoagulation

After the acute phase, therapy is switched-over to oral anticoagulation. The INR target is 2.0–3.0. If CVST occurs during pregnancy, oral anticoagulation should be avoided because of its possible teratogenic effect and ability to pass the placenta. In these cases anticoagulation should be continued with heparin. Controlled data regarding the benefit and optimal duration of oral anticoagulation in patients with CVST are not available. An MRI follow-up study of 33 patients reported that recanalization occurred within the first 4 months after CVST irrespective of further anticoagulation [69].

According to European guidelines [63], anticoagulation may be given for 3 months if CVST was secondary to a transient risk factor, and for 6–12 months in patients with idiopathic CVST and in those with 'mild' hereditary thrombophilia. Indefinite anticoagulation should be considered in patients with two or more episodes of CVST and in those with one episode of CVST and 'severe' hereditary thrombophilia.

Symptomatic therapy

The prophylactic use of antiepileptic drugs is controversial. Two studies have identified focal sensory and motor deficits, the presence of parenchymal lesions and intracranial haemorrhage on admission CT/MRI, and cortical vein thrombosis as being independent predictors for early symptomatic seizures [70, 71]. According to European guidelines

[63], preventive antiepileptic drugs may be a therapeutical option in patients with focal neurological deficits and focal parenchymal lesion. Treatment could be maintained for 1 year.

Although brain swelling occurs in about 50% of CVST patients, minor brain oedema only needs heparin to restore venous outflow [72, 73]. In patients with isolated intracranial hypertension and threatened vision, a lumbar puncture with sufficient CSF removal should be done before starting heparin. There are no controlled data, but acetazolamide may be effective in persistent papilloedema. Steroids are not recommended for treatment of intracranial hypertension, because of their unproven efficacy. In severe cases with threatening transtentorial brain herniation, due to a unilateral large haemorrhagic infarct, decompressive surgery is reported to be the sole live-saving option [74].

Stroke occurring after cardiac surgery

Specificities

More than 800 000 patients undergo coronary artery bypass graft (CABG) surgery worldwide annually [75]. The incidence of stroke occurs in approximately 2% of post-CABG patients, with higher reported rates after valve replacement or other cardiac surgical procedures [76, 77]. Causes of stroke after cardiac surgery include perioperative heart or aortic arch embolism, systemic hypoperfusion, large-vessel occlusive disease induced ischaemia, or a combination of these [78–80]. One study identified risk factors for stroke after cardiac surgery as increasing age, history of previous stroke, hypertension, diabetes mellitus, and the presence of carotid bruit [81], while another identified history of stroke and hypertension, older age, systolic hypertension, bronchodilator and diuretic use, high serum creatinine, surgical priority, great vessel repair, use of inotropic agents after cardiopulmonary bypass, and total cardiopulmonary bypass time ($p < 0.05$ for all comparisons) [82].

Treatment

At present, specific recommendations for CABG perioperative stroke do not exist. [83]. Even so, CABG stroke patients are treated like acute stroke patients with a loading dose of aspirin (160–325 mg) [83].

Stroke occurring after carotid surgery

Carotid endarterectomy (CEA) became the standard method for treating symptomatic carotid stenosis upon the publication of large randomized trials [84]. It is recommended for patients with 70–99% symptomatic stenosis. Although trials for asymptomatic carotid stenosis have shown that surgery reduces the incidence of ipsilateral stroke the absolute benefit is small [85], provided the perioperative stroke or death rate is 3%. The outcome comparison of any stroke or death within 30 days of treatment compared to stenting favoured surgery (fixed-effects OR 1.35). Thus, presently, stenting is not recommended for carotid revascularization.

The pathophysiological mechanism causing stroke during carotid revascularization can be due to haemodynamic cerebral ischaemia or to artery–artery embolism. This latter mechanism seems to be more frequent during stenting because of its intravascular approach.

Stroke occurring at the acute stage of coronary syndromes

Specificities

ICH is a serious side effect of thrombolytic use in ACS. The risk of ICH is dependent on previous episode of ICH, age, and the thrombolytic regimen that is being used. In general, the risk of ICH due to thrombolytic use for the treatment of an acute MI is between 0.5 and 1 %. The other condition that could occur during ACS could be ischaemic stroke due to reduced cardiac output or embolic complications.

Treatment

The treatment of ICH complications is described under specific management of ICH. There are no specific indications from guidelines for treatment of ischaemic stroke during ACS. In the presence of an ACS, the European Stroke Organization guidelines recommend lowering blood pressure [6]. Anticoagulation is not recommended, while a combination therapy of clopidogrel and aspirin is recommended for cardiac reasons [6].

Stroke occurring in patients with atrial fibrillation

Specificities

Heart embolisms account for at least 20% of ischaemic strokes of which nonvalvular atrial fibrillation (AF) is the most common cause, associated with a fivefold increased risk of stroke, and constitutes around 25% of strokes in patients older than 80 years [86, 87]. Long-term antithrombotic prophylaxis is essential for the prevention of stroke in

AF patients. Clinical trials of stroke prevention in AF have demonstrated the benefit of warfarin; risk reduction of 66% and mortality reduction of 26% with an acceptable risk of bleeding [88], while aspirin (325 mg/day), reduces the rate of stroke by 26% and mortality by 10% [89]. Recently, patients with AF for whom vitamin K antagonist therapy was unsuitable were studied and it was seen that clopidogrel plus aspirin reduced the risk of major vascular events, especially stroke, and increased the risk of ICH [90]. Oral direct thrombin inhibitors, such as dabigatran which has been recently shown to be associated with lower rates of stroke and systemic embolism while having similar rates of ICH compared to warfarin [91].

Stroke in patients with AF can be divided into three groups:

◆ Ischaemic stroke in patients who are not properly treated, i.e. who are not receiving oral anticoagulation despite a CHADS2 score of 2 or more [92].

◆ Ischaemic stroke occurring despite an adequate treatment with warfarin.

◆ ICH occurring in patients with anticoagulation. The reported incidence of ICH is 7- to 10-fold higher than in patients who are not receiving oral anticoagulation, and is as high as 1.8% per year in stroke risk patients [93].

Treatment

In the acute stroke phase heparin is not recommended: it is associated with a nonsignificant in recurrence reduction, no substantial reduction in death and disability, and an increased incidence of ICH [94].

Cardiac changes secondary to stroke ('neurocardiology')

Cardiac arrhythmias, particularly AF, are relatively common after stroke and heart failure, while MI and sudden death are also recognized complications, especially in insular strokes [95]. Sometimes stroke patients show raised blood troponin levels indicative of cardiac damage.

Personal perspective

Stroke is a heterogeneous disorder that can be prevented and is treatable provided patients reach hospital shortly after symptom onset. All stroke patients benefit from general stroke management provided in stroke units. Depending on the mechanism (ischaemic or haemorrhagic) and other factors (underlying cause, pre-existing state, coexisting therapies, etc.) more specific treatments are sometimes necessary, such as thrombolytic therapy or preventive decompressive surgery. An appropriate diagnosis of stroke, of its nature and of its cause, are needed in emergency to provide the most appropriate therapeutic strategy. Stroke unit care has allowed the development of effective evidence-based specific treatments and has contributed to the overall decline in stroke mortality in Western countries.

Further reading

Adams HP Jr, Bendixen BH, et al. Classification of subtype of acute ischemic stroke. Definitions for use in a multicenter clinical trial. TOAST. Trial of Org 10172 in Acute Stroke Treatment. *Stroke* 1993;**24**(1):35–41.

Cordonnier C, Leys D. Stroke: the bare essentials. *Pract Neurol* 2008;**8**(4):263–272.

European Stroke Organization Working Group. Guidelines for management of ischaemic stroke and transient ischaemic attack 2008. *Cerebrovasc Dis* 2008;**25**(5):457–507.

Georgiadis D, Schwab S. Hypothermia in acute stroke. *Curr Treat Options Neurol* 2005;**7**:119–127.

Hacke W, Brott T, et al. Thrombolysis in acute ischemic stroke: controlled trials and clinical experience. *Neurology* 1999;**53**(7): S3–14.

Hacke W, Kaste M, et al. Thrombolysis with alteplase 3 to 4.5 hours after acute ischemic stroke. *N Engl J Med* 2008;**359**(13):1317–1329.

Hankey GJ, Warlow CP. Treatment and secondary prevention of stroke: evidence, costs, and effects on individuals and populations. *Lancet* 1999;**354**(9188):1457–1463.

Rothwell PM, Coull AJ, et al. Change in stroke incidence, mortality, case-fatality, severity, and risk factors in Oxfordshire, UK from 1981 to 2004 (Oxford Vascular Study). *Lancet* 2004;**363**(9425):1925–1933.

Steiner T, Kaste M, et al. Recommendations for the management of intracranial haemorrhage—part I: spontaneous intracerebral haemorrhage. The European Stroke Initiative Writing Committee and the Writing Committee for the EUSI Executive Committee. *Cerebrovasc Dis* 2006;**22**(4):294–316.

Vahedi K, Hofmeijer J, et al. Early decompressive surgery in malignant infarction of the middle cerebral artery: a pooled analysis of three randomised controlled trials. *Lancet Neurol* 2007;**6**(3): 215–222.

Warlow C, van Gijn J, Dennis M, *et al. Stroke: practical management*, 3rd edition, Blackwell Science, 2008.

Training in use of the NIH Stroke Scale. http://www.ninds.nih.gov/doctors/NIH_Stroke_Scale.pdf

Online resources

National Institute of Health (NIH) Stroke Scale .http://www.strokecenter.org/trials/scales/nihss.html

➲ For additional multimedia materials please visit the online version of the book (🔗 http://www.esciacc.oxfordmedicine.com).

CHAPTER 66

Acute kidney injury

Sean M. Bagshaw, John Prowle,
and Rinaldo Bellomo

Contents

Summary

Acute kidney injury (AKI) is serious complication of critical illness in general and a major complication of acute decompensated heart failure (ADHF), acute coronary syndromes (ACS), cardiac surgery, and radiocontrast administration in particular. New consensus definitions of this syndrome have enabled a more detailed understanding of its epidemiology. Some degree of AKI is seen in up to 60% of critically ill patients, depending on the characteristics of the population of critically ill patients being studied, and its development is independently associated with an increased risk of death. Its pathogenesis is complex and probably changes according to the aetiology of the underlying condition. However, in most conditions, it is likely that neurohumoral factors, haemodynamic factors, and immunological/inflammatory processes all play important roles in its development. Prevention of AKI requires attention to general patient care, prompt resuscitation, avoidance of excessive fluid administration, maintenance of an adequate cardiac output, maintenance of an adequate mean arterial pressure, avoidance of a markedly raised right atrial pressure, avoidance of intravascular volume depletion, maintenance of an adequate haemoglobin, and avoidance of nephrotoxins. No pharmacological agents have been shown to be consistently effective as preventive agents. If AKI is severe enough to require the application of renal replacement therapy, several dialytic techniques are now available to support patients to recovery, if the primary disease can be effectively treated. Worldwide, continuous renal replacement therapy (CRRT) is now more commonly used than intermittent dialysis, while peritoneal dialysis is all but absent from the treatment of adult patients with severe AKI. The advantages of CRRT (gentle and steady fluid removal, haemodynamic stability, steady acid–base control) are particularly important in critically ill patients and in patients with myocardial dysfunction. However, no sufficiently powered studies have yet demonstrated that one technique is superior to another in terms of outcome. Once AKI has become severe enough to require CRRT, no pharmacological agents have been consistently shown to accelerate recovery. The prognosis of AKI requiring renal replacement therapy remains unfavourable in up to 50% of patients, mostly because of the underlying disease.

Introduction

Acute kidney injury (AKI), formerly called acute renal failure, remains a major diagnostic and therapeutic challenge for the cardiologist, the nephrologist, and the critical care physician. The term AKI describes a syndrome characterized by a rapid (hours to days) decrease in the kidney's ability to eliminate waste products. Such loss of function is clinically manifested by the accumulation of end products of nitrogen metabolism such as urea and creatinine. Other typical clinical manifestations include decreased urine output (not always present), accumulation of nonvolatile acids, and an increased concentration of potassium and phosphate.

Definition of acute kidney injury

The primary functions of the kidney are to eliminate water-soluble waste products of metabolism and other potentially toxic substances (e.g. drugs), control fluid and electrolyte balance, maintain acid–base homeostasis, help control blood pressure, modulate erythropoiesis, help maintain calcium and phosphate homeostasis, and, in part, participate in the excretion of small proteins that participate in immune function (cytokines and β_2-microglobulin). AKI is a rapid (over hours to days) (and usually reversible) failure of the kidneys to perform its many functions and, in particular, to excrete nitrogenous and other waste products causing loss of detoxification homeostasis and retention of toxins within the body. Depending on the criteria used to define its presence, AKI has been reported in up to 60% or more of critically ill patients with most reports showing an incidence around 30–40% in large case series [1–5]. Recently a consensus definition and classification for AKI has been developed and validated in hospitalized and critically ill patients [6–8]. This definition, which goes by the acronym of RIFLE, divides renal dysfunction across a continuum of severity from Risk to Injury and Failure (➲Fig. 66.1) and is likely to be a major approach to defining AKI in intensive care units (ICU) for the next 5–10 years. Using this classification, the incidence of at least some degree of renal dysfunction has been reported as high as 67% in a recent study of more than 5000 critically ill patients [8]. The development of renal dysfunction with a maximum RIFLE category of Failure has been reported in up to 28% of critically ill patients and is associated with a several-fold increased risk of in-hospital death [7, 8].

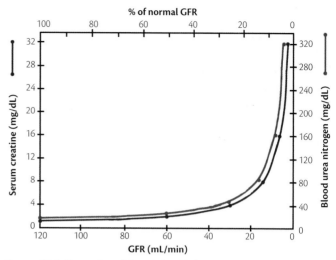

Figure 66.1 Illustration of the relationship between serum creatinine and urea and glomerular filtration rate (GFR). Both of these biomarkers do not increase until more than 50% of GFR is lost.

Epidemiology

The occurrence of AKI is dependent on its definition. However, a degree of AKI (manifested by either release of neutrophil gelatinase associated lipocalin (NGAL), albuminuria, or loss of small tubular proteins, or inability to excrete a water load or a sodium load or amino acid load or any combination of the above) can be demonstrated in most ICU patients.

The syndrome of AKI occurs in 5–8% of all hospitalized patients [9, 10]. The incidence is even greater in ICU patients depending on the operative definition and specific populations (where sepsis and multiorgan failure occur) being studied [1–5].

Several risk factors for AKI in ICU patients have been identified including older age, male sex, pre-existing comorbid illness (e.g. diabetes, hypertension, cardiac failure, chronic liver disease), a diagnosis of sepsis, major surgery (specifically cardiac surgery), cardiogenic shock, hypovolaemia, and exposure to nephrotoxic drugs [1, 4]. In addition, multiorgan dysfunction, specifically concomitant acute circulatory, pulmonary, and hepatic organ dysfunction, is commonly associated with AKI [2, 11].

Assessment of kidney function

Kidney function is complex. In the clinical context, however, monitoring of kidney function is reduced to the indirect assessment of glomerular filtration rate (GFR) by the measurement of serum creatinine and urea. These waste products are insensitive markers of GFR and are heavily modified by numerous factors. Furthermore, they become abnormal only when GFR is reduced by generally more than 50% (➜ Fig. 66.1), fail to reflect dynamic changes in GFR, and can be grossly modified by aggressive fluid resuscitation. The use of creatinine clearance or the calculation of estimated GFR might increase the accuracy of biochemical assessment, but has not been validated in the acute setting and rarely changes clinical management.

Urine output is another commonly measured parameter of renal function but it is often more sensitive to changes in renal haemodynamics than GFR and patients can develop severe AKI while maintaining normal urine output (so-called nonoliguric AKI). Since nonoliguric AKI has a lower mortality rate than oliguric AKI, urine output is frequently used to differentiate AKI [9]. The recent RIFLE classification has incorporated oliguria as an important measure for categories of severity of AKI (➜ Fig. 66.2).

Aetiology and clinical classification

The most practically useful approach to the aetiological diagnosis of AKI is to divide its causes according to the probable source of renal injury: prerenal, renal (parenchymal), and postrenal.

Prerenal acute kidney injury

This form of AKI is by far the most common in the ICU. The term indicates that the kidney malfunctions predominantly because of systemic factors that decrease GFR, such as decreased cardiac output, hypotension (➜ Fig. 66.3), or raised intra-abdominal pressure. If the systemic cause of AKI is rapidly removed or corrected, renal function improves and relatively rapidly returns to near normal levels. However, if intervention is delayed or unsuccessful, AKI becomes established and several days or weeks are then necessary for recovery. Several tests (measurement of urinary sodium, fractional excretion of sodium, and other derived indices) have been promoted to help clinicians identify the development of such 'established' AKI and differentiate it from so-called prerenal uraemia, which can be reversed over a few days. Unfortunately, their accuracy and significance is questionable [13, 14]. In particular, the clinical value of these tests in ICU patients, coronary care patients, or patients after cardiac surgery who receive vasopressors, massive fluid resuscitation, and loop diuretics is low. Furthermore, it is important to observe that prerenal AKI/prerenal uraemia and established AKI are part of a continuum, and their separation has limited clinical implications. The principles of management are essentially the same: treatment of the cause while promptly resuscitating the patient using invasive haemodynamic monitoring to guide therapy.

Parenchymal acute kidney injury

This term is used to define a syndrome where the principal source of damage is within the kidney and where typical

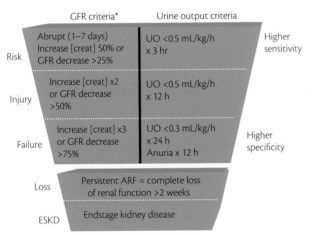

Figure 66.2 Risk Injury Failure Loss Endstage (RIFLE) classification scheme for acute renal failure. The classification system includes separate criteria for creatinine and urine output. The criteria, which lead to the worst possible classification should be used. Note that RIFLE-F (F = failure) is present even if the increase in serum creatinine concentration (S_{Creat}) is less than threefold so long as the new S_{Creat} is more than 4.0 mg/dL (350 μmol/L) in the setting of an acute increase of at least 0.5 mg/dL (44 μmol/L). The designation RIFLE-FC should be used in this case to denote 'acute-on-chronic' disease. Similarly, when RIFLE-F classification is reached by urine output criteria only, a designation of RIFLE-FO should be used to denote oliguria. The shape of the figure denotes the fact that more patients (high sensitivity) will be included in the mild category, including some without actually having 'renal failure' (less specificity). In contrast, at the bottom, the criteria are strict and therefore specific, but some patients with renal dysfunction might be missed. AKI, acute kidney injury; ARF, acute renal failure; GFR, glomerular filtration rate; UO, urine output.
* GFR estimated using the modification of diet in renal disease (MDRD) equation.

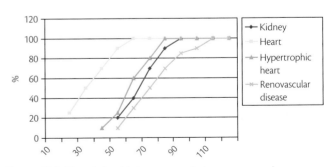

Figure 66.3 The relationship between perfusion pressure and organ blood flow. The kidney is uniquely sensitive to pressure, more than the heart. Renal perfusion pressure (RPP) equals mean arterial pressure (MAP) minus tissue pressure. Renal blood flow begins to fall at mean arterial pressures less than 80 mmHg. If there is significant renovascular disease, such decreases in blood flow begin at higher levels of pressure

---

Box 66.1 Causes of parenchymal acute kidney injury

- Glomerulonephritis
- Vasculitis
- Renovascular
- Cholesterol emboli
- Interstitial nephritis
- Nephrotoxins
- Tubular deposition/obstruction
- Renal allograft rejections
- Trauma
- Haemolytic–uraemic syndrome
- Thrombotic thrombocytopenic purpura

---

structural changes can be seen on microscopy. Numerous disorders that affect the glomerulus or the tubule may be responsible (◗ Box 66.1). Among these, nephrotoxins are particularly important, especially in hospitalized patients [10]. The most common nephrotoxic drugs affecting ICU patients are listed in ◗ Box 66.2.

More than one-third of patients who develop AKI in the ICU have chronic renal dysfunction due to factors such as age-related changes, long-standing hypertension, diabetes

---

Box 66.2 Drugs that may cause acute kidney injury in the critically ill

- Radiocontrast media
- Aminoglycosides
- Amphotericin
- Nonsteroidal anti-inflammatory drugs
- β-Lactam antibiotics (interstitial nephropathy)
- Sulphonamides
- Aciclovir
- Methotrexate
- Cisplatin
- Ciclosporin A
- Tacrolimus (FK-506)
- Sirolimus
- Mannitol
- Glycopeptides

---

mellitus, or atheromatous disease of the renal vessels. Such chronic renal disease may be manifest by a raised serum creatinine, but this is not always the case. Often, what may seem to the clinician to be a relatively trivial insult, which does not fully explain the onset of AKI in a normal patient, is sufficient to unmask lack of renal functional reserve in those patients with chronic renal disease.

Postrenal acute kidney injury

Obstruction to urine outflow is the most common cause of functional renal impairment in the community [15], but is uncommon in the ICU or coronary care unit (CCU). The clinical presentation of obstruction may be acute or acute-on-chronic in patients with long-standing renal calculi. It may not always be associated with oliguria. If obstruction is suspected, ultrasonography can be easily performed at the bedside. However, not all cases of acute obstruction have an abnormal ultrasound and, in many cases, obstruction occurs in conjunction with other renal insults (e.g. stag-horn calculi and severe sepsis of renal origin). Assessment of the role of each factor and overall management should be conducted in conjunction with a urologist. Finally, the sudden and unexpected development of anuria in an ICU patient should always suggest obstruction of the urinary catheter as the cause.

Major specific syndromes

Hepatorenal syndrome

This condition is a form of AKI, which typically occurs in the setting of severe liver dysfunction [16]. It can occur rapidly and be severe (type I) or slowly and be moderate in severity (type II). Several potential mechanisms that may contribute to hepatorenal syndrome (HRS) [16, 17]. While HRS can occur spontaneously in patients with advanced cirrhosis, it is important to recognize that other precipitants are much more common. These include sepsis, specifically spontaneous bacterial peritonitis (SBP), raised intra-abdominal pressure due to tense ascites, gastrointestinal bleeding, and hypovolaemia due to paracentesis, diuretics, and/or lactulose, or any combination of these factors. Likewise, other contributing factors to AKI should be routinely assessed for including cardiomyopathy due to alcoholism, nutritional deficiencies, viral infection, or exposure to nephrotoxins.

Typically, HRS develops in patients with advanced cirrhosis and evidence of portal hypertension with ascites in the absence of other apparent causes of AKI. It generally presents as oligoanuria with progressive increases in serum creatinine and/or urea and bland urinary sediment. These patients develop profound sodium and water retention with evidence of hyponatraemia, a urine osmolality higher than that of plasma, and a very low urinary sodium concentration (<10 mmol/L).

The principles of management are the same as in other causes of AKI (see below). Specifically, however, albumin administration in patients with SBP has been shown to decrease the incidence of AKI in a randomized controlled trial [18] and vasopressin derivatives (terlipressin) may improve GFR in this condition [19, 20]. The life expectancy of patients with this syndrome is measured in months. Successful liver transplantation is the only viable therapy to improve long-term prognosis.

Rhabdomyolysis-associated acute kidney injury

The incidence of rhabdomyolysis-induced AKI is estimated at 1% in hospitalized patients but it may account for close to 5–7% of cases of AKI in critically ill patients depending on the setting [10, 23]. Its pathogenesis involves the interplay of prerenal, renal, and postrenal factors [24]. The causes of rhabdomyolysis are listed in ➲ Box 66.3.

The clinical manifestations include an elevated serum creatine kinase, evidence of pigmented granular casts, and red to brown colouring of the urine. Patients can also have various electrolyte disorders as a result of muscle breakdown including hyperphosphataemia, hyperkalaemia, hypocalcaemia, and hyperuricaemia.

Box 66.3 Causes of rhabdomyolysis

- Major trauma
- Drug overdose (i.e. narcotics, cocaine, or other stimulants)
- Vascular embolism
- Prolonged seizures
- Malignant hyperthermia
- Neuroleptic malignant syndrome
- Infections (i.e. pyomyositis, necrotizing fasciitis, influenza, HIV)
- Severe exertion
- Alcoholism
- Agents that can interact to induce major muscle injury (i.e. combination of macrolide antibiotics or ciclosporin and statins).

Treatment includes prompt and aggressive fluid resuscitation, maintenance of polyuria, and urine alkalinization in order to reduce the renal toxicity of myoglobin [24].

Drug-induced acute kidney injury

Particular drugs (see ➲ Box 66.2) can often invoke a variety of pathophysiological effects on the kidney that collectively contribute to AKI [25–28]. Radiocontrast media and aminoglycosides are leading agents contributing to nephrotoxin-induced AKI [29, 30]. In cardiology and cardiac surgery patients, radiocontrast-induced renal injury is particularly important [10]. It presents with an acute rise in serum creatinine within 24–48 h following injection of radiocontrast media. The serum creatinine level generally peaks within 3–5 days and returns towards baseline within 7–10 days; however, in some patients kidney function may not return to baseline and a persistent reduction in function may occur.

Radiocontrast nephropathy is often associated with pre-existing risk factors, in particular pre-existing chronic kidney disease (GFR <60 mL min^{-1} 1.73 m^{-2}) and a diagnosis of diabetes mellitus [10].

There are few effective prophylactic or therapeutic interventions [31]. Strategies for prevention include early identification of patients at risk, consideration of delay of the investigation, or using alternative modality until kidney function can be optimized. Likewise, every effort should be made correct volume depletion and discontinue potential nephrotoxins. There is no evidence to support the routine use of diuretics, mannitol, or dopamine. Periprocedure hydration and use of nonionic iso-osmolar (i.e. iodixanol) radiocontrast media can reduce the risk [32–35]. Several randomized trials and meta-analyses have suggested potential benefit with use of *N*-acetylcysteine [36, 37] (➲ Fig. 66.4). Considering that these preventive measures have minimal risk, their use should be considered whenever a patient is scheduled for the administration of intravenous radiocontrast media.

Sepsis-associated acute kidney injury

Sepsis is a leading predisposing factor to AKI in critically ill patients [4] Epidemiological studies estimate between 45–70% of all AKI encountered in the ICU is associated with sepsis [1, 4, 23] Septic AKI may be characterized by a unique pathophysiology [38–48] which involves systemic and local neurohormonal changes, toxic and immune-mediated mechanisms (cytokines, arachidonic acid metabolites, and thrombogenic agents), and renal tubular cell apoptosis in response to inflammatory mediators in

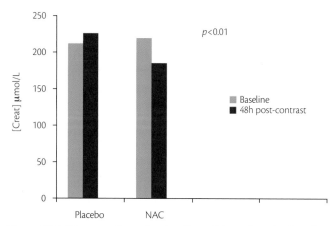

Figure 66.4 Histogram illustrating the effect of *N*-acteylcysteine (NAC) on renal function compared to placebo after exposure to radiocontrast in a recent randomized controlled trial. There appears to be a moderate protective effect.

endotoxaemia [45, 47–50] (for more detail see 📇 66.1) No studies exist to tell us which of the above mechanisms are most important and when they might be active in the course of an episode of septic AKI. However, interventions with antiapoptotic properties, such as intensive insulin therapy, human recombinant activated protein C, or selective caspase inhibitors, may aid in attenuating renal injury and promote recovery of function [46]. To date, however, no human randomized controlled trials have assessed the impact of these interventions on kidney function and their value is unknown.

Major surgery-associated acute kidney injury

AKI is a common complication following major surgery [4] The incidence is variable and dependent on the prevalence of pre-existing comorbid illnesses, preoperative kidney function, and the type and urgency of surgery being performed. Numerous intraoperative events can act to negatively affect kidney function including haemodynamic instability (i.e. intravenous or inhaled anaesthetic agents), hypovolaemia due to blood loss or third spacing, details of operative field (i.e. aortic cross-clamping in major vascular surgery), increases in intra-abdominal pressure (i.e. laparoscopic insufflation of CO_2), concomitant sepsis, and use of nephrotoxic drugs. Any of these factors, alone or in combination, may contribute to critical reductions in renal blood flow (RBF) and ischaemia, impaired oxygen delivery, and toxin or inflammatory-mediated injury. Postoperative AKI is believed to be mediated in part by proinflammatory mechanisms such as increased endothelial cell adhesion, tubular cell infiltration, generation of reactive oxygen species, proinflammatory cytokines, and reperfusion injury [51, 52].

Cardiorenal syndromes

Recently, there has been growing interest in the clinical importance of syndromes which reflect the simultaneous consequences and interactions of heart and kidney failure. These syndromes have been classified under the term of cardiorenal syndromes (CRS) [53]. Among such syndromes, two are particularly relevant to AKI (➲ Fig. 66.5).

Acute cardiorenal syndrome (type 1)

This syndrome is characterized by an initial abrupt change in cardiovascular function that leads to AKI. The common clinical scenarios include acutely decompensated heart failure (ADHF) and acute coronary syndromes (ACS) [54–60]. The incidence of AKI associated with ADHF and ACS ranges between 24–45% and 9–19% respectively, and is associated with greater mortality and morbidity [61–65]. Venous congestion seems to be an important haemodynamic factor driving AKI in ADHF [66]. In the setting of ACS and developing cardiogenic shock, the risk of acute CRS (type 1) is high and can be only partially managed with prompt revascularization and haemodynamic support with inotropic agents, vasopressors, and intra-aortic balloon counterpulsation (IABP).

Acute renocardiac syndrome (type 3)

This syndrome is characterized by AKI that leads to cardiac failure in susceptible patients, most of whom probably have underlying subclinical heart disease. The clinical problem in many cases is sodium and water retention. In this setting, prompt aggressive avoidance of hypervolaemia prevents cardiac decompensation. Prototypical scenarios for acute renocardiac syndrome type 3 include contrast-induced AKI, AKI after bypass or other major surgery, and other less common forms of isolated AKI (e.g. rapidly progressive glomerulonephritis) that secondarily lead to left ventricular dysfunction.

Acute kidney injury associated with cardiac surgery

Acute renal injury associated with cardiac surgery (CSA-AKI) (➲ Fig. 66.6) is common. CSA-AKI carries a mortality of between 40–70% in cases requiring artificial renal support [67–70]. AKI after cardiac surgery is multifactorial in aetiology and pathogenesis [70–72].

Haemodynamic management to maintain adequate perfusion should be routinely applied to all CSA patients and close monitoring should continue in all patients at risk of CSA-AKI. Furthermore, if possible, nephrotoxic agents

Syndromes	Acute cardiorenal (Type 1)	Acute renocardiac (type 3)
Organ failure sequence	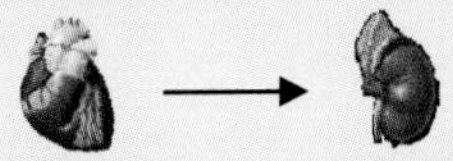 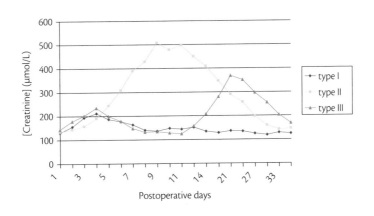	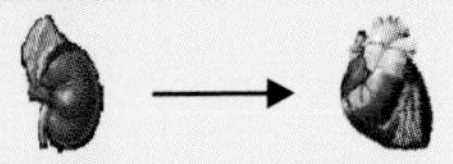
Definition	acute worsening of heart function leading to kidney injury and/or dysfunction	Acute worsening of kidney function leading to heart injury and/or dysfunction
Primary events	ADHF ACS Cardiogenic shock	AKI
Criteria for primary events	ESC, AHA/ACC	RIFLE -AKIN
Secondary events	AKI	ADHF, ACS, arrythmias, shock
Criteria for secondary events	RIFLE -AKIN	ESC, AHA/ACC
Cardiac biomarkers	Troponin, BNP, MPO	BNP, CRP
Renal biomarkers	Serum cystatin, creatinine, NGAL. Urinary KIM-1, IL-18, NGAL, NAG	Serum cystatin, creatinine, NGAL. Urinary KIM-1, IL-18, NGAL, NAG
Pathophysiology	ADHF and ACS are most common scenarios. Inciting event may be acute coronary ischemia, poorly controlled blood pressure, and noncompliance with medication and dietary sodium intake.	Acute sodium and volume overload are part of the pathogenesis. Volume control may be a very important aspect of cardiac protection
Management strategies	Specific—depends on precipitating factors General supportive—oxygenate, relieve pain and pulmonary congestion, treat arrhythmias appropriately, differentiate left from right heart failure, treat low cardiac output, avoid nephrotoxins, closely monitor kidney function	Follow ESC guidelines for acute CHF. Management may depend on underlying etiology, may need to exclude renovascular disease and consider early renal support, if patient is diuretic resistant

Figure 66.5 Summary of the major characteristics of two acute cardiorenal syndromes relevant to acute kidney injury. ACS, acute coronary syndrome; ADHF, acute decompensated heart failure; AKI, acute kidney injury; BNP, brain-type natriuretic peptide; CHF, congestive heart failure; CRP, C-reactive protein; MPO<,myeloperoxidase; NAC, N-acteylcysteine, NGAL, neutrophil gelatinase associated lipocalin.

should be avoided. Renal replacement therapy (RRT) plays an important supportive role for the patient. Although early initiation of RRT may be associated with better outcomes, no specific recommendations can be made on the dosing of therapy. Treatment of CSA-AKI should therefore be individualised to the clinical status of the patient.

Figure 66.6 Three types of renal impairment syndromes seen after cardiac surgery, with an illustration of their natural time course.

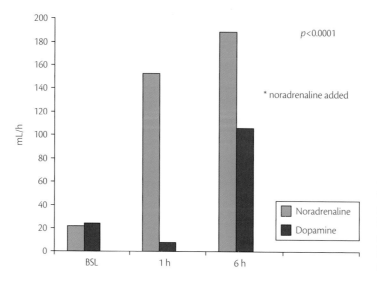

Figure 66.7 Comparison of the effect of noradrenaline (norepinephrine) infusion with high-dose dopamine infusion on urinary output in patients with hypotensive vasodilatory septic shock.

Prevention and treatment of acute kidney injury

The most common clinical picture seen in the ICU is that of a patient who has sustained or is experiencing a major systemic insult (i.e. trauma, sepsis, myocardial infarction, severe haemorrhage, cardiogenic shock, major surgery). When the patient arrives in the ICU, resuscitation is typically well under way or surgery may just have been completed. Despite such efforts, the patient is already anuric or profoundly oliguric, the serum creatinine is rising, and a metabolic acidosis is developing. Potassium and phosphate levels may be rapidly rising as well. Potassium levels can be rapidly lowered by the administration of intravenous glucose (50 mL of 50% glucose) with insulin (10 units) Accompanying multiple organ dysfunction (need for mechanical ventilation and vasoactive drugs) is common. Fluid resuscitation is typically undertaken under the guidance of invasive haemodynamic monitoring. Vasoactive drugs are often used to restore mean arterial pressure (MAP) to 'acceptable' levels (typically >65–70 mmHg) [73–75] (⊃ Fig. 66.7). The patient may improve over time and urine output may return with or without the assistance of diuretic agents. If urine output does not return, however, RRT must be considered. Slow recovery typically occurs, if the cause of AKI has been removed and the patient has become physiologically stable (from 4–5 days to 3–4 weeks). In some cases, urine output can be above normal for several days. If the cause of AKI has not been adequately remedied, the patient remains gravely ill, the kidneys do not recover, and death from multiorgan failure may occur.

The fundamental principles of AKI management are presented in ⊃ Box 66.4.

Resuscitation

Intravascular volume must be maintained or rapidly restored, and this is often best done using invasive haemodynamic monitoring (central venous catheter, arterial cannula, and pulmonary artery catheter or pulse contour cardiac output catheters in some cases). Oxygenation must be maintained. An adequate haemoglobin concentration (at least >70 g/L) must be maintained or immediately restored (see ⊃ Fig. 66.8). Once intravascular volume has been restored, some patients remain hypotensive (MAP <70 mmHg). In these patients, autoregulation of RBF may be lost. Restoration of MAP to near normal levels may increase GFR [73–75]. Such elevations in MAP, however, require

---

Box 66.4 Principles of management of acute kidney injury

- Identify cause and treat it
- Prompt fluid resuscitation
- Monitor adequacy of resuscitation by appropriate measures of intravascular filling depending on the severity of illness (physical examination, central venous pressure monitoring, cardiac output monitoring, echocardiography)
- Restore and/or maintain an adequate cardiac output
- Restore and/or maintain an adequate mean arterial pressure
- Remove or avoid nephrotoxins
- Rapidly start antibiotics if sepsis is suspected
- Consider relieving intra-abdominal pressure
- Exclude urinary tract obstruction

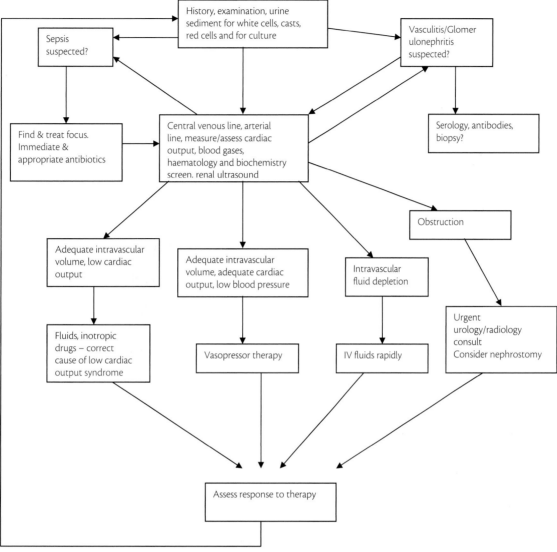

Figure 66.8 Diagnostic and treatment approach to an ICU patient presenting with acute kidney injury.

the addition of vasopressor drugs [73–75]. In patients with pre-existing hypertension or renovascular disease, a MAP of 75–80 mmHg may still be inadequate. The renal protective role of additional fluid therapy in a patient with a normal or increased cardiac output and blood pressure is questionable. Despite these resuscitation measures, renal failure may still develop if cardiac output is inadequate. This may require a variety of interventions from the use of inotropic drugs to the application of ventricular assist devices.

Fluid therapy

Fluid therapy is the cornerstone in the resuscitation of the critically ill patient. Fluid resuscitation is a primary strategy for preservation of kidney function in the setting of increases in serum creatinine and/or urea and oliguria. However, evolving evidence has suggested that overly aggressive fluid therapy has serious negative consequences for both renal and nonrenal organ function.

A large multicentre study found no significant difference in the incidence of AKI when comparing fluid resuscitation with crystalloid to albumin in critically ill patients [76] However, some synthetic colloid therapies (i.e. hydroxyethyl starches) have been associated with higher rates of AKI in critically ill patients after resuscitation for severe sepsis [77] The exact mechanism remains uncertain; however, the hydroxyethyl starches may influence intrarenal haemodynamics or glomerular filtration through alterations in vascular oncotic pressure.

In critically ill patients, once apparent optimization of haemodynamics and intravascular volume status has been achieved, there is little evidence to support continued aggressive fluid resuscitation to improve kidney function [78–80]. Rather, there is evidence from recent studies to suggest that such continued fluid administration and a positive cumulative balance can contribute to notable deteriorations in nonrenal organ function, in particular in oxygenation [65, 66]. The ARDS Clinical Trials Network has completed the largest randomized trial assessing fluid therapy in patients with lung injury [81]. This trial compared restrictive and liberal strategies for fluid management in 1000 critically ill patients, mostly with pneumonia or sepsis, and evidence of with acute lung injury. At 72 h those receiving a restrictive fluid strategy had a near neutral fluid balance, whereas those in the liberal strategy were positive by more than 5 L. Although the study failed to show a difference in mortality between the strategies, a restrictive strategy improved lung function, increased in ventilator-free days, and reduced ICU length of stay. Moreover, those in the restrictive group had a trend towards a reduced need for RRT.

Renal protective drugs

Following haemodynamic resuscitation and removal of nephrotoxins, it is unclear whether the use of additional pharmacological measures is of further benefit to the kidneys.

'Renal dose' or 'low-dose' dopamine

Evidence of the efficacy or safety of dopamine administration in critically ill patients is lacking. Furthermore, a recent large phase III trial in critically ill patients showed low-dose dopamine to be no better than placebo in the prevention of renal dysfunction [82].

Mannitol

A biological rationale exists for its use, as is the case for dopamine. However, no controlled human data exist to support its clinical use.

Loop diuretics

These agents may protect the loop of Henle from ischaemia by decreasing its transport-related workload. There are no double-blind randomized controlled studies of suitable size to prove that these agents reduce the incidence of renal failure. However, there are some studies supporting the view that loop diuretics may decrease the need for RRT in patients developing AKI [83]. They appear to achieve this by inducing polyuria, which allows for easier control of volume overload, acidosis, and hyperkalaemia, the three major triggers for RRT in the ICU. Because avoiding dialysis simplifies treatment and reduces cost of care, loop diuretics are occasionally used in patients with renal dysfunction, especially in the form of a continuous infusion.

Other agents

Other agents such as theophylline, urodilatin, anaritide (a synthetic atrial natriuretic factor), and fenoldopam have failed to show a consistently protective effect [84–87]. Many more investigations are urgently needed in this field.

Diagnostic investigations

An aetiological diagnosis of AKI must always be established. Investigations include microscopic examination of the urinary sediment. Urinalysis is a simple and noninvasive test that can yield important diagnostic information and patterns suggestive of specific syndromes. The finding of dysmorphic red blood cells (RBC) or RBC casts is virtually diagnostic of active glomerulonephritis or vasculitis. Heavy proteinuria suggests some form of glomerular disease. White blood cell casts can suggest either interstitial nephropathy or infection. Similarly, a normal urinalysis can provide important information and suggest that AKI is due to a prerenal or obstructive aetiology. Finally, examination of urine will provide evidence of whether a urinary tract infection is present.

In patients with a possible mechanism for muscle injury, creatine kinase and free myoglobin for possible rhabdomyolysis should be determined. If an elevated anion gap metabolic acidosis is present with suggestion of a toxic ingestion, ethylene glycol, methanol, and salicylates should be measured.

Measurements of specific autoantibodies or cryoglobulins are extremely useful screening tests to support the diagnosis of vasculitis or of certain types of collagen vascular diseases or glomerulonephritis. Imaging by renal ultrasonography is a rapid, noninvasive investigation principally designed to assess for evidence of obstruction, stones, cyst or mass, or overt renovascular disease. A chest radiograph may be important both to assess for pulmonary complications of AKI and if a diagnosis of systemic vasculitis is considered. In a few rare patients, a percutaneous renal biopsy becomes necessary [88].

Biomarkers of renal injury

An exciting development of the last decade in the field of AKI has been the identification and study of novel biomarkers for the early diagnosis of AKI [89–107].

- NGAL, a 25-kDa protein covalently bound to gelatinase from neutrophils, seems to be one of the earliest kidney markers of injury and may be detected in the blood and urine of humans within hours. A single measurement can differentiate those with AKI from other categories, with a sensitivity and specificity of 90% and 99% respectively.

◆ Cystatin C is a cysteine protease inhibitor that is synthesized and released into the blood at a relatively constant rate by all nucleated cells. It is freely filtered by the glomerulus, completely reabsorbed by the proximal tubule, and not secreted into urine. Its blood levels are not affected by age, gender, race, or muscle mass; thus it appears to be a better predictor of glomerular function than serum creatinine in patients with CKD.

◆ Kidney injury molecule 1 (KIM-1) is a protein detectable in the urine after ischaemic or nephrotoxic insults to proximal tubular cells. Urinary KIM-1 seems to be highly specific for ischaemic AKI and seems to represent an interesting additional marker for AKI adding specificity to the high sensitivity displayed by NGAL in the early phases of AKI.

◆ N-acetyl-β-(D)-glucosaminidase (NAG) is a lysosomal brush border enzyme found in proximal tubular cells. It is a relatively large molecule (>130 kDa), and is therefore not filtered through the glomerular membrane. NAG has been shown to function as a marker of AKI, reflecting particularly the degree of tubular damage.

◆ Interleukin-18 (IL-18) is a proinflammatory cytokine detected in the urine after acute ischaemic proximal tubular damage. It displays sensitivity and specificity for ischaemic AKI with an AUC greater than 90%, with increased levels 48 h prior to increase of serum creatinine.

Of the biomarkers listed above, NGAL (urine and plasma) and cystatin C are most likely to be integrated into clinical practice in the near future.

Management of established acute kidney injury

The principles of management of established AKI should always include confirmation of probable aetiology, elimination of potential contributors, institution of disease specific therapy if applicable, and prevention and management of the complications of AKI with maintenance of physiological homeostasis while recovery takes place. Complications such as encephalopathy, pericarditis, myopathy, or neuropathy should never occur in a modern ICU. Their prevention may include several measures, which vary in complexity from fluid restriction to the initiation of extracorporeal RRT.

Nutrition support must be started early and must contain adequate calories (25–35 kcal kg^{-1} day^{-1}) as a mixture of carbohydrates and lipids. Adequate protein (at least 1–2 g kg^{-1} day^{-1}) must be administered. Hyperkalaemia (>6 mmol/L) must be promptly treated either with insulin and dextrose administration, the infusion of bicarbonate if acidosis is present, the administration of nebulized salbutamol, or all of the above together. If the 'true' serum potassium is greater than 7 mmol/L or ECG signs of hyperkalaemia appear, calcium gluconate (10 mL of 10% solution IV) should also be administered. The above measures are temporizing actions while RRT is being arranged. The presence of hyperkalaemia is a major indication for the immediate institution of RRT.

Metabolic acidosis is almost always present but in itself rarely requires treatment. Anaemia requires correction to maintain a haemoglobin of at least 70 g/L. More aggressive transfusion needs individual patient assessment. Drug therapy must be adjusted to take into account the effect of the decreased clearances associated with loss of renal function.

Fluid overload can be prevented by the use of loop diuretics in polyuric patients. However, if the patient is oliguric, the only way to avoid fluid overload is to institute RRT at an early stage (see ◗ Chapter 28). Marked uraemia (urea >40 mmol/L or creatinine >400 μmol/L) is undesirable and should probably be treated with RRT unless recovery is imminent or already under way and a return toward normal values is expected within 24–48 h.

Renal replacement therapy

Issues relating to RRT are discussed in detail elsewhere (see ◗ Chapter 28). However, some aspects require discussion because of their direct relevance to therapeutic options in AKI. Many aspects of these therapies have been extensively reviewed [108–114].

In the critically ill patient, RRT should be initiated early, prior to the development of complications. A set of modern criteria for the initiation of RRT in the ICU is presented in ◗ Box 66.5. Once RRT is started with either intermittent haemodialysis (IHD) or CRRT, maintenance of homeostasis at all levels and better uremic control may translate into better survival. An appropriate target urea is at least under 20 mmol/L, with a protein intake of at least around 1.5g kg^{-1} day^{-1}. This can be easily achieved using CRRT at urea clearances of 30–40 L/day depending on patient size and catabolic rate. If IHD is used, daily treatment and extended treatment become desirable.

Box 66.5 Modern criteria for the initiation of renal replacement therapy in the intensive care unit

If one criterion is present, RRT should be considered. If two criteria are simultaneously present, RRT is strongly recommended.

- Anuria (no urine output for 6 h)
- Oliguria (urine output <200mL/12 h)
- [BUN] >75 mg/dL or urea >25 mmol/L
- [Creatinine] >3 mg/L or >265 µmol/L
- [K$^+$] >6.5 mmol/L or rapidly rising
- Pulmonary oedema unresponsive to diuretics
- Uncompensated metabolic acidosis (pH <7.1)
- Temperature >40° C
- Uraemic complications (encephalopathy/myopathy/neuropathy/pericarditis)
- Overdose with a dialysable toxin (e.g. lithium)

^{a} If one criterion is present, RRT should be considered. If two criteria are simultaneously present, RRT is strongly recommended.

Box 66.6 Strategies for circuit anticoagulation during continuous renal replacement therapy

- No anticoagulation
- Low-dose prefilter heparin (<5–8 IU kg^{-1} h^{-1})
- Medium-dose prefilter heparin (8–10 IU kg/h)
- Full anticoagulation with heparin (APTT 60–80 s)
- Regional heparin/protamine anticoagulation
- Regional citrate anticoagulation
- LMWH
- Prostacyclin
- Heparinoids
- Combination of prostacyclin with low-dose heparin

Using the above criteria, CRRT and slow low-efficiency daily dialysis (SLEDD) offer many advantages over peritoneal dialysis (PD) and conventional IHD (3–4 h/day, 3–4 times/week). However, in some settings, they may be more expensive. In order to make informed decisions, clinicians need to appreciate several technical and practical aspects of each approach to RRT (see ⊃ Chapter 28).

Continuous renal replacement therapy

CRRT is now typically performed with double-lumen catheters and peristaltic blood pumps in continuous venovenous haemofiltration (CVVH), haemodiafiltration (CVVHDF), or haemodialysis (CVVHD) mode.

Anticoagulants are frequently used during CRRT. However, the risks and benefits of more or less intense anticoagulation and alternative strategies (⊃ Box 66.6) must be considered.

In the vast majority of patients, low-dose heparin (5–10 IU kg^{-1} h^{-1}) is sufficient, and easy and cheap to administer with almost no effect on the patient's coagulation tests. In other cases (pulmonary embolism, myocardial ischaemia) full heparinization may be concomitantly indicated. Regional citrate anticoagulation is very effective but requires a special dialysate or replacement fluid and the monitoring of ionized calcium. Regional heparin/protamine anticoagulation is also somewhat complex but

may be useful in selected patients. Low-molecular-weight heparin must be used with caution as it may accumulate in AKI. Heparinoids or prostacyclin and citrate may be useful if the patient has developed heparin-induced thrombocytopenia and thrombosis. Finally, in some patients ant-coagulation is best avoided because of endogenous coagulopathy or recent surgery.

Continuous versus intermittent therapies

Continuous therapies are widely used for renal support. The broad use of continuous therapies is based on a satisfactory profile of haemodynamic safety, high capacity for solute and fluid removal, dynamic adjustment of parameters, rapid control of acid–base state, early start of nutrition support, and decreased of cerebral oedema. In particular, these therapies are highly suited to patients with acute heart failure or AKI after cardiac surgery because of their ability to deliver dialysis over 24 h with no haemodynamic instability. Whatever the choice of therapy, awareness of its effects on drug clearance is vital for safe patient treatment (⊃ Table 66.1). Finally the issue of dose of RRT has been extensively investigated in large multicentre trials and doses equivalent to approximately 25 mL kg^{-1} h^{-1} of effluent flow are now considered optimal [115–116].

The role of ultrafiltration

One of the most common conditions of patients with heart failure and CRS is reduced diuretic responsiveness. This diuretic resistance has resulted in the development of new technologies based on slow ultrafiltration. For example, slow ultrafiltration in patients with acute heart failure refractory to diuretics can remove up to remove 5 L without

Table 66.1 Drug dosage during renal replacement therapy[a]

Drug	CRRT[b]	IHD[c]
Gentamicin/tobramycin/amikacin	Normal dose every 36 h	50% normal dose every 48 h; 2/3 redose after IHD
Cefotaxime or Ceftazidime	1 g every 8–12 h	1 g every 12–24 h after IHD
Imipenem	500 mg every 8 h	250 mg every 8 h and after IHD
Meropenem	500 mg every 8 h	250 mg every 8 h and after IHD
Metronidazole	500 mg every 8h	250 mg every 8 h and after IHD
Co-trimoxazole	Normal dose every 18 h	Normal dose every 24 h after IHD
Amoxicillin/ampicillin	500 mg every 8 h	500 mg daily and after IHD
Vancomycin	1 g every 24 h	1 g every 96–120 h
Piperacillin (with or without sulbactam)	3–4 g every 6 h	3–4 g every 8 h and after IHD
Ticarcillin	1–2 g every 8 h	1–2 g every 12 h and after IHD
Ciprofloxacin	200 mg every 12 h	200 mg every 24 h and after IHD
Fluconazole	200 mg every 24 h	200 mg every 48 h and after IHD
Aciclovir	3.5 mg/kg every 24 h	2.5mg/kg per day and after IHD
Ganciclovir	5 mg/kg per day	5 mg/kg in 48 h and after IHD
Amphotericin B	Normal dose	Normal dose
Liposomal amphotericin	Normal dose	Normal dose
Ceftriaxone	Normal dose	Normal dose

CRRT, continuous renal replacement therapy; IHD, intermittent haemodialysis.

[a] The values in this table represent approximations and should be used as a general guide only. Critically ill patients have markedly abnormal volumes of distribution for these agents which will affect dosage. CRRT is conducted at variable levels of intensity in different units also requiring adjustment.

[b] The values reported here relate to CVVH at 2 L/h of ultrafiltration. Vancomycin is poorly removed by CVVHD.

[c] The values reported here relate to standard IHD with low-flux membranes for 3–4 h every second day.

haemodynamic instability. Oedema is thus reduced with an improvement in cardiac function, increased diuretic responsiveness, and haemodynamic stability. The advent of new technologies that allow peripheral venous access, exact volumetric control, avoidance of haemodynamic instability, and improved safety, have made ultrafiltration easier and more accessible in the CCU.

In this regard, the 'Relief for Acute fluid overload Patients with Decompensated CHF' (RAPID) trial [117] randomly assigned patients to either receive diuretic management or ultrafiltration for 8 h. Fluid removal during the first 24 h was higher in the ultrafiltration group (4.6 L vs 2.8 L) and occurred without renal functional deterioration or haemodynamic instability. In the larger UNLOAD trial [118], 200 patients were randomly assigned to receive either diuretic therapy or ultrafiltration. All patients with signs of fluid overload independent of the ejection fraction were included. The weight loss was greater in the ultrafiltration group (5.0±3.1 kg vs 3.1±3.5 kg). The requirement for inotropic support was also decreased in the ultrafiltration group (3% vs 12%). The 90-days follow-up showed a lower rehospitalization rate for heart failure in the ultrafiltration group (18% vs 32%), without renal functional deterioration.

Fluid removal is essential in treatment of symptomatic heart failure and diuretic resistance relatively common in CCU patients; opportunities for the use of slow ultrafiltration are therefore likely to increase. ⊃ Figures 66.9 and 66.10 show the changes in chest radiograph appearance in a patient presenting with CRS type 1 before and after ultrafiltration.

Prognosis

Acute renal failure can independently influence both short- and long-term prognosis. In hospitalized patients, mortality is estimated at 20% among all those developing AKI. The in-hospital mortality for critically ill patients with AKI is estimated at 40–55% [115, 116]. It is frequently stated that patients die *with* renal failure rather than *of* renal failure. However, better uraemic control and more intensive artificial renal support may improve survival. Thus, a careful and proactive approach to the treatment of critically ill patients with AKI, based on the prevention of uncontrolled uraemia and the maintenance of low urea levels throughout the patient's illness, is desirable. Renal recovery occurs in more than 90% of survivors [116].

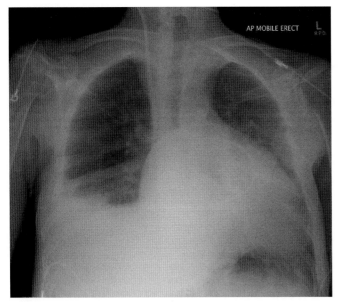

Figure 66.9 Chest radiograph of a patient presenting with diuretic resistant type 1 cardiorenal syndrome.

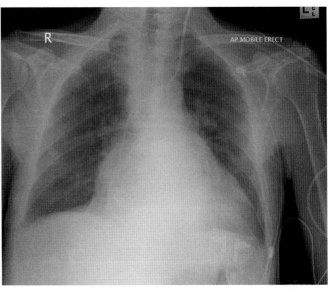

Figure 66.10 Chest radiograph of a patient presenting with diuretic resistant type 1 cardiorenal syndrome after treatment with ultrafiltration and the removal of 5.6 L over 3 days.

In those who survive AKI of critical illness, quality of life is generally perceived as acceptable, despite being lower than that of the general population.

Conclusion

AKI is a common syndrome in critically ill patients and recent developments and consensus criteria for its definition have facilitated a better understanding of its epidemiology. Growing evidence confirms that its pathogenesis is likely different according to the triggering disease or pathophysiological state. As our understanding evolves, it is likely that novel strategies to achieve prevention or attenuation of AKI will become condition specific. Moreover, the evolution of early and novel biomarkers of AKI will make such interventions possible at an earlier stage. Until that time, early intervention should remain focused on rapidly treating the underlying condition, restoring or maintaining haemodynamic homeostasis, and avoiding or removing nephrotoxins. If AKI becomes severe enough to warrant intervention with artificial renal replacement technology, continuous renal replacement therapy remains the preferred approach in all haemodynamically unstable patients.

Personal perspective

Although it is common and important, AKI remains a poorly understood syndrome from a pathogenetic point of view and is likely heterogeneous in mechanisms of injury. Lack of a clear understanding of the dominant mechanism(s) by which GFR is lost under situation of major physiological stress has so far made it impossible to develop effective pharmacologically based preventive or therapeutic interventions. Such failure may continue for years to come. Preservation of kidney function is best achieved by restoring and maintaining normal organ perfusion, avoiding nephrotoxic drugs, and instituting effective treatment of the primary disease process. Prophylactic approaches administered before injury with cardiac surgery or radiocontrast administration appear more likely to meet with success than postinjury interventions. However, the discovery of biomarkers like NGAL which allow the early diagnosis of AKI in a manner similar to the use of troponin in coronary syndromes may open the door to interventions which, using creatinine alone as diagnostic tool, were delivered too late to have chance of success. The technology of artificial renal support will continue to evolve and will increasingly be directed toward earlier intervention with continuous therapies. Ultrafiltration will likely become more common in the treatment of acute congestive decompensated heart failure.

Further reading

Bellomo R, Palevsky PM, Bagshaw SM, *et al.* Recent trials in critical care nephrology. *Contrib Nephrol* 2010;**164**:299–309.

Haase M, Bellomo R, Devarajan P, *et al.* Accuracy of neutrophil gelatinase associated lipocalin (NGAL) in diagnosis and prognosis in acute kidney injury: a systematic review and meta-analysis. *Am J Kidney Dis* 2009;**54**:1012–1024.

Haase M, Bellomo R, Haase-Fielitz. Novel biomarkers, oxidative stress, and the role of labile iron toxicity in cardiopulmonary bypass-associated acute kidney injury. *J Am Coll Cardiol* 2010;**55**:2024–2033.

Jun M, Heerspink HJ, Ninomiya T, *et al.* Intensities of renal replacement therapy in acute kidney injury: a systematic review and meta-analysis. *Clin J Am Soc Nephrol* 2010;**5**:956–63.

Prowle J, Echeveri JE, Ligabo EV, *et al.* Fluid balance and acute kidney injury. *Net Rev Nephrol* 2010;**6**:107–115.

Ronco C, McCullogh P, Anker SD, *et al.* Cardiorenal syndromes: report from the consensus conference of the acute dialysis quality initiative. *Eur Heart J* 2010;**31**:703–711.

Additional online material

- 66.1 Sepsis-associated acute kidney injury
- 66.2 Typical animal preparation for the measurement of vital organ blood flow
- 66.3 Induction of sepsis
- 66.4 Changes after induction of sepsis
- 66.5 Tissue flow Doppler technology
- 66.6 Implantation of phosphate detection coil
- 69.7 Transponder devices
- 69.8 Characteristics of the flow over time pattern of the renal arterial flow as acquired by ciné phase-contrast MRI

⮕ For additional multimedia materials please visit the online version of the book (🔗 http://www.esciacc.oxfordmedicine.com).

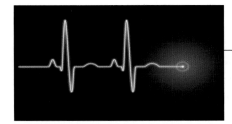

CHAPTER 67

Hyperglycaemia and diabetes

Marijke Gielen, Yoo-Mee Vanwijngaerden, Dieter Mesotten, and Greet Van den Berghe

Contents

Summary

In normal subjects blood glucose levels are tightly regulated within a relatively narrow range. This requires a coordinated interaction of glucose, insulin, and glucagon. All types of diabetes mellitus (DM) are characterized by hyperglycaemia. The morbidity and mortality of DM stem from acute metabolic derangements and from long-term complications that affect small and large vessels, resulting in retinopathy, nephropathy, neuropathy (microvascular disease), ischaemic heart disease, and arterial vasculopathy (macrovascular disease).

Hyperglycaemia, as part of the adaptive stress response, is also frequently present in patients suffering from acute stress such as myocardial infarction, even in the absence of a pre-existing diagnosis of diabetes.

The importance of glycaemic control has been confirmed in several large-scale controlled clinical trials. The Diabetes Control and Complications trial (DCCT) reported that intensive glycaemic treatment of type 1 DM was superior to conventional therapy in preventing the development of microvascular and neurological complications. Long-term follow-up data showed that intensive therapy beneficially affected the risk of cardiovascular disease in these patients. In the United Kingdom Prospective Diabetes Study (UKPDS) intensive blood glucose control by either sulphonylureas or insulin substantially decreased the risk of microvascular complications, but not macrovascular disease in patients with type 2 diabetes. The control of other risk factors in addition to tight glycaemic control decreased the risk of cardiovascular events. More recent trials on intensive glucose control in well-established type 2 diabetic patients revealed somewhat conflicting results, but irreversible damage, caused by long-time persisting hyperglycaemia, may be a possible explanation for these diverging results.

In critically ill patients, the Leuven studies showed that tight glycaemic control with intensive insulin therapy during critical illness improved outcome. Subsequent large multicentre studies failed to show the benefit of the Leuven studies, probably because they used an intermediate target for the control group and did not succeed in reaching the normoglycaemic target in the intervention group.

Introduction

Morbidity and mortality in diabetes is related to the development of microvascular and macrovascular complications as a consequence of sustained or transient hyperglycaemia. Several epidemiological studies have showed a graded relationship between the glycated haemoglobin (HbA_{1c}) level (as a measure of the degree of hyperglycaemia during the past 3 months) and the incidence of microvascular disease in diabetes. The benefit of strict glycaemic control on microvascular complications is now well-established (DCCT for type 1 DM, UKPDS for type 2 DM) but its cardiovascular benefit is more debatable since three recent trials (ACCORD, ADVANCE, VADT) did not at first glance show a cardiovascular benefit of strict glycaemic control [1–5].

Of course in the prevention of cardiovascular events strict glycaemic control is part of a broader treatment approach including correction of non-glycaemic risk factors and should always outweigh the risk of hypoglycaemia. The American Diabetes Association, the American Heart Association, and the American College of Cardiology therefore recommend achieving HbA_{1c} levels of less than 7.0%, in general, and for some patients a lower target may be more appropriate [6–7].

Numerous studies have shown a relationship between hyperglycaemia and increased morbidity and mortality, even in the absence of a pre-existing diagnosis of diabetes. More precisely, the statistical association in large observational studies between blood glucose level and risk of mortality follows a J or U-shaped curve with the nadir roughly between 90 and 140 mg/dL [8]. Also in patients with an acute coronary syndrome (ACS) a similar association has been observed, with the lowest risk of mortality with blood glucose levels between 81 and 99 mg/dL [9–11]. In patients with established diabetes mellitus (DM) prior to an acute life-threatening insult, the relationship between hyperglycaemia and mortality is blunted and shifted to the right. Whether preventing hyperglycaemia in the set-

ting of critical illness could also improve outcome has been the focus of several studies, which resulted in inconsistent results and fuelled the debate. Most of the concerns are about the increased incidence of hypoglycaemia. In their consensus statement on inpatient glycaemic control, the American Association of Clinical Endocrinologists and American Diabetes Association recommend maintaining glucose levels between 140 and 180 mg/dL, and for selected patients more stringent targets may be appropriate. For the moment, the evidence for tight glycaemic control (TGC) to achieve normoglycaemia is the strongest for adult and paediatric surgical intensive care (ICU) patients [6–7].

Pathophysiology of hyperglycaemia

In normal subjects blood glucose levels are tightly regulated within a relatively narrow range from 60 to 140 mg/dL. This requires a coordinated interaction of glucose, insulin, and glucagon.

All types of DM are characterized by hyperglycaemia, both fasting hyperglycaemia and larger increases in postprandial elevations of the plasma glucose level. Increased gluconeogenesis, accelerated glycogenolysis, and impaired glucose utilization by peripheral tissues, as a consequence of insulin deficiency or insulin insensitivity, lead to a state of sustained hyperglycaemia in diabetes. The different pathogenic processes leading to hyperglycaemia classify the type of DM (⊙ Box 67.1)[12]. Criteria for the diagnosis of DM are summarized in ⊙ Box 67.2 [12].

Non-diabetics may also develop hyperglycaemia. In non-diabetic patients who sustain an acute myocardial infarction (MI), the reported rate of stress hyperglycaemia varies from 3% to 71% [13]. Approximately 50% of non-diabetic ICU patients with sepsis have marked hyperglycaemia [14]. The stress imposed by any type of acute illness or injury triggers a response, which involves several neuro-endocrine and proinflammatory mediators affecting glucose metabolic pathways. This leads to dysregulation of glucose homeostasis, resulting in the development of hyperglycaemia, also referred to as 'diabetes of injury' [15–16]. Insulin resistance, characterized by hyperinsulinaemia, elevated hepatic glucose production, and impaired peripheral glucose uptake, plays a central role [16–17] (⊙ Fig. 67.1).

During the acute phase of critical illness hepatic glucose production is enhanced, as a result of ungoing gluconeogenesis and glycogenolysis, despite hyperglycaemia and hyperinsulinaemia. Insulin is abundantly released, while a state of hepatic insulin resistance prevails.

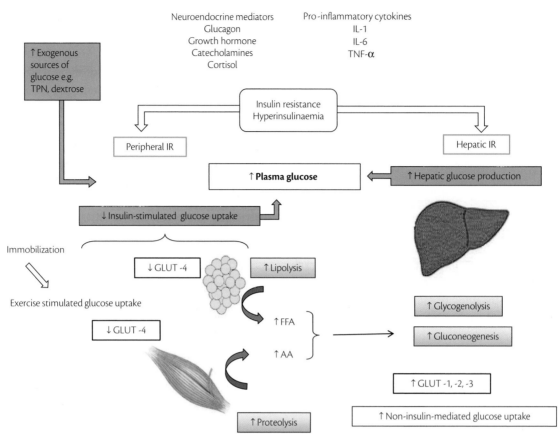

Figure 67.1 Mechanisms leading to hyperglycaemia during critical illness. IR, insulin resistance; FFA, free fatty acids; AA, amino acids; GLUT, glucose transporters; TPN, total parenteral nutrition.

Normally hyperinsulinaemia would inhibit endogenous glucose production, but in critical illness, despite the elevated blood glucose levels and abundance of insulin, hepatic glucose production is increased.

Besides stimulation of glucose production, significant changes in glucose uptake take place. The important exercise-stimulated glucose uptake in skeletal muscle is probably abolished in view of the immobilization of the critically ill patient. Insulin-stimulated glucose uptake by glucose transporter-4 (GLUT-4), present in heart, skeletal muscle, and adipose tissue, is impaired. Nevertheless, whole-body glucose uptake in critically ill patients is increased. This is caused by insulin-independent glucose uptake, facilitated by GLUT-1, GLUT-2, or GLUT-3, e.g. in the nervous system and the blood cells [18–19].

Several neuroendocrine and inflammatory mediators are involved in this process. In the acute phase of the stress response, neuroendocrine stimulation yields high circulating levels of glucagon, growth hormone (GH), catecholamines and cortisol, which are all inhibitors of insulin action. These hormonal changes (also known as the counter-regulatory response) and an increase in pro-inflammatory cytokines such as interleukin-1 (IL-1), interleukin-6 (IL-6),

tumour necrosis factor α (TNF-α), and macrophage migration inhibitory factor will lead to a state of insulin resistance. This is associated with increased proteolysis and lipolysis, hence providing substrates for the up-regulated gluconeogenesis pathway. Furthermore, both endogenous and exogenous catecholamines promptly inhibit insulin secretion from β-cells, resulting in a lowering of blood insulin levels later on during critical illness [20].

Clinical impact of hyperglycaemia

Diabetes mellitus

Diabetes mellitus results from a deficiency of insulin secretion or its action and it occurs when insulin secretion and/or insulin sensitivity are inadequate to prevent hyperglycaemia and its clinical consequences of polyuria, polydipsia, and weight loss [12].

The morbidity and mortality of DM stem from acute metabolic derangements and from the long-term complications, occurring within 10–15 years from the onset of diabetes, that affect small and large vessels, resulting in

---

Box 67.1 Classification of diabetes mellitus (DM)

Type 1 DM (insulin-dependent DM)

Characterized by

+ insulin deficiency
+ tendency to develop ketosis

Type 2 DM

Heterogeneous group of disorders characterized by variable degrees of

+ insulin resistance
+ impaired insulin secretion
+ increased glucose production

DM caused by

+ genetic defects (maturity onset diabetes of the young, MODY)
+ diseases of the exocrine pancreas (chronic pancreatitis, cystic fibrosis, hemochromatosis)
+ endocrinopathies (acromegaly, Cushing's syndrome, glucagonoma, pheochromocytoma, hyperthyroidism)
+ drugs (nicotinic acid, glucocorticoids, thiazides, protease inhibitors)
+ pregnancy (gestational DM)

Box 67.2 Criteria for the diagnosis of diabetes mellitus

1 Symptoms of diabetes (polyuria, polydipsia, and unexplained weight loss) and a casual plasma glucose concentration ≥11.1 mmol/L (≥200mg/dL), or

2 fasting plasma glucose ≥7.0 mmol/L (≥126 mg/dl), or

3 2-h plasma glucose ≥11.1 mmol/L (≥200 mg/dL) during a 75-g oral glucose tolerance test.

These criteria should be confirmed by repeat testing on a different day, unless unequivocal hyperglycaemia with acute metabolic decompensation is present.

Two intermediate categories have also been designated:

+ fasting plasma glucose between 6.1 and 7.0 mmol/L (110 and 126 mg/dL): impaired fasting glucose
+ plasma glucose levels between 7.8 and 11.1 mmol/L (140 and 200 mg/dL) 2 h after a 75-g oral glucose load: impaired glucose tolerance.

Individuals in these categories do not have DM but are at substantial risk for developing type 2 DM and cardiovascular disease in the future.

---

retinopathy, nephropathy, neuropathy, ischaemic heart disease, and arterial vasculopathy [21].

Chronic complications

An overview of the chronic complications of DM is given in ➲ Box 67.3.

Although cardiovascular disease is not specific to diabetes, it is more prevalent among patients with type 1 or type 2 diabetes than among those without diabetes. Type 1 diabetes is associated with at least a 10-fold increase in cardiovascular disease as compared with an age-matched non-diabetic population [22, 23].

Acute complications

The most serious, acute complications of diabetes are diabetic ketoacidosis (DKA) and non-ketotic hyperosmolar hyperglycaemic state (HHS). They both represent extremes in the spectrum of hyperglycaemia [24].

+ DKA exists when there is hyperglycaemia (blood glucose >250 mg/dL), ketonaemia, acidosis (pH ≤7.30 and bicarbonate ≤18 mEq/L), glucosuria, and ketonuria in addition to the clinical features of tachypnoea (Kussmaul

---

Box 67.3 Chronic complications of diabetes mellitus

Microvascular complications

+ Ophthalmological: nonproliferative or proliferative diabetic retinopathy
+ Renal: proteinuria, end-stage renal disease, type IV renal tubular acidosis
+ Neurological: distal symmetric polyneuropathy, polyradiculopathy, mononeuropathy, autonomic neuropathy

Macrovascular complications

+ Cardiovascular-atherosclerotic: coronary artery disease, congestive heart failure, peripheral vascular disease, stroke

Other

+ Gastrointestinal: gastroparesis, diarrhoea, constipation
+ Genitourinary: cystopathy, erectile dysfunction, female sexual dysfunction
+ Lower extremity: foot deformity (hammer toe, claw toe, Charcot foot), ulceration, amputation

respiration) and altered mental status in severe DKA (⊃ Table 67.1) [24]. Precipitating factors, even for the initial presentation, include stress (e.g. trauma), infections, vomiting, and major psychological disturbances.

DKA is the most common cause of death in children and adolescents with type 1 diabetes and accounts for half of all deaths in diabetic patients younger than 24 years of age. In adult subjects with DKA, the overall mortality is less than 1%; however, a mortality rate greater than 5% has been reported in elderly patients and those with concomitant life-threatening illnesses [24].

◆ HHS is a syndrome characterized by severe hyperglycaemia (blood glucose concentration >600 mg/dL), high serum osmolarity (commonly >320 mOsm/kg), absence of or only very slight ketosis, non-ketotic acidosis, severe dehydration, decreased consciousness or coma, and various neurological signs that may include focal or generalized seizures, hemianopia, and hemiparesis (⊃ Table 67.1) [24]. Respiration is usually shallow.

The key difference between DKA and HHS appears to be the degree of insulinopenia. Insulinopenia is nearly absolute in ketoacidosis, while there is sufficient residual activity in HHS to limit lipolysis in adipose tissue but not enough to permit normal peripheral glucose utilization at a time of increased glucose production induced by the stress hormones.

Mortality attributed to HHS is considerably higher than that attributed to DKA, with recent mortality rates of 5–20%. The prognosis of both conditions is substantially worsened at the extremes of age in the presence of coma, hypotension, and severe comorbidities [24].

DKA and HHS are medical emergencies as they represent a life-threatening decompensation of metabolism that requires prompt recognition and appropriate treatment (for a flow-chart of treatment, see ⊃ Fig. 67.2).

Critical illness

Diabetes of injury used to be interpreted as an adaptive stress response, and as such important for survival. The overall increase in glucose turnover and the fact that hyperglycaemia persists despite abundantly released insulin were considered arguments in favour of tolerating elevated blood glucose levels during critical illness [25]. Indeed, if one considers hyperglycaemia of injury as beneficial in promoting cellular glucose uptake in non-insulin-dependent tissues, tolerating hyperglycaemia is beneficial. Consequently, blood glucose concentrations of 160–200 mg/dL were hypothesized to maximize cellular glucose uptake while avoiding hyperosmolarity [17]. In addition, moderate hyperglycaemia was often viewed as a buffer against hypoglycaemia-induced brain damage.

Many studies nevertheless suggest that diabetes of injury may not be benign and that stress-induced hyperglycaemia is associated with a high risk of morbidity and mortality. The association between hyperglycaemia and mortality may even be stronger in critically ill patients without known diabetes. A strong association has been shown between stress hyperglycaemia after acute MI and increased risk of in-hospital mortality in patients with and without diabetes; the risk of congestive heart failure or cardiogenic shock was also increased in patients without diabetes [13]. Intraoperative hyperglycaemia appeared to be an independent risk factor for adverse outcome after cardiac surgery and in ST- and non-ST- segment elevation ACS [26, 27]. Short-term and 6-month mortality were also increased significantly with higher fasting glucose levels.

Table 67.1 Diagnostic criteria for diabetic ketoacidosis (DKA) and hyperosmolar hyperglycemic state (HHS)

	DKA			HHS
	Mild (plasma glucose >250 mg/dL)	Moderate (plasma glucose >250 mg/dL)	Severe (plasma glucose >250 mg/dL)	Plasma glucose >600 mg/dL
Arterial pH	7.25–7.30	7.00 to <7.24	<7.00	>7.30
Serum bicarbonate (mEq/L)	15–18	10 to <15	<10	>18
Urine ketone[a]	Positive	Positive	Positive	Small
Serum ketone[a]	Positive	Positive	Positive	Small
Effective serum osmolality[b]	Variable	Variable	Variable	>320 mOsm/kg
Anion gap[c]	>10	>12	>12	Variable
Mental status	Alert	Alert/drowsy	Stupor/coma	Stupor/coma

[a] Nitroprusside reaction method.
[b] Effective serum osmolality: $2[\text{measured Na}^+ \text{ (mEq/l)}] + \text{glucose (mg/dl)}/18$.
[c] Anion gap: $(\text{Na}^+) - [(\text{Cl}^- + \text{HCO}_3^- \text{ (mEq/l)}]$

Reproduced from Kitabchi AE, *et al.* Hyperglycemic crises in adult patients with diabetes. *Diabetes Care* 2009; **32** :1335–1343, with permission from The American Diabetes Association..

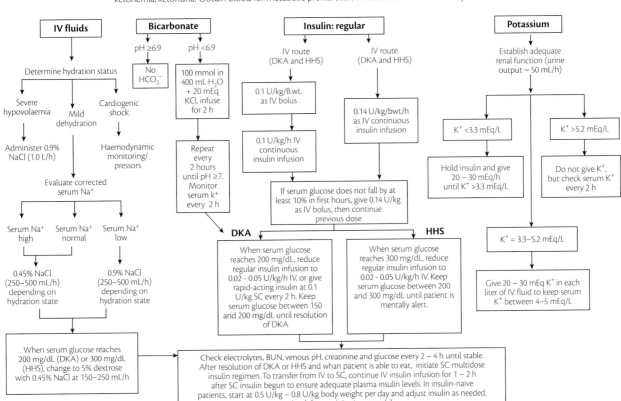

Complete initial evaluation. Check capillary glucose and serum/urine ketones to confirm hyperglycemia and ketonemia/ketonuria. Obtain blood for metabolic profile. Start IV fluids: 1.0 L of 0.9% NaCl per hour.

Figure 67.2 Management of adult patients with diabetic ketoacidosis (DKA) or hyperosmolar hyperglycaemic state (HHS). Reproduced from Kitabchi AE, *et al*. Hyperglycemic crises in adult patients with diabetes. *Diabetes Care* 2009; **32**:1335–1343, with permission from The American Diabetes Association.

Similarly, hyperglycaemia predicted an increased risk of in-hospital mortality after ischaemic stroke in non-diabetic patients and increased risk of poor functional recovery in stroke survivors [28].

In trauma patients, elevated blood glucose levels predicted mortality and length of stay and were associated with infectious morbidity and prolonged need for mechanical ventilation [29–32]. A strong link has also been described between increased blood glucose levels and the risk of critical illness polyneuropathy in sepsis and the systemic inflammatory response syndrome (SIRS) [33].

The above-mentioned observational evidence pointed to an association between hyperglycaemia and morbidity and mortality in critically ill patients. Randomized controlled trials assessing the impact of a treatment that prevents hyperglycaemia were required to identify hyperglycaemia as a causative factor of adverse outcome and not just as a marker of more severe illness. In 2001, a large randomized study demonstrated that maintenance of normoglycaemia with intensive insulin therapy substantially prevents morbidity and reduces mortality in surgical ICU patients. This landmark trial clearly undermined the dogma of hyperglycaemia as a beneficial response in critically ill patients [34].

Clinical evidence for tight glycaemic control

Diabetes mellitus

The importance of glycaemic control has been confirmed in several large-scale controlled clinical trials. In 1993, the 'Diabetes Control and Complications Trial' (DCCT) investigators reported that intensive glycaemic treatment of patients with type 1 DM was superior to conventional therapy in preventing the development of microvascular and neurological complications [1]. The intensive-therapy regimen was designed to achieve blood glucose values as close to the normal range as possible with three or more daily insulin injections or treatment with an insulin pump. Conventional therapy consisted of one or two insulin injections per day. During the DCCT, fewer cardiovascular events occurred in the intensive-treatment group than in the conventional-treatment group, but the small number of events in the relatively young cohort precluded a determination of whether the use of intensive diabetes therapy affected the risk of cardiovascular disease. Using long-term follow-up data of the 'Diabetes Control and Complications

Trial/Epidemiology of Diabetes Interventions and Complications' (DCCT/EDIC) cohort, researchers showed that intensive diabetes therapy beneficially affected the risk of cardiovascular disease in patients with type 1 diabetes [35].

In patients with type 2 diabetes, intensive blood glucose control by either sulphonylureas or insulin substantially decreases the risk of microvascular complications, but not macrovascular disease (UKPDS group) [2]. Steno-2, which was a study of intensive intervention in multiple cardiovascular risk factors in type 2 diabetic individuals with microalbuminuria, showed that in addition to the intensive glycaemic control, the control of other risk factors frequently observed in these individuals such as hypertension, dyslipidaemia, and microalbuminuria, significantly decreased the risk of cardiovascular events and microangiopathy [36].

More recent trials on intensive glucose control in well established type 2 diabetic patients revealed somewhat conflicting results. In the 'Action to Control Cardiovascular Risk in Diabetes' (ACCORD) trial, the finding of higher mortality in the intensive therapy group led to the termination of the study 17 months before the scheduled end [3]. The 'Action in Diabetes and Vascular Disease: Preterax and Diamicron Modified Release Controlled Evaluation' (ADVANCE) trial reported favourable effects on microvascular complications but not on macrovascular events [4]. In the 'Veterans Affairs Diabetes Trial' (VADT), in which poorly controlled type 2 diabetes patients were enrolled, intensive glucose control (with a HbA_{1c} value less than <7% vs 8–9% for the group undergoing standard therapy) had no significant effect on the rates of major cardiovascular events, death, or microvascular complications, with the exception of progression of albuminuria [5].

Irreversible damage, caused by long-time persistent hyperglycaemia, may be a possible explanation for these diverging results. Adaptive changes to protect the cells against elevated extracellular glucose may have been induced and the time window for prevention of toxicity may have passed, such that lowering of blood glucose with newly started intensive therapy may no longer be beneficial [37].

Critical illness

The first Leuven study showed that preventing hyperglycaemia during critical illness substantially improved outcome [34]. TGC with intensive insulin therapy (IIT) in critically ill surgery patients, started within 24 h after admission to an intensive care unit (ICU), resulted in a 3.4% absolute risk reduction of ICU mortality and 3.7% of in-hospital mortality, as compared with tolerating hyperglycaemia as an adaptive response. TGC positively affected the morbidity of the patients, as illustrated by earlier weaning from mechanical ventilation, shorter ICU and hospital stay, lower incidence of acute renal failure and critical illness polyneuropathy, and reduced inflammation. A greater benefit was shown for patients who were treated for at least 3 days, for whom mortality was reduced from 20.6% to 13.6%.

In the medical ICU, IIT also significantly reduced morbidity but not mortality among all patients [38]. In all large diagnostic subgroups of mixed medical/surgical patients in the pooled database of the two Leuven studies, including patients with cardiovascular, respiratory, gastrointestinal/hepatic disease or surgery, patients with active malignancy, and those with sepsis on ICU admission, IIT reduced mortality and morbidity [39]. Only in the group of patients with a history of diabetes was no survival benefit observed, but morbidity also tended to be reduced in these patients. The absence of survival benefit in this patient group, might also be explained by persistent diabetic vascular stress after glucose normalization, or the so-called 'metabolic memory'[37].

Subsequent large multicentre studies failed to show the benefit of the Leuven studies, probably because they used a much lower target range for blood glucose in the control group and did not succeed in reaching the normoglycaemia target in the intervention group, creating an important overlap between the two groups. The GLUCONTROL study was stopped prematurely because the normoglycaemic target was not reached and because of the increased incidence of hypoglycaemia (9.8%) [40]. Hospital mortality did not differ between the IIT group (19.5%) and the control group (16.2%). The insulin arm of the 'Volume Substitution and Insulin Therapy in Severe Sepsis' (VISEP) study was also stopped early, because the rate of hypoglycaemia in the IIT group (12.1%) was considered unacceptably high [41]. NICE-SUGAR, the largest trial to date, showed a 3% absolute mortality risk increase, mirroring the Leuven studies [42]. Lower target blood glucose range in the control group, lack of standardization in blood glucose measurements, different nutritional strategies, and lack of expertise in the regulation of glycaemia may all have contributed to the increased mortality in the intervention arm of the study [43].

In the context of acute MI a similar story can be told. The DIGAMI 1 study studied the effects of intensive in-hospital insulin treatment (insulin–glucose infusion for at least 24 h followed by a multidose subcutaneous insulin regimen) versus usual care in 620 acute MI patients with established diabetes and/or admission glucose of more than 200 mg/dL [44]. This study achieved significantly lower glucose levels in the intervention arm compared with the control group and demonstrated a survival benefit associated with better glucose control. Two other studies on the combined infusion of glucose, insulin, and potassium (GIK) could not show any beneficial effect on outcome after acute MI (DIGAMI 2 and CREATE-ECLA), as these trials never achieved normoglycaemia in the intervention group of the study [45, 46].

An overview of randomized outcome studies on IIT in cardiac ICU patients is given in ⊃ Table 67.2 [44–50].

Mechanisms of action of tight glycaemic control by intensive insulin therapy

Diabetes mellitus

In diabetes, avoiding prolonged exposure to hyperglycaemia, i.e. glucose toxicity, is crucial to prevent complications.

Intracellular hyperglycaemia causes mitochondrial overproduction of superoxide, which via inhibition of glyceraldehyde-3-phosphate dehydrogenase (GAPDH) activates four major pathways of hyperglycaemic damage: increased flux through the polyol pathway, intracellular production of advanced glycation end product (AGE) precursors, phospokinase C (PKC) activation, and increased hexosamine pathway activity. For the development of diabetic macrovascular disease, insulin resistance even before hyperglycaemia is present, can lead to increased oxidative stress. Increased flux of free fatty acids (FFA) into endothelial cells, as a consequence of insulin resistance leads to overproduction of reactive oxygen species (ROS) by increased β-oxidation of FFA. Maintaining normoglycaemia, will avoid oxidative stress and mitochondrial overproduction of ROS, which initiates the major damaging pathways leading to accelerated atherosclerosis, which is responsible for the majority of deaths in diabetes [51].

Critical illness

In stress hyperglycaemia, strict glycaemic control by IIT will also avoid cellular glucose overload. Most cells reduce their glucose transport rate on exposure to hyperglycaemia, but due in part to the stress response this protective response is

Table 67.2 Publications of randomized outcome studies on intensive insulin therapy in cardiac patients

Study	Patient no.	Patient type	Glycaemia (mg/dL)	Results	Type of study
DIGAMI, 1995	620	AMI with either diabetes (any type) or admission glucose >200 mg/dL	210 → 173	↓ mortality at 1 year	Single centre, randomized
Lazar, 2004	141	Diabetic patients undergoing CABG	260 → 138	Improved perioperative outcomes Enhanced survival ↓ incidence of ischaemic events and wound complications	Single centre, randomized
DIGAMI-2, 2005	1253	AMI with either diabetes or admission glucose >200 mg/dL	No TGC achieved	No difference in mortality at 2 years	Multicentre, randomized
HI-5, 2006	244	AMI with either type 2 diabetes or admission glucose >140 mg/dL	162→ 150; no TGC achieved	No difference in mortality, but lower rate of post-MI heart failure and reinfarction	Multicentre, randomized
CREATE-ECLA, 2006	20 201	STEMI; no requirement for diabetes or hyperglycaemia on admission	135→ 155; no TGC achieved	No difference in 30-day mortality	Multicentre, randomized
Ingels et al., 2006 (subanalysis of Van den Berghe et al., 2001)	970/1548	High risk cardiac surgery patients	157→ 104	↓ICU and in-hospital mortality ↓ morbidity ↑ 4-year survival	Single centre, randomized
Gandhi, 2007	400	IIT during cardiac surgery	157→ 114 intraoperatively only; 2 groups identical glucoses in the ICU	No reduction of perioperative death or morbidity	Single centre, randomized

AMI, acute myocardial infarction; CABG, coronary artery bypass graft; STEMI, ST-segment elevation myocardial infarction; IIT, intensive insulin therapy; TCG, tight glycemic control.

overruled, making hyperglycaemia even more acutely toxic. Experimental data and data from animal models have also unravelled beneficial non-glycaemic metabolic and non-metabolic effects of insulin. They include improvement in lipid and protein metabolism, inflammatory response, endothelial function, and coagulopathy [52–55].

Potential harm of tight glycaemic control

Diabetes mellitus

In the DCCT, the chief adverse event associated with intensive therapy was a two-to-threefold increase in severe hypoglycaemia [1]. Also in the UKPDS, ACCORD, ADVANCE, and VADT trials, hypoglycaemia was the most common adverse event, with significantly more episodes in the intensive therapy group than in the standard therapy group [2–5].

Severe or prolonged hypoglycaemia is known to cause convulsions, coma, and irreversible brain damage as well as cardiac arrhythmias.

According to the DCCT results published in 1993, with the first patient recruited in 1983 and an average follow-up of 6.5 years, relatively few patients required hospitalization or medical attention for hypoglycaemia or resultant injuries. However, the effects on cognition of repeated severe hypoglycaemia were the main long-term concern. Reassuringly, later published follow-up results showed that neither the frequency of hypoglycaemia nor the treatment group assignment were associated with cognitive decline 18 years after DCCT recruitment, either in the treatment group as a whole or in the adolescent participants, who were thought to be particularly vulnerable. Moreover, higher HbA_{1c} values were associated with declines in motor speed and psychomotor efficiency [1, 56, 57].

Critical illness

Intensive insulin therapy and the risk of hypoglycaemia

The risk of hypoglycaemia (glucose ≤40 mg/dL) with IIT increased from 0.8% to 5.1% in the surgical ICU study and from 3.1% to 18.7% in the medical ICU study [34, 38]. These brief episodes of biochemical hypoglycaemia were not associated with obvious clinical problems. Indeed, hypoglycaemia did not cause early deaths;, only minor immediate and transient morbidity was seen in a minority of patients,

and no late neurologic sequelae occurred among hospital survivors [39].

Nevertheless, the risk of hypoglycaemia coincided with a higher risk of death, equally in both conventional and intensive insulin groups. A higher mortality, however, was observed with spontaneous hypoglycaemia than with hypoglycaemic events during insulin infusion. Moreover, in a nested-case-control study in which case and control subjects were matched for baseline risk factors and time in the ICU before the hypoglycaemic event, no causal link was found between hypoglycaemia in the ICU and death [58]. These observations suggest that hypoglycaemia in ICU patients who receive IIT may merely identify patients at high risk of dying rather than representing a risk on its own [59].

Intensive insulin therapy, hypokalaemia, and large glucose fluctuations

Insulin therapy induces a shift of potassium from the extracellular to the intracellular compartment. This may induce hypokalaemia. By using arterial blood and an accurate point-of-care blood gas analyser for glucose monitoring, with each blood glucose check, potassium levels are also measured and corrected when needed. Hence, hypokalaemia-induced arrhythmia is carefully avoided. This may be particularly important with bolus injections of insulin, and with the use of volumetric pumps that deliver varying amounts of insulin over time.

Repeated large (undetected) fluctuations in blood glucose with hypoglycaemia alternating with hyperglycaemia in ill patients may also be worse than tolerating constant moderate hyperglycaemia [60].

Challenges for tight glycaemic control in the intensive care unit

TGC by IIT in the ICU is a complex intervention and should be carefully implemented. Differences in the practical implementation of TGC may partly explain the discrepant results between the initial proof-of-concept studies and the subsequent large multicentre trials. Therefore the focus of new clinical trials should first be on the improvement of the 'modus operandi' of IIT before embarking on large multicentre outcome trials. As an initial step an exploratory meta-analysis, preferably on a per patient basis, may assist in unravelling the mechanisms behind the different outcomes of TGC in critically ill patients.

The first challenge for the ICU community regarding TGC is finding a consensus on the accuracy which blood glucose meters should meet. It has become clear that capillary blood samples and most hand-held blood glucose meters are not reliable enough for glucose measurements for TGC in critically ill patients. [61]. Currently only on-site blood gas analysers seem appropriate for TGC in the ICU.

Secondly, computer algorithms to assist ICU nurses in the safe execution of TGC need to be further developed and tested in clinical studies. They should be able to drastically decrease the incidence of hypoglycaemia while at the same time steering blood glucose levels within the narrow range of normality.

Nevertheless, settling the debate on the impact of hypoglycaemia on long-term outcome will be the most important challenge. Until then it will remain hard to weigh the risks of prolonged hyperglycaemia against the risks of brief hypoglycaemia. So far long-term follow-up studies on the neurocognitive function of patients who were exposed to the varying blood glucose levels in the randomised clinical trials have been lacking.

critical illness hyperglycaemia is not a magic bullet but should always be seen as part of a broader treatment approach. The administration of insulin in order to strictly normalize blood glucose levels is a powerful strategy to improve patient outcome. However, one should be wary of the complications of IIT, notably hypoglycaemia and large blood glucose fluctuations. Hence, all precautions should be taken to safely implement TGC. This includes accurate and frequent blood glucose measurements, a reliable administration of insulin and a thorough training of the health care providers.

The contradicting results between proof-of-concept studies and the multicentre repeat trials do not permit clear-cut, evidence-based recommendations for one optimal blood glucose target in heterogeneous ICU populations and settings. In general, blood glucose levels should be controlled as close to normal fasting glucose concentrations (80–110 mg/dL). However, taking into account the variability in the health care providers' experience with IIT and the availability of state-of-the-art blood glucose measurement devices, one could recommend to keep blood glucose levels below 130 mg/dL. Frequent and reliable measurements of blood glucose remain mandatory in order to avoid hypoglycaemia and large glucose fluctuations.

Conclusion

Lowering blood glucose by intensive insulin therapy in the management of established diabetes mellitus and of

Personal perspective

The future development of accurate, continuous blood glucose monitoring devices, in combination with computer-based blood glucose control algorithms, will likely help to avoid hypoglycaemia and large blood glucose fluctuations.

Further reading

Capes SE, Hunt D, Malmberg K, Gerstein HC. Stress hyperglycemia and increased risk of death after myocardial infarction in patients with and without diabetes: a systematic overview. *Lancet* 2000;**355**:773–782.

Ceriello A, Ihnat MA, and Thorpe JE. The '"metabolic memory"': is more than just tight glucose control necessary to prevent diabetic complications? *J Clin Endocrinol Metab* 2009;**94**:410–415.

Deedwania P, Kosiborod M, Barrett E, *et al.* Hyperglycemia and acute coronary syndrome. A scientific statement from the American Heart Association Diabetes Committee of the Council on Nutrition, Physical Activity, and Metabolism. *Circulation* 2008;**117**:1610–1619.

The Diabetes Control and Complications Trial/Epidemiology of Diabetes Interventions and Complications (DCCT/EDIC) Study Research Group. Nathan DM, Cleary PA, Backlund JC *et al.* Intensive diabetes treatment and cardiovascular disease in patients with type 1 diabetes. *N Engl J Med* 2005;**353**(25): 2643–2653.

Malmberg K, Ryden L, Wedel H, *et al.* Intense metabolic control by means of insulin in patients with diabetes mellitus and acute myocardial infarction (DIGAMI 2): effects on mortality and morbidity. *Eur Heart J* 2005;**26**:650–661.

Mizock BA. Alterations in fuel metabolism in critical illness: hyperglycemia. *Best Pract Res Clin Endocrinol Metab* 2001;**15**(4):533–551.

The NICE-SUGAR Study Investigators. Finfer S, Chittock DR, Su SY *et al*. Intensive versus conventional glucose control in critically ill patients. *N Engl J Med* 2009;**360**:1283–1297.

Van den Berghe G, Schetz M, Vlasselaers D, *et al*. Intensive insulin therapy in critically ill patients: NICE-SUGAR or

Leuven blood glucose target? *J Clin Endocrin Metab* 2009; **94**(9):3163–3170.

Van den Berghe G, Wouters P, Weekers F, *et al*. Intensive insulin therapy in the critically ill patients. *N Engl J Med* 2001;**345**:1359–1367.

➔ For additional multimedia materials please visit the online version of the book (🕮 http://www.esciacc.oxfordmedicine. com).

CHAPTER 68

Endocrine emergencies

Yves Debaveye, Jeroen Vandenbrande,
and Greet Van den Berghe

Contents

Summary

The classical endocrine (nondiabetic) emergencies—thyroid storm, myxo-edema coma, acute adrenal crisis, and pheochromocytoma—are potentially life-threatening disorders that pose diagnostic and therapeutic challenges to the physician. Although these endocrine emergencies are mostly encountered in patients in whom the diagnosis of endocrine dysfunction has already been made, they are occasionally the presenting manifestation in undiagnosed patients. The patient's outcome in these endocrine emergencies is influenced predominantly by the ability of the alert physician to promptly recognize, or at least suspect, the diagnosis and to quickly institute adequate therapy. If these endocrine disorders are overlooked, however, specific treatment such as endocrine replacement or blockage therapy will be delayed and calamitous complications or death may ensue.

We also briefly discuss the approach to patients with amiodarone-induced thyroid dysfunction, because overt thyroid dysfunction occurs in up to one-fifth of patients treated with the commonly used antiarrythmic drug amiodarone.

Introduction

Although endocrine pathology is usually treated in the outpatient clinic, intensive care may be required when endocrinopathies are associated with other medical illnesses or reach a state of decompensation. Although endocrine emergencies are quite rare, they are potentially life-threatening if not recognized promptly and managed effectively. Therefore, every clinician should always be attentive for the probable diagnosis of these complex disorders.

Life-threatening thyreotoxicosis: thyroid storm

Thyrotoxicosis is a hypermetabolic clinical syndrome resulting from increased circulating levels of thyroid hormone. In the acute care setting, of greatest concern is thyroid storm (TS), a life-threatening thyrotoxicosis which occurs in patients with untreated or undertreated hyperthyroidism.

TS is mostly precipitated by an acute event such as infections, (thyroid) surgery, withdrawal of antithyroid drugs, radioiodine therapy or iodinated radiocontrast dyes, trauma, labour, and delivery. It is important to recognize that the diagnosis must be made on the basis of the clinical examination since rapid thyroid function tests are not universally available and do not distinguish between symptomatic hyperthyroidism and TS. As TS carries a high mortality (10–75%), early recognition and initiation of adequate therapy are crucial.

Clinical manifestations and diagnosis

Cardiovascular symptoms include sinus or supraventricular tachycardia (out of proportion to fever) and congestive heart failure, which may be rate-related or high output failure. Other clinical hallmarks of TS important to the diagnosis include profuse diaphoresis, severe thermoregulatory dysfunction (fever >38.5°C), gastrointestinal symptoms (nausea, vomiting, diarrhoea, rarely jaundice) and mental status changes (confusion, delirium, coma). Thyroid function tests are in generally straightforward with undetectable TSH (<0.001 mU/L) and raised total and free T_4 and T_3 levels. T_3 is typically more increased than T_4 as a result of enhanced peripheral thyroid hormone conversion. Because of the high risk of concurrent adrenal insufficiency and the common use of corticosteroids in the acute management of TS, it is advisable to obtain a serum sample for cortisol measurement before therapy is initiated.

Treatment

Treatment of TS is complex and generally requires an intensive care (ICU) environment. The acute therapy is multifaceted and may be thought as a four-pronged approach: (1) interventions to decrease thyroid hormone synthesis and release, (2) strategies to reduce effects of thyroid hormone on peripheral tissues, (3) supportive measures, and (4) cure of the precipitating illness (see ⟳ Box 68.1).

A nearly complete and rapid blockage of de novo thyroid hormone synthesis is achieved by the thionamides propylthiouracil (PTU) and methimazole (MMI). Although PTU is traditionally the preferred thionamide, because it inhibits peripheral T_4 to T_3 conversion, many authors prefer the more potent drug MMI in combination with other drugs that block the conversion of T_4 to T_3. Thionamides are given orally, rectally, or by nasogastric tube since they are unavailable for parenteral administration. High dosage is advisable because of possibly concurrent gastrointestinal dysfunction.

Blocking of thyroid hormone release of thyroid hormone from the thyroid gland can be accomplished by a saturated solution of potassium iodine or Lugol's solution. An initial dose of a thionamide must be given at least 1 h before iodine administration, to prevent iodine-induced thyroid hormone synthesis. Use of lithium should be considered only in patients with contraindications for iodine and thionamide, because of its renal and neurologic toxicity.

β-Blockers are important in the symptomatic treatment of peripheral adrenergic hyperactivity, although known contraindications must be taken into account. Propanolol has been used with greatest success as it also impairs peripheral thyroid hormone conversion.

Glucocorticoids also reduce T_4 to T_3 conversion, may have a direct effect on the underlying autoimmune process of Graves' disease, and apparently improve outcome. Cholestyramine binds to thyroid hormones in the gastrointestinal tract, resulting in a modest reduction of circulating thyroid hormone levels. Haemodialysis, plasmapheresis, and charcoal haemoperfusion should only be considered if progression occurs despite aggressive therapy.

Hyperthermia should be treated aggressively with antipyretics and peripheral cooling. Because salicylates affect the binding or displace thyroid hormone from binding proteins, paracetamol (acetaminophen) is the first-choice antipyretic agent.

Large fluid losses due to sweating, vomiting, and diarrhoea need to be adequately replaced to prevent cardiovascular collapse. Patients with underlying cardiac disease should be invasively monitored. To prevent hypoglycaemia, caused by rapid depletion of hepatic glycogen stores during TS, intravenous fluids should contain 5–10% glucose in addition to the required electrolytes. Vitamin supplements, especially thiamine, should be given to replace a possible coexisting deficiency. When sedation is required, phenobarbital may be preferred to benzodiazepines as the former stimulates hepatic clearance of thyroid hormone.

In most patients, clinical improvement is expected within the first 12–24 h of adequate therapy.

As infection is the most common precipitating cause of TS, a vigorous search for an infectious process is warranted in every febrile thyrotoxic patient. However, empirical antibiotics are not recommended in the absence of an identified focus of infection.

Once the acute event is controlled, consideration must be given to long-term treatment and control of hyperthyroidism. Nowadays most patients are treated with radioactive iodine therapy; however, this therapy must be

---

Box 68.1 Treatment of thyroid storm

Decrease of thyroid hormone synthesis and release

Inhibition of new hormone synthesis

- Propylthiouracil (PTU): load 600–1000 mg, then 200–300 mg by mouth every 4–6 h

- Methimazole: load 60–100 mg, then 20–30 mg by mouth every 6–8 h

Inhibition of thyroid hormone release

- Inorganic iodine

  - Saturated solution of potassium iodide (SSKI): 5 drops (250 mg) by mouth every 6–12 h

  - Lugol's solution: 4–8 drops by mouth every 6 h

- Lithium carbonate: 300 mg by mouth every 6 h (serum level <1 mEq/L)

Inhibition of T_4 to T_3 conversion

- PTU

- Corticosteroids: hydrocortisone 100 mg IV every 8 h (or equivalent)

- Propanolol

Reduction of peripheral effects of thyroid hormone

- β-blockade:

  - Propanolol: 0.5–1.0 mg IV every 2–3 h; or 40–80 mg by mouth every 4–8 h

  - Esmolol: load 250–500 μg/kg, then 50–100 μg kg^{-1} min^{-1} IV

- Corticosteroids

- Removal of excess circulating thyroid hormone:

  - Gastrointestinal clearance

    - Cholestyramine

  - Blood clearance

    - Haemodialysis

    - Haemoperfusion

    - Plasmapheresis

General supportive measures

- Antipyretics (paracetamol)

- Cooling

- Correction of dehydration

- Nutrition, vitamins

- Oxygen, mechanical ventilation

- Treatment of congestive heart failure

- Treatment of hyperkinesis: benzodiazepines, barbiturates

Cure of precipitating illness

- Search for potential source of infection

- Aetiology-dependent therapy (e.g. diabetic ketoacidosis, myocardial infarction)

---

appropriately delayed if iodine was used in the emergency management of TS.

Critical hypothyroidism: myxedema coma

Myxedema coma (MC) is an uncommon but life-threatening decompensated state of longstanding untreated or unrecognized hypothyroidism, whereby the homeostatic adaptations to cope with prolonged thyroid hormone deficiency are no longer sufficient. MC is classically encountered in elderly women and often triggered by an acute event, such as infection, trauma, cold exposure, or medications such as sedatives and anaesthetics. The term is largely a misnomer as most patients reveal neither myxoedema nor a comatose state. Rather, MC is characterized by progressive parallel dysfunction of the cardiovascular, respiratory, and central nervous systems. If not recognized rapidly and treated adequately, MC may carry a 60% risk of mortality.

Clinical manifestations and diagnosis

The diagnosis of MC is triggered by the presence of three key diagnostic features: (1) altered mental status, (2) defective thermoregulation, and (3) a precipitating illness or event. Altered mental status may manifest itself as disorientation, confusion, lethargy, frank psychosis, and, rarely, coma. Additional neurological features include seizures and delayed reflex relaxation. Defective thermoregulation is either expressed by absolute (usually <35.5°C) or relative hypothermia, such as (pseudo)normal body temperature during sepsis. Hypothermia in the absence of shivering is also indicative of the diagnosis. Since hypothyroidism itself does not bring on MC, one should always search for precipitating events. Pneumonia and urosepsis are among the most common events and should be considered as presumptive cause until proven otherwise. Furthermore, as severe hypothyroidism blunts normal leucocyte response to infection, even a subtle alteration in infectious parameters should be considered as highly suspicious for sepsis. The most common cardiovascular symptoms include bradycardia, hypotension, and decreased myocardial contractility with low cardiac output; however, congestive heart failure is uncommon in absence of pre-existing cardiac disease. Additional clinical features include hypoventilation, constipation, paralytic ileus, megacolon, and bladder atony.

The clinical diagnosis requires conformation by low or undetectable serum levels of T_4 and T_3. TSH levels are elevated in most patients, but may be normal or low in cases of hypothalamic-pituitary disease or advanced critical illness (e.g., nonthyroidal illness). As the degree of abnormality of the thyroid function tests does not correlate with the level of consciousness, rapid treatment must be instituted on the basis of clinical suspicion without awaiting laboratory confirmation. Additional laboratory hallmarks include hyponatraemia, hypoglycaemia, and normocytic anaemia.

Treatment

Patients with suspected MC should be admitted to the ICU for vigorous treatment that includes: (1) general supportive measures, (2) treatment of infections and metabolic complications, and (3) thyroid hormone replacement (see ⤷ Box 68.2). The overall goal is to resuscitate and stabilize the patient in the first 24–48 h, the time required for thyroid hormone therapy to start reversing the underlying metabolic state of hypothyroidism.

Mechanical ventilation is indicated at the first sign of respiratory failure, and haemodynamic deterioration must be treated aggressively. Vasopressors should be used with caution as they may induce arrhythmias in the setting of IV thyroid replacement. Passive rewarming with blankets is preferred, as active warming may induce peripheral vasodilatation and cardiovascular collapse. Glucocorticoid therapy should be administered until coexisting adrenal insufficiency is excluded.

A careful search for an underlying infection is essential, and broad-spectrum antibiotic coverage is advised pending the receipt of culture results. Monitoring and treatment of hyponatraemia must be considered. However, as hyponatraemia results in most case from excessive antidiuretic hormaone (ADH) secretion, the restoration of free water clearance with thyroid hormone treatment usually suffices to normalize sodium levels. Hypoglycaemia may occur in

---

Box 68.2 Management of myxoedema coma

General supportive measures

- Hypothermia
  - Passive rewarming with blankets, no heating devices
- Cardiac support
  - Correct hypotension
  - Cautious use of inotropes and vasopressors: glucocorticoids (stress doses); anticipate and treat heart failure; correct anaemia
- Pulmonary support
  - Ventilatory support
  - Monitoring of arterial blood gases
  - Treat pneumonia
- Slowed drug metabolism: avoid medication such as
  - Sedatives, narcotics, anesthetics
  - Digitalis
- Intestinal atony
  - Preferentially IV administration

Metabolic complications and infections

- Antibiotics
- Hydration and electrocytes
  - Maintain adequate blood volume
  - Avoid water intoxication
  - Hypertonic saline if serum sodium <120 mEq/L
- Nutrition: glucose, vitamins
- Glucocorticoids

Thyroid hormone replacement

- T_4 alone
  - Initial dose: 300–500 µg T_4 IV bolus
  - Maintenance: 50–100 µg T_4 IV bolus/day
- Combination $T_4 + T_3$
  - Initial dose: 200–300 µg T_4 IV bolus + 5–20 µg T_3 IV slow infusion
  - Maintenance: 50–100 µg T_4 IV bolus/day + 7.5–30 µg T_3 IV continuous infusion/day

the setting of secondary hypothyroidism and should be treated with intravenous glucose infusion. Seizures should be treated with standard anticonvulsants after correction of hyponatraemia, hypoglycaemia, and hypoxia.

Thyroid hormone therapy is crucial for survival and patients should be treated with a parenteral form of thyroid hormone as gastrointestinal absorption may be impaired. The drug selection (T_4 and/or T_3) and its optimal dose remain controversial. Many clinicians prefer a loading dose of 300–500 µg intravenous T_4 to quickly restore circulating levels of T_4 to approximately 50% of the euthyroid value, followed by 50–100 µg of intravenous T_4 daily until oral medication can be given. Administration of T_3 may be useful because of its greater biologic activity and the failure of the body to convert T_4 into T_3 during severe hypothyroidism. Since T_3 can potentially induce myocardial infarction and arrhythmias, monotherapy is not recommended. We prefer the combination of T_4 and T_3, using a loading dose of T_4 (200–300 µg IV bolus) and T_3 (5–20 µg slow IV injection) followed by a maintenance dose of T_4 (50–100 µg IV bolus daily) and T_3 (7.5–30 µg/day via continuous IV infusion) until oral therapy is initiated. Haemodynamics and diuresis typically improve within 24 h after initiation of treatment, whereas the restoration of body temperature takes 2–3 days.

Amiodarone-induced thyroid dysfunction

Because of its high iodine content, amiodarone can cause changes in thyroid function that result in either hypothyroidism (5–25%) or hyperthyroidism (2–10% of treated patients).

Amiodarone-induced hypothyroidism occurs rather early after starting treatment, especially in patients with pre-existing autoimmune thyroiditis, mainly due to an enhanced susceptibility to the inhibitory effect on thyroid hormone synthesis. Clinical presentation is usually subtle. In most cases amiodarone can be continued while T_4 is used to normalize TSH, as T_4 treatment does not impair the antiarrhythmic effect.

Amiodarone-induced hyperthyroidism (AIH) occurs at any time of the treatment and is frequently heralded by a worsening of the underlying cardiac disease, with tachyarrhythmias or angina. The management of patients with AIH is a major challenge and can be difficult. β-Blockade, if not already in place, is appropriate. Because of the long lifetime of amiodarone and high intrathyroidal iodine content, the stopping of amiodarone and the use of antithyroid drugs have only a marginal short-term effect. Prednisone (40–60 mg) may be considered. In rare cases, surgical thyroidectomy under local anaesthesia may be required.

Pheochromocytoma

Pheochromocytoma is a rare, catecholamine-secreting neoplasm (0.2% of patients with hypertension) that occurs in certain familial syndromes (e.g. multiple endocrine neoplasia type 2, von Hippel–Lindau disease, von Recklinghausen's neurofibromatosis) and other endocrinopathies (e.g. ACTH excess syndrome and hyperparathyroidism).

Clinical manifestations

The clinical manifestations are highly variable and result from excessive, either intermittent or continuous, catecholamine secretion by the tumour. Classically, patients present with sustained or paroxysmal hypertension and the 'classic triad' of headache, palpitations, and diaphoresis. Although this triad has a high specificity, most patients reveal only two of these three classic symptoms.

Upon admission to the ICU, the clinical picture is dominated by cardiovascular symptoms such as shock, myocarditis, dilatative cardiomyopathy, arrhythmias, pulmonary oedema, and heart failure; by neurological consequences such as altered mental status, stroke, seizures, and focal neurological pathology; by endocrine and metabolic consequences such as hyperglycaemia, hypercalcaemia, and lactic acidosis; or by surgical complications such as acute abdomen. Diagnosis is thus often missed. Pheochromocytoma should be suspected in patients with a paradoxical response to antihypertensive therapy, especially β-blockers, and a hypertensive response to anaesthesia, naloxone, metoclopramide, thyrotropin-releasing hormone (when used as diagnostic agent), tricyclic antidepressants, glucagon, voiding, or pregnancy. The differential diagnosis, including other clinical conditions associated with increased plasma and urinary catecholamine metabolites in the range of those observed with pheochromocytoma, is summarized in ⊃ Box 68.3.

Diagnosis

The diagnosis depends mainly on the documentation of catecholamine overproduction by measurements of 24-h urinary and levels of plasma fractionated catecholamines and metanephrine. Repeated testing is recommended since trade-offs between test sensitivity and specificity are

Box 68.3 Differential diagnosis of elevated catecholamines in plasma [P] and elevated catecholamine metabolites in urine [U]

- Pheochromocytoma [P, U]
- Cocaine abuse [P, U]
- Acute alcohol withdrawal [P, U]
- Acute myocardial ischaemia or infarction [P, U]
- Congestive heart failure [P, U]
- Acute cerebrovascular accident [P, U]
- Monotherapy with pure arterial vasodilators, hydralazine, or minoxidil [P, U]
- Dopamine IV, dopaminergic drugs [P]
- Acute hypoglycaemia [P]
- Labetalol [P]

a recurrent problem. This could lead to a false-positive diagnosis in the case of catecholamine secretion secondary to stress. Imaging studies to locate the tumour should be performed only after biochemical confirmation of the diagnosis. MRI is preferred to CT scanning. If abdominal and pelvic MRI or CT fails to localize the tumour, the diagnosis should first be reassessed. Only if the clinical suspicion remains high is it advisable to request additional imaging, such as total body MRI or nuclear medicine scan (e.g. meta-iodobenzylguanidine, PET, or octreotide).

Treatment

Definitive treatment of phaeochromocytoma requires surgical excision. Perioperative management is crucial to prevent hypertensive crises and to reduce the incidence and severity of postoperative hypotension.

The exact choice of drugs remains controversial. Most authors recommend the long-acting nonspecific α-blocker phenoxybenzamine. The starting dose of 10 mg orally twice a day should be gradually increased, usually up to 1 mg kg^{-1} day^{-1} given in three or four separate doses. Beta-blockers are needed to prevent reflex tachycardia only after adequate α-blockade, as they may otherwise precipitate a hypertensive crisis. Although selective $α_1$-blockers such as prazosin, terazosin, and doxazosin have a more attractive side-effect profile, they are not advised in the acute setting because of the incomplete α-blockade. As an alternative approach, calcium channel blockers can be used to control blood pressure and other adrenergic symptoms.

To treat acute hypertensive crises, repeated intravenous bolus of phentolamine (2.5–5 mg at 1 mg/min) or continuous infusion of nitropusside (0.5–10 µg kg^{-1} min^{-1} IV, not exceeding 800 µg/min) are the drugs of choice. Esmolol (50–200 µg kg^{-1} min^{-1} IV) and lidocaine (50–100 mg IV) can be used to manage tachyarrhythmias.

After tumour removal optimal fluid replacement is crucial to avoid postoperative hypotension, keeping in mind that pheochromocytoma patients mostly require large amounts of volume after tumour resection. Additionally, stress doses of glucocorticoids should be administered if bilateral adrenalectomy is planned. Since the inhibitory effect of catecholamines on insulin secretion is suddenly removed after surgery, hypoglycaemia occurs in up to 15% of patients. All patients should be monitored for blood glucose levels for at least 48 h postoperatively since β-blockers may mask the clinical manifestations of hypoglycaemia.

Acute adrenal crisis

Acute adrenal insufficiency (AI) is the manifestation of the failure of adrenal glands to cope with current, mostly elevated, physiological needs of the body. This life-threatening disorder can be due either to an acute decompensation of chronic process or the acute onset of a new pathology. In both conditions, the secretory inability of the adrenal gland leads to a deficiency of the steroid hormones androgens, glucocorticoids, and mineralocorticoids. The latter two are of importance in acute crisis.

Functionally, underlying reasons for AI can be divided into primary and secondary AI (⊃ Fig. 68.1). The majority of acute AI are observed in patients under chronic glucocorticoid treatment mainly after rapid withdrawal of glucocorticoids or when exposed to a major stressor, such as surgery, trauma, infection, or dehydration.

Clinical manifestations and diagnosis

The major clinical manifestation of acute AI is volume depletion with haemodynamic instability and shock. Other less specific clinical features include myalgia, joint or back pain, various mental stages (weakness up to coma), and gastrointestinal alterations (diarrhoea, vomiting, and abdominal pain) and fever.

In a critically ill patient, the clinical presentation of an adrenal crisis may mimic that of septic shock, with hypotension refractory to fluids and requirement of vasopressors.

The most important factor in diagnosing adrenal crisis is a high index of suspicion in cases of unexplained hypotension, especially in patients on prior glucocorticoid therapy or with conditions known to cause an acute AI (⊃ Fig. 68.1).

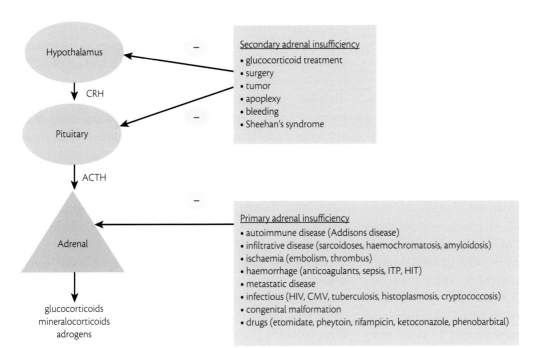

Figure 68.1 Precipitating factors for adrenal insufficiency. ACTH, adrenocorticotropic hormone; CRH, adrenocorticotropin-releasing hormone; HIT, heparin-induced thrombocytopenia; ITP, idiopathic thrombocytopenic purpura.

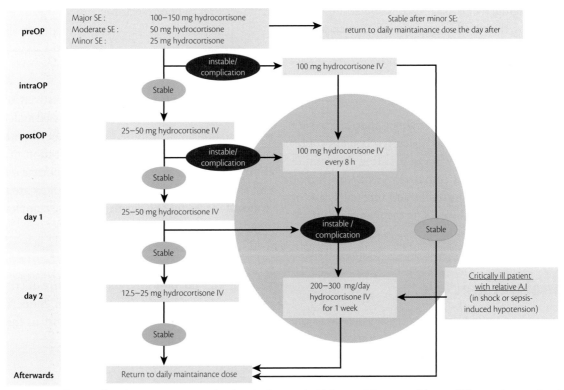

Figure 68.2 Prevention of acute adrenal crisis in patients under chronic glucocorticoid therapy. Minor stressful event (SE), e.g. coloscopy, inguinal hernia repair, mild–febrile illness, mild–moderate nausea/vomiting, gastroenteritis; moderate stressful event, e.g. open cholecystectomy, hemicolectomy, significant febrile illness, pneumonia, severe gastroenteritis; severe stressful event, e.g. Whipple's procedure, liver resection, cardiothoracic surgery, pancreatitis.

Laboratory abnormalities like hyponatraemia, hyperkalaemia, eosinophilia, and hypoglycaemia further strengthen the suspicion.

The definite diagnosis of acute AI relies on the demonstration of inadequate cortisol production via measurement of plasma corticotropin (ACTH) and the performance of a short ACTH (250 µg IV) stimulation test, before starting glucocorticoid therapy. A baseline cortisol level below 3 µg/dL (83 nmol/L) confirms the diagnosis of AI. Patients with primary AI have plasma ACTH concentrations that exceed 100 pg/mL (22 pmol/L) and thus do not respond to exogenous ACTH. In typical secondary AI, plasma cortisol levels increase after administration of ACTH, but due to adrenocortical atrophy this increase may be small or even absent.

Besides this classical presentation of AI, there is increasing attention to relative adrenal insufficiency (also known as critical-illness-related corticosteroid insufficiency, CIRCI) in critically ill patients, especially in those with severe sepsis of septic shock. In CIRCI the severely stressed adrenals appear unable to control the exaggerated inflammatory response because of lack of adrenocortisol reserve, which may be confirmed by consensus by a random total cortisol of less than 10 µg/dL (276 nmol/L) or by a change in total serum cortisol of less than 9 µg/dL (250 nmol/L) after a 250 µg ACTH stimulation test.

Diagnostic imaging, by CT and MRI, is sometimes helpful in determining the underlying cause of AI such as infarctions, bleeding, or others lesions in hypothalamus, pituitary, or adrenal glands.

Treatment

Acute AI is a true endocrine emergency that has a very poor prognosis if left untreated. However, when appropriate and immediate therapy—without awaiting the definite diagnostic confirmation—is initiated, AI has no major additional impact on the morbidity and mortality risk of the underlying disease. The 'five S's' in the management are saline, sugar, steroids, support, and search for a precipitating event. Volume should be rapidly restored by several litres of saline solution with 5% glucose (to correct possible hypoglycaemia). After a diagnostic blood sample has been obtained, most authors recommend a 100 mg intravenous bolus of hydrocortisone followed by 100 mg every 8 h. No additional mineralocorticoids are needed with these high doses of glucocorticoids. If the precipitating event or illness—frequently an infection—has been controlled, glucocorticoids should be tapered gradually to a maintenance dose. In addition, drugs that accelerate glucocorticoid metabolism (e.g. phenytoin, barbiturates, rifampicin) should be avoided if possible.

During therapy, electrolyte and glucose levels must always be carefully monitored and corrected, particularly if concomitant diabetes insipidus is suspected. As absence of cortisol inhibits free water clearance (i.e. polyuria) in these patients, glucocorticoid administration may induce or aggravate diabetes insipidus.

To prevent adrenal crisis in patients under chronic glucocorticoid treatment or with known AI, maintenance doses of steroids should be augmented when these patients undergo surgery or suffer from an acute illness (◑ Fig. 68.2). In addition, one should also be attentive for the high vulnerability of patients with Cushing's disease to develop acute AI after hypophysectomy.

Conclusion

Although endocrine emergencies are relatively uncommon, the clinical diagnosis should never be missed as delay can lead to devastating complications and often death. A high degree of clinical suspicion and prompt institution of aggressive, comprehensive treatment including supportive measures and endocrine replacement or blockage therapy are the cornerstones of successful management of these complex disorders.

Personal perspective

As understanding the pathophysiology is essential to the optimal treatment of these complex alterations and in keeping with the multidisciplinary nature of critical care medicine, it is advisable to consult an endocrinologist to help confirm the diagnosis and assist in the patient management.

Further reading

Arlt W, Allolio B. Adrenal insufficiency. *Lancet* 2003;**361**:1881–1893.

Bouillon R. Acute adrenal insufficiency. *Endocrinol Metab Clin North Am* 2006;**35**:767–775.

Bravo EL, Tagle R. Pheochromocytoma: state-of-the-art and future prospects. *Endocr Rev* 2003;**24**:539–553.

Burch HB, Wartofsky L Life-threatening thyrotoxicosis. Thyroid storm. *Endocrinol Metab Clin North Am* 1993;**22**:263–277.

Coursin DB, Wood KE. Corticosteroid supplementation for adrenal insufficiency. *JAMA* 2002;**287**:236–240.

Eskes SA, Wiersinga WM. Amiodarone and thyroid. *Best Pract Res Clin Endocrinol Metab* 2009;**23**:735–751.

Lenders JW, Eisenhofer G, Mannelli M, Pacak K. Phaeochromocytoma. *Lancet* 2005;**366**:665–675.

Marik PE, Pastores SM, Annane D, *et al.* Recommendations for the diagnosis and management of corticosteroid insufficiency in critically ill adult patients: consensus statements from an international task force by the American College of Critical Care Medicine. *Crit Care Med* 2008;**36**:1937–1949.

Nayak B, Burman K. Thyrotoxicosis and thyroid storm. *Endocrinol Metab Clin North Am* 2006;**35**:663–686.

Wartofsky L. Myxedema coma. *Endocrinol Metab Clin North Am* 2006;**35**:687–698.

➲ For additional multimedia materials please visit the online version of the book (🖱 http://www.esciacc.oxfordmedicine.com).

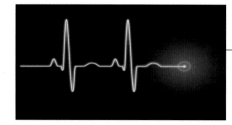

CHAPTER 69

Bleeding and haemostasis disorders

Pier Mannuccio Mannucci

Contents

Summary

The main cause of the haemostasis defects and related bleeding complications in patients with acute coronary syndromes (ACS) is the use of multiple antithrombotic drugs, alone or in association with invasive procedures such as percutaneous coronary intervention (PCI) with stent deployment. These drugs act on several components of haemostasis (platelet function, coagulation, fibrinolysis) and may be associated with major bleeding, particularly in elderly patients, those who are underweight and with cormobid conditions such as renal insufficiency, diabetes, malignancy, and hypertension. Identification of patients at higher risk of bleeding is the most important preventive strategy. Transfusions of red blood cells and platelets may become necessary in patients with severe bleeding but should be used with caution, because massively transfused patients with ACS have a high rate of adverse outcomes (death, myocardial infarction, and stroke). To reduce the need for transfusion, the general haemostatic agents that decrease blood loss and transfusion requirements in cardiac surgery (antifibrinolytic amino acids, desmopressin, recombinant factor VIIa) might be considered. However, efficacy of these agents in the control of bleeding complications in ACS is not unequivocally established, and there is concern for an increased risk of thrombosis. A low platelet count is another cause of bleeding in the intensive cardiac care unit (ICCU). The main aetiologies are drugs (unfractionated heparin and anti-IIb/IIIa inhibitors), thrombotic thrombocytopenic purpura, and disseminated intravascular coagulation, often paradoxically associated with thrombotic manifestations. In conclusion, evidence-based recommendations for the management of bleeding in patients admitted to the ICCU are lacking. Accurate assessment of the risk of bleeding and prevention are the most valid strategies.

Introduction

When the integrity of the blood vessel wall is altered, blood loss is stopped by the action of the haemostasis system, ultimately leading to clot formation and vascular sealing. Haemostasis is in turn assured by three phases that, acting in synergy, lead to the arrest of bleeding: (1) the platelet phase, (2) blood coagulation, and (3) fibrinolysis.

Haemostasis: the platelet phase

Vascular injury exposes circulating blood to subendothelial layers to which blood platelets tether and adhere by interacting with collagen fibres and the adhesive multimeric glycoprotein von Willebrand factor. The ultimate result of these reactions is platelet aggregation and formation of the primary haemostatic plug. Quantitative or qualitative defects of platelets lead to the inadequate or delayed formation of this plug and may cause bleeding, which occurs mainly in the skin and mucosal tracts (petechiae, epistaxis, menorrhagia, melena). Platelet defects can generally be controlled by replacement therapy through the transfusion of allogeneic platelets.

Blood coagulation

The primary platelet plug is frail and unable to stop bleeding (particularly from large vessels) unless it is strengthened by a mesh of fibrin. Fibrin formation is the final event of blood coagulation, and results from the sequential activation of coagulation factors ultimately leading to the transformation of the soluble plasma protein fibrinogen into fibrin. Congenital or acquired defects of coagulation factors cause a bleeding tendency, usually more clinically severe than that due to platelet defects. Bleeding mainly occurs in soft tissues, joints, from trauma- or surgery-induced wounds, at venous access sites, and, more rarely, in such life-threatening sites as the central nervous system, the retroperitoneal space and the gastrointestinal tract. When bleeding is due to single defects of coagulation factors (as in the haemophilias), the best therapeutic approach is specific replacement of the deficient factor. More often, particularly in acquired coagulation defects, more than one factor is deficient in plasma. A typical example is the defect induced by vitamin K antagonists used for therapeutic anticoagulation.

Fibrinolysis

The fibrinolytic system is made of enzymes that ultimately activate the proenzyme plasminogen to plasmin, which has the property to lyse clots. The most frequent clinical condition associated with hyperfibrinolysis is the therapeutic administration of tissue plasminogen activators or other fibrinolytic drugs to obtain thrombolysis in patients with acute coronary syndromes (ACS) or with arterial or venous thrombosis in other sites.

Haemostasis defects and bleeding in the intensive cardiac care unit

In the intensive cardiac care unit (ICCU), excessive bleeding typically occurs in patients with multiple haemostasis defects owing to the inhibition of coagulation by anticoagulants and platelet function by such drugs as aspirin, clopidogrel, and inhibitors of glycoprotein IIb/IIIa (GPIs). Thrombolytic therapy also causes hyperfibrinolysis. Multiple haemostasis defects that sometime lead to excessive blood loss typically develop after cardiac surgery, for several reasons: the large size of surgical wounds, decrease of platelet number during the circulation of blood in the extracorporeal oxygenator, hypocoagulability owing to incomplete neutralization of heparin after pump discontinuation, and complex defects of platelet function often accompanied by hyperfibrinolysis.

In this chapter the general measures that help to stop bleeding and/or reduce transfusion requirements when major blood loss occurs, irrespective of the nature and degree of the haemostatic defect, are first described. Cardiac surgery is taken as a proxy of the potential clinical efficacy of these measures, because haemostatic agents have been extensively investigated only in this context. Major bleeding and its management in patients with ACS treated with multiple antithrombotic drugs, often in association with the use of invasive procedures, is then discussed. Finally, the thrombocytopenic states that sometime occur in the ICCU, which may cause bleeding but also very severe thrombotic manifestations, are reviewed.

General haemostatic measures

The drugs that have been evaluated clinically are the antifibrinolytic amino acids aminocaproic acid and tranexamic acid, obtained by chemical synthesis; the broad-spectrum protease inhibitor aprotinin, extracted from bovine lung; the synthetic analogue of the antidiuretic hormone desmopressin and the activated form of coagulation factor VII (FVIIa) produced by recombinant DNA technology [1, 2]. Local measures should also be considered.

Antifibrinolytic amino acids

6-Aminohexanoic acid (ε-aminocaproic acid, aminocaproic acid) was the first drug of this category to be introduced and evaluated therapeutically [3]. 4-Aminomethyl cyclohexane-carboxylic acid (tranexamic acid) was subsequently developed: it is approximately 10 times more potent and has a longer half-life that permits dosing at more widely spaced intervals [4]. Both drugs inhibit fibrinolysis by saturating the lysine-binding sites on the plasminogen molecule, which are essential for binding of this precursor of plasmin to fibrin clots [5]. In cardiac surgery, both tranexamic and aminocaproic acid reduce the need for perioperative blood transfusion by approximately 30–40% [6]; there is also a reduction in the need for reoperation due to bleeding [6]. The main perceived risk of these drugs is thrombosis, owing to their inhibition of such an important antithrombotic system as fibrinolysis. For dosages and schedules of administration, see ❍ Table 69.1.

Aprotinin

This broad-spectrum protease inhibitor inhibits the fibrinolytic enzyme plasmin [7, 8]. In cardiac surgery, a Cochrane systematic review [6] demonstrated a reduction by 30% of

Table 69.1 General strategies for management of excessive bleeding

Strategy	Principles of management
Conservative measures	Compression only, where the site of minor bleeding is accessible
	Fibrin glue application to active bleeding sites where accessible
Antifibrinolytic amino acids	Tranexamic acid: oral 10–25 mg/kg every 8 h; intravenous 10–15 mg/kg every 8 h
	Aminocaproic acid: oral/intravenous 50–60 mg/kg every 4 h
Desmopressin	IV infusions of 30 min duration (0.3–0.4 μg/kg) at 12–24-h intervals, maximum 3–4 doses
Recombinant factor VIIa	Bolus injections: 80–100 μg/kg at intervals of 3 h, ≥3 doses. After bleeding stops, additional consolidation doses may help to decrease recurrence
Platelet transfusion	Only for severe bleeding or cases in which the aforementioned haemostatic drugs fail and before invasive procedures
	Dosage: one single-donor apheresis unit (or 6–8 random-donor units) is the standard dose for adult patients
	Use HLA-compatible and leucocyte-depleted platelets where available and when possible
	Continue until resolution of bleeding

the need for allogeneic transfusion of red cells, platelets, and fresh-frozen plasma, and a 60% reduction in the need for reoperation following excessive peri- and postoperative bleeding. Unfortunately the recent BART trial [9], carried out in 2331 patients undergoing complex cardiac operations at particularly high risk of excessive bleeding [9], had to be prematurely interrupted because of a higher 30-day mortality in patients receiving aprotinin (6.0%), compared with with 3.9% in the tranexamic acid and 4.0% in the aminocaproic acid treated patients [9]. The death excess observed in aprotinin-treated patients was mainly due to cardiac causes. In all, the BART study has shown that antifibrinolytic amino acids are perhaps somewhat less effective than aprotinin in reducing blood loss and transfusion requirements [6], but much safer and much less expensive.

Desmopressin

This agent is currently licensed only for the treatment of patients with mild to moderate haemophilia and von Willebrand's disease [1, 2]. In these conditions the efficacy of desmopressin is well established, owing to its property to increase the plasma levels of factor VIII and ultralarge von Willebrand factor multimers that are hyperactive in primary haemostasis [1, 2]. This drug has also been used to reduce blood loss and transfusion requirements in cardiac surgery and in other medical and surgical situations associated with excessive bleeding. Recommended dosages are shown in ❍ Table 69.1.

Recombinant activated factor VII

Produced by recombinant DNA technology, this activated form of coagulation factor VII promotes haemostasis by binding to tissue factor exposed on the damaged vessel wall and in the extravascular space and generating small amounts of thrombin [10–12]. In turn, thrombin acts mainly through further generation of thrombin on the platelet surface. The platelet reactions triggered by FVIIa and thrombin ultimately generate enough thrombin to transform plasma fibrinogen to fibrin at the site of vascular injury. FVIIa is also prohaemostatic through the inhibition of fibrinolysis [13]. Recombinant FVIIa was initially developed to bypass the coagulation defect in patients with haemophilia A complicated by anti-FVIII antibodies, and is licensed for the treatment of bleeding in these patients. The drug is also licensed to control bleeding in patients with Glanzman thrombasthenia, a rare but severe defect of platelet function due to the deficiency or dysfunction of platelet GPIIb/IIIa. The clinical use of FVIIa has also been proposed for treatment of haemorrhages caused by the use of anticoagulant or antiplatelet agents [14–17]. For recommended dosages, see ⊃ Table 69.1.

At the moment, recombinant FVIIa is not licensed for indications other than haemophilia and thrombasthenia, and can only be administered on a named patient basis. There is no randomized clinical trial showing its efficacy beyond haemophilia and thrombasthenia, the drug is very expensive, and the risk of thrombotic complications looms very large, particularly in patients with ACS already at high risk of this complication.

Local haemostatic measures

Finally, it must be pointed out that when there is excessive bleeding, before considering the use of the aforementioned haemostatic agents and of transfusional products, simple conservative measures should be considered such as the application of pressure to any accessible bleeding site, with or without the adoption of adjunctive local measures such as fibrin glue. ⊃ Table 69.1 summarizes the strategies that can be adopted for the management of excessive bleeding.

Bleeding complications in acute coronary syndromes

In patients treated in the ICCU for ACS, bleeding may range from minor (e.g. epistaxis) to life-endangering gastrointestinal, intracranial, and retroperitoneal haemorrhages. Bleeding at the vascular access site after percutaneous coronary intervention (PCI) is the most common complication in patients with ACS. PCI with stenting is carried out in 60–70% of patients with ACS who undergo diagnostic coronary angiography, the remainder being treated medically or with urgent coronary artery bypass surgery (CABG). These invasive procedures, carried out in patients taking multiple anticoagulant and antiplatelet agents, dramatically increase the risk of bleeding. Excessive bleeding is particularly frequent in ACS patients at high preprocedural risk such as those who are elderly, underweight, or with renal insufficiency [18]. It is also more frequent in women, because of their smaller weights on average and often older age of ACS occurrence than in men.

Categorization of bleeding severity

There have been attempts to categorize the severity of bleeding, but there is no uniform definition, leading to significant variations in the reported incidence of bleeding in patients with ACS, which ranges from as little as 0.2% to as high as 11.5% [19]. Originally bleeding was classified as major when it was intracranial, retroperitoneal, or associated with anaemia severe enough to warrant blood transfusion [20]. Other criteria have subsequently been developed in the attempt to define the severity of bleeding more accurately in nonsurgical cardiac patients [21]. The criteria adopted in the framework of the TIMI clinical trials of antithrombotic therapies are based on clinical and laboratory measurements that identify four categories of bleeding (major, minor, minimal, none) [22]. The criteria adopted by the GUSTO trialists also identify four categories (severe or life-threatening, moderate, mild, none), on the basis of the need of transfusion and the presence of haemodynamic compromise [23]. The evaluation of the risk of bleeding with these criteria does not give identical results. Even though some believe that the GUSTO criteria give more reliable and clinically relevant results (⊃ Table 69.2) [24], alternative criteria are being used, adding to the existing confusion. For instance, the sensitive ACUITY criteria identify major bleeding on the basis of a full clinical assessment, changes in haemoglobin levels, haematomas greater than 5 cm, and the need for blood transfusion.

Blood transfusion and clinical outcomes

Major or moderately severe bleeding has a negative effect on prognosis, as established by results of meta-analyses, large registries, and clinical trials. Overall, major bleeding in patients with ACS is associated with an approximately fivefold increased risk of death at 30 days, a fivefold increase in myocardial infarction (MI), and a threefold increase in ischaemic stroke [25, 26]. Even though some maintain that

Table 69.2 Bleeding classifications

TIMI	
Major	ICH or ↓ Hb ≥5 g/dL or ↓ Hct ≥15%*
Minor	Observed blood loss: ↓ Hb ≥3 g/dL or ↓ Hct ≥10%*No observed blood loss: ↓ Hb ≥4 g/dL or ↓ Hct ≥12%*
Minimal	Any clinically overt sign of haemorrhage (including imaging) associated with ↓ Hb ≤ 3 g/dL or ↓ Hct <9%*
GUSTO	
Severe or life threatening	ICH or bleeding causing haemodynamic compromise and intervention
Moderate	Bleeding requiring blood transfusion but without haemodynamic compromise
Mild	bleeding without the previous criteria

Hb, haemoglobin; Hct, haematocrit; ICH, intracerebral haemorrhage; ↓, reduction; *, absolute values.
Modified from Rao *et al.* [24].

the relationship between bleeding and these adverse outcomes is not causal and that excess mortality is accounted for more frequent comorbidities in bleeders [27], the perceived clinical relevance of this complication has led bleeding to be added to the traditional triad of events (death, MI, urgent revascularization) employed to evaluate the benefits of antithrombotic drugs in ACS patients undergoing PCI [28].

Because of the negative prognostic role of bleeding, it would be logical to assume that the early and liberal use of blood transfusion, and particularly of red cells and platelets, should benefit patients and decrease the rate of unfavourable events associated with bleeding. However, a number of studies indicate that clinical responses to blood transfusion are not favourable. A meta-analysis of 3 large clinical trials enrolling a total of 24 112 ACS patients showed that transfusion was associated with an approximately fourfold increased risk for 30-day mortality, even after adjustment for factors such as baseline and nadir haematocrit and the type of invasive procedures [29]. Even though contrasting data show a favourable effect of blood transfusion on the rates of adverse outcomes [31], the intensive and liberal use of transfusions should be adopted with caution in order to maintain normal levels of haemoglobin. Blood products should preferably be leucocyte-depleted, because multiply transfused patients undergoing cardiac surgery have a higher mortality if nondepleted transfusion products are preferred (whole blood, red cells, and platelets).

Prevention of bleeding and transfusion requirements

The concerns on the adverse effects of blood transfusion in patients with ACS emphasize the role of prevention. The aforementioned haemostatic agents have the potential to prevent or stop bleeding and to avoid transfusion. On the other hand, they may increase the risk of recurrent or novel thrombotic events in ACS patients. No randomized study has so far attempted to establish whether or not haemostatic drugs of established efficacy in cardiac surgery help to prevent or stop bleeding in patients with ACS or, most importantly, to avoid or at least reduce potentially dangerous transfusions of allogeneic blood products. At the moment available evidence on the clinical impact of the off-label use of haemostatic agents in ACS stems from case reports or small case series with no adequate control [15–17]. Furthermore, the frequent parallel use of other agents with a potentially favourable impact on haemostasis (such as fresh-frozen plasma and platelet concentrates) confuses our understanding of the efficacy of these drugs.

Hence, the best strategy in the ICCU is to accurately evaluate the risk of bleeding in the individual patient and to tailor the choice and dosages of antithrombotic drugs on risk magnitude. Evaluation of the patient's individual risk is based on the well-established knowledge that there are comorbid conditions and/or patient features that increase the risk of bleeding during antithrombotic therapy for ACS. There have been efforts to combine risk factors in the attempt to develop scores of bleeding risk intended to help clinicians in the choice and dosage of antithrombotic drugs for the medical treatment of ACS, with or without PCI. For instance, a bleeding score validated in patients with ACS is that proposed in the frame of CRUSADE [31], which includes eight parameters (♣ 69.1). According to CRUSADE, the risk of bleeding ranges from very low (score <20, predicted rate of major bleeding 3.1%), low (21–30, 5.5%), moderate (score 31–40, 8.6%) to high (score 41–50, 11.2%) and very high (>50, 19.5%) [31].

Bleeding risk of different antithrombotic drugs

The relationships between different antithrombotic drugs, their dosage, characteristics of the patient population, clinical conditions that led to use of antithrombotics, and the risk of haemorrhagic complications were recently reviewed in the framework of the American College of Chest Physicians (ACCP) guidelines [32]. In general, the new anticoagulants fondaparinux and bivalirudin cause a reduction in bleeding events, in comparison with unfractionated heparin (UFH) and low-molecular-weight heparins (LMWHs), and this reduction translates into a reduction in major adverse cardiac events (MACEs), both non-ST ACS (NSTE-ACS) [33] and ST-elevation myocardial infarction (STEMI) [34]. However, comparisons of between-drug safety are jeopardized by such uncontrolled variables as the selected dosages of antithrombotic drugs and other characteristics and risk factors in the patients actually treated [35].

Bleeding due to anticoagulation with vitamin K antagonists

Vitamin K antagonists such as warfarin and related drugs are efficacious in reducing arterial and venous thromboembolic events through the induction of a complex coagulation defect due to the abnormal biosynthesis of factors II, VII, IX, and X. In spite of improved laboratory control introduced by the widespread adoption of the international normalized ratio (INR), elevated INR values (whether or not associated with bleeding complications), may still occur in patients on vitamin K antagonists. If the patient admitted to ICCU while on vitamin K antagonists is not bleeding, and no invasive procedure is planned (e.g. coronary angiography or PCI), and no other antithrombotic drugs are added (e.g. fibrinolytic or antiplatelet agents), it is usually sufficient to stop warfarin until INR values return to the therapeutic range (in most clinical situations, between 2.0 and 3.0). Following this approach, the risk of bleeding is small (particularly if INR values are below 6.0), and there is no need to give supplemental vitamin K.

When INR values are above 6.0 and/or the nonbleeding patient warrants rapid reversal of anticoagulation because of the need of invasive procedures or powerful antithrombotic treatment (e.g. fibrinolysis followed or not by PCI), intravenous vitamin K_1, at dosages varying between 1.0 and 2.0 mg depending on patient weight, usually reverses the anticoagulant effect almost completely within 12–16 h. Similar effects can also be obtained with oral vitamin K_1 (the aforementioned dosages should be doubled), but the time until reversal is obviously somewhat longer (up to 24 h).

When the warfarin-treated patient is bleeding and/or there are clinical reasons demanding urgent reversal (e.g. emergency cardiac surgery) the approach differs depending on bleeding severity. If bleeding is minor (haematuria, oozing from venous access sites), the administration of vitamin K_1 as indicated above is usually sufficient and efficacious. When bleeding is major or occurs in life-threatening sites (the central nervous system or the retroperitoneal space) and major surgery cannot be deferred by 24–48 h, replacement therapy of the defective coagulation factor becomes necessary. The simplest method is the infusion of fresh-frozen plasma, which at a dose of 15–20 ml/kg usually obtains the almost complete reversal of the coagulation defect. The limits of this approach are the need of prolonging the infusion to 2–3 h to avoid transfusion reactions and volume overload, and that correction is not always complete in patients with very high INR values. The alternative weapon is plasma concentrates containing all the vitamin-K dependent coagulation factors (prothrombin complex concentrates, PCC), which achieve more rapid and complete normalization of the INR and stop bleeding more quickly. A dose of 20–30 IU/kg is usually adequate but if necessary it can be repeated at least once until normal INR values are obtained. There are several commercial brands of PCC; some contain all the vitamin-K dependent

factors but others do not contain factor VII. However, this does not apparently affect the reversal of the anticoagulant action.

Causes of thrombocytopenia in the intensive cardiac care unit

A low platelet count is sometime related to the use of drugs [35], but can also develop as a consequence of massive transfusion and of hypovolaemic shock after major blood loss. Some thrombocytopenias may be accompanied by a bleeding tendency, such as those occurring within the first 24 h after the use of GPIs. The most frequently implicated is abiciximab (incidence 0.5–1.0%), which lowers platelet counts through the formation of antibodies directed against the murine component of the monoclonal antibody and the subsequent removal from the circulating blood of antibody-loaded platelets. Other GPI inhibitors such as tirofiban and eptifibatide much less frequently (0.2–0.5%) cause thrombocytopenia, which develops due to the formation of neoantigens and antiplatelet antibodies following binding of drugs to their target, i.e. the platelet GPIIb/IIIa. The rate of occurrence of thrombocytopenia is much higher after drug re-exposure. The clinical manifestations of thrombocytopenia ensuing after the intake of these drugs are seldom severe and usually do not warrant replacement therapy with platelet concentrates, nor the intake of corticosteroids to block the production and action of antibodies.

Heparin-induced thrombocytopenia

Heparin-induced thrombocytopenia (HIT) typically develops 5–10 days after the onset of a first therapeutic course of UFH, and is due to autoantibodies reacting with complexes that form on the platelet surface between heparin and platelet factor 4. UFH is much more immunogenic than LMWHs and fondaparinux [36–38]. The risk associated with these drugs is much smaller but not trivial, because they both share the pentasaccharide structure with UFH. Complexes that form between autoantibodies, heparin, and factor 4 activate platelets and heighten thrombin generation leading to a strong hypercoagulable state. Hence the most serious clinical consequence of HIT is the occurrence, in up to 75% of patients, of venous or arterial thrombosis [36], often developing at the same vascular district that initially made the therapeutic use of heparin necessary. Mortality from HIT can be as high as 20% and major complications such as limb loss or stroke are not rare. Some serological tests detect antiplatelet antibodies, but they are useful only for their negative predictive value, because there may also be positivity in heparin-treated patients who are and may remain symptom-free [34–36]. The most important therapeutic measure is to stop UFH if HIT is asymptomatic, and to treat thrombotic symptoms with anticoagulants structurally unrelated to heparin, such as the direct thrombin inhibitors lepirudin, bivalirudin, or argatroban, and the heparinoid danaparoid. Vitamin K antagonists such as warfarin should not be used in the acute phase of HIT-associated thrombosis, because the onset of the anticoagulant effect of these drugs is delayed and the early treatment of thrombotic manifestations is compelling.

Box 69.1 lists the cornerstones of management in patients with or without thrombosis admitted to ICCU.

Thrombotic thrombocytopenic purpura

Thrombotic thrombocytopenic purpura (TTP) is a rare disease that may occur in patients with ACS treated with antiplatelet agents of the thienopyridine family (ticlopidine and, less frequently, clopidogrel). It is also a rare complication of cardiac surgery. TTP is associated with a decrease of platelet count accompanied by haemolytic anaemia due to *in vivo* fragmentation of red cells [39–41]. Low platelet

count is due to their *in vivo* consumption following the intravascular formation of platelet-rich thrombi in the microcirculation, leading in turn to ischaemia in multiple organs (most often the brain, followed by the kidney, myocardium, and gastrointestinal tract). Platelet-rich thrombi are in turn due to *in vivo* platelet aggregation induced by the ultralarge thrombogenic forms of von Willebrand factor (VWF), which are not cleaved to the less thrombogenic physiological forms because of the deficiency or dysfunction of the plasma metalloprotease ADAMTS13 [39, 40]. The thienopyridine-associated forms of TTP, which usually develop 10–15 days after the intake of ticlopidine or clopidogrel, should be treated with daily sessions of plasma exchange (4–6 L plasma) associated with the administration of corticosteroids (1.0–1.5 mg/kg, tapered off over 35–45 days). The outcome of TTP after thienopyridine intake is usually favourable, provided the complication is promptly diagnosed, implicated drugs are stopped and plasma exchange is initiated early and continued for 7–10 days or more. ADAMTS13 assays are useful but not essential for diagnosis, because there are TTP cases with normal levels of the VWF-cleaving protease [41].

Disseminated intravascular coagulation

Disseminated intravascular coagulation (DIC) may develop in the ICCU for two main reasons: bacterial infections (often related to infected catheters and other devices used for venous access) and posthaemorrhagic hypovolaemic shock. Bleeding symptoms may be prominent (oozing from venous lines, gastrointestinal bleeding, soft-tissue haematomas) but ischaemic symptoms due to microvascular thrombosis may also occur as a result of the impairment of the microcirculation of several organs (mainly the kidney) [40]. Thrombocytopenia varies from moderate to severe and there are signs of heightened activation of the coagulation system, the most typical being the presence of marked elevations of the fibrin degradation product D-dimer, a marker of fibrin formation, usually in excess of 3000–4000 µg/mL [42, 43]. More rarely, there are laboratory signs of consumption coagulopathy, with prolongations of the prothrombin time, low plasma levels of fibrinogen and other coagulation factors and inhibitors (FV, FVIII, antithrombin, protein C).

The mechanistic approach to the treatment of DIC is based principally on the removal of the underlying condition, such as bacterial infections and haemorrhagic shock, and the correction of an often present acidosis (Box 69.2).

Box 69.1 Cornerstones of management of heparin-induced thrombocytopenia in the intensive cardiac care unit

In patients without thrombosis

- Suspect HIT in patients treated with heparin with an unexplained >50% reduction of platelet count, >5 days after starting the drug

- Suspect HIT earlier (within 48 h after starting heparin) if there was previous exposure to this anticoagulant

In patients with thrombosis

- Heparin should be discontinued immediately

- As anticoagulants use direct thrombin inhibitors (e.g. lepirudin) or heparinoids (e.g. danaparoid).

- Recommended dosages: for danaparoid, 2000 units as intravenous bolus, followed by 2000 units subcutaneously twice daily; for lepirudin, 0.1–0.4 mg/kg bolus, followed by 0.1–0.15 mg/kg per hour intravenously

- Avoid warfarin until platelet count is normal

Box 69.2 Management of disseminated intravascular coagulation in the intensive cardiac care unit

- Identification and removal of the underlying cause (i.e. antibiotics for bacterial infections and restoration of haemodynamic stability due to hypovolaemic shock by means of whole blood transfusion)

- Basic support measures, with close attention to circulatory volume status, gas exchange, pH, electrolyte balance

- Platelet transfusion to maintain the platelet count >20 $\times 10^9$/L: only if the patient is bleeding or a procedure is planned

- Fresh-frozen plasma (15–20 mL/kg): only if bleeding is accompanied by prolonged coagulation tests (prothrombin time, partial thromboplastin time or thrombin time)

- Unfractionated heparin (80 U/kg IV bolus, followed by continuous infusion of 15–20 U/kg/hr) only in the presence of thrombotic symptoms

- Antithrombin and activated protein C concentrates: considered only in cases associated with sepsis and thrombotic symptoms

Box 69.3 Sequential steps for the management of bleeding associated with the use of antithrombotic drugs in the intensive cardiac care unit

Minor bleeding

- Measure global coagulation tests (prothrombin time, activated partial thromboplastin time, thrombin time) and complete blood count

- Watch the evolution by assessing and monitoring vital signs and complete blood count

- Avoid withdrawing antithrombotic drugs for as long as possible

Major bleeding

- Measure global coagulation tests (prothrombin time, activated partial thromboplastin time, thrombin time) and complete blood count

- Withdraw antithrombotic drugs

- Consider red cell and platelet transfusions (see ⊃ Table 69.1 for recommended dosages)

- Consider administration of haemostatic drugs (antifibrinolytic amino acids) (see ⊃ Table 69.1 for recommended dosages)

Replacement of the deficient factors and platelets by means of the infusion of fresh-frozen plasma or platelet concentrates is usually advisable when bleeding is associated with abnormal coagulation tests, even though there is some concern that the exogenous supply of factors and platelets may help to maintain the DIC process. Replacement therapy with naturally occurring anticoagulants, such as large doses of antithrombin concentrates or recombinant activated protein C, has been advocated but evidence of clinical efficacy is weak [43].

Conclusion

The combined use of multiple antithrombotic drugs has dramatically improved the prognosis of ACS, but has also increased the risk of bleeding, even though the overall balance is definitely in favour of the use of antithrombotic agents. The most important approach is prevention, which can be realized through the scrutiny of the pattern of risk factors in each patient. We do not recommend withdrawing the antithrombotic strategies and invasive procedures that are of proven efficacy in ACS in patients at high risk of bleeding.

However, the combination of drugs and their dosage may be tailored and modified for individual patients and their category of risk (see ⊃ Personal perspectives for examples).

If bleeding is severe, transfusion of blood products should be considered. However, the concept that patients with coronary artery disease should be aggressively transfused because of the putative adverse effects of anaemia on their heart disease has been challenged by the accumulating evidence that intense transfusional regimens may increase mortality and cause more cardiovascular events. Haemostatic drugs are definitely capable of reducing blood loss and transfusion requirements in cardiac surgery, particularly in complex operations. Antifibrinolytic amino acids and desmopressin should be preferred for their greater safety and lower cost. However, it remains to be established whether or not these drugs are also efficacious when bleeding occurs in patients with ACS treated with antithrombotic drugs. This question should be answered by means of controlled clinical trials.

⊃ Box 69.3 summarizes sequential steps to be considered for the general management of bleeding in patients with ACS admitted to the ICCU and treated with multiple antithrombotic drugs.

Personal perspective

Bleeding complications are unlikely to diminish in the near future, owing to the increasing age of the patient population, as well as to the development of more and more potent antithrombotic drugs and revascularization procedures. Hence, prevention is crucial, and this goal can only be achieved through the careful evaluation of the bleeding risk in each patient, e.g. using the CRUSADE score. In patients at high risk, the currently recommended combinations of multiple antithrombotic drugs and their dosages can perhaps be tailored and modified. For instance, fondaparinux or bivalirudin may be considered instead of heparin in ACS, while GPIs, which are recommended in addition to aspirin and clopidogrel in high-risk patients with ACS undergoing PCI, may be withdrawn. By the same token, double loading and maintenance doses of clopidogrel (600 and 150 mg daily), which are sometime used to circumvent poor responsiveness to this antiplatelet drug, should be avoided in patients at high risk of bleeding. In general, it is better to reduce dosages rather than to have to stop all antithrombotic drugs after the patient has bled. Haemostatic drugs that have proved their efficacy in cardiac surgery, and particularly antifibrinolytic amino acids, should be considered for prophylactic administration in patients at high risk of bleeding as well as for treatment of actual bleeders, with the goal of avoiding or reducing the need for blood transfusion and the corresponding risks. It is unlikely that randomized clinical trials will be conducted to provide definite evidence of efficacy, because there is little pharmaceutical interest in evaluating these drugs in the clinical context of ACS. Furthermore, there is the as yet unsubstantiated fear that haemostatic agents may increase the risk of thrombosis.

Further reading

Allford SL, Hunt BJ, Rose P, Machin SJ. Guidelines on the diagnosis and management of the thrombotic microangiopathic haemolytic anaemias. *Br J Haematol* 2003;**120**(4):556–573.

Arepally GM, Ortel TL. Clinical practice. Heparin-induced thrombocytopenia. *N Engl J Med* 2006;**355**(8):809–817.

Aster RH, Bougie DW. Drug-induced immune thrombocytopenia. *N Engl J Med* 2007;**357**(6):580–587.

De Luca L, Casella G, Lettino M, *et al.* Clinical implications and management of bleeding events in patients with acute coronary syndromes. *J Cardiovasc Med* 2009;**10**(9):677–686.

Levi M. Disseminated intravascular coagulation. *Crit Care Med* 2007;**35**(9):2191–2195.

Levi M. Epidemiology and management of bleeding in patients using vitamin K antagonists. *J Thromb Haemost* 2009;**7** (Suppl 1):103–106.

Levi M, Peters M, Buller HR. Efficacy and safety of recombinant factor VIIa for treatment of severe bleeding: a systematic review. *Crit Care Med* 2005;**33**(4):883–890.

Levi M, Toh CH, Thachil J, Watson HG. Guidelines for the diagnosis and management of disseminated intravascular coagulation. British Committee for Standards in Haematology. *Br J Haematol* 2009;**145**(1):24–33.

Makris M. Management of excessive anticoagulation or bleeding. *Semin Vasc Med* 2003;**3**(3):279–284.

Mannucci PM, Levi M. Prevention and treatment of major blood loss. *N Engl J Med* 2007;**356**(22):2301–2311.

Mannucci PM. Hemostatic drugs. *N Engl J Med* 1998;**339**(4):245–253.

Roberts HR, Monroe DM, White GC. The use of recombinant factor VIIa in the treatment of bleeding disorders. *Blood* 2004;**104**(13):3858–3864.

Schulman S, Beyth RJ, Kearon C, Levine MN. Hemorrhagic complications of anticoagulant and thrombolytic treatment: American College of Chest Physicians Evidence-Based Clinical Practice Guidelines (8th Edition). *Chest* 2008;**133**(6 Suppl):257S–298S.

Additional online material

69.1 Components of the CRUSADE bleeding score

➲ For additional multimedia materials please visit the online version of the book (✍ http://www.esciacc.oxfordmedicine.com).

CHAPTER 70

Anaemia and transfusion

Jean-Pierre Bassand, Francois Schiele,
and Nicolas Meneveau

Contents

Summary

Bleeding, anaemia, and transfusion impact greatly on prognosis in acute coronary syndromes (ACS). Bleeding is associated with a three- to five-fold higher rate of death, and death/myocardial infarction at 30 days and 6 months. Anaemia at admission is associated with a stepwise increase in the rate of death and myocardial infarction with decreasing levels of admission haemoglobin below 15–16 g/dL, and is also an independent predictor of bleeding complications, with a stepwise increase in the risk of major bleeds with declining admission haemoglobin.

Transfusions should be given in patients with haemodynamic instability. In stable patients, blood transfusion has deleterious effects if administered for haematocrit levels greater than 25%, but beneficial effects if given for haematocrit less than 25%. Iron therapy is necessary, irrespective of the cause of anaemia. Erythropoietin derivatives are contraindicated because of adverse side effects. A thorough search for the cause of anaemia is an essential part of the management strategy.

Introduction

Bleeding, anaemia and transfusion are three factors that impact greatly on prognosis in acute coronary syndromes (ACS) but also in percutaneous coronary interventions (PCI) [1–4]. Bleeding actually has a strong impact on outcome, with a four- to fivefold increase in the rate of death, myocardial infarction (MI), or stroke at 30 days and 6 months [2, 4]. Anaemia at admission has also been recently identified as a strong marker of the risk of both further ischaemic events and bleeding complications in ACS [1, 5]. The negative impact of anaemia at admission was also observed in PCI, cardiac surgery, heart failure, and in several noncardiac settings, such as diabetes and chronic kidney disease, as well as in elderly patients [6–18]. Both bleeding and anaemia at admission may trigger the use of blood transfusion, that has been shown to have deleterious effects, depending on the level of haematocrit at which transfusion is prescribed [19]; blood transfusion policies have therefore been reconsidered [20].

Bleeding complications in acute coronary syndromes (see also ⊃ Chapter 69)

Several concordant reports have shown that bleeding at the initial phase of ACS leads to a three- to fivefold increase in the risk of death and also of MI and stroke at 30 days and 6 months [2, 4]. Although several hypotheses exist, the mechanisms by which bleeding influences outcome are as yet poorly understood. Indeed, bleeding may lead to haemodynamic compromise through hypovolaemia, triggering a hyperadrenergic state, which can have deleterious consequences on an already ischaemic myocardium. Discontinuation of antithrombotics and more particularly, dual antiplatelet therapy in this context can also have catastrophic consequences [21]. In addition, bleeding is known to stimulate inflammation, which can trigger plaque instability [22] and may require blood transfusion that may under certain circumstances have a negative impact on outcome [19].

Bleeding rates depend mainly on the clinical setting and also on the definition of bleeding events. Indeed, several definitions, each categorizing bleeding events differently, are used to grade severity of bleeding complications (see also ⊃ Chapter 69). The rate of major bleeding in ACS patients varies from 1% to 5%, and the rate of minor bleeding from 2% to 8%, depending on the source of the data (trials or registries) [22, 23].

Age, low body weight, female gender, renal failure, use of glycoprotein IIb/IIIa inhibitors, use of invasive procedures and previous history of bleeding are the most powerful predictors of bleeding in ACS patients [23]. In addition, baseline anaemia has also recently been identified as a risk factor for bleeding complications [1]. Furthermore, inadequate dosage of drugs may lead to an excess of bleeding, particularly among elderly patients, women, and patients with impaired renal function, all groups that are known to be already at a particularly high risk of bleeding [24].

Actually, the predictors of bleeding and ischaemic risks largely overlap. In a substudy of the OASIS-5 trial, a tight relationship was shown between the GRACE risk score, predictive of outcome, and the rate of bleeding throughout the study [25].

In practical terms, risk stratification for both ischaemic and bleeding events should now be part of the evaluation process in ACS. Treatments and procedures known to minimize risk of bleeding should be favoured (see below). A range of validated risk scores exist to stratify ischaemic risk among ACS patients [26–28]. The GRACE risk score

(see 🎥 Online resources) makes it possible to quantify the risk of death in the whole spectrum of ACS, on the basis of a series of simple baseline characteristics, including age, systolic blood pressure, serum creatinine, presence or absence of biomarker release, ST deviation, cardiac failure, or a history of resuscitated cardiac arrest.

Anaemia at baseline

Low baseline haemoglobin at admission was shown to be associated with worse prognosis in ACS. In a metanalysis involving 39 922 patients with both non-ST-elevation ACS (NSTE-ACS) and ST-elevation MI (STEMI), outcome at 30 days was significantly influenced by baseline haemoglobin level. The probability of major adverse cardiac events (MACEs) increased as admission haemoglobin decreased below 16 g/dL with odds ratio (OR) of 1.21 for STEMI, and 1.45 for NSTE-ACS per 1 g/dL decrement in haemoglobin. The rate of cardiovascular events increased with admission haemoglobin levels higher than 16 g/dL [5] (⊃ Fig. 70.1). The same curvilinear relationship was observed in other studies [18, 29–33] including a recent pooled analysis of the OASIS-5 and OASIS-6 trials [1].

Is anaemia at admission a marker of comorbidities that may have an impact on the prognosis as suggested in one report [29], or is it truly a risk factor that impairs prognosis? Anaemia may be present in 5–10% of patients with NSTE-ACS [19] according to the WHO criteria (haemoglobin <13 g/dL in men and <12 g/dL in women) [30]. Higher rates were found in many reports, from 19.4% [1] to 43% in elderly patients [35]. However, baseline haemoglobin level less than 10 g/dL was observed in only 2.5% of patients in the pooled analysis of OASIS-5 and OASIS-6 [1]. Indeed, anaemia is associated with risk factors, such as older age [31–33], female sex, presence of diabetes [9, 34], renal failure [6], and heart failure [7, 16, 35], but also with noncardiovascular conditions such as haemorrhagic diathesis or malignancies [11], which may account for the adverse prognosis. However, after adjustment for a broad array of baseline characteristics, a proportional relationship across the whole spectrum of ACS has been shown: the lower the baseline haemoglobin levels, the worse the prognosis [1, 5, 18]. In the pooled analysis of OASIS-5 and OASIS-6, the OR for death per 1 g/dL admission haemoglobin increment was 0.94 (0.90–0.98) below 15.9 g/dL and 1.19 (0.98–1.43) above this value [1] (⊃ Table 70.1).

Anaemia is not included in the risk stratification of ACS, in particular in the GRACE risk score. However, adding baseline haemoglobin to the GRACE risk score improved

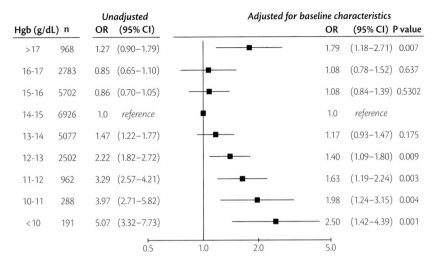

Hgb (g/dL)	n	Unadjusted			Adjusted for baseline characteristics		
		OR	(95% CI)			OR	(95% CI) P value
>17	968	1.27	(0.90–1.79)			1.79	(1.18–2.71) 0.007
16-17	2783	0.85	(0.65–1.10)			1.08	(0.78–1.52) 0.637
15-16	5702	0.86	(0.70–1.05)			1.08	(0.84–1.39) 0.5302
14-15	6926	1.0	reference			1.0	reference
13-14	5077	1.47	(1.22–1.77)			1.17	(0.93–1.47) 0.175
12-13	2502	2.22	(1.82–2.72)			1.40	(1.09–1.80) 0.009
11-12	962	3.29	(2.57–4.21)			1.63	(1.19–2.24) 0.003
10-11	288	3.97	(2.71–5.82)			1.98	(1.24–3.15) 0.004
<10	191	5.07	(3.32–7.73)			2.50	(1.42–4.39) 0.001

Figure 70.1 Unadjusted and adjusted odds ratios and 95% confidence intervals for association between baseline haemoglobin concentration and cardiovascular mortality through 30 days in patients with STEMI. Reproduced from Sabatine MS, Morrow DA, Giugliano RP, et al. Association of hemoglobin levels with clinical outcomes in acute coronary syndromes. *Circulation* 2005; **111**:2042–2049. With permission from Wolters Kluwer Health..

both the discriminatory capacity and the calibration of the prediction models, making it possible to reclassify 9%, 43%, 47%, and 22% of patients respectively into new risk categories, and confirming anaemia as an independent predictor of mortality [36].

There may be a causal link between anaemia and cardiovascular death. Indeed, anaemia increases heart rate and cardiac output, leading to development of left ventricular hypertrophy, and an imbalance between oxygen demand and supply to the myocardium [37, 38], particularly in patients with coronary artery stenosis; this can lead to increased infarct size, development of arrhythmias, heart failure, or hypotension, and eventually worsen prognosis. In addition, the inflammatory state may also play a role in the deterioration of the prognosis associated with low haemoglobin levels/anaemia [39, 40]. Furthermore, low

admission haemoglobin may lead to more frequent use of transfusions.

On the other hand, the reason why baseline haemoglobin levels of less than 15.9 g/dL are associated with a higher risk of ischaemic events remains speculative. Increased viscosity [41] and smoking status but also increased procoagulant or decreased fibrinolytic activities may account for the worse prognosis [50, 51].

Anaemia at baseline was shown to independently predict bleeding [19, 52]. In the pooled analysis of OASIS-5 and OASIS-6, irrespective of the type of bleeding, as well as of the clinical setting, NSTE-ACS, or STEMI, an inverse relationship between baseline haemoglobin and bleeding was observed: the lower the baseline haemoglobin level, the higher the bleeding risk. After adjustment, baseline haemoglobin was shown to be a strong independent predictor of bleeding risk [1] (❍ Table 70.2, ❍ Fig. 70.2). The rate of transfusion was higher in patients with low rather than high admission haemoglobin, indicating that the trigger for transfusion may have been lower in patients with lower haemoglobin levels. As transfusion was part of the definition of bleeding, particular attention was paid in this report to avoid classifying as bleeding events patients who may have been transfused merely because of anaemia at admission [1]. It is also noteworthy that the risk of major bleeding sharply increased for baseline haemoglobin levels below 12–13 g/dL (the lower limit of normal, according to the WHO definition of anaemia), as shown in ❍ Fig. 70.2. This implies that even modestly low baseline haemoglobin levels should be factored into the therapeutic decisions in patients with ACS and lead clinicians to select procedures or treatments with known reduced risk of bleeding.

Iron deficiency, occult gastrointestinal bleeding, inflammatory state, or haemorrhagic diathesis, which may be

Table 70.1 Independent predictors of death and death/MI at 30 days in the pooled analysis of OASIS-5 and OASIS-6 trials [1]

	Death at 30 days (OR, 95%CI)	Death/MI at 30 days (OR, 95%CI)
Treatment allocation	0.83, 0.75–0.93	0.86, 0.79–0.94
Baseline haemoglobin <15.9 g/dL[a]	0.94, 0.90–0.98	0.96, 0.93–0.99
Baseline haemoglobin >15.9 g/dL[a]	1.19, 0.98–1.43	1.15, 0.99–1.34
Age[b]	1.03, 1.02–1.04	1.03, 1.02–1.04
Heart failure	2.04, 1.81–2.31	1.71, 1.54–1.90
PCI	0.52, 0.41–0.67	0.84, 0.71–0.99
Diabetes	1.19, 1.06–1.34	1.18, 1.07–1.30
Creatinine clearance[c]	0.97, 0.97–0.98	0.98, 0.98–0.99

[a] Per increment of 1 g/dL in baseline haemoglobin level >10 g/dL.
[b] Per increase of 1 year
[c] Per decrease of 5 units.

Table 70.2 Independent predictors of overall, procedure-related, major, and non-procedure-related bleeding at 30 days, in the pooled analysis of OASIS-5 and OASIS-6 trials

Effect	Odds ratio estimates	
	Point estimate	95% Wald confidence limits
Overall major bleeding		
Baseline haemoglobin	0.94[a]	0.90–0.98
Treatment allocation	0.67	0.59–0.77
Age[b]	1.02	1.01–1.03
Male sex	0.82	0.72–0.95
Diabetes	1.17	1.0–1.35
Creatinine clearance[c]	0.93	0.92–0.94
Procedure-related bleeding		
Baseline haemoglobin	0.94[a]	0.90–0.99
Treatment allocation	0.70	0.60–0.83
Age[b]	1.02	1.01–1.03
Heart failure	0.62	0.47–0.80
Creatinine clearance[c]	0.93	0.92–0.95
Non-procedure-related bleeding		
Baseline haemoglobin	0.89[a]	0.83–0.95
Treatment allocation	0.64	0.52–0.78
Age[b]	1.04	1.03–1.05
Heart failure	1.55	1.21–1.99
Creatinine clearance[c]	0.92	0.90–0.94

[a] Per increment of 1 g/dL in baseline haemoglobin level >10 g/dL.
[b] Per increase of 1 year
[c] Per decrease of 5 units.

causal factors of low haemoglobin level/anaemia, may account for propensity to bleeding in such situation. In addition, haematocrit level has an influence on primary haemostasis. Increasing haematocrit levels were shown to lead on the one hand to increased platelet deposition to the arterial wall, and on the other hand to increased blood viscosity and increased shear forces, which may lead in turn to activation of platelet functions through ADP release by erythrocytes [41–43]. Use of aggressive antiplatelet and antithrombin treatments as well as invasive procedures may play the role of precipitating factor.

Management of anaemia

Anaemia may be observed at admission, or can be due to or worsened by bleeding. In unstable patients who remain symptomatic or who are in a critical haemodynamic situation, it needs to be corrected rapidly. Blood transfusion, iron therapy, and treatment of the cause of anae-

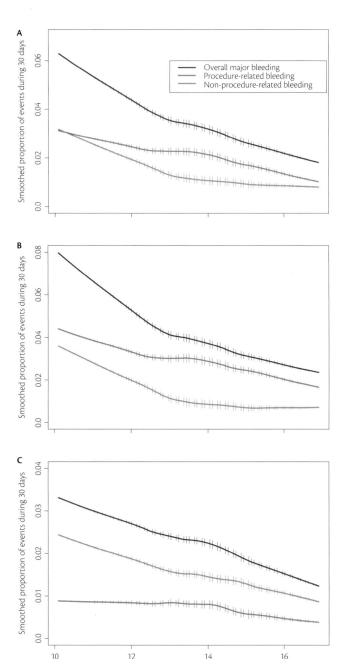

Figure 70.2 Relationship between baseline haemoglobin and overall, procedure-related, and non-procedure-related bleeding at 30 days in the overall population (A), in NSTE-ACS (B), and in STEMI (C).
Reproduced with permission from Bassand JP, Afzal R, Eikelboom J, et al. Relationship between baseline haemoglobin and major bleeding complications in acute coronary syndromes. *Eur Heart J* 2010;**31**(1):50–58.

mia are the most important measures. Erythropoietin or derivatives have no indications in ACS.

Blood transfusion

There is an ongoing controversy about the utility and efficacy of correcting anaemia by blood transfusion, and there are no clear indications about the level of haemoglobin at which transfusion should be started, or about the target level of haemoglobin to reach after transfusion [19, 44].

The potential impact of blood transfusion on outcome cannot be separated from the impact of bleeding. Both are intricately linked, not least because transfusion is included as a part of the definition of bleeding events in many bleeding scales. The rate of blood transfusion in ACS patients is highly variable and ranges from a low 2% to a high 12–15% depending on hospitals and countries [45, 46]. Nevertheless, blood transfusion has been shown to have detrimental effects in many clinical settings, including ACS and PCI, but also cardiac surgery and acute critical care among others [47–52]. The excess of death and MI thought to be linked to blood transfusion persisted after adjustment on all patient confounders [19]. Actually, the negative impact of blood transfusion on outcome depends largely on the nadir haematocrit or haemoglobin level at which transfusion was administered. Blood transfusion had a favourable impact if given for haematocrit values below 25%; above this value, blood transfusion had deleterious effects [19, 53] (➲Table 70.3). In patients undergoing PCI, there was a two- to fourfold increase in the risk of death in transfused versus nontransfused patients [54–58]. A similar deleterious effect of transfusion has also been reported in the setting of coronary artery bypass graft (CABG) surgery [59] and acute (noncardiac) care [44]. An increased risk of infection, especially lung infections, and an increased risk of ischaemic events was observed in transfused patients in

the setting of CABG, with a stepwise increase in the hazard ratio with the number of units of blood transfused [59]. The duration of storage of the blood transfused during open heart surgery has an influence on immediate and long-term outcome: patients who received newer blood (<14 days of storage) had much better outcome than those who received older blood (>14 days storage) [60].

However, the level of haematocrit or haemoglobin at which transfusion should be given, and the appropriate haematocrit or haemoglobin level to achieve with blood transfusion, have not yet been adequately defined. A haemoglobin level below 10 g/dL is the generally accepted trigger for transfusion [44, 53], but lower triggers are still debated [44, 61]. A restrictive blood transfusion strategy tested in the context of acute (noncardiac) care was shown to lead to better results than a more liberal policy [61, 62]. In the setting of acute care, a liberal transfusion policy, with a trigger for transfusion set at haemoglobin level less than 10 g/dL, and a target haemoglobin level post-transfusion of 10–12 g/dL, failed to demonstrate any superiority to a more restrictive policy, with a trigger set at 7 g/dL and a target haemoglobin level of 9–10 g/dL [62]. It is noteworthy that except for the report by Hebert et al. [63], there is a paucity of randomized data in this area, particularly in the setting of ACS. Most of the data reported in the ongoing debate about transfusion stem from retrospective post hoc analyses of registries, or meta-analyses of trials [47]. However, the data are concordant and suggest that clinicians be cautious when considering indications for blood transfusion. It is now increasingly recommended to consider transfusion in haemodynamically stable patients only for baseline haemoglobin levels less than 7 g/dL and to limit transfusion to patients in seriously unstable haemodynamic situations [20].

Storage of blood might be the problem. 2,3-diphosphoglycerate (2,3DPG) is depleted in stored red blood cells, which increases the haemoglobin affinity for oxygen, thereby reducing the capacity for oxygen delivery at tissue level. Tissue oxygenation is either decreased or not influenced by the transfusion of stored red blood cells. The membrane and the shape of preserved red blood cells is also dramatically modified, hampering their deformability and therefore impairing microvascular circulation by plugging of red blood cells in the capillaries [64–67].

Nitric oxide (NO), physiologically bound to haemoglobin in the form of S-nitrosothiol (SNO), is delivered at microvascular level, thus leading to vasodilation. SNO linked to haemoglobin is rapidly depleted during storage. As a result, transfusion of stored blood cells may cause vasoconstriction [68–70].

Table 70.3 Mortality associated with blood transfusion in each nadir haematocrit group

Nadir HCT	Unadjusted OR (95% CI)[a]	Adjusted OR (95% CI) for clinical factors, baseline HCT, and transfusion by nadir HCT interaction[b]
≤24%	0.76 (0.52–1.11)	0.67 (0.45–1.02)
24.1–27%	1.03 (0.81–1.31)	1.01 (0.79–1.30)
27.1–30%	1.21 (0.96–1.54)	1.18 (0.92–1.50)
>30%	4.97 (3.36–7.34)	3.47 (2.30–5.23)

BMI, body mass index; BO, blood pressure; CABG, coronary artery bypass grafting; CHF, chronic heart failure; CI, confidence interval; HCT, haematocrit; OR, odds ratio; PCI, percutaneous coronary intervention.

[a] Odds of mortality for transfused (nontransfused is reference) when adjusted for clinical factors including age, sex, BMI, race, family history of coronary artery disease, hypertension, diabetes, current/recent smoking status, hypercholesterolaemia, prior MI, prior PCI, prior CABG, prior CHF, prior stroke, renal insufficiency, ECG changes (ST-segment depression, transient ST-segment elevation), positive cardiac markers, signs of CHF at presentation, heart rate, and systolic BP at admission.

[b] Adjusted for clinical factors above as well as baseline HCT and transfusion by nadir HCT interaction.

Adapted with permission from Alexander KP, Chen AY, Wang TY, et al. Transfusion practice and outcomes in non-ST-segment elevation acute coronary syndromes. Am Heart J 2008;**155**:1047–1053.

Other potentially deleterious effects of blood transfusion have been reported, such as a prothrombotic effect, an increase in PAI-1 in packed red blood cells, or immunomodulation. Blood transfusion may have immunosuppressive effects due to various mechanisms, predisposing to infection and/or acute lung injury [71–77]. White blood cells in erythrocyte transfusion are present even in leucocyte-depleted blood [83] and can lead to a range of physiological and immunological dysfunctions in the recipients. Various soluble bioactive substances, including histamine and cytokines, may play an important role in transfusion-induced immunomodulation (TRIM) [72, 78]. Indeed, allogenic blood transfusion introduces many foreign antibodies which may trigger an immune response and be responsible for subclinical transfusion-associated graft versus host disease, or transfusion-related lung injury (TRALI) [72, 74]. In addition, microchimerism has also been proposed as a possible mechanism for TRIM [77]. Last but not least, numerous transfusion-transmitted infections may have an impact on prognosis.

Treating the cause of anaemia

Anaemia at admission can be due to multiple causes such as occult gastrointestinal bleed, genital bleeding in women, undiscovered malignancy, haemopathy, chronic renal failure, or heart failure, to mention but a few. It is appropriate to ask for consultation with other specialists, consider anticoagulant and antiplatelet therapies with caution, and defer invasive strategies whenever possible.

When overt bleeding is the cause of anaemia, interventions may be required to keep the situation under control, such as vascular repair, use of closure devices, or use of thrombin to stem bleeding at puncture site; or specific interventions depending on the location of bleeding, such as endoscopy in case of a gastrointestinal bleed. Other interventions may be required, such as interruption and neutralization of anticoagulants, interruption of antiplatelet agents and platelet transfusion, or use of substitutes such as cryoprecipitates or recombinant factor VII. These interventions are not inconsequential, and may all have an impact on outcome or result in untoward events. Platelet transfusion has been shown to lead to an excess of deep vein thrombosis in cancer patients with anaemia [79]. Reports have suggested that there is an excess of adverse thromboembolic events after use of recombinant human factor VII in various clinical situations [80]. In the setting of cardiac surgery, recombinant factor VII was shown to reduce the risk of bleeding, but was associated with a higher

risk of stroke [80, 81]. In the same setting aprotinin has long been used to reduce the risk of bleeding, but was recently shown to be associated with a higher risk of ischaemic events, and is therefore contraindicated in this setting [82]. This could indicate that, more generally speaking, manipulation of the coagulation system and platelet function in the aim of reducing bleeding risk may induce side effects in the form of excess ischaemic events, on the venous or arterial side, or both.

Iron therapy

Iron therapy is required in the presence of anaemia associated with iron deficiency, or bleeding with massive blood loss. Assessment of iron metabolism is useful to guide iron therapy. Serum ferritin level reflects iron reserves, transferrin saturation reflects iron transfer, and haemoglobin content of reticulocytes mirrors utilization of iron at the level of the bone marrow. Ferritin levels lower than 15 mg/L are considered as serious, absolute iron deficiency (normal values 20–100 mg/L in females, 30–300 mg/L in males). Transferrin saturation less than 20% means that there is insufficient transfer of iron to the bone marrow. Lastly, haemoglobin content of reticulocytes below normal values is an indicator of iron-deficient erythropoiesis.

The treatment of iron deficiency consists of long-term oral administration of iron supplements. However, these compounds are often poorly tolerated in the gastrointestinal tract, and have been accused of inducing inflammatory reactions. Intravenous iron administration can be used if oral administration is poorly tolerated. Among available products, ferric carboxymaltose has been shown to be well tolerated and to restore iron reserves quickly [83, 84]. Monitoring of serum ferritin and transferrin saturation makes it possible to ascertain that iron reserves have been adequately restored. Concomitant administration of erythropoietin or derivatives cannot be given in the setting of ACS because of side effects (see below).

Erythropoietin and derivatives

Erythropoietin has been used to compensate for anaemia in the setting of chronic kidney disease with or without diabetes and heart failure. Erythropoietin derivatives have been shown to be efficacious in increasing haemoglobin levels and correcting anaemia, but have never been shown to improve outcome, irrespective of the clinical setting. On the contrary, side effects have been described, particularly excess of deep vein thrombosis, stroke, and ACS [85–90]. In the setting of ACS or coronary artery disease in general, these compounds cannot be recommended to compensate for anaemia.

Practical implications

Several measures should be taken without delay if anaemia is present at admission. Great attention must be paid to the dose and duration of antiplatelet and anticoagulant therapy. There is also a need for expert opinion to identify and correct the cause of anaemia. Irrespective of the cause (be it pre-existing anaemia or bleeding), correction of anaemia with blood transfusion may be necessary if patients are symptomatic with persisting anginal attacks, despite appropriate therapy, or in the presence of haemodynamic instability. For haemoglobin values less than 7 g/dL or haematocrit lower than 25%, blood transfusion is mandatory, while the need for blood transfusion above these values is not compelling in a stable situation and should be discussed on a case-by-case basis. Target haemoglobin levels to be achieved after transfusion remain ill defined, and it may not be necessary to target values above 10 g/dL.

Prevention of bleeding is an important component of the treatment of anaemia, leading to a risk reduction for ischaemic events, particularly death. In the OASIS-5 study, fondaparinux reduced bleeding risk by 50% in comparison to enoxaparin, which turned in a significant risk reduction for death at 30 days and 6 months [91]. The same findings were observed in the HORIZON trial in the setting of primary PCI, where bivalirudin reduced bleeding and lead to improved outcome [92]. In both studies, the only plausible explanation for this risk reduction for death is the reduction of bleeding. These are the only two trials to date to demonstrate that a significant risk reduction for bleeding could lead to an improvement in outcome. More trials may replicate these findings in the future.

The loop is therefore closed—an increased risk of bleeding leads to an increased risk of death, but a risk reduction for bleeding leads to a risk reduction for death. The paradigm in the treatment of patients suffering from ACS is now shifting, and prevention of bleeding has become equally important as the prevention of ischaemic events. The most appropriate therapeutic strategy should be chosen depending on the proven capacity of a drug, treatment, or procedure to reduce bleeding risk.

Characterization of ischaemic and bleeding risks is therefore part of the decision-making process. It has been greatly facilitated in recent years, and is based on a combination of clinical judgement and use of risk calculators (GRACE risk calculator for ischaemic risk and CRUSADE score for bleeding risk) (see ➲ Online resources and see also ➲ Chapter 69). The therapeutic approach must be adapted on a case-by-case basis, particularly with frailer patients. A very careful approach has to be taken when selecting drugs and their dosage, and interventions. Since many of the drugs used in the treatment of ACS are eliminated by the renal route, extreme attention has to be paid to renal function. Creatinine clearance (CrCl), or preferably glomerular filtration rate (GFR), should be systematically measured for every single patient and monitored during treatment to guide the choice of drug and dose, particularly for CrCL less than 60mL/min or GFR greater than 60 mL min^{-1} 1.73m^{-2} [93]. As a result, inappropriate dosage or unnecessary prolongation of treatment may lead to accumulation of the drug in the organism, and thereby to a higher risk of bleeding, even for moderate renal dysfunction. Drugs known to reduce the risk of bleeding should be favoured.

In addition, the need for an invasive strategy has to be evaluated according to the balance between ischaemic and haemorrhagic risk, and the appropriate vascular access route must be chosen, favouring radial access where possible [58, 94].

Conclusion

Anaemia, irrespective of the cause, whether linked to or worsened by bleeding, has an unfavourable impact on outcome in terms of death and MI in ACS. In addition, it is an independent predictor of the risk of bleeding. The treatment of anaemia includes a search for the cause, blood transfusion, and iron therapy. Erythropoietin derivatives are contraindicated. Blood transfusion should be considered with caution. It is indicated in case of haemodynamic or ischaemic instability. However, in stable patients, blood transfusion should not be administered in patients with haematocrit greater than 25% since deleterious effects of transfusion have been described in this situation. Below 25% haematocrit, blood transfusion should be administered. Target post-transfusion haemoglobin levels remain to be defined. In practical terms, the risks of further ischaemic events and bleeding have to be assessed on a case-by-case basis in every patient admitted for ACS. Pharmacotherapy and invasive strategies have to be customized depending on ischaemic and bleeding risk, bearing in mind that the patients at highest risk of further ischaemic events are often the same patients who are at highest bleeding risk.

Personal perspective

Anaemia, irrespective of the cause—whether linked to or worsened by bleeding—is a risk factor for further ischaemic events, and a predictor of bleeding risk. The instinctive reaction of the clinician confronted with bleeding and/or anaemia is to prescribe a blood transfusion. However, blood transfusion has been shown to have potentially deleterious effects, particularly when administered to patients in stable condition with haematocrit above 25%. Currently, all information collected about the potential risks of transfusion is derived from *post hoc* analysis of clinical trials or registries. Few clinical trials have been carried out to identify the best transfusion policy, restrictive or liberal. To date, it would appear that a restrictive transfusion policy leads to better outcome than a more liberal policy. The message about the potentially deleterious effects of blood transfusion will be difficult to get across to clinicians unless there is a clinical trial specifically in the setting of ACS and/or PCI to test these two transfusion policies head-to-head. There is no doubt that further research will be carried out to identify the risk incurred by blood transfusion, to determine the mechanisms that mediate the adverse effects and the factors that lead to untoward events. It is likely that blood storage has an impact, but the exact mechanisms by which blood transfusion exerts a negative effect remain to be elucidated. This issue could be solved over the coming 5–10 years.

Further reading

Bassand JP, Afzal R, Eikelboom J, *et al*. Relationship between baseline haemoglobin and major bleeding complications in acute coronary syndromes. *Eur Heart J* 2010;**31**(1):50–58.

Bassand JP, Hamm CW, Ardissino D, *et al*. Guidelines for the diagnosis and treatment of non-ST-segment elevation acute coronary syndromes. The Task Force for the Diagnosis and Treatment of Non-ST-Segment Elevation Acute Coronary Syndromes of the European Society of Cardiology. *Eur Heart J* 2007;**28**:1598–1660.

Budaj A, Eikelboom JW, Mehta SR, *et al*. Improving clinical outcomes by reducing bleeding in patients with non-ST-elevation acute coronary syndromes. *Eur Heart J* 2009;**30**:655–661.

Hebert PC, Wells G, Blajchman MA, *et al*. A multicenter, randomized, controlled clinical trial of transfusion requirements in critical care. Transfusion Requirements in Critical Care Investigators, Canadian Critical Care Trials Group. *N Engl J Med* 1999;**340**:409–417.

Hill SR, Carless PA, Henry DA, *et al*. Transfusion thresholds and other strategies for guiding allogeneic red blood cell transfusion. *Cochrane Database Syst Rev* 2002:CD002042.

Lyseng-Williamson KA, Keating GM. Ferric carboxymaltose: a review of its use in iron-deficiency anemia. *Drugs* 2009;**69**:739–756.

Raghavan M, Marik PE. Anemia, allogenic blood transfusion, and immunomodulation in the critically ill. *Chest* 2005;**127**:295–307.

Rao SV, Eikelboom JA, Granger CB, *et al*. Bleeding and blood transfusion issues in patients with non-ST-segment elevation acute coronary syndromes. *Eur Heart J* 2007;**28**:1193–1204.

Rao SV, Jollis JG, Harrington RA, *et al*. Relationship of blood transfusion and clinical outcomes in patients with acute coronary syndromes. *JAMA* 2004;**292**:1555–1562.

Sabatine MS, Morrow DA, Giugliano RP, *et al*. Association of hemoglobin levels with clinical outcomes in acute coronary syndromes. *Circulation* 2005;**111**:2042–2049.

Stone GW, Witzenbichler B, Guagliumi G, *et al*. Bivalirudin during primary PCI in acute myocardial infarction. *N Engl J Med* 2008;**358**:2218–2230.

Yusuf S, Mehta SR, Chrolavicius S, *et al*. Comparison of fondaparinux and enoxaparin in acute coronary syndromes. *N Engl J Med* 2006;**354**:1464–1476.

Online resources

- CRUSADE score for bleeding risk. http://www.crusadebleedingscore.org/
- GRACE risk score. http://www.outcomes-umassmed.org/grace

➲ For additional multimedia materials please visit the online version of the book (🔗 http://www.esciacc.oxfordmedicine.com).

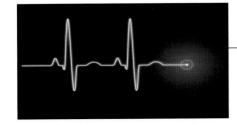

CHAPTER 71

Infection, sepsis, and multiple organ dysfunction syndrome

Julian Arias Ortiz, Raphaël Favory, and Jean-Louis Vincent

Contents

Summary

Sepsis is the main cause of multiple organ failure and remains a concern because of the associated high morbidity and mortality. In recent years, important advances have been made in the understanding of the pathophysiology of sepsis and its treatment. Severe sepsis and septic shock are the end result of complex interactions between infecting organisms and various elements of the host response. A key feature of the common sequence of organ failure is dysfunction of the cardiovascular system, involving the macrovascular (heart and vessels) and microcirculatory elements of the circulation.

Outcome improvement in sepsis is based on recognizing the process early, and instituting effective therapies. The time window for intervention is short and treatment must promptly control the source of infection and restore haemodynamic homoeostasis.

Introduction

Sepsis is the main cause of multiple organ dysfunction syndrome (MODS) and remains a concern because of the associated high morbidity and mortality [1]. Outcome improvement is based on understanding the pathophysiology, recognizing the process early, and instituting effective therapies.

Definition/epidemiology

Sepsis is defined as the systemic response to infection (➲ Box 71.1). Severe sepsis is sepsis complicated by organ dysfunction, and septic shock refers to a state of acute circulatory failure characterized by arterial hypotension despite adequate

Box 71.1 Currently proposed definitions of infection and sepsis

- **Infection:** a pathological process caused by the invasion of normally sterile tissue or fluid or body cavity by pathogenic or potentially pathogenic microorganisms
- **Sepsis:** the systemic response to infection
- **Severe sepsis:** sepsis complicated by organ dysfunction
- **Septic shock:** refers to a state of acute circulatory failure characterized by arterial hypotension despite adequate fluid resuscitation, so that vasopressor therapy is necessary to restore a minimally acceptable arterial pressure. Hypotension is defined by a systolic arterial pressure below 90 mmHg or a reduction of more than 40 mmHg from baseline, and it is associated with signs of altered tissue perfusion and metabolic markers (i.e. increased blood lactate levels).

Signs of sepsis

General signs and symptoms

- Rigor—fever (sometimes hypothermia)
- Tachypnoea/respiratory alkalosis
- Positive fluid balance—oedema

General inflammatory reaction

- Altered white blood cell count
- Increased CRP, IL-6, PCT concentrations

Haemodynamic alterations

- Arterial hypotension
- Tachycardia
- Increased cardiac output/low SVR/high Svo_2
- Altered skin perfusion
- Decreased urine output
- Hyperlactataemia—increased base deficit

Signs of organ dysfunction

- Hypoxaemia
- Coagulation abnormalities
- Altered mental status
- Hyperglycaemia
- Thrombocytopenia, DIC
- Altered liver function (hyperbilirubinaemia)
- Intolerance to feeding (altered GI motility)

Adapted from Vincent J-L, Korkut H. Defining sepsis. *Clin Chest Med* 2008;**29**:585–590.

fluid administration, so that vasopressor therapy is necessary to restore an acceptable arterial pressure. Hypotension is usually defined by a systolic arterial pressure below 90 mmHg or a reduction of more than 40 mmHg from baseline, and is associated with signs of altered tissue perfusion such as oliguria, altered mental status, or altered skin perfusion. The diagnosis is confirmed by increased blood lactate levels reflecting abnormal oxygen metabolism [2].

Severe sepsis and septic shock are major health care problems, affecting millions of individuals around the world each year, killing one in four (and often more), and increasing in incidence [3]. Sepsis and septic shock are the tenth most common cause of death in the United States [4]. A recent study from the United Kingdom documented a 46% in-hospital mortality rate for patients presenting with severe sepsis on admission to the intensive care unit (ICU) [5]. The incidence of sepsis and sepsis-related deaths appears to be increasing by about 1.5% per year [6]. In one study, the total national hospital cost invoked by severe sepsis in the United States was estimated at approximately $16.7 billion on the basis of an estimated severe sepsis rate of 751 000 cases per year with 215 000 associated deaths annually [6].

Pathophysiology of sepsis and multiple organ dysfunction syndrome

Regional hypoperfusion

Sepsis-induced vasodilation is quite variable in different vascular beds. The autoregulatory mechanisms that control the perfusion of the microcirculation, via multiple neuroendocrine, paracrine, and mechanosensory pathways, are altered in sepsis. Normally these mechanisms adapt to the balance between locoregional tissue oxygen transport and metabolic needs to ensure that supply matches demand. Alteration of these processes in sepsis leads to blood flow heterogeneity within organs.

The coronary response is vasodilation with an increase in coronary blood flow, even in septic shock. The mesenteric circulation is typically altered as a result of increased sympathetic tone and renin–angiotensin activation inducing vasoconstriction of the mesenteric territory [7], whereas down-regulation of endothelial nitric oxide (NO) synthase (eNOS) can decrease the endothelium-dependent vasodilation [8]. β-Adrenergic stimulation increases mesenteric perfusion in animal models [9] and in septic shock patients [10]. Hepatic blood flow has been shown to be diminished or increased, depending on the model. In humans, hepatic flow generally increases in parallel with cardiac output [11] but hepatic venous saturation (Sho_2) can decrease.

Renal blood flow is generally increased in hyperkinetic models but the repartition between medullar and cortical flows is altered probably largely because of an increased release of NO [12].

Cerebral blood flow is typically preserved, even in hypokinetic models. However, autopsy findings suggest ischaemic and apoptotic lesions in patients with septic shock [13].

Inflammation/thrombosis

During systemic inflammation, the activation of coagulation is due to tissue factor-mediated thrombin generation, down-regulation of physiological anticoagulant mechanisms, and inhibition of fibrinolysis. Proinflammatory cytokines play a pivotal role in the coagulation and fibrinolysis pathways. The clinical relevance of this cross-talk between inflammation and coagulation is suggested by the beneficial effects of activated protein C in severe sepsis and septic shock [14], although the mechanism of action may involve other pathways [15].

Septic shock is a form of distributive shock

The pump: septic myocardial depression

Pathophysiology

Initial characterization of sepsis-associated cardiovascular dysfunction was based on clinical patterns identified by physical examination in patients with septic shock.

Waisbren was the first to describe cardiovascular dysfunction due to sepsis [16]. He recognized a hyperdynamic state with full bounding pulses, flushing, fever, oliguria, and hypotension (so-called 'warm' shock). In addition, he described a second, less common pattern in which patients were clammy, pale, and hypotensive with low volume pulses. The latter, so-called 'cold' shock, reflected a hypokinetic pattern that might well have been volume under-resuscitated. With the ability to measure cardiac output and other haemodynamic variables at the bedside, the view of septic shock as a typically hyperdynamic state emerged.

Under conditions of adequate volume resuscitation, the profoundly reduced systemic vascular resistance typically encountered in sepsis [17] is associated with a high cardiac index that obscures the myocardial dysfunction that also occurs.

Although a number of mediators and pathways has been shown to be associated with myocardial depression in sepsis, the pathophysiology is multifactorial and involves multiple pathways (● Fig. 71.1).

Global ischaemia

Early theories of myocardial dysfunction in sepsis included the hypothesis of global myocardial ischaemia. However, this theory has been dismissed on the basis of studies in animals and humans showing that septic patients have high coronary blood flow and diminished coronary artery–coronary sinus oxygen difference [18]. Also there is no evidence supporting global ischaemia as an underlying cause of myocardial dysfunction in sepsis.

However, in septic patients with coexistent and possibly undiagnosed coronary artery disease (CAD), regional myocardial ischaemia or infarction secondary to CAD can occur. The manifestation of myocardial ischaemia due to CAD might even be facilitated by tachycardia, as well as by generalized microvascular dysfunction in sepsis [19]. Additional CAD- aggravating factors encountered in sepsis are inflammation and activation of the coagulation system that may promote thrombosis of the coronary circulation.

The absence of significant myocardial cell death and the reversible nature of myocardial dysfunction in sepsis support a prominent role for functional rather than anatomical abnormalities in the underlying pathophysiology.

Myocardial depressant substances

A circulating myocardial depressant factor in septic shock was first proposed more than 50 years ago. Parker *et al.* [20] demonstrated myocardial depression in isolated myocytes exposed to serum obtained from septic patients with clinical manifestations of sepsis-induced myocardial dysfunction. Many substances can have myocardial depressant effects, including NO, tumour necrosis factor-α (TNF), interleukin (IL)-1, platelet activating factor (PAF), and oxygen free radicals.

Cytokines

Further studies identified cytokines, such as IL-1 and IL-6, as circulating causative factors of myocardial depression in sepsis [21]. Lysozyme C, a bacteriolytic agent believed to originate mainly from disintegrating neutrophilic granulocytes and monocytes, can mediate cardiodepressant effects in animal models of sepsis [22]. Furthermore, competitive inhibition of lysozyme C in these animal models was protective and prevented sepsis-induced myocardial dysfunction [22].

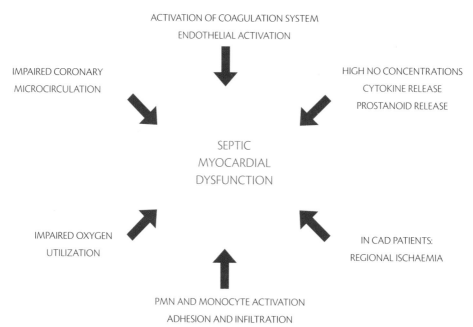

Figure 71.1 Potential mechanisms implicated in septic myocardial dysfunction. CAD, coronary artery disease; NO, nitric oxide; PMN, polymorphonuclear cells.

Prostanoids

The enzyme cyclooxygenase (COX) produces prostanoids through the metabolism of arachidonic acid. COX-1 is expressed constitutively, but the expression of COX-2 is induced, among other stimuli, by endotoxin (lipopolysaccharide, LPS) and cytokines. Elevated levels of prostanoids, such as thromboxane and prostacyclin, have the potential to alter coronary autoregulation, coronary endothelial function, and intracoronary leucocyte activation [23].

Endothelin-1

Endothelin-1 (ET-1) up-regulation has been demonstrated within 6 h of LPS-induced septic shock [24]. Cardiac overexpression of ET-1 triggers an increase in inflammatory cytokines (TNFα, IL-1, and IL-6), interstitial inflammatory infiltration, and an inflammatory cardiomyopathy that results in heart failure [25]. Although the pathophysiological importance of ET-1 has been demonstrated in a wide array of cardiac diseases, its biosynthesis, receptor-mediated signalling, and functional consequences in septic myocardial dysfunction warrant further investigation to assess the therapeutic potential of ET-1 receptor antagonists.

Nitric oxide

NO is produced by all types of cardiac cells and has many biological effects in the cardiovascular system [26]. It has been shown to modulate cardiac function under physiological and a multitude of pathophysiological conditions.

The effects of NO relevant to sepsis-induced myocardial dysfunction include vasodilatation, depression of mitochondrial respiration, and enhanced release of proinflammatory cytokines, which may exert their own cardiovascular effects [27]. NO is produced from conversion of L-arginine to L-citrulline by NOS. NOS has two forms: constitutive (cNOS) and inducible (iNOS). Early myocardial dysfunction in sepsis may occur through overproduction of NO and resultant cyclic guanosine monophosphate (cGMP) through cNOS activation in cardiac cells. Through the expression of iNOS, massive release of NO contributes to myocardial dysfunction, in part through the generation of cytotoxic peroxynitrite, a product of the reaction of NO with the superoxide anion [28].

NO can also contribute to the alterations in myocardial mitochondria during sepsis [29, 30]. Increased levels of NO and superoxide can lead to the inhibition of oxidative phosphorylation and decreased production of ATP. This 'cytopathic hypoxia', inability of the cells to utilize oxygen and produce ATP, can contribute to the development of MODS in sepsis [30]. Hearts from septic animals show reduced activity of electron transport chain enzyme [31]. The role of mitochondrial dysfunction in sepsis-induced myocardial depression is further supported by animal studies showing that inhibition of this process can improve cardiac function and reduce mortality [32].

A provocative theory regarding the myocardial depression in sepsis suggests that it may play a protective role in the heart similar to the phenomenon of hibernation in coronary ischaemia [33]. Myocardial depression may represent a protective adaptation by reducing cellular energy expenditure in the heart during a situation of decreased energy production.

Calcium is also thought to play an important role in the development of sepsis-induced myocardial depression. Current evidence suggests reductions in cytosolic calcium levels during sepsis leading to reduced contractility [34]. Calcium signalling and metabolism are linked to mitochondrial function. The relationship of intramyocyte calcium homeostasis with NO in sepsis is still not fully understood.

Adhesion molecules

Surface-expression up-regulation of intercellular adhesion molecule-1 (ICAM-1) and vascular cell adhesion molecule-1 (VCAM-1) has been demonstrated in murine coronary endothelium and cardiomyocytes after LPS and TNF-α administration [35]. VCAM-1 blockade with antibodies has been shown to prevent myocardial dysfunction and decrease myocardial neutrophil accumulation [35]. However, neutrophil depletion does not protect against septic cardiomyopathy, suggesting that the cardiotoxic potential of neutrophils infiltrating the myocardium is of lesser importance [35].

Role of apoptosis

There is increasing evidence that apoptosis is involved in sepsis-induced cardiovascular dysfunction [36]. Increased release of various substances implicated in the initiation of apoptosis, such as caspases and mitochondrial cytochrome c, has been shown in sepsis. Therapeutic strategies aimed at inhibition of apoptosis have resulted in improved cardiovascular function in animal models of sepsis [37]. However, the natural evolution of sepsis-induced myocardial dysfunction with recovery of cardiac function in survivors (after 7–10 days) suggests perhaps a less critical pathogenic role for apoptosis.

Echocardiographic findings

Echocardiographic evaluation at the bedside can be very useful in the evaluation of sepsis-related myocardial dysfunction, as it can reveal right or left systolic ventricular dysfunction, as well as left diastolic dysfunction. Many septic shock patients are treated with mechanical ventilation, so that transoesophageal echocardiography is the preferred approach, although technical improvements enable good images to be obtained using transthoracic views, even in mechanically ventilated patients. The incidence of cardiac dysfunction in septic shock may be higher than suspected [38, 39] and may vary between 45% and 60%, depending on the criteria used. The development of acute ventricular dilation is still debated [40]. However, it seems that acute left ventricular dilation is observed only when septic myocardial injury results in acute systolic left ventricular dysfunction, defined by reduced ejection fraction, reduced stroke volume, or both [40]. Whether dilation occurs or not, left ventricular dysfunction is transient and entirely reversible in surviving patients, lasting typically less than 1 week.

Troponin levels

Most of the cardiac troponin T and cardiac troponin I is bound to myofilaments; the remainder is free in the cytosol. When myocyte damage occurs, the cytosolic pool is released first, followed by a more protracted release from stores bound to deteriorating myofilaments [41]. Direct effects of endotoxin, oxidative stress, and cytokines, or their effects on downstream pathways, can reduce myocyte integrity, explaining an increase in plasma troponin levels. For example, executioners of apoptotic pathways, caspases, can induce sarcomere disarray and cleave α-actin, α-actinin, and troponin T [42]. The role of global coronary ischaemia is minor [18, 43], but microcirculatory derangements can be present [44]. The increase in blood troponin levels may result from myocardial ischaemia secondary to these microcirculation abnormalities, but an increase in myocyte permeability is another option. Cytokines, like TNF-α or IL-6, may be good candidates to explain this phenomenon since they can induce increased membrane permeability *in vitro* and their plasma levels have been found to be more elevated in troponin-positive than troponin-negative patients [45].

The correlation between left ventricular dysfunction and increased troponin levels is not a universal finding in patients with septic shock [46], probably because the diagnosis of myocardial depression is not easy at the bedside. Elevation of troponin levels is correlated with a worse outcome.

The vessels

Alterations in vascular tone

Sepsis and septic shock are characterized by a decrease in vascular reactivity. Both vasodilation (endothelium-dependent and independent) and vasoconstriction (receptor-dependent and independent) mechanisms are altered. The principal mechanisms that explain the altered vascular tone in sepsis are the activation of iNOS with massive release of NO [47], increased levels of prostaglandins [48], and hyporeactivity to catecholamines due to relative adrenal insufficiency in some patients and to vasopressin deficiency [49, 50]. Oxidative stress can also accelerate the degradation of catecholamines.

Microcirculatory alterations

The microcirculation, a network of vessels less than 150 μm in diameter—arterioles, capillaries, and venules—is critical for supplying tissues with substrates and removing metabolites. The microcirculation is the principal site of oxygen exchange between blood and underlying tissues, and in sepsis there is profound disruption of microcirculatory homeostasis.

Microcirculatory alterations are a hallmark of the maldistributive defect characterizing sepsis. After aggressive resuscitation of the septic patient, a normal or high cardiac output is typically achieved, yet tissue perfusion can remain markedly impaired. Clinically, this may manifest with persistent acidosis, mottled skin, or progressive multiorgan failure. Limiting goal-directed resuscitation solely according to macrocirculatory perfusion indices alone (e.g. cardiac filling pressure, mean arterial pressure, cardiac output, or even mixed/central venous oxygen saturation) may therefore not be sufficient to optimize blood flow to the tissues in many patients.

It has been proposed that the failure of the microvasculature is the key event that leads to MODS [51].

The microcirculatory unit is the landscape where most of the pivotal events of sepsis pathogenesis take place, including loss of vasomotor reactivity, endothelial cell injury leading to capillary leakage, and interstitial oedema which increase the diffusion distance of oxygen to cells [52] (➲ Fig. 71.2), activation of coagulation, and disordered leucocyte trafficking. Stiff leucocytes and red blood cells (RBCs), platelet/fibrin clots, and endothelial cell swelling are proposed to be responsible for capillary occlusion.

As an example, circulating blood cells are thought to occlude capillaries, resulting in a decrease in perfused capillary density [53]. The activation of circulating mature leucocytes or the release of immature leucocytes from bone marrow may result in a population of less deformable cells that can be entrapped in the capillaries [53]. Decrease in RBC deformability may contribute also to the loss of perfused capillaries. Disseminated intravascular coagulation (DIC) and cell aggregates can be involved in the decrease in perfused capillaries. Finally, capillary endothelial swelling and the formation of pseudopod extensions are thought to reduce the capillary lumen, thus contributing to the trapping of blood cells [54].

An obvious consequence of the microvascular abnormalities in sepsis is that both diffusive and convective oxygen transport are impaired in sepsis. Diffusive oxygen transport may be compromised in the lung, due to pulmonary oedema, or in the peripheral microcirculation.

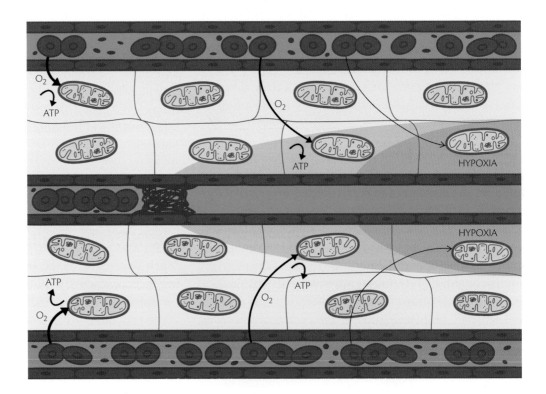

Figure 71.2 Mitochondrial and microcirculation dysfunction. Arrows show the increase in the diffusion distance of oxygen to cells that results from the loss of perfused capillaries.

Convective transport may be impaired because of myocardial dysfunction, blood flow maldistribution, and inadequate capillary perfusion.

An objective and reliable method of monitoring microcirculatory organ perfusion is still not available. A new, minimally invasive video microscopy technique (orthogonal polarization spectral (OPS) or side-stream dark field (SDF) imaging) permits direct visualization of the microcirculatory network beneath thin mucosal surfaces using a hand-held instrument [55]. The sublingual site has emerged as the preferred site for microcirculatory assessment in patients with overt or impending shock. Monitoring sublingual blood flow can yield important information for use in clinical studies of circulatory shock because (1) the sublingual mucosa shares the same embryologic (and therefore anatomic) origin as the splanchnic mucosa; (2) derangements in sublingual perfusion can reflect derangements in splanchnic blood flow [55]; and (3) the sublingual space is easily accessible. Despite the advantages of these techniques, there are still many limitations for their practical use at the bedside, so at the moment their use remains investigational.

Cellular and metabolic failure

The redox potential of mitochondria is decreased in sepsis [56]. This phenomenon is associated with ATP depletion and is correlated with a poor outcome in septic shock patients [29]. Various mechanisms can contribute to the altered mitochondrial function. NO and nitrosative stress derivates (peroxynitrite, $ONOO^-$), the production of which are increased during sepsis, inhibit cytochrome oxidase (complex IV) [57]. The inhibition by NO is reversible, but peroxynitrite irreversibly inhibits F0F1 ATPase complex I and II. The nuclear enzyme poly(ADP-ribose) polymerase (PARP-1) is activated by ADN breaks caused by oxidative stress. This activation decreases the cellular NAD^+/NADH content. In endotoxic shock models, inactivation of PARP-1 can prevent vascular contractile dysfunction [58]. Both the alterations in oxidative phosphorylation and a decrease in antioxidant defences (notably catalase activity [59]) can explain an increase in oxidative stress. Stress hormones (cortisol, catecholamines, vasopressin, growth hormone) are released in greater amounts in sepsis and can impact on cellular respiration. For example, acute glucocorticoid stimulation in rats leads to increased complex IV activity whereas chronic exposure seems to diminish mitochondrial function [60].

Cytosolic and mitochondrial apoptotic pathways are both activated during sepsis. The phenomenon known as mitochondrial permeability transition leads to the transition of the cytochrome c from the mitochondria to cytosol and the activation of caspases. A positive impact of inhibition of permeability pore transition has been shown in several models [32, 60, 61].

Mitochondrial biogenesis is altered during sepsis. TNF-α can promote mitochondrial autophagy [62]. Thyroid, sex hormones, insulin, and glucocorticoids are able to modulate mitochondrial biogenesis. The expression of complexes I and IV is decreased 6–24 hrs after injection of LPS [63]. A positive impact of carbon monoxide (CO) on mitochondrial biogenesis in parallel with a reduction of mortality has been shown during rodent sepsis [64].

Management

Antibiotic therapy and source control

Because the type of infecting organism(s) is usually unknown at the time of antibiotic initiation, empiric antibiotic therapy is based on clinical presentation and epidemiologic factors, including local flora, resistance patterns, and previous antibiotic exposure (⊃ Fig. 71.3).

As stated in the Surviving Sepsis Campaign Guidelines [65], the initial empirical anti-infective therapy should include one or more drugs that have activity against all likely pathogens and that penetrate in adequate concentrations into the presumed source of sepsis. Combination therapy is preferred for patients with known or suspected *Pseudomonas* infections as a cause of severe sepsis and for neutropenic patients with severe sepsis.

Intravenous antibiotic therapy should be started as early as possible in severe sepsis. Timing of initial administration of effective antimicrobial therapy is the most important predictor of survival [65]. Appropriate cultures should be obtained before initiating antibiotic therapy whenever possible, but should not prevent prompt administration of antimicrobial therapy. When used empirically, combination therapy should not be administered for more than 3–5 days. De-escalation to the most appropriate single therapy should be performed as soon as the susceptibility profile is known.

Source control is a critical issue in the optimal management of infection associated with severe sepsis. All patients presenting with severe sepsis should be evaluated for the presence of a focus of infection amenable to source control measures, specifically the drainage of an abscess or local focus of infection, the debridement of infected necrotic tissue, the removal of a potentially infected device, or the

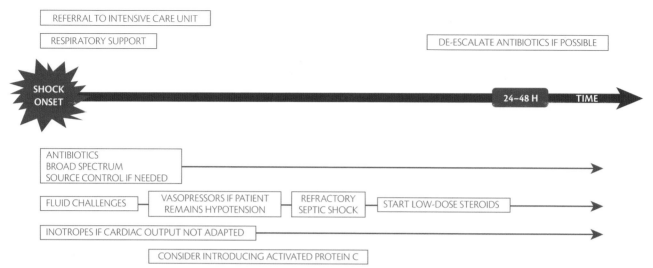

Figure 71.3 Basic principles of treatment in septic shock. The time window for starting effective therapies is short (<6 h); most important is to promptly control the source of infection and restore haemodynamic homeostasis.

definitive control of a source. Time lapse from hypotension to implementation of source control was found to correlate highly with outcome [66].

Haemodynamic management

Fluid therapy/transfusion strategies

Efficient restoration of circulating blood volume is the primary goal of resuscitation in septic patients [67]. Although controversy persists in the literature for the preferential use of crystalloids or colloids, at the moment there is no evidence-based support for one type of fluid over another, but some general recommendations can be made. According to the Surviving Sepsis Campaign Guidelines [65] an initial strategy may consist in the rapid administration of 20 ml/kg of fluids. Then a fluid challenge technique [68] should be applied with administration of at least 1000 mL of crystalloids or 300–500 mL of colloids over 30 min. The rate of fluid administration should be reduced substantially when cardiac filling pressures (central venous pressure (CVP) or pulmonary artery balloon-occluded pressure (PAOP)) increase without concurrent haemodynamic improvement.

The likelihood of fluid responsiveness can be evaluated by pulse pressure or stroke volume variation in patients treated by mechanical ventilation, who are well sedated and without significant arrhythmias.

To summarize, although infusing fluids is a cornerstone of supportive care during sepsis, optimal modalities and volumes are difficult to determine and choices should be driven by objectives in the individual patient.

Concerning transfusion strategies, once tissue hypoperfusion has resolved and in the absence of extenuating circumstances, such as myocardial ischaemia, severe hypoxaemia, acute haemorrhage, or lactic acidosis, the recommendation is that red blood cell transfusion should be considered when haemoglobin decreases to less than 7.0 g/dL [65]. This transfusion threshold of 7 g/dL contrasts with the early goal-directed resuscitation protocol, which uses a target haematocrit of 30% in patients with low central venous oxygen saturation ($Scvo_2$) during the first 6 hr of resuscitation of septic shock [69]. A similar transfusion trigger of 8–10 g/dL could be considered in early septic shock (<6 h), particularly if there is evidence of inadequate oxygen delivery (e.g. low mixed venous saturation) after fluid resuscitation [70]. For critically ill patients with acute ischaemic heart disease, a haemoglobin concentration of 8–10 g/dL is recommended. The need for a RBC transfusion should be individualized based on a patient's clinical circumstances rather than an arbitrary haemoglobin concentration.

Early goal-directed therapy

In 2001, a trial of early haemodynamic resuscitation to normal physiological parameters, or early goal-directed therapy (EGDT), was conducted in emergency department patients with severe sepsis/septic shock and was associated with a significant mortality reduction [69]. EGDT is an algorithmic approach within the first 6 h of disease recognition that diverges from standard management primarily by increasing oxygen content (with fluids including blood transfusions) and cardiac contractility (with inotropes) to optimize oxygen delivery so as to obtain an oxygen saturation of at least 70% in the superior vena cava ($Scvo2$, measured through a central venous catheter). Specifically, patients were managed by (1) fluid resuscitation with either crystalloid or colloid to achieve a CVP goal of 8–12 mmHg; (2) vasoactive agents to achieve a MAP goal of 65 mmHg; (3) blood transfusion to a haematocrit of 30% or greater; and (4) inotropic therapy with dobutamine. The primary outcome variable, in-hospital mortality, was 46.5% in the control group versus 30.5% in the EGDT group (relative reduction in mortality rate of 34.4%; relative risk [RR] 0.58; 95% CI 0.38–0.87; $p = 0.009$). The value of this protocol has been debated, in terms of the liberal use of packed RBCs, the use of CVP and $Scvo_2$ to evaluate attainment of physiological goals, barriers to applying the concept in emergency departments, among others. Three studies are currently ongoing to evaluate this particular strategy at the multicentre level, but it is clear that early and complete haemodynamic resuscitation is of paramount importance.

Which arterial pressure and choice of vasopressor

International guidelines propose an initial target value of mean arterial pressure of 65 mmHg in septic shock [71]. These recommendations are based on observational data relating mean arterial pressure to outcome and on a few interventional studies testing, in a very small number of patients, the impact of an increase in blood pressure on tissue perfusion or organ dysfunction. Increasing arterial pressure in septic shock may improve tissue perfusion pressure, although vasoconstrictor agents may impair cardiac output as a result of increased afterload. In addition, vasopressor agents may further impair hepatosplanchnic perfusion as well as microcirculatory perfusion. Studies testing an increase in mean arterial pressure from 60–65 mmHg to 85–90 mmHg have tested noradrenaline (norepinephrine) only on a short-term basis [72, 73]. In parallel with an increase in cardiac index, there was sometimes an improvement in tissue perfusion and organ function, as evidenced by clinical variables, such as urine output [72, 73], and technical measures like gastric tonometry, microvascular blood flow [74, 75], and lactate levels [72, 73], but sometimes no effect or even a deleterious effect has been shown. Moreover, significant interindividual differences were reported in two studies [74, 76]. The target arterial pressure should be higher in patients with chronic hypertension or advanced arteriosclerosis.

The choice of vasopressor is important. Depending on its receptor modulation, the vasopressor agent may have an impact on myocardial function, different organ perfusion (renal, hepatosplanchnic), and microcirculatory perfusion.

Dopamine can increase hepatosplanchnic and renal blood flows, but protective effects on organ function have not been demonstrated. Because of its stronger vasopressor effects, noradrenaline has become the most commonly used agent. Adrenaline is not superior to the combination of dobutamine and noradrenaline [77].

Vasopressin administration has been suggested on the basis of inadequate blood levels in septic shock. The VASST study showed a similar survival rate with vasopressin compared to noradrenaline in septic shock, with perhaps a decreased mortality in patients with less severe forms of shock [78]. Vasopressin administration may be of interest in the context of renal failure because it acts on V_1 receptors that are located at the efferent arterioles and not on afferent arterioles as for α_1 receptor agonists (dopamine, noradrenaline, adrenaline). A *post hoc* analysis of the VASST study [79] indicated that vasopressin was associated with a trend to a lower rate of progression to renal failure, and a lower rate of use of renal replacement therapy (RRT) compared to noradrenaline.

The reduction in cardiac output and the decrease in hepatosplanchnic and coronary blood flows induced by vasopressin are of concern.

In summary, noradrenaline is now the preferred first-line vasopressor agent. The place of vasopressin is still not well defined.

When to use inotropes/calcium sensitizers (levosimendan)

Despite a lack of randomized data demonstrating its efficacy, dobutamine is the first-choice inotropic agent for patients with measured or suspected low cardiac output in the presence of adequate filling pressures [80]. The challenge in interpreting myocardial dysfunction in sepsis is that the most important physiological variable is cardiac output. Patients with pre-existing cardiac dysfunction, who may have decreased cardiac output, are candidates for inotropic therapy to improve oxygen delivery (Do_2). Even patients without underlying cardiomyopathy may have an inadequate cardiac output to meet the oxygen demands of the cells. The presence of a low $Svo_2/Scvo_2$ or persistent hyperlactataemia may suggest inadequate cardiac output (❯Fig. 71.4) and an indication for dobutamine.

In any case a strategy of routinely increasing cardiac index or Do_2 to predefined 'supranormal' levels has not been shown to improve outcome, and may be deleterious.

Phosphodiesterase inhibitors, such as milrinone, can be considered as an adjunct to adrenergic agents, although their vasodilating effects and their prolonged half-life complicate their routine use.

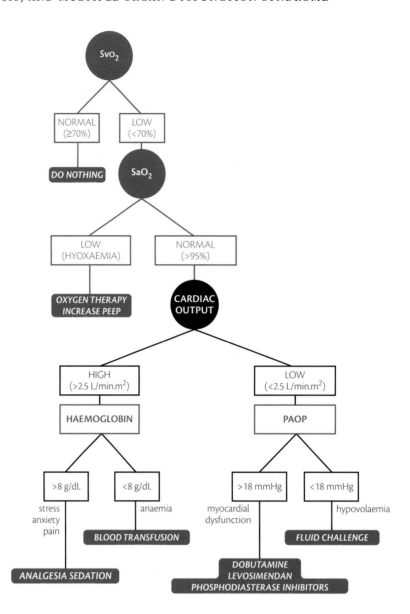

Figure 71.4 Diagnostic and therapeutic algorithm based on mixed venous oxygen saturation (SvO$_2$) measurements. PAOP, pulmonary artery occlusion pressure; PEEP, positive end-expiratory pressure; SaO$_2$, arterial oxygen saturation.

Levosimendan exerts beneficial effects on the left and right ventricles, which are independent of β-adrenergic signalling or changes in intracellular calcium concentration, by increasing contractile myofilament sensitivity to calcium.

As administration of adrenergic agents may be associated with tachyarrhythmia or increase in myocardial oxygen demand, levosimendan may represent an alternative in the setting of sepsis-induced myocardial dysfunction [81]. Although some data suggest that the use of levosimendan is safe and effective, the vasodilating effects, the long half-life, and the cost of the drug remain important issues.

General management

FAST HUG

Checklists can help to enhance the efficiency, safety, and efficacy of care. One suggested approach is to 'Give your

patient a FAST HUG at least once a day'. This FAST HUG is an acronym for simple interventions in the critically ill patient, that can contribute to the quality of care and may improve outcomes [82] (➲ Box 71.2).

Ventilator settings for acute lung injury/acute respiratory distress syndrome

In patients with sepsis-induced acute lung injury/acute respiratory distress syndrome (ALI/ARDS), ventilator settings should be limited to maintain a so-called 'gentle ventilation': one can start with a tidal volume of around 6 mL/kg (predicted) body weight and an upper limit of plateau pressure of 30 cmH$_2$O or less (considering the chest wall compliance). Positive end-expiratory pressure (PEEP) should be set to avoid extensive lung collapse at end-expiration. There is some evidence that higher PEEP levels may be associated with improved survival rates [83]. One may allow $Paco_2$ to increase above normal (so called 'permissive hypercapnia'), if needed to minimize tidal volume and plateau pressures [65].

Glucose control

Following initial stabilization, patients with severe sepsis and hyperglycaemia who are admitted to the ICU should receive intravenous insulin therapy to reduce blood glucose levels. With the current evidence, a validated protocol for insulin dose adjustments must be applied, targeting a glucose level between 110 and 150 mg/dL range with minimal glucose variability [65, 84].

Renal replacement therapy

Although there is no definitive evidence that supports superiority of continuous RRT over intermittent haemodialysis, the use of continuous therapies facilitates management of fluid balance in haemodynamically unstable septic patients [65]. Because, there is no evidence to support an early RRT strategy systematically, decisions have to be made on an individual basis for each patient. However, since acute renal failure and its associated metabolic alterations appear to increase the risk of severe extrarenal complications, the initiation of RRT should not be retarded in patients with severe, rapidly developing, and oliguric forms of acute renal failure. The 'optimal dose' of renal support is still a matter of debate, but the last published trials did not show a benefit of high doses compared to conventional doses of RTT.

The use of polymyxin haemoperfusion to reduce blood levels of endotoxin has also been proposed, with promising results in a recent trial by Cruz *et al.* [85].

Immunomodulatory therapies

The use of steroids in septic shock is still controversial. According to the Surviving Sepsis Campaign, use of intravenous hydrocortisone is recommended only in adult septic shock patients after blood pressure is identified to be poorly responsive to fluid resuscitation and vasopressor therapy [65]. The ACTH stimulation test is not indicated to identify the subset of patients with septic shock who should receive hydrocortisone. The dose of intravenous hydrocortisone administered should be 50 mg every 6 h or 100 mg every 8 h. The addition of fludrocortisone is optional. The patient should be weaned from the steroids when the vasopressor support is no longer required [65].

There is, however, no contraindication to continuing maintenance steroid therapy or to using stress dose steroids if the patient's endocrine or corticosteroid administration history warrants.

The only sepsis drug that has been proven to decrease mortality in patients with severe sepsis in a well-conducted randomized controlled trial, is recombinant human activated protein C (APC). In 2001, the PROWESS trial of APC for severe sepsis reported a 6.1% absolute reduction in mortality and a 19.4% relative reduction in the risk of mortality at 28 days [14]. The ENHANCE trial, which had inclusion and exclusion criteria similar to those of PROWESS, was able to demonstrate a similar reduction in 28-day mortality in patients with severe sepsis treated with APC within the first 24 h of their organ dysfunction regardless of disease severity [86].

The use of activated protein C can, therefore, be considered, if there are no contraindications, in the first 24 h in patients with sepsis-induced organ dysfunction associated with a clinical assessment of high risk of death, most of whom will have shock or multiple organ failure [65].

Personal perspective

There has been a strong focus on improving our understanding of the pathophysiology of septic shock and MODS during the last decade. As a result, multiple potential therapeutic targets have been identified. However, many questions remain unanswered and there has been no great breakthrough in terms of therapeutic intervention. The importance of early intervention ('time is tissue') has come to the fore with EGDT and early, effective antibiotic treatment being associated with improved outcomes. Optimal resuscitation targets remain unclear: Systemic haemodynamic parameters may be inadequate targets as microcirculatory inadequacies can remain even when the macrocirculation is apparently restored, and persistent microcirculatory abnormalities are associated with poor prognosis. However, monitoring of the microcirculation remains a research tool at present and further study is needed to determine whether this approach, using direct visualization of the microcirculation with hand-held cameras and/or assessment of tissue oxygenation, can be used to guide therapy. Many drugs can impact on the microcirculation, including vasoactive drugs (with beneficial or detrimental effects), vasodilators (nitroglycerine, dobutamine), and modulators of coagulation, such as activated protein C. One of the major questions for the near future is whether we actually need to treat the microcirculation and/or the mitochondria, and if so with which drugs? Moreover, how should we monitor their effects? Finally, as our understanding of how different patients respond to sepsis improves and our ability to measure this response with techniques such as proteomics and genomics increases, targeting of therapeutic choices and targets to individual patients will be a fascinating challenge for ICU physicians over the next few years.

Further reading

Antonelli M, Levy M, Andrews PJ, *et al*. Hemodynamic monitoring in shock and implications for management. International Consensus Conference, Paris, France, 27–28 April 2006. *Intensive Care Med* 2007;**33**:575–590.

Dellinger RP, Levy MM, Carlet JM, *et al*. Surviving Sepsis Campaign: international guidelines for management of severe sepsis and septic shock: 2008. *Intensive Care Med* 2008;**34**:17–60.

Hebert PC, Tinmouth A, Corwin HL. Controversies in RBC transfusion in the critically ill. *Chest* 2007;**131**:1583–1590.

Hollenberg SM. Inotrope and vasopressor therapy of septic shock. *Crit Care Clin* 2009;**25**:781–802, ix.

Rivers E, Nguyen B, Havstad S, *et al*. Early goal-directed therapy in the treatment of severe sepsis and septic shock. *N Engl J Med* 2001;**345**:1368–1377.

Rudiger A, Singer M. Mechanisms of sepsis-induced cardiac dysfunction. *Crit Care Med* 2007;**35**:1599–608.

Trzeciak S, Cinel I, Phillip DR, *et al*. Resuscitating the microcirculation in sepsis: the central role of nitric oxide, emerging concepts for novel therapies, and challenges for clinical trials. *Acad Emerg Med* 2008;**15**:399–413.

Vincent JL. Give your patient a fast hug (at least) once a day. *Crit Care Med* 2005;**33**:1225–1229.

Vincent JL, Gerlach H. Fluid resuscitation in severe sepsis and septic shock: an evidence-based review. *Crit Care Med* 2004;**32**:S451–S454.

Vincent JL, Weil MH. Fluid challenge revisited. *Crit Care Med* 2006;**34**:1333–1337.

➲ For additional multimedia materials please visit the online version of the book (🔗 http://www.esciacc.oxfordmedicine.com).

CHAPTER 72

Acute pain in the intensive cardiac care unit

S. Curac, A. Ricard-Hibon, and V. Belpomme

Contents

Summary

Pain is the most frequent symptom encountered by practitioners. Pain may be defined as 'an unpleasant sensory and emotional experience associated with actual or potential tissue damage' associated with surgery, trauma, and acute illness.

Pain may be considered a physiological phenomenon: the process of pain transmission is multifaceted, and research continues to provide further understanding of these mechanisms. Pain transmission is triggered by tissue injury or the treatment of tissue damage; protective mechanisms are elicited to prevent or minimize injury. However, at some stage, especially in postoperative or post-trauma acute pain, these mechanisms, which are designed to protect, are detrimental to the patient.

This chapter reviews the neurobiology of pain and focuses on the adequate treatment of pain in the acute cardiac and intensive care setting, emphasizing the favourable impact of acute pain control and discussing treatment options to maximize patient benefit. Inadequately treated pain is a major public health problem and a particular problem in emergency departments. Patients usually present to the emergency department when other medical help is not accessible or when symptoms, often including pain, are most severe. Emergency department visits therefore represent high-risk encounters in which assessment and treatment of pain should receive careful attention [1]. Despite traditional inadequacies and the development of nonopioid pain therapy modalities, systemic morphine may still be considered the mainstay for acute pain control in diverse settings, and is recommended particularly for ischaemic chest pain. The titration, size of doses, timing of doses, and use of escape doses has to be well organized.

Introduction

Pain is the cardinal symptom in many conditions typically encountered in critical care departments, including many cardiological conditions involving tissue injury: myocardial infarction (both ST-segment elevation and non-ST-segment elevation), pericarditis/myocarditis, and aortic dissection (see also ➲ Chapter 17 of *The ESC Textbook of Cardiovascular Medicine*: Chronic ischaemic heart disease).

Although useful as a warning sign and in the initial diagnostic work-up, pain may hamper vital functions, and must be treated without further delay. For ischaemic chest pain, although reperfusion is the fundamental treatment, residual acute pain is frequent despite conventional acute coronary syndrome (ACS) therapy, and needs adequate analgesia straight away.

Inadequate acute pain relief from tissue injury can have detrimental physiologic effects that are additive to the original insult. Accelerated catecholamine release increases systemic vascular resistance, increases cardiac stroke work, and worsens myocardial oxygen supply–demand ratios. In addition, pain related to therapeutic procedures in the intensive cardiac care unit (ICCU) is frequent and must be prevented by procedural analgesia or sedation. The patient's anguish and suffering may lead to agitation, making it difficult to provide adequate medical care.

Optimal pain management in the ICCU requires precise pain assessment, efficient analgesic therapy, and careful monitoring. The incorrect choice of medications represents a dramatic example of misconceptions that result in inadequate pain control.

Neurobiology of acute pain

The gate control theory of pain proposed by Melzack and Wall has led to much research in the field of pain [2]. A brief synopsis of acute pain is helpful here to delineate steps targeted by analgesic interventions.

As defined by the International Association for the Study of Pain, pain is an unpleasant sensory and emotional experience associated with actual or potential tissue damage, or described in terms of such damage. Five different types of pain are described, the two main ones being nociceptive and neuropathic pain.

When stimulated, nociceptors transmit signals, via the Aδ and the C fibres, to the spinal cord and then up to the brain. Within the brain the signal is transformed into a conscious unpleasant experience. The dorsal horn of the spinal cord has a central role; ascending pathways relay nociceptive information rostrally to thalamic, limbic, and cortical structures responsible for affective and sensory-discriminative responses. The dorsal horn integrates incoming signals through multiple mechanisms and quickly adapts to them. Many molecules that take part in peripheral nociceptive processing also function in spinal nociceptive integration. Agents that impair the synthesis release or effects of such substances within the dorsal horn include morphine, blockers of the N-methyl-D-aspartate (NMDA) receptor or of sodium or calcium channels, α_2-adrenergic agonists, α-aminobutyric acid (GABA), and antagonists of substance P. The essential property of any agent that can control acute pain is its ability to induce dorsal horn amnesia, i.e. to regress the dorsal horn from any injury-induced state to its previous state, and if possible back to the basal state.

Nociception is not synonymous with pain; this process may be necessary for pain to occur, but it is not sufficient to account for pain as a clinical presentation. Nociception is a physiological phenomenon, whereas pain is a perceptual one that involves higher central nervous system mechanisms. Note that neuropathic pain is caused by a primary lesion or dysfunction of the nervous system. Conventional and opioid analgesics are usually ineffective against neuropathic pain.

Endogenous analgesia also commences promptly at the onset of painful processes, such as inflammation or burn injury, and persists for hours. Stress-induced analgesia reflects bilateral descending inhibition of neural activity from the brainstem to multiple spinal levels ('diffuse noxious inhibitory controls') and the analgesic and anti-inflammatory effects of humoral agents (e.g. β-endorphin).

Pain is a stressor with global endocrinological, immunological, and inflammatory consequences. Limbic input to the hypothalamus, integrated by the paraventricular nucleus, drives classic pituitary–adrenal and sympathomedullary stress responses.

Principles of pain management

Guidelines for acute pain management that can be implemented through various models share key strategies [3]:

◆ Assess options for pain control with each patient and provide instruction in simple cognitive behavioural techniques.

◆ Assess pain routinely, just as one monitors vital signs to discern trends before they became catastrophic.

- Treat pain as early as possible.
- Use nondrug and drug interventions together.
- Select treatment according to the clinical setting and modify it promptly according to the patient's response.
- Provide continuity of pain control after discharge (post surgery).

Pain assessment

Valid and reliable assessment of pain is essential for effective pain management. A patient's attempt to communicate pain and distress may not succeed when the patient and physician have different languages, experiences, expectations, or frames of reference. Measurements of pain rely on patients' self-reports, or the inferences physicians make on the basis of the patient's behaviour [4, 5].

Patients can quantify their pain by rating the intensity of pain, e.g. 'Is your usual pain mild, moderate, or severe?' or 'Rate your typical pain from 0 (no pain) to 10 (the worst pain you can imagine)'. In this context, the patient must quantify and average their pain retrospectively. Pain, however, is likely to vary over time and with different activities. In addition, ratings of 'unusual' pain tend to use current pain as their reference point. Thus, asking about usual or typical pain may not accurately reflect pain severity over time. More valid information may be obtained by asking about the current level of pain.

Several simple methods can be used to assess current intensity of pain: numeric scales, descriptive rating scales, visual analogue scales, and box scales. In the numeric rating scale (NRS), the patient is asked to rate the pain from 0 to 10, 0 being 'no pain at all', 10 being 'the worst pain imaginable'. In the visual analogue scale (VAS), the scale is usually a horizontal line measuring 100 mm, where the left end represents 'no pain at all' and the right 'very severe pain'. The patient is asked move the cursor on the line which represents their current pain. The distance in millimetres between the left extremity of the line (0) and the patient's mark is quantified from 0 to 100.

Some patients, e.g. elderly people or those with language problems, may not be capable of using the NRS or VAS. To these patients, the practitioner can propose the simpler but less precise, five-point verbal rating scale (VRS):

- 0 no pain
- 1 mild pain
- 2 moderate pain
- 3 severe pain
- 4 very severe pain.

Ultimately, for cognitive or communication impaired patients, the use of behavioural pain assessment tools is recommended [6, 7] (Abbey Rating Scale [8], Algoplus scale, Doloplus-2 scale).

In sedated, mechanically ventilated patients, pain can be assessed using the Behavioural Pain Scale [9], which is based on the sum of three behavioural expressions: facial expressions, upper limb movements, and compliance with mechanical ventilation, a score of 3 meaning no pain, and 12 being the highest pain score possible.

Pain levels and analgesic therapy

The World Health Organization (WHO) three-step analgesic ladder, originally developed for cancer pain, is applicable to every nociceptive pain.

- Step 1 of the ladder is for mild pain (NRS <3, VAS <30 mm, VRS <2). Nonopioid analgesics such as paracetamol (or if necessary, nonsteroid anti-inflammatory drugs and aspirin) are recommended.
- Step 2 is employed for persisting or worsening pain (NRS <6, VAS <60, VRS <3). A weak opioid such as codeine or tramadol is added to step 1 analgesics. Step 2 analgesics cannot be used in combination; if the analgesia is insufficient, step 3 analgesics should be employed.
- Step 3 is for severe pain (NRS ≥6, VAS ≥60, VRS ≥3) which require a strong opioid analgesia in first intention treatment. The dose is titrated according to response. Nonopioid analgesics can still be used in association with opioids in order to reduce morphine consumption.

The objectives of analgesia are a VRS of less than 3 and/or a VAS of less than 30 mm, i.e. NRS less than 3.

When analgesia must be administered, especially opioids, side effects must be carefully monitored.

Opioid analgesia in the intensive cardiac care unit

Opioids are our most powerful analgesics, but politics, prejudice, and our continuing ignorance still impede optimum prescribing. Opioids act on injured tissue to reduce inflammation, in the dorsal horn to impede transmission of nociception, and supraspinally to activate inhibitory pathways that descend to the spinal segment.

Pros

Opioid and especially morphine analgesia is widely recommended in ACS [10–13]. Morphine is the analgesic of choice in both ST-elevation myocardial infarction (STEMI, class I) and non-STEMI (class II) pain management. It is a strong analgesic, with an onset time of 5–20 min [14–16]. At low doses, morphine is an analgesic and an anxiolytic; at higher doses, it induces sedation.

Although morphine has some side effects, these are limited and seldom serious if the recommended administration protocols are respected (5.5% incidents reported, 2.5% involving minor cardiovascular or respiratory side effects [17]. Paying strict respect to administration protocols and close monitoring may prevent these side effects, and the use of antagonists (naloxone) can treat them if necessary.

The physiological effects of pain have been widely studied, and it is well known that pain induces emotional stress, which increases heart rate and blood pressure by increasing adrenaline levels [18]. Release of adrenaline increases arterial vasoconstriction and the risk of rhythm abnormalities (atrial fibrillation, ventricular tachycardia or fibrillation). Catecholamines have also been reported to be responsible for transient left ventricular ballooning in patients with takotsubo-like left ventricular dysfunction [19].

Adequate analgesia reduces adrenergic stress and minimizes arterial spasm; in particular, it may reduce radial artery spasm, improving chances of success of transradial angioplasty in women [20].

Alongside these cardiac beneficial effects through stress reduction, experimental studies indicate that opioid receptor stimulation in rats results in a reduction in infarct size [21, 22].

Being a dilator of venous capacitance vessels, morphine may have a beneficial effect in patients with pulmonary congestion.

Scientific data have established harmlessness of morphine use in critically ill patients, and ethical considerations must also be taken into account: quality care is impossible to achieve with a suffering patient. Every practitioner should also consider the psychological side effects of medium-term or long-term pain, which include hyperalgesia, allodynia, and fear of health care.

Cons

Pain is the main symptom in acute coronary diseases; the absence of pain may misguide the practitioner and/or underestimate the emergency or severity of coronary disease, even though diagnosis is usually decided on ECG findings and not on persistent pain.

Side effects related to opioid use in analgesia are limited and seldom serious if the recommended administration protocols are respected. Adverse effects and analgesic action are dose-dependent, therefore a cautious titration will provide the best balance between adequate analgesia and side effects. Higher doses may be associated with pruritus, histamine liberation, respiratory depression, nausea, vomiting, and hypotension. Morphine and other opioids have cardiovascular depressant effect, may induce mild hypotension [23–25], and theoretically hamper coronary blood flow and increase the size of myocardial infarction [26]. However, this hypothesis has not yet been demonstrated in patients. Hypotension seems to occur in 1% of spontaneously breathing patients receiving morphine, which could be prevented by correct prescription, careful monitoring, and adequate vascular fluid administration.

A large retrospective study conducted across the United States (CRUSADE Initiative) showed that use of morphine either alone or in combination with nitroglycerine is associated with higher mortality in patients presenting with non-STEMI [27]. However, this retrospective analysis has several methodological limits which do not allow any conclusion on this topic and only emphasize the need for double-blind randomized studies.

The risk–benefit balance favours the use of morphine in acute pain management in the ICCU. Aetiologic treatment is essential, especially reperfusion in STEMI in the 90 min after the onset of pain, but acute pain relief is an important factor in quality care and has beneficial effects.

Choice of opioid

Morphine [36] is a strong μ agonist and is widely used for acute pain relief in both prehospital and in-hospital care. It is the analgesic of choice for management of pain associated with acute coronary disease [10–12]. Its efficacy and safety are widely demonstrated either in emergency care and/or in postoperative analgesia and/or in the intensive care unit [17, 28, 29].

Morphine provides pain and anxiety relief but induces sedation at higher doses. It has no respiratory depressant effect in a patient who is still experiencing pain. At normal analgesic doses, morphine has minimal cardiovascular effects, but at higher doses, it may produce bradycardia by a specific stimulant effect on the central nuclei of vagus nerves. It also produces peripheral vasodilatation by depressing vasomotor centres in the medulla and by histamine liberation. These cardiovascular effects may be prevented by cautious titration.

Severe side effects may occur, such as respiratory depression or sedation, but these can be reversed by naloxone as an antagonist to morphine (and other opioids). It must be administered cautiously (0.04 mg IV repeatedly) in order to maintain a certain analgesic level (see ➲ Intravenous morphine titration). Naloxone has poor efficacy when given by the oral route and a short duration of action (1–4 h) when given by injection.

Morphine is the standard opioid against which others are judged. Beliefs that other drugs act faster, last longer, or have a better balance between beneficial and adverse effects for a particular patient often have little empirical credibility. A list of opioid derivatives is provided in ➲ Table 72.1.

There is little difference in onset time and duration of effect: a faster onset and a longer effect are often achieved by changing the route of administration or formulation.

Intravenous morphine titration

Morphine titration is essential because there is an intra- and an interindividual variation of opioid effects: the relation between opioid dose and analgesia is not predictable for each patient, nor for the same patient in different pain experiences. The main principle of titration (and also of patient-controlled analgesia) is the minimum effective analgesic concentration. Repeated administration of low doses of morphine should allow pain relief but limit side effects. The necessary analgesic dose of morphine varies with time and is different for every patient. Also, the onset time, the duration, and the quality of analgesia are different.

Intravenous morphine titration is widely recommended and used for acute pain analgesia. This initial dose is still debated, as various other schemes have been proposed: no initial bolus but repeated small doses (1–4 mg), or an initial dose of 0.05 mg/kg [17, 30] or 0.1 mg/kg [31–33]. In both out-of-hospital and in-hospital emergency care, as in medical or surgical conditions, the benefit–risk balance does not favour a large initial bolus. The historical first bolus of 0.1 mg/kg or more is no longer recommended [29, 34, 35]. Most European studies recommend small boluses of 2–3 mg every 5 min until pain is relieved [29] or an initial bolus of 0.05 mg/kg [17, 28, 34]. The interval between boluses

should be 5 min [36], and boluses should be repeated until pain is relieved (NRS <3, VAS <30 mm). There is no limited maximal dose, the titration should be pursued as long as the patient is suffering and no major side effects occur. Nevertheless, after a certain number of boluses, which are called 'alarm' doses, the practitioner should reconsider the analgesic protocol: after the fifth bolus medical staff should be advised, and after the tenth, another analgesic or analgesic method (epidural analgesia, peripheral nerve block, etc.) should be considered.

Although titration is a safe way of administering morphine, side effects may exist and patient should be monitored for:

◆ mental status

◆ respiratory status

◆ vital signs (heart rate, respiratory rate, blood pressure, saturation)

◆ pain relief (using the same scale as prior to onset of morphine)

◆ other side effects: nausea, vomiting, urinary retention, etc.

Morphine titration must be stopped if sedation or respiratory depression occurs (Ramsay score >2, respiratory rate <10, Spo_2 <95%) and when pain level is less than 3 on the NRS, 30 mm on the VAS (➲ Fig. 72.1).

Patient-controlled analgesia

After successful titration, analgesia must be pursued. In postsurgical care, patient-controlled analgesia (PCA) has shown better efficiency than conventional systematic prescription of intramuscular or subcutaneous morphine [37]. PCA procures a higher level of comfort; adequate analgesia even if residual pain with a VAS score of 30 mm is sometimes observed, and a global satisfaction score higher than 90%.

Usual settings are:

◆ bolus 1 mg

Table 72.1 Characteristics of opioids

Opioid	Equianalgesic doses (mg)	IV bolus (mg)	Onset time (min)	Average dose (mg)	Duration of action (h)	Side effects
Morphine	1	1–4	5–7	5–15	1–2	Respiratory depression, nausea, vomiting, pruritus, sedation, acute urinary retention
Nalbuphine	2	4–6	5–7	10–20	1–2	As for morphine + limited by a ceiling effect
Fentanyl	0.01	0.02–0.03	5	0.05–0.1	0,5	As for morphine
Sufentanil	0.001	0.002–0.003	3–5	0.008–0.04	4	As for morphine

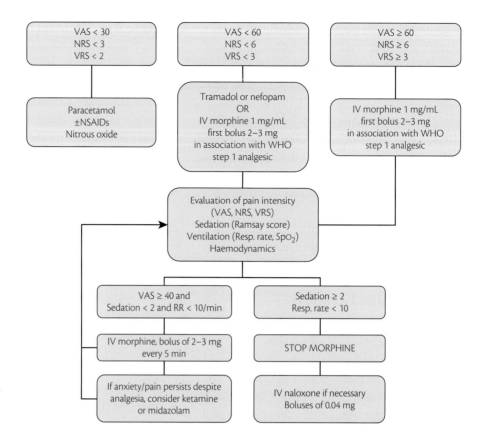

Figure 72.1 Evaluation of pain intensity: visual analogue scale (VAS, mm); numerical rating scale (NRS, 0–10), verbal rating scale (VRS).

+ lockout time 7 min

+ no continuous infusion

Although PCA is recommended for postsurgical analgesia, it is inefficient for procedure-related care.

Besides the usual monitoring when opioids are used, close attention must be paid to the number of boluses required versus delivered. Ineffective pain control (VAS >40, NRS >4, VRS >2/3, or difference between required/delivered boluses >3) must be assessed to determine whether the problem stems from inadequate dosage/settings or from inability or unwillingness of the patient to carry out their own pain management. If ineffective, PCA must be re-explained or adapted (shorter lockout time, greater boluses) or associated with other analgesic therapies (step 1 analgesics, regional analgesia techniques). Morphine PCA cannot be associated with other opioid or sedative therapies.

Fentanyl and derivatives are opioids stronger than morphine. Fentanyl is not a potent histamine liberator but, like all its derivatives, can induce thoracic rigidity. In hypovolaemic patients, intravenous boluses of fentanyl induce hypotension. Fentanyl is not recommended in spontaneously breathing patients, but it is recommended in intubated and ventilated patients. The adult dosage is 2–5 μg/kg per hour intravenously in ventilated patients.

Sufentanil is a fentanyl derivate and, as such, it is not recommended in spontaneously breathing patients, but in intubated and ventilated patients. The adult dosage is 0.15–0.6 μg/kg per hour intravenously in ventilated patients.

Other analgesics

+ Paracetamol is a 'weak', widely used [38] peripheral analgesic with rare side effects and few contraindications (allergy, severe hepatic disease). Efficiency is achieved in 20–30 minutes when administered intravenously. It can be associated with other analgesics. The dosage is 1 g in a 15-min infusion every 6 h.

+ Nefopam is a strong central nonopioid analgesic which inhibits serotonin, dopamine, and noradrenaline reuptake, and has no respiratory depressant effect [39]. In postsurgical care, nefopam reduces morphine consumption by 30–50% [40]. Its principal side effects (nausea, sweats, and tachycardia) may be prevented by a slow infusion (30 min). It may be associated with any other analgesic. Nefopam may be administered intravenously, intramuscularly, or by mouth, at the dose of 20 mg, every 4 h.

- Tramadol is an opioid μ agonist with weak action (10 times less than morphine) [36]. Its usefulness in acute pain in the ICCU is limited in comparison with that of morphine.

- Nalbuphine is primarily a κ agonist that causes sedation and analgesia. It causes mild analgesia on the μ receptor, but a high affinity with this receptor causes antagonism if another opioid was bound to it previously. Its ceiling effect limits analgesia [41], while the respiratory effect has been reported as similar to that of morphine for equivalent analgesia. The sedative effect can be reversed by naloxone. Adult dosage is 0.3 mg/kg intravenously.

- Ketamine is a NDMA receptor inhibitor [42, 43]. At low doses it has a analgesic effect (0.1–0.3 mg/kg). it can be used in association with morphine, particularly in post-operative pain management, where it has an antihyperalgesic effect. Low doses of ketamine have been found to reduce consumption of opioids. It has a low sedative, cardiovascular, and respiratory depressant effect, but its psychotropic effects must be taken into account. Ketamine may be used in small doses (0.1–0.3 mg/kg·per hour) as a local anesthetic, particularly for the treatment of neuropathic pain.

- Nitrous oxide and oxygen is a mixture of equal volumes of these gases, with very low cardiovascular and respiratory effects. It provides analgesia rapidly and with fast recovery after cessation. Nitrous oxide should be self-administered and can be used during a painful procedure (arterial punctures, kinaesitherapy, debridement of cutaneous ulcer, bandages, etc.). It should not be used in patients with thoracic injury, pneumothorax, or in patients requiring more than 50% of oxygen.

- Midazolam can be used at low doses as an anxiolytic agent, with extreme caution in spontaneously breathing patients due to its side effects (sedation, respiratory depressant effect). In this case the dose is intravenous boluses of 1 mg. Its use must be reserved for persistent pain despite a adequate analgesic protocol. When used in association with opioid analgesics, side effects tend to multiply. Midazolam is the sedative drug of choice in ventilated patients in association with fentanyl or sufentanil; the adult dosage is 0.1 mg/kg per hour.

Psychological interventions

Surgery or trauma not only damages tissue, but also elicits psychological responses similar to post-traumatic stress disorder. Anxiety and agitation are often due to incomprehension, inadequate information, and insufficient empathy.

Giving more information and empathy can help in treating acute pain. Psychological resilience and preparedness help the patient to control pain.

Specific conditions

Ischaemic chest pain and use of nitrates (see also ◉ Chapter 17 of *The ESC Textbook of Cardiovascular Medicine*)

Nitroglycerine is an effective treatment for ischaemic chest pain and is recommended in both STEMI and non-STEMI patients, if no contraindications exist [10–12]. Although the use of nitrates is controversial, it can be beneficial for patients with acute myocardial infarction through their vasodilatative and analgesic effect. However, nitrates can also be deleterious by inducing hypotension, particularly in inferior or right location of STEMI. Nitroglycerine is particularly indicated as a vasodilator in patients with left ventricular failure.

Nitrates should be avoided in patients with systolic blood pressure less than 90 mmHg or 30 mmHg below baseline, patients with marked bradycardia or tachycardia, and patients with suspected right ventricle infarction and probably in inferior ischaemia. Nitrates should not be administrated to patients who have received phosphodiesterase inhibitor (e.g. sildenafil) for erectile dysfunction within 24–48 h.

In ischaemic pathology, analgesic treatment must not be delayed, in order to obtain pain relief as soon as possible. When ischaemic pain persist despite the initial dose of nitrates, analgesic treatments should be employed straightaway.

Patients with organ failure

Pulmonary failure

Pain must be treated in patients with pulmonary failure [44]. Multimodal analgesia including regional analgesic techniques must be used whenever possible in the postoperative period and/or in traumatic injury. Medullar regional anaesthesia and/or local infiltration are the postsurgical analgesia techniques of choice.

In acute respiratory failure, morphine has a positive effect on respiratory function. When respiratory failure is due to pain, adequate analgesia improves ventilation. Even if nonopioid analgesics must be preferred, morphine may be used with extreme caution and in association with nonopioid analgesics in order to reduce consumption of morphine. PCA is therefore preferred to other administration modalities.

If administration of morphine is necessary, the patient must be monitored cautiously (sedation and respiratory status). Other sedative and respiratory depressant molecules are proscribed (benzodiazepine) in spontaneously breathing patients.

If sedation or respiratory depression occurs, it must be treated by naloxone.

Acute heart failure

Effective analgesia is essential, as pain and its sympathomimetic effects are deleterious [45]. Morphine is the recommended analgesic. In postoperative care, optimal analgesia is multimodal, involving loco-regional anaesthesia, paracetamol, low dose of ketamine, nefopam, and morphine.

Tramadol can be used with extreme caution. nonsteroidal anti-inflammatory agents (NSAIDs), including COX-2 inhibitors, are proscribed in coronary patients (prothrombotic effect, hypertension, renal injury, etc.).

Liver failure

There is a distinction between chronic liver patients and acute liver patients. Liver failure is associated with coagulopathy (coagulation factor V <50%). Liver disease globally increases volumes of distribution and biological half-life, therefore use of opioids may require a dose adaptation and close monitoring [46].

NSAIDs are contraindicated in cirrhotic patients, while paracetamol, tramadol, and NSAIDs are contraindicated in case of acute hepatitis. Ketamine may be used.

Renal failure

NSAIDs and tramadol are proscribed in case of severe renal failure [47]. Paracetamol and ketamine may be used. Opioid analgesia must be used cautiously. Although the titration protocol can be identical to the initial pain relief in the ICCU, opioid analgesia requires dose adaptation and a longer delay for readministration in renal patients. PCA is preferred. Whenever applicable, regional anaesthesia techniques must be preferred.

Post-thoracotomy analgesia

Patients undergoing thoracotomy may suffer from severe postoperative pain if analgesia is not managed appropriately. In addition, the impaired pulmonary function as a result of thoracotomy may be worsened by the effects of pain. Studies have shown that acute postoperative pain is a predictor of long-term pain after thoracotomy, and early and aggressive treatment may help to reduce the chronic pain.

In post-thoracotomy patients, systemic analgesia has often proven to be insufficient for pain relief when used alone.

Thoracic epidural analgesia and paravertebral block are commonly used regional techniques. Although thoracic epidural analgesia is commonly considered as the 'gold standard' for postoperative pain treatment, it may be contraindicated or not efficient enough. The Procedure-Specific Postoperative Pain Management (PROSPECT) working group recommends either thoracic epidural local anesthetic plus opioid or paravertebral block with local anesthetic, and, if contraindicated, intercostal local anesthetic [48].

Iatrogenic neuropathic pain is probably the most common type of postsurgical persistent pain and, as such, surgical techniques that avoid nerve damage should be used wherever possible [49].

Despite advances in the understanding of the processes that lead to persistent pain and the increasing ease of identification of patients at risk of developing such pain, the management and prevention of postsurgical persistent pain often remains inadequate.

Management of neuropathic pain

Neuropathic pain is caused by neural injury, and the symptoms experienced by the patient with neuropathic pain differ from those with nociceptive pain. Many patients with neuropathic pain exhibit persistent or paroxysmal pain that is independent of a stimulus. This stimulus-independent pain can be shooting, lancinating, or burning and may depend on activity in the sympathetic nervous system. Pain is normally elicited only when intense or damaging noxious stimuli activate high-threshold nociceptor primary sensory neurons. Peripheral neuropathic pain manifests as spontaneous pain (stimulus-independent pain) or pain hypersensitivity elicited by a stimulus after damage to or alterations in sensory neurons (stimulus-evoked pain).

Spontaneous activity in nociceptor C fibres is thought to be responsible for persistent burning pain and the sensitization of dorsal horn neurons. Similarly, spontaneous activity in large myelinated A fibres (which normally signal innocuous sensations) is related to stimulus-independent paraesthesias and, after central sensitization, to dysaesthesias and pain.

Neuropathic pain is currently classified on the basis of the aetiology of the insult to the nervous system or the anatomical distribution of the pain. Although this classification has some use for the differential diagnosis of the neuropathy, and for disease-modifying treatment if available, it offers no framework for clinical management of the pain.

Opioids are less effective in neuropathic [50] than in nociceptive pain while other agents (i.e. tricyclic antidepressants [51], anticonvulsivants [52, 53], nefopam, ketamine) can relieve neuropathic pain. Anticonvulsants have differing modes of action, so ineffectiveness of one does not imply that others may not work.

Recommendations for treatment are based on degrees of evidence of analgesic efficiency, safety, ease of use, and cost-effectiveness. Analgesic agents recommended for first-line treatments are antidepressants (tricyclics) and anticonvulsants (gabapentin and pregabalin) and for second-line treatments, tramadol and opioid agents. Third line treatments (serotonin noradrenaline reuptake inhibitors and topical lidocaine) can be considered as second-line treatments under certain circumstances [54]. Analgesic selection should be individualized for each patient, considering side effects, potential beneficial or deleterious effects on comorbidities, and whether prompt onset of pain relief is necessary.

Conclusion

In critical care patients, pain is a frequently encountered symptom, which can have multiple aetiologies. Although useful as a warning sign and sometimes pathognomonic of ischaemic heart disease, pain is deleterious for vital functions and therefore must be treated efficiently and systematically without delay. Intravenous morphine titration is still the 'gold standard' for acute pain analgesia, especially for ischaemic chest pain. The development and use of multimodal analgesia and regional techniques must be encouraged whenever possible, and particularly for postsurgical pain.

Personal perspective

The prevalence of pain in the ICCU is significant. Acute pain must be treated aggressively, without any delay, supporting opioid analgesia in multimodal analgesic protocols according to international recommendations.

Optimal pain management, especially in the ICCU requires pain intensity evaluation, clear and written protocols widely distributed to all ICCU staff, staff training, patient monitoring, and care quality control.

Further reading

Arntz H-R, Bossaert L, Filippatos GS. European Resuscitation Council Guidelines for Resuscitation 2005 Section 5. Initial management of acute coronary syndromes. *Resuscitation* 2005;**67**S1:S87–S96.

Joshi G, Bonnet F, Shah R, *et al.* A systematic review of randomized trials evaluating regional techniques for postthoracotomy analgesia. *Anesth Analg* 2008;**107**:1026–1040.

Puntillo K, Pasero C, Li D, *et al.* Evaluation of pain in ICU patients. *Chest* 2009;**135**:1069–1074.

Online resource

🖰 Société Française d'Anesthésie et de Réanimation (SFAR) Expert conference on sedation and analgesia in spontaneously breathing patients in emergency structures SFAR 2010, in process. http://www.sfar.org

➲ For additional multimedia materials please visit the online version of the book (🖰 http://www.esciacc.oxfordmedicine.com).

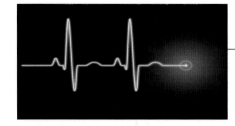

CHAPTER 73

Acute cognitive disorders: recognition and management of delirium in the intensive cardiac care unit

John A. McPherson, Chad E. Wagner, and E. Wesley Ely

Contents

Summary

Delirium is the most common acute cognitive disorder seen in critically ill patients in the intensive cardiac care unit. It is defined as a disturbance of consciousness and cognition that develops suddenly and fluctuates over time. Delirious patients can become hyperactive, hypoactive, or both. The occurrence of delirium during hospitalization is associated with increased in-hospital and long-term morbidity and mortality. The cause of delirium is multifactorial, and may include imbalances in neurotransmitters, inflammatory mediators, metabolic disturbances, impaired sleep, and use of sedatives and analgesics. Patients with advanced age, dementia, chronic illness, extensive vascular disease, and low cardiac output are at particular risk of developing delirium. Specialized bedside assessment tools are now available to rapidly diagnose delirium, even in mechanically ventilated patients. Increased awareness of delirium risk factors, in addition to nonpharmacological and pharmacological treatments for delirium, can be effective in reducing the incidence of delirium in cardiac patients, and in minimizing adverse outcomes once delirium occurs.

Introduction

Delirium is a disturbance of consciousness and cognition associated with increased in-hospital morbidity and mortality. In an executive summary of medical injury in hospitalized patients, delirium was considered as one of the six leading causes of preventable injury in those over 65 [1]. The diagnosis and treatment of delirium is particularly challenging in cardiac surgery and cardiology patients where the primary focus is on life-threatening issues. Patients diagnosed with delirium in the coronary care unit (CCU) may have increased time of mechanical ventilation, increased CCU length of stay, prolonged neuropsychological dysfunction, and increased mortality. This chapter seeks to define delirium and describe delirium subtypes, pathophysiology, and risk factors. The chapter relays strategies for assessment, prevention, and treatment of the delirious cardiac patient.

Definition

Delirium is defined by *The Diagnostic and Statistical Manual of Mental Disorders* (DSM IV) [2] as a disturbance of consciousness with inattention, accompanied by a change in cognition or perceptual disturbance that develops over a short period of time (hours to days) and fluctuates over time. Though many different terms have been used, the current consensus of many is to use the unifying term delirium and subcategorize according to level of alertness (hyperactive, hypoactive, or mixed) [3].

Prevalence and subtypes of delirium

In a 1975 review of the psychiatric aspects of cardiac intensive therapy, Bourden stated 'The post cardiotomy state is typically delirious and although organic factors are important it is multi-determined [4].' Over the past 30 years, the prevalence of delirium in several cohort studies has been reported to range between 20% and 80% [5–8]. There are few studies in nonsurgical cardiac patients, but one study observed an incidence of delirium of 28% in patients more than 90 years old after myocardial infarction [9].

There is more data on the incidence of delirium after cardiac surgery, with rates ranging from 3% to 70%, but this may be an underestimation due to the difficulty in diagnosing hypoactive delirium with lack of frequent assessments and standardized criteria for diagnosis [10]. Delirium rates may also vary according to type of surgery, with valve replacement surgery having a higher incidence of delirium than coronary bypass grafting [11]. A recent study evaluated delirium subtypes from a cohort of ventilated and nonventilated medical intensive care unit (ICU) patients and found the rates of these subtypes in the ICU to be 1.6% hyperactive, 43.5% hypoactive, and 54.1% mixed [12]. Hyperactive delirium, rare in the pure form, is characterized by agitation, restlessness, attempting to remove catheters or tubes, hitting, biting, and emotional lability [3, 13]. This subtype is often referred to as 'ICU psychosis' and is associated with a better overall prognosis. Hypoactive delirium is very common and may lead to a more deleterious outcome [14]. This delirium subtype is characterized by withdrawal, flat affect, apathy, lethargy, and decreased responsiveness [14–16].

Unfortunately, delirium remains unrecognized and misdiagnosed in 66–84% of patients because of its short onset, fluctuating course, and manifestations similar to those of depression and dementia [17]. Delirium is clearly linked to increased morbidity and its prevalence is significant even if underestimated in the cardiac literature. It is therefore recommended that all CCUs and cardiothoracic surgical ICUs employ a valid and reliable diagnostic instrument to screen for delirium.

Prognostic significance of delirium

Among medical ICU patients, delirium has been shown to be a strong predictor of increased time on mechanical ventilation, increased ICU length of stay, increased hospital costs, prolonged neuropsychological dysfunction, and even mortality [18–21]. A prospective study of 112 cardiac surgical patients found that delirious patients had more postoperative respiratory insufficiency, longer hospitalization, longer CCU stay, and higher mortality [22]. Ely and coworkers studied 275 medical ICU patients and found the development of delirium is associated with a threefold increase in risk of death after controlling for pre-existing comorbidities, severity of illness, coma, and the use of sedative and analgesic medications [19]. Additionally, in a recent study of 98 medical ICU patients [23], neuropsychological testing 3 months after ICU discharge demonstrated that the duration of delirium was associated with an increased risk of long-term cognitive impairment. In cardiac surgery patients, Koster *et al.* showed that delirium was related to an increased incidence of nursing home placement and reduced cognitive and functional recovery for up to 1.5 years after surgery [22]. Preliminary data suggests there is a significant association between ICU delirium and long-term cognitive impairment; future prospective work may help further define the prognostic significance of delirium in the cardiac patient.

Pathophysiology of delirium

It is likely that multiple factors play a role in the development of delirium. Further, these factors are also likely associated with long-term cognitive impairment in many patients seen in the CCU and following cardiac surgical procedures.

Neurotransmitters

Imbalances in the synthesis, release, and inactivation of neurotransmitters modulating the control of cognitive function, behaviour, and mood can lead to delirium [14, 15]. Three of the neurotransmitter systems involved in the pathophysiology of delirium are dopamine, γ-aminobutyric acid (GABA), and acetylcholine [24–26]. While dopamine increases the excitability of neurons, GABA and acetylcholine decrease it [26]. As a result, dynamic changes in one or more of these neurotransmitters can result in neuronal instability and unpredictable neurotransmission. In particular, an excess of dopamine and depletion of acetylcholine are two major physiological problems believed to be central to delirium. In addition to these neurotransmitter systems, others that are thought to be involved in the development of delirium are serotonin imbalance, endorphin hyperfunction, and increased central noradrenergic activity [14, 24]. During and after cardiopulmonary bypass surgery, levels of all of these neurotransmitters may be affected, thus increasing the risk of postoperative delirium.

Inflammatory mediators

Abnormalities induced by endotoxin and cytokines [27–30] in critically ill cardiac patients can also lead to acute cognitive disorders. Mediators such as tumour necrosis factor α (TNF-α) and interleukin-1 (IL-1) initiate an inflammatory cascade that leads to endothelial damage, thrombin formation, and microvascular compromise [31], and are commonly elevated in acute coronary syndromes (ACS). Animal models reveal that these inflammatory mediators cross the blood–brain barrier [32], increase vascular permeability in the brain [33], and result in electroencephalographic (EEG) changes consistent with those seen in septic patients with delirium [34, 35]. Potential mechanisms include (1) decreased cerebral blood flow; (2) formation of microaggregates of fibrin, platelets, neutrophils, and erythrocytes in the cerebral microvasculature; (3) cerebral vasoconstriction occurring in response to α_1-adrenoceptor activity [36]; and (4) interference with neurotransmitter synthesis and neurotransmission [37]. Intraoperative cerebral embolization during cardiac surgery can precipitate an inflammatory response to ischaemic injury; cerebral emboli have long been implicated as a cause of cognitive disorders following cardiac surgery [38].

Impaired oxidative metabolism

Others have speculated that delirium is a behavioural manifestation of a 'widespread reduction of cerebral oxidative metabolism resulting in an imbalance of neurotransmission [39].' Based on various EEG evaluations of delirious patients, Engel and Romano postulated that delirium is a state of 'cerebral insufficiency,' i.e. a global failure of cerebral oxidative metabolism [40]. Their work demonstrated that delirium is associated with diffuse slowing on the EEG, a finding thought to represent a reduction in brain metabolism.

Cholinergic deficiency

Blass *et al.* [41] suggested that impaired oxidative metabolism in the brain results in a cholinergic deficiency. The finding that hypoxia impairs acetylcholine synthesis supports this hypothesis [42]. This reduction in cholinergic function results in an increase in the level of glutamate, dopamine, and noradrenaline (norepinephrine) in the brain. Additionally serotonin and GABA are reduced, all contributing to delirium.

Large neutral amino acids in delirium

Disturbances in the amount of amino acids, the precursors of cerebral neurotransmitters, may contribute to the development of delirium [43]. The large neutral amino acid transporter type1 (LAT1) regulates the cerebral uptake of amino acids [44]. The essential amino acid tryptophan, the precursor for serotonin, competes with several large neutral amino acids (LNAA) such as tyrosine, phenylalanine, valine, leucine, and isoleucine for transport across the blood–brain barrier via LAT1 [44]. Another amino acid that may play an important role in the pathogenesis of delirium is phenylalanine [39]. Like tryptophan, phenylalanine competes with various LNAAs for transport across the blood–brain barrier. An increase in the cerebral uptake of tyrosine and phenylalanine, compared to the other LNAAs, leads to increased availability of precursors for both dopamine and noradrenaline, which has been implicated in the pathogenesis of delirium [39].

Inflammatory response

While delirium may occur as a result of perturbations in other organ systems, the brain responds to systemic illness with an inflammatory response of its own that also includes the production of cytokines, cell infiltration, and tissue damage [45–46]. Conversely, local inflammation in the brain and subsequent activation of central nervous system immune responses can lead to manifestations of systemic inflammation [12, 47, 48] including increased systemic levels of TNF-α, IL-10, and interferon-γ [45, 49–51]. Thus, the brain can potentially become an engine of inflammation driving the development and/or resolution of multiple organ dysfunction syndrome.

Risk factors for delirium

Only a few studies have examined the risk factors of delirium in cardiac patients. In general, delirium is more prevalent in patients with pre-existing dementia, chronic illness, advanced age, and depression [7, 26, 52, 53]. Dubois et al. [54] found that pre-existing hypertension and smoking (presumably due to relative hypoperfusion and nicotine withdrawal, respectively) were significantly associated with the development of ICU delirium. Following cardiac surgery, the risk of postoperative delirium is increased in patients with a history of myocardial infarction, prior stroke, decreased cardiac output, diabetes, and extensive peripheral arterial disease [55].

Precipitating and iatrogenic risk factors represent areas of potential modification and thus intervention for delirium prevention and/or treatment. Precipitating factors include hypoxia, metabolic disturbances, electrolyte imbalances, withdrawal syndromes, acute infection (systemic and intracranial), seizures, dehydration, hyperthermia, sleep deprivation, head trauma, vascular disorders, and intracranial space-occupying lesions [26, 52, 53].

Risk factors for delirium can be divided into three categories: (1) host factors; (2) the acute illness itself; and (3) iatrogenic or environmental factors (⊃ Table 73.1). While delirium may be a function of the patient's specific underlying illness, it may also be due to their medical management and thus be preventable in many cases. In particular, sedative and analgesic medications and sleep deprivation appear to be the most common iatrogenic, and potentially preventable, risk factors for delirium. Data on the association of anticholinergics, corticosteroids, histamine-2 receptor antagonists, and anticonvulsants on the development of delirium in critically ill patients is conflicting and will not be discussed further [56–59].

Sedatives and analgesic agents contributing to delirium

Sedative and analgesic medications remain fundamental in the treatment of acutely ill cardiac patients. However, continuous intravenous sedation is associated with prolonged mechanical ventilation and increased morbidity [60]. Similarly, associations between psychoactive medications and worsening cognitive outcomes in postsurgical patients have been published. Marcantonio et al. [61] studied postoperative patients with delirium, and found a positive association with concomitant benzodiazepine and meperidine use. Others [54] have shown that opiates (morphine and meperidine) administered either intravenously or via an epidural catheter may be associated with the development of delirium in medical/surgical ICU patients. Recently our group has studied the temporal relationship of administration of sedatives and analgesics and delirium [62]. In our study, lorazepam, but not fentanyl, morphine, and propofol, was found to be an independent risk factor for daily transition to delirium [62]. Similar associations between midazolam and transition to delirium have been found in trauma and postsurgical patients [8].

GABA-receptor sparing agents may help reduce some of the cognitive dysfunction seen in critically ill patients. As indicated above, the data on opioids and delirium is not as consistent as that with the benzodiazepines. While meperidine has been associated with delirium in most of the published studies, the data regarding fentanyl and morphine are less convincing [54, 61, 63]. A recent prospective observational trial found that patients with well-controlled pain on morphine following hip surgery were less likely to develop delirium than those who received other opioids [63]. These investigations also point to the importance of judicious use of these psychoactive medications, with focus on adequate analgesia.

Table 73.1 Risk factors for delirium in coronary care unit patients

Patient factors	Acute illness	Iatrogenic or environmental
Age	Low cardiac output	Metabolic disturbances [a]
Baseline comorbidities/ vascular disease	Hypoxaemia [a]	Anticholinergic medications [a]
Baseline cognitive impairment	Global severity of illness score	Sedative and analgesic medications [a]
Genetic predisposition (?)	Metabolic disturbances	Sleep disturbances [a]

[a] Potentially modifiable factors.

Sleep disturbances contributing to delirium

Critically ill patients typically have severe sleep deprivation with disruption of sleep architecture. The average amount of sleep in ICUs is as low as 2 h out of 24 h, with less than 6% of it spent in REM sleep [64]. The causes of sleep deprivation in the ICU are legion, including excessive noise and lighting, patient care activities such as procedures and baths, metabolic consequences of critical illness, mechanical ventilation, and sedative and analgesic medications administered to the patients [65]. Any disturbance in duration and quality of sleep can have detrimental effects on protein synthesis, cellular and humoral immunity, and energy expenditure resulting in respiratory alterations, haemodynamic effects and cognitive function [65, 66]. Studies have demonstrated that only about 30% of sleep arousals in the CCU are a result of environmental factors such as noise, patient activities, and light, suggesting that other patient factors or management issues significantly alter natural sleep patterns [67]. It is worth noting that psychoactive medications are common risk factors for both delirium and sleep disturbances, while sleep deprivation can itself lead to delirium.

Diagnosis of delirium in intensive care unit patients

The development of tools such as the Intensive Care Delirium Screening Checklist [68] and the Confusion Assessment Method for the ICU (CAM-ICU) [6, and see ➲ Online resource] have allowed for the rapid diagnosis of delirium by nonpsychiatric physicians and other health care personnel, even in mechanically ventilated patients. As a result, the Society of Critical Care Medicine has proposed guidelines [69] for more standardized monitoring of delirium using the CAM-ICU. Applying this assessment tool to acutely ill cardiac patients is both straightforward and practical.

Diagnosis of delirium is a two-step process (➲ Box 73.1). The level of arousal is first measured by using a standardized sedation scale, such as the Richmond Agitation-Sedation Scale (RASS) [70, 71]. The RASS is a 10-point scale ranging from + 4 to –5, with a score of 0 denoting a calm and alert patient. Positive RASS scores denote active or aggressive symptomology ranging from +1 (mild restlessness) to + 4 (dangerous agitation). Negative RASS scores indicate progressive sedation with response to verbal commands

(RASS score –1 to –3) and physical stimuli (RASS score –4 and –5). If the RASS score is –4 or below, no further evaluation for delirium is performed, as the patient is comatose. For patients with a RASS score of –3 and above, delirium can be assessed by the CAM-ICU in about 60–90 s [72]. The CAM-ICU assesses the following four features: acute change or fluctuation in mental status (Feature 1), inattention (Feature 2), disorganized thinking (Feature 3), and an altered level of consciousness (Feature 4). To be diagnosed as delirious, the patient needs to have a RASS score of –3 or higher, with an acute change or fluctuation in mental status (Feature 1), accompanied by inattention (Feature 2) and either disorganized thinking (Feature 3) or an altered level of consciousness (Feature 4).

Prevention and management of delirium

Primary prevention and nonpharmacological approaches

In a large study of 852 older general medical patients [73], strategies for primary prevention of delirium resulted in a 40% reduction in the odds of developing delirium (15% in controls vs 9.9% in the intervention patients). The protocol addressed multiple risk factors for delirium via the following methods: repeated reorientation of the patient by trained volunteers and nurses; provision of cognitively stimulating activities for the patient three times a day; a nonpharmacological sleep protocol to enhance normalization of sleep/wake cycles; early mobilization activities and range of motion exercises; timely removal of catheters and physical restraints; institution of the use of eyeglasses and magnifying lenses, hearing aids, and earwax disimpaction; and early correction of dehydration. However, this intervention did not show sustained benefit when the patients were followed to 6 months [74]. Other prevention studies of delirium prevention either demonstrated benefit only in subgroups such as those without underlying dementia [75] or did not show any benefit at all [76]. In contrast, when multidisciplinary delirium-specific education is provided for medical staff, studies have demonstrated a decrease in the duration and severity of delirium in their patients [77, 78].

Given the clinical characteristics of patients in the CCU, delirium is often likely to be inevitable. In these cases, the basic tenets of patient care such as restoring sleep/wake cycles, timely removal of catheters, early mobilization,

---

Box 73.1 The Richmond Agitation–Sedation Scale (RASS) and the Confusion Assessment Method for the ICU (CAM-ICU)

This sedation scale and delirium instrument can be used together as a two-step approach to assess consciousness and diagnose delirium. Patients are considered to have delirium if they have RASS scores of –3 and above and are CAM-ICU positive by having Features 1 and 2 and either Feature 3 or Feature 4 positive.

Step 1: Sedation assessment

The Richmond Agitation and Sedation Scale (RASS)

Score	Term	Description	
+4	Combative	Overtly combative, violent, immediate danger to staff	
+3	Very agitated	Pulls or removes tube(s) or catheter(s); aggressive	
+2	Agitated	Frequent nonpurposeful movement, fights ventilator	
+1	Restless	Anxious, but movements not aggressive; vigorous	
0	Alert and calm		
–1	Drowsy	Not fully alert, but has sustained awakening (eye opening/eye contact) to voice (≥10 s)	Verbal stimulation
–2	Light sedation	Briefly awakens with eye contact to voice (<10 s)	
–3	Moderate sedation	Movement or eye opening to voice (but no eye contact)	Physical stimulation
–4	Deep sedation	No response to voice, but movement or eye opening to physical stimulation	
–5	Unarousable	No response to voice or physical stimulation	

* If RASS is –4 or –5, then stop and reassess patient at later time.

* If RASS is above –4 (–3 through +4) then proceed to Step 2

Step 2: Delirium assessment

* Feature 1: Acute onset of mental status changes or a fluctuating course
and

* Feature 2: Inattention
and
EITHER

* Feature 3: Disorganized thinking
OR

* Feature 4: Altered level of consciousness
= DELIRIUM

Data From Ely EW, Inouye S, Bernard G, *et al.* Delirium in mechanically ventilated patients: validity and reliability of the confusion assessment method for the intensive care unit (CAM-ICU). *JAMA* 2001;**286**:2703–2710; and Ely EW, Margolin R, Francis J, *et al.* Evaluation of delirium in critically ill patients: validation of the Confusion Assessment Method for the Intensive Care Unit (CAM-ICU). *Crit Care Med* 2001;**29**:1370–137.

---

minimization of unnecessary noise/stimuli, and frequent reorientation should be applied liberally. While sedative and analgesics have a very important role in patient comfort, particularly in patients with acute cardiovascular disease, providers must strive to achieve the proper balance of administering these drugs and avoiding unnecessary or overzealous use. Instituting daily interruption of sedatives and analgesics, protocolizing their delivery, and instituting target-based sedation have all been shown to improve patients' outcomes [60, 79–81]. Family involvement can also be very helpful in reorienting and soothing some

delirious patients. It is important to teach family members of the fluctuating course of delirium as well as how they can detect delirium. Preventive and management strategies for delirium in the CCU represent an important area for future investigation.

Pharmacological therapy

Medications to treat delirium should be used only after efforts have been made to correct modifiable contributing factors (e.g. sleep disturbance, restraints, etc.) as discussed above. It is important to recognize that delirium can be a manifestation of an acute, life-threatening problem that requires immediate attention (such as hypoxia, hypercarbia, hypoglycaemia, metabolic derangements, or cardiogenic shock). These conditions should be ruled out prior to the institution of drug therapy. While agents used to treat delirium are intended to improve cognition, they all have psychoactive effects which may further cloud the sensorium and promote a longer overall duration of cognitive impairment. As a result, these drugs should be used judiciously in the smallest possible dose and for the shortest time necessary, a practice infrequently adhered to in most CCUs. In addition, some patients will prove refractory to all 'cocktail' approaches to sedation and delirium therapy, and these patients should be considered for a trial of complete cessation of all psychoactive drugs. A prospective, randomized, but unblinded trial in postoperative cardiac surgical patients showed that sedation with dexmedetomidine at sternal closure had an 8% incidence of delirium postoperatively compared to 50% in those sedated with either propofol or benzodiazepines [82]. Similarly, in a recently completed double-blind randomized controlled trial in ICU patients, a sedation strategy with dexmedetomidine versus lorazepam resulted in fewer coma days and more days free of delirium [83]. While these are small pilot studies, they form the basis for the design of larger interventional studies targeting α_2 receptors in order to spare the GABA receptors.

Benzodiazepines, commonly used in the CCU for sedation, are not recommended for the management of delirium due to the likelihood of oversedation, exacerbation of confusion, and respiratory suppression. However, they remain the drugs of choice for the treatment of delirium tremens (and other withdrawal syndromes) and seizures. The amnesic qualities of benzodiazepines can be useful during painful or unpleasant procedures. However, the accumulation of these drugs may lead to prolonged delirium long after the drugs have been discontinued. In certain populations, particularly elderly patients with underlying dementia, benzodiazepines may lead to increased confusion and agitation. In such cases, one may try to take advantage of the sedative effects of haloperidol in lieu of continued benzodiazepines.

Currently, haloperidol is the drug of choice in the treatment of delirium, although this is based on limited data from nonrandomized case series and anecdotal reports [69]. Haloperidol is a butyrophenone 'typical' antipsychotic, and is the most widely used neuroleptic agent for delirium [84]. It does not suppress the respiratory drive and works as a dopamine receptor antagonist by blocking the D_2 receptor,

which effectively treats positive symptomatology (hallucinations, unstructured thought patterns, etc.) and produces a variable sedative effect.

In the CCU, a recommended starting dose would be 2–5 mg every 6 to 12 h (IV or oral), with maximal effective doses approaching 20 mg/day. This dose range is usually adequate to achieve the 'theoretically optimal' 60% D_2 receptor blockage [85], while avoiding complete D_2 receptor saturation associated with the adverse effects cited below. The critical nature of care in cardiac patients—due to the potential for inadvertent removal of central lines, endotracheal tubes, or aortic balloon pumps—frequently requires the use of much higher doses of haloperidol or another sedative. Unfortunately, there is little evidence-based data to guide dosage recommendations in the CCU. Once calm, the patient can usually be managed with much lower maintenance doses of haloperidol.

Neither haloperidol nor similar agents (i.e. droperidol and chlorpromazine) have been extensively studied in the CCU [69]. Newer 'atypical' antipsychotic agents (e.g. risperidone, ziprasidone, quetiapine, and olanzapine) may also prove helpful for delirium [86]. The theoretical basis for such agents (especially in hypoactive/mixed subtypes of delirium) is derived from their effect on other potentially important neurotransmitters such as serotonin, acetylcholine, and noradrenaline [86–89]. The use of haloperidol has been associated with a mortality benefit in a retrospective analysis of critically ill patients with delirium [90]. Kalisvaart [91] also showed that low-dose haloperidol prophylaxis reduced the duration and severity of delirium in elderly hip surgery patients, even though the actual prevalence of delirium was not reduced. Similarly, Skrobik [86] reported that olanzapine and haloperidol were equally efficacious in treating delirium in both medical and surgical patients, but that olanzapine was associated with fewer side effects. Kato [92] has suggested that genotyping may affect the choice of antipsychotic drugs used to treat delirium. His group described a patient with the CYP2D6 genotype who had persistent delirium and developed severe extrapyramidal symptoms when treated with risperidone. The patient was then switched to quetiapine (metabolized by CYP3A4) and the patient's delirium cleared within 2 days without side effects. This case report is interesting and hypothesis-generating in that pharmacogenetics may play an important role in the future management of delirium. Adequately powered prospective randomized controlled trials of these agents are not yet available but are needed in order to provide clinicians with evidence-based guidelines for preventing and treating delirium.

Adverse effects of typical and atypical antipsychotics include hypotension, acute dystonias, extrapyramidal effects, laryngeal spasm, malignant hyperthermia, glucose and lipid dysregulation, and anticholinergic effects such as dry mouth, constipation, and urinary retention. Perhaps the most immediately life-threatening adverse effect of antipsychotics is torsades de pointes, and these agents should be avoided whenever possible in patients with prolonged QT intervals. Patents who receive substantial quantities of typical or atypical antipsychotics or coadministered arrhythmogenic drugs should be monitored closely with daily ECGs. In 2005, the United States Food and Drug Administration issued an advisory that the outpatient use of atypical antipsychotic medications is associated with a mortality risk among elderly patients [93]. Similar associations with increased stroke risk and mortality have been reported by other investigators [94, 95]. Subsequently, investigators have reported that such an increased risk of death in elderly patients treated with antipsychotics may not be limited to the atypical class, as they found that the conventional antipsychotic haloperidol had an even higher mortality risk than atypical antipsychotics [94].

Personal perspective

While delirium is very common in cardiovascular ICU patients, it remains poorly understood and under-recognized by cardiologists, anaesthetists, and cardiac surgeons. Given the nature of our patients' illnesses and our procedure-based approach to them, our patients are at particularly high risk of developing this condition, which

Conclusion

Acute cognitive disorders are a ubiquitous problem seen in all critical care units, including the CCU. Delirium is the most common manifestation of these disorders, characterized by a sudden, dynamic disturbance of consciousness. Patients suffering from delirium during a cardiovascular illness are at a significantly increased risk of complications, including in-hospital and long-term mortality. There are many different causes of delirium in this setting, including neurotransmitter imbalances, inflammatory mediators, metabolic disturbances, abnormal sleep patterns, and the use of certain sedatives and analgesics. There are now specific bedside assessment tools available to diagnose delirium across the complete spectrum of critically ill cardiovascular patients. Once diagnosed, the implementation of both pharmacologic and nonpharmacological treatments for delirium can be effective in minimizing adverse outcomes. Further, increased awareness of the prevalence of acute cognitive disorders in the CCU and recognition of the specific risk factors for delirium may lead to prevention of this complication and improved overall cardiovascular care.

is clearly associated with adverse in-hospital and long-term outcomes. Fortunately, based on ongoing studies, protocols and evidence-based strategies for prevention and treatment of delirium in the CCU will undoubtedly emerge; randomized clinical trials of both nonpharmacological and pharmacological strategies have been planned which should ultimately result in improved clinical outcomes in countless future cardiac patients.

Further reading

Dubois MJ, Bergeron N, Dumont M, *et al*. Delirium in an intensive care unit: a study of risk factors. *Intensive Care Med* 2001;27(8):1297–1304.

Ely EW, Inouye SK, Bernard GR, *et al*. Delirium in mechanically ventilated patients: validity and reliability of the confusion assessment method for the intensive care unit (CAM-ICU). *JAMA* 2001;286(21):2703–2710.

Ely EW, Inouye S, Bernard G, *et al*. Delirium in mechanically ventilated patients: validity and reliability of the confusion assessment method for the intensive care unit (CAM-ICU). *JAMA* 2001;286:2703–2710.

Ely EW, Truman B, Shintani A, *et al*. Monitoring sedation status over time in ICU patients: reliability and validity of the Richmond Agitation-Sedation Scale (RASS). *JAMA* 2003;289(22):2983–2991.

Jacobi J, Fraser GL, Coursin DB, *et al*. Clinical practice guidelines for the sustained use of sedatives and analgesics in the critically ill adult. *Crit Care Med* 2002;30(1):119–141.

Pandharipande PP, Shintani A, Peterson J, *et al*. Lorazepam is an independent risk factor for transitioning to delirium in intensive care unit patients. *Anesthesiology* 2006;104:21–26.

Sockalingam S, Parekh N, Bogoch II, *et al*. Delirium in the postoperative cardiac patient: a review. *J Cardiac Surg* 2005;20:560–567.

Online resource

Confusion Assessment Method for the ICU (CAM-ICU) (complete description and training materials, including translations and clinical vignettes). http://www.icudelirium.org.

➲ For additional multimedia materials please visit the online version of the book (⌕ http://www.esciacc.oxfordmedicine.com).

CHAPTER 74

Special considerations in immunosuppressed patients

Alain Durocher and Raphaël Favory

Contents

Summary

Many patients encountered in the intensive care unit (ICU) are immuno-suppressed. Immunosuppression may be caused by an underlying disease (e.g. haematological disease), by treatment (drugs to prevent organ rejection), or as a side effect of chemotherapy.

The immune system is generally plays a successful role in maintaining the integrity of the individual. It is made up of integumental function, the innate immune response, and the adaptive immune response. Immune function is not static and can change over the period of illness in some patients. Immunosuppression in itself does not cause pathology, but leaves the patient prone to infection, which is the cause of morbidity and mortality in immunosuppressed patients. This highlights the importance of infection control, the most important aspect of which is prevention.

The most important intervention is the timely initiation of appropri-ate antimicrobial therapy. Sending adequate and appropriate samples to the microbiology laboratory is also important in the management of an infected immunosuppressed patient.

In organ recipients, the required immunosuppression increases the risk of infection and can also make the onset of symptoms insidious.

Introduction

The incidence of patients with compromised host defences encountered in criti-cal care services, emergency departments, and the intensive care unit (ICU) has increased dramatically over recent decades. Reasons include HIV infection; greater use of solid-organ and haematological transplantation strategies; treat-ment of cancer with conventional chemotherapy and immunotherapy; and the introduction of new monoclonal antibody therapy (e.g. anti-tumour necrosis fac-tor) for common conditions, such as Crohn's disease or rheumatoid arthritis.

Despite significant advances in the prevention, diagnosis, and treatment of infection in immunocompromised patients it remains a major cause of morbid-ity, increased length of stay, and mortality in hospital, particularly in the ICU.

Investigation of immune deficiency status

Full blood count and differential white cell count

Each cell type has different functions. Dividing the count into its constituent parts may reveal abnormalities and assist in the diagnosis of specific disorders.

- Neutrophils play an important role in the defence against bacteria in particular, but also against fungi and viruses. The absolute neutrophil count (ANC) is the best single predictor of infection risk. As the ANC drops below 1×10^6/L, susceptibility to infection increases.

- The differential WBC count. The total lymphocyte count may point to immune suppression in the setting of AIDS or bone marrow depression. However, it may also be depressed e.g. in patients receiving steroids, with adrenal suppression, severe malnutrition. The T-helper cell count can be used to quantify the risk of opportunistic infections. In HIV infection and AIDS the CD4 count is used as a prognostic indicator, along with the viral load.

Biochemical markers of infection

- C-reactive protein (CRP) is a nonspecific marker of inflammation. Some physicians use daily CRP as an early warning of impeding infection. Its usefulness is matter of debate.

- Procoalcitonin is used as a bedside marker of impeding sepsis.

- Soluble triggering receptor on myeloid cells (TREM-1) is a hallmark of both infectious and noninfectious inflammation, and conflicting results can be found in literature concerning its diagnostic accuracy compared with other biomarkers like CRP; in one study, immunocompromised patients were excluded [1]. Ventilator-associated pneumonia (VAP) seems to be the more interesting context for this new biomarker [2].

Causes and consequences of immunosuppression

The immunosuppressed patient has an increased susceptibility to develop infection by organisms with minimal virulence. Any deficiency in the layers of the immune system potentially increases the likelihood of infection. There are three layers of the immune system that invading microorganisms must breach in order to cause infection:

- Physical barriers (e.g. skin and epithelial covering of mucosa, stomach acidity, normal flora).

- Innate immune response (phagocytic cells, natural killer cells (a subset of lymphocytes), complement system, acute phase proteins, cytokines). The innate immune system is capable of rapid reaction to foreign antigen without having previously been exposed. It is a nonspecific first line of defence; it lacks memory and subsequent responses are the same as the first. It is only when the innate immune system is overwhelmed, bypassed, or evaded that the adaptive immune system is needed.

- Adaptive immune response (humoral, cell-mediated). The adaptive response has memory, and subsequent responses are quantitatively and qualitatively superior.

However, depending on the nature of the immunosuppression, other complications, such as drug side effects and complications of the underlying disease, may also occur.

Neutrophil dysfunction

Neutrophil dysfunction is mainly represented in adult patients by quantitative defects. Neutropenia is defined as less then 1000 granulocytes/mm^3 and absolute neutropenia as less than 500 cells/mm^3. It is mainly seen in the context of myelogenous leukaemias, myoloproliferative disorders, and 7–10 days after administration of chemotherapy that is toxic for bone marrow. The risk of infection depends on the depth and duration of neutropenia. The risk is high for bacterial infections after 10 days and for fungal infections after 3 weeks of neutropenia.

Defects in humoral immunity

Defects in humoral immunity include disorders in immunoglobulin production (multiple myeloma, Waldenström's macroglobulinaemia, chronic lymphocyte leukaemia, B-cell lymphomas), hypo- or asplenia and hypocomplementaemia. Encapsulated microorganisms are most commonly encountered (e.g. *Streptococcus pneumoniae* and *Haemophilus influenzae*).

Defects in cellular immunity

Defects in cellular immunity includes HIV infections, immunosuppressive therapy, antirejection therapy for transplantation, corticosteroids, lymphomas and T-cell malignancies, and solid tumours. Cellular-mediated immunity is important in defending against viruses, protozoa (e.g. *Strongyloides*), and most fungi, especially intracellular pathogens.

Risk factors for infection

In HIV-infected patients the main risk factor is a low CD4 count (<400) whereas for other immunosuppressed patients the type, dosage, and duration of immunomodulating medications are important. Significant granulocytopenia (<200 polymorphonuclear leucocytes/mL) is the most important risk factor for developing severe bacterial and fungal infections. Granulocytopenia of more than 10 days duration is associated with a marked increase in morbidity and mortality from infectious causes. Moreover, the qualitative capacities of white cells can be adversely affected by chemotherapy, corticosteroids, or radiation. The dermis and the intestinal mucosa are the primary barriers to infection and can be affected by chemotherapy and radiation. This shows in the integrity of the skin, the gastrointestinal mucosa (mucositis), and abnormal intestinal motility, which promotes the overgrowth of some species and facilitates their translocation.

Approach to the immunocompromised patient with infection

General truths and clinical presentations

The general presentation of infected immunosuppressed patients may be altered by the decrease in inflammation [3]. Indeed, some usual signs or symptoms can be absent, rendering a diagnosis more difficult. Patients in the ICU may also have a different presentation for many other reasons: chest radiographs in supine position, sedation with difficult clinical examination or anamnesis, etc. The difference between infection and colonization is subtle.

The patient who is immunocompromised and requires ICU care for respiratory failure and pulmonary infiltrates is a common complication and associated with high mortality rates (30–90%) [4]. Although noninfectious causes (e.g. radiation, chemotherapy, sirolimus, diffuse alveolar haemorrhage, idiopathic pneumonitis, acute respiratory distress syndrome, pulmonary oedema, pulmonary emboli, or lung transplant rejection) are not uncommon, infectious aetiologies remain the prime concern and require primary diagnostic and empirical treatment considerations. Delays in

source control or anti-infectious therapies are poorly tolerated by immunosuppressed patients.

Unfortunately, no radiographic pattern is pathognomic for a specific pathogen in any host category. Chest CT scans can reveal lesions not visualized on plain radiographs in up to 50% of immunosuppressed patients, which can guide fibreoptic bronchoscopy with bronchoalveloar lavage (BAL) [5]. Because of higher organism loads, *P. jiroveci* and mycobacterial infection are more easily detected with BAL in patients infected with HIV-1. The diagnostic sensitivity for *Aspergillus* and other fungi is lower, but superior to that of sputum or endotracheal aspirates [6]. Transbronchial biopsy may improve diagnostic sensitivity in patients with diffuse infiltrates that were negative with BAL, with fungal and mycobacterial infection, and for the diagnosis of non-infectious causes of pulmonary infiltrates. However, the risk of pneumothorax is always a concern, especially if the patient is under mechanical ventilation. Open lung biopsy is a possibility, but is accompanied by a very high complication rate without significant changes in management [7].

Diagnostic strategy

Imaging

In case of respiratory distress with bilateral infiltrates on chest radiograph, a CT scan has to be done before BAL because the injection of saline into the lungs will cause artefacts on the lung CT scan.

Although imaging may make it possible to identify a source of infection, it will not allow identification of the pathogen in most cases. However, it may trigger management for further microbiological sampling, such as drainage of an abscess.

In-hospital or interhospital transport of haemodynamically unstable or hypoxaemic patients can be dangerous, and the risk/benefit ratio has to be assessed for each individual patient.

Microbiological examination

Microbiological examination of either fluid or tissue specimens consists of qualitative culture results and in many cases quantitative analysis. Sending appropriate samples to the microbiology laboratory is an important part of managing the immunosuppressed patient, in order to guide therapy. In the diagnosis of VAP, quantitative analysis is often performed on BAL samples. BAL can be performed under noninvasive ventilation with an adapted face mask or helmet. The need for tracheal intubation is then not a prerequisite for BAL in unstable patients, even if the risks are increased. Fibreoptic bronchoscopy can have negative consequences for pulmonary and haemodynamic function. The bronchoscope occupies about 10% of the cross-sectional area of the trachea, thus decreasing tidal volume, increasing the work of breathing, and inducing hypercapnia. These changes can last for 2 h and BAL can induce a desaturation of 15% of Sao_2. When suction is applied during bronchoscopy, end-expiratory volume decreases tidal volume, inducing alveolar collapse and increasing venous admixture. It must also be borne in mind that BAL can induce a temporary inflammatory syndrome in up to 10% of patients.

Serological investigations

Difficulties in reaching microbiological diagnosis with conventional cultures have led to newer approaches. These include antigen testing for cyomegalovirus (CMV), reverse transcriptase polymerase chain reaction (rtPCR) for RNA (HIV), and PCR for DNA (CMV, herpes simplex).

Investigations are summarized in ❯ Table 74.1.

Specific treatment or pre-emptive therapy

Anti-infectious agents

The initiation of an antibiotic regimen will depend on local practice, guidelines and regional infectious epidemiology. The following elements should be considered (see ❯ Table 74.2):

◆ Potential sites of infection

◆ The most likely infecting organism(s)

◆ Local resistance patterns

◆ Pre-existing organ dysfunction

◆ Allergies

◆ Previous antibiotic exposure

◆ Broad spectrum coverage

Depending on the context, initial antibiotic treatment must include extended spectrum antibiotics covering Gram-negative bacilli. In some situations, meticillin-resistant staphylococcus (MRSA) must be covered. Antifungal therapy depends on the context. Whatever is chosen, a de-escalation strategy must be the rule (for guidelines, see ❯ Online resources.) The best initial empirical therapy includes a β-lactamine, and in patients with severe sepsis and septic shock this should be given in association with an aminoside. In this case, the daily dose of aminoside should be the same as usual but with serial measurements of serum levels. In all cases, the efficacy of antibiotic therapy must be checked at 48–72 h. If there is a persistent febrile state or if the procalcitonin level is still high, a change of antibiotic and the addition of an antifungal agent is recommended. Anti-MRSA must be considered in cases of septic shock, if there is a previous colonization with MRSA, or in cases of catheter-related infection or skin portal of entry.

How to deal with immunosuppressive agents

Withdrawal or rapid tapering of iatrogenic immunosuppression, particularly corticosteroids, is a well-described option particularly in organ transplant recipients with rapid deterioration caused by life-threatening infection or post-transplant lymphoproliferative disease. This decision needs careful consideration:

◆ Can the allograft be sacrificed with fallback on artificial support? (Possibly for kidney transplants, but the situation is not clear for heart and lung transplants.)

◆ Will withdrawal of corticosteroids culminate in adrenal insufficiency, especially in the context of septic shock?

◆ Sometimes corticosteroids can be useful for pneumocystis, cerebral oedema, etc.

Cardiac infections in the immunosuppressed patient

Congestive heart failure is the most significant manifestation. When unexplained heart failure occurs in an

Table 74.1 Diagnostic approach in the immunosuppressed patient with infection.

Investigation	Neurological signs	Respiratory signs	Abdominal signs	Cardiac signs
Radiology	Cerebral CT scan	Lung CT scan (halo sign)		Echography
Microbiological examination (peripheral blood cultures, central line cultures)	Lumbar puncture *Cryptococcus* antigen, PCR VZV, PCR CMV	Fibreoptic bronchoscopy + BAL *Nocardia*, actinomycosis, virus, *Aspergillus* (antigen), *Cryptococcus*, *Pneumocystis* (±PCR)	Rectosigmoidoscopy ± biopsy (CMV) Parasitology exam *Clostridium* toxin	Pericardiocentesis in some cases
Serological examination	Toxoplasmic serology	*Aspergillus* antigen (galactomannan)		Toxoplasmic serology

BAL, bronchoalveolar lavage; CMV, cytomegalovirus; PCR, polymerase chain reaction; VZV, varicella zoster virus.

Table 74.2 Elements of antibiotic regimen

Initially	+ Aminoglycoside	+ Anti-MRSA	+ Antifungal
β-Lactam antibiotic: 3rd generation cephalosporin or ureidopenicillin or penem	Septic shock In documented cases if needed	At 48–72 h if unsuccessful initial treatment Central line, skin MRSA colonization PCT values still high	At 48–72 h if unsuccessful initial treatment, PCT values still high Galactomannan in BAL + CT scan signs (halo) Several noncontiguous sites of colonization of *Candida*, or candidaemia

BAL, bronchoalveolar lavage; MRSA, methicillin-resistant *Staphylococcus aureus*; PCT, procalcitonin.

immunosuppressed patient, an infectious process must be ruled out by appropriate means.

Infectious endocarditis

Infectious endocarditis (IE) is seen primarily in intravenous drug abusers, but may be a nosocomial infection (usually in ICU patients). It is the most common clinically relevant cardiac infection in immunosuppressed patients [8]. However, clinical presentation is more frequently an association of nonspecific signs of sepsis (e.g. hypotension) than fever or leucocytosis (*c.*50%). It is defined as a valvular infection that becomes apparent either 48 h after hospitalization or within 3–4 weeks following the performance of a hospital-based invasive procedure. Immunomodulating viruses (such as CMV) can play a significant role in determining endocarditis. CMV can also induce leucopenia and significantly suppresses the function of natural killer cells and macrophages.

Central venous catheters are the primary cause of nosocomial endocarditis, with the skin tract as main portal of entry. The most common catheter-associated organisms are coagulase-negative staphylococcus, *S. aureus*, fungi, and the microbial flora endogenous to the particular patient care area. *Candida* does not survive in these mixtures, but does in the solutions used for total parenteral nutrition. Most bacteria are not able to survive in such hypertonic environments.

Blood cultures remain the gold standard for diagnosing IE. Unfortunately, up to 50% of blood cultures may be contaminated [9]. The type of organism, multiple positive cultures, and a short growth period favour the validity of a positive blood culture. Echocardiography should not be used as an initial screening test because almost 20% of IE shows no valvular vegetations and, conversely, 50% of valvular thrombi detected by echocardiography are sterile. Candida is the most frequent cause of fungal endocarditis (80% of those with detectable fungaemia). Usually, it produces endocarditis in prosthetic valves but it can infect native valves.

(See also ⊃ Chapter 57, and ⊃ Chapter 22 (Infective endocarditis) in *The ESC Textbook of Cardiovascular Medicine.*)

Myocarditis

The signs and symptoms of myocarditis range from the asymptomatic through fulminant congestive heart failure (see also ⊃ Chapter 56, and ⊃ Chapter 18 (Myocardial disease) in *The ESC Textbook of Cardiovascular Medicine.*)

Viral myocarditis

Coxsackie A and B are the most common causes of viral myocarditis, and significant antibody titres appear within the first 3 weeks of infection [10]. CMV is the most common definable cause of myocarditis in patients with AIDS, in whom it is usually asymptomatic. In non-AIDS immunosuppressed patients, CMV seems to be significant only in heart-transplanted patients, in whom it may contribute to rejection of the transplant. Serological tests or the detection of PP 65 immediate-early antigen or viral DNA in peripheral blood white cells is useful in patients with AIDS and in organ transplant recipients. The presence of the virus in sputum or urine is not sufficient to make the diagnosis of active CMV disease. Epstein–Barr virus is rarely clinically relevant, but may induce myocarditis.

Toxoplasma gondii

Hodgkin's disease is the main risk factor, with reactivation of latent infection in most cases [11]. Congestive heart failure, pericarditis, and bundle branch block are possible clinical scenarios. Rejection of the transplanted heart can also occur. Most patients with disseminated toxoplasmosis have cardiac involvement. Serial serology is required to rule out a reactivation.

Chagas' disease

The risk of reactivation of quiescent *Trypanosoma cruzii* infections is especially high for recipients of cardiac and renal transplants, and is directly proportional to the dosage and duration of ciclosporin therapy [12]. The cardiomyopathy is often accompanied by either expanding intracerebral masses or meningoencephalitis. Fever, myalgias, congestive heart failure, and meningoencephalitis are the main clinical manifestations. The ECG may show heart block or arrhythmias. Diagnosis is made primarily by detecting the parasite on examination of fresh blood or of the buffy coat. Various serological tests are unreliable.

Pericarditis

Viral pericarditis

CMV is the most common cause of viral pericarditis. In patients with AIDS, idiopathic pericarditis may well be caused by various enteroviruses, especially Coxsackie strains [13]. The signs and symptoms of pericarditis in the immunosuppressed patient are similar to those in the normal host.

Tuberculous pericarditis

This diagnosis should be considered in immunosuppressed patients who present with cardiomegaly and fever [14]. A definitive diagnosis depends on recovering the organism from either pericardial tissue or fluid. Elevated adenosine deaminase in pericardial fluid is quite sensitive and specific for tuberculous disease; a tuberculin skin test is not discriminant.

Bacterial pericarditis

This is most commonly seen as a consequence of cardiothoracic surgery or of IE [15]. Compared with patients with viral or idiopathic pericarditis, those with suppurative pericarditis appear quite toxic with systemic symptoms but lack the typical type of chest pain.

(See also ➲ Chapter 19 (Pericardial disease) in *The ESC Textbook of Cardiovascular Medicine*.)

Infections in heart and heart–lung transplant recipients

Infection and rejection are the major causes of death after cardiac transplantation. One-third of patients get an infection in the first year. This may be viral (especially CMV), fungal (up to 7% of the patients, especially *Candida*), or protozoal (*Pneumocystis jiroveci*) (➲ Table 74.3).

Diagnosis of infection in post-transplant patients may be difficult. A vigorous search for infection is needed in all transplant patients appearing even mildly unwell. Procalcitonin (PCT) dosage can be useful in the context of post-transplant patients because it can differentiate acute rejection and infection [16], but it must be borne in mind that PCT can increase for 1 week after uncomplicated cardiac surgery. In various studies, the diagnostic value of PCT for the diagnosis of proven infection has a sensitivity ranging from 50% to 60% and a specificity ranging from 89% to 100%. The dynamics of PCT over time are probably the most relevant factor in ensuring the efficacy of anti-infectious treatment.

Heart transplant recipients are at high risk for pneumonia caused by bacteria (including *Legionella*, discussed below) and fungi, including *Aspergillus* and *Pneumocystis jiroveci*. Infection of the sternal wound or incisional surgical site may also be a problem after heart transplantation, and may be complicated by mediastinitis, the incidence of which is up to 3%. The initial clinical presentation may be poor, with low-grade fever or an elevated leucocyte count being the only manifestation. Later, more specific signs develop, such as erythema, tenderness, or drainage along the sternal incision. Positive cultures from blood and temporary epicardial pacing wires can be helpful in suggesting the presence of mediastinitis. Surgical drainage appears to be crucial to the successful treatment of mediastinitis in transplant patients. Vacuum-assisted closure and hyperbaric oxygen have been proposed in some cases. One must also be alert to the possible presence of unusual pathogens such as *Mycoplasma hominis*, *Legionella pneumophila*, *Aspergillus*, and *Nocardia*.

HIV and the heart

Infectious complications

Most cardiac infections in HIV-positive patients are an infectious consequence of the various types of immunosuppression caused by the virus. However, since the introduction of highly active antiretroviral therapy (HAART) and other infection prophylaxis, the incidence of non-HIV-associated infection (e.g. non-pneumocystis pneumonia) as a cause of ICU admission is increasing.

Pericarditis is the most frequent clinical cardiac manifestation [17]. It is often complicated by effusion related

Table 74.3 Infections commonly found in the first year after cardiac tranaplantation

<1 month	1–6 months	>6 months
Nosocomial or donor-derived pathogens	Opportunistic infections	Community acquired infection and
Bacteria: MRSA, *Clostridium difficile*	Bacteria: *Listeria, Mycobacterium tuberculosis*	*Aspergillus*
Fungi: *Candida, Aspergillus*	Virus: HSV, CMV, HBV, HCV, EBV	CMV
	Parasites : *Pneumocystis, Toxoplasma, Strongyloides, Leishmania*	

CMV, cytomegalovirus; EBV, Epstein–Barr virus; HBV, hepatitis B virus; HCV, hepatitis C virus; HSV, herpes simplex virus; MRSA, meticillin-resistant *Staphylococcus aureus* directly to the stage of HIV disease (10% of these produce tamponade). In AIDS, the pericardium is the target of a variety of processes (lymphoma, Kaposi's sarcoma, fungi, mycobacteria, and many types of viruses).

Myocarditis may be either caused by primary infection or secondary to concurrent involvement with opportunistic organisms or neoplasms. The pathological picture seen in HIV myocarditis is consistent with a viral myocarditis (maybe CMV). It may be a virus-induced narrowing of the coronary arteries that leads to ischaemic changes and eventually to cardiac dysfunction. In patients without clinical heart disease, many of the focal myocardial lymphocytic collections reflect a bacteraemia, fungaemia, or viraemia arising from an extracardiac source. The most common identified cardiac pathogens are *Toxoplasma gondii* (1%) and CMV (2%). Toxoplasmosis often coexists with other pathogens, most commonly with CMV (24% of cases). In patients with AIDS, toxoplasma of the heart is almost always associated with encephalitis.

Noninfectious complications

Tumoral complications

Kaposi's sarcoma and lymphoma occur more commonly in people with HIV than in immunocompetent individuals [18], generally in the setting of widespread mucocutaneous disease [19]. The heart is only very rarely the sole site of involvement and is usually asymptomatic. Primary cardiac lymphomas are typically aggressive B-cell lymphomas involving the right atrium. As well as symptoms and signs of heart failure, patients may also present with atrioventricular block caused by infiltration of the conduction system [20], or the ECG simulation of infarction caused by myocardial infiltration. Other potential manifestations include ventricular tachycardia and pericardial effusion. Conduction disturbances are potentially reversible with treatment of lymphoma. However, patients receiving chemotherapy should be closely monitored for arrhythmia induced by tumour necrosis.

Coronary artery disease

Sporadic case reports raising concerns about premature coronary artery disease (CAD) in patients treated with HAART led to retrospective analysis of large cohort studies. Combination antiretroviral therapy was independently associated with a 26% increase in rate of myocardial infarction (MI) per year of exposure over the first 4–6 years of use [21]. The risk of MI seems to increase in patients with HIV infection receiving HAART. However, the absolute risk is small, and the marked overall benefits of antiretroviral therapy are evident. HIV infection causes profound functional alterations of the endothelium, resembling the subclinical inflammation in atherosclerosis.

Metabolic changes associated with HIV infection and HAART

HIV infection itself is associated with dyslipidaemia. Protease inhibitors (PI) can cause hyperlipidaemia, hyperglycaemia, and central obesity [22]. Insulin resistance occurs in as much as 25–60% of patients [23]. Moreover, PIs directly impair endothelium-dependent vasodilation. Patients receiving PIs should be screened for hyperlipidaemia, hyperglycaemia, and hypertension. They may be candidates for lipid-lowering therapies, depending on their long-term prognosis and individual risk of cardiovascular disease. The invasive treatment of acute MI does not differ from that in patients who are not infected with HIV. However, the restenosis rates after percutaneous coronary intervention (PCI) are unexpectedly high [24]. Atazanavir is a PI which may have less impact on lipid elevation in treated patients, whereas both nucleoside and non-nucleoside reverse transcriptase inhibitors may also contribute to lipid elevation in treated patients. The lipid-lowering therapy must be considered according to the antiretroviral therapies. When initiating lipid-lowering therapy, interactions between statins and HIV PIs affecting cytochrome P450 (CYP) function must be considered [25]. Simvastatin, atorvastatin, and lovastatin, but not pravastatin or fluvastatin, are metabolized by CYP3A4 and should thus be avoided in patients taking PIs such as ritonavir, atazanavir, and saquinavir. Pravastatin does not alter the pharmacokinetics of nelfinavir and thus appears to be safe for concomitant use. However, dose adjustment of pravastatin may be necessary with concomitant use of ritonavir, atazanavir, and saquinavir.

Cardiovascular toxicities of immunosuppressive agents and chemotherapy

Hypertension

Hypertension occurs in up to 50–100% of patients treated with immunosuppressant agents [26]. Recognized risk factors include greater age, family history of hypertension, and male gender [27]. Beyond the risk of decrease of survival of allograft, one must be aware of the possibility of cardiac hypertrophy and a shift to the right of the autoregulation blood flow curve of some organs (especially the brain). Calcineurin inhibitors (tacrolimus and ciclosporin) are the main agents responsible for induced hypertension.

Ciclosporin-induced hypertension can resolve at the discontinuation of the treatment and generally develops within weeks or months after its introduction. The mechanisms involved in ciclosporin-associated hypertension are (1) the release from endothelium of endothelin, which is a very potent vasoconstrictor, and (2) ciclosporin-induced nephropathy [28]. Immunosuppressive effects [29, 30]) and particularly the inhibition of the calcineurin pathway have also been suggested to be implicated.

Tacrolimus (FK-506) can lead to hypertension by the same mechanisms as ciclosporin, but in fewer cases [31]. There is no data suggesting that either azathioprine or mycophenolate mofetil (MMF) contributes to the development of clinically significant increases in hypertension.

Coronary artery disease

The incidence of CAD in heart transplant recipients, which ranges from 1% to 18% at 1 year and from 20% to 50% at 3 years [32], has not decreased in the past 25 years, despite improvements in immunosuppressive regimens. An unusually accelerated form of CAD, cardiac allograft vasculopathy (CAV), is a long-term complication following cardiac transplantation.

Ciclosporin

Although the addition of ciclosporin to immunosuppressive regimens has resulted in a significant decrease in the incidence of acute rejection in heart transplant recipients, ciclosporin also appears to protect the recipient from the development of comorbid factors resulting from CAV. Accelerated atherosclerosis is thought to be due, in part, to the effect of ciclosporin on the endothelium, causing endothelial cell damage that leads to the accumulation of inflammatory cells and release of endothelin and other growth factors, which in turn mobilize smooth muscle cells to proliferate [33]. Moreover, ciclosporin has also been shown to increase the plasma levels of plasminogen activator inhibitor 1 (PAI-1) [34], leading to decreased fibrinolytic activity.

Tacrolimus

Vasculitis has been reported in humans receiving tacrolimus. These findings may be related to effects on calcium channels in cardiac and striated muscle. Significant cardiomyopathy with progression to severe hypertrophic obstructive cardiomyopathy and congestive heart failure in some patients has also been noted in liver and/or bowel transplant recipients receiving tacrolimus [35]. The hypertrophy was partially reversed by lowering the dose or discontinuing tacrolimus.

Sirolimus

Sirolimus increases endothelium-dependent vasodilation and inhibits the development of intimal hyperplasia and transplant arteriosclerosis in aortic grafts by allowing endogenous gene expression of nitric oxide synthase [36]. Vasculitis was also increased by the immunological events of rejection. However, the combination of sirolimus and ciclisporin reduced the frequency and severity of vasculitis compared with sirolimus alone [37]. It remains to be seen if the effect of sirolimus on hyperlipidaemia will lead to an increase in CAD when it is used for longer periods.

Azathioprine and mycophenolate mofetil

These have the lowest adverse cardiovascular toxicities. Clearly, if these findings are sustained over the long term, MMF represents a potential advantage in the control of CAV [38].

Cardiomyopathy induced by chemotherapy

Cardiotoxicity includes a wide range of cardiac effects. Different mechanisms of cardiotoxicity are postulated, including cellular damage due to the formation of reactive oxygen species, induction of immunogenic reactions, and effects on cardiolipin. These effects can be seen several weeks after treatment but also several years later.

Anthracyclines

The use of anthracyclines usually leads to a dilated symptomatic cardiopathy [39]. Anthracyclines have been reported to cause cardiomyopathy, congestive heart failure, and ECG alterations (nonspecific ST-T changes, decreased QRS voltage, and prolongation of QT interval). Both early (within 1 year) and late onset (20 years) cardiac effects are reported. Acute effects can occur during perfusion, are generally transient, and attenuate when the treatment is stopped. Cumulative dose, age, prior irradiation, concomitant administration of other chemotherapeutic agents, and underlying heart disease are the main risk factors [40]. Cumulative dose is the predominant factor, but there are some interindividual differences. Routine cardiac imaging studies (echocardiography and multiple gate acquisition CT) can be used to follow or detect subclinical dysfunctions. Endomyocardial biopsy directly shows the presence and extent of fibrosis, but is limited by its invasiveness. Studies of troponin T measurements in adults have given conflicting results. B-type natriuretic peptide (BNP) might be a better tool to detect subclinical dysfunction, but its exact usefulness in this setting needs more study. The antioxidant and iron chelator dexrazoxane has been successfully applied to protect the heart from cardiotoxicity with high-dose anthracycline therapy [41], but further studies are still required.

5-Fluorouracil

Cardiotoxicity related to the use of 5-FU occurs in up to 20% of patients, more often after continuous infusion than bolus injection. Cardiac arrhythmias, silent myocardial ischaemia (vasospasm, direct toxicity?), angina, congestive heart failure, and sudden death can occur with this drug. Risk factors include pre-existing CAD and concurrent radiotherapy [42]. There is no preventive therapy.

Cyclophosphamide

This can lead to acute cardiotoxicity, such as cardiac decompensation with reversible systolic dysfunction or fatal cardiomyopathy [43].

Cisplatin

Several cases of acute MI have been described during cisplatin treatment [44].

Herceptin (trastuzumab)

This drug, used for breast cancer treatment, usually leads to asymptomatic cardiopathy in 15% of patients and to symptomatic cardiopathy in 5% of patients [45]. Herceptin is a monoclonal antibody directed against the HER2 receptor protein on breast cancer cells and it has been used alone or in combination with other chemotherapeutic agents. Cardiac toxicity associated with herceptin seems to be similar to the congestive heart failure observed with anthracycline therapy. Concomitant anthracycline therapy and age appear to be independent risk factors.

Preventing infection and superinfection in the immunosuppressed patient

Protective isolation and specific precautions

Hand hygiene is of paramount importance in preventing infection and superinfection in all patients in the ICU, but of course especially in immunosuppressed patients. The use of alcoholic gels has transformed prevention, providing a more efficient and easier way to improve hand hygiene.

Despite the higher prevalence of multidrug-resistant bacteria in the ICU, and the greater severity of illness in immunocompromised patients requiring intensive care, the vast majority of immunocompromised patients in the ICU do not routinely require protective or reverse isolation. The intention of protective isolation is to prevent patients acquiring exogenous organisms by nursing them in their own room, with controlled entry to limit access, and ambient positive pressure. This practice has usually been limited to neutropenic patients and pre-engraftment bone marrow transplant recipients. However, most infections in these patients arise from their endogenous colonizing microflora. Thus, although reverse isolation remains a common and traditional practice even in the ICU, its use is not strongly evidence-based. Airborne fungal spores, particularly *Aspergillus*, are a notable exception; however, only laminar-flow rooms with high-efficiency particulate air-filtration filters have been shown to reduce the incidence of aspergillosis in patients with haematological or oncological bone marrow transplant [46]. Most ICUs have such dedicated technology. However, special isolation precautions are frequently indicated in immunocompromised patients, both on an empirical basis and for definitive isolation of specific organisms that are potentially transmissible to other patients. Negatively pressurized ICU rooms with an anteroom are required for suspected or documented airborne infections including *Mycobacterium tuberculosis* and influenza and varicella zoster viruses. Delayed respiratory isolation has resulted in catastrophic spread of *M. tuberculosis*, particularly from source patients infected with HIV-1.

An antibiotic restriction policy and a de-escalation strategy is important to decrease the emergence of multidrug-resistant bacteria. Screening of multidrug-resistant colonization is mandatory. The routine surveillance of biomarkers is probably of some interest in the context of immunosuppression because of the poor clinical signs of infection. Procalcitonin seems to be one of the more useful markers at present. Some data suggest that the duration of use of anti-infectious agents could be guided by procalcitonin kinetics.

Decontamination of the digestive tract and oropharynx has a long history. The encouraging data from a recent study [47] have been mitigated by the effects, shown by the same authors [48], of a marked impact on ceftazidime resistance in their population. The debate concerning this strategy is still open.

In general, minimally invasive procedures are preferred whenever possible, and this is particularly true for immunosuppressed patients. Noninvasive ventilation (NIV) is probably one of the most useful. NIV or laryngeal mask [49] can allow BAL in better conditions, avoiding tracheal intubation. Echo-guided placement of central venous or arterial lines may also help to reduce the risk not only of mechanical complications but also of infectious complications, because of the shorter time required for the procedure [50].

Personal perspective

The management of patients with immunosuppression represents a significant challenge to the ICU team. As our understanding of the mechanisms has developed, clinical recognition of signs and or symptoms has improved; however, better laboratory tests for immunosuppression would be welcome.

Better diagnosis and treatment strategies and opening the field to new diseases explain the higher incidence of complications in immunosuppressed patients. This trend will probably increase in the future, so we need to have some basis for the better care for these patients (who are often young) in developing new strategies of prevention and treatments.

A growing body of evidence suggests that morbidity and mortality of these patients are not so high and not so different if they are treated aggressively in the ICU, but 'aggressively' is not synonymous with 'invasively'. For example, less invasive procedures such as NIV have been tested with good results in this population.

The downside is that NIV failures greatly increase mortality. So efforts must still be made to detect patients who will or will not benefit from this therapy. One reason for a better prognosis is less need for sedation; the immune effects of sedation have recently been underlined. Moreover, the more recognized complications of sedation, such as neuromuscular weakness, prolonged unconsciousness, and maybe more post-traumatic stress disorders are a controversial topic. Moreover, when a patient is intubated, a pavlovian reflex seems to incite physicians to place central venous lines and maybe an arterial catheter, and these two invasive devices increase the risk of nosocomial infection.

The development of echographically guided procedures (central venous lines, arterial lines, punctures, etc.) is needed to develop a better preventive strategy. Obviously, the use of alcohol gels must increase further in the ICU even if the workload is high in this kind of unit: it is a key step for decreasing nosocomial infections. In addition, depending on the turnover of patients, at least one air purification system should be available in the ICU.

Conclusion

In infected immunocompromized patients, the most important intervention in is the timely initiation of appropriate antimicrobial therapy. Clinical presentation is often poor and microbiological isolation is quite often difficult. A diagnostic and therapeutic strategy is required with keeping in mind the most frequent microorganisms in specific situations and/or timing (after transplantation e.g.). Prevention is very important: non invasive procedures (non invasive ventilation) are preferred, de escalation antibiotic policy are paramount to avoid emergence of multiresistant strains.

Hypertension and coronary artery disease are the most common cardiovascular complications of immunosuppressive agents whereas cardiomyopathy is the most frequent side effect in patients receiving chemotherapy (anthracycline e.g.).

Further reading

Adda M, Coquet I, Darmon M, et al. Predictors of noninvasive ventilation failure in patients with hematologic malignancy and acute respiratory failure. *Crit Care Med* 2008;**36**(10):2766–2772.

Adelberg DE, Bishop MR. Emergencies related to cancer chemotherapy and hematopoietic stem cell transplantation. *Emerg Med Clin North Am* 2009;**27**(2):311–331.

Currier JS. Update on cardiovascular complications in HIV infection. *Top HIV Med* 2009;**17**(3):98–103.

Fink MP, Abraham E, Vincent JL. *Textbook of critical care*, 5th edition. WB Saunders, Philadelphia, 2005.

Larche J, Azoulay E, Fieux F, et al. Improved survival of critically ill cancer patients with septic shock. *Intensive Care Med* 2003;**29**(10):1688–1695.

Linden PK. Approach to the immunocompromised host with infection in the intensive care unit. *Infect Dis Clin North Am* 2009;**23**(3):535–556.

Mandell GL, Bennett JE, Dolin R (eds) *Mandell, Douglas, and Bennett's principles and practice of infectious diseases*, 7th edition, Churchill Livingstone, Philadelphia, 2010.

Miller LW. Cardiovascular toxicities of immunosuppressive agents. *Am J Transplant* 2002;**2**(9):807–818.

Mordente A, Meucci E, Silvestrini A, *et al.* New developments in anthracycline-induced cardiotoxicity. *Curr Med Chem* 2009;**16**(13):1656–1672.

Rhee J, Al Mana N, Freeman R. Immunosuppression in high-risk transplantation. *Curr Opin Organ Transplant* 2009;**14**(6):636–642.

Online resources

- Infectious Diseases Society of America. Practice guidelines. http://www.idsociety.org
- International Immunocompromised Host Society. Guidelines for the management of bacterial, fungal and viral infections. http://www.ichs.org/ecilslides.htm

↪ For additional multimedia materials please visit the online version of the book (☘ http://www.esciacc.oxfordmedicine.com).

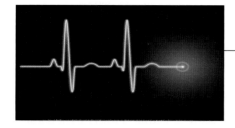

CHAPTER 75

Perioperative management of the high-risk noncardiac surgical patient

Don Poldermans and Sanne Hoeks

Contents

Summary

The cardiac high-risk surgical patient can be defined as an individual with an increased probability of suffering excess event rates including mortality following surgery as a result of the underlying disease necessitating the surgical intervention, comorbid medical factors, or the nature of the surgical intervention itself, or a combination of these.

Several scoring systems have been developed with the specific aim of evaluating cardiac risk prior to noncardiac surgery. The following risk factors are associated with an increased risk of mortality and morbidity following surgery: age, ischaemic heart disease, heart failure, stroke, diabetes mellitus, high-risk surgery, chronic obstructive pulmonary disease, and renal dysfunction; particularly when pathology impacts the cardiorespiratory function and type of surgery.

Perioperative management should be guided by preoperative risk assessment and test outcomes. Several studies have suggested that the use of perioperative β-adrenoreceptor blockade in patients with risk factors for ischaemic cardiac disease reduces the incidence of postoperative cardiac events and mortality of cardiac causes. It is also known that withdrawing long-standing β-blockade preoperatively increase the risk of perioperative adverse cardiac events. Recently it has been shown that statins improve postoperative outcome in patients with risk factors for, or proven coronary artery disease.

Introduction

Patients undergoing noncardiac surgery are at increased risk of cardiovascular morbidity and mortality. Hertzer's landmark study in 1000 consecutive patients undergoing operations for peripheral arterial disease (PAD) who underwent preoperative cardiac catheterizations reported that only 8% of their patients (who were roughly divided into thirds—aortic, infrainguinal, and carotid disease) had normal coronary arteries, and approximately one-third had severe–correctable or severe–inoperable coronary artery disease (CAD) [1]. More recent studies using functional tests for CAD such as dobutamine stress echocardiography confirmed these findings. In a study population of 1097 vascular surgical patients, the incidence of rest wall motion abnormalities was nearly 50%, while one-fifth of patients had stress-induced myocardial ischaemia [2]. Careful management of patients undergoing surgery is therefore mandatory in the perioperative setting.

In general, the risk of perioperative complications depends on the clinical condition of the patient prior to surgery, the prevalence of comorbidities, and the impact of the surgical procedure. Cardiac complications are especially suspected in patients with documented or hidden CAD undergoing procedures that are associated with prolonged haemodynamic and cardiac stress. Importantly, the first European guidelines on perioperative cardiac evaluation and management for noncardiac surgery have now been published [3].

The global ageing phenomenon will have a major impact on perioperative management in future years. Ageing of the world's population can be seen as an indicator of improving global health but also enforces a change in health care toward the elderly population. Furthermore, the burden of cardiovascular disease will increase even further in future years. It is estimated from primary care data that in the 75–84 year age group 19% of men and 12% of women have some degree of cardiovascular disease (CVD) [4]. Major surgical interventions are increasingly performed in elderly people, which did not happen in the past. Demographics of patients undergoing surgery indeed show a trend toward an greater number of preoperative risk factors, including increasing age and more comorbidities [5].

With the growing elderly population, increased incidence of CVD, and the availability of advanced surgical techniques, preoperative cardiac risk assessment and perioperative cardiac management continue to be major challenges.

Pathophysiology of myocardial infarction (see also ⮌ Chapters 39, 41, 44)

Perioperative myocardial infarction (PMI) is one of the most important predictors of short- and long-term morbidity and mortality associated with noncardiac surgery. The highest incidence of PMI is within the first 3 days after surgery (±5%) [6–8].

Unfortunately the exact underlying mechanism of PMI is still not clear, but seems to be the same as in other settings. Coronary plaque rupture, leading to thrombus formation and subsequent vessel occlusion, is considered to be an important cause of acute perioperative acute coronary syndromes (ACS). This is similar to myocardial infarctions occurring in the nonoperative setting. Surgery itself is a significant stress factor leading to an increased risk of plaque rupture. The perioperative surgical stress response includes a catecholamine surge with associated haemodynamic stress, vasospasm, reduced fibrinolytic activity, platelet activation, and consequent hypercoagulability [6]. [Factors that impact perioperative myocardial oxygen balance and listed in ⮌ Box 75.1.

Two retrospective studies investigated the coronary pathology of fatal PMI. As demonstrated in the autopsy study by Dawood and colleagues, 55% of the fatal perioperative MIs have direct evidence of plaque disruption, defined as fissure or rupture of plaque and haemorrhage into the plaque cavity [9]. Similar autopsy results were found in the study of Cohen and Aretz; a plaque rupture was found in 46% of patients with PMI [10].

Box 75.1 Understanding perioperative pathophysiology

Myocardial ischaemia leading to the risk of arrhythmia, MI, and new heart failure (worsening)

- Factors that increase myocardial oxygen demand:
  - tachycardia
  - shivering
  - systemic inflammatory response syndrome
  - sepsis
  - magnitude of tissue injury
  - endogenous cathecholamines
  - exogenous catecholamines
- Factors that reduce myocardial oxygen supply:
  - hypoxaemia
  - anaemia
  - hypotension
  - critical coronary stenosis
  - endogenous vasoconstrictors
  - exogenous vasoconstrictors

Hypovolaemia leading to inadequate tissue perfusion and subsequent organ dysfunction
Impaired cardiorespiratory performance

In patients with significant CAD, PMI may also be caused by a sustained myocardial supply/demand imbalance due to tachycardia and increased myocardial contractility [6]. Episodes of perioperative ST-depression, indicating subendocardial myocardial ischaemia, has been described in up to 41% of vascular surgery patients mostly occurring within the first 2 days after operation [11].

Preoperative risk stratification

Risk score

The first question arising in perioperative care is which patients are at risk for perioperative cardiac events. In this context, adequate risk stratification of patients undergoing noncardiac surgery is of utmost importance. Several risk indices have therefore been developed in the past decades for noncardiac surgery patients [12–13]. Nowadays, the Lee Index is considered by many clinicians and researchers to be the best currently available cardiac risk prediction model in noncardiac surgery [14]. This risk index was developed in 1999 on a cohort of 2893 consecutive patients who underwent a wide spectrum of procedures. The Lee Index consists of six independent predictors of major cardiac complications (Fig. 75.1):

- high-risk surgery
- ischaemic heart disease

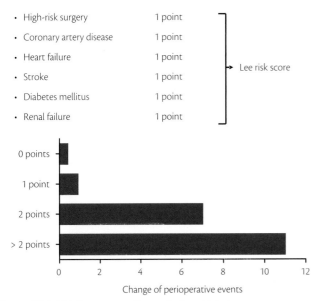

Figure 75.1 Risk factors according to the Lee risk index.
Reproduced with permission from Carroll K, Majeed A, Firth C, Gray J. Prevalence and management of coronary heart disease in primary care: population-based cross-sectional study using a disease register. *J Public Health Med* 2003;**25**(1):29–35.

- congestive heart failure
- cerebrovascular disease
- insulin-dependent diabetes mellitus
- renal failure.

All factors contribute equally to the index with each factor assigned 1 point. The incidence of major cardiac complications in the validation cohort (n = 1422) was estimated at 0.4%, 0.9%, 7%, and 11% in patients with an index of 0, 1, 2, or 3 or more points, respectively. Evidence exists in 108 593 patients undergoing all types of noncardiac surgery that this revised cardiac risk index was indeed predictive of cardiovascular mortality but could be substantially improved by adding age and an extensive description of the type of surgery (C-statistic improved from 0.63 to 0.85).

Surgery

The extent of preoperative cardiac evaluation will also depend on the type and the urgency of surgery in question [15–17]. Every operation will elicit a stress response to injury. This response is initiated by tissue injury and mediated by neuroendocrine factors inducing tachycardia and hypertension. Fluid shifts in the postoperative period add to the surgical stress. This stress will influence the balance between myocardial oxygen supply and demand.

Surgery will also cause alterations in the balance between prothrombotic and fibrinolytic factors resulting in hypercoagulability (elevation of fibrinogen and other coagulation factors, increased platelet aggregation and activation, reduced fibrinolysis). This is relative to the extent and duration of the intervention. Other factors that can influence cardiac stress are blood loss, perioperative fluid shifts, and body core temperature. These may cause haemodynamic changes and/or cardiac depression and are related to an increased cardiac risk.

With regard to cardiac risk, surgical interventions can be divided into a high, intermediate and low-risk group with estimated event rates of <1%, 1–5%, and >5%, respectively [18]. The urgency of the surgery determines the weight of cardiac evaluation.

Noninvasive testing

PMI occurs in 2–15% of patients undergoing vascular surgery, with great impact on postoperative cardiovascular outcome [19]. When the preoperative risk assessment identifies a patient with an increased cardiac risk, or if there is a suspicion of CAD on examination, further cardiac testing is warranted in this patient [17, 20]. The goals of noninvasive risk stratification are:

- to identify patients at extremely high risk in whom surgery should be cancelled, or another less hazardous procedure should be considered

- to identify those patients in whom the optimization of medical therapy or a coronary revascularization before surgery might reduce the risk of the surgical procedure

- to identify those patients in whom an invasive and intensive monitoring might reduce the risk of perioperative events

- to assess the long-term risk of a future cardiac event.

Treadmill or cycle ergometer test

Several noninvasive and (non-) exercise stress tests are available for perioperative risk assessment. The most commonly used stress test for detecting myocardial ischaemia is the treadmill or cycle ergometer test. These tests provide an estimate of the functional capacity and haemodynamic response, and detect myocardial ischaemia by ST-segment changes. The accuracy varies widely among studies [21].

Nonphysiological stress tests

An important limitation in patients undergoing noncardiac surgery is the frequently limited exercise capacity in elderly people, and the presence of claudication, arthrosis, or chronic obstructive pulmonary disease. Consequently, nonphysiological stress tests such as dobutamine stress echocardiography (DSE) and dipyridamol myocardial perfusion scintigraphy (MPS) are recommended in patients with limited exercise capacity.Many reports have demonstrated that DSE predicts perioperative events in patients undergoing vascular surgery [22–25]. The negative predictive value of dobutamine stress tests is high but the positive predictive value is much lower. Kertai et al. reported a weighted sensitivity of 85% (95% CI 74–97%) and a specificity of 70% (95% CI 62–69%) for DSE in 850 patients from 8 studies [21]. A recent meta-analysis by Beattie et al. analysed the predictive value of pharmacological stress testing compared to MPS [26]. This report included 25 studies (3373 patients) of mainly dobutamine and several DSE. The likelihood ratio of a perioperative event with a positive stress echocardiogram was 4.09 (95%CI 3.21–6.56).

Myocardial perfusion scintigraphy

To evaluate myocardial viability, MPS is performed during rest, exercise, or pharmacological induced stress. Nuclear imaging differs from other imaging techniques by focusing on physiological processes in the left ventricular myocardium rather than anatomy [27]. The detection of CAD is based on a difference in blood-flow distribution through the left ventricular myocardium. These perfusion abnormalities can be explained by insufficient coronary blood flow based on coronary stenosis. Pharmacological agents such as adenosine, dipyridamole, and dobutamine are used to obtain maximal vasodilatation, needed to evaluate perfusion abnormalities during stress. Results derived from stress and rest MPS should be compared with distinct viable and irreversible myocardial abnormalities [28].

Different patterns of wall motion or perfusion responses to a graded infusion of dobutamine can be assessed, such as:

- a normal wall motion or perfusion response

- a biphasic response, with initial improvement of wall motion or perfusion at low doses of dobutamine followed by worsening at higher infusion rates (ischaemic viable myocardium)

- lack of initial improvement in wall motion or perfusion response (nonviable myocardium).

Previous studies indicate that MPS is highly sensitive in predicting cardiac complications, but the positive predictive value of MPS remains less satisfactory. A meta-analysis conducted by Kertai et al. reported a sensitivity of 83% (95% CI 77–89%) and a much lower specificity of 47% (95% CI 41–57%) for thallium-201 MPS in predicting perioperative cardiac events [21]. Although MPS demonstrated lower diagnostic accuracy than DSE they conclude that MPS is a valuable test for cardiac risk assessment, especially in patients with contraindications to DSE. Using several specific analyses Beattie et al. conclude that DSE has a superior negative predictive value in preoperative cardiac assessment compared to MPS [26]. This meta-analysis identified 75 studies of preoperative noninvasive testing, including 25 MPS and 50 DSE studies involving vascular surgery patients over a 20-year period. They demonstrated that the likelihood ratio of a postoperative cardiac event was higher for DSE (LR 4.09; 95% CI 3.21–6.56, $p = 0.001$) compared to MPS (LR 1.83; 1.59–2.1, $p = 0.001$).

Invasive testing

Coronary angiography is a well-established invasive diagnostic procedure for the evaluation of cardiac patients. However, in patients scheduled for noncardiac surgery there is paucity of information focusing on the efficacy of this procedure. Nevertheless, as already extensively discussed, most of the patients scheduled for noncardiac surgery present with underlying ischaemic heart disease. Invasive testing should only be done if test results will alter preoperative or perioperative management. In patients with known CAD, indications for perioperative coronary angiography and revascularization should be similar to angiography indications for the nonoperative setting [29–32].

Preoperative coronary revascularization

The number of patients with CAD undergoing noncardiac surgery is steadily increasing. These patients may either have documented symptomatic involvement or be fully asymptomatic. The main goal of preoperative coronary revascularization is the prevention of the occurrence of PMI in patients with significant CAD scheduled for noncardiac surgery. Importantly, the cumulative risk of prophylactic coronary revascularization and noncardiac surgery needs to be weighted against the risk of the surgical procedure performed without preoperative interventions. Faced with a medical emergency, there is no other choice but to proceed with surgery and to postpone cardiac evaluation until afterwards. If not, the need for diagnostic evaluation and subsequent revascularization will have to be questioned, in particular in those patients requiring surgery within weeks or a few months.

After the presence of severe CAD is confirmed by angiography, coronary revascularization via percutaneous coronary intervention (PCI) or coronary artery bypass grafting (CABG) can be considered as prophylactic therapy in these patients prior to noncardiac surgery. In recent years two randomized controlled trials have hinted that prophylactic coronary revascularization of cardiac-stable patients provides no benefit for postoperative outcome. There are no trials investigating the role of prophylactic revascularization in patients with unstable angina pectoris requiring noncardiac surgery. If noncardiac surgery can safely be postponed, diagnosis and treatment for these patients should be in line with the recent guidelines on management of unstable angina [30]. The 'Coronary Artery Revascularization Prophylaxis' (CARP) trial randomized 510 patients with significant artery stenosis of 5859 screened patients at 18 Veterans Affairs hospitals in the United States to either revascularization or no revascularization before surgery [33]. The main finding of this study was that there was no difference in the primary outcome of long-term mortality (median follow-up 2.7 years) in patients who underwent preoperative coronary revascularization compared to patients who received optimized medical therapy (22% vs 23%, relative risk 0.98, 95% CI 0.70–1.37). To address the issue of generalizability of this trial to patients with multivessel disease, the CARP investigators recently studied the long-term outcome of all screened patients (randomized + registry) who underwent coronary angiography before vascular surgery from the original population [34]. No long-term survival benefit was observed in patients with two- and three-vessel disease. In contrast, in the cohort of 48 patients (4.6%) with left main coronary artery stenosis, patients who had undergone preoperative revascularization did seem to have an improved 2.5-year survival (84% vs 52%).

In a recent study evaluating vascular surgery patients with predominantly three-vessel disease, similar findings were obtained [35]. Cardiac-stable, elective vascular surgery patients were screened for risk factors, and those with three or more clinical risk factors underwent cardiac stress testing. All patients with extensive stress-induced ischaemia were randomly assigned for additional revascularization. All patients received optimized medical therapy including β-blockers aiming at a heart rate of 60–65 beats/min, and continued antiplatelet therapy. Of 430 high-risk patients, 101 (23%) showed extensive ischaemia and were randomly assigned to revascularization (N = 49) or no revascularization (N = 52). Coronary angiography showed two-vessel disease in 12 (24%), three-vessel disease in 33 (67%), and left main in 4 (8%). Revascularization did not improve perioperative outcome: the incidence of cardiac death and MI was 43% versus 33% (OR 1.4, 95% CI 0.7–2.8, $p = 0.30$). Also no benefit during 1-year follow-up was observed after coronary revascularization (49% vs 44%, OR 1.2, 95% CI 0.7–2.3, $p = 0.48$).

Perioperative medical management

Pharmacological risk reduction is one of the most important elements of perioperative management. Data from observational studies and registries, however, show poor compliance with guidelines in pharmacological treatment [36–38].

β-Blockers

Randomized controlled trials investigating the effect of β-blockers in the perioperative period have shown divergent results. There are different explanations regarding this conflicting evidence for perioperative β-blocker use. In particular, the initiation time and dose of β-blocker therapy, dose adjustments for heart rate control, and the patient's underlying cardiac risk are important factors that may relate to the effectiveness of therapy [39]. Monitoring of the heart rate and consequent adjustment of β-blocker dose is of critical importance for the likelihood that a patient will benefit from β-blockade [40, 41].

Evidence supporting the use of β-blockers is based mainly on two small, prospectively randomized clinical trials and several observational studies. In the first study, Mangano *et al.* randomized 200 patients with either known or suspected CAD undergoing high-risk noncardiac surgery to receive atenolol (50 mg or 100 mg) or placebo just before the induction of anaesthesia [42]. Atenolol therapy was not associated with an improved in-hospital outcome (cardiac death or MI), but it was associated with a 50% reduction in ECG evidence of myocardial ischaemia detected with continuous three-lead Holter monitoring during the first 48 h after surgery. Furthermore, although the study of Mangano *et al.* did not demonstrate a perioperative effect, atenolol use was associated with significantly lower mortality rates at 6 months after discharge (0% vs 8%; *p* = 0.005), and after 2 years (10% vs 21%; *p* = 0.019).

The other trial, the Dutch Echocardiographic Cardiac Risk Evaluation Applying Stress Echocardiography Study (DECREASE)-I trial, randomized 112 vascular surgery patients with evidence of myocardial ischaemia on preoperative DSE. The DECREASE-I trial started bisoprolol at an average of 37 (range 7–89) days before surgery and careful titration was performed. Poldermans *et al.* showed a 10-fold reduction in the incidence of perioperative cardiac death and MI with perioperative bisoprolol use compared with placebo (3.4% vs 34%; *p* <0.001) [43].

Several trials also showed evidence that did not support the use of perioperative β-blockade [44–46]. The MAVS trial and DIPOM trial both included many patients at low risk for complications. In the MAVS trial almost 60% had a Lee risk index of only 1. This is in contrast to the DECREASE study which randomized vascular surgery patients with a positive dobutamine echocardiography. In a large retrospective cohort study of 782 969 patients undergoing major noncardiac surgery a relationship between the effect of β-blocker use and the patient risk profile was observed [47]. β-Blocker use was associated with a significant beneficial effect in high-risk patients but showed no effect or possible harm in low-risk patients.

Recently the results of the large randomized POISE trial were published. A total of 8351 patients were randomized to controlled-release oral metoprolol succinate or placebo. Patients older than 45 years and were included if they had known cardiovascular disease, at least three out of seven clinical risk factors, or should undergo major vascular surgery. The POISE trial initiated randomized treatment of controlled-release metropolol just before surgery, and the maximum recommended therapeutic dose (400 mg) could already be achieved within the first day of surgery. The primary endpoint of cardiac death, MI, or cardiac arrest was reduced in the metoprolol group, compared to placebo (5.8% vs 6.9%, hazard ratio 0.83, 95% CI 0.70–0.99, *p* = 0.04). However, the 30% decrease of non-fatal MI (3.6 vs 5.1%, *p* = 0.0008) was accompanied by a 33% increase in total mortality (3.1% vs 2.3%, *p* = 0.03) and a twofold increase risk in stroke (1.0 vs 0.5%, *p* = 0.0005). Stroke was associated with perioperative bradycardia, hypotension, and bleeding in patients randomized to metoprolol with a diseased cerebrovascular tree. *Post hoc* analysis also showed that hypotension had the largest population-attributable risk for death and stroke. Importantly, hypotension can be related to the use of a high dose of metoprolol without dose titration.

Statins

Statins are widely prescribed in patients with or at risk for CAD because of their effectiveness in lowering serum cholesterol concentrations through inhibition of 3-hydroxy-3-methylglutaryl coenzyme A reductase. Reduction of low-density lipoprotein (LDL) cholesterol is one of the primary objectives of cardiovascular disease prevention. Beyond the lipid lowering effect of statins alone, evidence suggests that the more immediate benefits are related to the so-called pleiotropic effects of statins. These pleiotropic effects are thought to include improved endothelial function, enhanced stability of atherosclerotic plaques, decreased oxidative stress, and decreased vascular inflammation [48]. These effects of statins may consequently prevent plaque rupture and subsequent MI in the proinflammatory and prothrombotic environment of the perioperative period.

Two randomized controlled clinical trials have been performed so far evaluating the effect of statins in patients undergoing noncardiac surgery, i.e. vascular surgery. Durazzo *et al.* randomized 100 vascular surgery patients to either 20 mg atorvastatin or placebo [49]. After 6 months cardiovascular events had occurred in 26% of the placebo group but only in 8% of the statin group (*p* = 0.03). Though the trial was not powered to assess 30-day postoperative outcome, there was a clear trend for the beneficial effect of statins (OR 0.23, 95% CI 0.09–1.30). A large retrospective cohort study of 780 591 patients undergoing major noncardiac surgery showed that the 70 159 statin users had a 1.4-fold reduced risk of in-hospital mortality (adjusted OR 0.62, CI 0.58–0.67). The recently reported DECREASE III study is the first adequately powered randomized controlled trial that could address the role of statins in the perioperative period. This trial randomized 497 vascular surgery patients to either fluvastatin extended-release 80 mg once daily or placebo [50]. The incidence of MI in the fluvastatin and placebo allocated groups respectively was 10.8% versus 19.0% (OR 0.55; 95%CI 0.34–0.88). With respect to intermediate-risk surgical patients, the DECREASE IV trial assessed the effectiveness and safety of β-blockers, statins, and their combination, on the incidence of perioperative cardiac death and MI. Patients randomized to fluvastatin experienced a lower incidence of the primary endpoint than those randomized to fluvastatin-control therapy (3.2% vs 4.9% events, HR 0.65, 95% CI 0.35–1.10), but statistical significance was not reached ($p = 0.17$).

Antiplatelet therapy

Aspirin (acetylsalicylic acid, ASA) is one of the cornerstones in the primary and secondary prevention of cardiovascular diseases. Furthermore, dual antiplatelet therapy, the combination of aspirin and clopidogrel, has proved to be effective for the prevention of stent thrombosis. The evidence of aspirin in the perioperative period in patients undergoing noncardiac surgery is less clear. Trials of patients undergoing carotid surgery showed some evidence in favour of aspirin, although the evidence was inconclusive for all endpoints [51–52]. The meta-analysis of Robless et al. in 2001 demonstrated a reduction of serious vascular events and vascular death in patients with peripheral vascular disease [53]. However, the benefit of antiplatelet therapy did not reach statistical significance for the combined endpoint of vascular events (OR 0.76, 95% CI 0.54–1.05) in this vascular surgery population.

An important issue is how to manage patients with antiplatelet therapy in the perioperative period. Concerns of promoting perioperative haemorrhagic complications often withheld continuation of aspirin in the perioperative period. In their extensive review on the impact of antiplatelet therapy on perioperative bleeding complications, Harder et al. concluded that monotherapy with aspirin or clopidogrel alone usually does not have to be discontinued in the perioperative period [54]. This conclusion was confirmed in the meta-analysis of Burger et al. [55]. In 41 studies including a total of 49 590 patients undergoing a variety of noncardiac surgical procedures (14 981 on perioperative aspirin and 34 609 not on aspirin) they found that aspirin continuation led to a 1.5 times increased risk of bleeding complication, but not to a higher level of the severity of bleeding complications.

Conclusion

Perioperative cardiac complications remain an area of clinical interest and concern in patients undergoing noncardiac surgery. In order to reduce the risk of developing perioperative complications, risk stratification tools such as the Lee Index are widely used to identify patients in clinical practice who are at relatively high risk of adverse outcomes. Together with the surgical risk, this risk assessment guides clinicians when to conduct additional testing and when to initiate pharmacological treatment (β-blockers, statins, and aspirin) The preoperative hospital visits related to the intended procedure can be considered as a golden opportunity to initiate medical therapy and lifestyle changes with achievement of treatment targets according to the guidelines.

Personal perspective

Preoperative cardiac risk assessment offers the treating physicians the unique opportunity to screen and identify cardiac risk factors and disease that will influence not only direct postoperative outcome, but also late survival after successful surgery. After surgery, the patient should live long enough to enjoy the benefits of surgery. The emphasis is on medical treatment of risk factors, similar to that in the general, nonsurgical population. As shown, the initiation of medical therapy such as β-blockers, statins, and aspirin not only improves postoperative outcome, but also late outcome. The treatment targets for the immediate perioperative period for statins are not yet determined. In patients treated with β-blockers heart rate control aims at a window between 60 and 80 beats/min, avoiding overtreatment with the risk of intraoperative hypotension in patients with hypovolaemia. Coronary revascularization immediately before surgery is complex and rarely indicated in cardiac-stable patients. The impact of in-stent thrombosis after PCIs, even during dual antiplatelet therapy has not yet been solved, and will become an increasing problem, as the population send for surgery will have more frequently coronary interventions than in the past. As in the nonsurgical population, only clinical randomized trials can answer questions on medication, revascularization, and optimal anaesthesia care.

Further reading

Fleisher LA, Beckman JA, Brown KA, *et al.* ACC/AHA 2007 Guidelines on Perioperative Cardiovascular Evaluation and Care for Noncardiac Surgery: Executive Summary: A Report of the American College of Cardiology/American Heart Association Task Force on Practice Guidelines. *J Am Coll Cardiol* 2007;**50**(17):1707–32.

McFalls EO, Ward HB, Moritz TE, *et al.* Coronary-artery revascularization before elective major vascular surgery. *N Engl J Med* 2004;**351**(27):2795–804.

Poldermans D, Bax JJ, Boersma E, *et al.* Guidelines for pre-operative cardiac risk assessment and perioperative cardiac management in non-cardiac surgery: The Task Force for Preoperative Cardiac Risk Assessment and Perioperative Cardiac Management in Non-cardiac Surgery of the European Society of Cardiology (ESC) and endorsed by the European Society of Anaesthesiology (ESA). *Eur Heart J* 2009;**30**:2769–2812.

Poldermans D, Hoeks SE, Feringa HH. Pre-operative risk assessment and risk reduction before surgery. *J Am Coll Cardiol* 2008;**51**(20):1913–24.

Rabbitts JA, Nuttall GA, Brown MJ, *et al.* Cardiac risk of noncardiac surgery after percutaneous coronary intervention with drug-eluting stents. *Anesthesiology* 2008;**109**(4):596–604.

Schouten O, Boersma E, Hoeks SE, *et al.* Fluvastatin and perioperative events in patients undergoing vascular surgery. *N Engl J Med* 2009;**361**:980–989.

⮕ For additional multimedia materials please visit the online version of the book (✎ http://www.esciacc.oxfordmedicine.com).

CHAPTER 76

Perioperative management of the high-risk cardiac surgery patient

Marco Ranucci, Serenella Castelvecchio, and Andrea Ballotta

Contents

Summary

During the last decade, as a result of continually improving surgical strategy and the technology which supports it (e.g. anaesthesia), cardiac surgery is offered to patients of advanced age and patients with increasingly complex coexisting conditions that were previously considered to be contraindications. In addition, an increasing number of patients have previously undergone angioplasty, thereby delaying their initial coronary artery bypass grafting (CABG) surgery to a more advanced age. In general, candidates for cardiac surgery may now be not only older than in the past but also more likely to have such health problems as hypertension and diabetes. Risk stratification may help to identify the 'high-risk' patient: forewarned is forearmed.

In high-risk cardiac surgery patients the surgical treatment options and perioperative care must be tailored to each patient in order to optimize the benefits and minimize the risk of detrimental effects. The perioperative anticoagulation practice is an important aspect, balancing the risk between ischaemic and bleeding complications.

High-risk cardiac surgery patients

Vital aspects of postoperative critical illness can often be predicted and ameliorated by appropriate perioperative assessment and intervention. Published estimates of risk for an individual patient may aid the operator in selecting or avoiding specific devices or adjunctive pharmacotherapy, but they are not substitutes for clinical judgement.

At present, the risk stratification models most widely used for the evaluation of procedural risk in cardiac surgery are the European system for cardiac operative risk evaluation score (EuroSCORE) [1] and the Society of Thoracic Surgeons (STS, STSWebRiskCalc) score [2] (see ➲ Online resources). Both provide a web-based calculator. Very recently, a parsimonious risk model for predicting operative mortality risk in patients undergoing elective cardiac operations using only three variables was introduced [3]. This score is based on age, creatinine value, and ejection fraction (ACEF) and is calculated by using the following formula:

$$\text{age (years)/ejection fraction (\%)} + 1$$
$$(\text{if creatinine} \geq 2\ \text{mg/dL})$$

So far, validation has only been performed in elective patients, where the score was shown to have similar sensitivity/specificity, and similar positive/negative predictive values compared to other risk models including the additive/logistic EuroSCORE. Recently, the ACEF score has been added to the Syntax Score for percutaneous catheter interventions (Clinical Syntax Score). The Clinical Syntax Score demonstrated a higher accuracy in predicting mortality than the Syntax Score or the ACEF alone.

The predictive accuracy of different risk scoring systems may be influenced by numerous factors, such as differences in variable definitions, management of incomplete data fields, surgical procedure selection criteria, and geographical differences in patient risk factors. An area under the curve greater than 70% is usually considered to be associated with a good predictive value. Predictive values for older scoring algorithms are usually poorer than more recent ones. Most algorithms overestimated the 30-day mortality in this patient population.

The EuroSCORE model, both logistic and additive, provides a high discriminatory power to predict 30-day mortality in many European countries and in the United States. Overall, and for coronary artery bypass grafting (CABG)-only surgery it compared favourably with the STS risk stratification algorithm [4]. However, in (high-risk) patients undergoing isolated aortic valve replacement, the EuroSCORE highly overestimates mortality and can only be used applying a correction factor, whereas the STS score actually seems to be more suitable in assessing perioperative mortality for these patients [5]. Patients at high risk for in-hospital mortality with percutaneous coronary intervention (PCI) are most often also high risk for CABG [6]. The most important surgical risk groups are listed in ⟳ Box 76.1.

Emergent procedures

Emergent surgical priority is associated with high risk within 7 days after surgery but with subsequent rapidly decreasing risk over time. Patients with evolving (non-) ST-segment elevation (STE) acute coronary syndrome (ACS) are a high-risk group in CABG surgery. The higher

---

Box 76.1 High-risk patients

- The elderly patient [16, 17].
- The patient with severe pulmonary disease. Chronic obstructive pulmonary disease (COPD) is associated with increased in-hospital mortality in patients undergoing CABG, especially when combined with one or more other comorbidities [18].
- The patient with chronic renal failure. CABG is associated with adverse outcome in patients with renal dysfunction. Renal dysfunction is an important factor for calculating CABG risk scores, according to ACC/AHA guidelines, Cleveland clinic score, and EuroSCORES [19–22].
- The patient with low ejection fraction (EF ≤30%) [23, 24].
- The obese patient. Increased body size is not a significant risk factor for CABG mortality [25], but there is a significant increased risk of morbidities and postoperative length of stay in obese patients compared to nonobese patients, and sternal wound infections are of concern [26]. The perioperative care of severely obese patients presents a number of unique challenges [27]. Potential arterial and venous access sites should be evaluated. Obesity is an independent risk factor for deep vein thrombosis and pulmonary embolism.
- The cachectic patient.
- The frail patient.

---

rate of particular major morbidities is related to processes of care before CABG (see ⟳ Chapter 46) [7, 8]. It may be advisable to delay surgical intervention whenever possible. However, in the presence of refractory symptoms, haemodynamic alterations not responsive to standard treatment, or in STE-ACS patients, emergency surgical treatment within the first hours is indicated. Emergent CABG following primary PCI for STE-ACS is consistently associated with higher mortality and higher incidence of stroke, renal failure, and postoperative bleeding [9]. Beating-heart CABG performs better than conventional cardioplegic cardiac arrest strategies in terms of in-hospital clinical outcome.

Balancing ischaemic and bleeding complications

About 10–15% of ACS patients will require CABG during their hospitalization. In these patients enhanced and irreversible platelet inhibition reduces ischaemic complications within 30 days but comes with a potential cost of increased bleeding [10]. The use of a thienopyridine in combination with aspirin within 5 days of CABG results in increased postoperative blood loss(mean chest tube output), increased use of blood products, and 10-fold increased re-exploration rates for bleeding [11, 12]. In contrast, if CABG was delayed for 5 days or more after stopping clopidogrel, bleeding was similar to that in those patients who had not received it [13, 14]. Individualized care is rapidly evolving, with new discoveries and innovations that go beyond traditional risk factors. Point-of-care platelet function assays may eventually enable physicians to tailor antiplatelet therapy to the individual patient. If validated, point-of-care assays may help tailor the management of ACS patients who go on to receive CABG by identifying those at low risk for surgical bleeding [15].

Perioperative care

Very high-risk procedures are of course sometimes inevitable because of the inherent risk of the underlying disease. A multidisciplinary approach to the care of the high-risk cardiac surgery patient is necessary, and a distinct care plan for these patients should be designed as soon as it is feasible. Many of these procedures are elective. However, even in the acute setting, the benefits of a specific procedure should be weighed against the risks involved, taking into account alternative treatment strategies, the individual operators, and overall experience of the institution (surgical and intensive care team). In some circumstances, a transfer to a major teaching hospital or high-volume centre that routinely performs complex surgical procedures may be the most effective and efficient course of action [28]. Standby or preoperative (supported) insertion of an intra-aortic balloon pump (IABP) or more extensive mechanical circulatory support (MCS) are some important safeguards.

Haemodynamic monitoring

Background

The primary physiological task of the cardiorespiratory system is to deliver adequate oxygen (Do_2:$Cao_2 \times CO \times 10$) to meet the metabolic demands of the body (Vo_2). An increase in oxygen demand is usually met by a combined increase in Do_2 and oxygen extraction ratio by the tissues (O_2ER). An increase in Do_2 can be accomplished by an increase in cardiac output, and arterial oxygen content:

$$Cao_2: (Sao_2 \times Hb \times 1.36) + (0.0031 \times Pao_2)$$

where Hb is the haemoglobin level and S_ao_2 the arterial oxygen saturation. Parameters reflecting a disturbance in the balance between oxygen demand and Do_2 (e.g. mixed venous saturation, lactate), at both global and regional level, could be of value to optimize tissue oxygen delivery. Manipulation of cardiac output is a common clinical intervention.

Conventional haemodynamic monitoring for cardiac surgery patients includes the positioning of a pulmonary artery catheter (PAC) and an arterial line as well as measurement of standard end-tidal CO_2 and transcutaneous oxygen saturation. Invasive haemodynamic and oxygen monitoring identifies correctable physiological deficiencies at an early stage. The purpose of monitoring is to obtain frequent, repeated measurements of circulatory variables so as to allow rapid recognition of circulatory problems, to evaluate physiological conditions, and to evaluate the therapeutic effect of corrective therapy (see also ➲ Chapter 18).

Pulmonary artery catheter

In critically ill patients, the impact of PAC use on outcome is debated. Also in (high-risk) cardiac surgery, the implementation of PACs into the monitoring protocol is matter of personal preference, with supporters [29] and detractors [30]. The haemodynamic variables easily measured by a PAC include mixed venous oxygen saturation (Svo_2), cardiac output, right ventricular ejection fraction (with some catheters), and intrapulmonary vascular pressures. Clearly, newer monitoring devices including oesophageal Doppler and arterial pulse contour analyses can be used to measure cardiac output. However, none measures Svo_2 nor can simultaneously assess intrathoracic vascular pressure, factors that may determine treatment options. Recent advances in catheter technology have produced impressive novel and innovative uses of monitoring devices requiring only central venous catheterization or central venous catheterization combined with arterial catheterization. Central venous fiberoptic technology also allows for the continuous measurement of superior vena caval oxygen saturation as a surrogate marker of Svo_2. Unfortunately, the central venous pressure does not reliably reflect left-sided filling pressures nor predict volume responsiveness, less invasive measurements of cardiac output are often approximate, and $Scvo_2$ is not a reliable reflection of Svo_2.

Potential indications for the use of PAC in perioperative monitoring include [31]:

♦ patients with preoperatively severely depressed left ventricular (LV) systolic function (LV ejection fraction ≤0.30–0.35).

- patients with LV ventricular diastolic dysfunction.
- patients with impaired right ventricular (RV) function.
- patients with acute ventricular septal defect.
- patients supported by an MCS.

Transoesophageal echocardiography (see also ⮕ Chapter 20)

Transoesophageal echocardiography (TOE) should not be though of as an alternative to PAC; they should be considered complementary. Each technique gives unique information and can guide diagnosis and therapy differently. Echocardiography is often limited by the quality of images (transthoracic) or patient comfort (transoesophageal) in the postoperative phase.

TOE provides continuous intraoperative but not postoperative monitoring; it is a semiquantitative tool, providing a comprehensive imaging of heart chambers and valve function, and can be used to assess both systolic and diastolic function of both ventricles. With adequate calculations, TOE may provide an indirect pressure measurement (pulmonary artery pressure), and an approximation of the cardiac output. Therefore, the information derived from these two devices is complementary rather than alternative, and patients with perioperative heart failure should be monitored with both PAC and TOE.

All cardiac surgery operations may be considered as suitable scenarios for the use of TOE. In high-risk coronary patients the routine intraoperative use of TOE resulted in major changes in surgery in 33% of the patients, and in major changes in the haemodynamic management in 51% [32]. Other studies have highlighted the role of intraoperative TOE in detection of new findings, changes in surgical planning, and the decision-making process in case of haemodynamic instability.

Mixed venous oxygen saturation (SVo_2)

SVo_2 and its surrogate, $ScVo_2$ (measured at the level of the superior vena cava with standard central venous catheters) are indices that may represent the adequacy of Do_2 with respect to the metabolic needs (Vo_2) (⮕ Box 76.2).

Blood lactate

When the oxygen delivery (Do_2) is inadequate to sustain the oxygen consumption (Vo_2), energy for cellular life is derived from anaerobic metabolism [33]. This generates blood lactates. Hyperlactataemia is a well-recognized index of inadequate cardiac output. Hyperlactataemia during and after cardiopulmonary bypass (CPB) is associated with

---

> **Box 76.2 Physiology of mixed venous and central venous oxygen saturation**
>
> O_2 delivery (Do_2) describes whole-body oxygen supply according to the following formulae:
>
> $$Do_2 = CO \times Cao_2 \qquad (1)$$
>
> $$Cao_2 = (Hb \times 1.36 \times Sao_2) + (Pao_2 \times 0.0031) \qquad (2)$$
>
> where CO is cardiac output and Cao_2 is arterial oxygen content, i.e. O_2 bound to haemoglobin (product of haemoglobin concentration (Hb) and arterial O_2 saturation (Sao_2)) + physically dissolved oxygen (arterial Po_2 (Pao_2)).
>
> Oxygen demand can be summarized in the whole-body oxygen consumption (Vo_2), which is expressed mathematically by the Fick principle as the product of CO and arteriovenous O_2 content difference (Cao_2–Cvo_2):
>
> $$Vo_2 = Cao_2 - Cvo_2 \qquad (3)$$
>
> $$Cvo_2 = (Hb \times 1.36 \times Svo_2) + (Pvo_2 \times 0.0031) \qquad (4)$$
>
> where Cvo_2 is the mixed venous O_2 content.
>
> Oxygen extraction (O_2ER):
>
> $$Vo_2/Do_2 = (Cao_2 - Cvo_2)/Cao_2$$
>
> Equation (3) may be transposed to:
>
> $$Cvo_2 = Cao_2 - Vo_2/CO \qquad (5)$$
>
> As physically dissolved oxygen can be neglected, Equation (5) may be written as:
>
> $$Hb \times 1.36 \times Svo_2 \approx (Hb \times 1.36 \times Sao_2) - Vo_2/CO \Leftrightarrow$$
> $$Svo_2 \sim Vo_2/CO$$
>
> This equation demonstrates that Svo_2 is directly proportional to the ratio of Vo_2 to CO. Thus Svo_2 reflects the relationship between whole-body O_2 consumption and cardiac output. Indeed, it has been shown that Svo_2 is well correlated with the ratio of O_2 supply to demand.

---

a poor outcome in cardiac surgery, with increased morbidity and mortality rates [34–36]. Blood lactate monitoring is valuable during perioperative heart failure. Rising values of blood lactates are a negative prognostic index, whereas stable and decreasing values may indicate that the cardiac output is recovering. However, this monitoring should be seen within a comprehensive context of clinical evaluation, haemodynamic parameters, and potentially other measures of tissue perfusion. Some potential limitations of lactate measurement must be considered in this setting:

- Liver dysfunction. The accumulation of any metabolite is dependent on the balance between production and elimination. Lactate overproduction is mainly the result of anaerobic production. Once lactates are formed, they are eliminated primarily (50%) by the liver, but the kidneys (25–30%), heart, and skeletal muscle are also involved, with variable kinetics. However, they always require a certain period of time to be cleared. Liver failure may contribute to hyperlactaemia, but is probably not enough to account for it altogether.

- Washout phenomenon. During (early) hypoperfusion, reduced blood flow may cause sequestration of lactate in regional tissues. A late blood lactate rise following cardiac operations may be simply the expression of a reperfusion phenomenon.

Pharmacological interventions

Myocardial protection

During cardiac operations the heart is susceptible to various kind of insults, such as ischaemic events and ischaemia–reperfusion injury. It is beyond the scope of this chapter to address the myocardial protection techniques related to cardioplegia solutions and temperature management. Actually, there is still no general agreement on the best myocardial protection during aortic cross-clamping, and the technique of choice basically depends on the surgeon's preferences. It is possible that some pharmacological strategies, targeting the principle of preconditioning, may be effective in exerting a myocardial protective effect [37–44].

Blood glucose control

For a detailed account, see ➲ Chapter 67.

Antiplatelet therapy

Therapy with antiplatelet agents such as aspirin, started within 24 h after CABG, reduces the risk of early occlusion of a saphenous vein graft and remains effective in reducing the risk of occlusion for 1 year, but not up to 3 years [45]. However, almost 50% of CABG patients had a previous infarction, and the benefit of aspirin in secondary prevention after myocardial infarction (MI) has been well established. Aspirin is a standard intervention for patients who have undergone CABG.

Nonpharmacological interventions

Surgical techniques (see also ➲ Chapters 46, 59)

Over the last two decades interest has emerged in performing CABG without the use of CPB (off pump), in order to reduce postoperative complications associated with the use of CPB. However, the short-term (before discharge or within 30 days after surgery) and long-term (beyond 12 months) benefit of off-pump surgery was questioned in a large randomized trial showing a significant increase in the primary short-term (death or complications: reoperation, new mechanical support, cardiac arrest, coma, stroke, or renal failure) and primary long-term (death from any cause, repeat revascularization procedure, or a nonfatal MI) composite endpoint. Similarly, off-pump CABG was not significantly different from on-pump CABG in neurocognitive outcomes [46].

Cardiac assist devices including intra-aortic balloon pump (see also ➲ Chapters 29–30]

The IABP is a circulatory support device operating on the principle of counterpulsation, in which arterial diastolic and coronary perfusion pressures are augmented and impedance to ventricular ejection (afterload) is reduced (➲ Chapter 29). An IABP could be used preoperatively or in the peri/postoperative period. The prophylactic insertion of an IABP in patients at high risk for postoperative heart failure is still a contentious issue [47]. Its use in the setting of postcardiotomy LV failure is established. Early implantation of an IABP together with pharmacological support may contribute to the successful weaning from cardiopulmonary bypass of 70–90% of all patients, with haemodynamic recovery and successful explantation of the IABP in 60–70% of patients. Treatment success should be assessed after 60 minutes based on simple haemodynamic parameters including left atrial pressure (<15 mmHg), mixed venous saturation (SV_{O_2} >60%) and diuresis (urine output >100 mL/h) [48].

Since IABP is incapable of supporting a patient with complete haemodynamic collapse, and for patients who are suffering from cardiac low-output syndrome despite IABP support, immediate triage to more advanced percutaneous (or implantable) circulatory support modalities may be warranted to achieve circulatory recovery. Percutaneous MCS can be provided by a variety of devices and modalities designed to increase forward blood flow and reduce filling pressures. A minimal flow rate of 70 mL/kg body weight per minute is required to provide adequate organ perfusion. Treatment options for MCS must be tailored to each patient in order to optimize the benefits and minimize the risk of detrimental effects; access site complications are of particular concern.

Peri- and postoperative complications

Despite its proven benefits, cardiac surgery (e.g. CABG) can occasionally result in devastating or debilitating outcomes (➲ Table 76.1). Some of these events represent a real challenge, because of either their relatively high incidence or their severe impact on mortality rate.

Perioperative myocardial infarction

Perioperative myocardial infarction (PMI) occurs in 7–15% of patients after cardiac surgery and is associated with increased hospital length of stay, costs, and reduced short- and long-term survival [49, 50]. MI is diagnosed with a combination of (markers of) myocardial necrosis (preferably troponin) in the presence of new clinical signs (e.g. an evolving ECG pattern which involves Q wave development) or symptoms of myocardial ischaemia [51–53]. The determination of PMI within the first 72 h after cardiac surgery may be problematic (type 5 of the 2007 universal definition of MI: see ➲ Chapter 39). Clinical symptoms are masked while the patient is intubated, sedated, or under

Table 76.1 Morbidity after cardiac operations

Event	Reported operative rate (%)	Associated morality rate (%)
Bleeding-related surgical re-exploration	2–6	10–12
Perioperative myocardial infarction	5–20	6–8
Perioperative heart failure	10–40	20–25
Stroke	1–3	12–14
Neuropsychological dysfunction	20–70	Unchanged
Acute kidney injury	8–12	8–12
Acute renal failure (renal replacement therapy)	1–2	40–50
Acute respiratory distress syndrome	0.4–1	12–16
Mesenteric ischaemia/infarction	0.2–0.4	60–80
Gastrointestinal bleeding, pancreatitis, cholecystitis	0.1–0.2	40–50
Mediastinitis	2–3	10–25
Sepsis	1–2	30–40

the intraoperative or postoperative effects of anaesthesia, and the sensitivity and specificity of postoperative ECG changes are poor. Periprocedural necrosis, within 72 h after CABG, is different from spontaneous infarction, and may be associated with the instrumentation of the heart, coronary dissection, global or regional ischaemia related to inadequate cardiac protection, microvascular events related to reperfusion, myocardial damage induced by oxygen free-radical generation, air embolism, or failure to reperfuse areas of the myocardium that are not subtended by graftable vessels [54].

Concentrations of cTnT after CABG are nearly universally elevated, are determined by numerous factors, and are independently prognostic for impending postoperative complications when used at appropriate cut points, while accounting for clinical risk [55]. Factors leading to periprocedural necrosis include direct myocardial trauma from sewing needles or manipulation of the heart. Many of these complications are at least partially attributable to the process of atherosclerosis, thrombosis, and haemostasis. If outcomes among CABG patients are to be improved, development of better strategies to reduce perioperative ischaemic events is imperative.

Perioperative MI may result in a wide spectrum of clinical consequences, ranging from minor patterns that are not hemodynamically relevant to severe perioperative heart failure. The haemodynamic conditions should be assessed immediately when a perioperative MI is suspected, through echocardiography and haemodynamic methods (see ➲ Fig. 76.1). The treatment of MI is addressed in the recent European Society of Cardiology (ESC) guidelines, which maintain their importance in the setting of perioperative MI following cardiac surgery [56] (see also ➲ Chapters 41–43 and 45).

There are no well-defined algorithms to guide the treatment of perioperative MI. According to the haemodynamic consequences, the treatment can either be conservative or require an early percutaneous or surgical revascularization. The risks and benefits of the following strategies should be considered in the light of the infarction site and area, and most importantly of the haemodynamic consequences of the lesion:

- Relief of pain, breathlessness, and anxiety. In patients under mechanical ventilation, oxygenation and level of sedation must be optimized.

- Haemodynamic stabilization. The heart function should be assisted with inotropic drugs (see ➲ Fig. 76.1), and mechanical assistance of the failing heart with an IABP may be indicated [57]. A ventricular assist device (VAD)

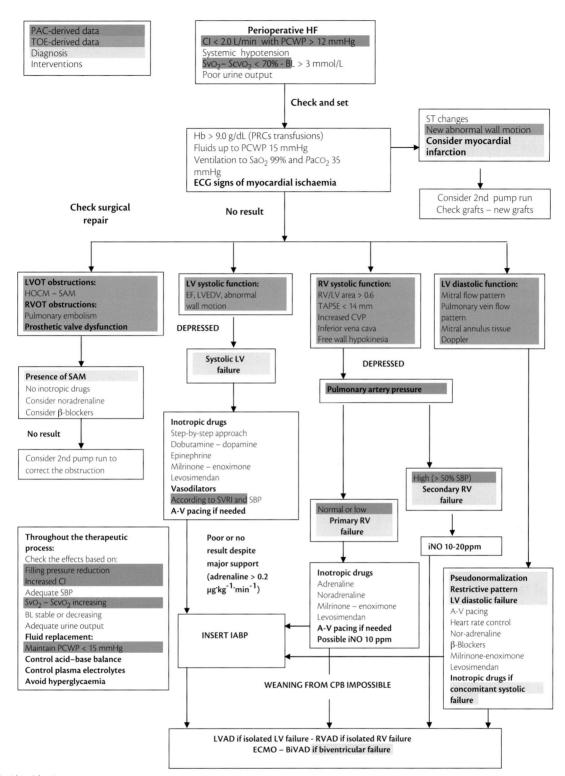

Figure 76.1 Algorithm?

BiVAD, biventricular assist device; CI, cardiac index; ECMO, extracorporeal membrane oxygenation; EF, ejection fraction; IABP, intra-aortic balloon pump; LV, left ventricle; LVAD, left ventricular assist device; LVEDV, left ventricular end-diastolic volume; LVOT, left ventricular outflow tract; PAC, pulmonary artery catheter; PCWP, pulmonary capillary wedge pressure; RVOT, right ventricular outflow tract; SAM, systolic anterior motion; SBP, systolic blood pressure; TAPSE, tricuspid annular plane systolic excursion; TOE, transoesophageal echocardiography.

GREEN: PAC-derived data
BLUE: TOE-derived data
YELLOW: diagnosis
WHITE: Clinical signs and interventions

may be considered when pharmacological therapy and IABP cannot achieve a satisfactory haemodynamic response.

- Restoration of coronary patency and myocardial tissue perfusion.

- Antithrombotic therapies. At all times the risks of ischaemic complications should be balanced against the risk of major bleeding. Heparin treatment may be established and modulated according to the activated clotting time and the bleeding tendency of the patient.

Heart failure (see also ➲ Chapters 49–52)

Postcardiotomy cardiogenic shock occurs in approximately 2–6% of patients who undergo open-heart surgery. Perioperative HF is often a very complex entity, with multifactorial patterns that can involve different aspects of cardiac function and may be isolated to the left (24%) or right (23%) ventricle, or involve both sides of the heart (25%) [58]. Mechanical factors, as well as systolic and/or diastolic ventricular dysfunction, may be involved. A diagnostic/therapeutic algorithm based on PAC and TEE data is shown in ➲ Fig. 76.1.

Respiratory failure

Respiratory failure is common (2–20%) and continues to be a major cause of potentially fatal morbidity after CABG. Respiratory function after CABG is readily influenced by postoperative occurrence of extracardiac organ or systemic complications [59].

Acute renal failure (see also ➲ Chapters 28, 66)

Acute kidney injury (AKI) is defined by the RIFLE criteria [60] as a peak postoperative creatinine value higher than 2.0 mg/dL and double the baseline value, sustained for more than 24 h within the first 72 h postoperatively. Acute renal failure (ARF) is a more severe condition, often requiring renal replacement therapy (RRT). Following cardiac surgery, AKI may be present in about 10% of the population, whereas ARF requiring RRT has an incidence of 1–2%, and is accompanied by a mortality rate of about 50% [61–64]. The occurrence of postoperative renal failure has risen over the past decade, most dramatically for those patients undergoing emergency CABG within 24 h of MI. The combination of radiopaque contrast for PCI, followed within 6 h by emergency CABG, has an obvious impact on renal function—but more so for patients with new MI, probably as a result of the notably higher rate of associated

preoperative cardiogenic shock. Independent predictors of ARF with RRT are listed in ➲ Box 76.3.

Specific aspects of AKI and ARF in the cardiac surgery setting rely mainly on the optimization of the circulating volume and renal perfusion pressure, especially in case of perioperative heart failure the limitation of inotropic and vasoconstrictive agents to the lower possible amount able to guarantee an adequate cardiac output and perfusion pressure; a fluid intake modulated on the basis of the urine output; restriction of potassium intake; discontinuation of

---

Box 76.3 Risk factors for postoperative acute renal failure

- Demographics
  - Age
  - Female gender
- Comorbidities and other preoperative factors
  - Peripheral vascular disease
  - Diabetes (on medication)
  - COPD
  - Elevated preoperative serum creatinine value/reduced creatinine clearance
  - Angiography performed within 24 h before the operation
- Heart function related factors
  - NYHA class 3–4
  - LVEF <0.35
  - Preoperative use of IABP
  - Cardiogenic shock
- Operative factors
  - Redo surgery
  - Complex surgery
  - Emergency surgery
  - Prolonged (>120 min) CPB
  - Severe haemodilution (nadir haematocrit during cardiopulmonary bypass <21%)
  - Inadequate oxygen delivery during cardiopulmonary bypass (<270 mL min^{-1}m^{-2})
- Postoperative factors
  - Allogeneic packed red cell transfusions
  - Low cardiac output syndrome

nephrotoxic drugs; and dose adjustment of drugs metabolized by the kidney.

Mesenteric infarction

Although a rare complication (0.2–0.5%), mesenteric infarction following cardiac surgery is a severe event associated with a mortality rate that exceeds 70% [65, 66]. Risk factors for mesenteric infarction include older age, intraoperative hypoperfusion, emergency operation, longer CPB time, need for high-dose vasopressor, IABP, and valve operations [66]. The pathogenesis of acute mesenteric infarction may be related to poor perfusion during CPB [67, 68]. Alternatively, mesenteric infarction may result from an acute perioperative thromboembolic event. This event is more common in patients with a prothrombotic state (history of smoking or chronic obstructive pulmonary disease, COPD) or a tendency to develop embolic events (previous heparin-induced thrombocytopenia, atrial fibrillation) [65].

The diagnosis of mesenteric infarction in cardiac surgery patients may be cumbersome and may be triggered by hyperlactataemia. Early laparotomy should be considered whenever acute mesenteric infarction is highly suspected [66].

Bleeding and transfusion

Cardiac surgery patients may experience excessive postoperative bleeding due to a number of factors (preoperative use of antiplatelet agents, CPB-induced platelet dysfunction, consumption of coagulation factors, hyperfibrinolysis). The incidence of severe bleeding in cardiac surgery exceeds 10%, and 5–7% of these patients experience blood loss in excess of 2 L within the initial 24 h after surgery [69].

As a consequence, allogeneic blood transfusions may be necessary, and in a certain proportion of patients (2–5%) surgical re-exploration is needed. Both these factors have deleterious effects on the quality of postoperative recovery. Transfusions are associated with increased morbidity and mortality [70], and surgical re-exploration is associated with a threefold increase of major complications and a fourfold increase in operative mortality [71]. In patients undergoing cardiac surgery, transfusion should be restricted and leucocyte depleted; 'young' red blood cells should preferred when available [72, 73]. There is no benefit from transfusion for haematocrits as low as 21% (haemoglobin 7 g/dL). Stored red blood cells are 2,3-DPG deficient and consequently less adept at unloading oxygen and less deformable, possibly leading to sludging and capillary occlusion. Transfusion of red cells that had been stored for more than 2 weeks was associated with a significantly increased risk of postoperative complications as well as reduced in-hospital and 12-month survival [72].

Every effort should be made to limit postoperative bleeding and transfusion. The most obvious and probably the most effective strategy is to improve surgical techniques and rule out abnormalities of haemostasis (see also ➲ Chapter 34). The approach to a patient with severe postoperative bleeding may be guided by specific algorithms based on point-of-care tests. This tests include thromboelastography or thromboelastometry, and platelet function analysis. Different algorithms have been proposed [74–76] and may be useful for suggesting the use of drugs, fresh frozen plasma, or platelet concentrates, as well as for deciding to surgically re-explore the patient.

Cases of excessive blood loss in which no surgical cause or abnormalities in haemostasis can be identified may require pharmacological strategies, which can be broadly divided into preoperative prophylaxis for operations that confer a high risk of bleeding and interventions for massive refractory bleeding. The medications that have been most extensively evaluated as haemostatic agents include the antifibrinolytic lysine analogues aminocaproic acid and tranexamic acid; aprotinin, a bovine-derived protease inhibitor; and desmopressin, a synthetic analogue of the antidiuretic hormone that raises the plasma levels of factor VIII and von Willebrand factor [77–81]. In addition, recombinant activated factor VII appears to be efficacious in an array of clinical situations associated with severe haemorrhage [82, 83]. The safety of aprotinin, the most widely used of these agents, has been questioned because of concerns about renal and cardiovascular adverse events [84]. Thrombotic complications constitute a major concern of agents that potentiate haemostasis.

Atrial fibrillation and supraventricular arrhythmia (see also ➲ Chapter 54)

Atrial fibrillation (AF) is the most common arrhythmia to occur after cardiac surgery. The incidence of AF has been reported to range between 20% and 40% depending on the risk profile and the type of surgery [85–87]. Most events occur within 6 days after the intervention. It is associated with increased morbidity, including increased risk of stroke (and decreased quality of life) and need for additional treatment, with prolonged hospital stay and increased health care resources [88, 89]. In addition to expected demographic factors (age, male sex, diabetes, history of AF, history of congestive heart failure, hypertension, COPD and a pre-CPB heart rate of >100 beats/min), certain surgical practices increase the risk of postoperative AF [90]. Preoperative treatment with β-blockers is the first choice in the prevention of postoperative AF. Also, the use of either an oral or intravenous amiodarone chlorhydrate load before surgery has been shown to decrease the postoperative risk of AF and proved cost-effective in the high clinical risk cohort [91–94]. When β-blockers are contraindicated, amiodarone pretreatment is recommended. Magnesium and potassium levels should be monitored and maintained during the early postoperative course [95]. Rate control may be a challenge in the postoperative setting, where adrenergic stress (either endogenous or secondary to inotropic drugs use) is present. Short-acting β-blockers such as esmolol may be used when haemodynamic instability is present. Direct-current cardioversion may be required, especially in the early phases after the operation, when AF affects the haemodynamics [96]. The usual anticoagulation precautions should be followed (see ➲ Chapter 54).

Stroke (see also ➲ Chapter 65)

Stroke following cardiac surgery is a relatively frequent (up to 2%) complication and long-term problem with important psychological implications for the patient [97]. Many risk factors have been identified for the development of stroke in cardiac operations: age, history of cerebrovascular disease, peripheral vascular disease, diabetes, hypertension, previous cardiac surgery, preoperative infection, active endocarditis, urgent operation, prolonged CPB time, transfusions, ARF, low cardiac output syndrome, and AF [98, 99]. The single most important cause of stroke is aortic atheromatous disease, which is detected with high reproducibility by intraoperative transoesophageal echocardiography or epiaortic scanning. In patients with large (>5 mm) or mobile aortic atheromas the rate of perioperative stroke is increased by a factor of 5–10, and they are likely to have a significantly increased long-term risk of stroke [100]. This finding highlights the role of surgical manoeuvres on the ascending aorta in the determining early postoperative stroke [101]. The treatment of perioperative stroke in cardiac surgery does not differ from the usual management of stroke.

Delirium (see also ➲ Chapter 73)

Postoperative delirium may be the manifestation of unrecognized preoperative disease, or the results of intra- or postoperative events [102].

Conclusion

The risk profile of cardiac surgery patients has increased dramatically during the last decade. The mean age of the patients is steadily increasing, and we can say that there are at present no age-related limitations for referring patients to cardiac surgery. This of course means that many age-related comorbidities and organ dysfunctions are more often seen now than in the past. In addition, the expanding role of PCI has greatly limited the number of low-risk coronary patients referred to surgery.

Taken together, these factors create a clinical scenario where high-risk cardiac patients are widely represented, with an increasing need for appropriate clinical measures to stratify and treat this specific subgroup of cardiac surgery patients.

Personal perspective

Haemostatic balance before and after cardiac operations is in a strategic position for the outcome of the patients. The great majority of the postoperative complications are either haemorrhagic or prothrombotic in nature (and sometimes both). CABG patients are now extensively treated with single, double, and even triple antiaggregation, and the new generation of platelet inhibitors (prasugrel) is associated with an increased perioperative bleeding tendency. However, the patient's response to these drugs is highly subjective, and the classically suggested withdrawal time may not be sufficient for many of them to restore an adequate platelet function. Point-of-care platelet function tests are presently widely available, but we are still lacking standard values and well-defined cut-off values to decide whether or not to postpone surgery. This is certainly a good topic for future clinical research. At the same time, postoperative complications related to thromboembolic events may account for up to 5–10% of the morbidity. In this setting, it is still not clear what may be the possible role of natural endothelial-derived anticoagulants (antithrombin, C-protein complex), which are extensively consumed during the operation but are rarely measured and even more rarely replenished. Finally, transfusions in the perioperative course are associated with a worse outcome, and every attempt should be applied to limit the use of allogeneic blood products. Even in this case, a rational approach should follow point-of-care based algorithms. Further studies incorporating the new platelet function tests within the existing algorithms are strongly suggested, in order to rationalize the use of allogeneic blood and derivatives.

Further reading

Bellomo R, Ronco C, Kellum JA, *et al*. Acute renal failure—definition, outcome measures, animal models, fluid therapy and information technology needs: the Second International Consensus Conference of the Acute Dialysis Quality Initiative (ADQI) Group. *Crit Care* 2004;**8**:R204–R212.

Cheitlin MD, Armstrong WF, Aurigemma GP, *et al*. ACC/AHA/ASE 2003 guideline update for the clinical application of echocardiography: summary article: a report of the American College of Cardiology/American Heart Association Task Force on Practice Guidelines (ACC/AHA/ASE Committee to Update the 1997 Guidelines for the Clinical Application of Echocardiography). *Circulation* 2003;**108**:1146–1162.

Dunning J, Treasure T, Versteegh M, *et al*. Guidelines for the prevention and management of de novo atrial fibrillation after cardiac surgery. *Eur J Cardiothorac Surg* 2006;**30**:852–872.

Mangano CM, Diamondstone LS, Ramsay JG, *et al*. Renal dysfunction after myocardial revascularization: risk factors, adverse outcomes, and hospital resources utilization. *Ann Intern Med* 1998;**128**:194–203.

Nashef SA, Roques F, Michel P, *et al*. European system for cardiac operative risk evaluation (EuroSCORE). *Eur J Cardiothorac Surg* 1999;**16**:9–13.

Ranucci M, Castelvecchio S, Menicanti L, *et al*. Risk of assessing mortality risk in elective cardiac operations: age, creatinine, ejection fraction, and the law of parsimony. *Circulation* 2009;**119**:3053–3061.

Roach GW, Kanchuger M, Mangano CM, *et al*. Adverse cerebral outcomes after coronary bypass surgery. Multicenter Study of Perioperative Ischemia Research Group and the Ischemia Research and Education Foundation Investigators. *N Engl J Med* 1996;**335**:1857–1863.

Ferraris VA, Ferraris SP, Saha SP, *et al*. Society of Thoracic Surgeons Blood Conservation Guideline Task Force Perioperative blood transfusion and blood conservation in cardiac surgery: the Society of Thoracic Surgeons and the Society of Cardiovascular Anesthesiologists clinical practice guideline. *Ann Thorac Surg* 2007;**83**:27–86.

Thygesen K, Alpert JS, White HD, *et al*. Universal definition of myocardial infarction. *J Am Coll Cardiol* 2007;**50**:2173–2195.

Vincent JL, Pinsky M. Let us use the pulmonary artery catheter correctly and only when we need it. *Crit Care* 2005;**33**:119–1122.

Online resources

- Euroscore (European system for cardiac operative risk evaluation score). http://www.euroscore.org/calc.html
- Society of Thoracic Surgeons. stswebriskcalc. http://209.220.160.181/STSWebRiskCalc261/

➲ For additional multimedia materials please visit the online version of the book (⧠ http://www.esciacc.oxfordmedicine.com).

Index

Page numbers in *italic* indicate boxes, figures and tables.